Mastering NEET Series

Second Edition

Volume-2
(Clinical Subjects)

- ENT
- General Surgery
- Obstetrics
- Anesthesia
- Radiotherapy
- Ophthalmology
- Orthopedics
- Gynecology
- Psychiatry
- General Medicine
- Pediatrics
- Dermatology
- Radiodiagnosis

Mastering NEET Series

Second Edition

Volume-2
(Clinical Subjects)

Kamal KV MBBS MS (Orthopaedics)
Ex-Senior Resident: Safdarjung, ESI-Okhla, Fortis-Noida
Ponseti and Ilizarov Techniques Fellow (Akola)
Madhya Pradesh – Indian Orthopaedic Association
Hand Surgery Fellow – Pune, Maharashtra, India

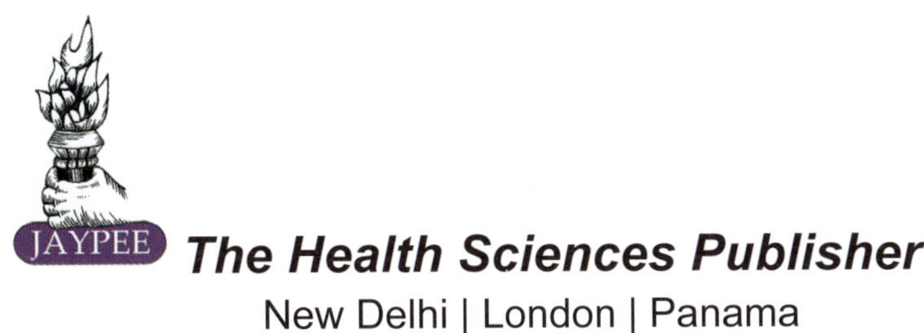

The Health Sciences Publisher
New Delhi | London | Panama

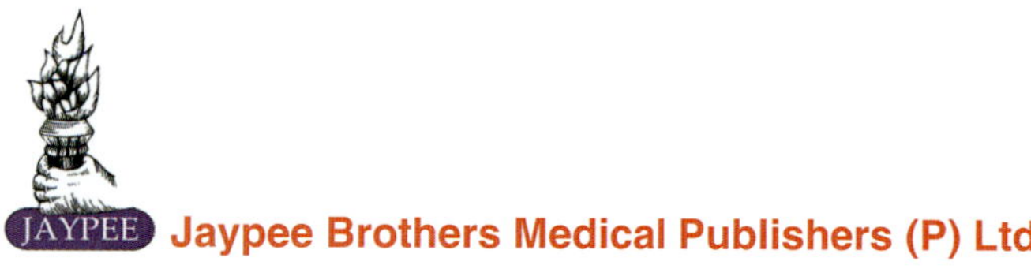

Jaypee Brothers Medical Publishers (P) Ltd

Headquarters

Jaypee Brothers Medical Publishers (P) Ltd
4838/24, Ansari Road, Daryaganj
New Delhi 110 002, India
Phone: +91-11-43574357
Fax: +91-11-43574314
Email: jaypee@jaypeebrothers.com

Overseas Offices

J.P. Medical Ltd
83 Victoria Street, London
SW1H 0HW (UK)
Phone: +44 20 3170 8910
Fax: +44 (0)20 3008 6180
Email: info@jpmedpub.com

Jaypee-Highlights Medical Publishers Inc
City of Knowledge, Bld. 235, 2nd Floor, Clayton
Panama City, Panama
Phone: +1 507-301-0496
Fax: +1 507-301-0499
Email: cservice@jphmedical.com

Jaypee Brothers Medical Publishers (P) Ltd
17/1-B Babar Road, Block-B, Shaymali
Mohammadpur, Dhaka-1207
Bangladesh
Mobile: +08801912003485
Email: jaypeedhaka@gmail.com

Jaypee Brothers Medical Publishers (P) Ltd
Bhotahity, Kathmandu, Nepal
Phone +977-9741283608
Email: kathmandu@jaypeebrothers.com

Website: www.jaypeebrothers.com
Website: www.jaypeedigital.com

Mastering NEET Series (Volume-2)

First Edition: 2017
Second Edition: **2018**

ISBN: 978-93-5270-437-8

Printed at Ajanta Offset & Packagings Ltd., Faridabad, Haryana

Dedication

Before you go through the main content of this book, it is my humble request to devote (at least) few minutes to this particular page and read the name of those brave soldiers who sacrificed their lives to make our lives secure and safe.

Being a son of Honorary Captain/Army Education Corps, I would like to dedicate this title to our brave soldiers who were martyred in Uri (Jammu & Kashmir) terror attack.

Located barely a few kilometres from the Line of Control (LoC) and some 70 km from Srinagar, the base was subjected to the brazen attack by four terrorists at around 5.30 AM, causing heavy casualties in the Dogra Regiment, which lost 17 of its men. About 20 more army personnel were injured, some critically, and were airlifted to the Army Base Hospital in Srinagar.

Here is the full list of jawans who died in the Uri terror attack:

1. Subedar Karnail Singh, r/o Vill Shibu Chak, Teh Bishnah, Dist Jammu, Jammu & Kashmir.
2. Havildar Ravi Paul, r/o Samba, Dist Jammu, Jammu & Kashmir.
3. Sepoy Rakesh Singh, r/o Vill Baddja, Dist Kaimur, Bihar.
4. Sepoy Javra Munda, r/o Vill Meral, Dist Khuti, Jharkhand.
5. Sepoy Naiman Kujur, r/o Vill Chainpur, Dist Gumla, Jharkhand.
6. Sepoy Uike Janrao, r/o Vill Nandgaon (Kh), Dist Amravati, Maharashtra.
7. Havildar NS Rawat, r/o Vill Rajawa, Dist Rajasmand, Rajasthan.
8. Sepoy Ganesh Shankar, r/o Vill Ghoorapalli, Dist Sant Kabir Nagar, Uttar Pradesh.
9. Naik SK Vidarthi, r/o Vill Boknari, Dist Gaya, Bihar.
10. Sepoy Biswajit Ghorai, r/o Vill Ganga Sagar, Dist South 24 Parganas, West Bengal.
11. Lance Naik G Shankar, r/o Vill Jashi, Dist Satara, Maharashtra.
12. Sepoy G Dalai, r/o Vill Jamuna Balia, Dist Howrah, West Bengal.
13. Lance Naik RK Yadav, r/o Vill Balia, Uttar Pradesh.
14. Sepoy Harinder Yadav, r/o Vill Ghazipur, Dist Ghazipur, Uttar Pradesh.
15. Sepoy TS Somnath, r/o Vill Khadangali, Dist Nashik, Maharashtra.
16. Havildar Ashok Kumar Singh, r/o Vill Raktu Tola, Dist Bhojpur, Bihar.
17. Sepoy Rajesh Kumar Singh, r/o Vill Jaunpur, Uttar Pradesh.

Preface to the Second Edition

As I always say, there is nothing more pleasant for an author to release a new edition of his book. This is an indirect indication that this title has been open heartedly accepted by the students. But at the same time it brings a challenge to come up to the expectations of readers in subsequent editions.

In the first edition, I have incorporated many images in the explanations. There were many books in the market, all of which were focussing mainly on explanations and less on illustrations. So I thought of presenting a title which did the reverse, I mean which focus more on illustrations and less on theoretical explanations. This concept was readily accepted by the students because it gave them an opportunity to correlate the theory with illustrations as this helps in understanding the facts clearly. But since the first edition was in single colour, so many images were not that impressive. Moreover at some places, where there were legends for colours (green, red or others), it was very difficult to understand which depiction is in which colour. So this time, we are presenting this title in full colour mode so that each and every image stands out clearly and adds to understanding of the concept.

Hope this title (like my other titles) would serve the purpose.

"To err is human" and being a human, I am bound to commit errors. If you find any such unintentional errors in the book, please do communicate with me on the below given modes of contact.

Since students are the best judge, please do shower me with your necessary feedbacks regarding improvement in the content and presentation of the text.

Good Luck

Kamal KV

drkamalkv's Classes, 116/3,
Near Sribalaji Restaurant, Sudarshan Road,
Gautam Nagar, New Delhi - 49, India

Web: www.drkamalkvgroup.co.in
Mail: drkamalkvgroup@gmail.com
Facebook: Drkamalkvgroup
Twitter handle: drkamalkvgroup
Whatsapp & Cell: 8470004333

Preface to the First Edition

There are many good titles available for PG-standard NBE exams, but the problem is that these are so bulky that the students are in a state of confusion when it comes to revision. They enjoy reading them during the initial few days of studies, but during the last few days, when the exams are near, the students find them very difficult to revise.

Keeping this fact in mind, I have compiled this title, which is comparatively easy to revise during the last few days.

Also earlier the students were always concerned about image-based questions. So, in the explanation part, I have liberally used plenty of images to help the students in this regard.

Related tables had been placed wherever necessity was felt.

MCQs have been categorized into different sections. The sections are the same as those in 'Self Assessment & Review of FMGE', so that the students can read both the titles together sectionwise.

An overall attempt has been made to accommodate much information in minimum space.

Hope this title (like my other titles) would serve the purpose.

"To err is human" and being a human, I am bound to commit errors. If you find any such unintentional errors in the book, please do communicate with me through the below given modes of contact.

Since the students are the best judge, please do shower me with your necessary feedback regarding the improvement in the content and presentation of the text.

Good luck

Kamal KV
116/3, Near A-1 Xerox Shop
Sudershan Road
Gautam Nagar
New Delhi – 110049
India
Web : www.drkamalkvgroup.co.in
Mail : drkamalkvgroup@gmail.com
Facebook : Drkamalkvgroup
Twitter handle : drkamalkvgroup
Whatsapp and Cell : 8470004333

How to Read this Title

This title should be revised thrice before the exams. The ideal way of reading this title is like this:

- First reading: 3 months
- Second reading: 2 months
- Third reading: 1 month

Content to be studied in different cycles:

- First reading: Read all MCQs with explanations with attached images/tables. Mark some images or tables which seem important and should be revised again.
- Second reading: Read MCQs with explanations only (no attached images or tables) plus marked images or tables.
- Third reading: MCQs and answers only (no explanations) plus marked images or tables.
- Rest of the content needs to be read in all cycles (keynotes, practice MCQs, image-based MCQs and MCQ points).

How to Solve Paper in Examination Hall

Divide the total duration of examination into 2 rounds: 1/3rd and 2/3rd of the time allotted.

1. First round is **'READ ALL QUESTIONS & MARK FEW'**. One should be able to mark the answer by just going through the MCQ statement. Do not try to search for the answers from the options. Read the MCQ statement, think of the answer and if you find any such option, mark it and go ahead. Obviously, ALL EXCEPT/FALSE statement kind of questions should not be attempted, as these questions demand some time to solve them. First reading of all the MCQs should be done within first round (1/3rd duration).
2. Second round is **'SOLVE USING ASSOCIATION/EXCLUSION PRINCIPLE'**. Here MCQs are not straightforward (ALL EXCEPT/FALSE statement kind of questions) and you have to apply your knowledge to choose the best answer. This stage demands a lot of concentration and ability to catch the hints given in the MCQ statement (2/3rd duration).

To minimize the errors, please discard the tendency of changing the answers frequently. Majority of the time, the students will replace a right answer with a wrong one. So, whatever you have marked once, let it be final. No second thoughts please.

Acknowledgments

Most the things (books, classes) I do by my own, singly. So I find it very difficult to write the acknowledgment section as there is no contribution from anyone.

Therefore, I try to pen down few persons/ incidences related to the title or any person who helped me (as a human) in one or other way.

Related to this particular title, I remember one incident.

One day me, Chairman JP Vij sir and Chetna madam were discussing on our FMGE title. In between, Chairman asked me "Kamal, I wish to publish a NBE pattern MCQs bank title. Can you suggest me any good author for the same". I smiled on this particular question. Chairman sir was little surprised as to why I am smiling on this serious question. I said "Sir, one of the best authors is sitting in front of you, and you are telling him to search somebody else". To this Chairman sir replied "I was expecting only this kind of reply from you. Definitely you and only you would be the best person to pen down this title". And that is how; this title was finalized all of a sudden.

So I would like to thank Chairman JP Vij sir for showering me with his blessing and giving me this wonderful opportunity to compile this title.

Chetna madam needs special mention as she never interfered in my work and accepted all my works without any objection. All my suggestions were duly considered and incorporated wherever necessary. Payal madam worked tirelessly to make sure that this title is finished well within the time limit.

I would also like to thank all my FMG (Foreign Medical Graduate) students, who constantly pressurized me to write a DNB/ NEET based title. With their blessings and unconditional support, my FMGE title was already a big hit and therefore they always wanted me to write a PG standard title as well. I would also love to thank them for supporting and promoting the first edition.

Special thanks to all the people who worked tirelessly in publishing the book. There are many, with whom I never met, but they all played a valuable role in putting this book to its final shape. I big thank to the entire unit.

For all my achievements till now, I will always bow my head in the feet of almighty.

Heartfelt thanks to Punit ji & Deepak ji (Arora Book Stall) for their timely help during my struggling days as an author, when they provided me necessary books for references. Words simply cannot pay back the help done by them during the need of hour.

Jain uncle (Jain stationery), Sanjay bhai & Chandarpal (A1 photocopy), and Sonu also need mention for all their timely help.

Special Thanks

I would extend my heartfelt thanks to:

- All the students of "**drkamalkv's classes**". Their faith helped me, survive in this competitive world of the coaching classes.
- My family members: Parents Hon. Capt./AEC ML Verma and Rati Devi, Brothers Ram Kishore and Anil, Sister Deepti, Wife Manju and my lovely daughters Kaakul and Kaavya.

Contents

CHAPTER

1

ENT

KEY POINTS

Boundaries of Suprameatal Triangle/Surface Marking for Mastoid Antrum Macewen's Triangle

- Anterior: Posterosuperior border of bony external auditory canal along with the Suprameatal spine of Henle
- Superiorly: Supramastoid crest
- Posteriorly: Vertical line drawn tangential to the posterior margin of the external auditory canal

Acceleration and Part of Ear Stimulated

- Angular acceleration: Semicircular canal
- Linear acceleration: Utricles and saccules
- Horizontal linear acceleration: Saccules
- Vertical linear acceleration: Saccules
- Gravity: Utricles and saccules
- Position of head in space: Utricle and saccules

Abscess Related to Ear

- Bezold's abscess: Deep to sternocleidomastoid
- Luc's abscess: Roof of bony canal, subtemporal
- Citelli's abscess: Digastric triangle, posterior belly of digastric

Terms Related with Lateral Sinus Thrombosis

- Griesinger's sign: Thrombosis of mastoid emissary vein, edema over posterior part of mastoid
- Tobey-Ayer test/Queckenstedt's test: Compression of vein on the thrombosed side produces no effect, while on healthy side it leads to rapid rise in CSF pressure

Hearing Loss

- Mild deafness: Hearing loss between 20-30 dB
- Moderate deafness: Hearing loss between 30-60 dB
- Severe deafness: Hearing loss above 60 dB

Rinne Test

- At least 15 dB of hearing loss should be present for it to become negative
- Positive: Normal and sensorineural deafness
- Negative: Conductive deafness

Weber Test

- At least 5 dB of hearing loss should be present for it to become lateralized
- Normal: Equal on both sides
- Conductive deafness: Lateralized to the affected ear
- Sensorineural deafness: Sound is lateralized to the better ear

Dangerous Area of Face

- Lower part of external nose and upper lip
- Infection may spread to the cavernous sinus through the inferior ophthalmic veins via the anterior facial vein

Dangerous Area of Nose

- Also olfactory area may infect the meninges along the pia mater and arachnoid mater sheath of the olfactory nerve passing through the cribriform plate of the ethmoid causing meningitis, encephalitis and brain abscess

Opening in the Lateral Wall of Nose

- Spheno-ethmoidal recess: Opening of sphenoid sinus
- Superior meatus: Opening of posterior ethmoidal sinus
- Middle meatus: Frontal sinus, maxillary sinus, anterior ethmoidal sinus, middle ethmoidal sinus
- Inferior meatus: Nasolacrimal duct

Antrochoanal Polyp

- From maxillary sinus
- Usually single
- Seen in children and adults
- Due to infection
- Extends backwards
- Recurrence unlikely

Ethmoidal Polyp

- Ethmoidal sinus
- Multiple and bilateral
- After puberty
- Allergy and infection
- Extends forwards
- Recurrence likely

Waldeyer's Ring

- Palatine tonsil
- Nasopharyngeal tonsil
- Tubal tonsils
- Lingual tonsils
- Lateral pharyngeal bands
- Pharyngeal nodules

Singer's Nodes/Vocal Nodules

- In persons who misuse or overuse their voice
- Excision by microlaryngoscopy

MCQs WITH SHORT EXPLANATIONS

EAR

1. Semicircular canal commonly affected in benign paroxysmal positional vertigo:

a. Lateral
b. Anterior
c. Posterior
d. All of the above

Pathology of benign paroxysmal positional vertigo

- Within the labyrinth of the inner ear lie collections of calcium crystals known as otoconia or otoliths.
- In patients with BPPV, the otoconia are dislodged from their usual position within the utricle and migrate over time into one of the semicircular canals (the posterior canal is most commonly affected due to its anatomical position)

2. In which condition, bones of ear are fused:

a. Chronic suppurative otitis media
b. Acute suppurative otitis media
c. Otitis media with effusion
d. Otosclerosis

Conductive hearing loss in otosclerosis is caused by two main sites of involvement of the sclerotic (or scar-like) lesions. The best understood mechanism is fixation of the stapes footplate to the oval window of the cochlea. This greatly impairs movement of the stapes and therefore transmission of sound into the inner ear ("ossicular coupling"). Additionally the cochlea's round window can also become sclerotic, and in a similar way impair movement of sound pressure waves through the inner ear ("acoustic coupling").

3. Regarding Eustachian tube, which of the following is FALSE:

a. Size is 3.75 cm
b. Cartilaginous 1/3rd & 2/3rd bony
c. Opens during swallowing
d. Tensor palate helps to open it

Eustachian tube

- The Eustachian tube extends from the anterior wall of the middle ear to the lateral wall of the nasopharynx, approximately at the level of the inferior nasal concha.
- A portion of the tube (1/3) proximal to the middle ear is made of bone; this bony part is about 12 mm in length.
- The cartilage of pharyngotympanic tube, about 24 mm. in length

4. In Bithermal Caloric test, hypoactive/absent response indicates:

a. Ossicles fixation
b. Otosclerosis
c. Acute otitis media
d. Meniere's disease

Less or no response from aparticular side is indicative of depressed function of the ipsilateral labyrinth, vestibular nerve or vestibular nuclei and is seen in Meniere's disease, acoustic neuroma, post-labyrinthetcomy or vestibular nerve section.

5. In which condition, Chemical labyrinthectomy is done:

a. Acute otitis media
b. Chronic otitis media
c. Meniere's disease
d. Acoustic neuroma

In Meniere's disease, the inner ear itself can be surgically removed via labyrinthectomy although hearing is always completely lost in the affected ear with this operation. Alternatively, a chemical labyrinthectomy, in which a drug (such as gentamicin) that "kills" the vestibular apparatus is injected into the middle ear can accomplish the same results while retaining hearing.

6. Inheritance of otosclerosis:

a. Autosomal dominant
b. Autosomal recerssive
c. X-linked dominant
d. X-linked recessive

The disease can considered to be hereditary, but its penetrance and the degree of expression is so highly variable that it may be difficult to detect an inheritance pattern. Most of the implicated genes are transmitted in an autosomal dominant fashion. One genome-wide analysis associates otosclerosis with variation in RELN gene.

7. In BERA, distal part of cranial nerve VIII near the brainstem generates which wave form:

a. Wave I
b. Wave III
c. Wave IV
d. Wave V

BERA waves neural generators

- **Wave I**: Distal part of CN VIII
- **Wave II**: Proximal part of CN VIII near the brainstem
- **Wave III**: Cochlear nucleus
- **Wave IV**: Superior olivary complex
- **Wave V**: Lateral lemniscus
- **Wave VI & VII**: Inferior colliculus

Ans. 1. **c.** Posterior 2. **d.** Otosclerosis 3. **b.** Cartilaginous 1/3rd & 2/3rd bony 4. **d.** Meniere's disease 5. **c.** Meniere's disease 6. **a.** Autosomal dominant 7. **a.** Wave I

8. Assessment of Vestibular function:

a. Rinne's test
b. Hallpike's test
c. Acoustic reflex
d. Impedance audiometry

The caloric test (Modified Kobrak test & Fitzgerald Hallpike's test) is an attempt to discover the degree to which the vestibular system is responsive and also how symmetric the responses are, between left and right ears. It is a test of the lateral semicircular canals alone — it does not assess vertical canal function or otolithic function.

9. In acoustic neuroma, cranial nerve to be involved earliest is:

a. 5th
b. 6th
c. 7th
d. 8th

The first extracanalicular nerve to be involved in acoustic neuroma is trigeminal. The tumour is in cerebellopontine angle/CPA and of about 2.5 cm. Patient present as reduced corneal sensitivity and numbness of paresthesia of face.

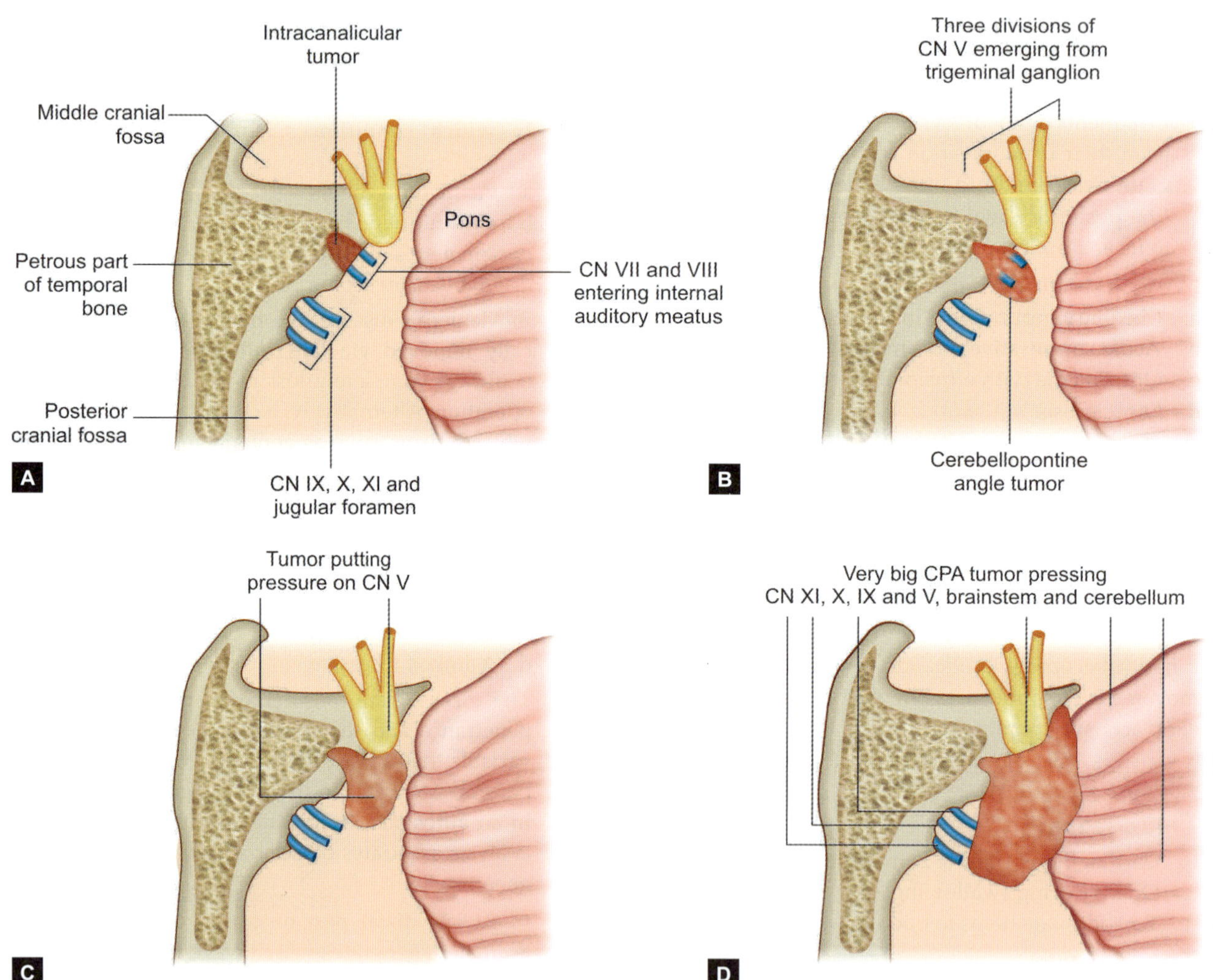

Acoustic neuroma. (A) Intracanalicular tumor; (B) Cerebellopontine angle tumor; (C) Tumor pressing trigeminal nerve; (D) Tumor pressing glossopharyngeal, vagus, and accessory nerves, brainstem and cerebellum

10. In the external auditory canal/EAC, the cartilaginous portion is:

a. Smaller than the bony portion
b. Larger than the bony portion
c. Both are equal
d. Devoid of ceruminous glands

EAC measures about 24 mm and extends from the concha to the tympanic membrane. Its outer one-third (8 mm) is cartilaginous and inner two-third (16 mm) is bony.

Ans. **8. b.** Hallpike's test **9. a.** 5th **10. a.** Smaller than the bony portion

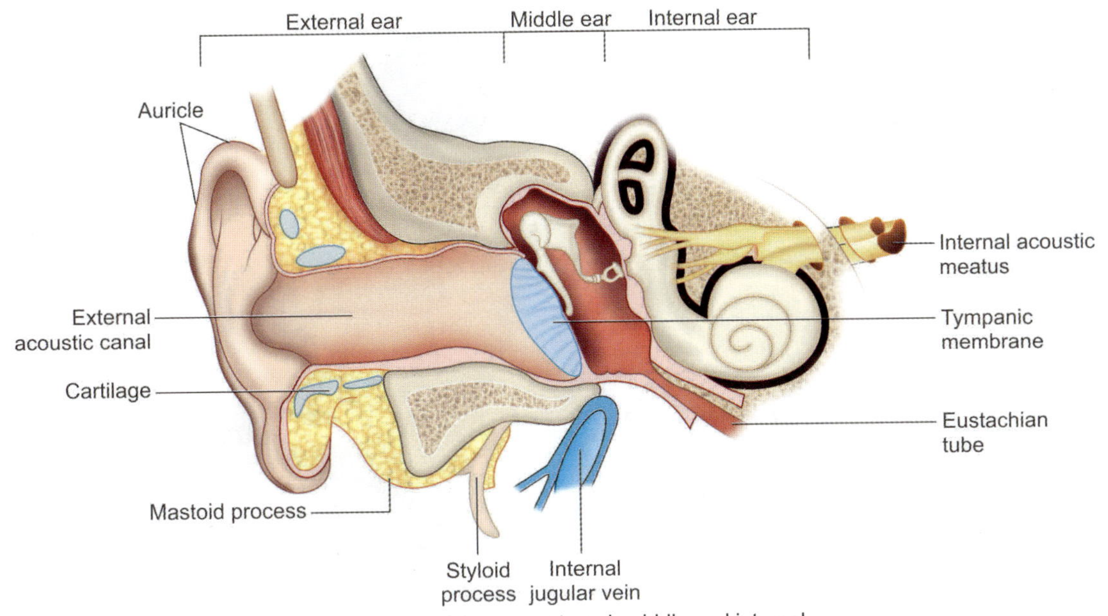

Three parts of the ear: external, middle and internal

11. Stapedius is supplied by:

a. Maxillary nerve b. Facial nerve

c. Auditory nerve d. Mandibular nerve

Stapedins muscle, on contraction dampens the loud sounds and prevents noise trauma to the inner ear. It is supplied by a branch of CN VII (nerve to stapedius of facial nerve).

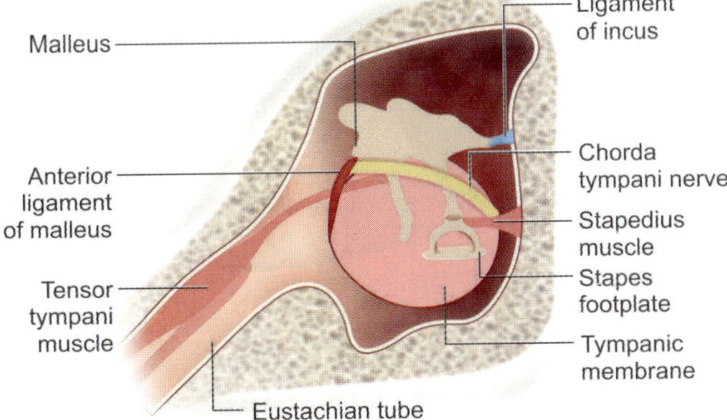

Right tympanic membrane, ossicles and Eustachian tube seen from medial side

12. Movement of stapes causes vibration in:

a. Semicircular canals b. Scala vestibuli

c. Scala tympani d. Scala media

Physiology of Hearing

- The pinna collects sound signals from the environment, which passes through EAC and vibrates the tympanic membrane
- Vibrations of the tympanic membrane are transmitted to the stapes footplate through chain of ossicles
- Vibrations of the stapes footplate result in the pressure changes in the labyrinthine fluids that make movement of the basilar membrane and thus stimulate the hair cells of the organ of Corti
- The IHC of cochlea acts as transducers and convert the mechanical energy into electrical impulses which travel along the auditory nerve.

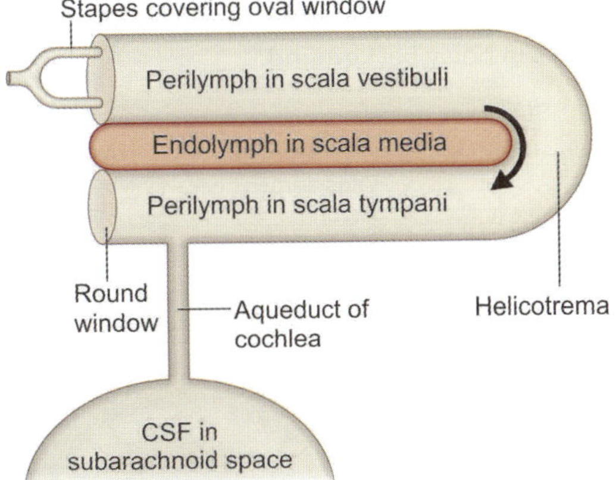

Cochlea: Peri- and endolymphatic systems relations with cerebrospinal fluid (CSF)

13. Hallpike maneuver is done for:

a. Vestibular function b. Audiometry

c. Cochlear function d. Corneal test

Dix-Hallpike maneuver has a positive predictive value of 83% and negative predictive value of 52% for the diagnosis of BPPV (benign paroxysmal positional vertigo). The causes of vertigo are categorized into two groups: peripheral (labyrinth and vestibular nerve) and central (vestibular nuclei and their central nervous system connections brainstem and cerebellum).

Ans. **11. b.** Facial nerve **12. b.** Scala vestibuli **13. a.** Vestibular function

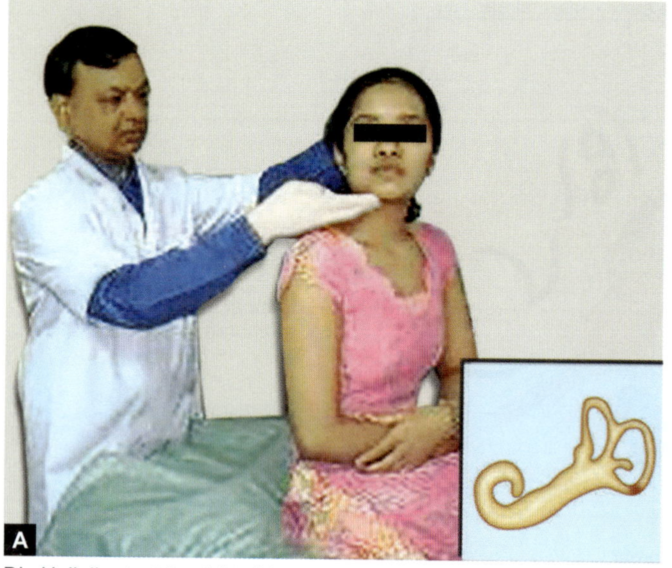

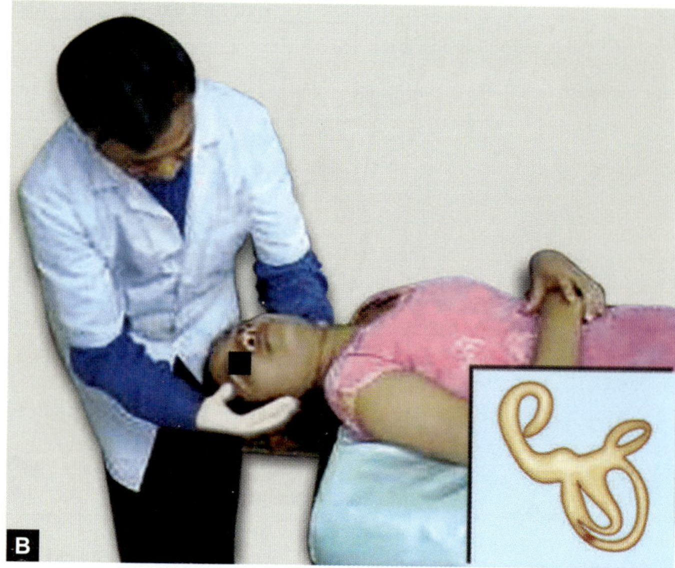

Dix Hallpike test for right side posterior canal BPPV. (A) First sitting position (inset shows debris near ampulla of posterior canal); (B) Second supine head hanging position (Inset shows debris moving away from the ampulla in the posterior canal

14. Hyperacusis is seen in all of the following EXCEPT:

a. Exposure to loud sounds
b. Otosclerosis
c. Meniere's disease
d. Severe head injury

Otosclerosis is characterized by gradually progressive conductive hearing loss with normal tympanic membrane. In paracusis Willisii, the patient's hearing improves in noisy background.

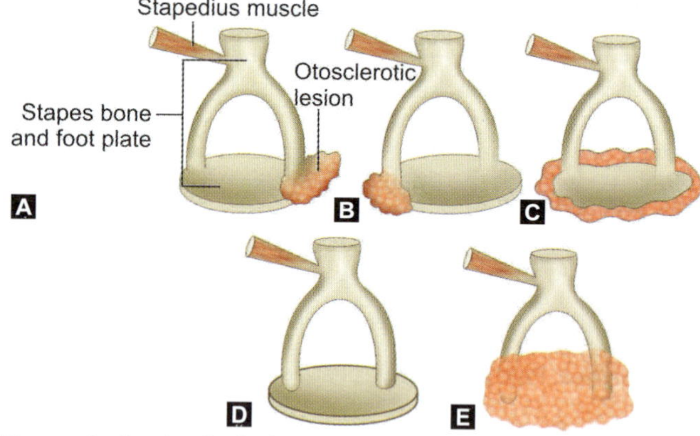

Types of otosclerotic lesions causing fixation of stapes footplate. (A) Anterior focus, the site of predilection "fissula ante fenestram"; (B) Posterior focus the lesion begins behind the oval window; (C) Circumferential, lesion begins around the margins of footplate; (D) Biscuit type lesion involves only footplate sparing the annular ligament; (E) Obliterative lesion completely obliterates the oval window niche

15. Meniere's disease is characterized by the triad of:

a. Deafness, nystagmus, tremors
b. Deafness, vertigo, nystagmus
c. Deafness, tinnitus, vertigo
d. Deafness, tremors, tinnitus

Symptom complex of Meniere's disease consists of spontaneous episodic vertigo, fluctuating sensorineural hearing loss (SNHL), tinnitus and often a sensation of fluctuating ear fullness.

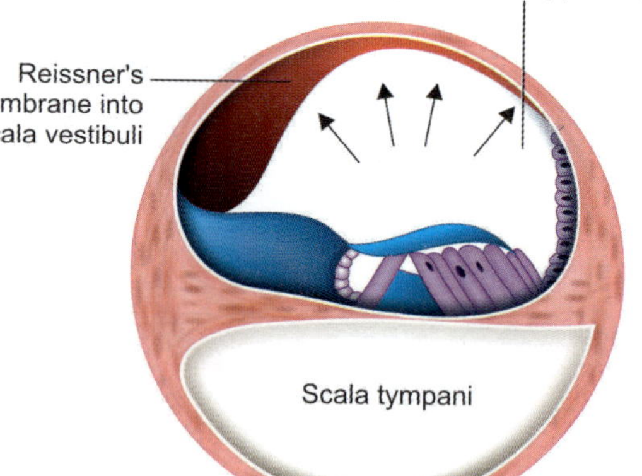

Ménière's disease. Distended cochlear duct pushing the Reissner's membrane into scala vestibuli

16. The most common clinical presentation of acoustic neuroma is feature of:

a. Brainstem involvement
b. Cerebellar involvement
c. Facial nerve involvement
d. Cochleovestibular symptoms

Progressive unilateral SNHL, which is often accompanied by tinnitus, is the most common presenting symptom.

Ans. 14. **b.** Otosclerosis
15. **c.** Deafness, tinnitus, vertigo
16. **d.** Cochleovestibular symptoms

Differential diagnoses of common causes of dizziness

Clinical features	*Meniere's disease*	*Vestibular neuritis*	*Benign paroxysmal positional vertigo*	*Acoustic neuroma*
Type of dizziness	*Whirling vertigo*	*Whirling vertigo*	*Whirling vertigo*	*Unsteadiness*
Duration of dizziness	Recurrent episodes (lasting for minutes to hours)	Acute prolonged attack (lasting for days)	Short spells (lasting for seconds) in certain positions	Recurrent Momentary or chronic
Tinnitus	Present	Absent	Absent	Present
Vomiting	Very common	Always	Uncommon	Rare
Sensorineural hearing loss	Moderate and fluctuating sensory type with recruitment	Absent	Absent	Progressive neural type with tone decay
Cranial nerve involvement (V, VII, VIII, IX, X and XI)	Absent	Absent	Absent	Present in late stages

17. Carhart's notch in audiogram is a dip at:

a. 0.5 kHz
b. 2 kHz
c. 4 kHz
d. 8 kHz

Carhart's notch is a dip (from 500-4,000 Hz) in bone conduction curve, which is maximum (15 dB) at 2,000 Hz (5 dB at 500 Hz, 10 dB at 1,000 Hz, 15 dB at 2,000 Hz and 5 dB at 4,000 Hz).

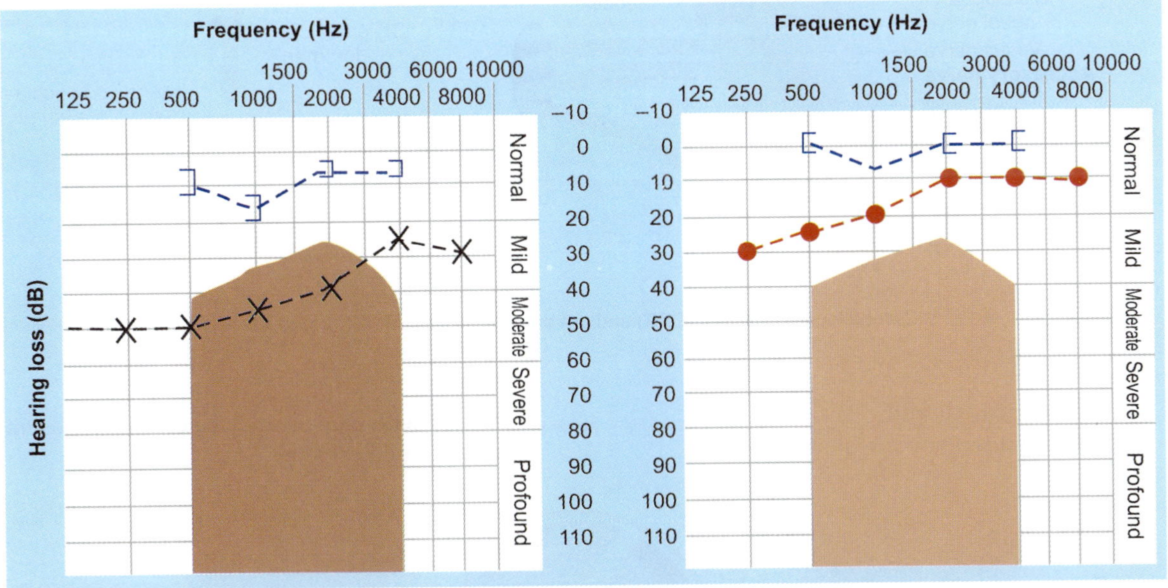

Audiogram otosclerosis. Bilateral predominantly low-frequency conductive hearing loss. Left ear stapes surgery planned

18. Meniere's disease is manifested by all of the following symptoms EXCEPT:

a. Tinnitus
b. Vertigo
c. Deafness
d. Otorrhea

Otorrhea refers to discharge from the ear. Infective diseases are the most common causes of otorrhea.

Classification and diagnosis of Ménière's disease. Committee of hearing and equilibrium. American Academy of Otolaryngology-Head and Neck Surgery

Certain: Confirmed by histopathology
Definite: Two or more episodes of spontaneous whirling vertigo lasting for 20 minutes or more
- Documented sensory hearing loss (HL) on audiometry on at least one occasion

Ans. 17. **b.** 2 kHz 18. **d.** Otorrhea

Contd...

Classification and diagnosis of Ménière's disease. Committee of hearing and equilibrium. American Academy of Otolaryngology-Head and Neck Surgery
❑ Tinnitus or aural fullness
❑ Other causes excluded
Probable:
❑ One episode of spontaneous whirling vertigo
❑ Documented sensory HL
❑ Tinnitus or aural fullness
❑ Other causes excluded
Possible:
❑ **Vestibular variant:** Episodes of spontaneous whirling vertigo without documented HL.

Contd...

Contd...

Classification and diagnosis of Ménière's disease. Committee of hearing and equilibrium. American Academy of Otolaryngology-Head and Neck Surgery
❑ **Cochlear variant:** Fluctuating or fixed with disequilibrium but without episodes of spontaneous whirling vertigo
❑ Other causes excluded.

19. Acoustic neuroma commonly affects the ..... cranial nerve:

a. 5th
b. 6th
c. 7th
d. 8th

Acoustic neuroma arises from the Schwann cells of the vestibular nerve twice as often as from the cochlear nerve. It reaches CPA after eroding and widening EAC.

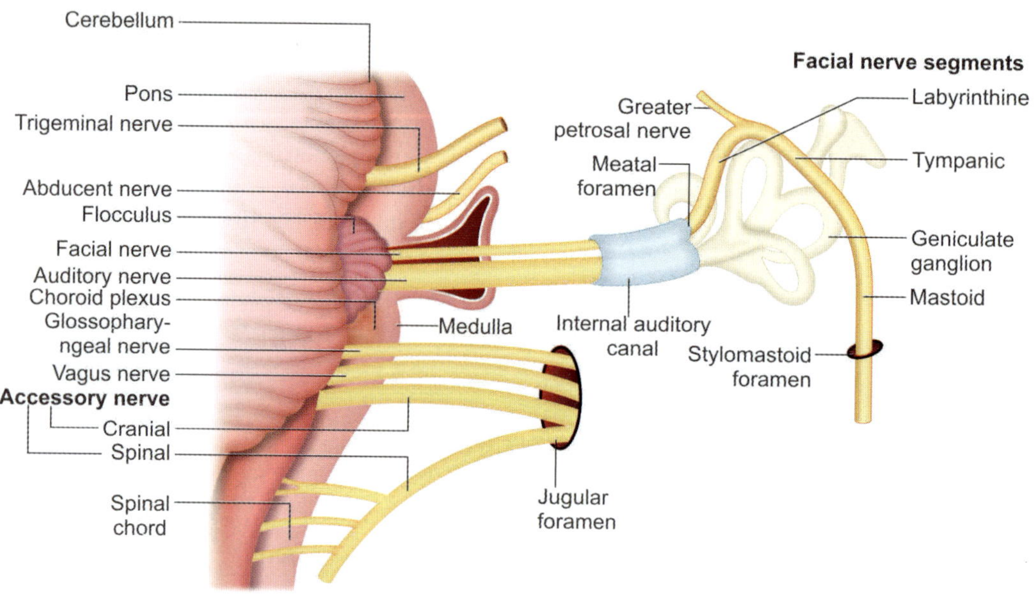

Cerebellopontine angle (CPA) and cranial nerves VII, VIII, IX, X and XI

20. True for glue ear:

a. Sodium fluoride is useful
b. Radical mastoidectomy is required
c. Painless
d. Painful

A child with glue ear may be completely asymptomatic and has mild earache.

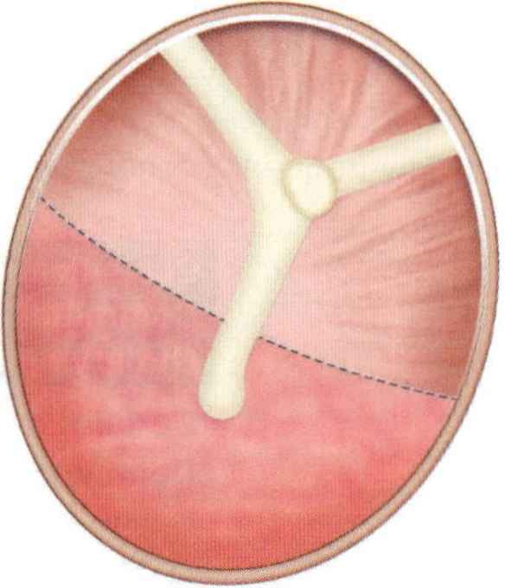

Otitis media with effusion. Otoscopy shows fluid level and air bubbles

Ans. 19. **d.** 8th   20. **c.** Painless

21. NOT a component of Gradenigo's syndrome:

a. Otorrhoea
b. VII cranial nerve palsy
c. VI cranial nerve palsy
d. V cranial nerve palsy

Gradenigo's triad consists of otorrhea, abducens palsy and retrobulbar pain, and is the classic presentation of petrous apicitis.

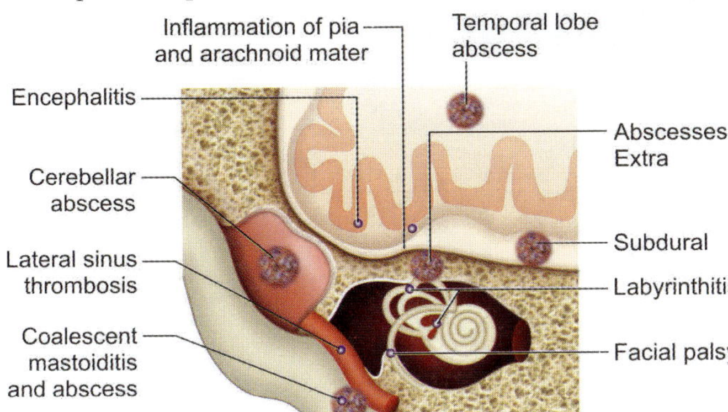

Complications of suppurative otitis media involving structures in relation with middle ear

22. Rinne test is positive in:

a. Normal ear
b. Otomycosis
c. CSOM
d. Wax in ear

Rinne test is said to be positive when AC is longer or louder than BC. The positive Rinne (AC > BC) is seen in cases of normal hearing or SNHL.

The interpretation of tuning fork tests (TFT)

Tests	*Normal*	*Conductive hearing loss*	*Sensorineural hearing loss*
Rinne	AC > BC (Rinne +)	BC > AC (Rinne -)	AC > BC (Rinne +)
Weber	Center	Lateralized to affected ear	Lateralized to better ear
Absolute bone conduction	Normal	Normal	Reduced
Schwabach	Normal	Lengthened	Shortened
Bing	Positive	Negative	Positive
Gelle	Positive	Negative (ossicular lesions)	Positive

23. CSF otorrhea is due to involvement/trauma of:

a. Cribriform plate
b. Petrous temporal bone
c. Parietal bone
d. Tympanic membrane

CSF otorrhea is seen in fracture temporal bone, tegmen defect, cochlea deformity or Hyrtl's disease.

Causes of otorrhea

- *External auditory canal:* Otitis externa (OE)*, otomycosis*, furunculosis*, keratosis obturans, malignant or necrotizing otitis externa, acute dermatitis (such as seborrheic, eczematous), parotid abscess, canal cholesteatoma, neoplasms (ceruminoma and malignancy)
- *Conditions predisposing to secondary otitis externa:* Osteoma, exostoses, canal dehiscence into the mastoid or glenoid fossa, otitis media with perforation, allergy to ear drops
- *Tympanic membrane*: Granulation tissue*, granular myringitis*, bullous myringitis, retraction pocket, cholesteatoma
- *Middle ear and mastoid*: Acute and chronic suppurative otitis media (ASOM and CSOM)* and mastoiditis, cholesteatoma*, granulomatous disease, neoplasms
- *CSF otorrhea*: Fracture temporal bone, tegmen defect, cochlea deformity, Hyrtl's disease

* Common causes of otorrhea

24. Angular movements are sensed by:

a. Cochlea
b. Utricle
c. Saccule
d. Semicircular canals

Semicircular canals respond to angular acceleration and deceleration. The one that lies at right angle to the axis of rotation is most stimulated. For example: The horizontal canal responds maximum to rotation on the vertical axis.

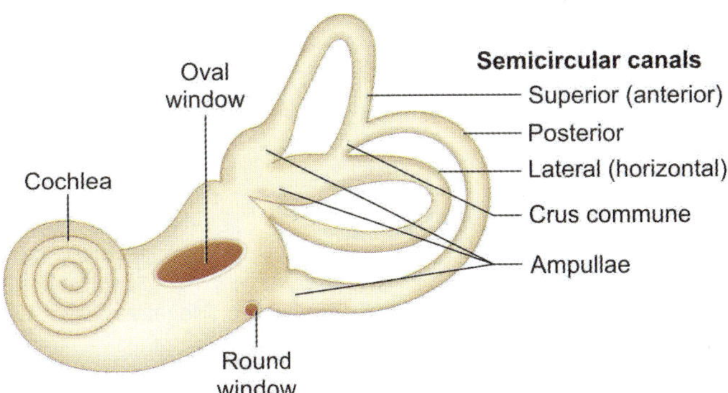

Bony labyrinth of left side. External features seen from lateral side

25. Weber's test in conductive deafness:

a. Sound louder in normal ear
b. Sound louder in diseased ear
c. Heard with intensity in both the ear
d. Inconclusive test

In conductive hearing loss, Weber test is lateralized toward the affected ear. If both the ears have CHL, Weber is lateralized to worst ear.

Ans. 21. **b.** VII cranial nerve... 22. **a.** Normal ear 23. **b.** Petrous temporal 24. **d.** Semicircular canals 25. **b.** Sound louder in diseased ear

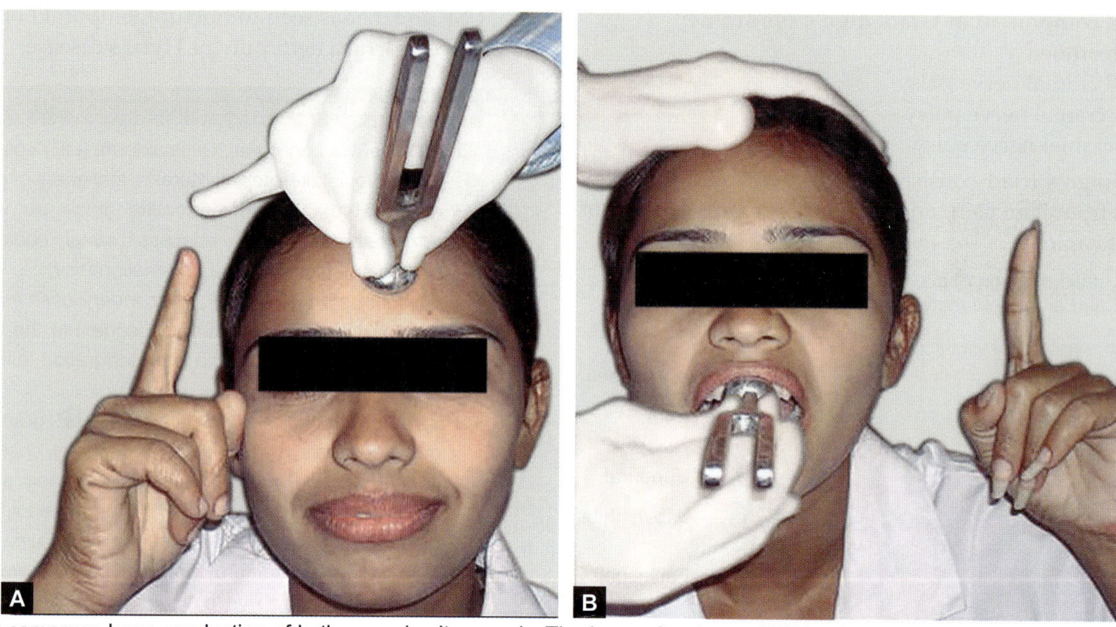

Weber Test compares bone conduction of both ears simultaneously. The base of a charged TF is placed in the center of the forehead (A); or upper central incisors (B). Patient raises finger on the side of better hearing (lateralization)

26. Most common cause of conductive deafness in children less than 12 yrs:

a. CSOM
b. Otosclerosis
c. Serous otitis media
d. Atresia of auditory canals on both sides

The most common causes of CHL include wax, otitis media (ASOM and CSOM), tympanosclerosis, and otosclerosis. In children, the most common cause is otitis media with effusion.

Differences between conductive hearing loss and sensorineural hearing loss

Features	*Conductive hearing loss*	*Sensorineural hearing loss*
Speech understanding	Good	Poor
Intolerance to loud sounds	Absent	Present in cochlear lesions
Speech of the patient	Low voice	Loud voice
Paracusis Willisii	Common	Absent
Common associated symptom	Otorrhea/earache	Tinnitus
Profound hearing loss	Never	Common
Rinne test	Negative (BC > AC)	Positive (AC > BC)
Weber test	Lateralized toward worst ear	Lateralized toward better ear
Absolute bone conduction	Normal	Reduced
Pure tone audiometry (PTA) Air-bone gap	Present	Absent
PTA: Recruitment	Absent	Present in cochlear lesions
PTA: Tone decay	Absent	Present in CN VIII lesion
PTA: Frequencies	Usually low tones involved	Usually higher tones involved
PTA: Thresholds	Never > 60–70 dB	Can be > 60–70 dB
Speech discrimination	Not affected	Poor
Site of lesion	External and middle ear	Internal ear, CN VIII and central auditory connections

Ans. **26. c.** Serous otitis media

27. Negative Rinne's test for 256 Hz tuning fork indicates a minimum air-bone gap of:

a. 10 dB
b. 15 dB
c. 20 dB
d. 25 dB

A negative Rinne with 256, 512 and 1,024 Hz shows air-bone gap of approximately 15, 30, 45 dB respectively.

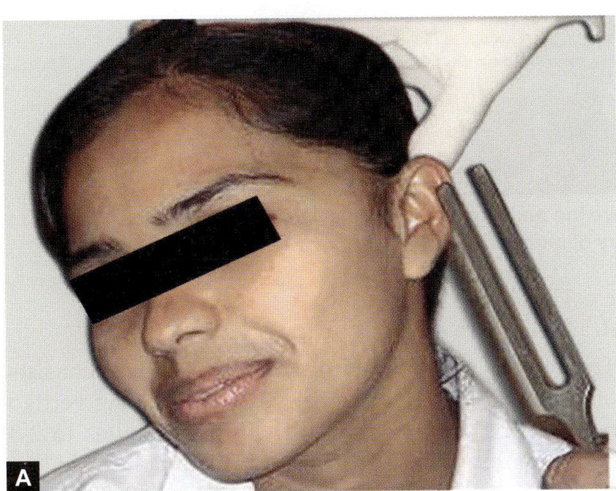

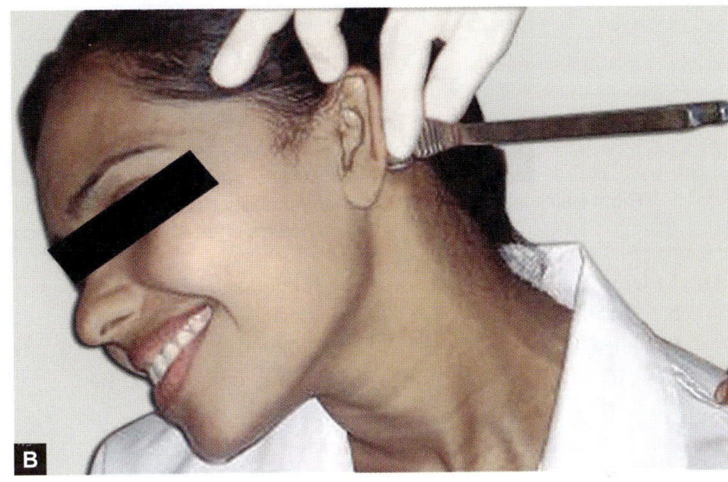

Rinne Test. It compares the loudness of sound of air conduction (A); Bone conduction (B)

28. Cauliflower ear seen in:

a. Hematoma of the auricle
b. Carcinoma of the auricle
c. Fungal infection of the auricle
d. Congenital deformity

Hematoma of the auricle refers to the collection of blood between the auricular cartilage and perichondrium due to blunt trauma. Cauliflower ear occurs when extravasated blood clots and gets organized.

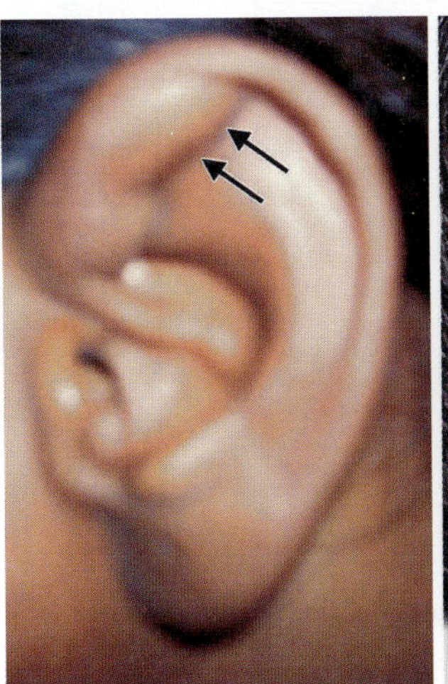

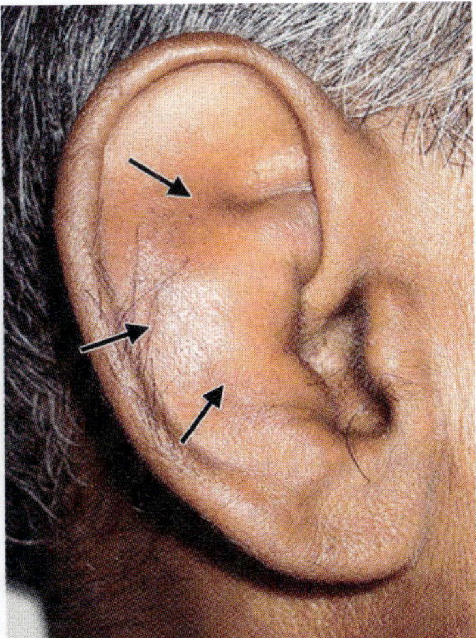

Auricular hematoma

29. Eustachian tube develops from:

a. 2nd and 3rd pharyngeal pouch
b. 1st pharyngeal pouch
c. 2nd pharyngeal pouch
d. 3rd pharyngeal pouch

The Eustachian tube, tympanic cavity, attic, antrum and mastoid air cells are derived from the endoderm of tubotympanic recess which arises from the first and partly from the second pharyngeal pouches.

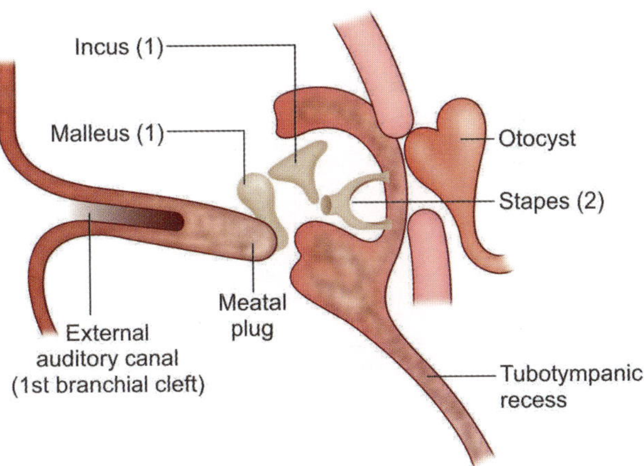

Development of external and middle ears. 1 (Meckel's cartilage) and 2 (Reichert's cartilage) branchial arches

30. Hyperacusis in Bell's palsy is due to the paralysis of:

a. Tensor tympani
b. Levator palatine
c. Tensor veli palatini
d. Stapedius

Hyperacusis is sensitivity to loud sounds and is due to stapedial palsy.

Ans. 27. **b.** 15 dB 28. **a.** Hematoma of the... 29. **b.** 1st pharyngeal pouch 30. **d.** Stapedius

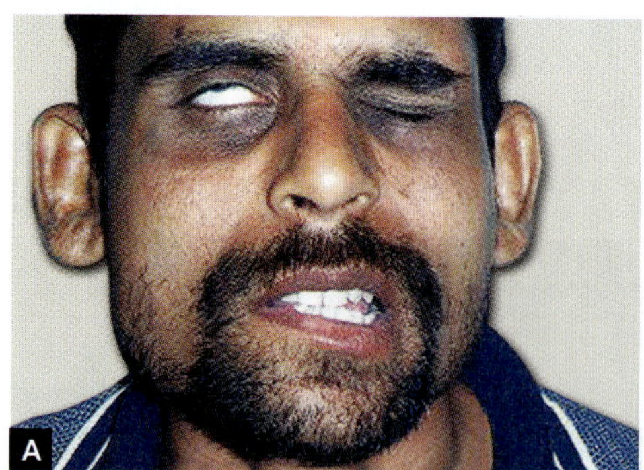

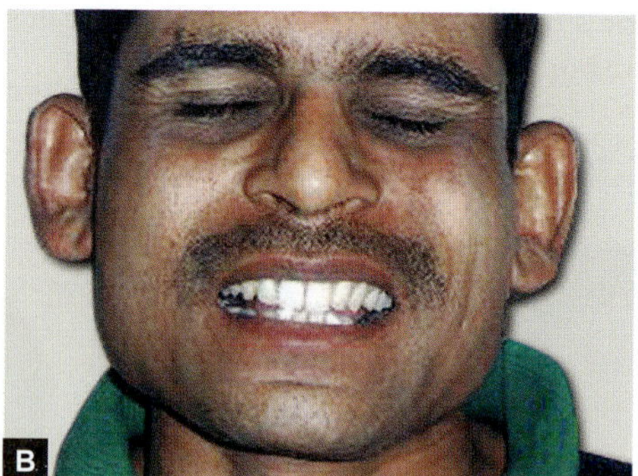

Right Bell's facial palsy. (A) Note the inability to close the eye and move the angle of mouth and upward rolling of eye ball (Bell's phenomenon); (B) Recovery of facial palsy

31. Myringitis bullosa is commonly caused by:

a. Viral
b. Bacteria
c. Fungal
d. Protozoan

Bullous otitis externa and myringitis is believed to be primarily viral.

32. NOT a feature of Meniere's disease:

a. Vertigo
b. Diplopia
c. Tinnitus
d. Pressure in ear

The typical presentation of Meniere's disease consists of recurring attacks (3-11 per year) of spinning vertigo (96.2%) in horizontal axis (usually for minutes to 2-3 hours) with tinnitus (91.1%) and ipsilateral hearing loss (87.7%). Attack lasting more than a day is inconsistent with the diagnosis.

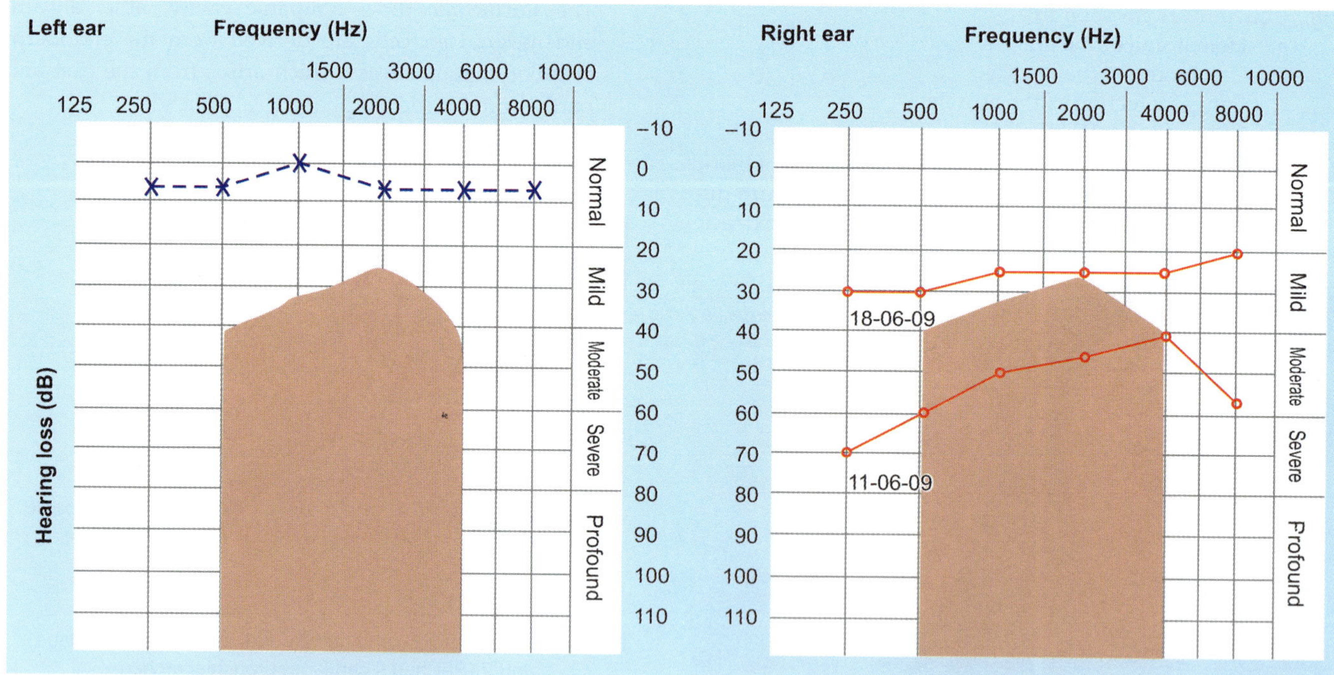

Audiogram Ménière's disease right ear. Low-frequency fluctuating (improvement after 1 week) sensorineural hearing loss in right ear

33. Causative organism for malignant otitis externa is:

a. Hemophilus
b. Staphylococcus
c. Streptococcus
d. Pseudomonas

Malignant otitis externa/MOE is a rare OE of immunocompromised patients is an aggressive and potentially fatal infection, which progressively spreads to skull base and intracranial structures. Pseudomonas aeruginosa is the most common cause. Staphylococcus aureus and Staphylococcus epidermidis are rare causes.

34. A patient with history of head injury developed unilateral conducting hearing loss. On examination, tympanic membrane is normal and mobile. The cause for deafness could be:

Ans. **31. a.** Viral **32. b.** Diplopia **33. d.** Pseudomonas **34. c.** Dislocation

a. Collection of fluid in the middle ear
b. Osteoma
c. Dislocation of the incudostapedial joint
d. ASOM

CHL with normal TM can be seen in temporal bone fracture, congenital fixity of ossicles, otosclerosis, congenital cholesteatoma or glomus tumour.

Flowchart for clinical diagnoses of causes of conductive hearing losses

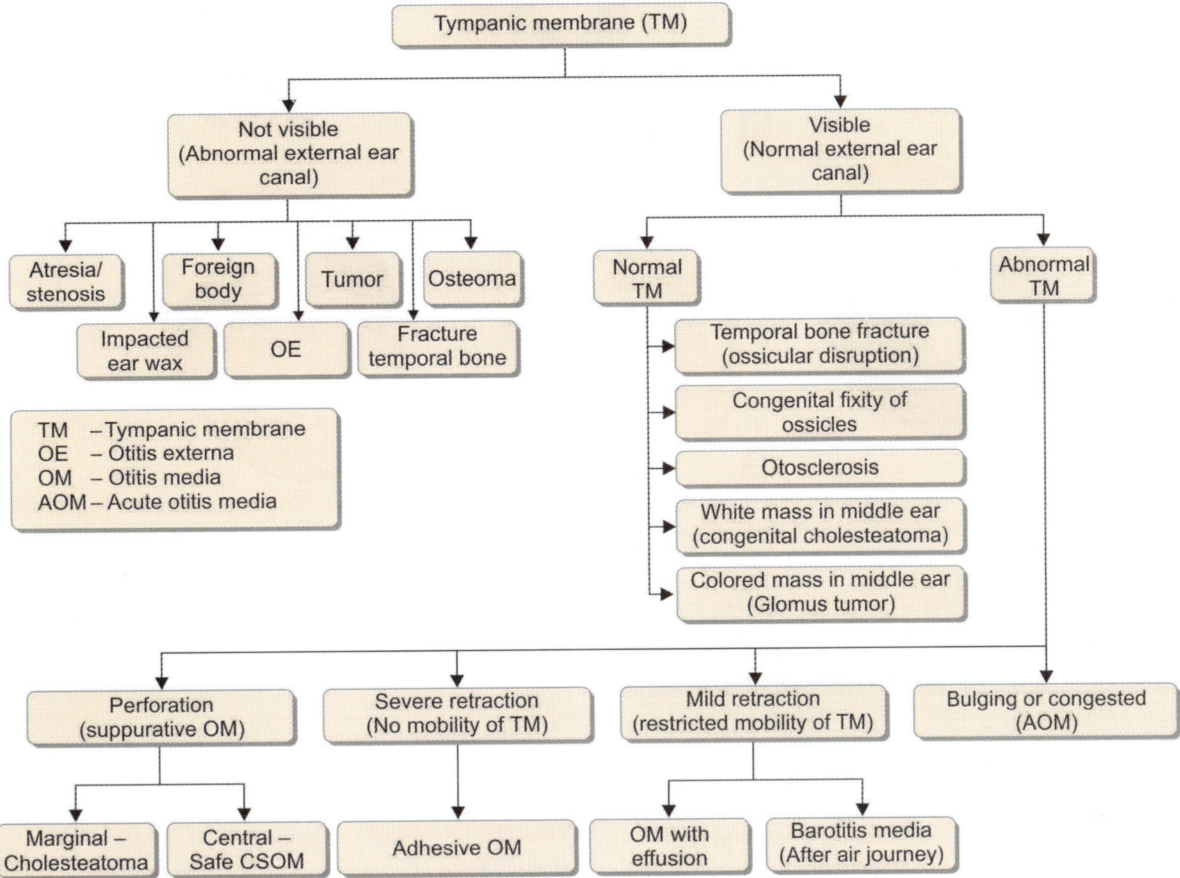

35. Most common cause of chronic ear infection in India is:

a. Syphilitic otitis media
b. TB otitis media
c. CSOM
d. Fungal otitis media

Chronic suppurative otitis media is a long-standing infection of the middle ear cleft. It is characterized by ear discharge and a permanent perforation of tympanic membrane. It is the MC cause of otorrhea.

(See Diagram on next page)

36. Otomycosis is commonly caused by:

a. Actinomycetes b. Aspergillus
c. Mucormycosis d. Candida

Fungal infection of ear is frequently seen in hot and humid climate of tropical and subtropical countries. Common fungal species are Aspergillus niger and Candida albicans.

37. External otitis is:

a. ASOM b. Telephonist's ear
c. Malignant otitis externa d. Glue ear

Diffuse Otitis Externa

- It is also called as Swimmer's ear or **Telephonist's ear**
- There is diffuse inflammation of external auditory meatal skin
- It is seen hot, humid climate and among swimmer's.

38. Which is the most pulsatile condition found in the external auditory meatus, which bleeds on touch:

a. CSOM
b. Chronic adhesive otitis media
c. Acute otitis media
d. Glomus tumour

On increasing the ear canal pressure with Siegle's speculum, glomus tumour pulsates vigorously and then blanches. Reverse happens with release of pressure (Brown's sign).

Ans. 35. **c.** CSOM 36. **b.** Aspergillus 37. **b.** Telephonist's ear 38. **d.** Glomus tumour

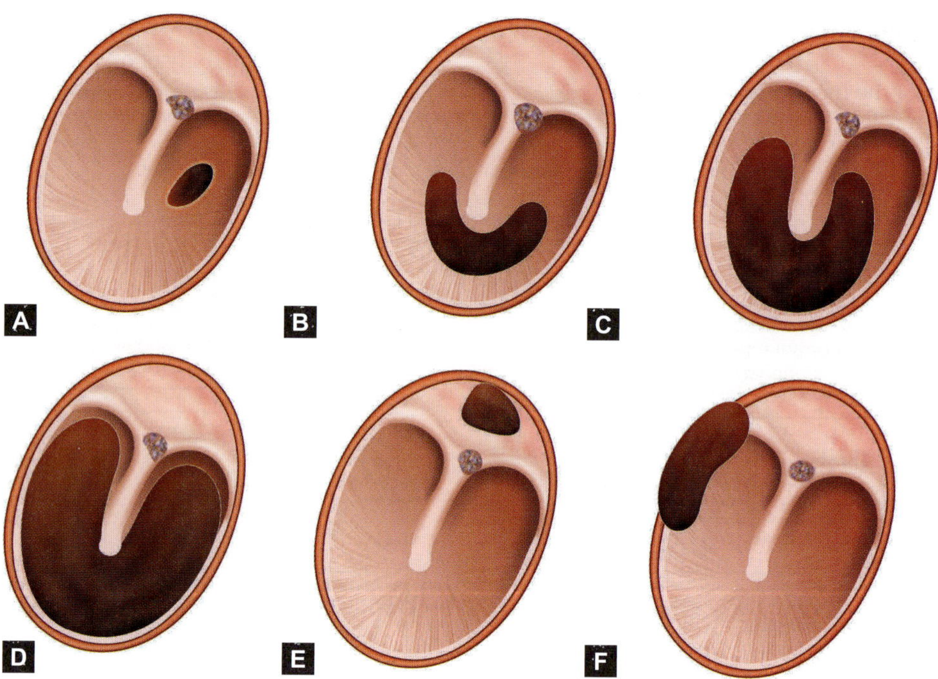

Types of perforations of tympanic membrane in cases of chronic suppurative otitis media (CSOM). (A) Small central perforation in anterosuperior quadrant; (B) Medium size kidney shaped central perforation; (C) Subtotal central perforation; (D) Total perforation with destruction of fibrous annulus; (E) Attic perforation of pars flaccida; (F) Posterosuperior marginal perforation. Note: A, B and C occur in tubotympanic CSOM. D, E and F seen in CSOM with cholesteatoma

Common causes of pulsatile tinnitus and their key clinical features

Causes	*Clinical features*
Benign Intracranial Hypertension (BIH) Syndrome (pseudotumor cerebri)	Young obese females complaining of headache, visual changes and dizziness, CSF pressure > 200 mm H_2O
Glomus Tumors, Persistent stapedial artery,	Reddish pulsatile mass medial to tympanic membrane
Dehiscent carotid, Aberrant carotid	Normal otoscopy
Vascular malformations Atherosclerotic Carotid Artery Disease	Risk factors of atherosclerosis, Carotid bruit
Dehiscent High-riding Jugular Bulb	Bluish mass medial to tympanic membrane and conductive hearing loss
Arterial dissection (carotid, vertebral)	Cerebral Ischemic Symptoms
Venous hum	Right-sided pulsatile tinnitus in women between the ages of 30 and 50 years

39. The most effective means of identifying site of sensorineural deafness is:

a. Stapedial reflex b. Audiometry
c. BERA d. CT scan

BERA finds out the threshold of hearing in infants, which are in high risk groups. It aids in the diagnosis of retrocochlear lesions.

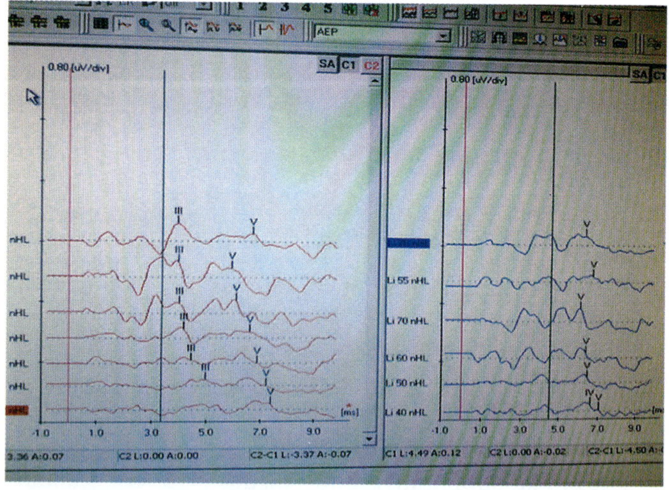

Normal BERA with normal latency and click stimulus from 80 to 40 dBnHL
Source: Dr Amit Anand and Dr Hemant Shah, Consultant Audiologists, Anand and Ahmedabad, Gujarat

40. Earliest symptom of acoustic neuroma:

a. Facial weakness
b. Vertigo
c. Tinnitus
d. Deafness

Progressive unilateral SNHL, which is often accompanied by tinnitus, is the most common presenting symptom.

Ans. **39. c.** BERA **40. d.** Deafness

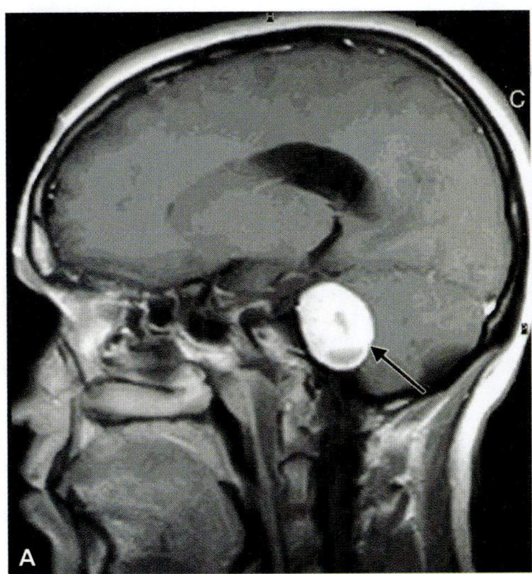

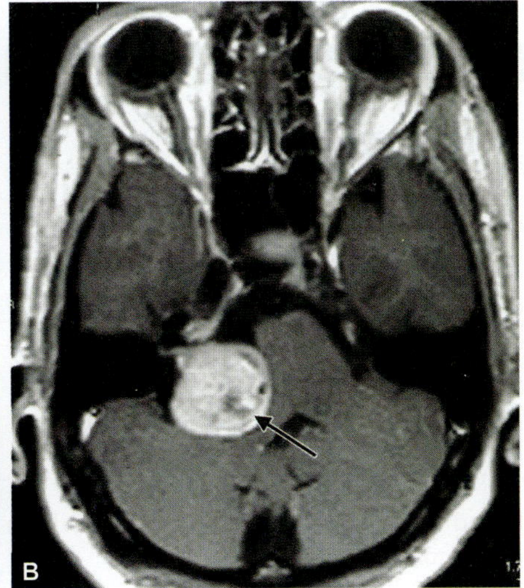

MRI of brain with gadolinium contrast in a case of cerebellopontine angle (CPA) tumor. (A) Sagittal section; (B) Axial section
Source: Dr Ritesh Prajapati, Consultant Radiologist, Anand, Gujarat

41. Referred pain in the ear is commonly from:

a. Maxillary carcinoma
b. Nasopharyngeal carcinoma
c. Carcinoma tongue
d. Malignant otitis externa

Referred otalgia. Common causes of referred otalgia and nerve supply of ear

Secondary otalgia is referred from the head and neck regions, which are innervated by the nerves that also supply to ear. Glossopharyngeal nerve also supplies to oropharynx, which include tonsil, soft palate, posterior pharyngeal wall and base of tongue.

42. Tuning fork frequency used for testing is:

a. 512 Hz
b. 1048 Hz
c. 248 Hz
d. All of the above

A tuning fork (TF) consists of a base (footplate), stem and two prongs. The tuning forks of 256, 512, 1,024 and 2,048 Hz[2] (cycles/second) are used. The tuning fork of 512 Hz is most important. The lower frequency TF produces sense of bone vibration while higher frequencies have shorter decay time.

Different types of hearing tests

1. *Traditional Screening Tests*
   a. Watch test
   b. Finger friction tests
   c. Voice tests (conversation and whisper)
2. *Tuning Fork Tests (TFT)*
   a. Air conduction
   b. Bone conduction
   c. Rinne test
   d. Weber test
   e. Absolute bone conduction (ABC)
   f. Schwabach's test
   g. Bing test
   h. Gelle's test
3. *Audiometric Tests*
   a. Pure tone audiometry (PTA)
      i. Air and bone conduction thresholds
      ii. Recruitment
         - Alternate binaural loudness balance test for recruitment
         - Short increment sensitivity index (SISI) test
      iii. Tone decay test

Contd...

Ans. **41. c.** Carcinoma tongue **42. a.** 512 Hz

Contd...

Different types of hearing tests

b. Speech audiometry
   i. Speech reception threshold (SRT)
   ii. Discrimination score
c. Impedance audiometry
   i. Tympanometry
   ii. Acoustic reflex measurement

4. *Evoked Response Audiometry*
   a. Brainstem Evoked Response Audiometry (BERA)
   b. Electrocochleography (EcoG)
5. *Otoacoustic emissions*
6. *Central auditory tests*
7. *Hearing evaluation in infants and children* (chapter Hearing Impairment in Infants and Young Children)

43. Calorie test based on thermal stimulation of which part of the semi circular canals:

a. Lateral b. Posterior
c. Anterior d. All of the above

Caloric test compares the labyrinthine (lateral SCC) functioning of two ears, however there are no absolute figures for normality. In rare cases only when genuinely needed, a strong stimulus (2 ml ice water) though unpleasant to patient can be used to know the presence or absence of vestibular function.

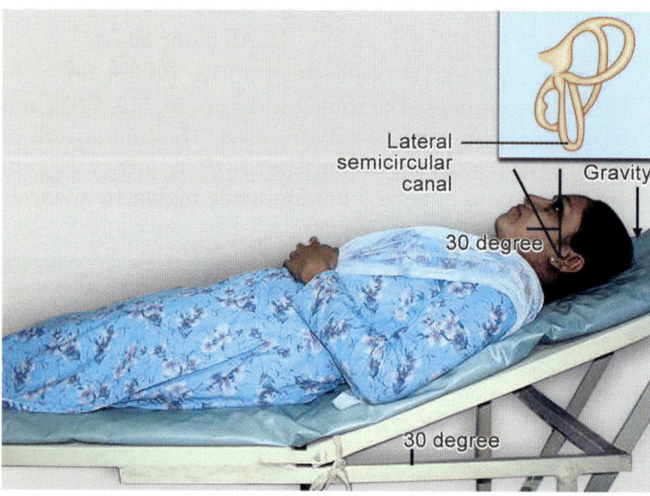

Caloric testing. In reclined position, 30° elevation of head end of table brings the lateral semicircular canal in vertical plane (inset)

44. Multiple perforation of the tympanic membrane is characteristic of .... otitis media:

a. Staphylococcal b. Streptococcal
c. TB d. Pneumococcal

TOM is a rare cause of chronic suppurative infection of the middle ear, ranging from 0.05 to 0.9% of the chronic otitis media TB. Because of similar symptoms and signs its differential diagnosis from non-TB chronic otitis media may be quite difficult TB. In addition, the clinical manifestations of this disease are not always in accordance with the description of the classical triad of painless otorrhea, multiple tympanic perforations, and facial palsy TB.

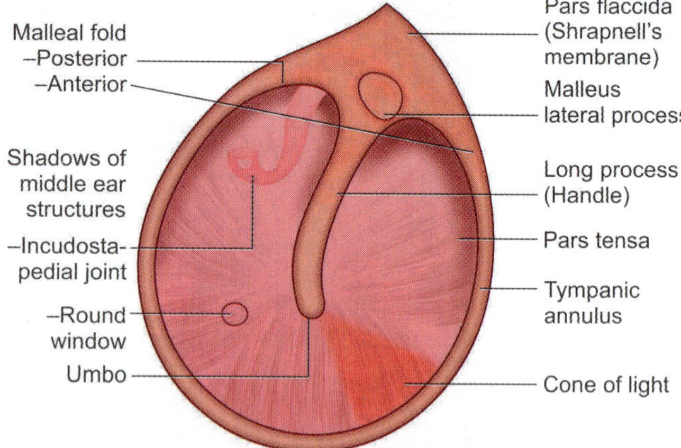

Tympanic membrane showing attic, malleus handle, umbo, cone of light and structures of middle ear seen through it on otoscopy

45. Commonest cause of suppurative otitis media:

a. Streptococcus
b. Pneumococcus
c. Staphylococcus
d. Pseudomonas

Most common cause of ASOM includes Streptococcus pneumoniae, Hemophilus influenzae, Branhamella catarrhalis (Moraxella catarrhalis).

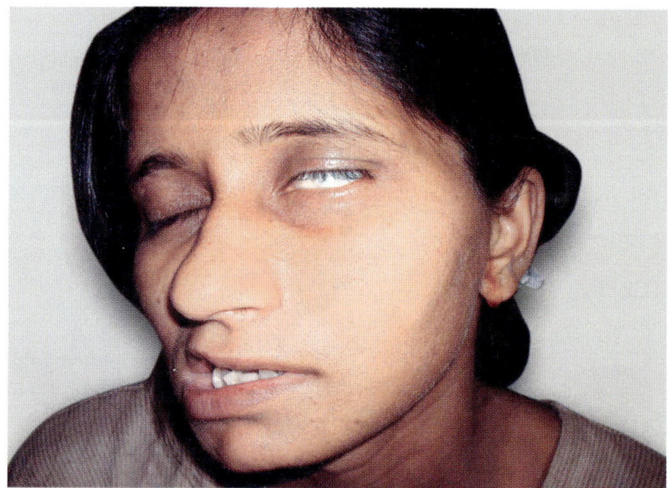

Left side facial palsy in a case of acute suppurative otitis media. Note the blood tinged discharge from left ear. Otoscopy showed subtotal central perforation

46. Schwartz operation is:

a. Myringotomy
b. Modified radical mastoidectomy
c. Radical mastoidectomy
d. Cortical mastoidectomy

Cortical mastoidectomy/simple or complete mastoidectomy or Schwartz operation refers to complete exenteration of all accessible mastoid air cells without removing the posterior meatal wall. Middle ear structures are not disturbed.

Ans. 43. a. Lateral **44. c.** TB **45. b.** Pneumococcus **46. d.** Cortical mastoidectomy

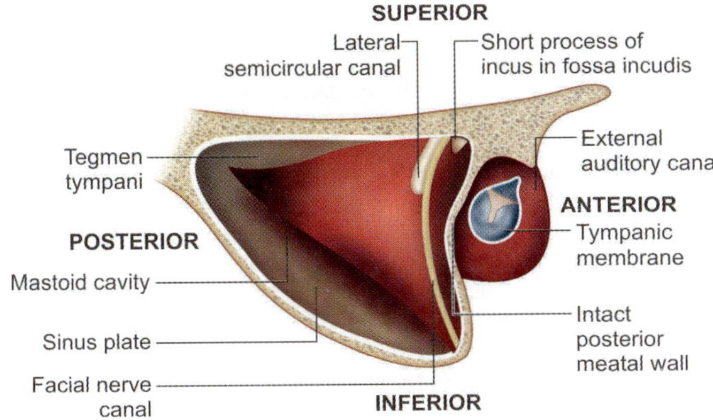

Simple cortical mastoidectomy with intact posterior meatal wall

47. **Narrowest part of facial nerve is in:**
    a. Labyrinthine canal
    b. Stylomastoid region
    c. Superior colliculus
    d. Pons

Labyrinthine segment of facial nerve is 3-5 mm and extends from internal auditory canal fundus (meatal foramen) to the geniculate ganglion (may be dehiscent) where facial nerve takes a posterior turn forming the first 'genu'. The bony fallopian canal in the labyrinthine segment is narrowest and more prone to compression in Bell's palsy.

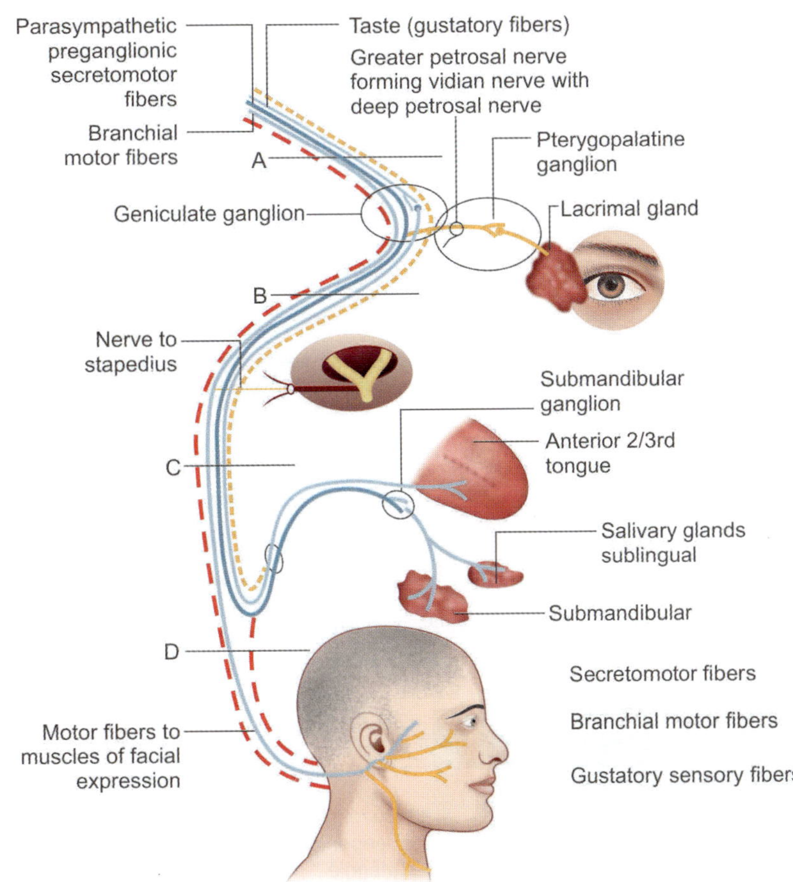

Topographical lesions of facial nerve. (A) Lesion above the geniculate ganglion damages the motor fibers to facial muscles and stapedius, secretomotor fibers to lacrimal and submandibular salivary glands, and taste fibers; (B) Lesion between the geniculate ganglion and nerve to stapedius spare secretomotor fibers to lacrimal gland; (C) Lesion between the nerve to stapedius and chorda tympani nerve spares stapedial reflex and lacrimation; (D) Lesion below chorda tympani nerve affects only muscles of facial expression

48. **Recruitment phenomenon is seen in:**
    a. Otitis media with effusion
    b. Acoustic nerve schwannoma
    c. Meniere's disease
    d. Otosclerosis

Hearing loss in Meniere's disease is fluctuating and progressive. Diplacusis (a difference in the perception of pitch between the ears) and recruitment (intolerance to loud sounds) may be present.

Ans. **47. a.** Labyrinthine canal **48. c.** Meniere's disease

49. Treatment of CSOM is:

a. Radical mastoidectomy
b. Modified radical mastoidectomy
c. Simple mastectomy
d. None of the above

In modified radical mastoidectomy, hearing mechanism and middle ear cleft structures are preserved as far as possible. Only irreversibly damaged tissues are removed. Preservation and conservation of middle ear structures help in reconstruction of the hearing mechanism.

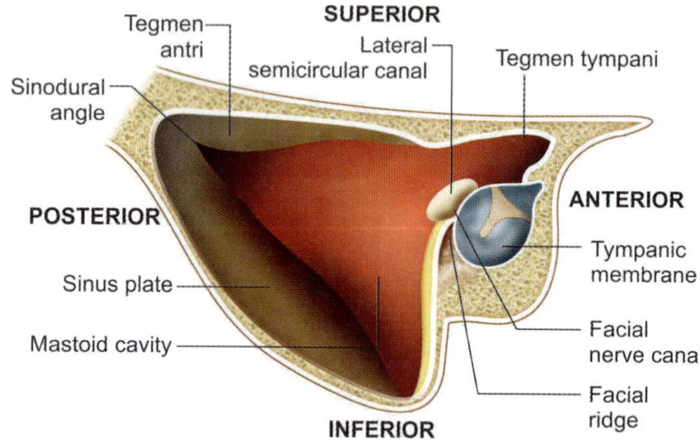

Modified radical mastoidectomy cavity after removing the posterior meatal wall and exteriorizing the diseased area of attic and mastoid antrum without removing the normal ossicles and tympanic membrane

50. Dangerous type of perforation refers to:

a. Marginal
b. Central
c. Multiple
d. All of the above

Atticoantral type (posterosuperior lesion or cholesteatoma) of CSOM is also known as unsafe or dangerous as it is often associated with risk of serious complications due to bone erosion nature of cholesteatoma.

Differences between atticoantral and tubotympanic types of CSOM

	Tubotympanic CSOM	*Atticoantral CSOM*
Nature	Safe and benign	Unsafe and dangerous
Otorrhea (ear discharge)		
Odor	Odorless	Malodorous (putrid)
Amount	Usually profuse	Usually scanty
Type	Usually mucoid	Usually purulent
Periodicity	Usually intermittent	Usually continuous
Perforation	Central	Attic or marginal
Granulations	Uncommon	Common
Polyp	Pale	Red and fleshy
Cholesteatoma	Absent	Present
Intracranial complications	Never	Not uncommon

Contd...

Contd...

51. Bezold's abscess is located in:

a. Submandibular region
b. Sternomastoid muscle
c. Digastric muscle
d. Infratemporal region

In acute coalescent mastoiditis, pus can break the thin medial side of the tip of the mastoid and present as upper neck swelling. The abscess may follow any of the following courses: (i) Lie deep to sternocleidomastoid muscle and pushing it laterally (ii) Lie in the digastric triangle (iii) Lie in the upper part of posterior triangle (iv) Lie in the parapharyngeal space (v) Lie along the carotid vessels.

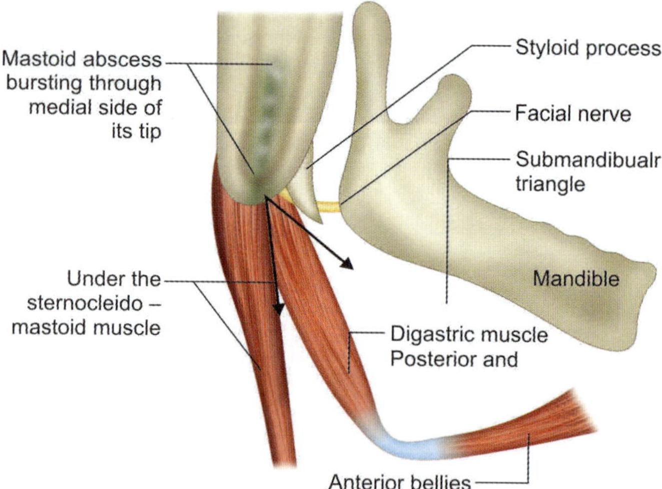

Bezold's abscess. Through the mastoid tip abscess extends either deeper to sternocleidomastoid muscle or into the submandibular triangle

52. Part commonly involved in otosclerosis is:

a. Malleus
b. Oval window
c. Round window
d. Tympanic membrane

Stapedial otosclerosis is the most common variety of otosclerosis. It causes stapes fixation and presents with conductive deafness. The fissula ante-fenestram, which lies in the front of the oval window, is the site of predilection.

Ans. **49. b.** Modified radical... **50. a.** Marginal **51. b.** Sternomastoid muscle **52. b.** Oval window

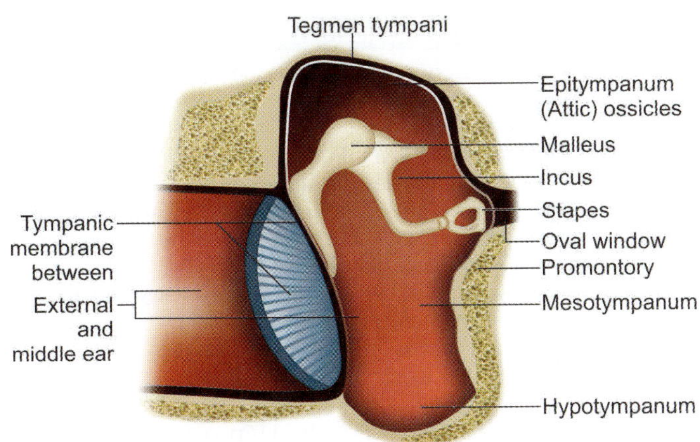

Parts of middle ear seen on coronal section

53. Otoacoustic emissions arise from:

a. Organ of corti
b. Both inner and outer hair cells
c. Outer hair cells
d. Inner hair cells

OAE are low-intensity sounds, which are produced by movements of the outer hair cells of the cochlea. Absence of OAE indicates disorders of outer hair cells.

54. A child with otitis media, not responding to ampicillin presents with bulging membrane with dull look. Treatment of choice is:

a. Ciprofloxacin
b. Mastoidectomy
c. Myringotomy
d. Grommet insertion

Indications of myringotomy in ASOM: (i) Bulging eardrum (ii) Acute excruciating pain (iii) Unresponsiveness to antibiotics (iv) Complications like facial paralysis, labyrinthitis or meningitis with bulging tympanic membrane.

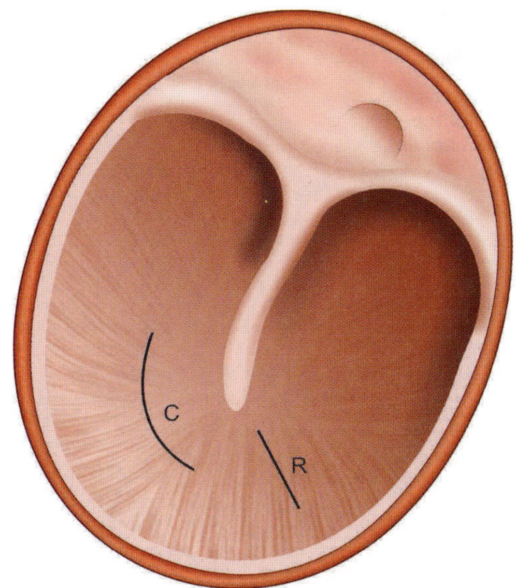

Myringotomy incisions. Circumferential (C) for acute suppurative otitis media (ASOM) and radial (R) for otitis media with effusion (OME)

55. Tobey-Ayer test is done for:

a. Acantholysis
b. Hemoglobinuria
c. Ketosis
d. Lateral sinus thrombosis

Queckenstedt's test or Tobey-Ayer test: In this test CSF pressure is recorded by manometer when one or both jugular veins are compressed manually. Compression of affected (thrombosis) side of the vein produces no effect. Compression of the opposite side internal jugular vein produces rapid rise in CSF pressure.

56. A patient presented with high fever and signs of raised intracranial tension. There is past history of CSOM. Likely diagnosis is:

a. Brain abscess
b. Pyogenic meningitis
c. Acute subarachnoid hemorrhage
d. Acute osteomyelitis of the skull

Fifty percent cases of brain abscesses in adults and 25% in children are otogenic. In adults, cholesteatoma and in children AOM are the most common causes. Cerebral abscess occurs more frequently than cerebellar abscess.

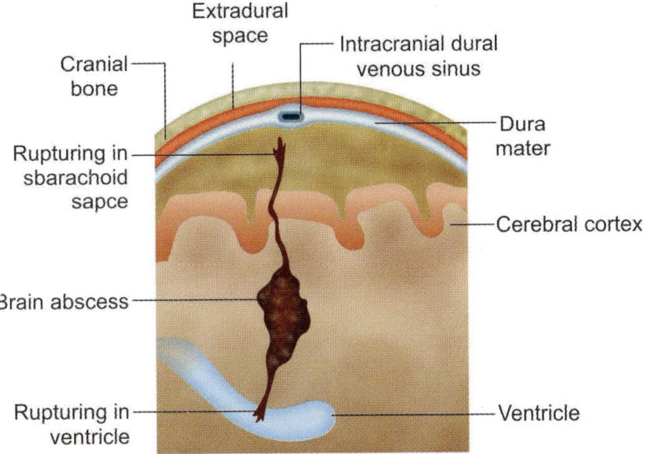

Brain abscess rupture in ventricle and subarachnoid space. Rupture usually occurs in the ventricle because encapsulation of abscess is more on outer side

57. Iatrogenic facial nerve palsy commonly occurs after:

a. Ossiculoplasty
b. Cortical mastoidectomy
c. Stapedectomy
d. Myringoplasty

Complications of cortical mastoidectomy include perioperative injuries to facial nerve, horizontal semicircular canal (patient develops vertigo and jerky nystagmus), sigmoid sinus (profuse bleeding), duramater of middle cranial fossa (CSF leak) and dislocation of incus (conductive hearing loss/CHL).

Ans. 53. **c.** Outer hair cells 54. **c.** Myringotomy 55. **d.** Lateral sinus throm... 56. **a.** Brain abscess
57. **b.** Cortical mastoidectomy

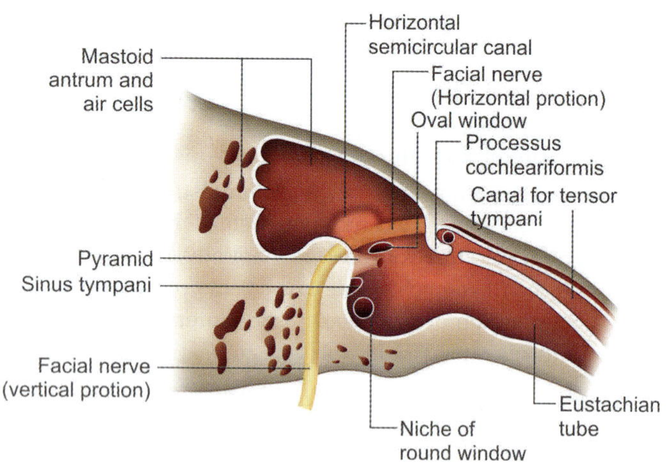

Medial wall of middle ear cleft

58. Tympanogram in osteogenesis imperfecta:

a. Low compliance b. Noncompliance
c. High compliance d. Flat

About 50% cases of type I osteogenesis imperfect develop hearing loss, histological changes and COL1A1 expression that are indistinguishable from otosclerosis. Otosclerosis shows normal curve with low compliance on tympanogram.

Different types of tympanogram

Type	*Characters of graph*	*Diseases of middle ear*
Type A	Normal Curve	Normal middle ear function
Type As	Normal curve with low compliance at or near normal ambient air pressure	Fixation of ossicles such as otosclerosis, malleus fixation
Type Ad	High compliance at or near normal ambient pressure	Ossicular discontinuity, thin and lax tympanic membrane
Type B	A flat or dome-shaped curve. No change in compliance with pressure changes	Middle ear fluid
Type C	Maximum compliance (peak) at negative pressure range < 150 mm of H_2O	Retracted tympanic mem- brane, negative pressure or some fluid in middle ear

59. Otospongiosis is inherited as:

a. Autosomal dominant
b. X-linked recessive
c. Autosomal recessive
d. X-linked dominant

About 50% of the cases of otosclerosis give positive family history. Remaining cases are sporadic. An autosomal dominant inheritance with penetrance in range of 20-40 has been reported.

Causes of conductive hearing loss

- *External auditory canal*: Wax, foreign bodies, otitis externa, congenital and acquired stenosis, exostoses, osteomas, tumors, cyst
- *Tympanic membrane*: Perforations (traumatic, ASOM, CSOM), tympanosclerosis, retraction
- *Ossicles*: Fixation (otosclerosis, tympanosclerosis, adhesive otitis media, congenital); discontinuity (traumatic, inflammatory, cholesteatoma)
- *Middle ear*: Otitis media with effusion, hemotympanum, cholesteatoma, tumors (benign and malignant); Eustachian tube dysfunction

60. A patient hears better in noise. The diagnosis is:

a. Hyperacusis b. Hypoacusis
c. Presbycusis d. Paracusis

In paracusis willisii the patient's hearing improves in noisy background.

61. Higher auditory centre determines:

a. Sound localization
b. Speech discrimination
c. Loudness
d. Sound frequency

Medial geniculate body and temporal lobe auditory cortex are organized into isofrequency layers arranged tonotopically from low frequency to higher frequency. Most cells respond to binaural stimulation. Their main function appears to be sound localization.

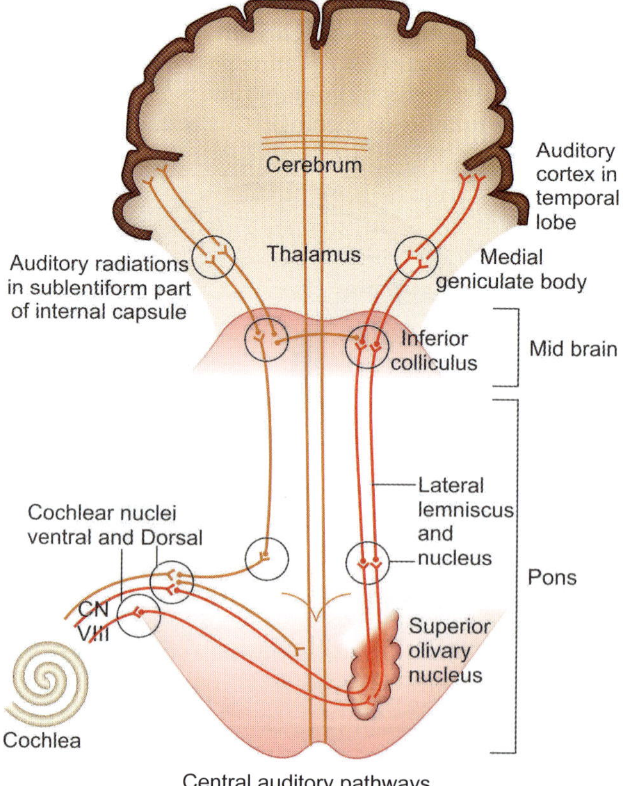

Central auditory pathways

Ans. 58. a. Low compliance 59. a. Autosomal dominant 60. d. Paracusis 61. a. Sound localization

62. Endolymph is secreted by:

a. Hensen cell
b. Cochlear duct
c. Basilar membrane
d. Stria vascularis

Stria vascularis contains vascular epithelium and secretes endolymph.

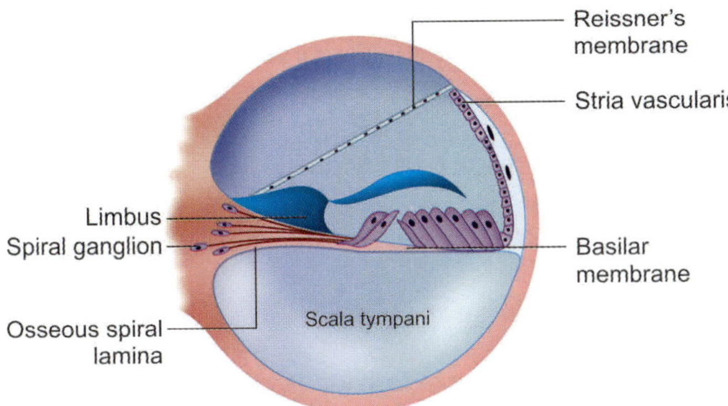

Structure of cochlear canal after its cut section

63. Which is NOT seen in Meniere's disease:

a. Tinnitus
b. Hearing loss
c. Loss of consciousness
d. Vertigo

Patient with Meniere's disease may have occasional sudden unexplained falls without loss of consciousness or associated vertigo. Patient feels pushing or moving during this shortlived spells (drop attacks/otolithic crises of Tumarkin).

64. Which of the following forms lateral wall of mastoid antrum:

a. Mastoid process
b. Suprameatal triangle
c. Petrous temporal bone
d. Tympanic cleft

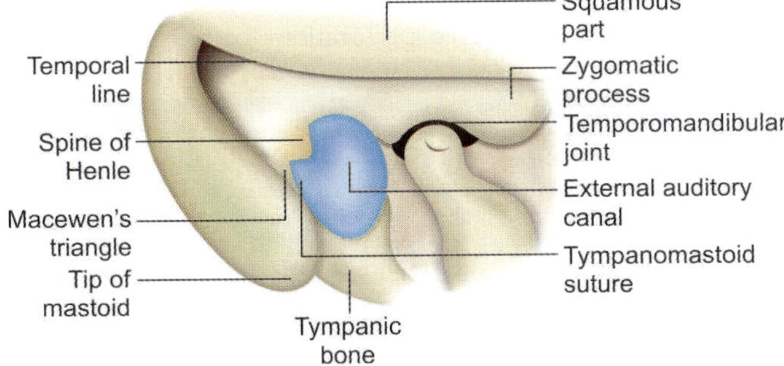

Macewen's triangle. Surface landmark for mastoid antrum

Lateral wall of mastoid antrum is formed by a 1.5 cm thick plate of squamous part of temporal bone which is marked on the lateral surface of mastoid by suprameatal (Macewen's) triangle. It is covered by postaural skin.

65. Bithermal caloric test stimulates which of the following:

a. Superior semicircular canal
b. Posterior semicircular canal
c. Horizontal semicircular canal
d. All of the above

Fitzgerald-Hallpike Bithermal Caloric test

- Patient lies in supine position with head flexed 30 degree (to bring horizontal SCC in vertical position).
- Ears are alternately irrigated for 40 seconds with water that is 7 degree above and below the normal body temperature, i.e. 30 degree C and 44 degree C.
- The eyes are observed for nystagmus
- A gap of 5 minutes is kept between each ear test.
- The time is recorded noted from the start of irrigation to the end of nystagmus on a calorigram.
- It is easy to remember the mnemonic COWS, which says that cold water will produce nystagmus on the opposite side while warm water on the same side.

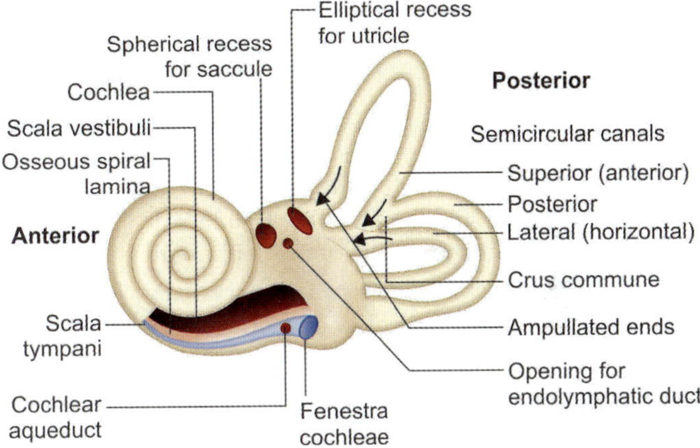

Medial wall of left bony labyrinth seen from lateral side after the removal of its lateral wall

66. Which of the following define vertigo:

a. Ringing of ears
b. Subjective sense of imbalance
c. Sense of pressure in the ear
d. Infection of the inner ear

Vertigo is defined as false sense of motion, such as rotation (spinning or whirling).

Common differential diagnoses of vertigo and their key features

Group/cause	*Key features*
Peripheral causes	
Suppurative labyrinthitis	Findings of middle ear infections (pain, discharge, deafness) or meningitis (headache, fever, neck rigidity)

Contd...

Ans. 62. **d.** Stria vascularis 63. **c.** Loss of consciousness 64. **b.** Suprameatal triangle 65. **c.** Horizontal semicircular... 66. **b.** Subjective sense of imbalance

Contd...

Group/cause	*Key features*
Vestibular neuritis	Acute prolonged isolated vertigo without any otological and neurological findings. Nystagmus is of peripheral type
Benign positional paroxysmal vertigo	Transient (for seconds) episodes of vertigo triggered by certain head positions, such as rolling in bed
Cholesteatoma	Chronic foul smelling ear discharge. Ear microexamination will reveal the cholesteatoma
Herpes zoster oticus (Ramsay Hunt syndrome)	Vesicular eruption in the posterior part of external ear and facial palsy
Ménière's disease	Recurrent episodes of vertigo, hearing loss, tinnitus or aural fullness
Perilymphatic fistula	Dizziness of variable duration after trauma, surgery, excessive straining. Spontaneous in profound congenital deafness. Episodes of dizziness triggered by pressure and noise
Central causes	
Cerebellopontine angle tumor	Unilateral gradually progressive sensorineural hearing loss with imbalance (usually not spinning vertigo)
Cerebrovascular disease such as transient ischemic attack or stroke	Sudden spontaneous attack of vestibular symptoms associated with motor or sensory deficits and central type of vertigo. Vascular risk factors present
Migraine	Episodic throbbing headaches, usually unilateral and accompanied by nausea, vomiting, photophobia or phonophobia
Multiple sclerosis	Sensory or motor deficits. Sudden hearing loss, facial palsy, blindness. CNS dysfunctions are disseminated in time and space
Other causes	
Cervical vertigo	Vertigo triggered by somatosensory input from head and neck movements
Drug-induced vertigo	H/o adverse reaction to medications, alcohol abuse
Psychological	Associated mood, anxiety, somatization, personality disorders

67. All are tests for vestibular function EXCEPT:

a. Galvanic stimulation b. Fistula test
c. Acoustic reflex d. Cold caloric test

Acoustic reflex is used for facial nerve palsy and differentiation between cochlear and 8th nerve hearing losses.

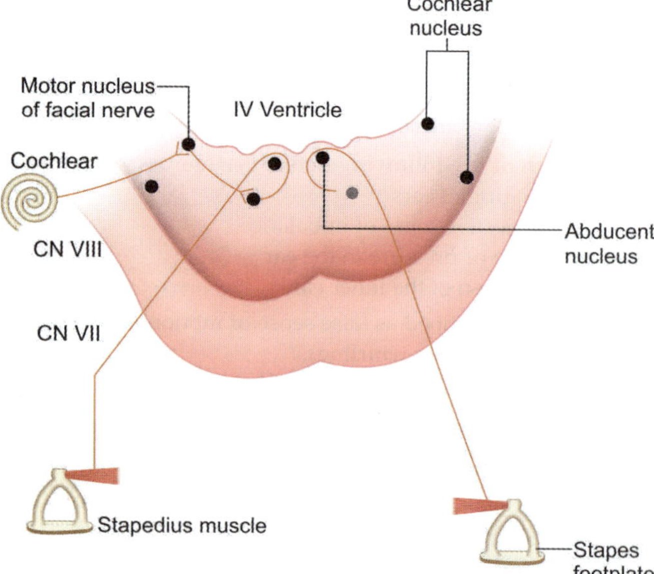

Cut section of the pons showing acoustic reflex pathways

68. Classical findings of tubercular otitis media:

a. Pain out of proportion to symptoms
b. Mastoiditis
c. Scanty discharge
d. Multiple perforation

In TB otitis, multiple perforations of tympanic membrane are seen.

Examination of ears: findings and their causes

Physical Examination

- *Pinna and surrounding area* (Chapter Diseases of External Ear)
  - Size, shape and position: Microtia/macrotia; cauliflower ear; bat ear
  - Swellings: Furuncle/hematoma/neoplasm; perichondritis, Abscesses (Mastoid or zygomatic abscess), lymph nodes
  - Ulcer: Malignancy, trauma, herpes zoster
  - Scar: Trauma/operation (endaural/postaural)
  - Sinus and fistula: Preauricular sinus, postauricular (mastoid) fistula
  - Palpation: Raised temperature and tenderness (perichondritis or abscess); thickness of tissues (perichondritis); fluctuation (hematoma, seroma or abscess). Painful movement of pinna (furunculosis of the external canal)
- *Examination of external auditory canal* (See chapter Diseases of External Ear)
  - Size of meatus: Atresia/narrow/wide
  - Contents of lumen: Wax, debris, discharge, granulations, polyp, and foreign body (FB)
  - Swelling: Furuncle, sagging of posterosuperior area (coalescent mastoiditis), exostosis, neoplasm (benign or malignant)

Contd...

Ans. 67. **c.** Acoustic reflex 68. **d.** Multiple perforation

Contd...

Examination of ears: findings and their causes
❑ *Examination of tympanic membrane (TM)* (See chapter of Otitis Media) – Color: Red and congested (acute otitis media), bluish (secretory otitis media or hemotympanum) and a chalky plaque (tympanosclerosis) – Retraction: General retraction (tubal occlusion), retraction pockets attic or posterosuperior region/collection of epithelial flakes, deeply retracted, fixed to promontory (adhesive otitis media) – Bulging: Acute otitis media, hemotympanum or neoplasm – Thickness and transparency: Opaque/thick; translucent/semitransparent/transparent/very thin – Vesicles or bullae: Herpes zoster or myringitis bullosa – Perforation (acute or chronic suppurative otitis media): Size (small, medium, subtotal or total in pars tensa), shape (oval, round or kidney), single or multiple (tuberculosis), site, central (Safe chronic suppurative otitis media) or marginal (at the periphery involving the annulus) or attic (in pars flaccida) with cholesteatoma – Mobility (siegalization): Mobile (normal), restricted (presence of fluid), fixed (adhesions in the middle ear), or hypermobile (an atrophic segment of tympanic membrane)
❑ *Examination of middle ear* (through the perforation, transparent TM, exploration): – Mucosa: Normal/atrophic/hypertrophic/polypoidal/granulations/in-growth/flaques of squamous epithelium (cholesteatoma) – Contents: Ossicles, growth, FB – Normal structures: Oval and round windows, Eustachian tube
❑ *Examination of mastoid (Chapter complicatory of Suppurative Otitis Media)* – Swelling: Abscess or enlarged nodes, furuncle (obliteration of retroauricular groove), fistula (burst abscess), scar (previous operation) – Palpation: Smooth (periosteal inflammation/subperiosteal abscess)/irregular/tenderness (mastoiditis) over antrum (just above and behind the meatus), tip, and between mastoid tip and antrum
❑ *Examination of Eustachian tube (See chapter Disorders of Eustachian Tube)* – Eustachian catheterization – Posterior rhinoscopy – Valsalva maneuver
❑ *Examination of facial nerve* (See chapter Facial Nerve Disorders) – Lower/upper motor neuron – Grade: Complete/partial
Functional Examination
❑ *Auditory function* (See chapter on Hearing Evaluation) – Voice test – Tuning fork tests – Rinne test – Weber test – Schwabach test – Absolute bone conduction test – Audiometry: Pure tone, speech and impedance

Contd...

Contd...

Examination of ears: findings and their causes
❑ *Vestibular function* (See chapter on Evaluation of Vertigo) – Spontaneous nystagmus – Fistula test – Positional tests

69. A 31-year-old female patient complains of bilateral impairment of hearing for the past 5 years. On examination, tympanic membrane is normal and audiogram shows a bilateral conductive deafness. Acoustic reflexes are absent. All constitute part of treatment EXCEPT:

a. Hearing aid
b. Stapedectomy
c. Sodium fluoride
d. Gentamicin

In aminoglycoside antibiotics group, streptomycin, gentamicin and tobramycin are primarily vestibulotoxic. So patients presents with dizziness/vertigo. In large doses, they can damage the cochlea also.

The site of action of ototoxic agents	
Ototoxic agent	Site of action
Aminoglycoside antibiotics	Destroy type1 hair cells of the crista ampullaris; destruction of outer hair cells
Vancomycin	Damage to cochlear hair cells initially of basal turn (high frequency)
Loop diuretics	Edema and cystic changes in the stria vascularis
Salicylates	Probably interfere at enzymatic level
Chloroquin and quinine	Vasoconstriction in the small vessels of the cochlea and stria vascularis
Cytotoxic drugs	Affect the outer hair cells

70. Tuning fork of 512 FPS is used to test the hearing because it is:

a. Better heard
b. Better felt
c. Produces overtones
d. Not heard

The commonly used tuning forks to test hearing are 256 Hz, 512 Hz and 1024 Hz. These frequencies correspond to the speech frequencies. Tuning forks of lower frequencies (like 128 Hz) produce vibrations that are felt more than they are heard, while those of higher frequencies produce more overtones.

71. Stylalgia may present with ear pain. Which nerve may refer the pain:

a. Auriculotemporal nerve
b. Posterior auricular nerve
c. Occipital nerve
d. Glossopharyngeal nerve

Ans. 69. **d.** Gentamicin 70. **b.** Better felt 71. **d.** Glossopharyngeal nerve

Elongated styloid process (Eagle's syndrome) or calcification of stylohyoid ligament can cause pain in tonsillar fossa and upper neck. Pain radiates to ear and gets aggravated on swallowing. The ear pain is secondary to stretching and irritation of glossopharyngeal nerve from elongated styloid process.

Causes of otalgia

A. Local causes (Primary otalgia)

- Auricle: Skin lesion, perichondritis/chondritis, trauma
- External auditory canal: Furuncle*, impacted wax*, otitis externa*, trauma*, foreign bodies especially live insects*, otomycosis*, myringitis bullosa, herpes zoster oticus (Ramsay Hunt Syndrome), and malignant neoplasms
- Middle ear: Acute otitis media*, Eustachian tube obstruction*, cholesteatoma*, mastoiditis*, Barotrauma, and malignancy middle ear
- Intracranial complications of otitis media: Extradural abscess

B. Referred causes (Secondary otalgia)

1. *Area supplied by CN V (trigeminal nerve)*
   - Dental and periodontal diseases*: Caries tooth, apical abscess, impacted 3rd molar, malocclusion. Erupting dentition in children.
   - Oral cavity: Infection, trauma, aphthous* or malignant ulcers of oral cavity*
   - Salivary glands: Parotid and submandibular inflammatory and malignant diseases
   - Periauricular lymphadenopathy from scalp or neck infections
   - Temporomandibular joint*: Myofascial pain dysfunction. bruxism, osteoarthritis, recurrent dislocation, ill-fitting denture, malocclusion, Costen's syndrome
   - Nose and paranasal sinuses: Trauma, infection, tumors and contact points between turbinates and septal spur
   - Nasopharynx: Infection and tumors and after adenoidectomy*
   - Sphenopalatine (Sluder's) neuralgia
   - rigeminal neuralgia
   - Headache: Tension type, traction and inflammatory headaches
   - Atypical facial pain
2. *Area supplied by Cn ix (glossopharyngeal nerve)*
   - Oropharynx*: Acute tonsillitis, peritonsillar abscess, post-tonsillectomy, benign and malignant ulcers of soft palate, tonsil and its pillars and base of tongue. Tuberculosis
   - Elongated styloid process (Eagle's syndrome)
   - Glossopharyngeal neuralgia
3. *Area supplied by CN X (vagus nerve)*
   - *Vallecula, larynx, laryngopharynx, esophagus*: Malignancy* or ulcerative lesions
   - *Thyroid*: Thyroiditis
   - *Cardiac/pulmonary*: Coronary Artery Disease (CAD), aneurysmal dilation of great vessels
   - *Esophagus*: Hiatus hernia with gastroesophageal reflux
4. *Area supplied by C2 and C3 spinal nerves*
   - Cervical arthritis/disc disease
   - Cervical spondylosis*, injuries of cervical spine, caries spine
5. *Facial nerve*: Geniculate neuralgia, Bell's palsy*, and herpes zoster oticus
6. *Psychogenic*

*Common causes of otalgia

72. Most common cause of necrotizing otitis externa:

a. Staphylococcus
b. Pseudomonas aeruginosa
c. Streptococcus
d. Influenza virus

Malignant or necrotizing otitis externa of immunocompromised patients is an aggressive and potentially fatal infection, which progressively spreads to skull base and intracranial structures.

73. Gradenigo's syndrome includes all EXCEPT:

a. Ear discharge
b. Retro-orbital pain
c. Superior oblique palsy
d. Lateral rectus palsy

Gradenigo's syndrome or triad (1904)

- Cranial nerve VI palsy
- Deep seated ear or retro-orbital pain (due to the involvement of CN V ganglion)
- Persistent ear discharge

74. Otalgia is not from:

a. Pharynx
b. Temporomandibular joint
c. Tooth
d. Nasal vestibule

Dental and periodontal diseases, oropharynx and temporomandibular joint problems are important cause of secondary otalgia.

Ans. **72. b.** Pseudomonas... **73. c.** Superior oblique palsy **74. d.** Nasal vestibule

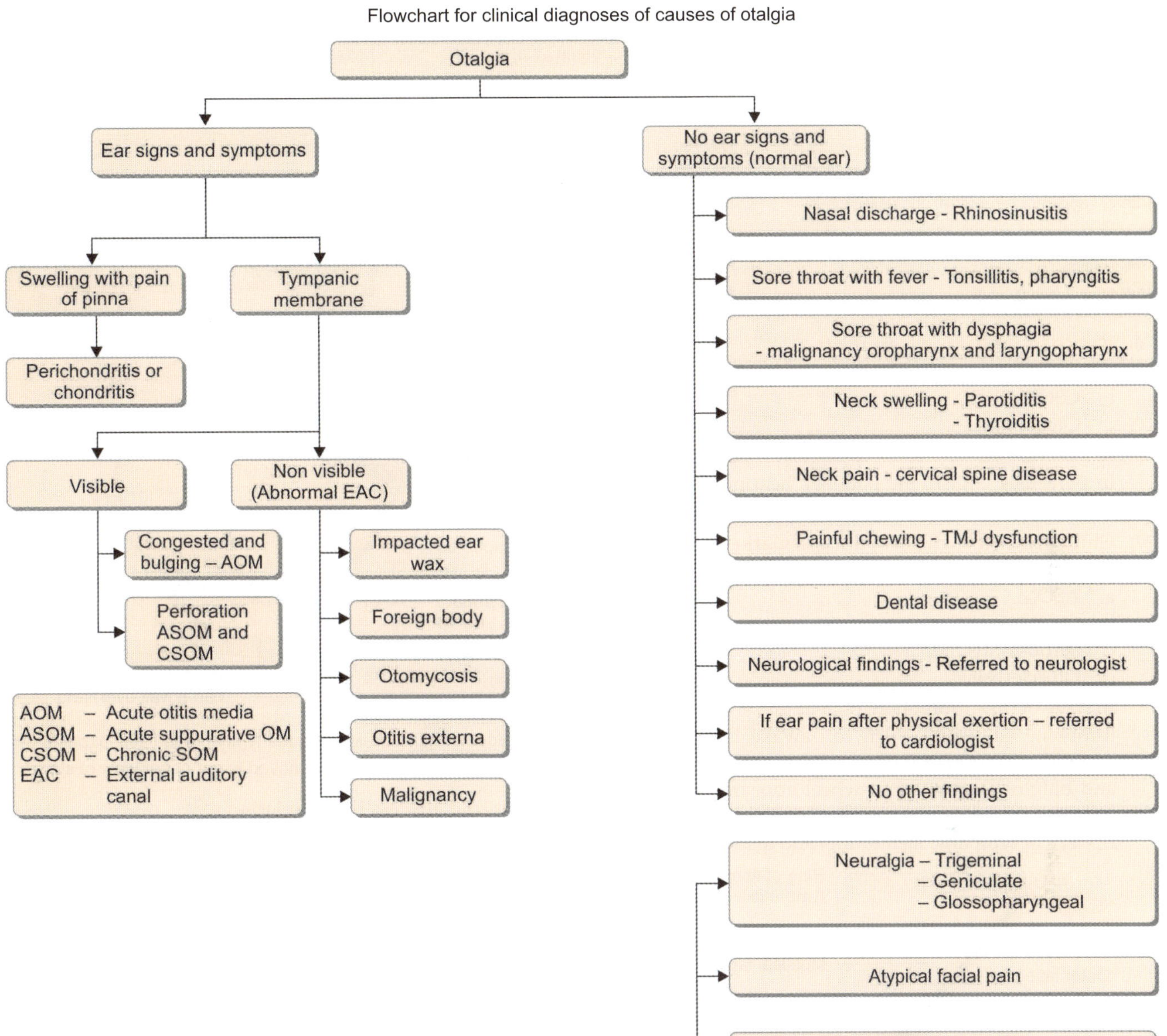

75. A patient is having scanty, foul smelling discharge from the ear and hearing loss. Treatment of choice in such a case:

a. Radical mastoidectomy
b. Modified radical mastoidectomy
c. Suction clearance
d. Cautery with trichloroacetic acid

Modified radical mastoidectomy eradicates diseases from the attic and mastoid and exteriorizes both into EAC by removal of the posterior meatal and lateral attic walls. The remnant of tympanic membrane, functioning ossicles and the reversible mucosa and function of the Eustachian tube, which are necessary to reconstruct hearing mechanism, are preserved.

Differences between canal wall up and canal wall down procedures

	Canal wall-up	*Canal wall down*
Examples	Combined approach tympanoplasty, posterior tympanotomy	Mastoidectomy: Simple, Radical, Modified radical, Bondy

Contd...

Ans. 75. **b.** Modified radical mastoidectomy

Contd...

	Canal wall-up	*Canal wall down*
Posterior canal wall	Not removed	Removed
Mastoid and ear canal	Remains separate	Merge with each other
Meatoplasty	Not required	Required
Postoperative regular cleaning under microscope	Usually not needed	Usually required
Rate of recurrence/residual cholesteatoma	High	Low
Second look surgery	Required after 6 months	Not required
Swimming	Allowed	Usually discouraged
Hearing aid fitting	Easy	Problematic

76. Paracusis willisi is a feature of:

a. ASOM
b. CSOM
c. Otosclerosis
d. Otomycosis

In paracusis willisii, the patient's hearing improves in noisy background.

77. Child presented with ear pain and markedly congested tympanic membrane. Diagnosis is:

a. ASOM
b. CSOM
c. Serous otitis media
d. Otosclerosis

In stage of presuppuration, patient present with marked throbbing ear pain, which can awake the child from sleep in night. On examination, pars tensa is congested and bulging out with cart-wheel appearance (leash of blood vessels along the handle of malleus and at the periphery of tympanic membrane) and loss of light reflex.

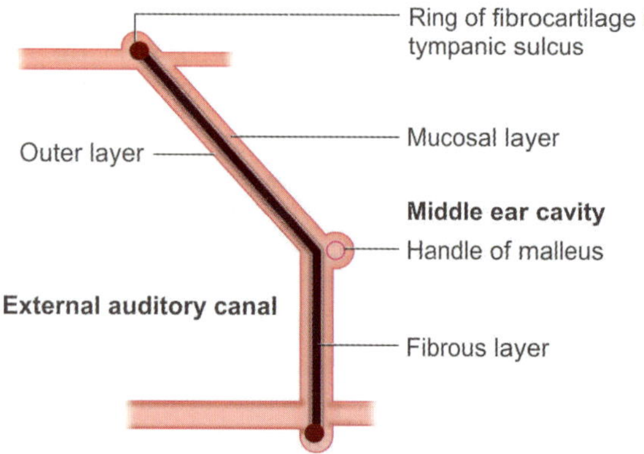

Three layers of tympanic membrane

78. Medication which may prevent rapid progression of cochlear otosclerosis is:

a. Steroids
b. Antibiotics
c. Fluorides
d. Vitamins

Sodium fluoride hastens the maturity of active focus and arrests further SNHL in otosclerosis.

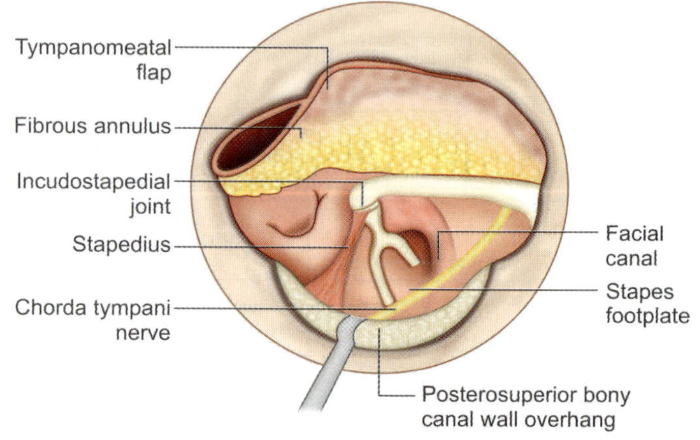

Stapedectomy. After elevating the tympanomeatal flap, posterosuperior bony canal wall is removed to get better view of stapes

79. Bezold abscess lies in relation to:

a. Sternocleidomastoid muscle
b. Behind the mastoid
c. Submandibular region
d. Bony meatus

Bezold's abscess may lie deep to Sternocleidomastoid muscle and pushing it laterally.

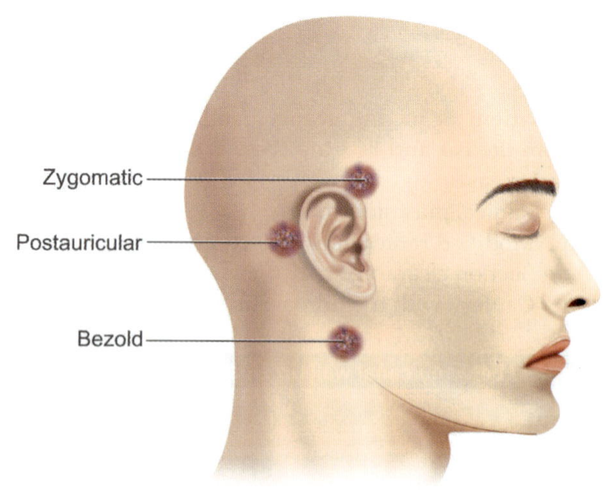

Type of mastoid abscesses

Ans. **76. c.** Otosclerosis **77. a.** ASOM **78. c.** Fluorides **79. a.** Sternocleidomastoid...

80. Frequency of tuning fork commonly used for performing Rinne's test is:

a. 256 Hz
b. 512 Hz
c. 1024 Hz
d. 2048 Hz

In ENT examination, the tuning fork of 512 Hz is most important.

81. An infant with a past history of ear infection is suspected to have meningitis. Organism commonly responsible for such a presentation would be:

a. Mycobacterium
b. Moraxella catarrhalis
c. Pseudomonas
d. Streptococcus pneumoniae

Meningitis is the MC intracranial complication of SOM. In infants and children, meningitis is often the complication of AOM, while in adults it occurs due to cholesteatoma. The one-third cases of meningitis are otogenic in origin. Major pathogens are Hemophilus influenza and Streptococcus pneumoniae.

82. The limit of loudness (expressed as decibels) that workers can tolerate without substantial damage to their hearing, during their work hours, is:

a. 55
b. 65
c. 75
d. 85

Noise can cause hearing impairment (occupational hearing loss) at long-term exposures of over 85 decibels (known as an exposure action value), and it also acts as a causal factor for stress and raises systolic blood pressure.

Intensities of different types of speech	
Whisper	30 dB
Normal conversation	60 dB
Shouting	90 dB
Discomfort in the ear	120 dB
Pain in the ear	130 dB

83. Maximum permissible noise level in hospital wards is:

a. 20-35 dBA
b. 35-40 dBA
c. 40-45 dBA
d. 50-60 dBA

Recommended loudness (in dB)

- Office: 35-45
- Conference: 40-45
- Industrial workshop: 40-60
- Hospital: 20-35

84. Amplification of sound in middle ear:

a. 14 times
b. 16 times
c. 18 times
d. 20 times

Amplification mechanism

- Ear canal: Resonates speech frequencies (2500-4000 Hz) and these amplify the sound 2-4 times
- Ossicular chain: Leverage power of ossicular chain multiplies tympanic vibration slightly
- Ear drum → stapes: Difference in size between tympanic membrane and footplate of stapes; amplifies sound upto 14 times.

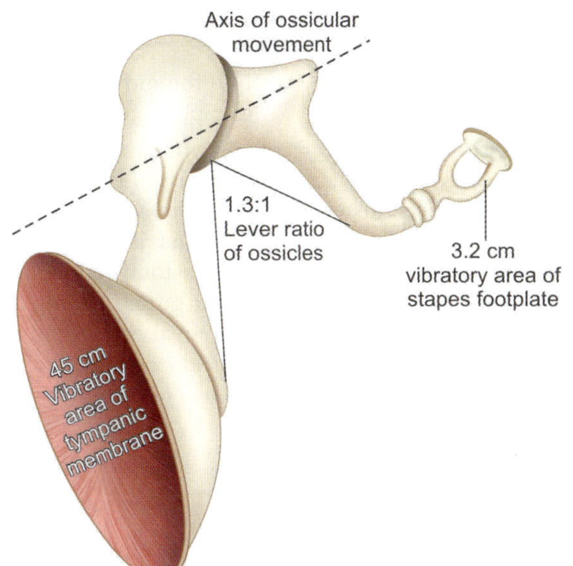

Transformer function of middle ear. Hydraulic effect of tympanic membrane (17:1) and lever action of ossicles (1.3:1)

NOSE

85. Nasolacrimal duct runs:

a. Downward, Forward, Medial
b. Downward, Forward, Lateral
c. Downward, Backward, Lateral
d. Downward, Backward, Medial

The **nasolacrimal duct** (sometimes called the **tear duct**) carries tears from the lacrimal sac into the nasal cavity. The opening of the nasolacrimal duct into the inferior nasal meatus is partially covered by a mucosal fold (valve of Hasner or *plica lacrimalis*). Excess tears flow through nasolacrimal duct which drains into the inferior nasal meatus. This is the reason the nose starts to run when a person is crying or has watery eyes from an allergy, and why one can sometimes taste eye drops.

86. What would be the appropriate management of a 6-year-old child with history of recurrent URTI has snoring, mouth breathing, decreased hearing & speech abnormalities:

a. Myringotomy
b. Myringoplasty
c. Adenoidectomy
d. Tonsillectomy

An enlarged adenoid, or adenoid hypertrophy, can become nearly the size of a ping pong ball and completely block airflow through the nasal passages. Even if the enlarged adenoid is not substantial enough to physically block the back of the nose, it can obstruct airflow enough so that breathing through the nose requires an uncomfortable amount of work, and inhalation occurs

Ans. 80. **b.** 512 Hz 81. **d.** Streptococcus... 82. **d.** 85 83. **a.** 20-35 dBA 84. **a.** 14 times 85. **c.** Downward... 86. **c.** Adenoidectomy

instead through an open mouth. The enlarged adenoid can also obstruct the nasal airway enough to affect the voice without actually stopping nasal airflow altogether.

87. Which of the following is approached in Caldwell Luc operation:

a. Frontal
b. Ethmoid
c. Maxillary
d. Sphenoid

For persistent symptoms of sinusitis or in patients who have failed medical and the functional endoscopic approaches for sinusitis, older techniques can be used to address the inflammation of the maxillary sinus, such as the Caldwell-Luc radical antrostomy. This surgery involves an incision in the upper gum, opening in the anterior wall of the antrum, removal of the entire diseased maxillary sinus mucosa and drainage is allowed into inferior or middle meatus by creating a large window in the lateral nasal wall.

88. Unilateral nasal obstruction with blood stained discharge in a child is commonly due to:

a. Foreign body
b. Choanal atresia
c. Polyps
d. Fungal infection

Causes of unilateral blood stained discharge

- Forgotten foreign body nose
- Rhinolith and sequestra
- Nasal diphtheria
- Nasal myiasis (maggots)
- Acute and chronic unilateral sinusitis
- Malignancy of nose and paranasal sinuses

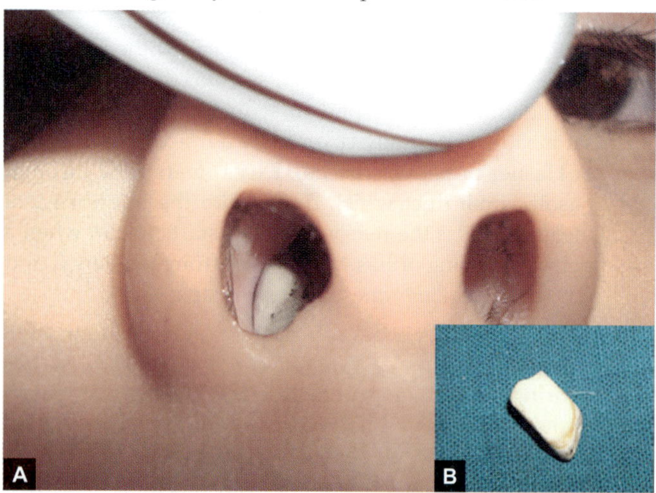

Foreign body (chalk writing stick) in right nose; (B) Removed piece of chalk writing stick.

89. CSF rhinorrhea is common with fractures of:

a. Cribriform plate
b. Frontal
c. Sphenoid
d. Maxilla

Fracture of middle turbinate can damage cribriform plate and cause CSF rhinorrhea and anosmia.

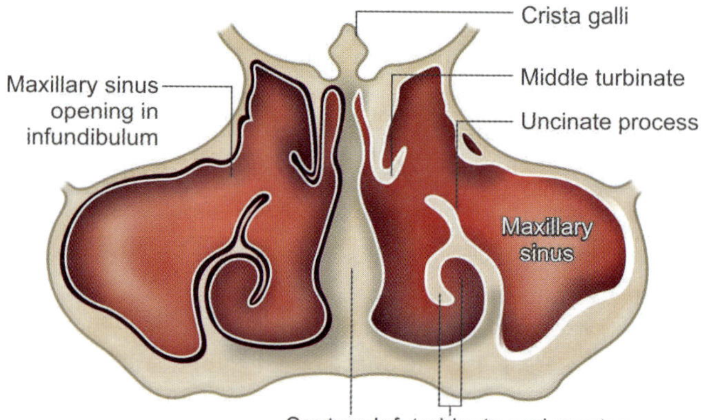

Osteomeatal complex. Coronal section of nose and paranasal sinuses at the level of osteomeatal complex. The uncinate process is in sagittal plane bounding the infundibulum in which opens the ostium of maxillary sinus.

90. Angiofibroma bleeds profusely because:

a. It has multiple sites of origin
b. It lacks a capsule
c. Vessels lack a contractile component
d. None of the above

Angiofibroma consists of varying amount of vascular and fibrous tissues. Vessels do not have muscle coat and are just endothelium lined. It results in severe bleeding which cannot be controlled by application of adrenaline.

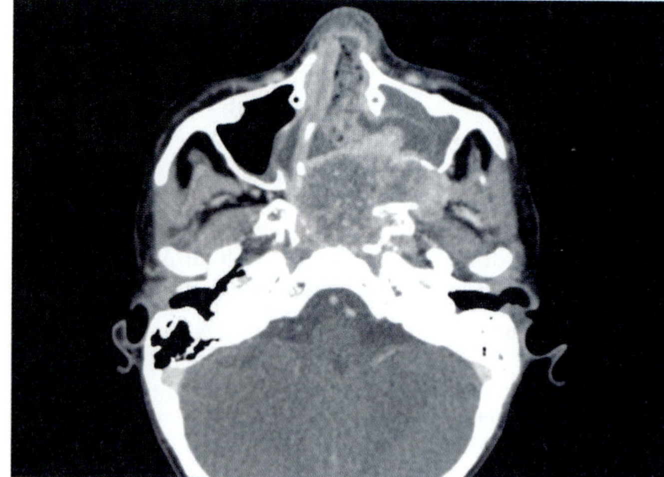

Contrast CT scan juvenile nasopharyngeal angiofibroma. Note the pterygopalatine fossa and infratemporal fossa extension
Source: Dr Amit Goyal, Shillong

91. Not an attachment of quadrilateral cartilage:

a. Maxilla
b. Sphenoid
c. Vomer
d. Ethmoid

Ans. 87. **c.** Maxillary 88. **a.** Foreign body 89. **a.** Cribriform plate 90. **c.** Vessels lack a contractile... 91. **b.** Sphenoid

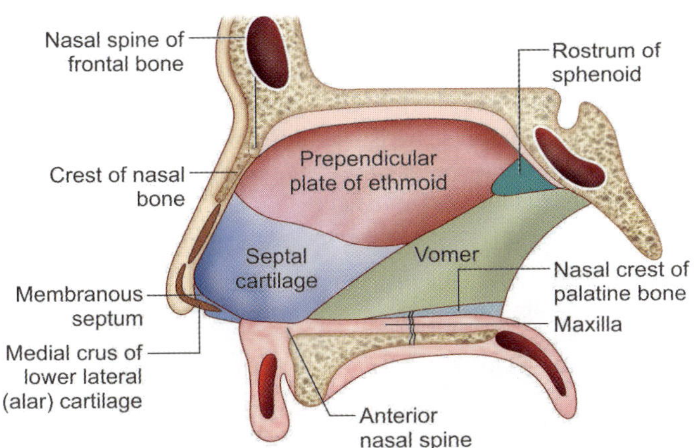

Structure of the nasal septum lateral view. Bony and cartilaginous part seen after removing the mucosa. Posterior triangular segment of cartilaginous septum generally overlaps the bony septum.

Septal cartilage is a large quadrilateral septal cartilage wedged between vomer and ethmoid bone. It rests anteriorly on anterior nasal spine of maxilla.

92. Does not drain into middle meatus:

a. Ethmoidal sinus
b. Maxillary sinus
c. Lacrimal duct
d. Frontal sinus

Nasolacrimal duct opens in the anterior part of inferior meatus.

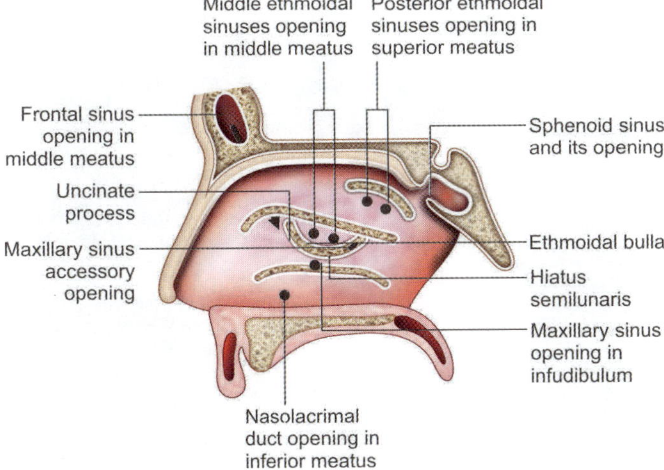

Openings of paranasal sinuses. Lateral wall of nose after removal of turbinates

93. Septal perforation is NOT seen in:

a. Trauma
b. Rhinophyma
c. Septal abscess
d. Leprosy

Rhinophyma is a slow growing benign tumour occurring due to the hypertrophy of sebaceous glands in the region of nasal tip.

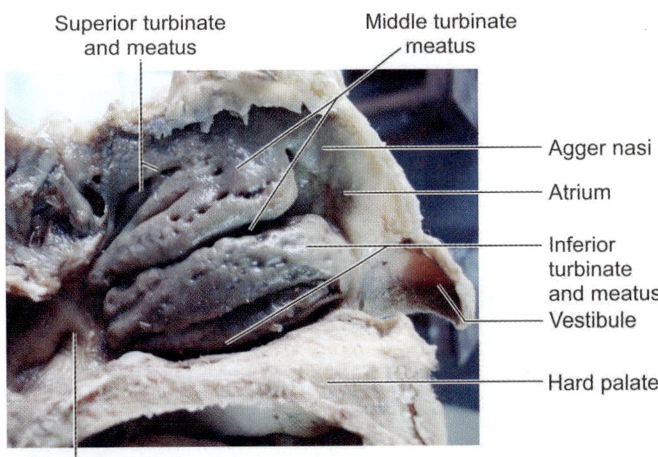

Nasal septum of a cadaver

94. CSF rhinorrhoea is due to the fracture of which of the following:

a. Nasal bones
b. Cribriform plate
c. Temporal bone
d. Maxillary bone

The most common site of CSF rhinorrhea is cribriform plate. Next common site is ethmoidal sinuses.

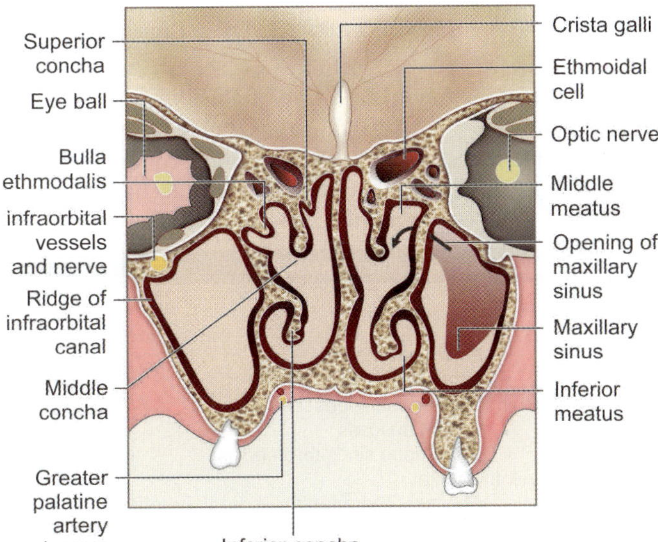

Coronal section of nose and paranasal sinuses seen from behind

95. Young's operation is done for:

a. Atrophic rhinitis
b. Vasomotor rhinitis
c. Antrochoanal polyp
d. Allergic rhinitis

In Young's operation (a plastic surgery) both the nostrils are completely closed within the nasal vestibule with flaps. Nasal mucosa may revert to normal and crusting is reduced. The nostrils are opened again after about 6 months or later. It is done for ozena.

Ans. **92. c.** Lacrimal duct **93. b.** Rhinophyma **94. b.** Cribriform plate **95. a.** Atrophic rhinitis

96. Treatment of choice for antrochoanal polyp:
a. Intranasal polypectomy
b. Caldwell-Luc operation
c. Endoscopic sinus surgery
d. Intranasal ethmoidectomy

Currently almost all the polyps, which do not respond to medical treatment (antihistamines, steroids), are managed by ESS.

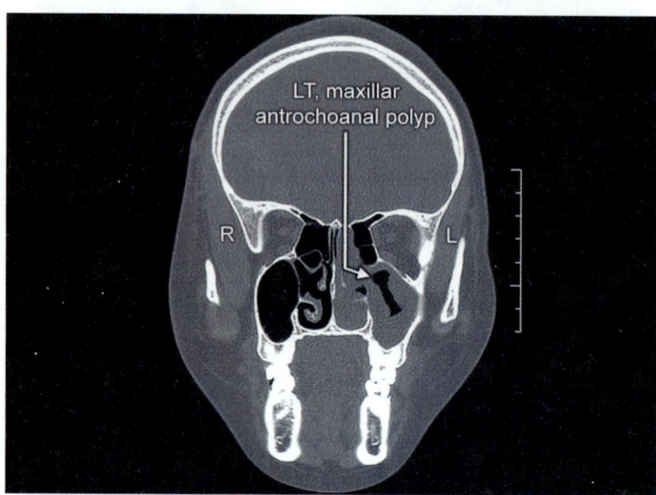

Plain CT scan paranasal sinuses coronal section. A case of left antrochoanal polyp obliterating left nasal cavity and showing mucosal thickening in left maxillary sinus
Source: Dr Ritesh Prajapati, Consultant Radiologist, Anand, Gujarat

97. Mucocele is commonest in:
a. Sphenoethmoidal
b. Sphenoid
c. Maxillary
d. Frontoethmoidal

Frontoethmoidal mucocele is the most common type of mucocele. It presents with frontal headache, proptosis, deep nasal or periorbital pain and diplopia.

Complications of rhinosinusitis

1. *Acute*
   a. Orbital
      i. Inflammatory edema
      ii. Orbital cellulitis
      iii. Subperiosteal abscess
      iv. Orbital abscess
      v. Cavernous sinus thrombosis
   b. Intracranial
      i. Abscess: Extradural, subdural, cerebral
      ii. Meningitis
      iii. Encephalitis
      iv Cavernous and superior sagittal sinus thrombosis
   c. Bony
      i. Osteitis/Osteomyelitis (Pott's puffy tumor)
   d. Dental
   e. Toxic shock syndrome
2. *Chronic*
   a. Mucocele/Pyocele
3. *Associated diseases*
   a. Otitis media
   b. Adenotonsillitis
   c. Bronchiectasis

98. Most appropriate management of antrochoanal polyp in children:
a. Wait and watch
b. Steroids
c. Intranasal polypectomy
d. Caldwell Luc operation

Krause's nasal snare is used for removal of nasal polyps and partial turbinectomy. The polyp mass is engaged in the wire loop and avulsed.

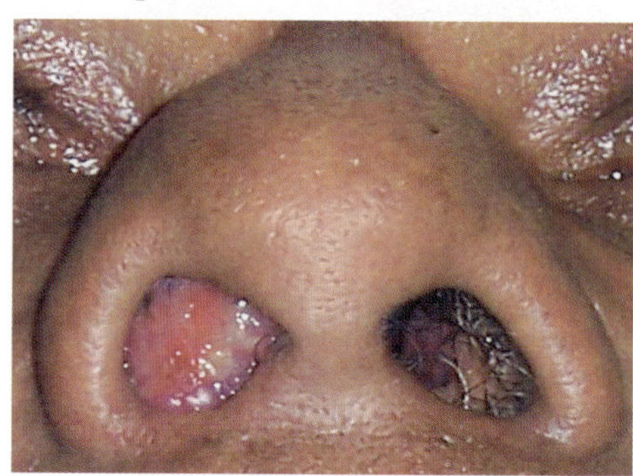

Big nasal polyp protruding out from right nostril appears pink and vascular and simulating neoplasm

99. Horner's syndrome is caused by:
a. Facial injury
b. Nasopharyngeal carcinoma with metastasis
c. Meniere's disease
d. All of the above

Nasopharyngeal carcinoma may lead to Horner's syndrome due to involvement of cervical sympathetic chain.

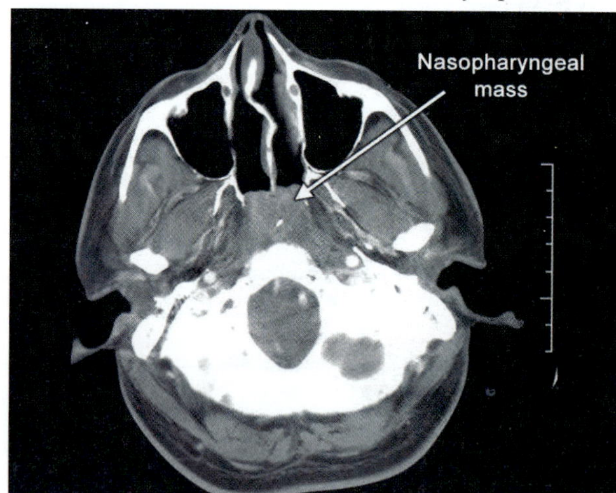

Contrast CT scan Nasopharyngeal mass axial section. Large soft tissue density mass causing complete obliteration of nasopharyngeal lumen. Laterally it is obliterating lateral recesses and openings of Eustachian tubes. It is also extending into both posterior choanae. Mass shows foci of calcification
Source: Dr Ritesh Prajapati, Consultant Radiologist, Anand, Gujarat

100. False regarding nasolabial cyst:
a. Usually seen in adults
b. Bilateral
c. Presents submucosally in anterior nasal floor
d. Arises from odontoid epithelium

Ans.
96. **c.** Endoscopic sinus surgery
97. **d.** Frontoethmoidal
98. **c.** Intranasal polypectomy
99. **b.** Nasopharyngeal carcinoma with metastasis
100. **d.** Arises from odontoid epithelium

Nasolabial/nasoalveolar/Klestadt's cyst is a squamous epithelium-lined cyst which arises from the epithelial rests situated at the junction of globular, lateral nasal and maxillary processes.

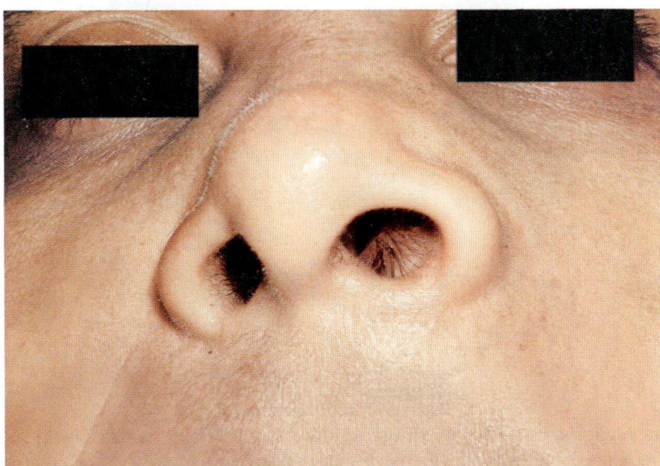

Left side nasolabial cyst. Note the smooth bulge in the floor and lateral wall of left nasal vestibule and upper part of upper lip. Cyst is obliterating the alar facial fold

101. Which radiological view is preferred for demonstration of maxillary sinus:

a. Skyline view b. Fergusson's view
c. Caldwell's view d. Water's view

Structure seen on Water's view (occipitomental view): Maxillary sinus (seen best), frontal and sphenoid sinuses, zygoma, zygomatic arch, nasal bones, frontal process of maxilla, superior orbital fissure and infratemporal fossa.

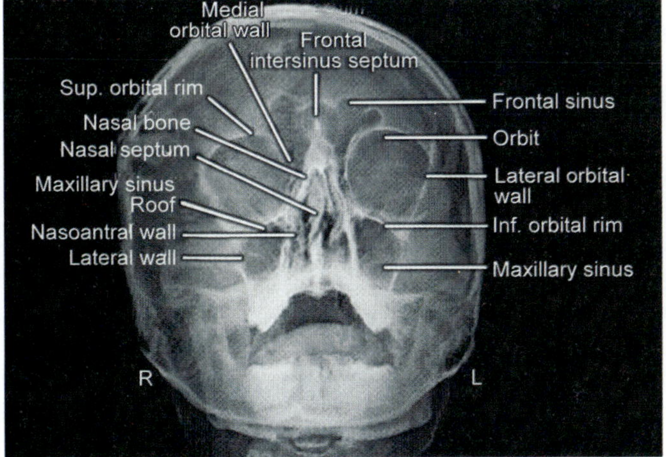

X-ray PNS Water's view–Normal

Source: Dr Jayesh Patel, Consultant Radiologist, Anand, Gujarat

102. Nasal angiofibroma of nose is common in:

a. Younger males b. Younger females
c. Young adults d. Adolescents of both sexes

Juvenile nasopharyngeal angiofibroma occurs exclusively in males of 10-25 years of age.

Radkowski classification of juvenile nasopharyngeal angiofibroma (JNA)	
IA	Tumor limited to nose and nasopharyngeal vault
IB	Extension to paranasal sinuses
IIA	Minimal extension to pterygomaxillary fissure (PMF)
IIB	Full extension to PMF and/or erosion of orbital bones
IIC	Extension to infratemporal fossa and/or cheek or posterior to pterygoid plates
IIIA	Erosion of skull base: minimal intracranial
IIIB	Extensive intracranial and/or cavernous sinus extension

Source: Radkowski D, Mcgill T, Healy GB, et al. Angiofibroma. Changes in staging and treatment. Arch Otolaryngol Head and Neck. 1996;122:122-9.

103. Malignant tumour is commonest in which of the following sinus:

a. Maxillary b. Frontal
c. Ethmoidal d. Sphenoidal

The MC site of malignancy of paranasal sinuses is the maxillary sinus followed in descending order by ethmoids, frontal and sphenoid.

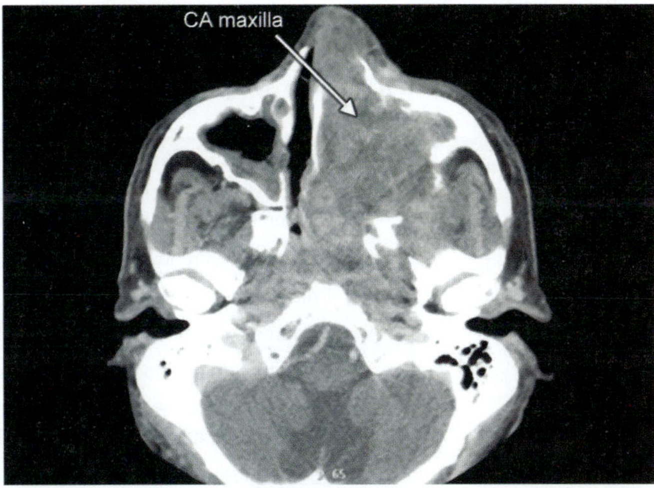

Contrast CT scan of nose and paranasal sinuses axial section. A large growth of left maxillary sinus. It is destructing the medial wall of maxillary sinus and extending into the left nasal cavity. It is destructing the posterolateral wall of maxillary sinus and pterygoid plates and extending into pterygopalatine fossa and pterygomaxillary fissure and involves lateral pterygoid muscle. Posteriorly the mass is extending into the nasopharynx through the choanal with complete obliteration of nasopharyngeal lumen

104. A child presents with unilateral, foul smelling nasal discharge. Most probable cause could be:

a. Acute sinusitis b. Foreign body
c. Rhinolith d. Nasal synechiae

A unilateral foul smelling purulent nasal discharge in a child is mostly due to forgotten foreign body nose.

Ans. **101. d.** Water's view **102. a.** Younger males **103. a.** Maxillary **104. b.** Foreign body

105. NOT true for adenoid hypertrophy:

a. Mouth breathing is seen
b. High arched palate present
c. There is failure to thrive
d. CT scan should be done to assess size

X-ray soft tissue nasopharynx lateral view reveals the size of adenoids, and extent of nasopharyngeal air space compromise.

Differences between palatine tonsils and adenoids

	Adenoids	*Palatine Tonsils*
Number	Single	One on each side
Site	Nasopharynx	Tonsillar fossa in oropharynx
Crypts or Furrows	Only furrows	Only crypts
Capsule	Absent	Present
Epithelium	Ciliated columnar	Squamous stratified
In adults after 20 years of age	Absent	Present

106. Early maxillary carcinoma presents as:

a. Bleeding per nose
b. Supraclavicular lymph node enlargement
c. Tooth pain
d. All of the above

Malignancy of maxillary sinus arises from the sinus mucosa and may remain silent for a long period, during which patient has vague symptoms of rhinosinusitis such as nasal stuffiness, blood stained nasal discharge, facial paraesthesia or pain and epiphora.

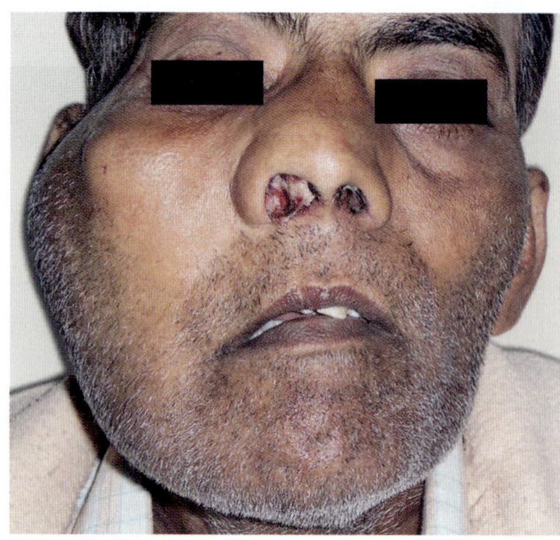

Malignancy maxillary sinus. Anterior spread towards face. Note swelling of infratemporal fossa region and mass in right nasal cavity

107. Regarding atrophic rhinitis, which is incorrect:

a. Common in females
b. Anosmia
c. Due to chronic use of nasal drops
d. None of the above

The long term use of cocaine and topical nasal decongestants (cause rebound congestion) leads to rhinitis medicamentosa.

Etiological classification of nonallergic rhinitis

Medicines: Local and systemic	Topical decongestants (rhinitis medicamentosa), antihypertensive, beta-blockers, aspirin, nonsteroidal anti-inflammatory drug (NSAID), oral contraceptive, psychotropic
Hormonal	Puberty, pregnancy, menstruation, postmenopausal, hypothyroidism, acromegaly
Irritant and corrosives	Irritant rhinitis due to dusts, fumes, smoke, gases, chemicals, pollution, acids, organophosphates
Smell	Perfumes, cosmetics, fragrances, deodorizers, cleaning agents
Taste	Gustatory rhinitis due to hot and spicy foods
Occupational	Occupational NAR due to pyrethrum (insecticide), acid anhydrides (adhesive industry), toluene (body spray), latex, grains, paint industries
Environmental	Temperature, humidity, barometric changes, weather, altitude, aviation
Local: Structural, infections, tumors and trauma	DNS, septal perforation, nasal valve collapse, choanal atresia, turbinate and adenoid hypertrophy, cleft palate, rhinosinusitis, rhinoscleroma, polyps, inverting papilloma, malignancies.
Substance abuse	Cocaine, alcohol and nicotine
Emotional	Anxiety, tension, hostility, humiliation, resentment and grief
Exercise	Sedentary lifestyle and recumbency
Decreased nasal airflow	Laryngectomy, tracheostomy
Atrophic changes	Surgery, aging, infections, atrophic rhinitis
Systemic diseases	Autoimmune systemic lupus erythematosus, Sjogren's, vasculitides (Wegener's granulomatosis, sarcoid), Ciliary dyskinesia (Young's and Kartagener's syndromes), cystic fibrosis, superior vena cava and Horner's syndrome
Idiopathic	Vasomotor rhinitis and nonallergic rhinitis with eosinophilia

Ans. **105. d.** CT scan should be done to assess size **106. a.** Bleeding per nose
107. c. Due to chronic use of nasal drops

108. All of the following statements about Nasopharyngeal carcinoma are true EXCEPT:

a. Bimodal age distribution
b. Nasopharyngectomy with radical neck dissection is the treatment of choice
c. IgA antibody to EBV is observed
d. Squamous cell carcinoma is the most common histological subtype

Irradiation is the primary treatment of choice for nasopharyngeal carcinoma. External radiation or intracavitary implants (brachytherapy) or both are used.

WHO classification of epithelial carcinoma based on histopathology	
Type 1	Keratinizing squamous cell carcinoma
Type 2	Nonkeratinizing carcinoma
	❑ Without lymphoid stroma
	❑ With lymphoid stroma
Type 3	Undifferentiated carcinoma
	❑ Without lymphoid stroma
	❑ With lymphoid strom

109. In sinus X-rays pictures, Water's view (Occipito-mental) provides good visualization of the following EXCEPT:

a. Maxillary sinus
b. Orbitofrontal sinus
c. Frontal sinus
d. Sphenoid sinus

Anterior and posterior extents of sphenoid sinus are best seen on lateral view (also seen in frontal and maxillary sinuses, sella turcica, ethmoid sinuses, alveolar process, condyles and neck of mandible).

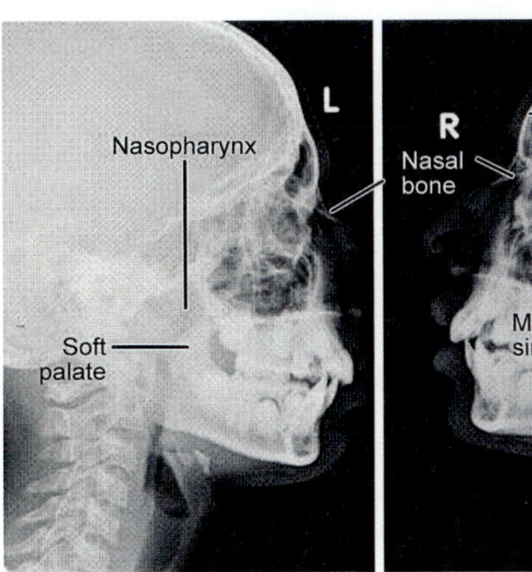

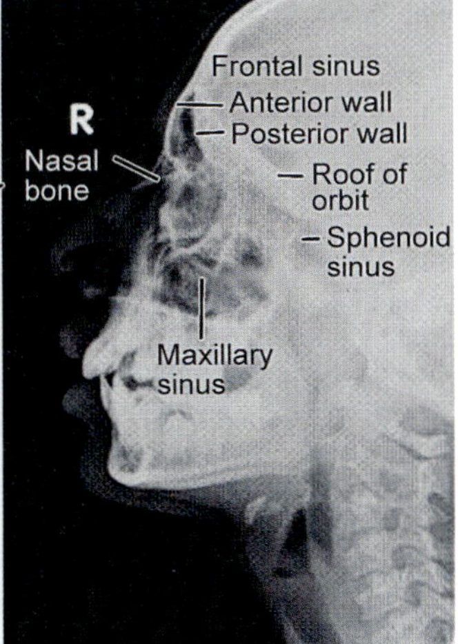

X-ray nasal bones lateral view left and right showing fracture of septal cartilage

Source: Dr Jayesh Patel, Consultant Radiologist, Anand, Gujarat

110. Bone involved in tripod fracture:

a. Zygomatic bone
b. Temporomandibular joint
c. Frontal bone
d. Maxilla

Zygoma (tripod) fracture (caused by direct trauma) is the second most common fracture (after nasal bones) of maxillofacial region. Fracture line involves zygomaticofrontal suture, orbital floor, infraorbital margin and foramen, anterior wall of maxillary sinus and the zygomaticotemporal suture.

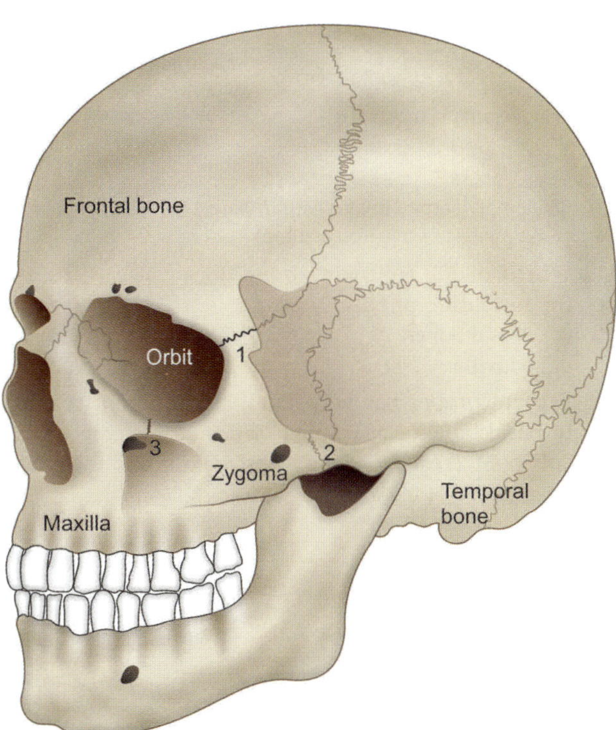

Left zygoma (tripod) fracture showing three sites of fracture. (1) Zygomaticofrontal; (2) Zygomaticotemporal; (3) Infraorbital

111. MC presentation of nasopharyngeal carcinoma:

a. Epistaxis
b. Neck mass
c. Nasal obstruction
d. Deafness

Patient of nasopharyngeal carcinoma may present with only cervical lump of nodes. It is usually seen between the angle of jaw and the mastoid. Nodal metastases during first consultation are seen in 75% and about half of them have bilateral nodes.

112. Immunoglobulin involved in allergic rhinitis:

a. IgA
b. IgE
c. IgM
d. IgG

Allergic rhinitis is a symptomatic disorder of nose induced by an IgE mediated inflammation after allergen exposure (ARIA). Demonstration of allergic hypersensitivity by in vivo or in vitro testing of specific-IgE antibody to aeroallergens is mandatory for confirming the diagnosis of allergic rhinitis.

Ans. 108. **b.** Nasopharyngectomy with radical neck...
109. **d.** Sphenoid sinus
110. **a.** Zygomatic bone
111. **b.** Neck mass
112. **b.** IgE

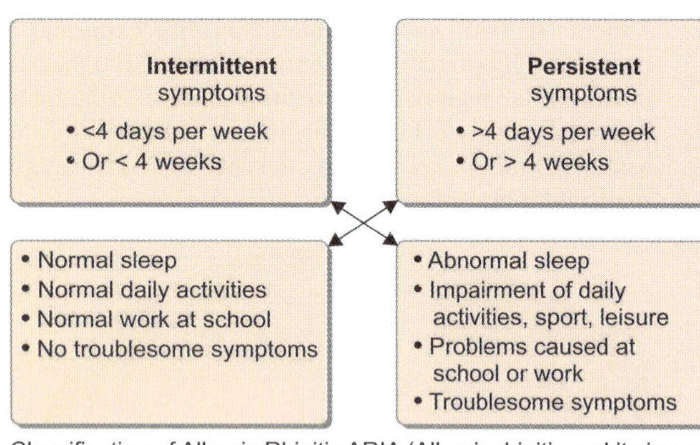

Classification of Allergic Rhinitis ARIA (Allergic rhinitis and its impact on asthma)

113. Which of the following bone does not contribute in the formation of nasal septum:

a. Nasal bones b. Frontal bone
c. Maxilla d. Lacrimal

Septum proper has very small contribution from crest of nasal bones, nasal spine of frontal bone, rostrum of sphenoid, crests of palatine and maxilla and the anterior nasal spine of maxilla.

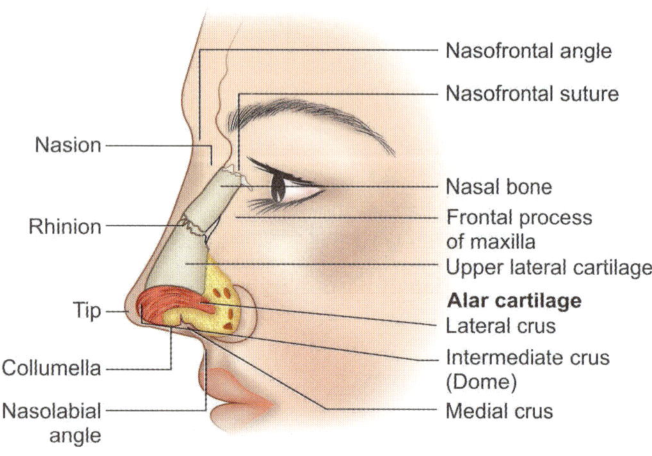

External nose structure—lateral view

114. Mikulicz cells and Russell bodies are seen in:

a. Rhinoscleroma b. Rhinosporidiosis
c. Rhinophyma d. Rhinitis

Biopsy of rhinoscleroma shows infiltration of submucosa with plasma cells, lymphocytes, eosinophils, Mikulicz cells and Russell bodies. The vacuolated Mikulicz cells (almost diagnostic), large foamy histiocytes with central nucleus, stains well with hematoxylin and eosin.

Systemic diseases involving nose

Group	Diseases
Vasculitides	Wegener's granulomatosis, sarcoidosis and Churg-Strauss syndrome
Bacterial	Rhinoscleroma, syphilis, tuberculosis, lupus and leprosy
Fungal	Rhinosporidiosis, aspergillosis, mucormycosis, histoplasmosis and blastomycosis
Lymphoma	Peripheral T-cell neoplasm (Nonhealing midline granuloma)

115. Which sinus is normally present at birth:

a. Maxillary sinus b. Ethmoid sinus
c. Both of the above d. None of the above

The paranasal sinuses, which develop as out-pouchings from the mucous membrane of nose, continue to grow during childhood and early adult-life. At the time of birth, only the maxillary and the ethmoidal sinuses are present.

Development and growth of paranasal sinuses

Sinus	At birth	Adult size	Growth	Radiological appearance (Age)
Maxillary	Present	15 years	Biphasic growth: Birth–3 years, 7–12 year	4–5 months
Ethmoid	Present	12 years	Size increases up to 12 years	1 year
Frontal	Absent	13–18 years	Invades frontal bone (2–4 yrs), size increases until teens	6 years
Sphenoid	Absent	12–15 years	Reaches sella turcica (7 yrs), dorsum sellae (late teens), basisphenoid (adult)	4 years

116. Adult patient presented with headache, epiphora and nasal obstruction, but there was no fever. Condition could be:

a. Meningitis
b. Foreign body obstruction
c. Cavernous sinus thrombosis
d. Carcinoma of maxillary sinus

Late features of maxillary carcinoma appear when tumour spreads and destroys the bony confines and involves surrounding structures. Medial spread towards nasal cavity result in nasal obstruction, discharge and epistaxis. Superior spread towards orbit result in facial paresthesia/anesthesia, proptosis, diplopia, ocular pain and epiphora.

Ans. 113. d. Lacrimal 114. a. Rhinoscleroma 115. c. Both of the above 116. d. Carcinoma of maxillary...

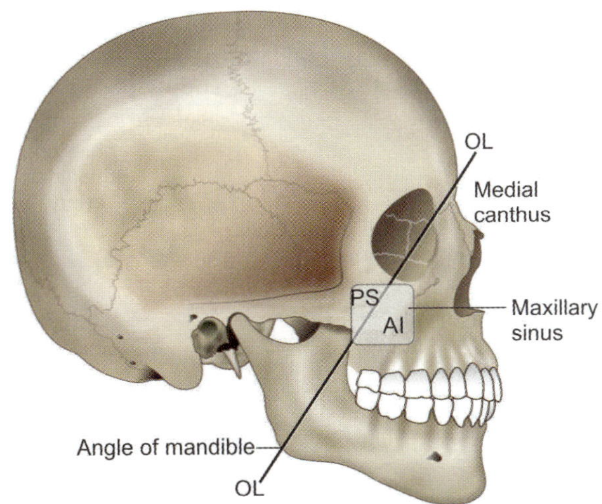

Ohngren's classification. Ohngren's line is an imaginary line (OL), which extends between medial canthus and the angle of mandible, divides the maxilla into two regions anteroinferior (AI) and posterosuperior (PS). AI growths are easy to manage and have better prognosis than PS tumors

117. EBV causes:

a. Maxillary carcinoma
b. Nasopharyngeal carcinoma
c. Glottic carcinoma
d. Carcinoma tongue

Epstein Barr virus (EBV) is usually associated with nasopharyngeal cancer. Specific viral markers are used to screen people in high-risk areas.

Viruses that cause ear, nose and throat disorders with their structure, transmission, diseases and antiviral agents

Virus	*Structure and types*	*Transmission*	*Diseases*	*Antiviral agents*
Coronavirus	RNA virus; strains 229E, OC4	Aerosol	Common cold, pneumonia, acute otitis media (AOM)	
Adenovirus	Double stranded DNA virus; Types 1,2,3,5,7	Aerosol	Pharyngitis, exudative tonsillitis, pneumonia, pharyngoconjunctival fever, AOM, keratoconjunctivitis	Ribavirin in childhood pneumonia
Rhinovirus	Nonenveloped RNA virus	Aerosol, contact (hands, utensils)	Common cold, pneumonia, AOM	
Influenza Incubation 1-3 days	RNA orthomyxovirus; Subtypes A,B,C; Avian H5N1, H1N1 (swine flu)	Droplets;	Flu, bronchiolitis, pneumonia, acute sensorineural hearing loss (SNHL) anosmia	Zanamivir, oseltamivir, amantadine, rimantadine
Mumps Incubation 2-3 weeks	RNA virus	Respiratory droplet, close contact	Mumps (parotitis), orchitis, pancreatitis, acute SNHL	
Respiratory syncytial virus; Incubation 2-8 weeks	RNA virus; Serotypes A, B	Contact with respiratory secretions	Croup, bronchiolitis, bronchitis, AOM, anosmia	Ribavirin aerosol inhalation
Parainfluenza virus	Types 1,2,3,4	Person to person	Common cold, croup, bronchiolitis, pneumonia, anosmia	
Herpes simplex virus (HSV); Incubation 2-14 days	Double stranded DNA virus; Types 1, 2	Direct contact with mucosal secretions; oral (HSV-1), genitourinary (HSV-2)	Pharyngitis, gingivostomatitis, recurrent labial herpes, Bell's palsy, acute SNHL, anosmia	Famciclovir, valacyclovir, acyclovir,
Epstein-Barr virus	DNA virus		Infectious mononucleosis, hairy oral leukoplakia, nasopharyngeal carcinoma, Burkitt's lymphoma, B-cell lymphoma	Acyclovir
Human papilloma virus	Double stranded DNA papovavirus	Perinatal (types 6, 11)	Papillomas and carcinoma of skin, genitalia, larynx, recurrent respiratory papillomatosis	

Ans. **117. b.** Nasopharyngeal carcinoma

118. MC site juvenile nasopharyngeal angiofibroma:

a. Roof of nasopharynx
b. Anterior wall of sphenoid
c. Sphenopalatine foramen
d. Posterior wall of sphenoid

The site of origin of JNA is a matter of dispute. Currently it is believed to arise close to the superior margin of sphenopalatine foramen (bounded by palatine bone, horizontal ala of vomer and root of pterygoid plexus). In past it was said to arise from the roof of nasopharynx or the anterior wall of sphenoid bone.

119. CSF rhinorrhea is due to fracture of:

a. Mastoid air cells
b. Parietal bone
c. Floor of posterior cranial fossa
d. Cribriform plate

Anterior cranial fossa CSF reaches the nose through the cribriform plate, ethmoid air cells or frontal sinus.

Differences between CSF rhinorrhea and nasal secretions

	CSF rhinorrhea	*Nasal secretions*
History	Surgery, injury and tumor	Sneezing, stuffiness, itching
Discharge flow	A few drops or a stream of fluid	Continuous
Aggravation	Straining and forward bending	Allergy, infection, crying
Sniffing back	Impossible	Possible
Character	Thin, watery and clear	Mucus, mucopurulent, tears
Taste	Sweet	Salty
Sugar content	Normally more than 30 mg/dl	Less than 10 mg/dl
β2 transferrin	Present	Absent

120. Nasopharyngeal carcinoma is most common in which country:

a. India
b. America
c. China
d. Russia

NPC is most common in southern states of China, Taiwan and Indonesia. In Guangdong Province of Southern China, NPC is the third MC malignancy among men. In India, NPC constitutes only 0.5% of all body cancers.

121. Source of epistaxis, below the level of middle turbinate:

a. Anterior ethmoidal artery
b. Sphenopalatine artery
c. Posterior ethmoidal artery
d. All of the above

Sphenopalatine and greater palatine branches of internal maxillary artery (branch of external carotid artery) supply posterior inferior part of internal nose.

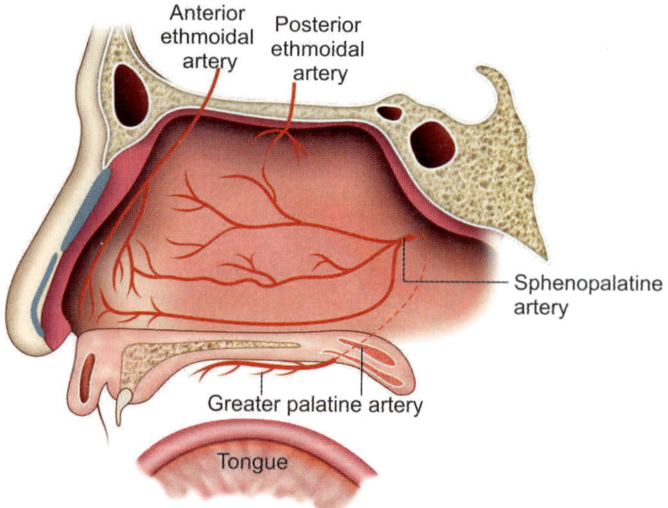

Blood supply of lateral wall of nose

122. NOT a component of Trotter's triad:

a. Ipsilateral soft palate immobility
b. VII nerve palsy
c. Trigeminal neuralgia
d. Conduction deafness

Trotter's triad of NPC includes conductive deafness, ipsilateral temporoparietal neuralgia (CN V) and palatal paralysis (CN X).

123. In Kiesselbach's plexus, which artery is a branch of internal carotid artery:

a. Sphenopalatine artery
b. Ethmoidal artery
c. Greater palatine artery
d. Posterior lateral nasal branches

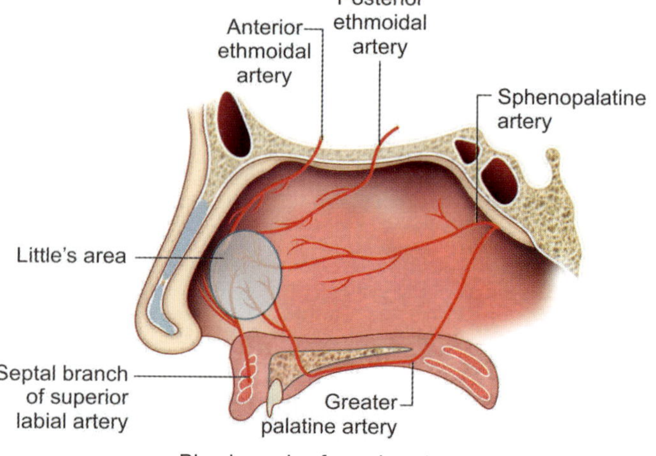

Blood supply of nasal septum

Ans. 118. **c.** Sphenopalatine... 119. **d.** Cribriform plate 120. **c.** China 121. **b.** Sphenopalatine artery 122. **b.** VII nerve palsy 123. **b.** Ethmoidal artery

Anterior and posterior ethmoidal branches of ophthalmic artery (branch of internal carotid artery) supply superior part of nasal cavity.

124. MC malignancy of maxillary antrum:
a. Mucoepidermoid ca
b. Adenoid cystic ca
c. Adeno ca
d. Squamous cell ca

More than 80% of the malignant tumours of nose and paranasal sinuses are squamous cell carcinoma. Others in descending order, are adenoid cystic carcinoma and adenocarcinoma. Melanoma and sarcomas are rare.

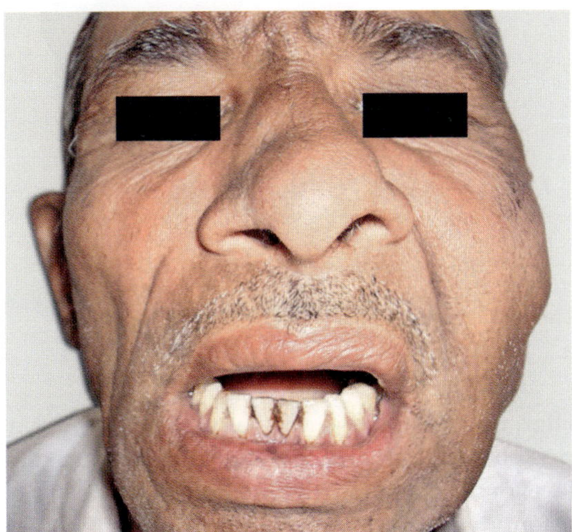

Carcinoma maxillary sinus with trismus indicating retromolar extension

125. Transnasal approach is NOT used in:
a. Lateral orbitotomy
b. Ethmoidectomy
c. Antrostomy
d. Hypophysectomy

In lateral orbitotomy, lateral half of the supraorbital margin with the quadrilateral piece of the bone forming the lateral orbital wall is temporarily removed. This approach provides an adequate exposure to the orbital contents and is particularly valuable for the retrobulbar lesions.

126. In endoscopic dacryo-cysto-rhinostomy, opening is made in:
a. Inferior meatus
b. Middle meatus
c. Superior meatus
d. None of the above

Steps in endoscopic DCR:
- Endoscopic identification of sac area in the middle meatus
- Opening created in the middle meatus
- Stenting of rhinostomy opening with fine silicon tubes

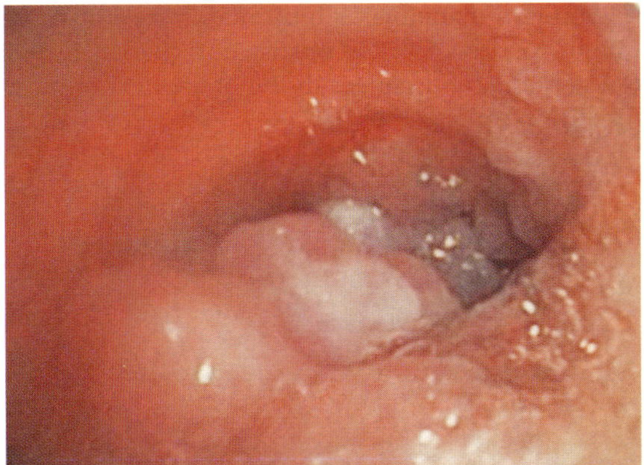

Lateral wall of nasal cavity of cadaver showing turbinates and meatuses

THROAT

127. Cartilage attached to true vocal cords:
a. Cricoid b. Thyroid
c. Arytenoid d. Hyoid

The **arytenoids** cartilages are a pair of small three-sided pyramids which form part of the larynx, to which the vocal folds (vocal cords) are attached. These allow and aid in the vocal cords' movement.

128. Which of the following cyst moves on swallowing movement:
a. Thymic cyst b. Branchial cyst
c. Thyroglossal cyst
d. Sublingual dermoid cyst

Thyroglossal duct cysts most often present with a palpable asymptomatic midline neck mass below the level of the hyoid bone. The mass on the neck moves during swallowing or on protrusion of the tongue because of its attachment to the tongue via the tract of thyroid descent.

129. True regarding Heimlich manoeuvre:
a. Peripheral circulation
b. Pulmonary function without heart lung machine
c. Cardiac function without pacemaker
d. For relieving airway obstruction

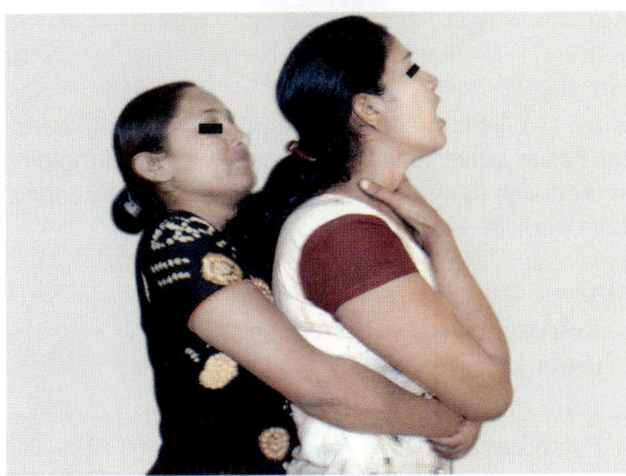

Heimlich's maneuver. Standing behind the standing patient, sudden upward and backward thrusts just below the epigastric region squeeze the lungs' air, and may dislodge laryngeal foreign body

Ans. 124. d. Squamous cell... 125. a. Lateral orbitotomy 126. b. Middle meatus 127. c. Arytenoids
128. c. Thyroglossal cyst 129. d. For relieving airway obstruction

Heimlich's maneuver is indicated in case of a large bolus of food completely obstructing the larynx with total aphonia, and patient dying of asphyxia (impending death).

130. Tonsillectomy is contraindicated in:
a. Tonsillolith
b. Poliomyelitis epidemic
c. Quinsy
d. Small atrophic tonsils

Contraindications of adenotonsillectomy
- Anemia
- Acute URTI/acute tonsillitis
- Overt or submucous cleft palate
- Bleeding disorders
- Epidemic of polio
- During the period of menses in females

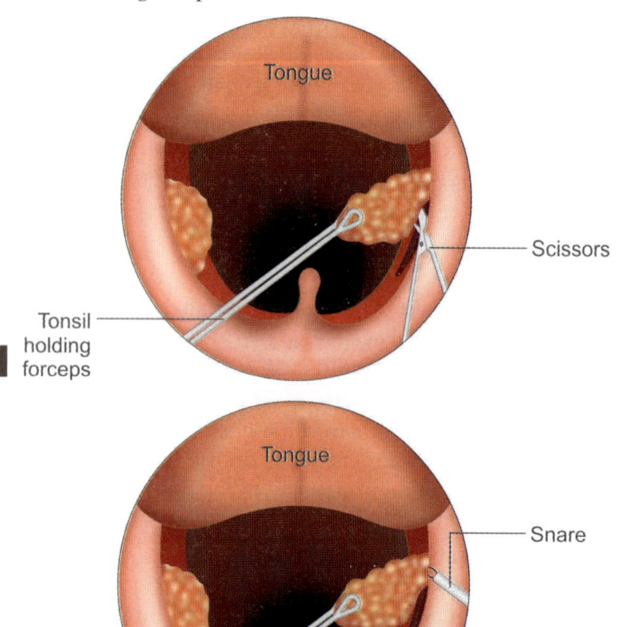

Tonsillectomy. (A) A blunt curved scissor is dissecting tonsil from the peritonsillar tissue while tonsil is grasped with tonsil holding forceps and pulled medially; (B) Wire loop of tonsillar snare threaded over the tonsil onto its pedicle and cut

131. Reinke's space is situated in:
a. Retropharyngeal space
b. Prelaryngeal space
c. True vocal cords
d. False vocal cords

Reinke's space is a potential space with scanty subepithelial connective tissues lies under the epithelium of vocal cords and superficial to its elastic layer.

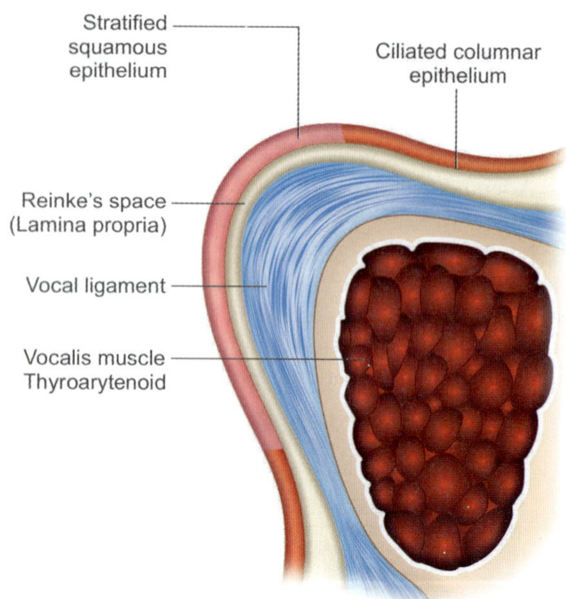

Structure of vocal fold. Cross-section

132. Indication of high tracheostomy:
a. Diphtheria
b. TB
c. Tetanus
d. Carcinoma

High tracheostomy is done at the level of first tracheal ring above the level of thyroid isthmus, which lies at the level of third and fourth tracheal rings. The high tracheostomy is generally avoided because of the postoperative risk of perichondritis of the cricoids cartilage and subglottic stenosis. In cases of carcinoma larynx with stridor when total laryngectomy would be done, high tracheostomy is indicated.

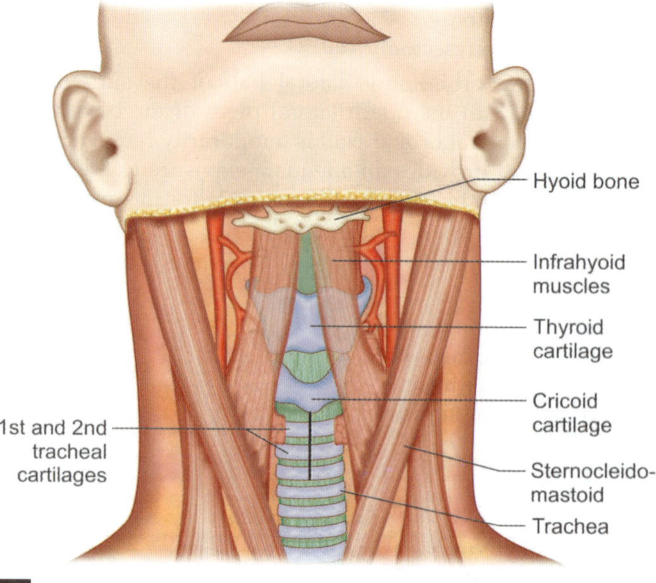

Ans. 130. **b.** Poliomyelitis epidemic
131. **c.** True vocal cords
132. **d.** Carcinoma

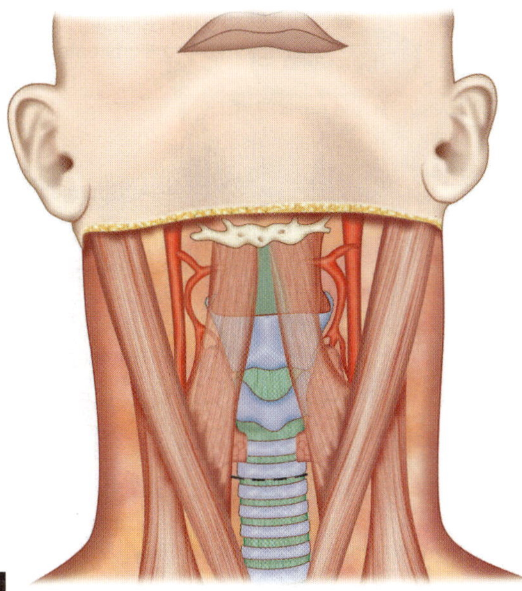

Incisions for tracheostomy. (A) Surface landmarks for the midline skin vertical incision for tracheostomy; (B) Horizontal skin incision for cricothyrotomy

133. Common location of singer's nodule:

a. Junction of anterior 2/3rd and posterior 1/3rd of vocal cords
b. Junction of posterior 2/3rd and anterior 1/3rd of vocal cords
c. Junction of middle 1/3rd and posterior 1/3rd of vocal cords
d. None of the above

Vocal nodules/singer's or screamer's nodules are bilateral and occur at the area of maximum vibration of the cord. It is at the junction of anterior one-third and posterior two-thirds of the free edge of vocal cord.

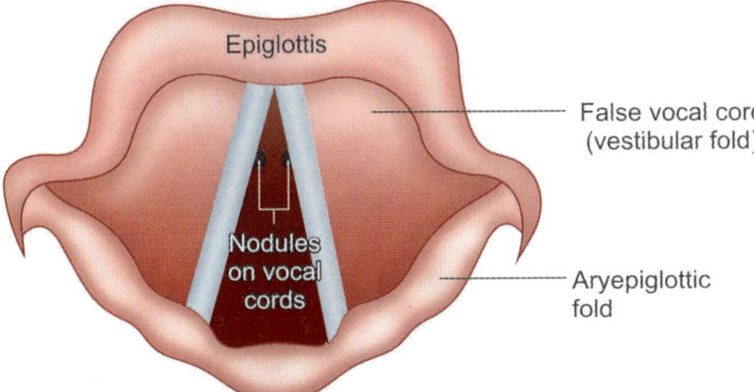

Bilateral vocal nodules at the junction of anterior one-third and posterior two-thirds of vocal cords

134. Structure preserved in radical neck dissection:

a. Sternocleidomastoid muscle
b. Internal jugular vein
c. Accessory nerve
d. Vagus nerve

Nerves preserved in RND are brachial plexus, phrenic nerve, vagus nerve, cervical sympathetic chain, marginal mandibular branch of facial, lingual and hypoglossal nerves.

Classification of neck dissection

- *Radical neck dissection (RND):* Removes I, II, III, IV and V level of lymph nodes, sternocleidomastoid muscle, internal jugular vein, spinal accessory nerve, submandibular salivary gland, tail of the parotid and omohyoid muscle.
- Modified radical neck dissection:
  - Type I: Preserves accessory cranial nerve (CN XI)
  - Type II: Preserves CN XI and internal jugular vein (IJV)
  - Type III: Preserves CN XI, IJV and sternocleidomastoid muscle (SCM)
- *Selective neck dissection:* Preserves CN XI, IJV and SCM.
  - Supra omohyoid (or anterolateral): Removes level I, II and III lymph nodes (cancer of oral cavity).
  - Lateral: Removes level II, III and IV lymph nodes (cancer of pharynx, hypopharynx and larynx)
  - Posterolateral: Removes level II, III, IV, V and suboccipital lymph nodes (cancer or melanoma of posterior scalp or posterior upper neck)
  - Anterior compartment: Removes level VI lymph nodes (cancer thyroid, subglottic, cervical trachea, hypopharynx)
- *Extended neck dissection*: Extended RND may include additional lymph node groups (retropharyngeal, parotid or level VI nodes) and nonlymphatic structures (external carotid artery, hypoglossal nerve, parotid gland, mastoid tip).

135. All of the following are true regarding tracheostomy tube EXCEPT:

a. Double lumen tube
b. Made of titanium silver alloy
c. Cuffed tube prevents aspiration of pharyngeal secretions
d. Ideally should be changed every 3rd day

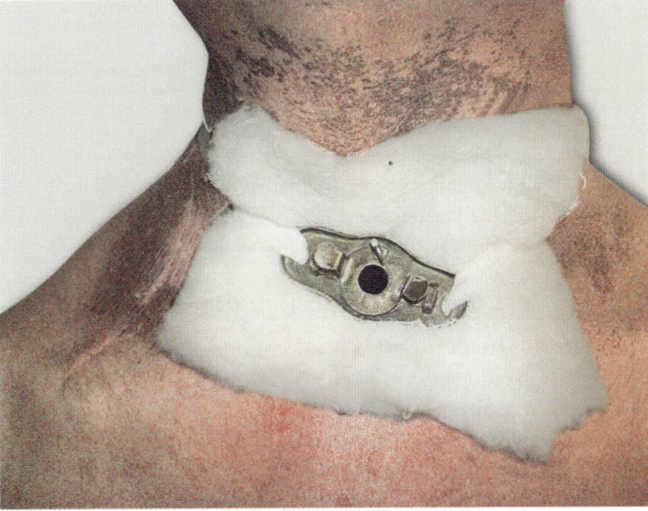

Tracheostomy tube inserted and secured by tapes

Ans. 133. **b.** Junction of posterior 2/3rd... 134. **d.** Vagus nerve
135. **d.** Ideally should be changed every 3rd day

Inner cannula is removed, and cleaned regularly for the first 3 days to prevent respiratory distress. Outer tube is changed daily after 3-4 days of tracheostomy when a track is formed that facilitates easy tube placement.

136. One of the most important complications of tracheostomy is:

a. Surgical emphysema
b. Hemorrhage
c. Recurrent laryngeal nerve palsy
d. Displacement of tube

The most common (MC) complications of tracheostomy include hemorrhage (3.7%), tube obstruction (2.7%) and tube displacement (1.5%). The common sites of hemorrhage are anterior jugular veins and thyroid isthmus.

Complications of tracheostomy	
1.	Immediate
	a. Hemorrhage b. Apnea c. Pneumothorax d. Vocal cord palsy e. Tracheoesophageal fistula f. Aspiration of blood g. False passage
2.	Intermediate
	a. Bleeding: Reactionary and secondary b. Displacement of tube c. Obstruction of tube d. Subcutaneous emphysema e. Pneumomediastinum and pneumothorax f. Crusting in trachea g. Tracheitis and stoma cellulitis h. Tracheobronchitis i. Severe infections: mediastinitis, clavicular osteomyelitis, and necrotizing fasciitis j. Atelectasis and lung abscess k. Local wound infection and granulations
3.	Late (with prolonged use of tube):
	a. Hemorrhage due to granulation tissue and innominate artery blowout b. Laryngeal stenosis c. Tracheal stenosis d. Tracheoesophageal fistula e. Difficult decannulation f. Persistent tracheocutaneous fistula g. Keloid or unsightly scar h. Corrosion of tracheostomy tube.

137. Stridor in an infant is most commonly due to:

a. Diphtheria
b. Acute epiglottitis
c. Foreign body aspiration
d. Laryngomalacia

Laryngomalacia is the MC cause of stridor in childhood and usually occurs within the first 2 weeks of life.

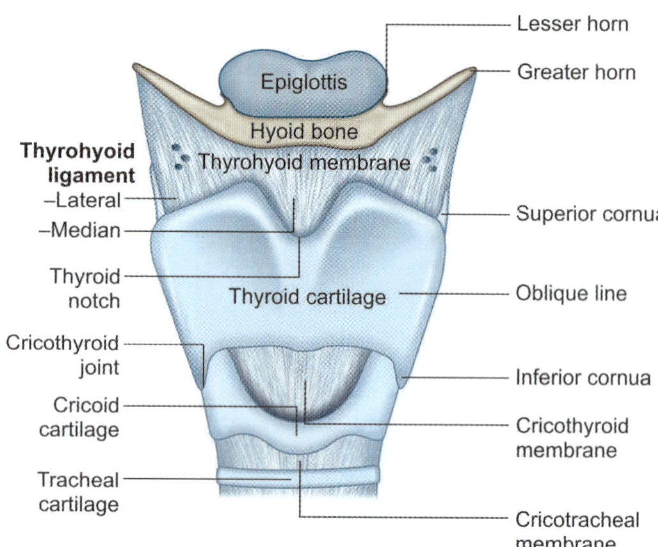

Laryngeal framework—anterior view

138. Laryngocele arises from:

a. Subglottis
b. Anterior commissure
c. Saccule
d. True glottis

Laryngocele is an abnormally enlarged and distended saccule containing air. Saccule is diverticulum of mucous membrane starting from the anterior part of ventricle and extends superiorly between vestibular folds and thyroid lamina.

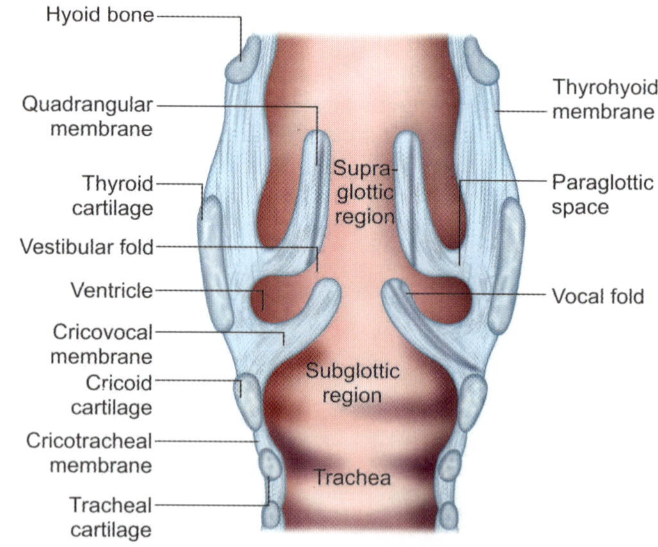

Coronal section of larynx

139. 'Gold standard' surgical procedure for prevention of aspiration:

a. Feeding gastrostomy/jejunostomy
b. Tracheal division and permanent tracheostomy
c. Tracheostomy
d. Thyroplasty

Ans. 136. b. Hemorrhage 137. d. Laryngomalacia 138. c. Saccule 139. b. Tracheal division and...

Indications of tracheostomy include easier management of secretions and an adjuvant procedure during chest surgery, and major head and neck operations. Cuffed tracheostomy tube protects the tracheobronchial tree against aspiration of secretions and blood.

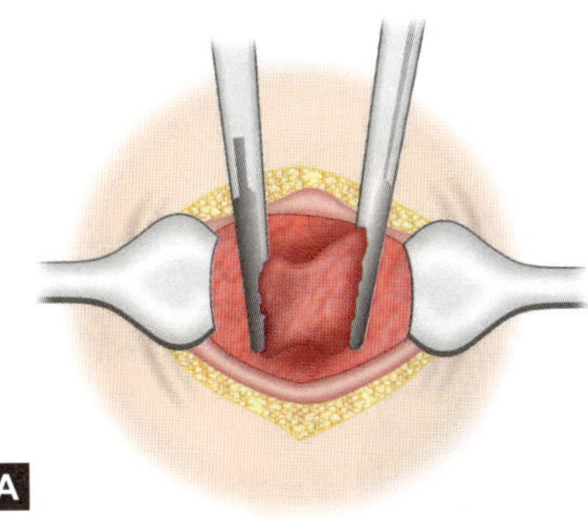

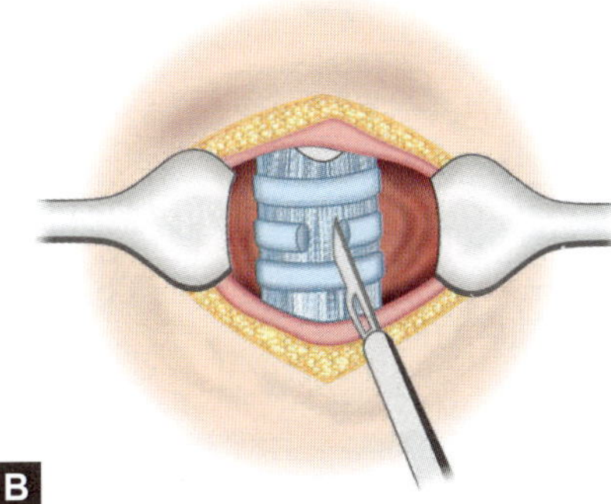

Thyroid isthmus and tracheostomy. (A) Thyroid isthmus may be retracted superiorly or inferiorly, or transected and suture ligated; (B) Anterior section of a tracheal ring can be removed or a round window spanning two tracheal rings can be created

140. Direct bronchoscopy cannot visualize:

a. Subcarinal lymph nodes
b. First segmental subdivision of bronchi
c. Vocal cords
d. Trachea

Bronchoscope can visualize the structure in the interior of respiratory pathway.

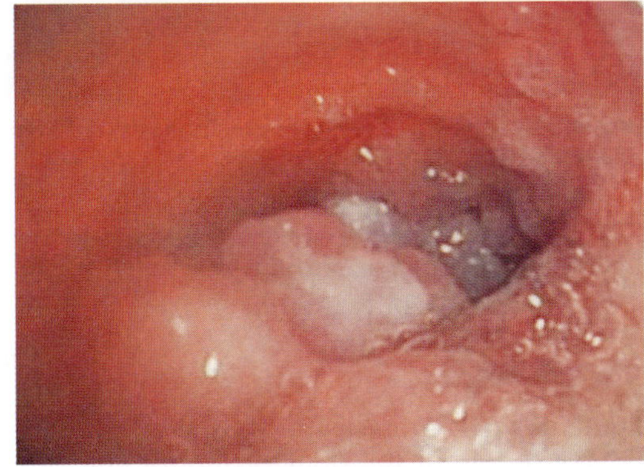

Endobronchial mass lesion
Source: Dr Rajiv Paliwal, Professor, Chest Medicine, Pramukh Swami Medical College, Karamsad, Anand, Gujarat

141. Middle superior alveolar nerve is a branch of:

a. Inferior alveolar
b. Mandibular branch of trigeminal nerve
c. Nasal branch of maxillary nerve
d. None of the above

The middle superior alveolar nerve drops from the infraorbital portion of the maxillary nerve to supply the sinus mucosa, the roots of the maxillary premolars, and the mesicobuccal root of the first maxillary molar.

142. Omega shaped epiglottis is seen in:

a. Laryngotracheobronchitis
b. Acute epiglottitis
c. Laryngomalacia
d. TB of larynx

Laryngomalacia has multiple anatomic abnormalities, which include exaggerated omega-shaped epiglottitis and short and inward collapse of aryepiglottic folds.

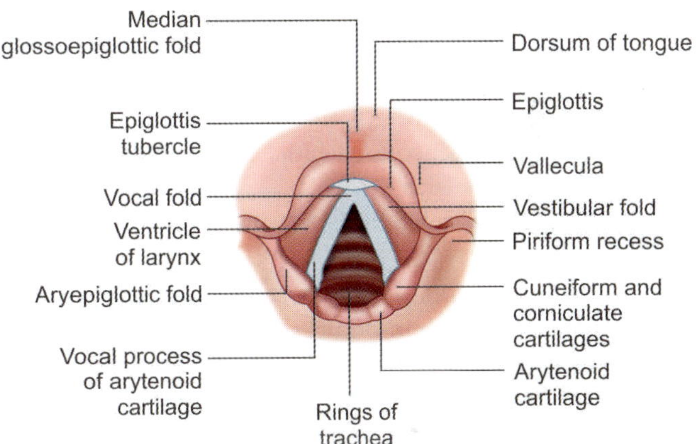

Superior view of the inside of the larynx as seen during laryngoscopic examination during moderate respiration. Some of the subsites of oropharynx and laryngopharynx can also be noticed

143. Quinsy is also known as:

a. Paratonsillar abscess
b. Peritonsillar abscess
c. Parapharyngeal abscess
d. Retropharyngeal abscess

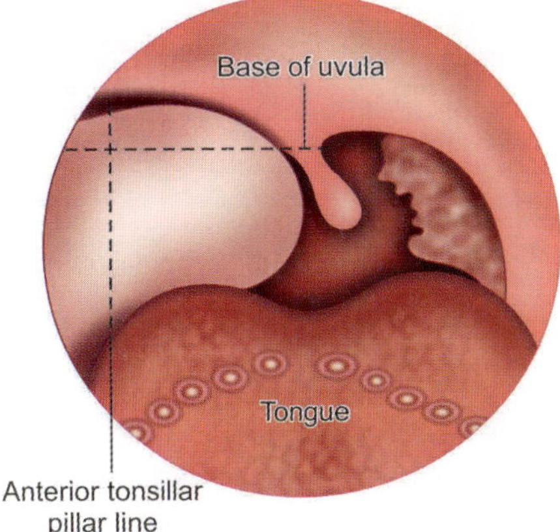

Peritonsillar abscess. Site of incision and drainage lies just lateral to the junction of vertical anterior faucial pillar line and horizontal base of uvula line

Ans. 140. **a.** Subcarinal lymph nodes
141. **d.** None of the above
142. **c.** Laryngomalacia
143. **b.** Peritonsillar abscess

Peritonsillar abscess (Quinsy) is a collection of pus in the peritonsillar space which lies between tonsil capsule and the superior constrictor muscle covered by the buccopharyngeal fascia.

144. NOT indicated in early glottic carcinoma-in-situ:

a. Radiotherapy
b. Partial laryngectomy
c. Transoral endoscopic CO_2 laser
d. Stripping of vocal cords

Management of carcinoma in situ includes endoscopic CO_2 laser application or stripping of vocal cord and tissue is sent for biopsy. If biopsy is reveals invasive carcinoma, radiotherapy is given. CIS needs regular follow-up.

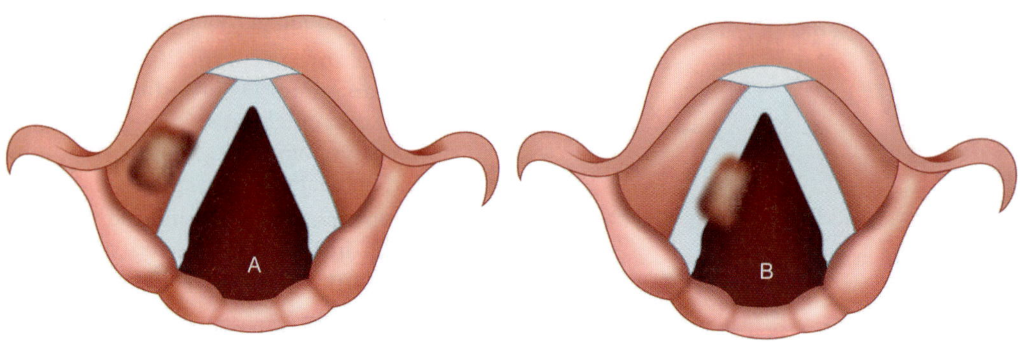

Carcinoma larynx. (A) Supraglottic; and (B) Glottic

145. MC cause of stridor in 3 months old:

a. Laryngo-tracheo-bronchitis
b. Laryngomalacia
c. Congenital subglottic stenosis
d. Laryngeal web

In laryngomalacia, the newborn develops intermittent, low-pitched inspiratory stridor within the first 2 weeks of life. The stridor usually starts resolving after 9 months, and disappears by 2 years of age.

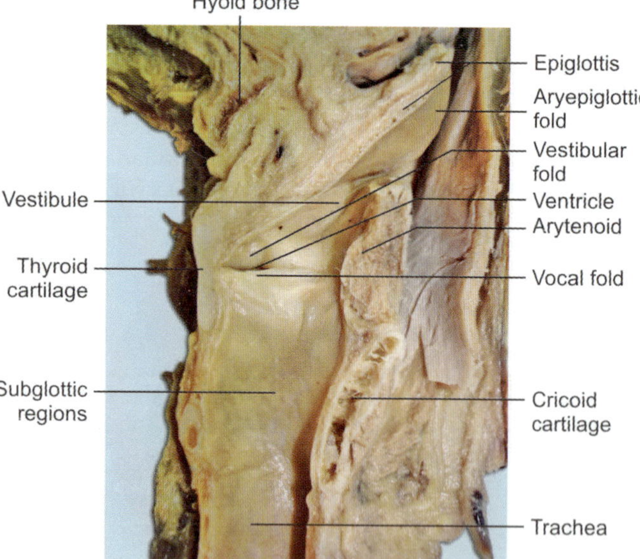

Sagittal section of larynx and laryngopharynx

146. Which of the following is premalignant:

a. Chronic glossitis
b. Submucous fibrosis
c. Hypertrophic glossitis
d. Aphthous stomatitis

Malignant transformation has been observed in 3-7.6% of cases of oral SMF.

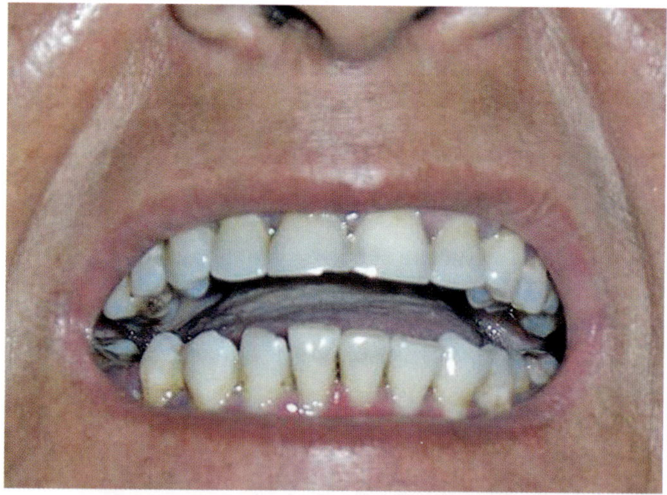

Oral submucous fibrosis. Severe trismus with 0.73 cm mouth opening

147. Ranula is:

a. Hypertrophied lymphoid tissue
b. Arises from floor of mouth
c. Hard and hemorrhagic
d. An abscess

Ranula, a cystic grayish translucent swelling occurs in the lateral part of the floor of mouth and pushes the tongue up. Ranula is the result of obstruction of the ducts of sublingual salivary glands.

Ans. **144. b.** Partial laryngectomy
145. b. Laryngomalacia
146. b. Submucous fibrosis
147. b. Arises from floor of mouth

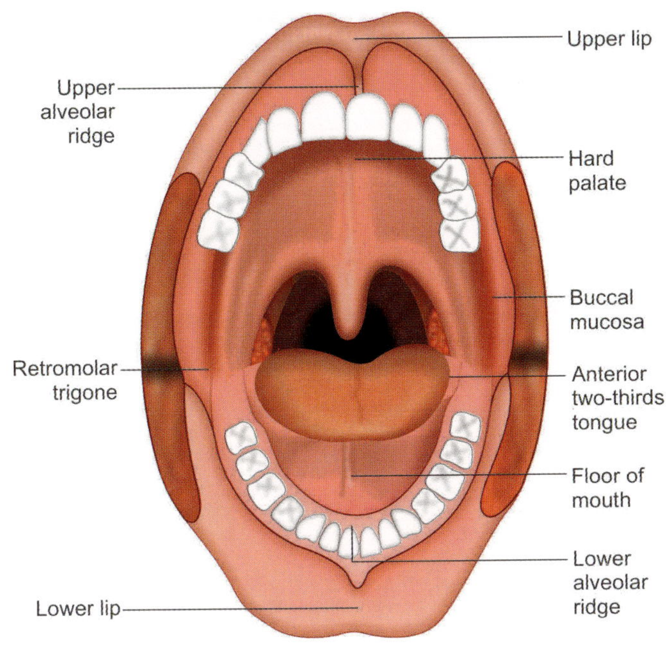

Oral cavity overview

148. A patient who had undergone tooth extraction for dental caries, presents with swelling in posterior part of middle 1/3rd of sternomastoid and tonsil is pushed medially. The diagnosis is:

a. Retropharyngeal abscess b. Parapharyngeal abscess
c. Ludwig's angina d. Vincent's angina

The parapharyngeal abscess collects medial to the medial pterygoid muscle. The otogenic parapharyngeal abscess is caused by petrositis. In other instances it occurs due to caries/extraction of molar tooth. Patient develops trismus, fever and swelling that pushes the tonsil medially and spreads laterally posterior to sternocleidomastoid.

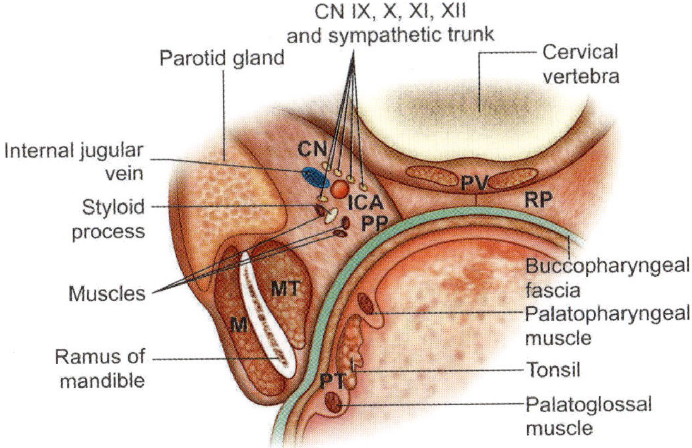

Deep neck spaces for abscesses

Abbreviations: CN, Cranial nerves IX, X, XI and XII and sympathetic trunk; IC, Internal carotid artery; IJV, Internal jugular vein; M, Masseter muscle; MT, Medial pterygoid muscle; PP, Parapharyngeal space; PT, Peritonsillar space; PV, Prevertebral space; RP, Retropharyngeal space.

MISCELLANEOUS

149. Which of the following nerve gives origin to Arnold nerve:

a. Facial b. Vestibulocochlear
c. Glossopharyngeal d. Vagus

Auricular branch of vagus nerve is known as Arnolds nerve, which supplies concha and corresponding eminence on the medial surface (pinna)

150. False regarding skull of newborn:

a. Mastoid process is not completely formed
b. Middle ear ossicles are of same size as in adults
c. Absent diploic spaces
d. All paranasal sinuses are absent

At birth, both frontal as well as sphenoid sinuses are absent and therefore not clinically significant in young children.

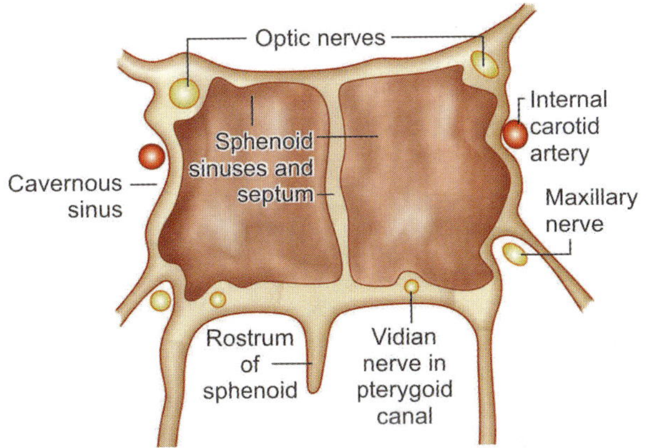

Sphenoidal sinuses coronal section showing important structures situated in relation with sphenoid sinus walls

151. Nerve of pterygoid canal is also known as:

a. Arnold's nerve
b. Vidian nerve
c. Nerve of kuntz
d. Criminal nerve of Grassi

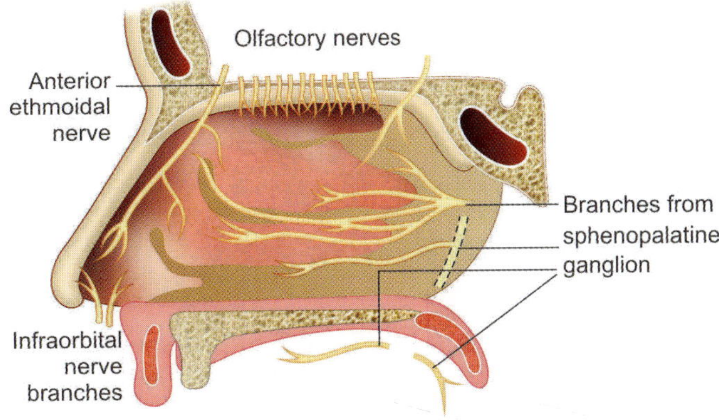

Nerve supply of lateral wall of nose

Ans. **148. b.** Parapharyngeal abscess
149. d. Vagus
150. d. All paranasal sinuses are absent
151. b. Vidian nerve

The greater superficial petrosal nerve, which carry preganglionic fibers from the parasympathetic nucleus situated in brain stem, joins deep petrosal nerve (postganglionic vasomotor sympathetic fibers) and forms nerve to pterygoid canal (vidian nerve), which reaches to the sphenopalatine ganglion where only parasympathetic fibers relay.

152. Absent at birth:

a. Malleus
b. Incus
c. Mastoid tip
d. Ethmoid sinus

Malleus and incus develops from mesoderm of first pharyngeal arch.

Development of ear (Timings shown in the week of gestation)**

Development	*Beginning*	*Completion*
Vestibule	3	20
Cochlea	3	20
Middle ear	3	30
Auricle	6	20
EAC	6	28

**Gulya AJ. Developmental anatomy of ear. Glasscock and Shambaugh. Surgery of Ear. WB Saunders (1990)

Ans. 152. c. Mastoid tip

ANSWERS WITH REFERENCES

EAR

1. **Ans. (c) Posterior**
Ref: Internet resources

2. **Ans. (d) Otosclerosis**
Ref: Dhingra's ENT, 4/e p86

3. **Ans. (b) Cartilaginous 1/3rd & 2/3rd bony**
Ref: Dhingra's ENT, 4/e p56

4. **Ans. (d) Meniere's disease**
Ref: Dhingra's ENT, 4/e p43

5. **Ans. (c) Meniere's disease**
Ref: Dhingra's ENT, 4/e p102

6. **Ans. (a) Autosomal dominant**
Ref: Dhingra's ENT, 4/e p86

7. **Ans. (a) Wave I**
Ref: Dhingra's ENT, 4/e p29

8. **Ans. (b) Hallpike's test**
Ref: Dhingra's ENT, 4/e p42

9. **Ans. (a) 5th**
Ref: Bansal's ENT 1/e p274

10. **Ans. (a) Smaller than the bony portion**
Ref: Bansal's ENT 1/e p3

11. **Ans. (b) Facial nerve**
Ref: Bansal's ENT 1/e p8

12. **Ans. (b) Scala vestibuli**
Ref: Bansal's ENT 1/e p14

13. **Ans. (a) Vestibular function**
Ref: Bansal's ENT 1/e p233

14. **Ans. (b) Otosclerosis**
Ref: Bansal's ENT 1/e p152

15. **Ans. (c) Deafness, tinnitus, vertigo**
Ref: Bansal's ENT 1/e p241

16. **Ans. (d) Cochleovestibular symptoms**
Ref: Bansal's ENT 1/e p276

17. **Ans. (b) 2 kHz**
Ref: Bansal's ENT 1/e p153

18. **Ans. (d) Otorrhea**
Ref: Bansal's ENT 1/e p242

19. **Ans. (d) 8th**
Ref: Bansal's ENT 1/e p273

20. **Ans. (c) Painless**
Ref: Bansal's ENT 1/e p204

21. **Ans. (b) VII cranial nerve palsy**
Ref: Bansal's ENT 1/e p217

22. **Ans. (a) Normal ear**
Ref: Bansal's ENT 1/e p140

23. **Ans. (b) Petrous temporal bone**
Ref: Bansal's ENT 1/e p131

24. **Ans. (d) Semicircular canals**
Ref: Bansal's ENT 1/e p13

25. **Ans. (b) Sound louder in diseased ear**
Ref: Bansal's ENT 1/e p141

26. **Ans. (c) Serous otitis media**
Ref: Bansal's ENT 1/e p150

27. **Ans. (b) 15 dB**
Ref: Bansal's ENT 1/e p141

28. **Ans. (a) Hematoma of the auricle**
Ref: Bansal's ENT 1/e p185

29. **Ans. (b) 1st pharyngeal pouch**
Ref: Bansal's ENT 1/e p20

30. **Ans. (d) Stapedius**
Ref: Bansal's ENT 1/e p262

31. **Ans. (a) Viral**
Ref: Bansal's ENT 1/e p191

32. **Ans. (b) Diplopia**
Ref: Bansal's ENT 1/e p242

33. **Ans. (d) Pseudomonas**
Ref: Bansal's ENT 1/e p191

34. **Ans. (c) Dislocation of the incudostapedial joint**
Ref: Bansal's ENT 1/e p151

35. **Ans. (c) CSOM**
Ref: Bansal's ENT 1/e p210

36. **Ans. (b) Aspergillus**
Ref: Bansal's ENT 1/e p189

37. **Ans. (b) Telephonist's ear**
Ref: Bansal's ENT 1/e p188

38. **Ans. (d)** Glomus tumour
Ref: Bansal's ENT 1/e p134

39. **Ans. (c)** BERA
Ref: Bansal's ENT 1/e p146

40. **Ans. (d)** Deafness
Ref: Bansal's ENT 1/e p275

41. **Ans. (c)** Carcinoma tongue
Ref: Bansal's ENT 1/e p129

42. **Ans. (a)** 512 Hz
Ref: Bansal's ENT 1/e p139

43. **Ans. (a)** Lateral
Ref: Bansal's ENT 1/e p234

44. **Ans. (c)** TB
Ref: Bansal's ENT 1/e p5

45. **Ans. (b)** Pneumococcus
Ref: Bansal's ENT 1/e p202

46. **Ans. (d)** Cortical mastoidectomy
Ref: Bansal's ENT 1/e p551

47. **Ans. (a)** Labyrinthine canal
Ref: Bansal's ENT 1/e p260

48. **Ans. (c)** Meniere's disease
Ref: Bansal's ENT 1/e p241

49. **Ans. (b)** Modified radical mastoidectomy
Ref: Bansal's ENT 1/e p553

50. **Ans. (a)** Marginal
Ref: Bansal's ENT 1/e p209

51. **Ans. (b)** Sternomastoid muscle
Ref: Bansal's ENT 1/e p220

52. **Ans. (b)** Oval window
Ref: Bansal's ENT 1/e p6

53. **Ans. (c)** Outer hair cells
Ref: Bansal's ENT 1/e p146

54. **Ans. (c)** Myringotomy
Ref: Bansal's ENT 1/e p548

55. **Ans. (d)** Lateral sinus thrombosis
Ref: Bansal's ENT 1/e p225

56. **Ans. (a)** Brain abscess
Ref: Bansal's ENT 1/e p223

57. **Ans. (b)** Cortical mastoidectomy
Ref: Bansal's ENT 1/e p8

58. **Ans. (a)** Low compliance
Ref: Bansal's ENT 1/e p145

59. **Ans. (a)** Autosomal dominant
Ref: Bansal's ENT 1/e p150

60. **Ans. (d)** Paracusis
Ref: Bansal's ENT 1/e p152

61. **Ans. (a)** Sound localization
Ref: Bansal's ENT 1/e p21

62. **Ans. (d)** Stria vascularis
Ref: Bansal's ENT 1/e p15

63. **Ans. (c)** Loss of consciousness
Ref: Bansal's ENT 1/e p242

64. **Ans. (b)** Suprameatal triangle
Ref: Bansal's ENT 1/e p11

65. **Ans. (c)** Horizontal semicircular canal
Ref: Bansal's ENT 1/e p14

66. **Ans. (b)** Subjective sense of imbalance
Ref: Bansal's ENT 1/e p230

67. **Ans. (c)** Acoustic reflex
Ref: Bansal's ENT 1/e p145

68. **Ans. (d)** Multiple perforation
Ref: Bansal's ENT 1/e p126

69. **Ans. (d)** Gentamicin
Ref: Bansal's ENT 1/e p159

70. **Ans. (b)** Better felt
Ref: Bansal's ENT 1/e p140

71. **Ans. (d)** Glossopharyngeal nerve
Ref: Bansal's ENT 1/e p129

72. **Ans. (b)** Pseudomonas aeruginosa
Ref: Bansal's ENT 1/e p191

73. **Ans. (c)** Superior oblique palsy
Ref: Bansal's ENT 1/e p220

74. **Ans. (d)** Nasal vestibule
Ref: Bansal's ENT 1/e p130

75. **Ans. (b)** Modified radical mastoidectomy
Ref: Bansal's ENT 1/e p214

76. **Ans. (c)** Otosclerosis
Ref: Bansal's ENT 1/e p152

77. **Ans. (a)** ASOM
Ref: Bansal's ENT 1/e p5

78. **Ans. (c)** Fluorides
Ref: Bansal's ENT 1/e p154

79. **Ans. (a)** Sternocleidomastoid muscle
Ref: Bansal's ENT 1/e p219

80. **Ans. (a)** 512 Hz
Ref: Bansal's ENT 1/e p140

81. **Ans. (d)** Streptococcus pneumoniae
Ref: Bansal's ENT 1/e p222

82. **Ans. (d)** 85
Ref: Bansal's ENT 1/e p138

83. **Ans. (a)** 20-35 dBA
Ref: Internet resources

84. **Ans. (a)** 14 times
Ref: Bansal's ENT 1/e p23

NOSE

85. **Ans. (c)** Downward, Backward, Lateral
Ref: Disease of sinuses: Diagnosis & treatment, 2/e p377

86. **Ans. (c)** Adenoidectomy
Ref: Dhingra's ENT, 4/e p385

87. **Ans. (c)** Maxillary
Ref: Dhingra's ENT, 4/e p366

88. **Ans. (a)** Foreign body
Ref: Bansal's ENT 1/e p349

89. **Ans. (a)** Cribriform plate
Ref: Bansal's ENT 1/e p34

90. **Ans. (c)** Vessels lack a contractile component
Ref: Bansal's ENT 1/e p437

91. **Ans. (b)** Sphenoid
Ref: Bansal's ENT 1/e p34

92. **Ans. (c)** Lacrimal duct
Ref: Bansal's ENT 1/e p33

93. **Ans. (b)** Rhinophyma
Ref: Bansal's ENT 1/e p34

94. **Ans. (b)** Cribriform plate
Ref: Bansal's ENT 1/e p37

95. **Ans. (a)** Atrophic rhinitis
Ref: Bansal's ENT 1/e p314

96. **Ans. (c)** Endoscopic sinus surgery
Ref: Bansal's ENT 1/e p309

97. **Ans. (d)** Frontoethmoidal
Ref: Bansal's ENT 1/e p305

98. **Ans. (c)** Intranasal polypectomy
Ref: Bansal's ENT 1/e p308

99. **Ans. (b)** Nasopharyngeal carcinoma with metastasis
Ref: Bansal's ENT 1/e p440

100. **Ans. (d)** Arises from odontoid epithelium
Ref: Bansal's ENT 1/e p292

101. **Ans. (d)** Water's view
Ref: Bansal's ENT 1/e p597

102. **Ans. (a)** Younger males
Ref: Bansal's ENT 1/e p438

103. **Ans. (a)** Maxillary
Ref: Bansal's ENT 1/e p356

104. **Ans. (b)** Foreign body
Ref: Bansal's ENT 1/e p349

105. **Ans. (d)** CT scan should be done to assess size
Ref: Bansal's ENT 1/e p52

106. **Ans. (a)** Bleeding per nose
Ref: Bansal's ENT 1/e p355

107. **Ans. (c)** Due to chronic use of nasal drops
Ref: Bansal's ENT 1/e p331

108. **Ans. (b)** Nasopharyngectomy with radical neck dissection is the treatment of choice
Ref: Bansal's ENT 1/e p439

109. **Ans. (d)** Sphenoid sinus
Ref: Bansal's ENT 1/e p597

110. **Ans. (a)** Zygomatic bone
Ref: Bansal's ENT 1/e p344

111. **Ans. (b)** Neck mass
Ref: Bansal's ENT 1/e p439

112. **Ans. (b)** IgE
Ref: Bansal's ENT 1/e p324

113. **Ans. (d)** Lacrimal
Ref: Bansal's ENT 1/e p32

114. **Ans. (a)** Rhinoscleroma
Ref: Bansal's ENT 1/e p311

115. **Ans. (c)** Both of the above
Ref: Bansal's ENT 1/e p39

116. **Ans. (d)** Carcinoma of maxillary sinus
Ref: Bansal's ENT 1/e p357

117. **Ans. (b)** Nasopharyngeal carcinoma
Ref: Bansal's ENT 1/e p95

118. **Ans. (c)** Sphenopalatine foramen
Ref: Bansal's ENT 1/e p437

119. **Ans. (d)** Cribriform plate
Ref: Bansal's ENT 1/e p348

120. **Ans. (c)** China
Ref: Bansal's ENT 1/e p438

121. **Ans. (b) Sphenopalatine artery**
Ref: Bansal's ENT 1/e p36

122. **Ans. (b) VII nerve palsy**
Ref: Bansal's ENT 1/e p439

123. **Ans. (b) Ethmoidal artery**
Ref: Bansal's ENT 1/e p36

124. **Ans. (d) Squamous cell ca**
Ref: Bansal's ENT 1/e p355

125. **Ans. (a) Lateral orbitotomy**
Ref: Khurana's Ophthalmology, 4th ed., p399

126. **Ans. (b) Middle meatus**
Ref: Bansal's ENT 1/e p32

THROAT

127. **Ans. (c) Arytenoids**
Ref: Dhingra's ENT, 4/e p261

128. **Ans. (c) Thyroglossal cyst**
Ref: Internet resources

129. **Ans. (d) For relieving airway obstruction**
Ref: Bansal's ENT 1/e p516

130. **Ans. (b) Poliomyelitis epidemic**
Ref: Bansal's ENT 1/e p570

131. **Ans. (c) True vocal cords**
Ref: Bansal's ENT 1/e p65

132. **Ans. (d) Carcinoma**
Ref: Bansal's ENT 1/e p511

133. **Ans. (b) Junction of posterior 2/3rd and anterior 1/3rd of vocal cords**
Ref: Bansal's ENT 1/e p485

134. **Ans. (d) Vagus nerve**
Ref: Bansal's ENT 1/e p77

135. **Ans. (d) Ideally should be changed every 3rd day**
Ref: Bansal's ENT 1/e p512

136. **Ans. (b) Hemorrhage**
Ref: Bansal's ENT 1/e p513

137. **Ans. (d) Laryngomalacia**
Ref: Bansal's ENT 1/e p62

138. **Ans. (c) Saccule**
Ref: Bansal's ENT 1/e p63

139. **Ans. (b) Tracheal division and permanent tracheostomy**
Ref: Bansal's ENT 1/e p512

140. **Ans. (a) Subcarinal lymph nodes**
Ref: Bansal's ENT 1/e p577

141. **Ans. (d) None of the above**
Ref: Internet resources

142. **Ans. (c) Laryngomalacia**
Ref: Bansal's ENT 1/e p64

143. **Ans. (b) Peritonsillar abscess**
Ref: Bansal's ENT 1/e p542

144. **Ans. (b) Partial laryngectomy**
Ref: Bansal's ENT 1/e p504

145. **Ans. (b) Laryngomalacia**
Ref: Bansal's ENT 1/e p56

146. **Ans. (b) Submucous fibrosis**
Ref: Bansal's ENT 1/e p375

147. **Ans. (b) Arises from floor of mouth**
Ref: Bansal's ENT 1/e p404

148. **Ans. (b) Parapharyngeal abscess**
Ref: Bansal's ENT 1/e p539

MISCELLANEOUS

149. **Ans. (d) Vagus**
Ref: Dhingra's ENT, 4/e p4

150. **Ans. (d) All paranasal sinuses are absent**
Ref: Bansal's ENT 1/e p38

151. **Ans. (b) Vidian nerve**
Ref: Bansal's ENT 1/e p36

152. **Ans. (c) Mastoid tip**
Ref: Bansal's ENT 1/e p19

PRACTICE QUESTIONS

EAR

1. Causative agent of acute suppurative otitis media:
a. Pseudomonas
b. Staphylococcus aureus
c. Pneumococcus
d. Neisseria

2. Endolymph is present in:
a. Scala tympani
b. Scala vestibuli
c. Scala media
d. All of the above

3. Prussak's space is seen in:
a. External ear
b. Middle ear
c. Mastoid process
d. Internal ear

4. Organ of Corti is present in:
a. Semicircular canal
b. Ossicles
c. Tympanic membrane
d. Cochlea

5. Cupula is present in:
a. Saccule
b. Utricle
c. Semicircular canal
d. Cochlea

6. BERA wave I originate from:
a. Cochlear nuclei
b. VIII nerve
c. Lateral lemniscus
d. Inferior colliculus

7. Bill's bar is present in:
a. External auditory canal
b. Semicircular canal
c. Ossicles
d. Internal acoustic canal

8. A patient presented with bilateral progressive facial palsy. Most probable site of lesion is:
a. Skull canal fractures
b. Parotid malignancy
c. Diabetes mellitus
d. ASOM

9. Which of the following is best to diagnose sensorineural deafness in a child?
a. Brainstem evoked auditory responses
b. Oto-acoustic emissions
c. Tympanometry
d. Tuning fork test

10. Location of ceruminous glands in external auditory canal:
a. Junction of outer 2/3rd and inner 1/3rd
b. Junction of outer 1/3rd and inner 2/3rd
c. Only in inner 2/3rd
d. Only in outer 1/3rd

11. True about auricle:
a. Skin only
b. Contains elastic cartilage
c. Skin with fat
d. Fat only

12. Site of attachment of tensor tympani:
a. Ear drum
b. Malleus
c. Stapes
d. Incus

13. Stria vascularis is related to which of the following?
a. Vestibule
b. Utricle
c. Saccule
d. Cochlea

14. Otoacoustic emissions/OAE are low intensity sounds produced by:
a. Ear drum
b. Middle ear ossicles
c. Cochlea
d. Vestibule

NOSE

15. Which of the following is true for antrochoanal polyp?
a. Seen in elderly
b. Recurrence is common
c. Unilateral
d. Allergic in nature

THROAT

16. A 40-year male, a chronic smoker presented with neck nodes, hearing loss, serous otitis media and epistaxis. He should be evaluated for:
a. Leukoplakia
b. Fibrous dysplasia
c. Nasopharyngeal angiofibroma
d. Nasopharyngeal carcinoma

Ans.
1. **c.** Pneumococcus
2. **c.** Scala media
3. **b.** Middle ear
4. **d.** Cochlea
5. **c.** Semicircular...
6. **b.** VIII nerve
7. **d.** Internal...
8. **a.** Skull...
9. **a.** Brainstem...
10. **d.** Only...
11. **b.** Contains...
12. **b.** Malleus
13. **d.** Cochlea
14. **c.** Cochlea
15. **c.** Unilateral
16. **d.** Naso..

17. Singer nodule is present at:
a. Midpoint of vocal cords
b. Anterior end of vocal cords
c. Posterior end of vocal cords
d. Junction of anterior one-third and posterior two-third of vocal cords

18. MC cause of tonsillitis:
a. Group A alpha haemolytic streptococci
b. Group B beta haemolytic streptococci
c. Group A beta haemolytic streptococci
d. Group B alpha haemolytic streptococci

19. In which of the following carcinoma, radiation therapy is most useful and prognosis overall is good?
a. Ca glottis b. Ca epiglottis
c. Ca subglottis d. Ca supraglottis

20. Which of the following condition does not present with hot-potato voice?
a. Peritonsillar abscess
b. Tongue malignancy
c. Tonsillar malignancy
d. Streptococcal pharyngitis

21. Which of the following has highest malignant potential?
a. Thin leukoplakia b. Erythroplakia
c. Speckled leukoplakia d. Verrucous leukoplakia

MISCELLANEOUS

22. Nerve involved in Frey's syndrome:
a. Facial b. Mandibular
c. Maxillary d. Auriculotemporal

23. Which of the following has no role in balancing of body?
a. Visual impulses
b. Olfactory impulses
c. Proprioceptive impulses
d. Vestibular impulses

24. Which of the following cranial nerve is present in fallopian canal?
a. V
b. VI
c. VII
d. VIII

25. NOT a derivative of branchial arch:
a. Ultimobranchial body
b. Meckel's cartilage
c. Laryngeal cartilage
d. Stapes

26. Which of the following is not derived from 3rd branchial arch?
a. Lesser cornu of hyoid
b. Greater cornu of hyoid
c. Stylopharyngeus
d. All of the above

27. Retromolar trigone is related to which of the following anatomical landmark?
a. Posterior part of mandible
b. Ascending ramus of mandible
c. Submandibular area
d. Digastric muscle

Ans. 17. **d.** Junction... 18. **c.** Group A beta haemol... 19. **a.** Ca glottis 20. **a.** Peritonsillar...
21. **b.** Erythroplakia 22. **d.** Auriculotemporal 23. **b.** Olfactory... 24. **c.** VII
25. **a.** Ultimobranchial... 26. **a.** Lesser cornu of hyoid 27. **b.** Ascending ramus of mandible

IMAGE-BASED QUESTIONS

1. Spot diagnosis:

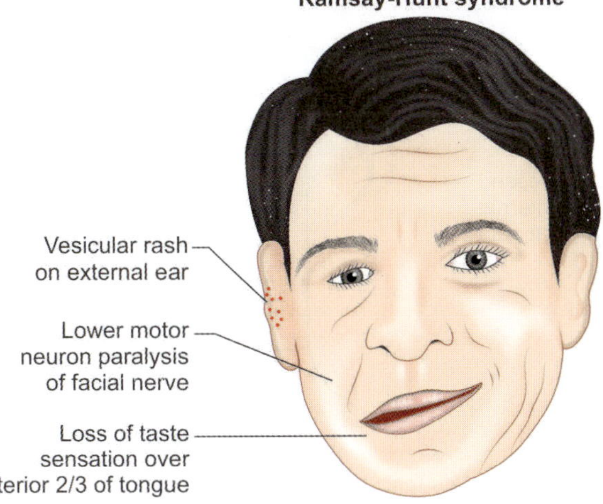

a. Alport's syndrome
b. Melkersson-Rosenthal syndrome
c. Ramsay-Hunt syndrome
d. Bell's palsy

Ramsay Hunt syndrome is a Herpes zoster virus infection involving geniculate ganglion of the facial nerve. Vesicular eruptions are seen in concha, posteromedial surface of pinna and soft palate.

2. Which sided tympanic membrane?

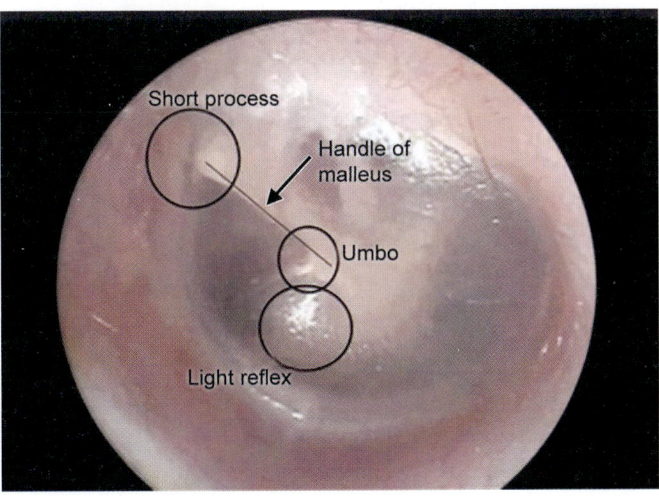

a. Left
b. Right
c. Variable
d. None of the above

A bright cone of light radiating from the tip of malleus to the periphery in the anteroinferior quadrant is usually seen during otoscopy. So this tympanic membrane is of left side.

3. Spot diagnosis:

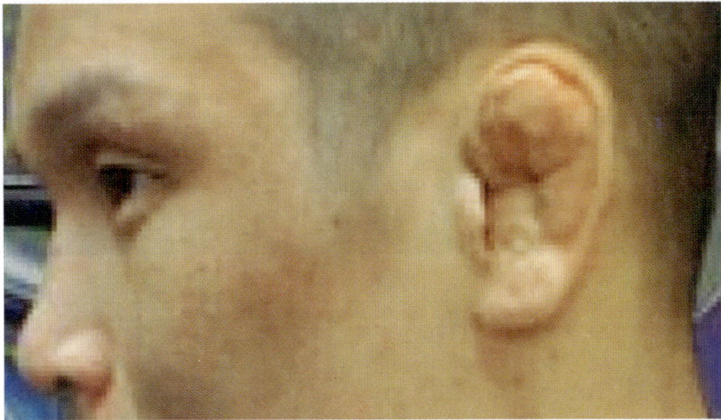

a. Carcinoma pinna
b. Cauliflower ear
c. Ear polyp
d. Microtia

Cauliflower ear is an auricular deformity seen when extravasated blood (hematoma) clots and gets organized.

4. Spot diagnosis:

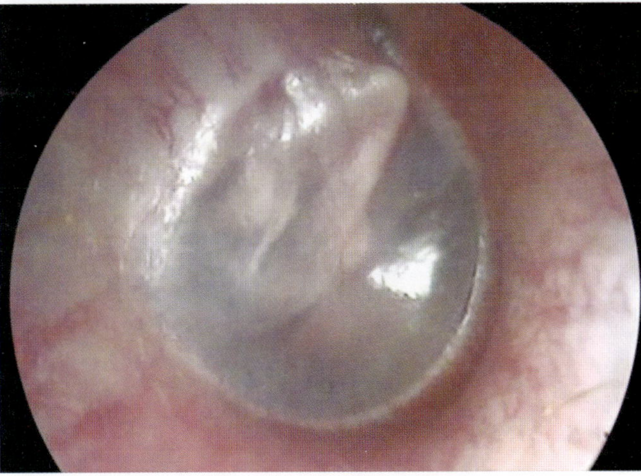

a. ASOM
b. CSOM
c. Otitis media with effusion
d. Tubercular OM

Otoscopic examination of OME shows dark, fluid filled middle ear which obscures the vision of long process of incus.

5. Management of which condition?

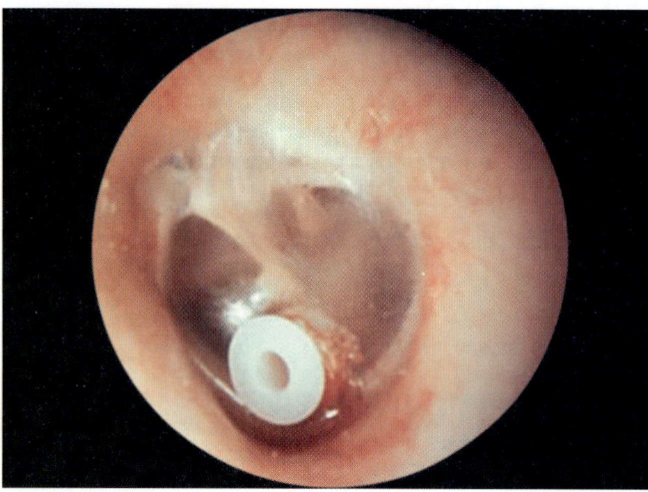

a. ASOM
b. CSOM
c. OME
d. Tubercular OM

Most widely used treatment option for OME when present for more than 3 months with associated hearing loss of more than 30 dB in better ear is tympanostomy tube (Grommet).

6. Spot diagnosis:

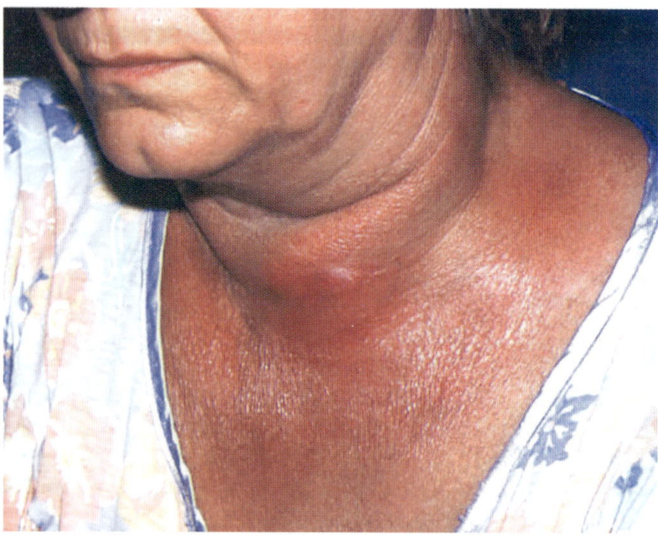

a. Citelli's abscess
b. Luc's abscess
c. Bezold's abscess
d. Zygomatic abscess

Bezold's abscess may lie deep to sternocleidomastoid muscle and pushing it laterally or it may lie in the digastric triangle.

7. Following figure illustrates:

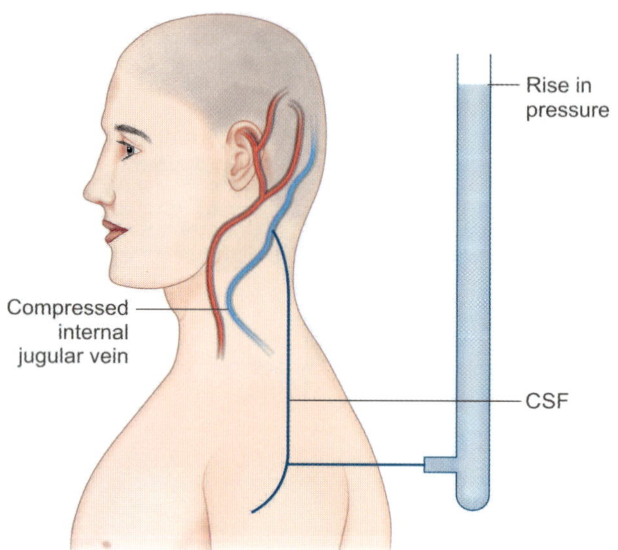

a. Fistula's test
b. Hennebert's sign
c. Tullio's phenomenon
d. Tobey-Ayer test

Tobey-Ayer test is done for lateral sinus thrombosis.

8. Spot diagnosis:

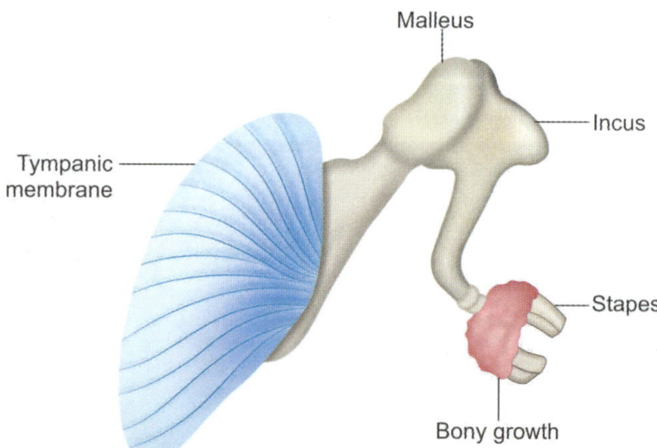

a. Van der Hoeve syndrome
b. Otospongiosis
c. Osteosclerosis
d. Carcinoma of stapes

Otosclerosis is a primary disease of the endochondral bony labyrinth. In this hard endochondral bone, some islands of cartilage remain unossified. This cartilage rests due to certain nonspecific factors, are activated to form new spongy bone (otospongiosis). The otosclerotic focus usually involves the stapes region and results in stapes fixation and conductive deafness.

9. Audiogram of which condition?

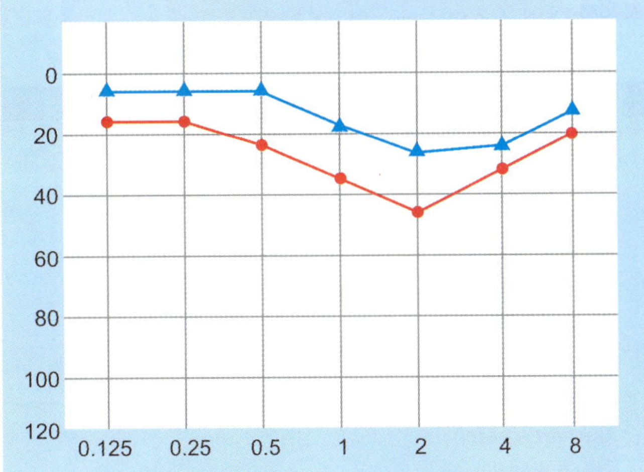

a. Meniere's disease
b. Otosclerosis
c. CSOM
d. Acoustic neuroma

Carhart's notch is a dip in bone conduction curve, which is maximum (15 dB) at 2,000 Hz.

10. Which investigation?

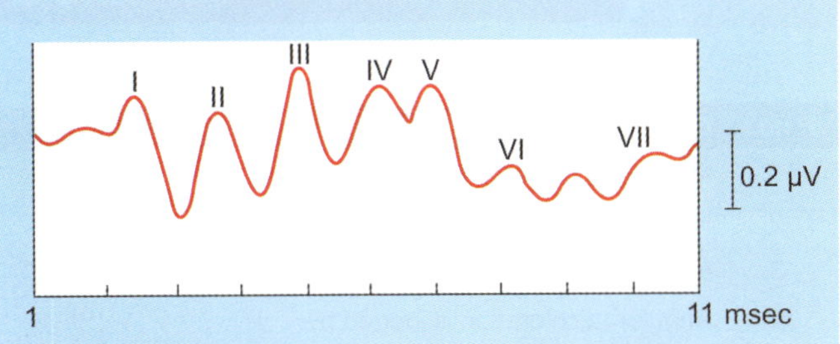

a. Rinne test
b. Pure tone audiometry
c. BERA
d. Electrocochleography

Brainstem evoked response audiometry is a non-invasive technique that finds the integrity of central auditory pathways, which consists of 8th nerve, pons, midbrain, and forebrain. BERA measures hearing in the range of 1,000-4,000 Hz. Seven waves are generated in the first 10 milliseconds.

MCQ POINTS

S. no.	Question statements	Answers
1.	MC cause of malignant otitis externa	***Pseudomonas aeruginosa***
2.	Hyperacusis is prevented by	***Stapedius***
3.	Eustachian tube develops from	***1st pharyngeal pouch***
4.	Angular acceleration is judged by	***Semicircular canals***
5.	Surgical procedure for serous otitis media	***Myringotomy with grommet tube insertion***
6.	MC complication of CSOM	***Mastoiditis***
7.	Bezolds abscess lies in relation to … muscle	***Sternocleidomastoid***
8.	Paracusis willisi is a feature of	***Otosclerosis***
9.	Audiometric finding of otosclerosis	***Carhart's notch***
10.	Triad of deafness, vertigo and tinnitus is suggestive of	***Meniere's disease***
11.	MC involves structure in acoustic neuroma	***Superior vestibular nerve***
12.	Sinus opening in sphenoethmoid recess	***Sphenoid sinus***
13.	Mikulicz cells are seen in	***Rhinoscleroma***
14.	Apple jelly nodules on nasal septum is seen in	***Lupus vulgaris***
15.	CSF rhinorrhoea is seen in fracture of	***Cribriform plate of ethmoid***
16.	MC site of epistaxis	***Little's area***
17.	MC cause of epistaxis in children	***Trauma***
18.	MC site of nasopharyngeal carcinoma	***Fossa of Rosenmuller***
19.	MC causative agent of quinsy	***Streptococcus pneumonia***
20.	Abductor of vocal cord	***Posterior cricoarytenoid***
21.	Epithelial lining of true vocal cords	***Stratified squamous non-keratinised***
22.	Nerve supply of cricothyroid	***External laryngeal nerve***
23.	MC cause of stridor of newborn	***Laryngomalacia***
24.	Management of laryngomalacia	***Observation***
25.	Virus causing nasopharyngeal carcinoma	***EBV***

CHAPTER 2

OPHTHALMOLOGY

KEY POINTS

Normal Values

- Refractory index of emmetropic eye = 60 D
- Normal intraocular pressure is 10-22 mm Hg

Pupil

- *Adie's pupil:* Due to degeneration of ciliary ganglion. Dilated pupil. Tonic reaction to light and accommodation. Associated with hyporeflexia (Holmes-Adie pupil)
- *Marcus-Gunn pupil:* Normal sized pupil. Relative afferent pupillary defect. Cause optic nerve/retinal disease.

Organisms Penetrating Intact Cornea

- *Neisseria gonorrhoea*
- *N. meningitidis*
- *Corynebacterium diphtheria*
- *Acanthamoeba*
- *Listeria monocytogenes*

Layers of Cornea

- Epithelium: Stratified squamous epithelium
- Bowman's membrane: Condensed collagen fibrils
- Stroma/substantia propia: Collagen fibrils
- Descemet's membrane/posterior elastic lamina
- Endothelium: Single layer

Causes of Neurotrophic Keratopathy

- Herpes zoster
- Herpes simplex
- Fifth nerve damage
- Diabetes
- Leprosy

Avascular Ocular Structures

- Vitreous
- Cornea
- Lens

Direct ophthalmoscopy	Indirect ophthalmoscopy
Erect	Inverted
Virtual	Real
15 times magnification	5 times magnification
Visualize slightly beyond equator	Can visualize up to ora serrata
Not useful in hazy media	Helpful (illumination is bright)
Stereopsis absent	Present
Distance of 15 mm from eye	At an arm's length's distance

Color Blindness

- *Protanopia:* Defective red color perception
- *Deuteranopia:* Defective green color perception
- Tritanopia: Defective blue color perception

Hirschberg Test (Used to Roughly Estimate the Angle of Deviation in Strabismus)

- *Edge of pupil:* 15 degree
- *Mid cornea:* 30 degree
- *Corneal margin:* 45 degree
- *Sclera:* 60 degree
- *1 mm from papillary center:* 7 degree
- *Nasal limbus:* 35 degree

The Plan followed in the Management of Squint (in Order)

- Refraction
- Orthoptic exercise
- Operative correction
- Prism for remaining error after operation

Conditions and Affected Glands

- *Chalazion:* Chronic inflammation of meibomian gland
- *Hordeolum externum:* Suppurative inflammation of glands of Zeiss

- *Hordeolum internum:* Suppurative inflammation of meibomian glands

Laws of Ocular Motility

- *Herring's law:* Yoke antagonist muscles and yoke agonist muscles receive equal innervation
- *Sherrington's law of reciprocal innervation:* Increased innervation of contacting agonist muscle is accompanied by simultaneous decreased innervation of its antagonist.

Jaw Winking of Marcus Gunn

- Due to aberrant regeneration of nerve fibers.
- Spasm of one Levator palpebrae occurs on movement of jaw
- Seen in congenital Ptosis.

Pre-Requisites for LASIK (Laser Assisted in Situ Keratomileusis)

- Age should be more than 21 years
- Stable refractory error
- Corneal thinning disorder should be ruled out
- It can correct myopia of range –6 to 30 diopters.

Acanthamoeba Infection

- Contact lens wearers who use distilled water and salt tablets instead of commercial saline solution
- Corneal scrapings are stained with calcofluor white dye/potassium hydroxide mount/lactophenol cotton blue
- Treated with polyhexamethylene biguanide or chlorhexidine with propamidine

Staphyloma

- *Anterior:* Ectasia of pseudocornea
- *Intercalary:* Localized bulge in limbal area lined by iris root
- *Ciliary:* 2–3 mm away from limbus, lined by ciliary body
- *Equatorial:* Choroidal incarceration at the equator
- *Posterior:* Lined by choroids behind the equator

Conditions Affecting Conjunctiva

- *Ophthalmia nodosa/caterpillar hair conjunctivitis:*
  - Granulomatous inflammation of conjunctiva,
  - Leading to formation of nodule on the bulbar conjunctiva in response to irritation caused by the retained hair of caterpillar
- *Pinguecula:* Yellowish white patch on the bulbar conjunctiva near the limbus
- *Pterygium:* Folds of conjunctiva encroaching upon the cornea.

Vernal Keratoconjunctivitis/Spring Catarrh

- Recurrent bilateral external ocular inflammation
- *Seasonal:* Summer
- *Cobblestone/pavement stone:* Hard, flat topped papillae in upper tarsal conjunctiva and
- *Tranta's spots:* Discrete whitish raised dots along the limbus.

Trachoma

- Caused by *Chlamydia trachomatis* serotypes A, Ba, and C, D and K
- The organism produces:
  - Intracytoplasmic inclusion bodies called H.P. bodies (Halberstaedter Prowazek bodies)
  - Arlt's line—linear scars present in sulcus subtarsalis
  - Herbert follicles—typical follicles present in the limbal area
  - Herbert pits—circular pitted scars left after healing of Herbert follicles

Diagnostic Criteria for Trachoma (at Least 2 of Following)

- Follicles on upper tarsal conjunctiva
- Limbal follicles or Herbert's pits
- Typical conjunctival scarring
- Vascular pannus most marked in the superior limbus

WHO Classification (1987): Meant to be used by Field Workers

- *TF (trachomatous inflammation follicular):* > 5 follicles
- (> 0.5 mm diameter) on upper tarsal conjunctiva
- *TI (Trachomatous Inflammation Intense):* Inflammation and papillary hypertrophy obscuring > ½ of tarsal vessels
- *TT (Trachomatous Trichiasis):* At least 1 trichiatic cilia rubbing on the globe or evidence of its recent removal
- *TS (Trachomatour Scarring):* Obvious trachomatous scarring of upper tarsal conjunctiva
- *CO (Corneal Opacity):* Trachomatous corneal opacity at least a part of which extends over the pupil

MacCallan's Classification of Trachoma Based on Conjunctival Characteristics

- Stage 1: Incipient trachoma; immature follicles on superior palpebral conjunctiva
- Stage 2: Established trachoma; mature follicles on superior palpebral conjunctiva
- Stage 3: Cicatrizing trachoma; follicles, scales, scarring on superior Tarsus
- Stage 4: Healed trachoma; no follicles, extensive conjunctival Scarring

Sequelae of Trachoma

- Distortion of lids
- Entropion
- Trichiasis
- Ectropion (hypertrophy of conjunctiva)
- Herbert's pits
- Ptosis (tylosis and infiltration of LPS)
- Madarosis
- Posterior symblepharon
- Parenchymatous xerosis
- Defective lid closure, lid deformity and deficient tear film, corneal damage. Cicatrization involving lacrimal drainage and dacryolith formation, epiphora, glaucoma (perilimbal fibrosis and infiltration of the outflow channels)
- *Secondary infection:* Haemphilus aegyptius (commonest)

Causes of Cloudy Cornea at Birth

- Glaucoma
- Trauma
- Intrauterine infections
- Mucopolysaccharidoses
- Mucolipidosis

Order of Less Visual Field in Glaucoma

- *First:* Isopter contraction
- *Second:* Baring of blind spot
- *Third:* Wing shaped paracentral scotoma (first clinically significant)
- *Second last:* Loss of temporal island
- *Last:* Macular fires lost

Epidemic Dropsy Glaucoma/Bengal Glaucoma

- Characterized by diarrhea, edema legs, myocarditis
- Visual field changes resemble those of chronic simple glaucoma

Sudden Painful Loss of Vision

- Acute congestive glaucoma
- Acute iridocyclitis
- Injuries

Causes of Tunnel Vision

- Glaucoma
- Retinitis pigmentosa
- High myopia
- High powered glasses
- CRAO with sparing of cilioretinal artery
- Luetic chorioretinitis

Sudden Painless Loss of Vision

- Central retinal artery occlusion
- Vitreous hemorrhage
- Retinal detachment
- Central retinal vein occlusion
- Central serous retinopathy
- Optic neuritis

Gradual Painless Loss of Vision

- Pterygium encroaching on papillary area
- Corneal degeneration
- Corneal dystrophies
- Senile cataract
- Optic atrophy
- Diabetic retinopathy
- Refractive errors

Gradual Painful Loss of Vision

- Chronic iridocyclitis
- Corneal ulceration
- Chronic simple glaucoma

Transient Loss of Vision/Amaurosis Fugax

- Migraine
- Carotid artery disease
- Raynaud's disease

Ectopia Lentis

- *Marfan's syndrome:* Most common cause of inheritable EL; bilateral upward and temporal displacement
- *Homocystinuria:* Second most common cause; downward nasal displacement
- *Weil-Marchesani syndrome:* Forward displacement

Other Conditions Causing Ectopia Lentis

- Sulfite oxidase deficiency
- Hyperlysinemia
- Ehlers-Danlos syndrome
- Refsum's disease
- Sturge-Weber syndrome
- Pierre Robin syndrome

Laser and Uses

- *ND-YAG:* After cataract
- *Excimer laser:* LASIK, keratotomy
- *Frequency doubled ND-YAG, Argon-green, diode, krypton:* Retinal photocoagulation

Special Types of Cataract

- *Christmas tree:* Myotonic dystrophy
- *Sunflower:* Wilson's disease
- *Rosette:* Concussion trauma
- *Oil drop:* Galactosemia
- *Snowflake/snowstorm:* Diabetes mellitus
- *Polychromatic luster:* Complicated cataract
- *Blue dot:* Cortical developmental cataract
- *Glassblower's:* Infrared radiation
- *Anterior subcapsular:* Anticholinesterase
- *Posterior subcapsular:* Radiation/steroids
- *Shield cataract:* Atopic dermatitis
- *Spoke like cataract:* Mannosidoses
- *Propeller cataract:* Fabry's disease

Stages of Maturation of Cortical Senile Cataract

- Stage of lamellar separation by fluid
- Stage of incipient cataract
- Immature senile cataract
- Mature senile cataract
- Hypermature senile cataract

Second Sight

- In nuclear cataract, refractive of lens increases so the light rays become more convergent and patient becomes more myopic. So, his near vision improves and presbyopia is corrected.

Foster Kennedy Syndrome

- Tumor of anterior cranial fossa
- Ipsilateral papilledema
- Contralateral optic atrophy

Iridocyclitis

- *Keratic precipitates:* Proteinaceous cellular deposits at the back of cornea
  - Mutton fat KP—occur in granulomatous iridocyclitis, composed of epithelioid cells and macrophages. Large, thick and fluffy
  - Granular KP—small and medium, of nongranulomatous origin, composed of lymphocytes
  - Red KP—along with lymphocytes, erythrocytes also take part in composition, seen in hemorrhagic uveitis
  - Old KP—healed uveitis; shrunken, lightly pigmented and crenated

Retinoblastoma Treatment

- *Small tumors:* Photocoagulation; transpupillary thermotherapy with laser or cryotherapy
- *Medium tumors:* Brachytherapy; external beam radiotherapy with cobalt chemotherapy
- *Large tumors:* Enucleation; chemoreduction
- Enucleation is most widely practiced modality of treatment in unilateral sporadic disease and in the more affected eye in bilateral disease

Causes of Leukocoria

- Retinoblastoma
- Congenital cataract
- Coloboma choroid
- Retinopathy of prematurity
- Persistent hyperplastic primary vitreous
- Toxocara endophthalmitis
- Coat's disease

Fundus

- *Candle wax spots:* Retinopathy of sarcoidosis
- *Salt and pepper fundus:* Congenital syphilis
- *Watered silk appearance of fundus:* Hypermetropia

Refsum's Syndrome

- Retinitis pigmentosa
- Peripheral neuropathy
- Cerebellar ataxia

Grading of Hypertensive Retinopathy

- *Grade 1:* Mild generalized arteriolar attenuation.
- *Grade 2:* Grading of hypertensive retinopathy—marked generalized narrowing and focal attenuation of arterioles, with deflection of veins at the arteriovenous junction
- *Grade 3:* Grade 2 plus copper wiring of arterioles, banking of veins, distal to A-V crossing. Flame shaped hemorrhages, cotton wool spots and hard exudates
- *Grade 4:* Grade 3 plus silver wiring of arterioles and papilledema

Signs of Hypertensive Retinopathy

- *Salu's sign:* Arteriovenous nipping
- *Bonnet's sign:* Dilated vein distal to A-V crossing
- *Gunn's sign:* Tapering of vein on either side of crossing, right angle deflection of vein
- *Elschnig's spots:* Ischemic Choroidal infarcts

Retinal Changes in Sickle Cell

- Sea fan neovascularisation
- Black sun bursts
- Salmon patch hemorrhage
- Angioid streaks

Causes of Cherry Red Spot in Macula are:

- CRAO
- Tay-sachs disease
- Niemann-Pick disease
- Gaucher's disease
- Sandhoff's disease
- Sialidosis

Hyperthyroidism

- Lid lag (Von Graefe's sign),
- Poor convergence (Mobius sign)
- External ophthalmoplegia
- Large extraocular muscles

Causes of Night Blindness

- Vitamin A deficiency
- Retinitis pigmentosa
- Myopia
- Peripheral cortical cataract
- Oguchi disease
- Goldmann-Favre disease
- Central nuclear cataract
- Central corneal opacities
- Central vitreous opacities

Blindness

- *Economic blindness:* Vision less than 6/60
- *Social blindness:* Inability to move around. Vision less than 3/60

Drugs

- *Tropicamide:* Shortest and quickest acting
- *Phenylephrine:* Only mydriatic
- *Cyclopentolate:* Only cycloplegic

MCQs WITH SHORT EXPLANATIONS

OPHTHALMOLOGY ANATOMY

1. **Which of the following is a synergistic muscle of right inferior oblique?**
   a. Right superior oblique b. Left superior rectus
   c. Left inferior rectus d. Right superior rectus

   Synergists muscle of inferior oblique are superior rectus and lateral rectus whereas antagonists are superior oblique and inferior rectus

2. **Which of the following muscle would be paralysed in a patient who is not able to look downward?**
   a. Superior oblique b. Inferior oblique
   c. Superior rectus d. Lateral rectus

   Patient will not be able to look downward if SO/ IR is paralyzed [depression of eye/ downward looking is an action of inferior rectus (primary action) and superior oblique (secondary action)]

3. **The corneal transparency is maintained by:**
   a. Keratocytes b. Bowman's membrane
   c. Descemet's membrane d. Endothelium

   The corneal endothelium are specialized, flattened, mitochondria-rich cells that line the posterior surface of the cornea and face the anterior chamber of the eye. The corneal endothelium governs fluid and solute transport across the posterior surface of the cornea and actively maintains the cornea in the slightly dehydrated state that is required for optical transparency.

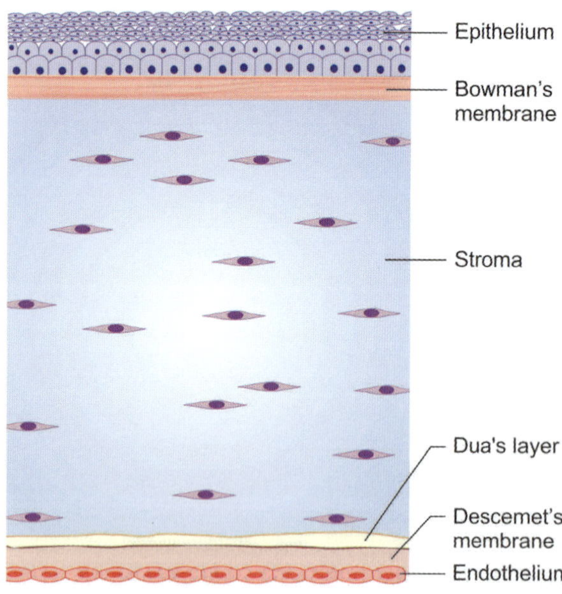

Microscopic structure of the cornea.

4. **Cornea derives its nutrition chiefly from:**
   a. Aqueous humor
   b. Mucous layer
   c. Corneal vessels
   d. Perilimbal vessels

   Because transparency is of prime importance the cornea does not have blood vessels; it receives nutrients via diffusion from the tear fluid through the outside surface and the aqueous humor through the inside surface, and also from neurotrophins supplied by nerve fibers that innervate it.

5. **Depth of the anterior chamber of the eye is:**
   a. 2–3 mm
   b. 3–4 mm
   c. 4–5 mm
   d. 6–8 mm

   The anterior chamber is about 2.5 mm deep in the centre in normal adults.

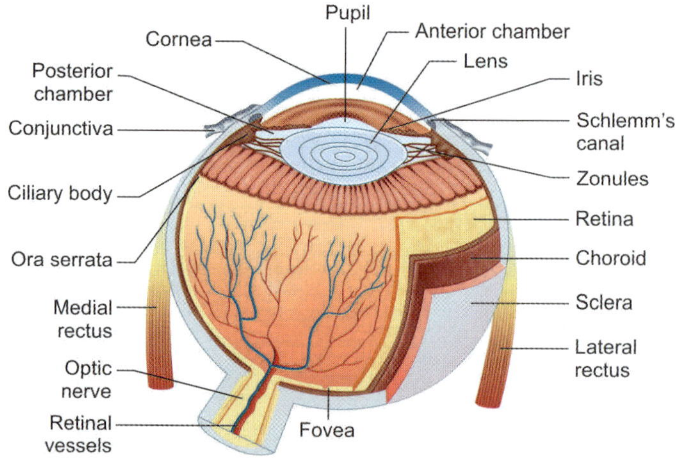

Gross anatomy of the eyeball

6. **Most sensitive part of the retina is:**
   a. Fovea centralis
   b. Macula lutea
   c. Blind spot
   d. Temporal retina

   The center of the fovea is the foveola—about 0.2 mm in diameter—or central pit where only cone photoreceptors are present and there are virtually no rods. The central fovea consists of very compact cones, thinner and more rod-like in appearance than cones elsewhere. These cones are very densely packed (in a hexagonal pattern).

Ans. 1. **d.** Right superior... 2. **a.** Superior oblique 3. **d.** Endothelium 4. **a.** Aqueous humor
5. **a.** 2–3 mm 6. **a.** Fovea centralis

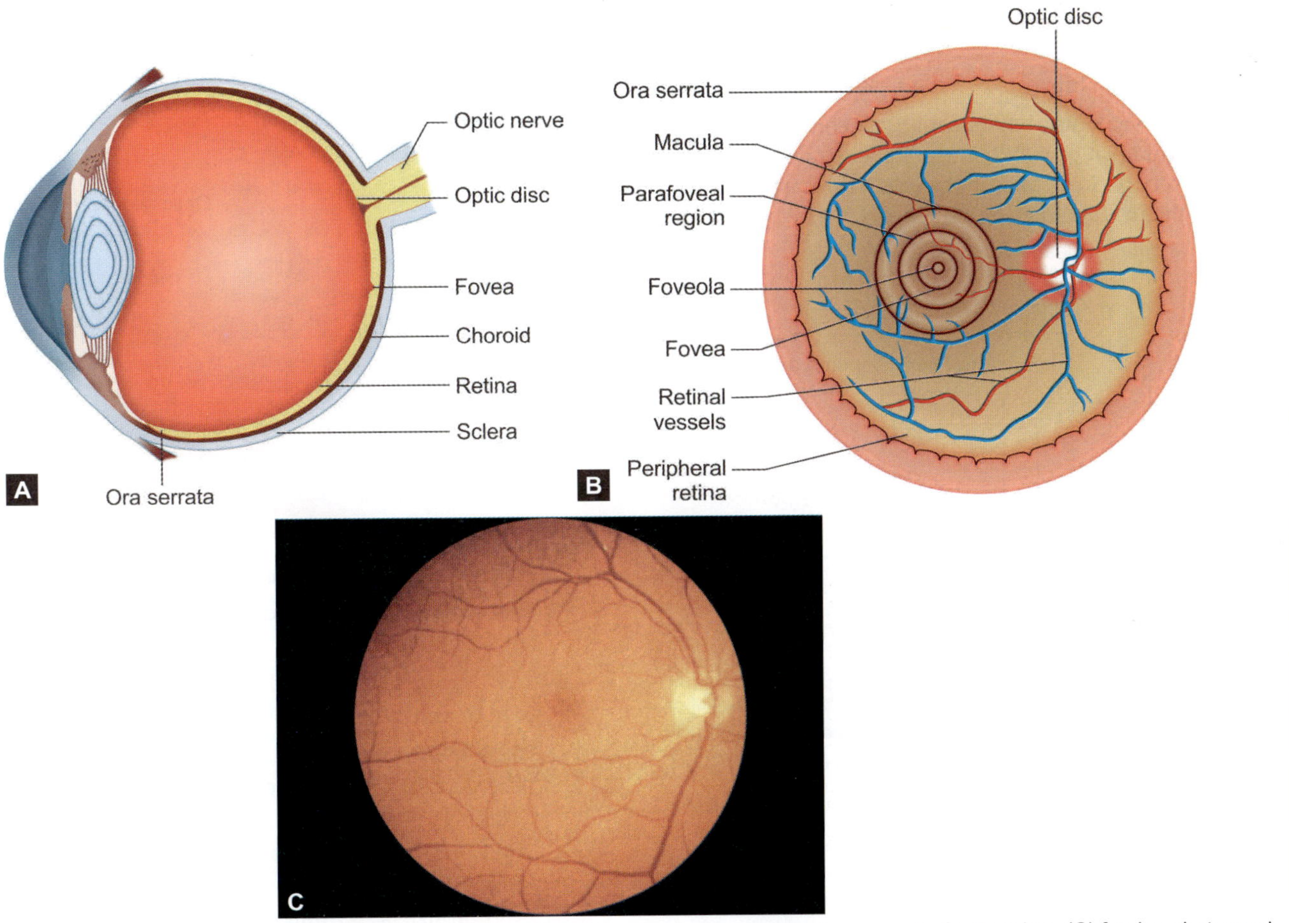

Gross anatomy of the retina: (A) parts of retina in horizontal section at the level of fovea, (B) diagrammatic fundus view, (C) fundus photograph

7. The conversion of CO_2 and H_2O into carbonic acid during the formation of aqueous humor is catalyzed by which one of the following enzymes:

a. Carboxylase
b. Carbamylase
c. Carbonic anhydrase
d. Carbonic deoxygenase

The formation of aqueous humor by the ciliary body is a complex process. Active transport of solutes by the ciliary process epithelium is an energy-dependent mechanism that selectively transports substances against an electrochemical gradient across the cell membranes. Water passively follows the active solute transport. In addition to these active transport processes, ultrafiltration contributes to the formation of aqueous humor. The ciliary epithelium contains enzyme systems that function in the production of aqueous humor. The enzymes sodium-potassium-activated adenosine triphosphatase [(Na+:K+)ATPase] and carbonic anhydrase participate in the active transport across this epithelium.

Flowchart depicting drainage of aqueous humor.

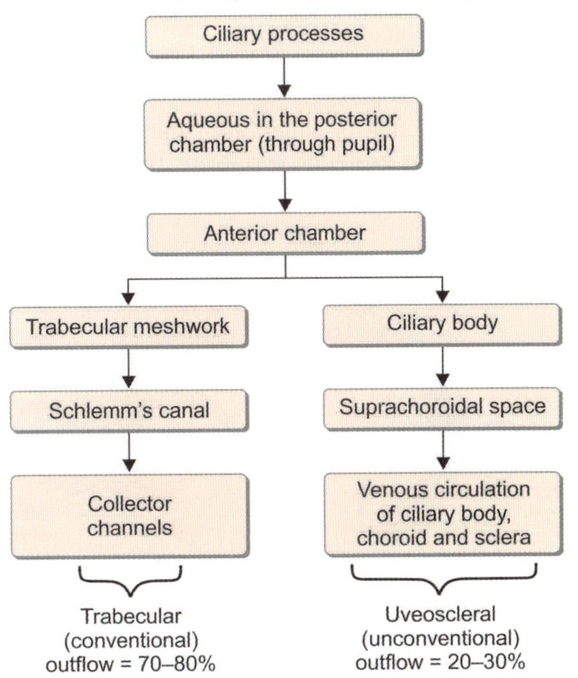

Ans. 7. **c.** Carbonic anhydrase

8. Maximum cones are seen in:

a. Limbus b. Fovea centralis
c. Macula lutea d. Blind spot

The **fovea centralis** (the term *fovea* comes from the Latin, meaning *pit* or *pitfall*) is a small, central pit composed of closely packed cones in the eye. It is located in the center of the macula lutea of the retina.

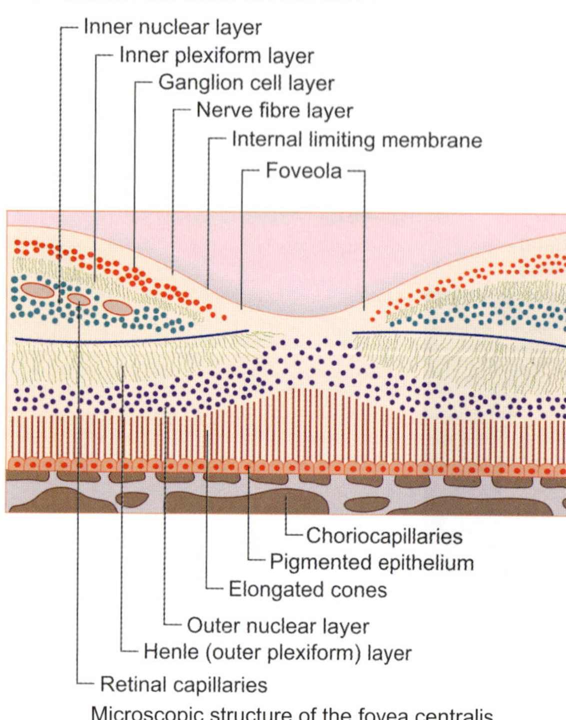

Microscopic structure of the fovea centralis

9. Wieger's ligament is seen at:

a. Junction of cornea and sclera
b. Suspension of ciliary body
c. Attachment of vitreous to posterior lens
d. Posterior chamber

The circular line of adhesion of the anterior vitreous cortex to the posterior surface of the lens is termed **Wieger's ligament** and has a diameter of about 8 mm.

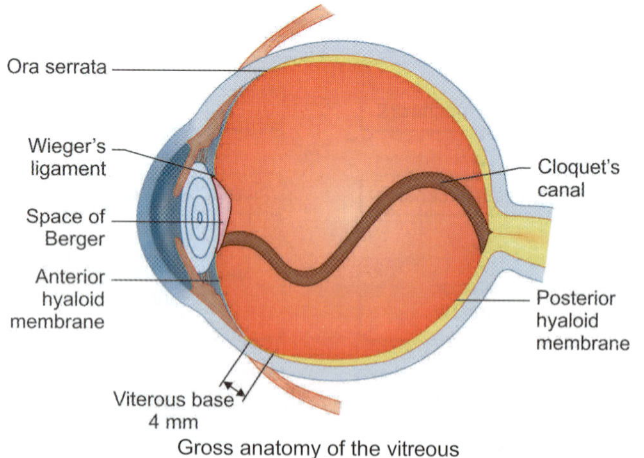

Gross anatomy of the vitreous

10. Superior oblique muscle is supplied by:

a. Third cranial nerve
b. Fourth cranial nerve
c. Fifth cranial nerve
d. Sixth cranial nerve

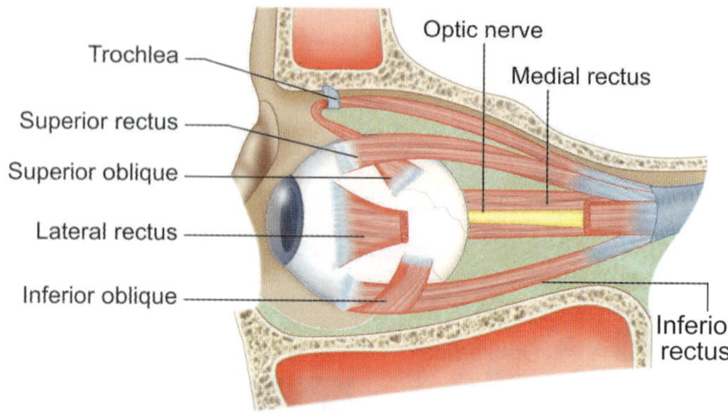

Extraocular muscles

Remember SO_4, LR6 and rest of the extraocular muscles by 3rd cranial nerve.

11. Axial length of eye ball is:

a. 16 mm b. 20 mm
c. 24 mm d. 28 mm

The vertical measure, generally less than the horizontal distance, is about 24 mm among adults, at birth about 16–17 millimetres (about 0.65 inch). The transverse size of a human adult eye is approximately 24.2 mm and the sagittal size is 23.7 mm with no significant difference between sexes and age groups.

12. Metabolically active layer of cornea is:

a. Endothelium b. Stroma
c. Descemet's membrane d. All of the above

Corneal endothelium is a simple squamous or low cuboidal monolayer, approx 5 μm thick, of mitochondria-rich cells. These cells are responsible for regulating fluid and solute transport between the aqueous and corneal stromal compartments. If the endothelium can no longer maintain a proper fluid balance, stromal swelling due to excess fluids and subsequent loss of transparency will occur and this may cause corneal edema and interference with the transparency of the cornea and thus impairing the image formed.

13. Corneal transparency is due to:

a. $Na^+ K^+$ pump
b. Normal IOT
c. Hypercellular stroma
d. Peculiar arrangement of lamella

Corneal Transparency is due to the following factors:

- Peculiar arrangement of corneal lamellae (Lattice Theory of Maurice)

Ans. 8. **b.** Fovea centralis 9. **c.** Attachment of vitreous... 10. **b.** Fourth cranial nerve 11. **c.** 24 mm
12. **a.** Endothelium 13. **d.** Peculiar arrangement of lamella

- Peculiar refractive index of corneal lamellae with variation less than 200 micrometers (Goldmann and Benedek theory)
- Avascularity of cornea
- Relative state of dehydration maintained by barrier effects of epithelium and endothelium and active bicarbonate pump of endothelium

14. Distance of macula from disc:

a. 1 mm
b. 2 mm
c. 3 mm
d. 4 mm

Optic disc is placed 3.4 mm nasal to the fovea.

15. The following structure is NOT derived from surface ectoderm:

a. Crystalline lens
b. Sclera
c. Corneal epithelium
d. Epithelium of lacrimal glands

Mesoderm contributes to the following ocular structures:

- Extraocular muscles
- Endothelial lining of blood vessels of the eye
- Blood vessels in sclera and choroid
- Sclera and choroid
- Vitreous
- Suspensory fibers
- Cornea: Bowman's membrane and stroma

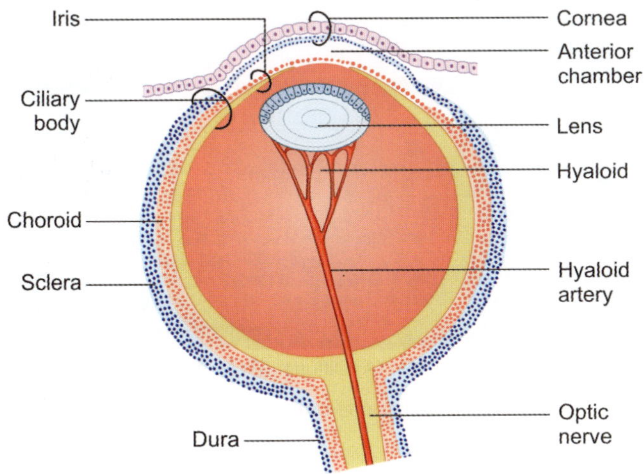

Derivation of various structures of the eyeball

16. Smooth muscles of the iris develop from:

a. Surface ectoderm
b. Mesoderm
c. Neural crest
d. Neural ectoderm

The stroma of the iris and the ciliary body develop from neural crest cells that migrate into the area. Within the stroma of the iris, the sphincter pupillae and dilator pupillae muscles develop from optic cup neuroectoderm. In contrast, the ciliary muscle, which is responsible for changing the shape of the lens, is derived from overlying mesenchyme.

17. Which of the following is known as dangerous zone of the eye:

a. Sclera
b. Retina
c. Optic nerve
d. Ciliary body

Owing to the extensive destruction which is apt to follow septic infection of the ciliary region, it has been termed the dangerous area of the eye.

18. No visual sensations are perceived on which part of the retina:

a. Optic disc
b. Ora serrata
c. Macula densa
d. Fovea

The **optic disc** or **optic nerve head** is the point of exit for ganglion cell axons leaving the eye. Because there are no rods or cones overlying the optic disc, it corresponds to a small **physiological blind spot** in each eye.

19. Blind spot of Mariotte is also known as:

a. Optic disc
b. Ora serrata
c. Macula
d. Fovea

The existence of a small blind region in the normal human eye was predicted in the seventeenth century by the French scientist Edmé **Mariotte**.

20. The eye in the newborn is:

a. Hypermetropic with regular astigmatism
b. Hypermetropic
c. Hypermetropic with irregular astigmatism
d. Myopia

Most normal infants when they are born have a hypermetropia of +2 to +3 dioptres. This is due to a variety of factors though the main reasons are a shorter eye and a forward-placed lens. As the child grows older, the length of the eyeball increases to normal and the hypermetropia usually goes away by the age of 5 years.

21. Kappa angle is the angle between the:

a. Pupillary and the visual axis
b. Visual and optical axis
c. Centre of eyeball rotation and line of fixation
d. None of the above

Ans. 14. **c.** 3 mm 15. **b.** Sclera 16. **b.** Mesoderm 17. **d.** Ciliary body
18. **a.** Optic disc 19. **a.** Optic disc 20. **b.** Hypermetropic
21. **a.** Pupillary and the visual axis

Angle kappa is the **angle** between the visual axis and the pupillary axis. It is clinically important to the refractive surgeon because patients, especially hyperopes, have a large **angle kappa** and the center of the pupil is no longer the point through which a fovea-centric ray of light passes.

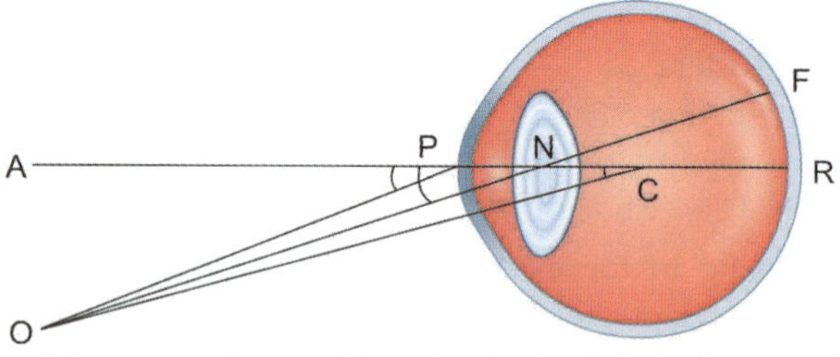

Axes of the eye: optic axis (AR); visual axis (OF); fixation axis (OC) and visual angles: angle alpha (ONA, between optical axis and visual axis at nodal point N); angle kappa (OPA, between optical axis and pupillary line–OP); angle gamma (OCA, between optical axis and fixation axis).

22. Alpha angle is the angle between:

a. Pupillary axis and optical axis
b. Visual axis and optical axis
c. Centre of eyeball rotation and line of fixation
d. None of the above

Angle alpha which is the **angle** formed by the intersection between the visual axis and optical axis. The optical axis is defined as a line passing through the nodal point that is normal to the surface of the cornea.

23. Refractive power of cornea is:

a. 15
b. 30
c. 45
d. 60

In humans, the refractive power of the cornea is approximately 45 dioptres (roughly 3/4th of the total refractive power of eye *i.e.* 60 dioptres). While the cornea contributes most of the eye's focusing power, its focus is fixed. The curvature of the lens, on the other hand, can be adjusted to "tune" the focus depending upon the object's distance.

24. Total diopteric power of eye is:

a. 23 D
b. 43 D
c. 15 D
d. 60 D

Total **dioptric power** is **+60** D, of which cornea contributes +43 D and the lens +17 D.

25. Sclera is thinnest at:

a. Equator
b. Posterior pole
c. Behind the insertion of recti
d. Limbus

Sclera is thicker in males than in females. Human sclera is thickest near the optic nerve, where it is approximately 1 mm in thickness and thinnest at the insertion of extra ocular muscles (0.3 mm). The tendon of the extra ocular muscles are of same thickness here at this point of insertion, so with merging of these tendons, the collective thickness of sclera reaches to 0.6 mm here. Sclera gradually thickens towards cornea and at limbus the thickness of sclera is 0.83 mm.

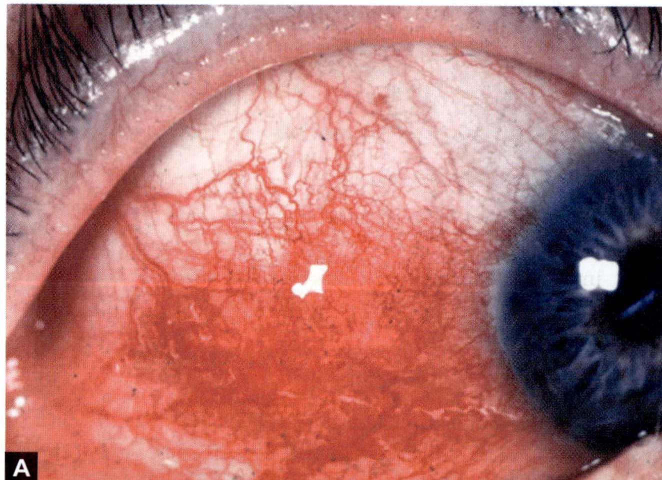

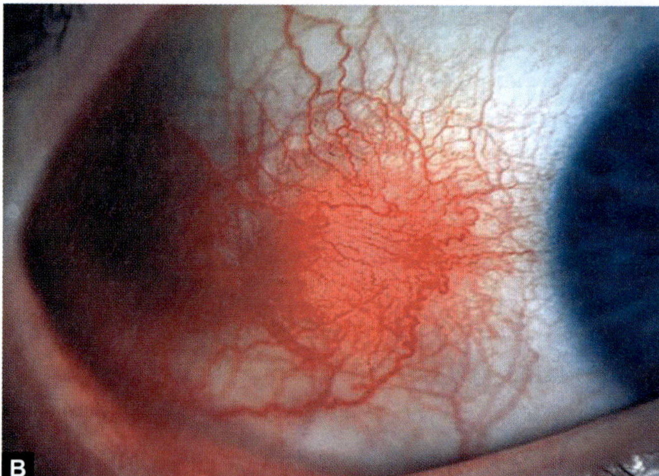

Episcleritis: (A) Diffuse; (B) Nodular.

26. Corneal endothelium is embryologically derived from:

a. Endoderm
b. Ectoderm
c. Mesoderm
d. Neural crest

The corneal endothelium is embryologically derived from the neural crest. The postnatal total endothelial cellularity of the cornea (approximately 300,000 cells per cornea) is achieved as early as the second trimester of gestation. Thereafter the endothelial cell density (but not the absolute number of cells) rapidly declines, as

Ans. **22. b.** Visual axis... **23. c.** 45 **24. d.** 60 D **25. c.** Behind the insertion... **26. d.** Neural crest

the fetal cornea grows in surface area, achieving a final adult density of approximately 2400–3200 cells/mm². The number of endothelial cells in the fully developed cornea decreases with age up until early adulthood, stabilizing around 50 years of age.

OPHTHALMOLOGY PROCEDURES

27. Purpose of doing Worth 4 dot test:

a. Cornea
b. Refractive errors
c. Intraocular pressure
d. Binocular vision

The **Worth Four Light Test**, also known as the **Worth's Four Dot test** or **W4LT**, is a clinical test mainly used for assessing a patient's degree of "binocular vision" and "binocular single vision". Binocular vision, involves an image being projected by each eye (simultaneously) into an area in space and being fused into a single image. The Worth's Four Light Test is also used in detection of suppression of either the right or left eye. Suppression occurs during binocular vision when the brain does not process the information received from either of the eyes. This is a common adaptation to strabismus, amblyopia and aniseikonia.

28. Use of Maddox rod:

a. Strabismus
b. Refractive error
c. Retinal hemorrhage
d. Color blindness

The **Maddox Rod Test** can be used to subjectively detect and measure a latent, manifest, horizontal or vertical strabismus for near and distance. The test is based on the principle of diplopic projection. Dissociation of the deviation is brought about by presenting a red line image to one eye and a white light to the other, while prisms are used to superimpose these and effectively measure the angle of deviation (horizontal and vertical).

29. Used in Schiotz tonometry:

a. 1–2% xylocaine
b. 2–4% xylocaine
c. 4–6% xylocaine
d. 6–8% xylocaine

For Schiotz **tonometry**, a drop of surface anaesthetic solution like **2-4% xylocaine** is enough. The patient is asked to lie down and look at his own thumb held above his face. It is important that patient keep both his eyes open. With the eyelid gently pulled apart, the tonometer with 5.5 gram

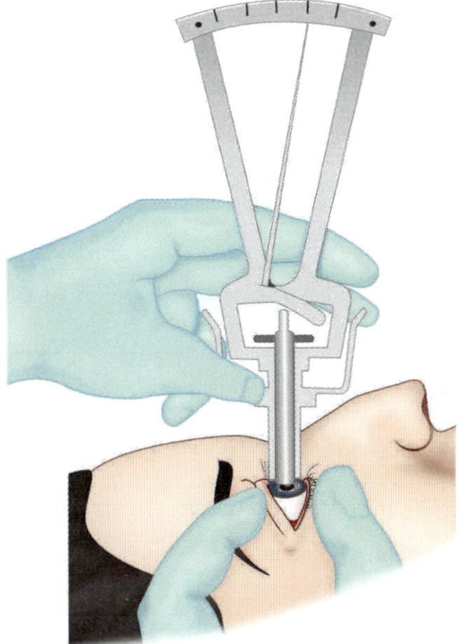

Technique of Schiotz tonometry.

weight is slowly brought down to rest on the center of cornea and held there by its own weight, without any pressure. The reading of the scale is noted.

30. Campimetry is used to measure:

a. Field of charting
b. Pattern of retina
c. Malignant melanoma
d. Squint

The **campimeter** is an instrument for examining the central visual field. Campimeters have been in clinical use since the mid-nineteenth century. Initially, examination of the visual field was concerned only with the outer limits, or 'perimeter' of the visual field, hence the term 'perimetry', which tends to be used interchangeably with 'campimetry'.

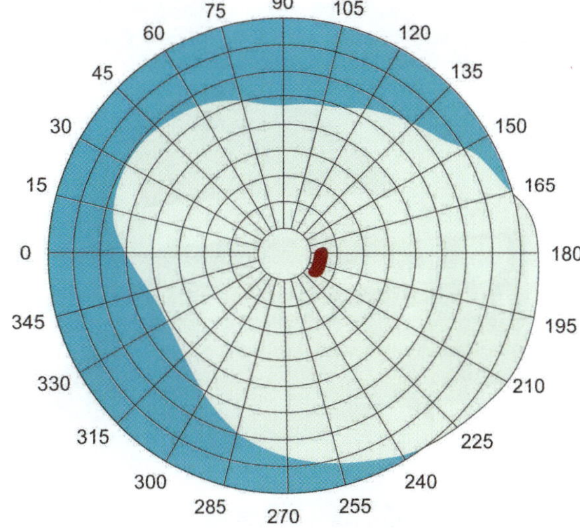

Extent of normal visual field.

Ans. 27. **d.** Binocular vision 28. **a.** Strabismus 29. **b.** 2–4% xylocaine 30. **a.** Field of charting

31. In direct ophthalmoscopy, image is magnified by:

a. 5 times
b. 10 times
c. 15 times
d. 20 times

Direct ophthalmoscopy one that produces an upright, or unreversed, image of approximately 15 times magnification.

Direct versus indirect ophthalmoscopy.

Sl. no.	Feature	Direct ophthalmoscopy	Indirect ophthalmoscopy
1.	Condensing lens	Not required	Required
2.	Examination distance	As close to patient's eye as possible	At an arm's length
3.	Image	Virtual,	Real,
		Erect	Inverted
4.	Magnification	About 15 times	2.5 times (with +20 D lens)
5.	Illumination	Not so bright; so not useful in hazy media	Bright; so, useful for hazy media
6.	Area of field in focus	About 2 disc diameter	About 8 disc diameter
7.	Stereopsis	Absent	Present
8.	Accessible fundus view	Slightly beyond equator	Up to ora serrata
9.	Examination through hazy media	Not possible	Possible

32. True about indirect gonioscopy are all EXCEPT:

a. Done under local anesthesia
b. A contact lens is inserted between the lids
c. Single mirror gonioscopes allows examination of 360 degrees of the angle
d. Better visualization of the anterior chamber angle

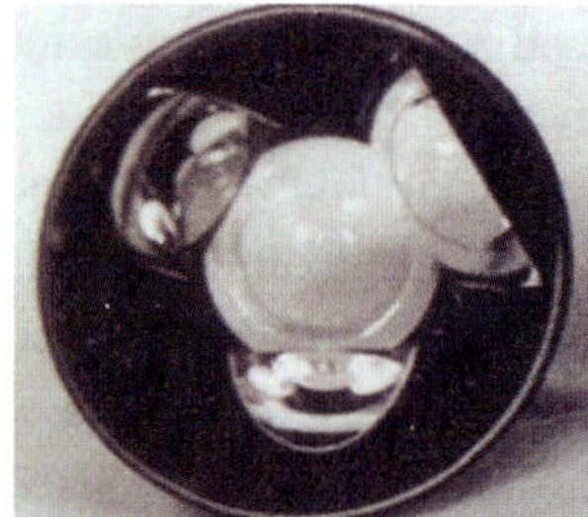
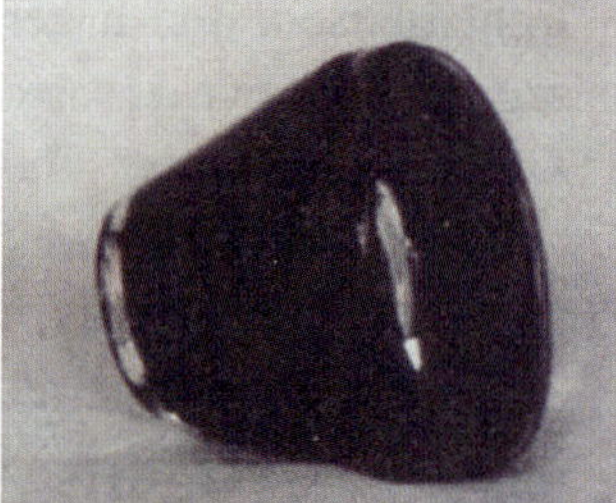
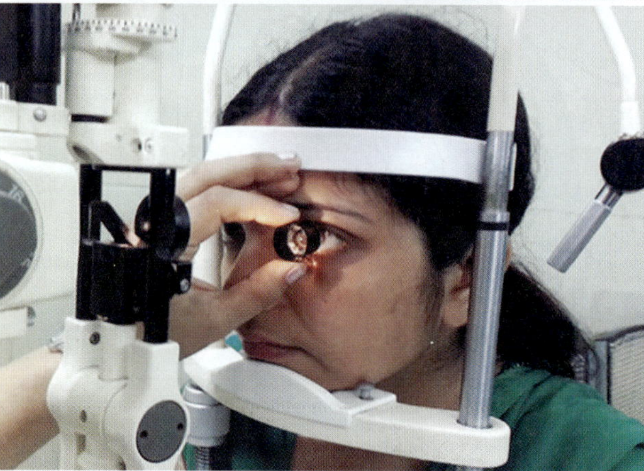

Goldmann goniolens (A) and technique of gonioscopy (B).

Indirect gonioscopy is more frequently used in the clinician's office. Indirect gonioscopy also eliminates the total internal reflection at the surface of the cornea. Light reflected from the chamber angle passes into the indirect gonioscopy lens and is reflected by a mirror within the lens. Indirect gonioscopy may be used with the patient in an upright position, with illumination and magnification provided by a slit lamp. A *goniolens,* which contains a mirror or mirrors, yields an inverted and slightly foreshortened image of the opposite angle. Although the image is inverted with an indirect goniolens, the right–left orientation of a horizontal mirror and the up–down orientation of a vertical mirror remain unchanged. The foreshortening, combined with the upright position of the patient, makes the angle appear a little shallower than it does with direct gonioscopy systems.

33. All are true regarding direct ophthalmoscopy EXCEPT:

a. Image is erect
b. Magnification is more than indirect ophthalmoscopy
c. Wide area of fundus with least magnification can be seen in hypermetropics
d. It has a large field of view

Binocular indirect ophthalmoscopy technique allows for viewing the fundus at a wider angle which allows examination of the peripheral retina and also a better view through lens opacities as well.

Ans. **31. c.** 15 times **32. c.** Single mirror gonioscopes allows examination of 360 degrees of the angle **33. d.** It has a large field of view

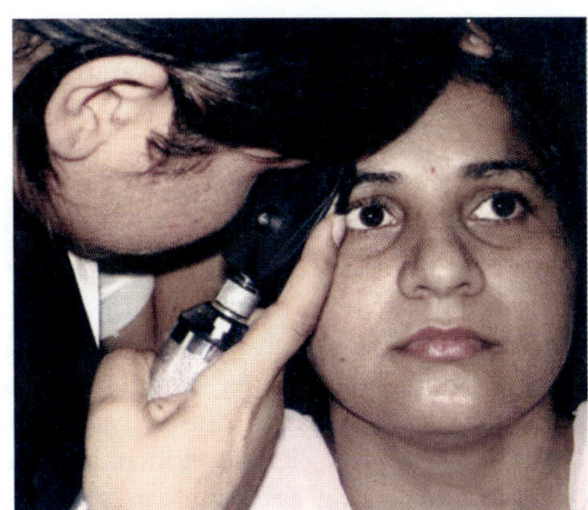

Technique of direct ophthalmoscopy.

34. Isochromatic charts are used for:

a. Contrast sensitivity
b. Testing color vision
c. Visual fields charting
d. Visual acuity testing

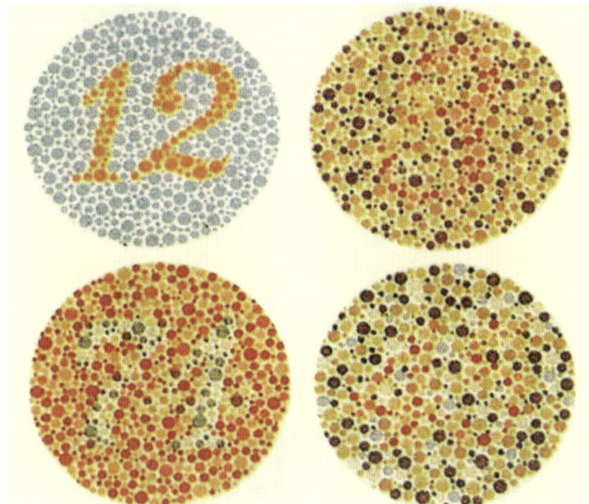

Ishihara's pseudoisochromatic chart.

The **Ishihara test** is a color perception test for red-green color deficiencies. It was named after its designer, Dr. Shinobu Ishihara, a professor at the University of Tokyo, who first published his tests in 1917.

The test consists of a number of colored plates, called **Ishihara plates**, each of which contains a circle of dots appearing randomized in color and size. Within the pattern are dots which form a number or shape clearly visible to those with normal color vision, and invisible, or difficult to see, to those with a red-green color vision defect, or the other way around. The full test consists of 38 plates, but the existence of a deficiency is usually clear after a few plates. There is also the smaller test consisting only 24 plates.

35. True regarding retinoscopy, are all of the following EXCEPT:

a. Helps in estimating the condition of the refraction
b. Usually performed at 1 m distance
c. Consists of a plane and a concave mirror
d. Hyperopes display an "against" movement

Static retinoscopy is a type of retinoscopy used in determining a patient's refractive error. It relies on Foucault's principle, which states that the examiner should simulate optical infinity to obtain the correct refractive power. Hence, a power corresponding to the working distance is subtracted from the gross retinoscopy value to give the patient's refractive condition, the working distance lens being one which has a focal length of the examiner's distance from the patient (e.g. +1.50 dioptre lens for a 67 cm working distance). Myopes display an "against" reflex, which means that the direction of movement of light observed from the retina is a different direction to that in which the light beam is swept. Hyperopes, on the other hand, display a "with" movement, which means that the direction of movement of light observed from the retina is the same as that in which the light beam is swept.

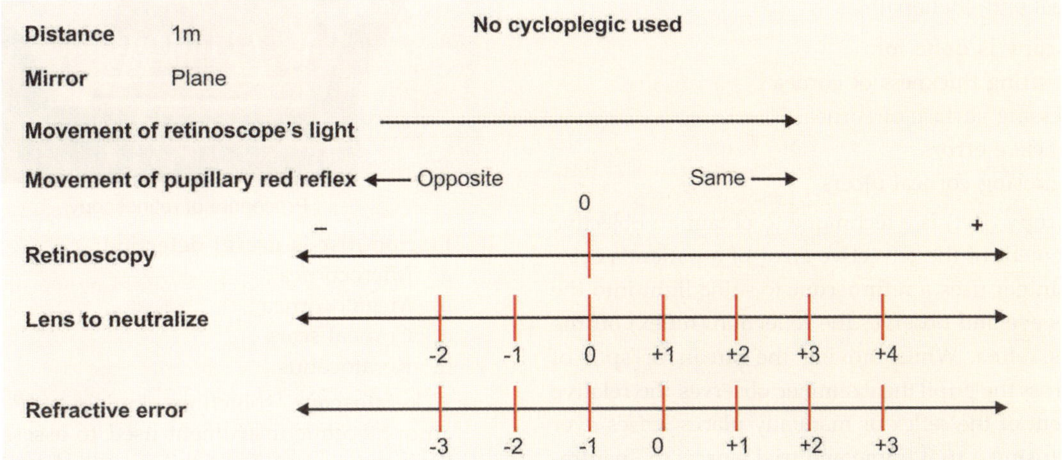

Diagrammatic depiction of the relation of movement of pupillary red reflex with the error of refraction.

Ans. **34. b.** Testing color vision **35. d.** Hyperopes display an "against" movement

36. Anomaloscope is used to detect is:

a. Squint
b. Retinopathy
c. Congenital glaucoma
d. Color blindness

An **anomaloscope** or **Nagel's anomaloscope** is an instrument used to test for color blindness. It is used to measure quantitative and qualitative anomalies in color perception. It can be used to determine whether a person is a tritanope, dichromat or achromatop. The apparatus was invented by the German ophthalmologist and physiologist Willibald A. Nagel (1870–1911) who named it "anomaloskop" in 1907.

37. Fincham test is used to differentiate:

a. Acute congestive glaucoma and chronic simple glaucoma
b. Chronic simple glaucoma and iridocyclitis
c. Acute congestive glaucoma and cataract
d. Simple glaucoma and cataract

The colored halos in glaucoma must be differentiated from those found in acute purulent conjunctivitis and early cataractous changes. In conjunctivit's, the halos can be eliminated by irrigating the discharge. The halos of glaucoma and immature cataract may be differentiated by Fincham's test in which a stenopaeic slit is passed across the pupil. During this test glaucomatous halo remains intact, while a halo due to cataract is broken up into segments. Emsley-Fincham stenopaeic-slit test demonstrating breaking up of halos due to immature cataract into different segments.

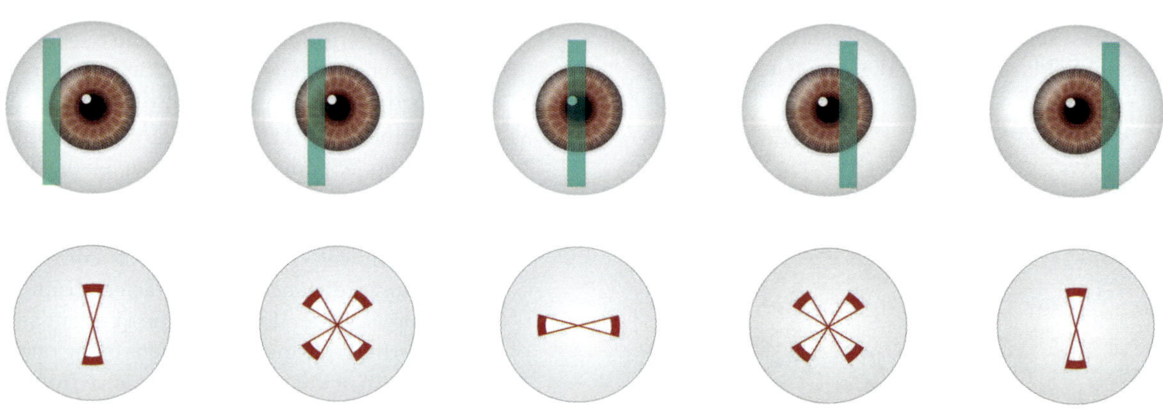

Emsley-Fincham stenopaeic-slit test demonstrating breaking up of halos due to immature cataract into different segments.

38. Used to examine corneal endothelium:

a. Pachymeter
b. Keratometer
c. Specular microscope
d. Tonometer

Specular microscopy is a noninvasive photographic technique that facilitates rapid and accurate diagnosis of corneal endotheliopathies

39. Retinoscopy is done for:

a. Measuring thickness of cornea
b. Assessing surface of cornea
c. Refractive errors
d. Diagnosing corneal ulcers

Retinoscopy (Ret) is a technique to obtain an objective measurement of the refractive error of a patient's eyes. The examiner uses a **retinoscope** to shine light into the patient's eye and observes the reflection (reflex) off the patient's retina. While moving the streak or spot of light across the pupil the examiner observes the relative movement of the reflex or manually places lenses over the eye (using a trial frame and trial lenses) to "neutralize" the reflex.

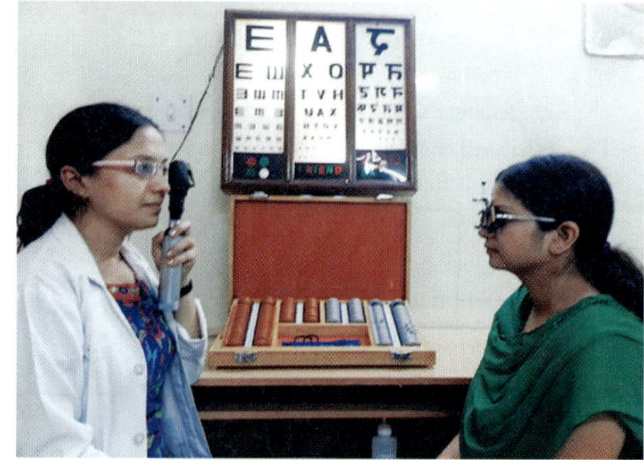

Procedure of retinoscopy.

40. Placido disc is useful detecting:

a. Microcornea
b. Megalocornea
c. Corneal scars
d. Keratoconus

A **keratoscope**, sometimes known as *Placido's disk*, is an ophthalmic instrument used to assess the shape of the anterior surface of the cornea. A series of concentric rings is projected onto the cornea and their reflec-

Ans. **36. d.** Color blindness **37. c.** Acute congestive glaucoma and cataract **38. c.** Specular microscope **39. c.** Refractive errors **40. c.** Corneal scars

tion viewed by the examiner through a small hole in the centre of the disk. A regular-shaped cornea should show equally spaced symmetric reflections. If the patient is suffering from astigmatism or from a corneal dystrophy, the rings will be distorted.

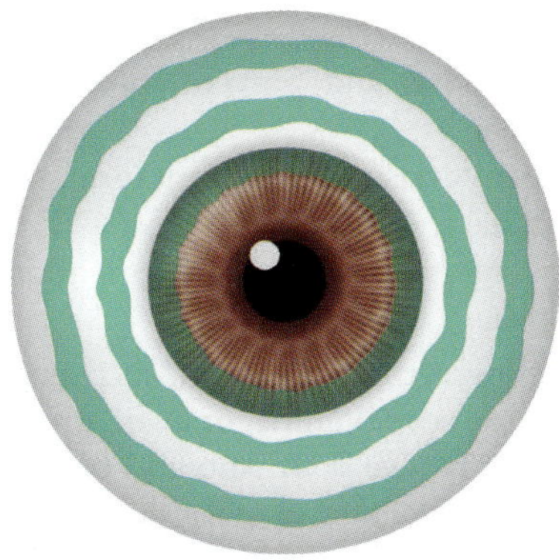

Placido's disc reflex from irregular corneal surface.

41. Keratometry is done to assess:

a. Corneal sensation
b. Corneal endothelium
c. Corneal thickness
d. Curvature of cornea

A **keratometer**, also known as an **ophthalmometer**, is a diagnostic instrument for measuring the curvature of the anterior surface of the cornea, particularly for assessing the extent and axis of astigmatism. It was invented by the German physiologist Hermann von Helmholtz in 1851, although an earlier model was developed in 1796 by Jesse Ramsden and Everard Home.

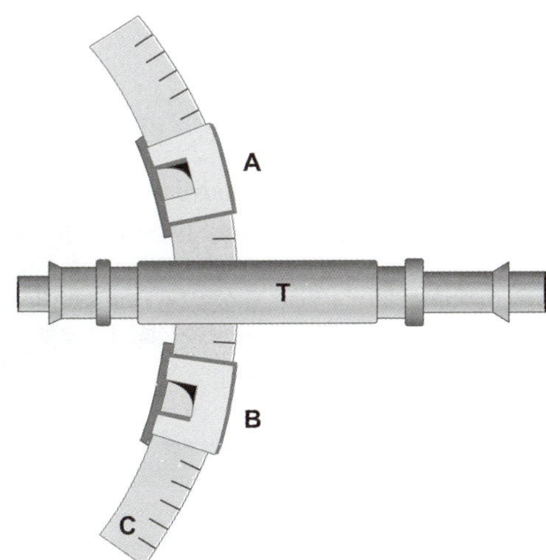

Basic structure of Javal and Schiotz keratometer.

42. Visual acuity is:

a. Refractive power of eye
b. Dividing denominator with distance at which the letters can be read on Snellen chart
c. Ability to increase converging power of eye
d. Ability to discriminate 2 points

Visual acuity is a measure of the spatial resolution of the visual processing system. **Visual acuity (VA)** commonly refers to the clarity of vision. Visual acuity is dependent on optical and neural factors, i.e., (i) the sharpness of the retinal focus within the eye, (ii) the health and functioning of the retina, and (iii) the sensitivity of the interpretative faculty of the brain.

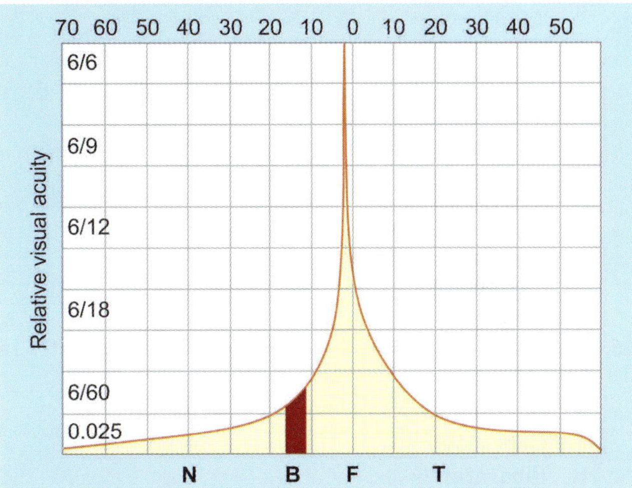

Visual acuity (form sense) in relation to the regions of the retina: N: Nasal retina; B: Blind spot; F: foveal region; T: temporal retina.

OPHTHALMOLOGY PHARMACOLOGY

43. Ethambutol toxicity can cause colour blindness for:

a. Red blue colour
b. Red green colour
c. Blue colour
d. Red green blue colour

Protanopia, deuteranopia, protanomaly, and deuteranomaly are commonly inherited forms of red-green color blindness which affect a substantial portion of the human population. Those affected have difficulty with discriminating red and green hues due to the absence or mutation of the red or green retinal photoreceptors.

44. NOT an antiglaucoma drug:

a. Brimonidine
b. Prednisolone
c. Dorzolamide
d. Timolol

Prednisolone is a synthetic glucocorticoid, a derivative of cortisol, used to treat a variety of inflammatory and autoimmune conditions and some cancers. It is the active metabolite of the drug prednisone

Ans. **41. d.** Curvature of cornea **42. d.** Ability to discriminate 2 points **43. b.** Red green colour **44. b.** Prednisolone

Corticosteroids: equivalent anti-inflammatory oral dose (mg) and relative anti-inflammatory potency.		
Drug	*Equivalent anti-inflammatory oral dose (mg)*	*Relative anti-inflammatory potency*
I. *Glucocorticoids*		
1. *Short-acting*		
Hydrocortisone (Cortisol)	20	1
Cortisone	25	0.8
Prednisolone	5	4
Prednisone	5	4
Methylprednisolone	4	5
2. *Intermediate-acting*		
Triamcinolone	4	5
Fluprednisolone	1.5	15
3. *Long-acting*		
Dexamethasone	0.75	26
Betamethasone	0.60	33
II. *Mineralocorticoids*		
Fludrocortisone	2	10

45. The drug of choice for cytomegalovirus retinitis in HIV patients:

a. Acyclovir
b. Ganciclovir
c. Ribavarin
d. Vidarabine

Ganciclovir is indicated for

- Sight-threatening CMV retinitis in severely immuno-compromised people
- CMV pneumonitis in bone marrow transplant recipients
- Prevention of CMV disease in bone marrow and solid organ transplant recipients
- Confirmed CMV retinitis in people with AIDS (intra-vitreal implant)

46. Which of the following drug can be used topically in eye:

a. Erythromycin
b. Ganciclovir
c. Clindamycin
d. Tetracyclines

The second-line treatment for trachoma is **topical tetracycline eye** ointment 1%. Topical tetracycline is applied to both eyes twice a day for 6 weeks.

47. One percent atropine is given in uveitis to:

a. Cause mydriasis and prevent formation of anterior synechiae
b. Cause miosis and prevent formation of posterior synechiae
c. Cause mydriasis and prevent formation of posterior synechiae
d. Cause miosis and prevent formation of posterior synechiae

A long-acting cycloplegic agent, such as cyclopentolate, homatropine, scopolamine, or even atropine, should be used to help relieve both pain and photophobia and to prevent the formation of posterior synechiae in acute symptomatic anterior uveitis

48. Topical antifungal for keratomycosis is:

a. Silver sulfadiazine
b. Flucytosine
c. Ketoconazole
d. Natamycin

A presumptive diagnosis of fungal keratitis requires immediate empirical therapy. Natamycin ophthalmic suspension is the drug of choice for filamentous fungal infection. Fluconazole ophthalmic solution is recommended for *Candida* infection of the cornea. Amphotericin B eye drops may be required for nonresponding cases, but can be quite toxic and requires expert pharmacist for preparation.

49. Mydriatic used for refraction in infants is:

a. Atropine ointment
b. Atropine drops
c. Homatropine
d. Eucatropine

Atropine is necessary to achieve adequate cycloplegia in some children. The usual dosage for cycloplegic refraction in children is one drop of 0.5% atropine solution bilaterally twice daily or one centimeter of a 1% ointment into the conjunctival sac once daily for 1-3 days prior to examination.

Salient features of common cycloplegic and mydriatic drugs.

Sl. no.	*Name of the drug*	*Age of the patient when indicated*	*Dosage of instillation*	*Peak effect*	*Time of performing retinoscopy*	*Duration of action*	*Period of postcyclo-plegic test*	*Tonus allowance*
1.	Atropine sulphate (1 % ointment)	< 5 year	TDS x 3 days	2–3 days	4th day	10–20 days	After 3 weeks of retinoscopy	1D

Contd...

Ans. 45. **b.** Ganciclovir 46. **d.** Tetracyclines 47. **c.** Cause mydriasis... 48. **d.** Natamycin 49. **a.** Atropine ointment

Contd...

Sl. no.	Name of the drug	Age of the patient when indicated	Dosage of instillation	Peak effect	Time of performing retinoscopy	Duration of action	Period of postcyclo-plegic test	Tonus allowance
2.	Homatropine hydrobromide (2% drops)	5–8 years	One drop every 10 min. for 6 times	60–90 min.	After 90 min. of instillation of first drop	48–72 hours	After 3 days of retinoscopy	0.5D
3.	Cyclopentolate hydrochloride (1% drops)	8–20 years	One drop every 15 min. for 3 times	80–90 min.	After 90 min. of instillation of first drop	6–18 hours	After 3 days of retinoscopy	0. 75D
4.	Tropicamide (0.5%, 1% drops)	Not used as cycloplegic for retino-scopy; used only as mydriatic	One drop every 15 min. for 3 to 4 times	20–40 min.		4–6 hours		
5.	Phenylephrine (5%, 10% drops)	Used only as mydriatic alone or in combination with tropicamide	One drop every 15 min. for 3 to 4 times	30–40 min.		4–6 hours		

50. Drug contraindicated in iridocyclitis:

a. Aspirin
b. Pilocarpine
c. Atropine
d. Steroids

Pilocarpine: Ocular adverse effects:

- Miosis
- *Brow ache:* Ciliary body (CB) contraction
- Globe and orbital pain
- Allergic reactions
- Increased myopia due to accommodative spasm
- *Vision reduction:* Especially with cataracts
- Posterior synechia in some cases
- *Retinal detachment:* Ciliary body contraction- not common, but be aware of the potential
- *Angle closure:* Due to pupil block with a changing cataractous lens
- Field constriction

51. First line drug for primary open angle glaucoma is:

a. Pilocarpine
b. Dorzolamide
c. Dipivefrine
d. Beta blockers

Beta antagonists (blockers):

- All forms block norepinephrine and thus blocks aqueous formation- considered aqueous suppressants
- May be selective
  - Beta 1 specific (blocks only beta 1 receptors)
  - Most are nonspecific and block both beta 1 and beta 2
- Reduced sympathetic activity
- Aqueous suppressant
- Bilateral effects when using in only one eye due to systemic absorption
- Short-term escape
  - After an initial decrease in IOP from several days to weeks, a rise in IOP will occur. After an additional 2-4 weeks, the IOP will stabilize, often below pre-treatment levels.
- Long-term drift
  - A slow steady rise in IOP after months to years of treatment.
  - Medications become ineffective
  - Common problem with beta blockers

CONJUNCTIVA

52. Effect of Chlamydia trachomatis A-C infection:

a. Ophthalmia neonatorum
b. Paratrachoma
c. Lymphogranuloma venerum
d. Trachoma

Trachoma is caused by Chlamydia trachomatis, serotypes (serovars) A, B, and C. It is spread by direct contact with eye, nose, and throat secretions from affected individuals, or contact with fomites (inanimate objects that carry infectious agents), such as towels and/or washcloths, that have had similar contact with these secretions. Flies can also be a route of mechanical transmission

Ans. 50. **b.** Pilocarpine 51. **d.** Beta blockers 52. **d.** Trachoma

53. Which of the following causes swimming pool conjunctivitis?

a. Pneumococcus
b. Chlamydia
c. Poxvirus
d. Staph. aureus

Adult inclusion conjunctivitis (swimming bath or swimming pool conjunctivitis) is caused by Chlamydia trachomatis serotypes D through K. In most instances, adult inclusion conjunctivitis results from sexual contact with a person who has a genital infection. Usually, patients have acquired a new sex partner in the preceding 2 mo. Rarely, adult inclusion conjunctivitis is acquired from contaminated, incompletely chlorinated swimming pool water.

54. Maxwell Lyon's sign is a feature of:

a. Angular conjunctivitis
b. Sympathetic ophthalmitis
c. Dendritic ulcerative keratitis
d. Spring catarrh

VKC is characterized by marked burning and itchy sensations which may be intolerable and accentuates when patient comes in a warm humid atmosphere. Associated symptoms include mild photophobia, lacrimation, stringy discharge and heaviness of eyelids.

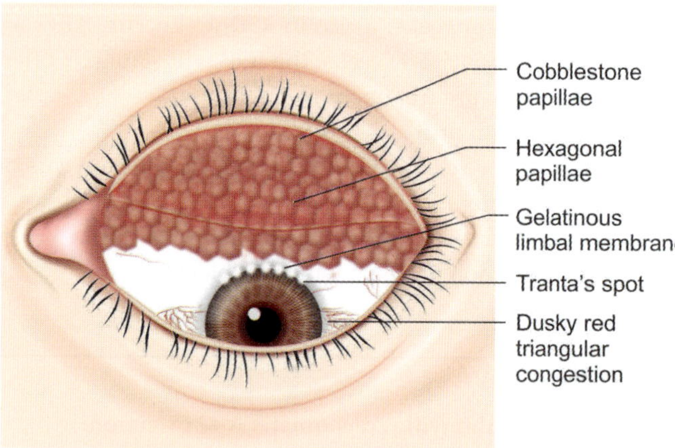

Diagram of mixed form of vernal keratoconjunctivitis.

55. Horner trantas spots are seen in:

a. Vernal keratoconjunctivitis/ VKC
b. Phlyctenular conjunctivitis
c. Angular conjunctivitis
d. Follicular conjunctivitis

Bulbar form of VKC is characterized by dusky red triangular congestion of bulbar conjunctiva in palpebral area, gelatinous thickened accumulation of tissue around limbus and presence of discrete whitish raised dots along the limbus (Tranta's spots).

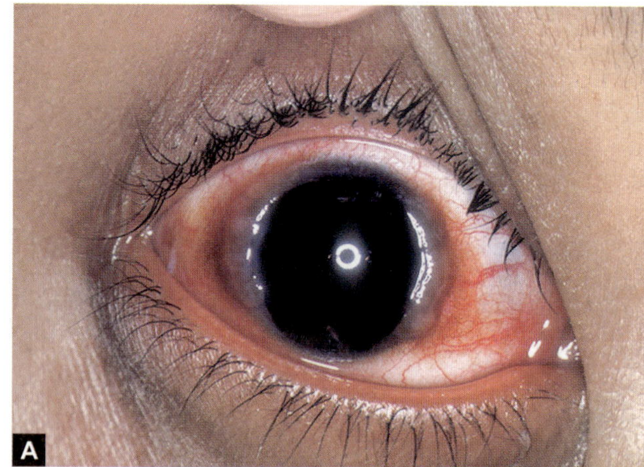

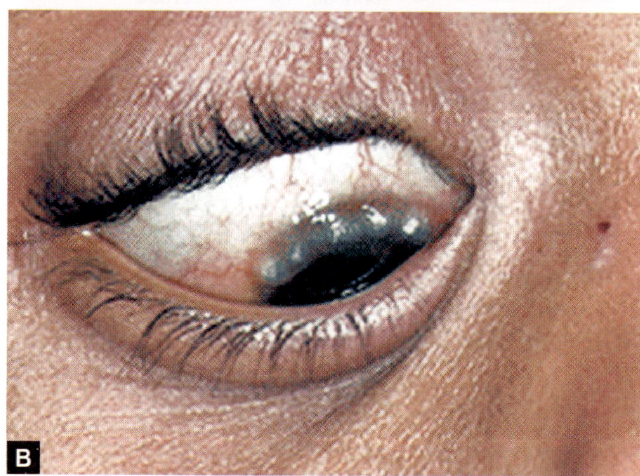

Bulbar form of VKC depicting: (A) Gelatinous membrane around limbus; (B) Tranta's spots at limbus.

56. Herbert's pit is seen in:

a. Vernal conjunctivitis
b. Atopic conjunctivitis
c. Gonococcal conjunctivitis
d. Chlamydial conjunctivitis

In trachoma, blood vessels and scar tissue can invade the upper cornea (pannus). Resolved limbal follicles may leave small gaps in pannus (Herbert's Pits).

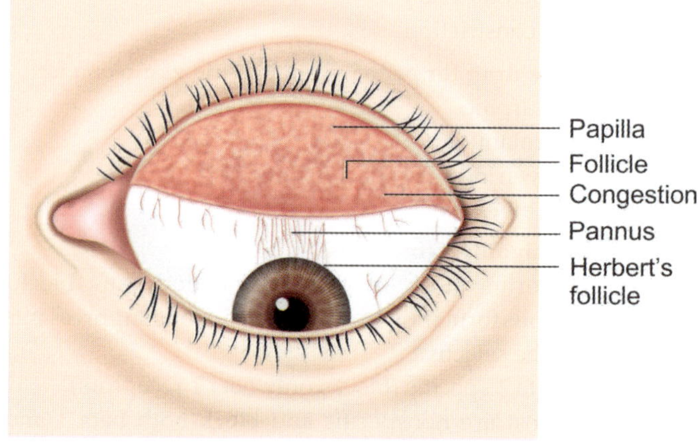

Signs of active trachoma (diagrammatic).

Ans. 53. **b.** Chlamydia 54. **d.** Spring catarrh 55. **a.** Vernal keratoconjunctivitis/VKC 56. **d.** Chlamydial conjunctivitis

57. Xerosis is seen in:

a. Vitamin A deficiency
b. Vitamin B deficiency
c. Vitamin C deficiency
d. Vitamin D deficiency

VAD (vitamin A deficiency) may produce xerophthalmia. Its ocular manifestations include conjunctival and corneal xerosis (drying), keratomalacia (corneal necrosis/ulceration), nyctalopia (night blindness), and Bitot spots (conjunctival lesions).

58. Arlt's line is seen in:

a. Ophthalmia neonatorum
b. Trachoma
c. Angular conjunctivitis d. Vernal catarrh

In trachomatous conjunctival scarring stage, linear scar present in the sulcus subtarsalis is called Arlt's line (named after Carl Ferdinand von Arlt).

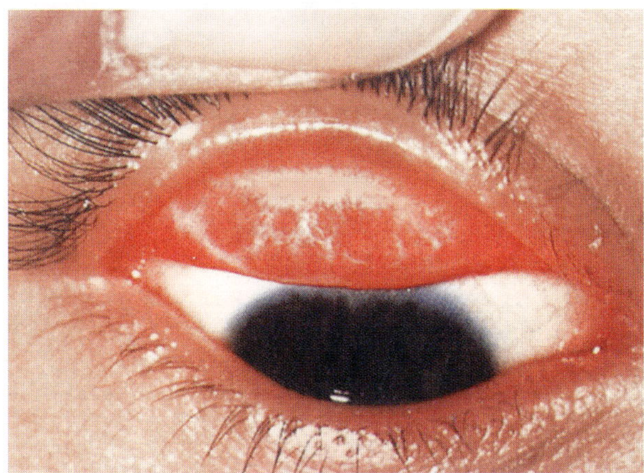

Trachomatous scarring (TS).

59. Type IV hypersensitivity to mycobacterium TB antigen may manifest as:

a. Iridocyclitis b. Polyarteritis nodosa
c. Phlyctenular d. Giant cell arteritis

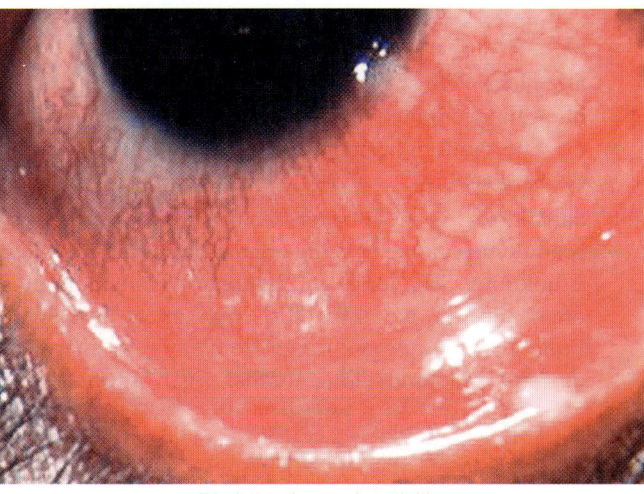

Phylctenular conjunctivitis.

Phlyctenular keratoconjunctivitis results from a delayed hypersensitivity (type IV cell mediated) reaction to bacterial antigens, primarily staphylococcal, but TB, *Chlamydia,* and other agents have been implicated. It is more common among children.

60. SAFE strategy has been developed for the control of:

a. Conjunctivitis
b. Trachoma
c. Refractive error
d. Ocular trauma

National governments in collaboration with numerous nonprofit organizations implement trachoma control programs using the WHO-recommended SAFE strategy, which includes:

- Surgery to correct advanced stages of the disease;
- Antibiotics to treat active infection, using azithromycin
- Facial cleanliness to reduce disease transmission;
- Environmental change to increase access to clean water and improved sanitation.

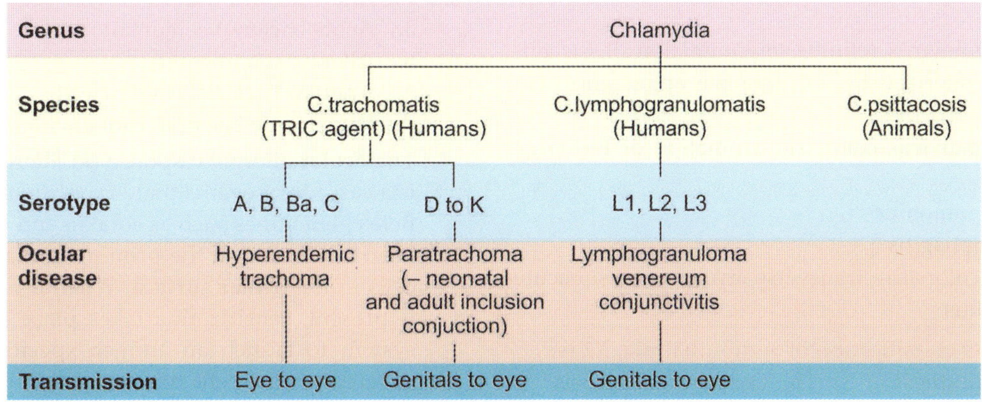

Genus	Chlamydia			
Species	C.trachomatis (TRIC agent) (Humans)		C.lymphogranulomatis (Humans)	C.psittacosis (Animals)
Serotype	A, B, Ba, C	D to K	L1, L2, L3	
Ocular disease	Hyperendemic trachoma	Paratrachoma (– neonatal and adult inclusion conjuction)	Lymphogranuloma venereum conjunctivitis	
Transmission	Eye to eye	Genitals to eye	Genitals to eye	

Summary of ocular infections caused by chlamydia.

Ans. **57. a.** Vitamin A def... **58. b.** Trachoma **59. c.** Phlyctenular **60. b.** Trachoma

61. Conjunctival xerosis is seen in all of the following EXCEPT:

a. Steven-Johnson syndrome
b. Keratoconjunctivitis sicca
c. Vitamin A deficiency
d. Sarcoidosis

Sarcoidosis is a disorder resulting in noncaseating granulomas in one or more organs and tissues; etiology is unknown. The lungs and lymphatic system are most often affected, but sarcoidosis may affect any organ. Pulmonary symptoms range from none to exertional dyspnea and, rarely, lung or other organ failure.

62. Xerophthalmia can be caused by:

a. Steven-Johnson syndrome
b. Vitamin A deficiency
c. Sulfa drugs
d. All of the above

Xerophthalmia is a term that usually implies a destructive dryness of the conjunctival epithelium due to dietary vitamin A deficiency—a rare condition in developed countries, but still causing much damage in developing countries. Other forms of dry eye are associated with aging, poor lid closure, scarring from previous injury, or autoimmune diseases such as rheumatoid arthritis and Sjögren's syndrome, and these can all cause chronic conjunctivitis. Radioiodine therapy can also induce xerophthalmia, often transiently, although in some patients late onset or persistent xerophthalmia has been observed.

63. Which of the following virus does NOT cause conjunctivitis:

a. CMV
b. Adenovirus
c. Herpes simplex virus
d. Picornavirus

Specific diseases caused by CMV

- CMV hepatitis, which may cause fulminant liver failure
- Cytomegalovirus retinitis (inflammation of the retina, characterized by a "pizza pie appearance" on ophthalmoscopy)
- Cytomegalovirus colitis (inflammation of the large bowel)
- CMV pneumonitis
- CMV esophagitis
- Polyradiculopathy, transverse myelitis, and subacute encephalitis

64. As per WHO classification of xerophthalmia, X2 is:

a. Night blindness
b. Conjunctival xerosis
c. Bitot's spots
d. Corneal xerosis

Different eye signs of vitamin A deficiency (VAD) in children, as graded by the WHO

- Night blindness (XN)
- Conjunctival xerosis (X1A)
- Bitot's spots (X1B)
- Corneal xerosis (X2)
- Corneal ulcer covering less than 1/3 of the cornea (X3A)
- Corneal ulcer covering at least 1/3 of the cornea, defined as keratomalacia (X3B)
- Corneal scarring (XS)
- Xerophthalmic fundus (XF)

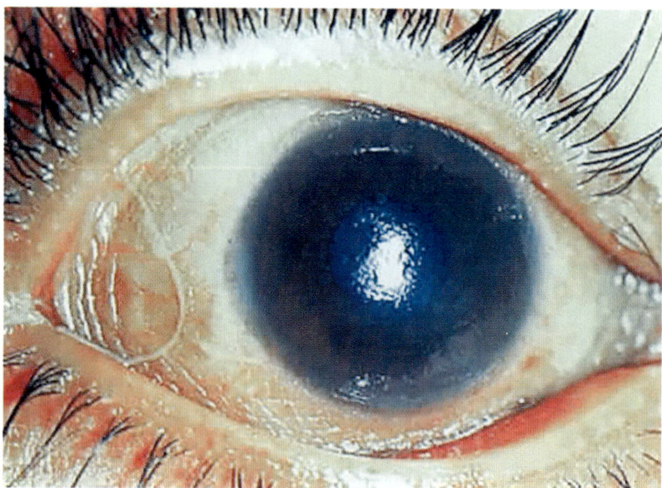

Xerophthalmia, stage X2: Corneal xerosis.

65. Ophthalmia nodosa (granuloma in the sclera) is seen in:

a. Caterpillar hair in the eye
b. Granulomatous uveitis
c. Leprosy
d. Syphilis

Ophthalmia nodosa is a cutaneous condition characterized by inflammation of the eye due to lodging of (for example) caterpillar hairs in the conjunctiva, cornea, or iris.

66. Polymorphic infiltration is NOT seen in:

a. Acute bacterial conjunctivitis
b. Allergic conjunctivitis
c. Angular bacterial conjunctivitis
d. Hyperacute bacterial conjunctivitis

The ocular allergic response (in allergic conjunctivitis) is a cascade of events that is coordinated by mast cells. Beta chemokines such as eotaxin and MIP-1 alpha have been implicated in the priming and activation of mast cells in the ocular surface. When a particular allergen is present, sensitization takes place and prepares the system to launch an antigen specific response. TH2 differentiated T cells release cytokines, which promote the production of antigen specific immunoglobulin E

Ans. 61. **d.** Sarcoidosis 62. **d.** All of the above 63. **a.** CMV 64. **d.** Corneal xerosis 65. **a.** Caterpillar hair... 66. **b.** Allergic conjunctivitis

(IgE). IgE then binds to IgE receptors on the surface of mast cells. Then, mast cells release histamine, which then leads to the release of cytokines, prostaglandins, and platelet-activating factor. Mast cell intermediaries cause an allergic inflammation and symptoms through the activation of inflammatory cells.

Differentiating features of common types of conjunctivitis.

	Bacterial	*Viral*	*Allergic*	*Chlamydial (TRIC)*
(A) CLINICAL SIGNS				
1. Congestion	Marked	Moderate	Mild to moderate	Moderate
2. Chemosis	++	±	++	±
3. Subconjunctival haemorrhages	±	±	–	–
4. Discharge	Purulent or mucopurulent	Watery	Ropy/ watery	Mucopurulent
5. Papillae	±	–	++	±
6. Follicles	–	+	–	++
7. Pseudomembrane	±	±	–	–
8. Pannus	–	–	– (Except vernal)	+
9. Preauricular lymph nodes	+	++	–	±
(B) CYTOLOGICAL FEATURES				
1. Neutrophils	+	+ (Early)	–	+
2. Eosinophils	–	–	+	–
3. Lymphocytes	–	+	–	+
4. Plasma cells	–	–	–	+
5. Multinuclear cells	–	+	–	–
6. Inclusion bodies:				
Cytoplasmic	–	+ (Pox)	–	+
Nuclear	–	+ (Herpes)	–	–
7. Micro-organisms	+	–	–	–

67. Angular conjunctivitis is caused by:

a. Staphylococcus
b. Coxsackie virus
c. Moraxella
d. Aspergillus

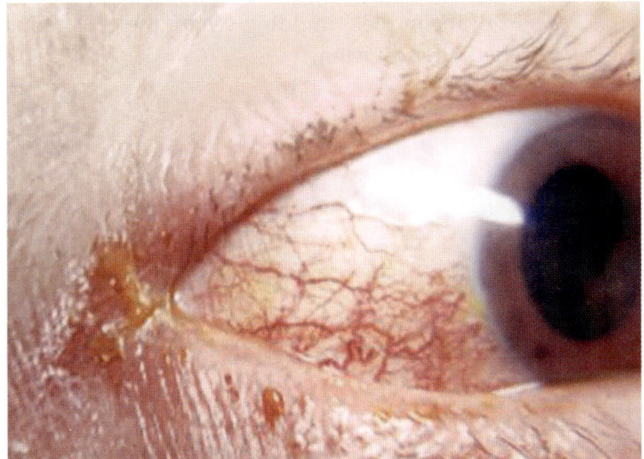

Signs of angular conjunctivitis.

Etiology of angular conjunctivitis

- Predisposing factors are same as for 'simple chronic conjunctivitis'.
- Causative organisms: Moraxella Axenfeld is the commonest causative organism. MA bacilli are placed end to end, so the disease is also called 'diplobacillary conjunctivitis'. Rarely, *staphylococci* may also cause angular conjunctivitis.
- Source of infection is usually nasal cavity.
- Mode of infection: Infection is transmitted from nasal cavity to the eyes by contaminated fingers or handkerchief.

68. Cobblestone appearance of conjunctiva is seen in:

a. Bacterial conjunctivitis
b. Spring catarrh
c. Ophthalmia neonatorum
d. Trachoma

Palpebral form of VKC

Usually upper tarsal conjunctiva of both eyes is involved. The typical lesion is characterized by the presence of hard, flat topped, papillae arranged in a 'cobble-stone' or 'pavement stone', fashion. In severe cases, papillae may hypertrophy to produce cauliflower like excrescences of 'giant papillae'. Conjunctival changes are associated with white ropy discharge.

Ans. **67. c.** Moraxella **68. b.** Spring catarrh

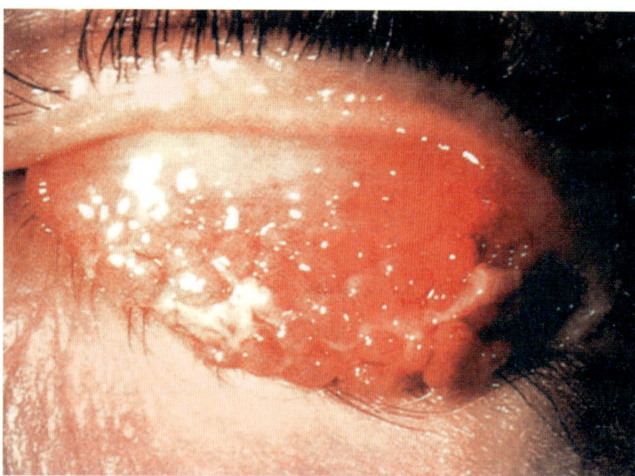

Palpebral form of vernals keratoconjunctivitis.

69. NOT a feature of trachoma:

a. Corneal opacity b. Chalazion
c. Herbert's pits d. Ectropion

The later structural changes of trachoma are referred to as "cicatricial trachoma". These include scarring in the eyelid (tarsal conjunctiva) that leads to distortion of the eyelid with buckling of the lid (tarsus) so the lashes rub on the eye (trichiasis). These lashes will lead to corneal opacities and scarring and then to blindness. There is also entropion, tylosis (thickening of lid margins), ptosis, madarosis and ankyloblepharon.

CORNEA

70. All of the followinga are true for keratoconus EXCEPT:

a. Progressive vision loss
b. KF rings
c. Scissoring reflex in retinoscopy
d. Munsen sign positive

Kayser Fleischer ring are seen in Wilson disease (Fleischer's ring are seen in keratoconus)

71. Which of the following can cause giant dendritic ulcers on cornea?

a. Fungal infection b. Chlamydial infection
c. HSV infection
d. Pneumococcal infection

Epithelial lesion is a classic herpetic lesion consists of a linear branching corneal ulcer (dendritic ulcer). During eye exam the defect is examined after staining with fluorescein dye. The underlying cornea has minimal inflammation.

72. Recurrent corneal erosions are seen in:

a. Corneal dystrophy b. Keratoconus
c. Keratoglobus d. Pateras anomaly

Recurrent corneal erosion (RCE) syndrome is a condition that is characterized by a disturbance at the level of the corneal epithelial basement membrane, resulting in defective adhesions and recurrent breakdowns of the epithelium. RCE syndrome may occur secondary to corneal injury or spontaneously. In the latter case, some predisposing factor, such as diabetes or a corneal dystrophy, may be the underlying cause.

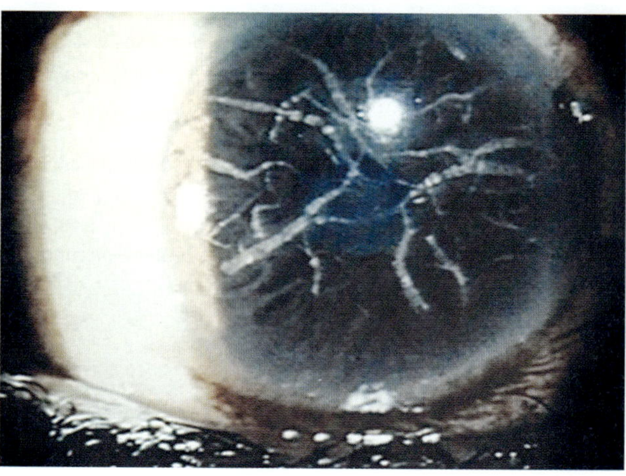

Lattice corneal dystrophy.

73. Microscopy of corneal ulcer showed branching septate hyphae. The probable diagnosis is:

a. Candida b. Mucormycosis
c. Aspergillus d. Histoplasma

Classification of fungi based on cell division

- Septate (with septa)
  - *Aspergillus* and many other species have septate hyphae.
- Aseptate or coenocytic (without septa)
  - Nonseptate hyphae are associated with Mucor, some zygomycetes, and other fungi.
- "Pseudohyphae" are distinguished from true hyphae by their method of growth, relative frailty and lack of cytoplasmic connection between the cells.
- Yeast can form pseudohyphae. They are the result of a sort of incomplete budding where the cells remain attached after division.

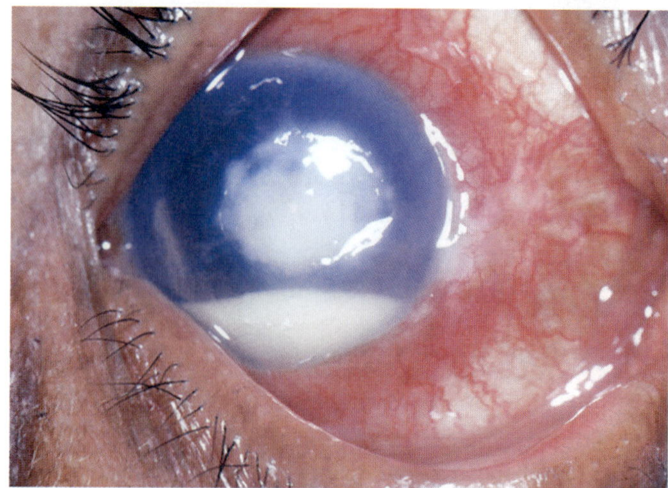

Fungal corneal ulcer.

Ans. 69. **d.** Ectropion 70. **b.** KF rings 71. **c.** HSV infection 72. **a.** Corneal dystrophy
73. **c.** Aspergillus

74. True about Moorens ulcer:

a. Painless condition b. Affects cornea
c. Sudden loss of vision
d. Bilateral in majority of cases

The location of the ulcer depends somewhat on the cause. Central ulcers are typically caused by trauma, dry eye, or exposure from facial nerve paralysis or exophthalmos. Entropion, severe dry eye and trichiasis (inturning of eyelashes) may cause ulceration of the peripheral cornea. Immune-mediated eye disease can cause ulcers at the border of the cornea and sclera. These include Rheumatoid arthritis, rosacea, systemic sclerosis which lead to a special type of corneal ulcer called **Mooren's ulcer**. It has a circumferential crater like depression of the cornea, just inside the limbus, usually with an overhanging edge.

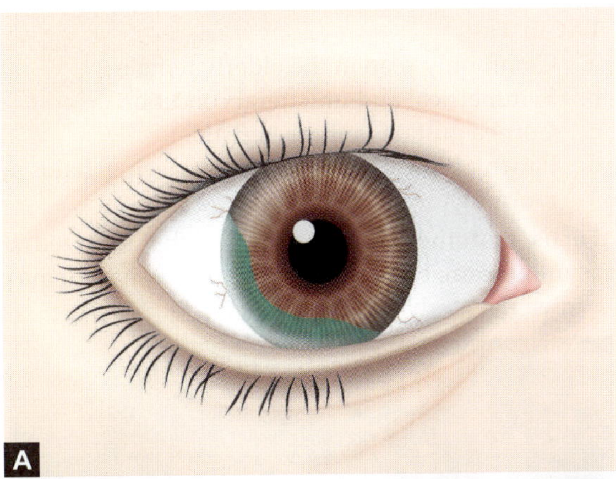

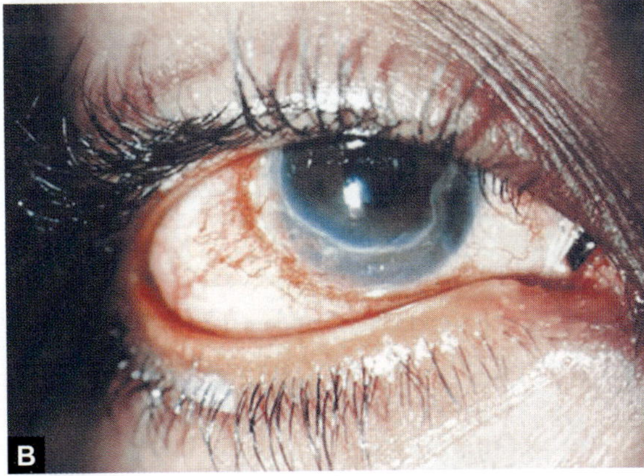

Mooren's ulcer: (A) diagrammatic depiction; (B) clinical photograph.

75. Dendritic ulcer is caused by:

a. Herpes simplex virus b. Bacteria
c. Trauma d. Fungi

Dendritic ulcer (Epithelial keratitis)

- This classic herpetic lesion consists of a linear branching corneal ulcer (dendritic ulcer). During eye exam the defect is examined after staining with fluorescein dye. The underlying cornea has minimal inflammation.
- Patients with epithelial keratitis complain of foreign-body sensation, light sensitivity, redness and blurred vision.
- Focal or diffuse reduction in corneal sensation develops following recurrent epithelial keratitis.

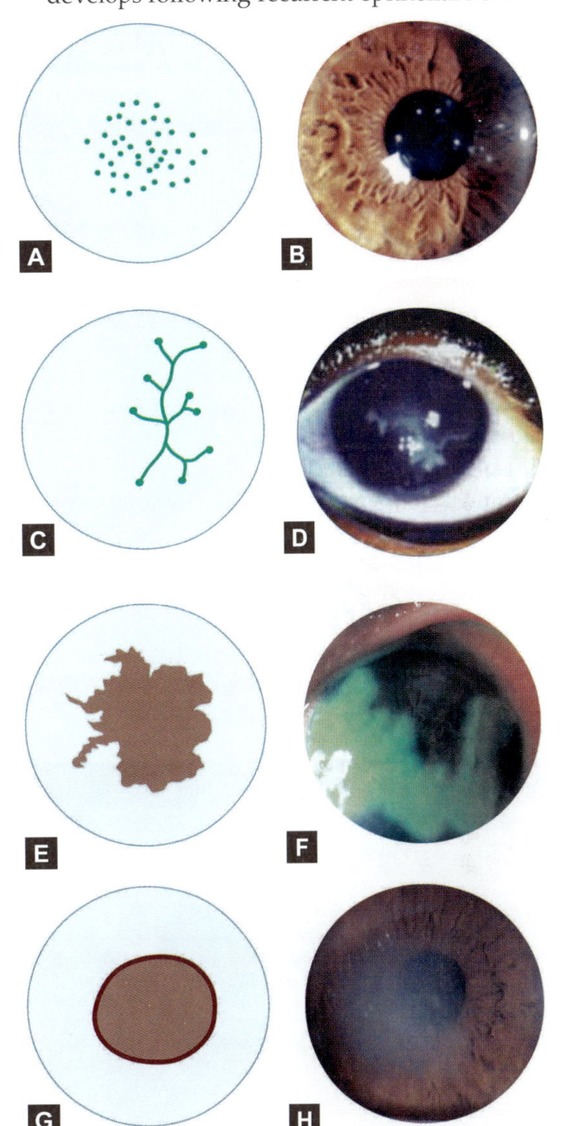

Lesions of recurrent herpes simplex keratitis; diagrammatic depiction and Clinical photograph; (A and B), Punctate epithelial keratitis; (C and D), Dendritic ulcer; (E and F), Geographical ulcer; and (G) and (H), Disciform keratitis.

76. The organism that penetrates normal cornea is:

a. Pneumococcus b. Pseudomonas
c. Gonococcus d. Chlamydia trachomatis

Only organisms which are able to invade normal intact epithelium of cornea are **Neisseria** (gonorrhoeae and meningitides both) and **Corynebacterium diphtheriae**. Many other bacteria are capable of producing ulceration especially *Streptococcus* pneumoniae when the epithelium is already damaged.

Ans. **74. b.** Affects cornea **75. a.** Herpes simplex virus **76. c.** Gonococcus

77. True about keratoconus are all of the following EXCEPT:

a. Can be seen in Down's syndrome
b. It manifests just after birth
c. Munsen sign is characteristic
d. Corneal transplantation is needed in severe cases.

Keratoconus (conical cornea) is a noninflammatory bilateral (85%) ectatic condition of cornea in its axial part. It usually starts at puberty and progresses slowly.

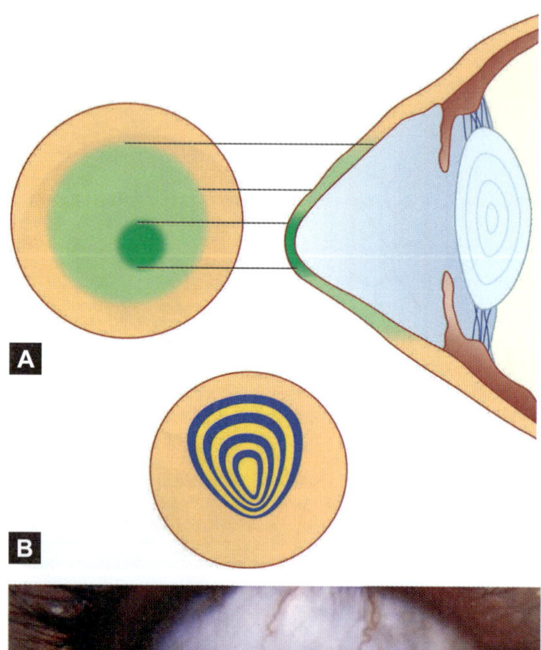

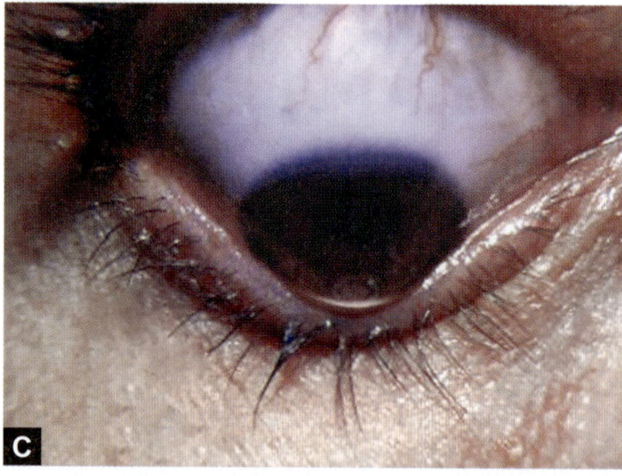

Keratoconus showing: (A) Diagrammatic depiction of configuration of cone-shaped cornea; (B) Irregular circles on Placido disc examination; (C) Clinical photograph (note Munson's sign).

78. Corneal lesion seen in Hutchinson triad associated with congenital syphilis is:

a. Disciform keratitis
b. Interstitial keratitis
c. Phlyctenular keratitis
d. Mooren ulcer

Interstitial Keratitis (IK) is corneal scarring due to chronic inflammation of the corneal stroma. Interstitial means space between cells i.e. corneal stroma which lies between the epithelium and the endothelium. By far the most common cause of IK is syphilitic disease.

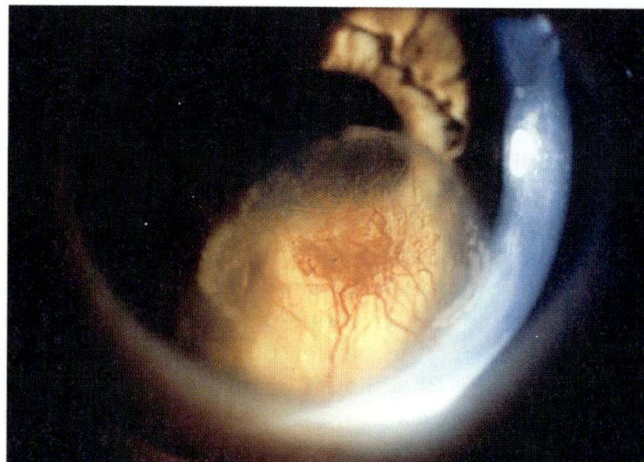

Interstitial keratitis: Salmon patch appearance.

79. True about Fuchs endothelial dystrophy are all EXCEPT:

a. Commonly seen in the elderly female
b. Symmetrical and unilateral condition
c. Cornea guttata is characteristic
d. Patient typically complains of seeing halos in the morning

Fuchs endothelial dystrophy is characterized by an asymmetrical, bilateral, slowly progressive edema of the cornea in elderly patients.

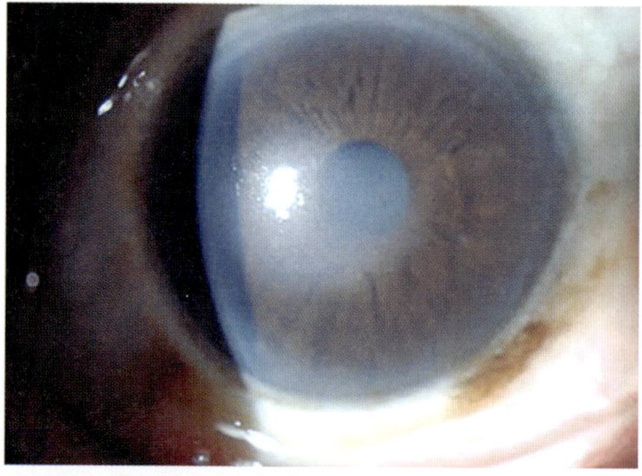

Fuch's endothelial corneal dystrophy.

80. A 28-year-old male complains of glare in both eyes. Examination of cornea showed whorl like opacities of epithelium. There is a past history of Amiodarone therapy. Most likely diagnosis is:

a. Arcus senilis
b. Band shaped keratopathy
c. Cornea verticillata
d. Terrain's marginal degeneration

Cornea verticillata, also called **Fleischer vortex**, **Vortex keratopathy** or **Whorl keratopathy**, is a condition characterised by corneal deposits at the level of the basal epithelium forming a faint golden-brown whorl pattern. It is seen in Fabry disease or in case of prolonged amiodarone intake.

Ans. 77. **b.** It manifests just after birth
78. **b.** Interstitial keratitis
79. **b.** Symmetrical and unilateral condition
80. **c.** Cornea verticillata

81. **Hypopyon is seen in:**
 a. Pneumococcal infection
 b. Fungal infection
 c. Gonococcus d. All of the above

Hypopyon is inflammatory cells in the anterior chamber of the eye.

It is a leukocytic exudate, seen in the anterior chamber, usually accompanied by redness of the conjunctiva and the underlying episclera. It is a sign of inflammation of the anterior uvea and iris, i.e. iritis, which is a form of anterior uveitis. The exudate settles at the dependent aspect of the eye due to gravity.

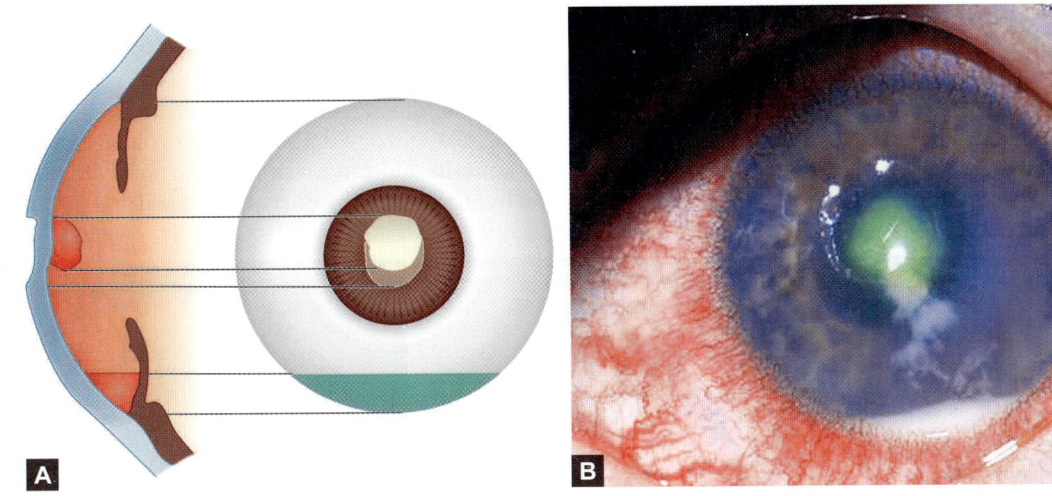

Hypopyon corneal ulcer: (A) Diagrammatic depiction; (B) Clinical photograph.

82. **Satellite nodules in the cornea are caused by:**
 a. Bacteria b. Virus
 c. Fungus d. Rickettsia

Fungal keratitis causes deep and severe corneal ulcer. It is caused by *Aspergillus sp., Fusarium sp., Candida sp.*, as also *Rhizopus, Mucor*, and other fungi. The typical feature of fungal keratitis is slow onset and gradual progression, where signs are much more than the symptoms. Small satellite lesions around the ulcer are a common feature of fungal keratitis and hypopyon is usually seen.

83. **Diagnostic test for corneal ulcer:**
 a. Methylene blue b. Sodium fluorescein dye
 c. Alcian blue d. Rose Bengal

Diagnosis of corneal ulcer is done by direct observation under magnified view of slit lamp revealing the ulcer on the cornea. The use of fluorescein stain, which is taken up by exposed corneal stroma and appears green, helps in defining the margins of the corneal ulcer, and can reveal additional details of the surrounding epithelium. Herpes simplex ulcers show a typical dendritic pattern of staining. Rose-Bengal dye is also used for supra-vital staining purposes, but it may be very irritating to the eyes. In descemetoceles, the Descemet's membrane will bulge forward and after staining will appear as a dark circle with a green boundary, because it does not absorb the stain. Doing a corneal scraping and examining under the microscope with stains like Gram's and KOH preparation may reveal the bacteria and fungi respectively. Microbiological culture tests may be necessary to isolate the causative organisms for some cases. Other tests that may be necessary include a Schirmer's test for keratoconjunctivitis sicca and an analysis of facial nerve function for facial nerve paralysis.

84. **Interstitial keratitis is commonly seen in:**
 a. Fungal keratitis b. Congenital syphilis
 c. Phlyctenular keratitis d. Trachoma

Symptoms of congenital syphilis:
- Blunted upper incisor teeth known as Hutchinson's teeth
- Inflammation of the cornea known as interstitial keratitis
- Deafness from auditory nerve disease
- Frontal bossing (prominence of the brow ridge)
- Saddle nose (collapse of the bony part of nose)
- Hard palate defect
- Swollen knees
- Saber shins
- Short maxillae
- Protruding mandible

85. **Important in Herpes simplex involvement of the eye are all EXCEPT:**
 a. Type of lesion b. Corneal anaesthesia
 c. Iridocyclitis d. Purulent discharge

It begins with infection of epithelial cells on the surface of the eye and retrograde infection of nerves serving the cornea. Primary infection typically presents as swelling

Ans. 81. **d.** All of the above 82. **c.** Fungus 83. **b.** Sodium fluorescein... 84. **b.** Congenital syphilis 85. **d.** Purulent discharge of the conjunctiva and eyelids (blepharoconjunctivitis), accompanied by small white itchy lesions on the corneal surface. The effect of the lesions varies, from minor damage to the epithelium (superficial punctate keratitis), to more serious consequences such as the formation of dendritic ulcers. Infection is unilateral, affecting one eye at a time. Subsequent recurrences may be more severe, with infected epithelial cells showing larger dendritic ulceration, and lesions forming white plaques. The epithelial layer is sloughed off as the dendritic ulcer grows, and mild inflammation (iritis) may occur in the underlying stroma of iris. Sensation loss occurs in lesional areas, producing generalized corneal anaesthesia with repeated recurrences.

86. Which of the following statement is true regarding *Acanthamoeba* keratitis:

a. For the isolation of the causative agent, corneal scraping should be cultured on a nutrient agar plate
b. The causative agent, *Acanthamoeba* is a helminth whose normal habitat is soil
c. Keratitis due to *Acanthamoeba* is NOT seen in the *immunocompromised* patient
d. *Acanthamoeba* does NOT depend upon a human host for the completion of its life-cycle

Species within the genus *Acanthamoeba* are generally free-living trophozoites. These trophozoites are relatively ubiquitous and can live in, but are not restricted to, tap water, freshwater lakes/rivers and soil.

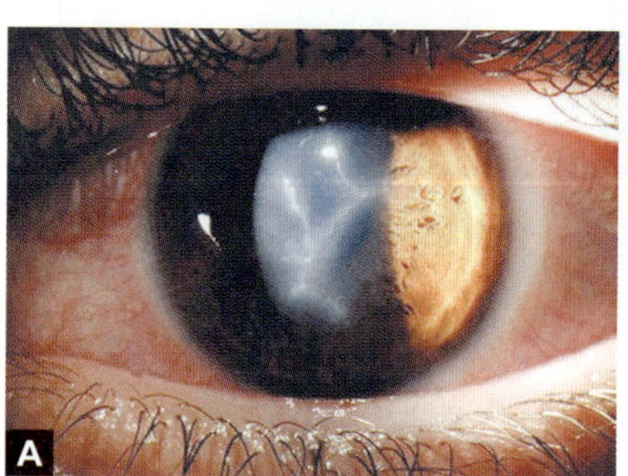

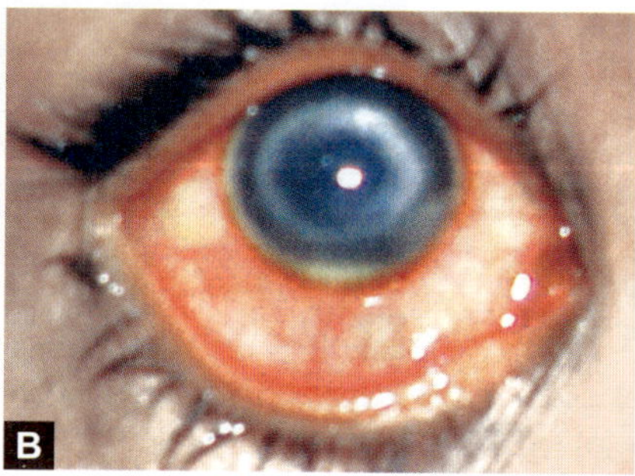

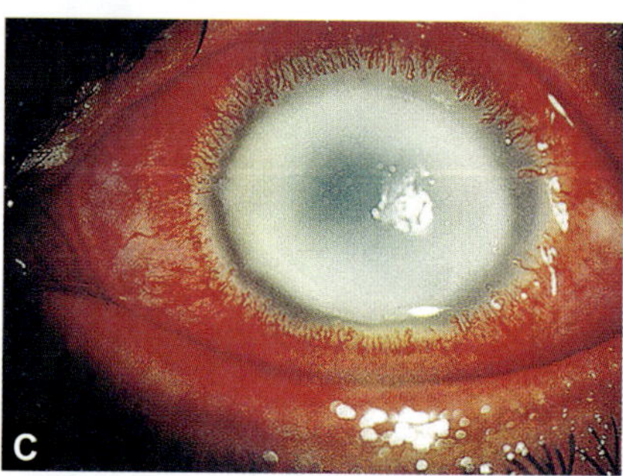

Acanthamoeba keratitis: (A) Radial keratoneuritis; (B) Ring infiltrate; and (C) Ring abscess.

87. Most important factor for corneal ulceration:

a. Virulent causative organism
b. Low immunity
c. Corneal epithelial damage
d. Local ocular predisposing diseases

Superficial ulcers involve a loss of part of the epithelium. Deep ulcers extend into or through the stroma and can result in severe scarring and corneal perforation. **Descemetoceles** occur when the ulcer extends through the stroma. This type of ulcer is especially dangerous and can rapidly result in corneal perforation, if not treated in time.

88. *Acanthamoeba keratitis* is:

a. Allergic reaction to tuberculoprotein
b. Seen in contact lenses users
c. Lesion of herpes zoster
d. Seen in congenital syphilis

Protozoa infection like *Acanthamoeba keratitis* is characterized by severe pain and is associated with contact lens users swimming in pools.

UVEAL TRACT AND GLAUCOMA

89. Which of the following condition does NOT present with coloured halos?

a. Cataract
b. Open angle glaucoma
c. Angle closure glaucoma
d. Purulent conjunctivitis

The coloured halos in glaucoma must be differentiated from those found in acute purulent conjunctivitis and early cataractous changes. In conjunctivits, the halos can be eliminated by irrigating the discharge. The halos of glaucoma and immature cataract may be differentiated by Fincham's test in which a stenopaeic slit is passed across the pupil. During this test glaucomatous halo remains intact, while a halo due to cataract is broken up into segments.

90. Which of the following is the surgery of choice in primary open angle glaucoma?

a. Peripheral iridectomy
b. Laser trabeculoplasty
c. Laser iridotomy
d. Trabeculectomy

Usually medical therapy is preferred for open angle glaucoma. Argon or diode laser trabeculoplasty can be used to control the IOP in glaucoma patients. It is not an substitute for medical therapy but may be an alternative to the filtration surgery, in most cases it can delay the surgical intervention.

91. Earliest field defect in primary open angle glaucoma:

a. Ring scotoma
b. Double Arcuate scotoma
c. Scotoma in Bjerrum's field
d. Nasal spur

Order of visual field defects/ VFD in POAG

- MC early VFDs are small isolated paracentral scotomas between 2–10 degrees

Ans. 86. d. *Acanthamoeba*... 87. c. Corneal epithelial... 88. b. Seen in contact... 89. b. Open angle glaucoma 90. b. Laser trabeculop... 91. c. Scotoma in Bjerrum's field

- In uncontrolled glaucoma, a sickle shaped extension of the blind spot, above or below, with the concavity towards the fixation point may develop (Seidel's sign)
- Simultaneously, isolated scotomas in Bjerrum's area may coalesce and form a classic arcuate scotoma (Bjerrum's scotoma)
- Double arcuate/ring scotoma (Arcuate scotomas both above and below the horizontal meridian)
- Roenne's nasal step (unequal contraction of peripheral isopters due to the loss of corresponding bundles of peripheral arcuate nerve fibres)

92. Rubeosis iridis is NOT seen in:

a. Neovascularization b. Diabetic retinopathy
c. CRAO d. CRVO

Rubeosis iridis is a condition of the iris of the eye in which new abnormal blood vessels (i.e. neovascularization) are found on the surface of the iris. This condition is often associated with diabetes in advanced proliferative diabetic retinopathy. Other conditions causing rubeosis iridis include central retinal vein occlusion, ocular ischemic syndrome, and chronic retinal detachment.

93. Argon laser trabeculoplasty is done in:

a. Angle closure glaucoma
b. Angle recession glaucoma
c. Secondary glaucoma d. Open angle glaucoma

A **trabeculoplasty** is a modification of the trabecular meshwork. **Laser trabeculoplasty** (LTP) is the application of a laser beam to burn areas of the trabecular meshwork, located near the base of the iris, to increase fluid outflow. LTP is used in the treatment of various open-angle glaucomas. The two types of laser trabeculoplasty are **argon laser trabeculoplasty** (ALT) and **selective laser trabeculoplasty** (SLT).

94. Sympathetic ophthalmitis results due to:

a. Penetrating injury of ciliary body
b. Uveitis
c. Glaucoma d. Trachoma

Sympathetic ophthalmia (SO) is a bilateral diffuse granulomatous uveitis (a kind of inflammation) of both eyes following trauma to one eye. It can leave the patient completely blind. Symptoms may develop from days to several years after a penetrating eye injury.

95. MC site for iris coloboma:

a. Inferonasal b. Superonasal
c. Inferotemporal d. Superotemporal

Colobomas of the uveal tract are often found in association with other ocular anomalies including those with systemic disease. They are usually located in the inferonasal quadrant as a result of defective closure of the embryonic fissure in the optic cup.

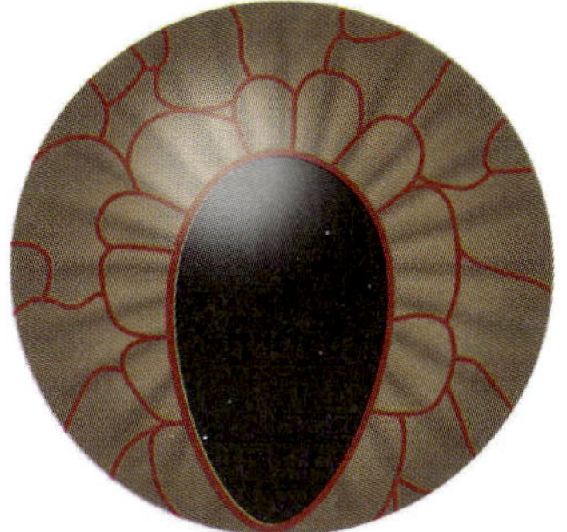

Typical coloboma of the iris.

96. Laser iridotomy done in:

a. Congenital glaucoma b. Open angle glaucoma
c. Angle closure glaucoma d. Neovascular glaucoma

In acute angle-closure glaucoma cases, surgical iridectomy has been superseded by Nd:YAG laser iridotomy, because the laser procedure is much safer. Opening the globe for a surgical iridectomy in a patient with high intraocular pressure greatly increases the risk of suprachoroidal hemorrhage, with potential for associated expulsive hemorrhage. Nd:YAG laser iridotomy avoids such a catastrophe by laser created hole in the iris, which facilitates flow of aqueous humor from the posterior to the anterior chamber of the eye.

97. Pupil in acute iritis:

a. Dilated b. Vertically oval
c. Normal d. Constricted

Iritis is characterized by a **miotic** constricted **pupil** and photophobia

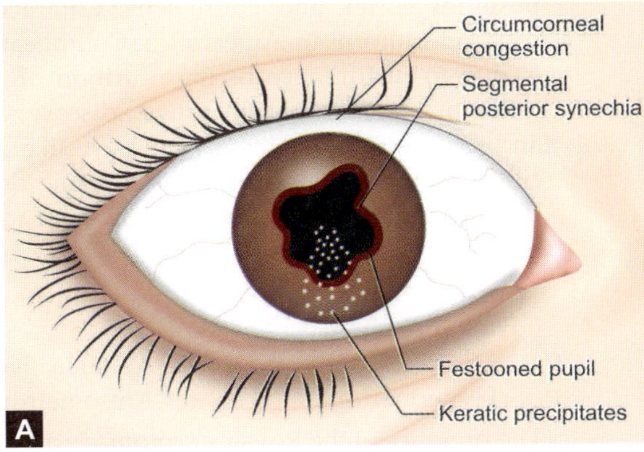

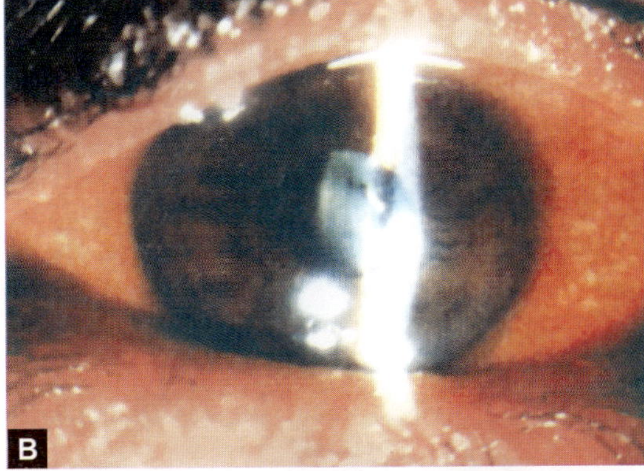

Signs of anterior uveitis: (A) diagrammatic depiction; (B) clinical photograph of a patient with acute anterior uveitis.

Ans. 92. **c.** CRAO 93. **d.** Open angle glaucoma 94. **a.** Penetrating... 95. **a.** Inferonasal
96. **c.** Angle closure... 97. **d.** Constricted

98. Most common etiolopathogenetic cause of glaucoma is:
a. Raised pressure in episcleritis veins
b. Decreased outflow
c. Increased formation of aqueous humor
d. Increased scleral outflow

In open/wide-angle glaucoma, flow is reduced through the trabecular meshwork, due to the degeneration and obstruction of the trabecular meshwork, whose original function is to absorb the aqueous humor. Loss of aqueous humor absorption leads to increased resistance and thus a chronic, painless buildup of pressure in the eye. In close/narrow-angle, the iridocorneal angle is completely closed because of forward displacement of the final roll and root of the iris against the cornea, resulting in the inability of the aqueous fluid to flow from the posterior to the anterior chamber and then out of the trabecular network. This accumulation of aqueous humor causes an acute increase of pressure and pain.

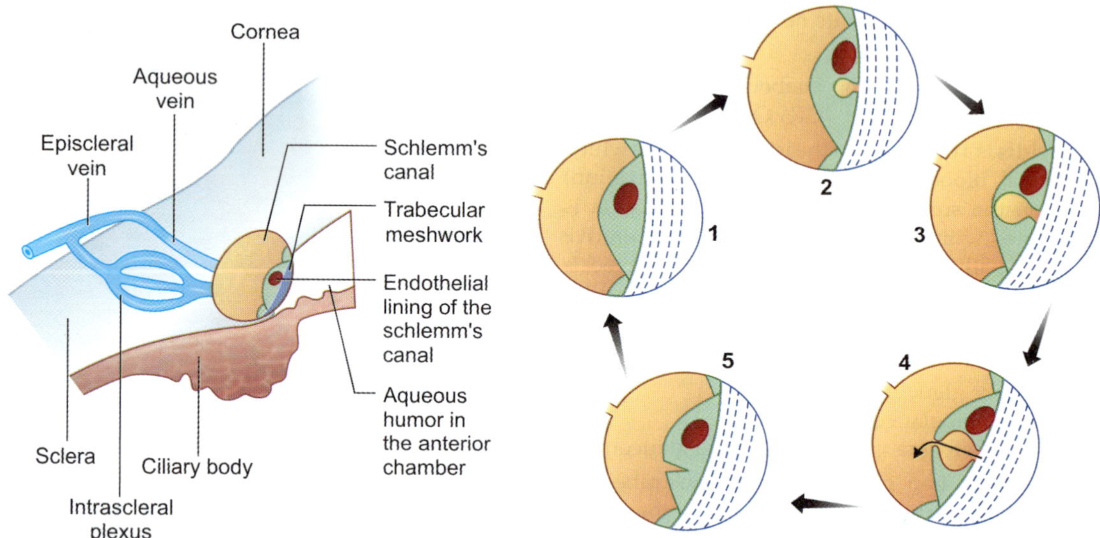

Vacuolation theory of aqueous transport across the inner wall of the Schlemm's canal: 1. Nonvacuolated stage; 2. Stage of early infolding of basal surface of the endothelial cell; 3. Stage of macrovacuolar structure formation; 4. Stage of vacuolar transcellular channel formation; 5. Stage of occlusion of the basal infolding.

99. True regarding buphthalmos are ALL EXCEPT:
a. Developmental anomaly of the angle of the anterior chamber
b. Bull like eyes
c. Unilateral
d. Photophobia is the initial sign

In most cases **buphthalmos** affects both eyes (*i.e.* it is **bilateral**), but the effect is not necessarily the same on each eye.

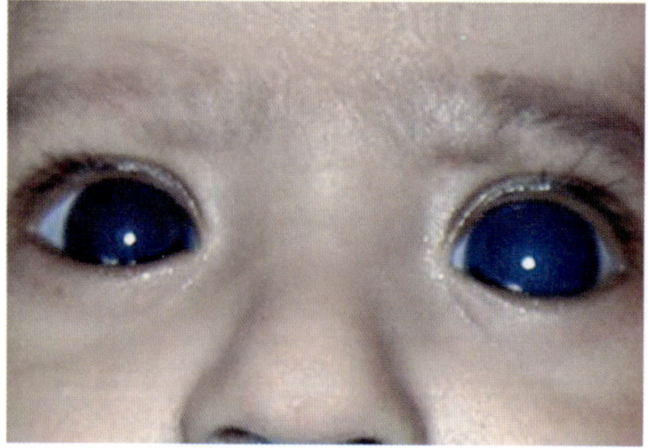
Corneal enlargement in a child with congenital glaucoma.

LENS

100. Complicated cataract can occur in all EXCEPT:
a. High myopia
b. Retinal detachment
c. Vitreous movement
d. Anterior uveitis

Complicated cataract has characteristic breadcrumb appearance and rainbow display of colours (polychromatic lustre). Cataract may remain stationary in posterior cortex or progress to involve the whole posterior cortex and entire lens. Cataract is usually soft and uniform in appearance. Complicated Cataract is due to disturbance of the nutrition of lens due to inflammatory or degenerative disease of anterior and /or posterior segment of the eye like iridocyclitis, cilitis, pars planitis, choroiditis, myopic degeneration, retinitis pigmentosa, retinal detachment, other retinal pigmentory dystrophies etc.

101. Which of the following condition shows Jack in the box phenomenon?
a. Myopia
b. Aphakia
c. Hypermetropia
d. Anisometropia

The presence of the Rovsing scotoma in aphakia leads to another interesting phenomenon. If an interesting object

Ans. **98. b.** Decreased out... **99. c.** Unilateral **100. c.** Vitreous movement **101. b.** Aphakia

appears in the periphery of the patients visual field, it appears blurred (because the light is passing from the side of the spectacle frame). The person tends to move his head towards the object in order to see it clearly. But as he turns the head the object comes to lie in the area of scotoma and thus disappears. As he turns his head further so that the object comes to lie in front of the spectacle in the visible area and so reappears again clear and sharp. This sudden disappearance and sharp reappearance of the objects is called **jack-in-the-box phenomenon**.

102. Commonest congenital cataract is:

a. Coralliform b. Capsular
c. Zonular d. Nuclear

Zonular cataract (lamellar cataract; perinuclear cataract) is the most common cataract in children presenting with visual impairment. It may be inherited through dominant genes, or caused by malnutrition during pregnancy or early infancy. This type of cataract occurs in both eyes, shortly before or after birth. The opacity is sharply delineated, and usually consists of two opaque rings. Partial blindness may possibly occur.

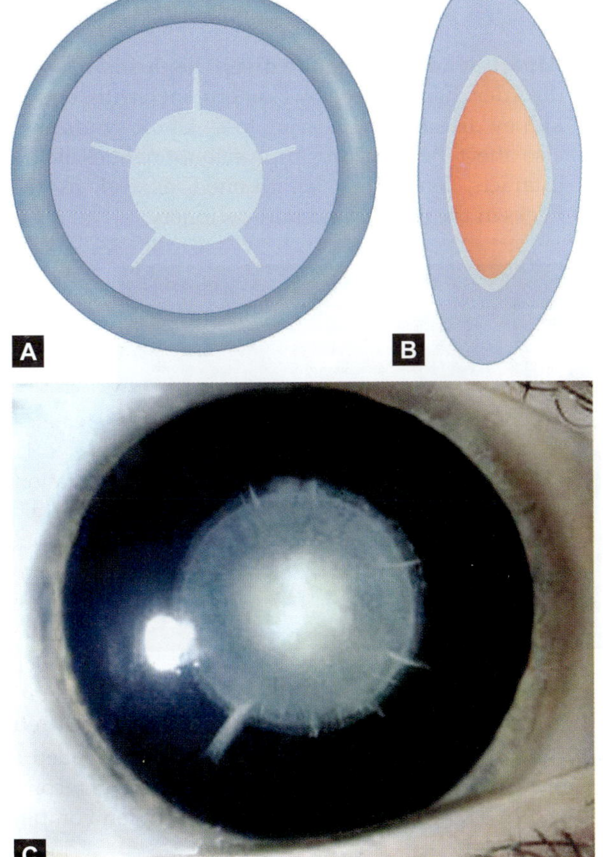

Lamellar cataract: (A and B) diagrammatic depiction as seen by oblique illumination and in optical section with the beam of the slit-lamp, respectively; (C) clinical photograph

103. Spectacles are prescribed in patients with aphakia after:

a. 1 week b. 2 weeks
c. 4 weeks d. 6 weeks

Spectacles in aphakia:

- *Advantages*
  - It is a cheap, easy and safe method of correcting aphakia.
- *Disadvantages*
  - Image is magnified by 30%, so not useful in unilateral aphakia (produce diplopia).
  - Problem of spherical and chromatic aberrations of thick lenses.
  - Field of vision is limited.
  - Prismatic effect of thick glasses.
  - 'Roving ring Scotoma' (Jack in the box phenomenon).
  - Cosmetic blemish especially in young aphakes.

104. Constantly changing refractive error is seen in:

a. Traumatic cataract b. Diabetic cataract
c. Morgagnian cataract d. Intumescent cataract

Diabetic cataract formation follows an increase in sugars in the lens. The excess sugar within the lens is reduced by aldose reductase to its alcohol, but the lens capsule is relatively impermeable to sugar alcohols. Because of the excess sugar alcohol (polyol), the lens imbibes water, causing osmotic imbalance. Eventually, increased sodium and decreased potassium levels and decreased glutathione levels lead to cataract formation.

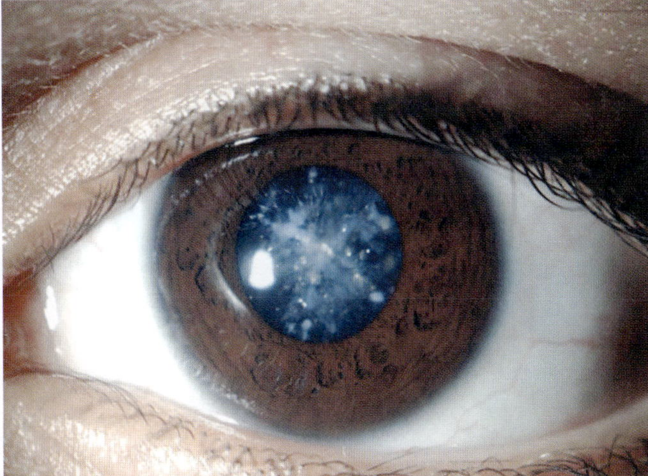

Snow-flake (diabetic) cataract.

105. Commonest cause of uniocular diplopia:

a. Rupture of superior oblique muscle
b. Third nerve palsy
c. Subluxated lens
d. Cataract

Monocular diplopia can occur when something distorts light transmission through the eye to the retina. There

Ans. 102. **c.** Zonular 103. **d.** 6 weeks 104. **b.** Diabetic cataract 105. **d.** Cataract

may be > 2 images. One of the images is of normal quality (e.g. brightness, contrast, clarity); the rest are of inferior quality. The most common causes of monocular diplopia are:

- Cataract
- Corneal shape problems, such as keratoconus or surface irregularity
- Uncorrected refractive error, usually astigmatism
- Other causes include corneal scarring and dislocated lens.
- Complaints also may represent malingering.

Signs of senile cataract.

Examination	*Nuclear cataract*	*ISC*	*MSC*	*HMSC (M)*	*HMSC (S)*
1. Visual acuity	6/9 to PL+	6/9 to CF+	HM+ to PL+	PL+	PL+
2. Colour of lens	Grey, amber, brown, black or red	Greyish white	Pearly white with sinking brownish nucleus	Milky white	Dirty white with hyper white spots
3. Iris shadow	Not seen	Seen	Not seen	Not seen	Not seen
4. Distant direct ophthalmoscopy with dilated pupil	Central dark area against red fundal glow	Multiple dark areas against red fundal glow	No red glow but white pupil due to complete cataract	No red glow milky white pupil	No red glow dirty white pupil
5. Slit-lamp examination	Nuclear opacity clear cortex	Areas of normal with cataractous cortex	Complete cortex is cataractous	Milky white cortex with sunken brownish nucleus	Shrunken cataractous lens with thickened anterior capsule

ISC: Immature senile cataract, MSC: Mature senile cataract, HMSC (M) Hypermature senile cataract (Morgagnian), HMSC (S): Hypermature senile cataract (Sclerotic), PL: Perception of light, HM: Hand movements, CF: Counting finger

106. Lenticonus is seen in:

a. Alstrom's syndrome
b. Avellis syndrome
c. Alport's syndrome
d. Down's syndrome

Alport syndrome or **hereditary nephritis**is a genetic disorder characterized by glomerulonephritis, end-stage kidney disease, and hearing loss. Alport syndrome can also affect the eyes, causing eye abnormalities including cataracts, lenticonus, keratoconus, as well as retinal flecks in the macula and mid-periphery.

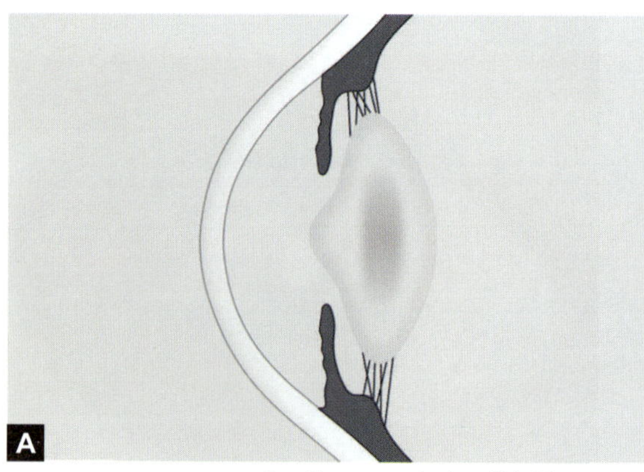

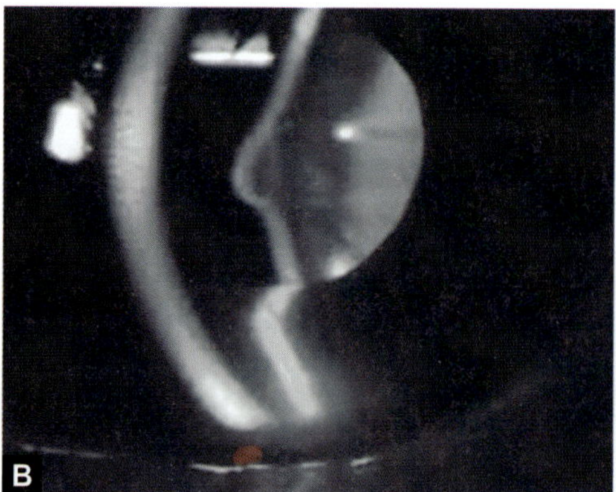

Lenticonus anterior: (A) Diagrammatic; (B) Slit-lamp photograph.

107. Spontaneous absorption of lenticular material is observed in:

a. Persistent hyperplastic primary vitreous
b. Aniridia
c. Hallermann Streiff syndrome
d. Myotonic dystrophy

Patients with Hallermann Streiff syndrome are shorter than the average person and may not develop hair in many places, including in the facial, leg and pubic areas. Patients also have eye problems including clouded eyes or reduced eye size, bilateral cataracts and glaucoma. It can be associated with sleep apnea. It can complicate intubation.

108. Sunflower cataract is associated with:

a. Chalcosis
b. Juvenile diabetes mellitus
c. Down syndrome
d. Trauma

Ans. **106. c.** Alport's syd... **107. c.** Hallermann Streiff... **108. a.** Chalcosis

Copper deposition in the lens leads to a '**sunflower**' or 'sunburst' **cataract** consisting of a greenish central disc in the anterior capsule with spoke-like radial.

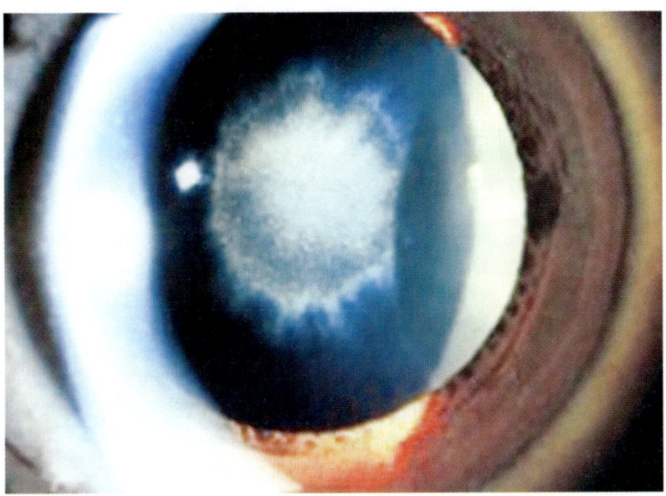

Sunflower cataract.

109. Cupuliform cataract involves which part of lens:

a. Posterior cortex b. Anterior cortex
c. Upper pole d. Lower pole

Cupuliform Cataract is a disc or saucer shaped area of the cortex beneath the posterior capsule undergo opacification. The opacity being central, the vision is worst in bright ambient illumination when the pupil is constricted.

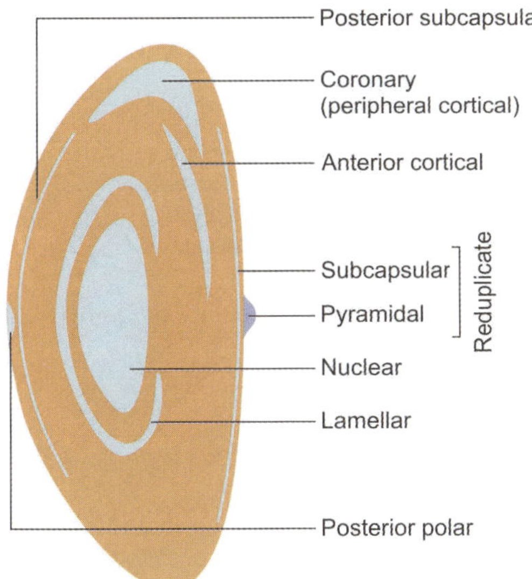

Morphological shapes of cataract.

110. Complicated cataract involves:

a. Anterior capsule b. Upper pole of lens
c. Lower pole of lens d. Posterior capsule

Complicated/secondary cataract a cataract, usually posterior subcapsular, that arises from other disease (especially iridocyclitis), degeneration (such as chronic glaucoma or retinal detachment), or surgery (such as glaucoma filtering or retinal reattachment).

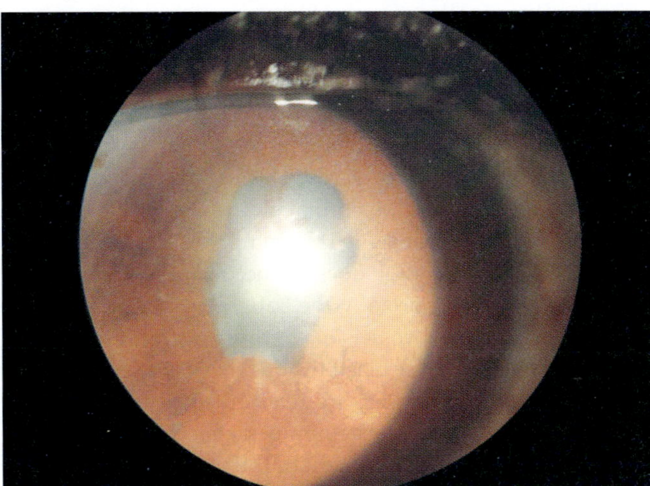

Complicated cataract with healed iridocyclitis.

111. Rehabilitation in removed cataractous lens is best done by:

a. Spectacles b. Intraocular lens
c. Contact lenses
d. Refractive corneal surgery

Intraocular lens implantation is the best available method of correcting aphakia. Therefore, it is the commonest modality being employed now a days.

RETINA

112. All of the following are associated with cherry red spots EXCEPT:

a. Trauma b. Tay Sachs disease
c. CRAO d. CRVO

Fundus examination in CRVO reveals engorged, tortuous retinal veins, oedema of the disc and retina, flame shaped and blot haemorrhages in the peripapillary and the macular area and cotton wool spots.

113. Cause of sudden painless loss of vision in diabetic patient:

a. Massive vitreous hemorrhage
b. Tractional retinal detachment
c. Diabetic retinopathy
d. Neovascularization

Trauma, diabetic and hypertensive retinopathy are common cause of vitreous hemorrhage. Small vitreous hemorrhage often is perceived as new multiple floaters, moderate vitreous hemorrhage is perceived as dark streaks, and dense vitreous hemorrhage tends to significantly decrease vision even to light perception. Usually, no pain is associated with vitreous hemorrhage. Exceptions may include cases of neovascular glaucoma, severe acute ocular hypertension secondary to ghost-cell glaucoma, or trauma.

Ans. **109. a.** Posterior cortex **110. d.** Posterior capsule **111. b.** Intraocular lens **112. d.** CRVO **113. a.** Massive vitreous hemorrhage

114. Cherry red spot on fundoscopy is NOT a feature of:

a. Generalized gangliosidoses
b. Retinopathy of prematurity
c. Sandhoff variant
d. Tay-Sachs disease

Changes in retinopathy of prematurity:

During development, blood vessels grow from the central part of the retina outwards. This process is completed a few weeks before the normal time of delivery. However, in premature babies it is incomplete. If blood vessels grow normally, ROP does not occur. If the vessels grow and branch abnormally the baby develops ROP. These abnormal blood vessels may grow up from the plane of the retina and may bleed inside the eye. When the blood and abnormal vessels are reabsorbed, it may give rise to multiple *band like* membranes which can pull up the retina, causing detachment of the retina and eventually blindness before 6 months.

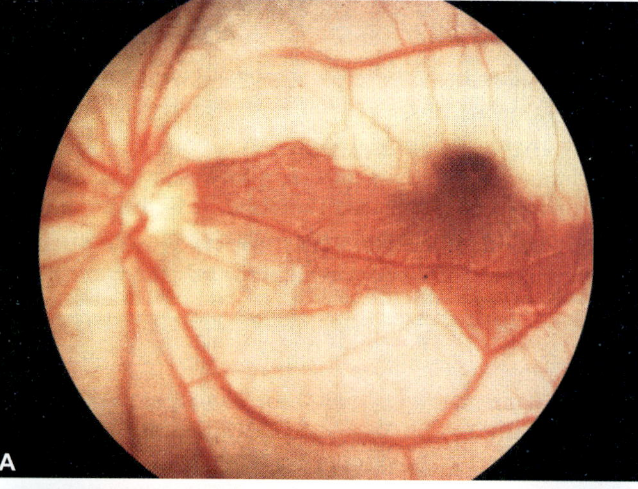

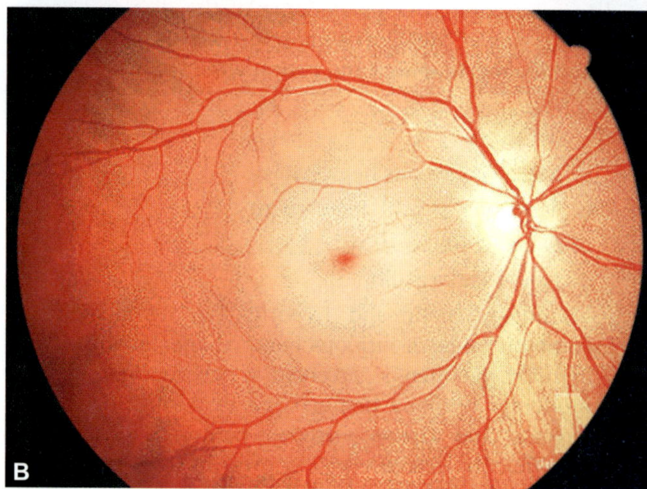

Fundus photograph showing marked retinal pallor in acute central retinal artery occlusion (CRAO): (A) with sparing of the territory supplied by cilioretinal artery; and (B) cherry-red spot in the absence of cilioretinal artery

115. Cause of sudden loss of vision in a diabetic patient:

a. Neovascular glaucoma
b. Central retinal artery block
c. Vitreous hemorrhage
d. None of the above

Diabetic retinopathy can cause blindness in 2 ways: Macular edema and proliferative retinopathy with vitreous hemorrhage.

Flowchart depicting pathogenesis of diabetic retinopathy.

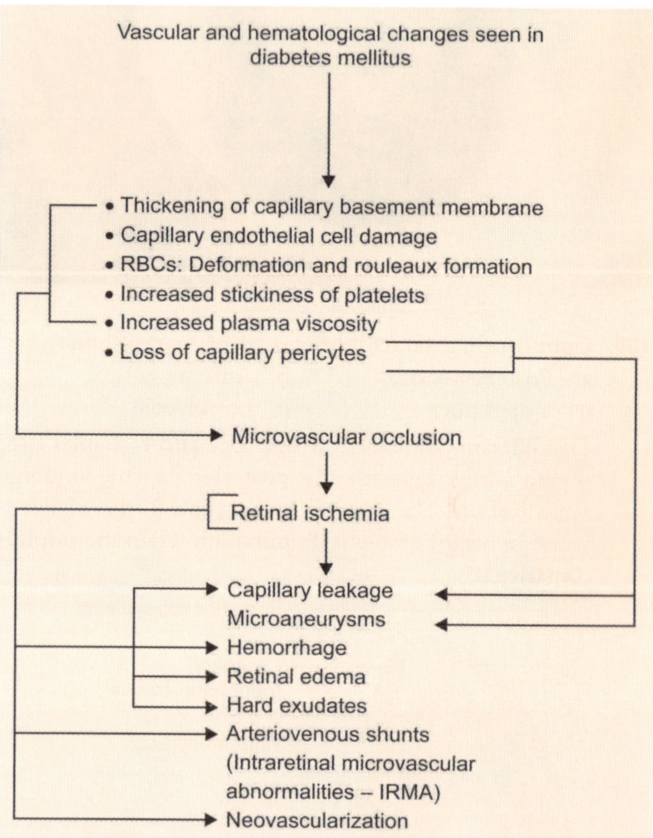

116. Cotton wool spots in diabetic retinopathy are due to:

a. Macular degenration
b. Retinal hemorrhage
c. Retinal holes
d. Retinal edema

Cotton wool spots are an abnormal finding on fundoscopic exam of the retina of the eye. They appear as fluffy white patches on the retina. They are caused by damage to nerve fibers and are a result of accumulations of axoplasmic material within the nerve fiber layer. There is reduced axonal transport (and hence backlog and accumulation of intracellular products) within the nerves because of the ischemia. This then causes the nerve fibers to be damaged by swelling in the surface layer of the retina.

Ans. **114. b.** Retinopathy of... **115. c.** Vitreous hemorrhage **116. d.** Retinal edema

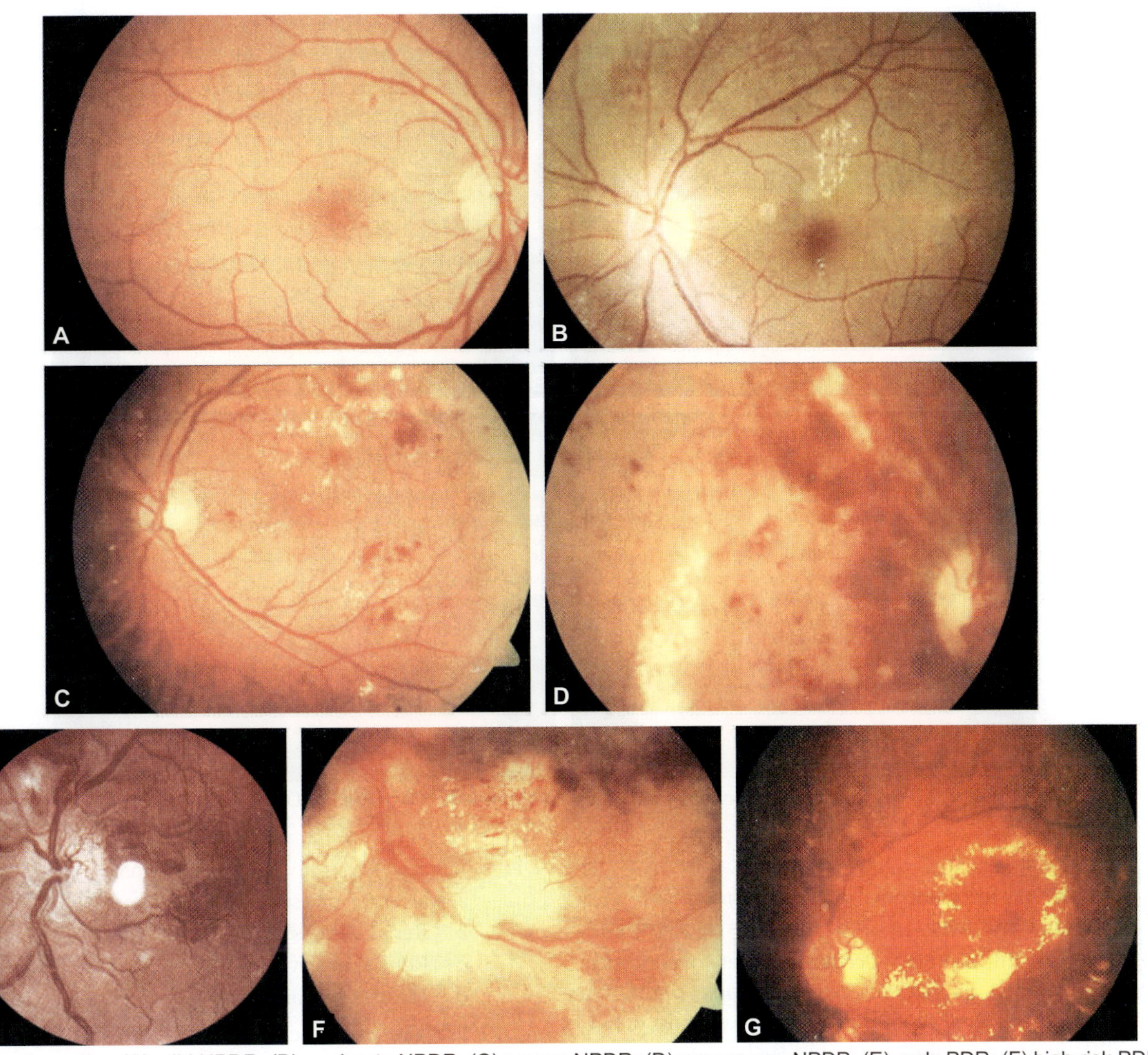

Diabetic retinopathy: (A) mild NPDR; (B) moderate NPDR; (C) severe NPDR; (D) very severe NPDR; (E) early PDR; (F) high-risk PDR; (G) focal exudative diabetic maculopathy.

117. Keith-Wagener classification is for:
a. Primary optic atrophy
b. Arteriosclerotic changes in retina
c. Hypertensive retinopathy
d. Diabetic retinopathy

Keith Wagener classification

Grade	Stage	Description	Ocular symptoms	Systemic involvement
1	Mild hypertension	Mild generalised arteriolar narrowing or sclerosis	No symptoms	None
2	More marked hyper-tension	Definite focal narrowing (arrows in figure) and arteriovenous crossings. Moderate to marked sclerosis of the retinal arterioles. Exaggerated arterial light reflex	No symptoms	None or minimal
3	Mild angiospatic retinopathy	Retinal haemorrhages, exudates and cotton wool spots. Sclerosis and spastic lesions of retinal arterioles	May be symptomatic	Cardiac, cerebral or renal dys-function are frequently identifi-able
4	Severe hypertensive retinopathy	Severe Grade III signs and papilledema. Elschning's spots are present in some	Symptomatic	Cardiac, cerebral and renal dysfunction are more severe

Ans. **117. c.** Hypertensive retinopathy

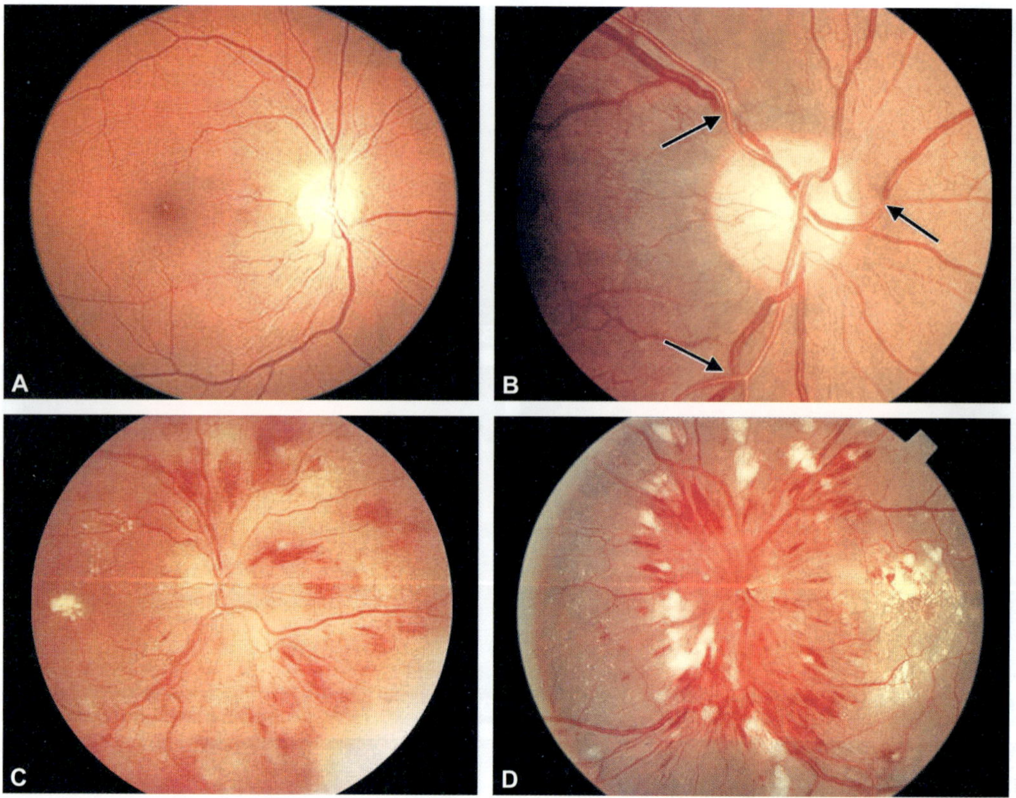

Hypertensive retinopathy: (A) grade I; (B) grade II; (C) grade III; (D) grade IV.

118. Ring scotoma is seen in:

a. Angle closure glaucoma b. Severe myopia
c. Night blindness d. Retinitis pigmentosa

Annular or ring scotomas occur in a variety of conditions, most notably in patients with various pigmentary retinopathies. Ring scotomas may also occur in patients with open angle glaucoma, but in such cases, the ring is actually caused by the coalescence of upper and lower arcuate scotomas originating from the physiologic blind spot and extending across the vertical midline into the nasal visual field.

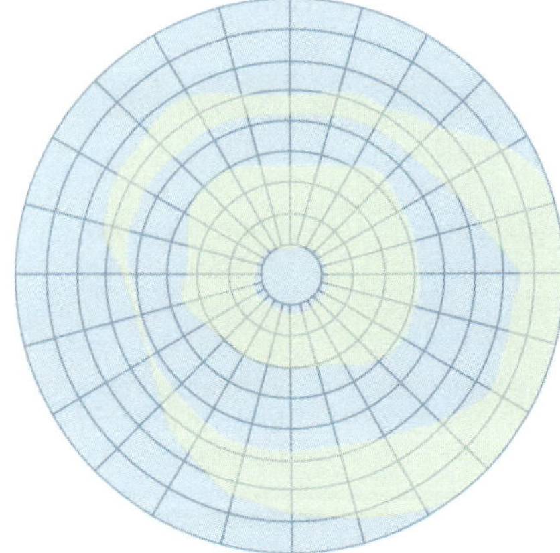
Field changes in retinitis pigmentosa.

119. Amaurosis fugax refers to occlusion of:

a. Mesenteric vessels
b. Renal vessels
c. Retinal artery
d. Middle cerebral artery

With respect to embolic and hemodynamic causes, this transient monocular visual loss ultimately occurs due to a temporary reduction in retinal artery, ophthalmic artery, or ciliary artery blood flow, leading to a decrease in retinal circulation which, in turn, causes retinal hypoxia. While, most commonly, emboli causing amaurosis fugax are described as coming from an atherosclerotic carotid artery, any emboli arising from vasculature preceding the retinal artery, ophthalmic artery, or ciliary arteries may cause this transient monocular blindness.

120. NOT a risk factor of rhegmatogenous retinal detachment:

a. Aphakia b. High myopia
c. Diabetes d. Pseudophakia

Diabetes causes Tractional retinal detachment (TRD), which occurs due to preretinal membrane formation and scarring that pulls the retina from its attachment. This may require surgery depending on the extent of the RD.

Ans. **118. d.** Retinitis pigm... **119. c.** Retinal artery **120. c.** Diabetes

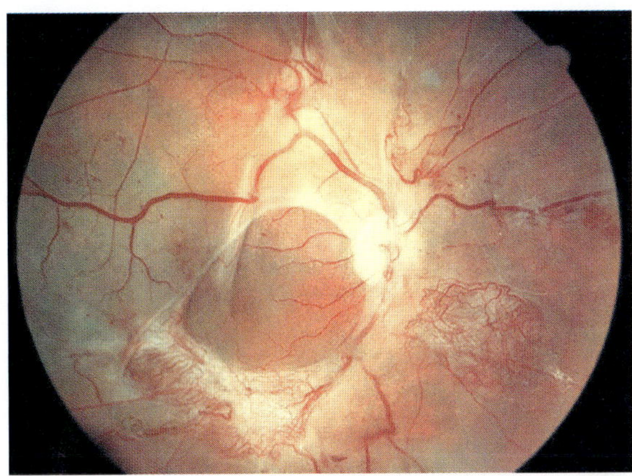
Tractional retinal detachment in a patient with advanced diabetic retinopathy.

121. Commonest early feature of diabetic retinopathy:
a. Dot and blot hemorrhages
b. Edema
c. Hard exudates
d. Neovascularization

In NPDR, the blood vessels in the retina are weakened causing tiny bulges called microaneurysms to protrude from their walls. This is the earliest feature followed by dot and blot hemorrhages

Differential diagnosis of ocular ischaemic syndrome

Condition		Similarities	Differences
1.	Nonischaemic CRVO	Unilateral retinal haemorrhages, venous dilatation and cotton wool spots	Veins are more tortuous, haemorrhages are more numerous, normal retinal arteriolar perfusion, disc oedema, and sometimes opticociliary shunt vessels can be seen on the disc.
2.	Diabetic retinopathy	Microaneurysms, dot and blot hemorrhages, venous dilatation, NVD and NVE, cotton wool spots	Usually bilateral, with characteristic hard exudates
3.	Hypertensive retinopathy	Arteriolar narrowing and focal constriction, retinal hemorrhages and cotton wool spots	Usually bilateral, no marked venous changes, and NVD and NVE.
4.	Aortic arch disease	Arteriolar narrowing, retinal hemorrhages, cotton wool spots, NVD and NVE	Usually bilateral, absent arm and neck pulses, cold hands, and spasm of arm muscles with exercise.

122. Characteristically associated with proliferative diabetic retinopathy:
a. Cotton wool spots
b. Papilloedema
c. Soft exudates
d. Neovascularization

Proliferative diabetic retinopathy (PDR) is the more advanced form of the disease. At this stage, new fragile blood vessels can begin to grow in the retina (neovascularization) and into the vitreous. The new blood vessel may leak blood into the vitreous, clouding vision.

123. FALSE statement regarding retinal detachment is:
a. Rhegmatogenous detachment is commonest type
b. May follow aphakia/ pseudophakia
c. Fellow eye is never involved
d. Surgery has good success rate

Because the abnormalities that caused the detachment are often bilateral, up to a third of patients may be blind in their other eye at presentation—often because of untreated retinal detachment

Flowchart depicting pathogenesis of rhegmatogenous retinal detachment.

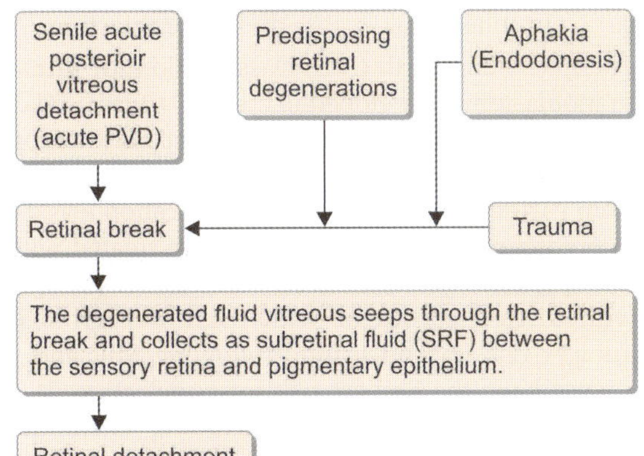

124. Optic disc changes of retinitis pigmentosa:
a. Consecutive optic atrophy
b. Blurring of optic disc margins
c. Hyperemia of disc
d. No significant change

In consecutive optic atrophy (e.g. retinitis pigmentosa, myopia, central retinal artery occlusion), the disc is waxy pale with a normal disc margin, marked attenuation of arteries, and a normal physiologic cup.

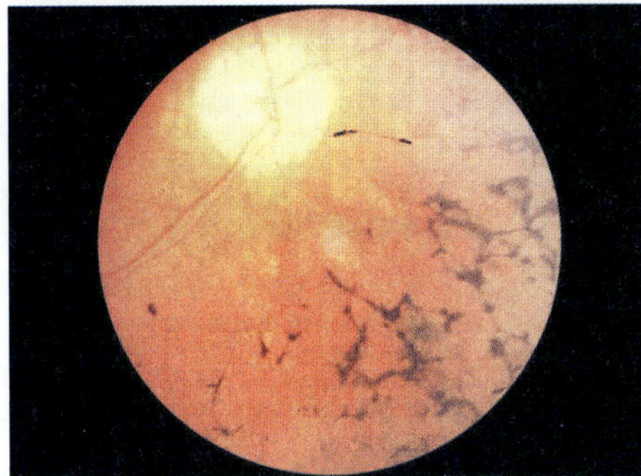
Fundus picture of retinitis pigmentosa with consecutive optic atrophy.

125. Eclipse burn/photoretinitis is due to:
a. Infrared rays
b. Ultraviolet light
c. Welding arc exposure
d. All of the above

Ans. 121. **a.** Dot and blot... 122. **d.** Neovascularization 123. **c.** Fellow eye is never... 124. **a.** Consecutive optic... 125. **d.** All of the above

Photoretinitis is another form that can occur due to infra-red rays (eclipse burn of retina), welding arc exposure, lightening retinopathy, etc. Photochemical effects are produced by UV and visible blue light and thermal effect is because of infra-red rays from the sun.

OPHTHALMIC ONCOLOGY

126. NOT seen in retinoblastoma:

a. Leucocoria
b. Reduced intraocular pressure
c. Esotropia
d. Secondary glaucoma

Pseudoglioma (non-neoplastic conditions having same clinical picture as that of retinoblastoma) have reduced IOP whereas in retinoblastoma, IOP is elevated.

127. Reese-Ellsworth classification is employed for:

a. Malignant melanoma
b. Retinoblastoma
c. Neuroblastoma
d. Nephroblastoma

The Reese-Ellsworth (R-E) classification for intraocular retinoblastoma, developed in the 1960s, was used during the last 40 years in assessing outcomes of therapy, and this classification facilitated the comparison of results from various studies. The R-E classification was devised to predict prognosis in eyes that were treated with EBR therapy. The classification scheme has five groups. Eyes with disease consistent with the lower groups have a lower risk for enucleation following EBR and group V eyes have the highest risk for enucleation. With the advent of other therapies, including chemotherapy, which has increasingly replaced EBR therapy in the treatment of intraocular disease, the usefulness of the R-E scheme is less apparent.

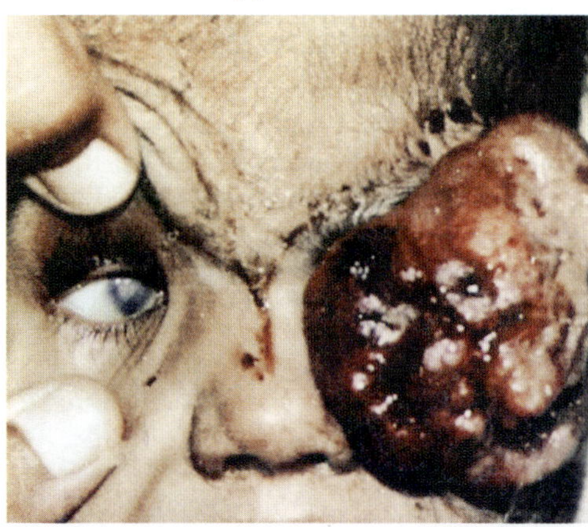

Fungating retinoblastoma involving the orbit.

128. All of the following are true for retinoblastoma EXCEPT:

a. Leucocoria is the most common presentation
b. Always unilateral
c. May have family history
d. Most common age group affected is 1-2 year

Bilateral retinoblastomas are commonly heritable, while unilateral retinoblastomas are commonly non-heritable. In about two-thirds of cases, only one eye is affected (unilateral retinoblastoma); in the other third, tumors develop in both eyes (bilateral retinoblastoma).

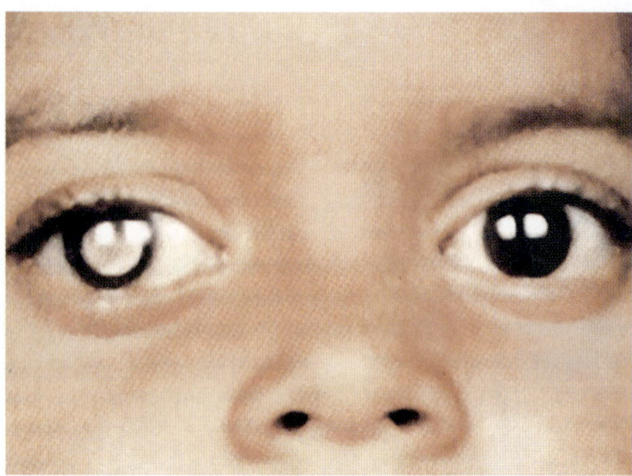

Leukocoria right eye in a patient with retinoblastoma.

129. Most common primary malignant tumor of orbit is:

a. Lacrimal gland carcinoma
b. Rhabdomyosarcoma
c. Lymphoma
d. Hemangioma

Rhabdomyosarcoma (RMS) is the **most common primary malignant orbital tumor** in children. The mean age at diagnosis is 8 years.

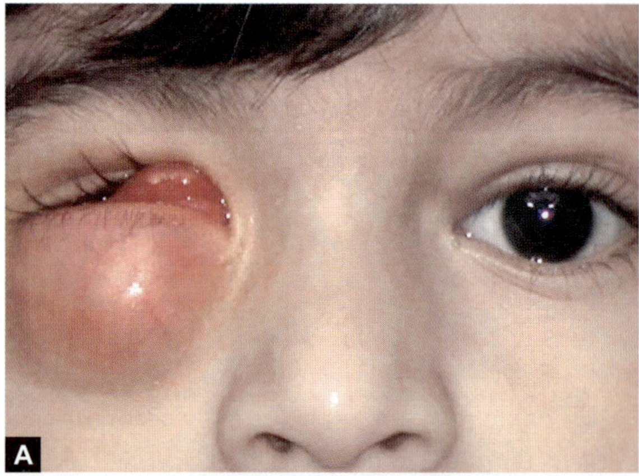

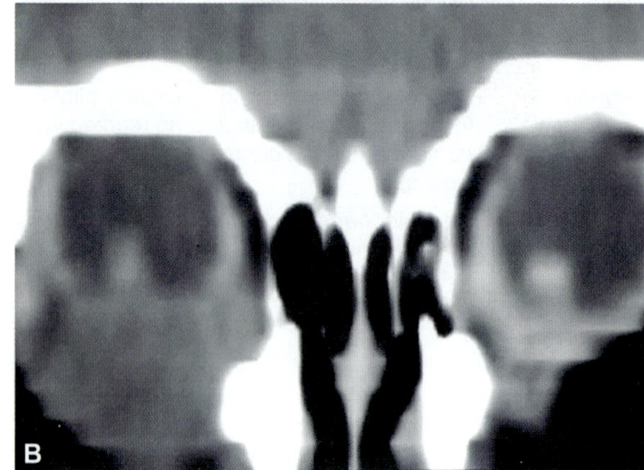

Rhabdomyosarcoma in inferior quadrant: (A) clinical photograph; (B) CT scan shows inferior orbital mass

Ans. **126. b.** Reduced intra... **127. b.** Retinoblastoma **128. b.** Always unilateral **129. b.** Rhabdomyosarcoma

130. In a child with retinoblastoma, which of the following is NOT a common finding in the X-ray:

a. Intraorbital calcification
b. Intracerebral calcification
c. Multiple cranial deposits
d. Widening of optic foramen

In areas of the world where ultrasonography and computerized tomography are not available, X-ray studies may be the only means of identifying intraocular (NOT intracerebral) calcium in patients with opaque media.

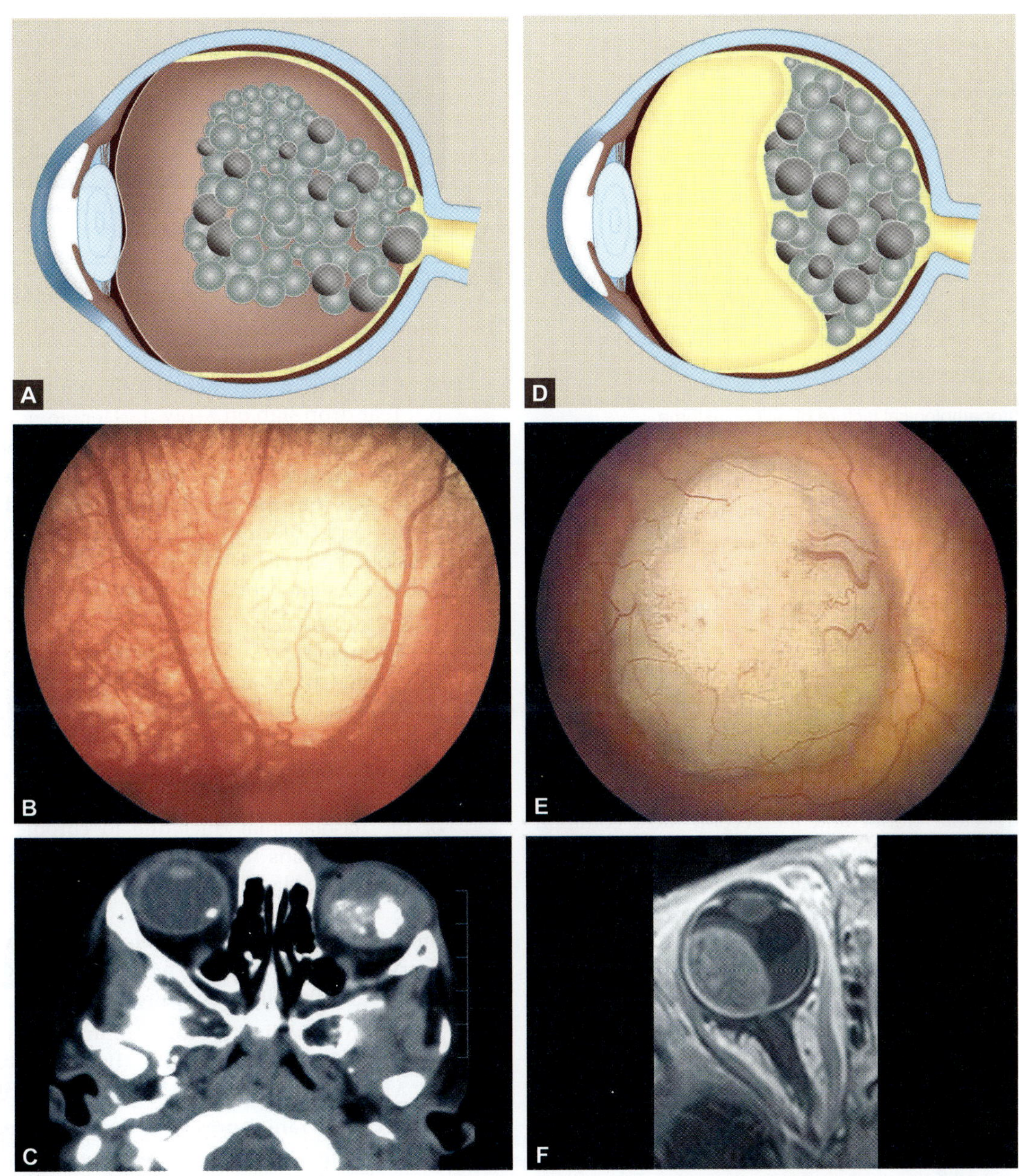

Diagrammatic depiction (A and D); Fundus photographs (B and E); CT scan/MRI scan (C and F) of endophytic and exophytic retinoblastoma, respectively.

131. Rosettes are a histological feature of:

a. Optic nerve glioma
b. Malignant melanoma
c. Retinoblastoma
d. Metastasis to eye

Macroscopically, viable tumor cells are found near blood vessels, while zones of necrosis are found in relatively avascular areas. Microscopically, both undifferentiated and differentiated elements may be present. Undifferentiated elements appear as collections of small,

Ans. **130. b.** Intracerebral... **131. c.** Retinoblas...

round cells with hyperchromatic nuclei; differentiated elements include Flexner-Wintersteiner rosettes, Homer Wright rosettes, and fleurettes from photoreceptor differentiation.

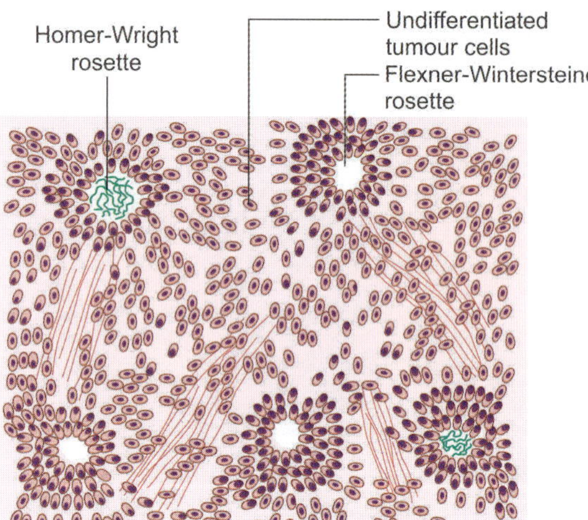

Histopathological picture of retinoblastoma.

132. Retinoblastoma gene is related to:

a. Chromosome 10 b. Chromosome 11
c. Chromosome 12 d. Chromosome 13

In children with the heritable genetic form of retinoblastoma there is a mutation in the RB1 gene on chromosome 13. RB1 was the first tumor suppressor gene cloned.

133. Most common primary intraocular tumour of adults:

a. Choroidal osteoma
b. Malignant melanoma of choroid
c. Retinoblastoma d. Neurofibroma

Choroidal melanoma is the most common primary malignant intraocular tumor and the second most common type of primary malignant melanoma in the body. It most often affects whites of northern European descent.

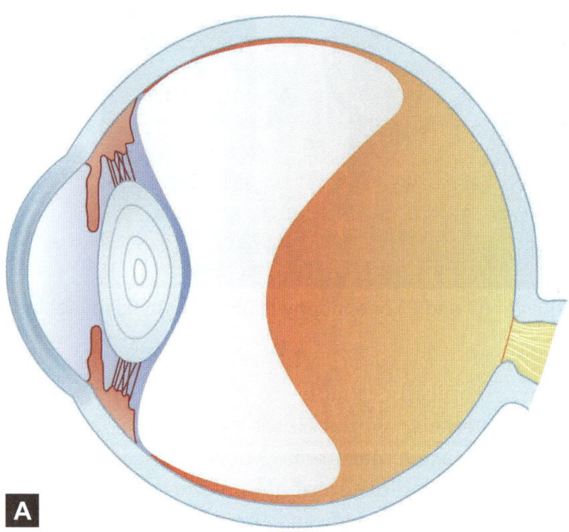

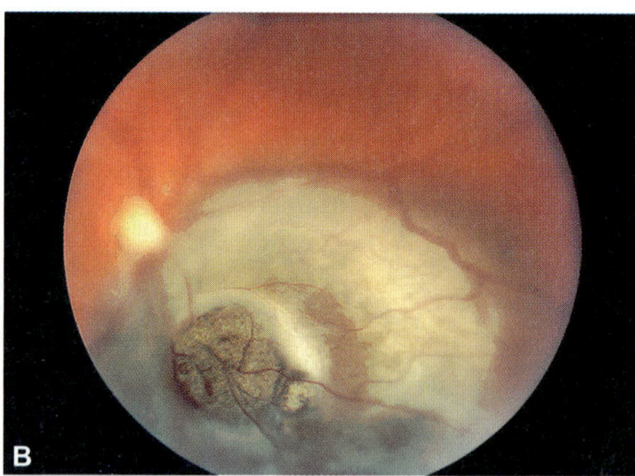

Malignant melanoma of the choroid causing exudative retinal detachment: (A) diagrammatic depiction in cut section; (B) fundus photograph.

MISCELLANEOUS

134. Blow-out fracture of orbit are associated with all EXCEPT:

a. Orbital floor and medial wall commonly injured
b. Tear drop sign on X-ray
c. Diplopia d. Normal vision

In the fracture of the floor of orbit, the eyeball is depressed into the maxillary antrum, and the inferior rectus and inferior oblique muscles are entrapped causing diplopia. There may be proptosis because of reactive oedema and intraorbital haemorrhage.

135. Chronic dacryocystitis is ideally managed by:

a. Syringing b. Dacryocystectomy
c. Conjunctivo-dacryo-cysto-rhinostomy
d. Dacryo-cysto-rhinostomy

Dacryocystorhinostomy (DCR) is a surgical procedure to restore the flow of tears into the nose from the lacrimal sac when the nasolacrimal duct does not function (obstruction of the nasolacrimal duct due to chronic obstruction). Atrophic rhinitis is an absolute contraindication. In case of acute dacryocystitis, this operation can not be done immediately, rather it is done after a period of time. In case of elderly patients (above 70 years of age), dacryocystectomy is preferred to dacryocystorhinostomy as old age naturally causes atrophy in nasal mucosa.

136. Raised intracranial tension commonly affects:

a. Inferior oblique b. Lateral rectus
c. Middle rectus d. Superior oblique

Raised intracranial pressure disproportionately affects the VI cranial nerve & lateral rectus is the muscle supplied by CN VI

137. NOT a complication of ulcerative blepharitis:

a. Trichiasis b. Tylosis
c. Madarosis d. Poliosis

Poliosis is the decrease or absence of melanin (or color) in head hair, eyebrows, or eyelashes. It can give rise to a "Mallen Streak" that can be hereditary.

Ans. 132. **d.** Chromosome 13 133. **b.** Malignant melanoma... 134. **d.** Normal vision 135. **d.** Dacryo-cysto-rhinostomy 136. **b.** Lateral rectus 137. **d.** Poliosis

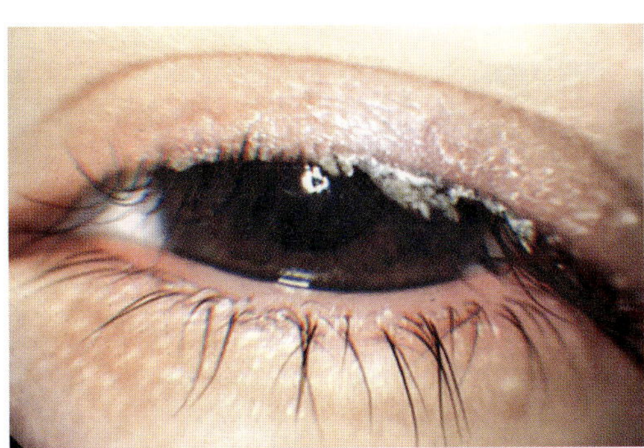

Bacterial blepharitis.

138. Feature of unilateral oculomotor nerve palsy:

a. Pupillary light reflex is completely absent
b. Visual loss
c. Accommodation reflex is absent
d. Drooping of eyelid

Ptosis occurs due to dysfunction of the muscles that raise the eyelid or their nerve supply (oculomotor nerve for levator palpebrae superioris and sympathetic nerves for superior tarsal muscle).

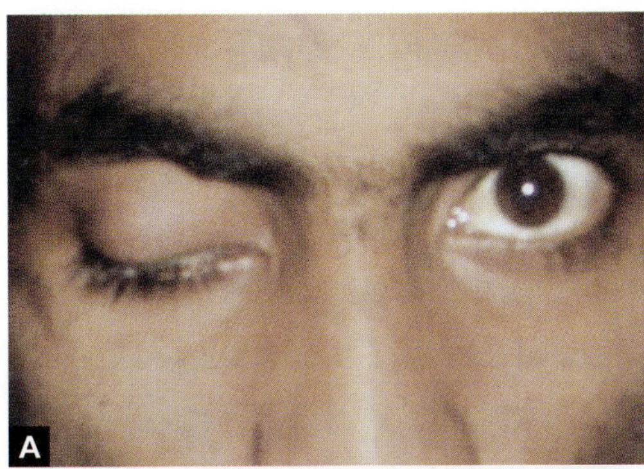

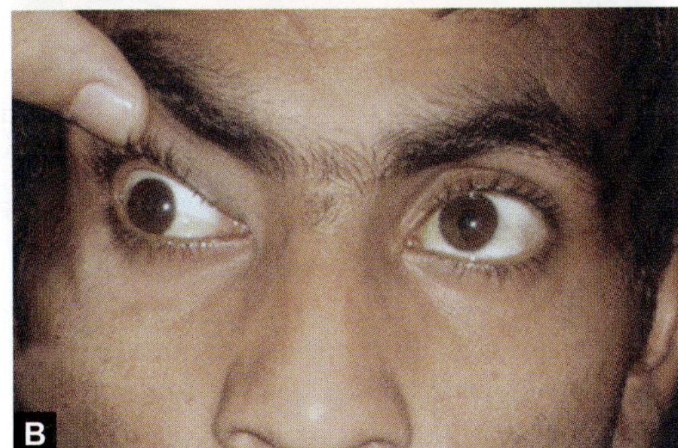

Patient with third cranial nerve paralysis showing: (A) ptosis; (B) divergent squint.

139. A boy complains of pain while reading. Diagnosis could be:

a. Uncorrected hypermetropia
b. Fully corrected hypermetropia
c. Spring catarrh
d. Glaucoma

A child with more severe farsightedness may

- Have headaches.
- Rub his or her eyes often.
- Have trouble reading or show little interest in reading.

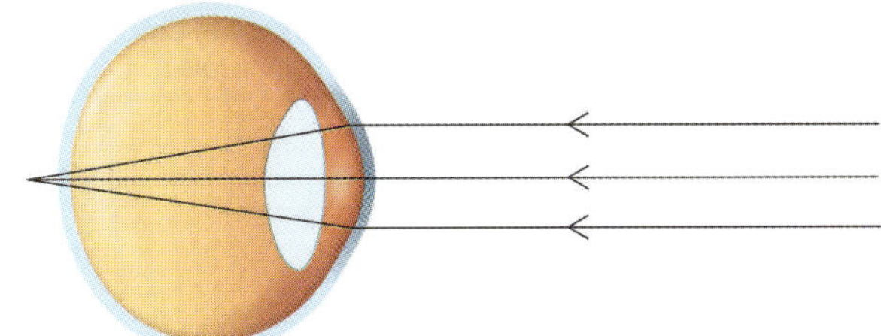

Refraction in a hypermetropic eye.

140. Cause of unilateral amblyopia:

a. High anisometropia
b. Hysteria
c. Meningitis
d. Uremia

Amblyopia has three main causes:

- Strabismic: By strabismus (misaligned eyes)
- Refractive: By anisometropia (high degrees of nearsightedness, farsightedness, or astigmatism in one or both eyes)
- Deprivational: By deprivation of vision early in life by vision-obstructing disorders such as congenital cataract

141. Anterior ischemic optic neuropathy (AION) is seen in case of:

a. Sarcoidosis
b. Chronic iridocyclitis
c. Giant cell arteritis
d. Chronic simple glaucoma

Anterior ischemic optic neuropathy(AION) is a medical condition involving loss of vision due to damage to the optic nerve from insufficient blood supply. AION is generally divided into two types: arteritic AION (or AAION) and non-arteritic AION (NAION or simply AION). AAION results from thrombotic and inflammatory occlusion of short posterior ciliary arteries caused by Giant cell arteritis/GCA.

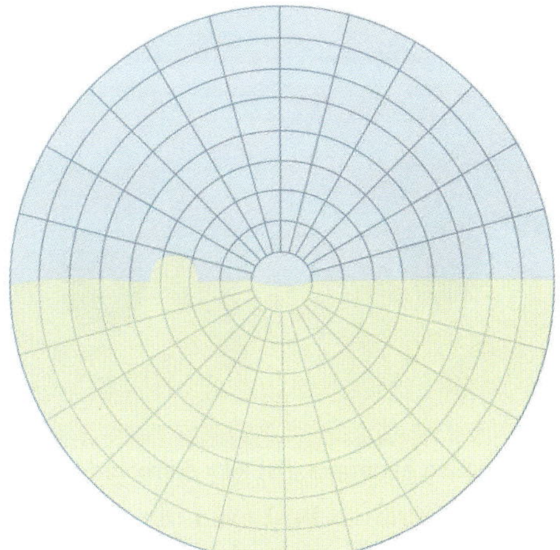

Altitudinal hemianopia in AION.

142. 1 mm change in the axial length of the eyeball produces a change in refractive index by:

a. 1D
b. 2D
c. 3D
d. 4D

Ans. **138. d.** Drooping of... **139. a.** Uncorrected hyper... **140. a.** High anisometropia **141. c.** Giant cell... **142. c.** 3D

Each 3 D of myopia corresponds to an increase in the **length** of the eye of **1 mm**.

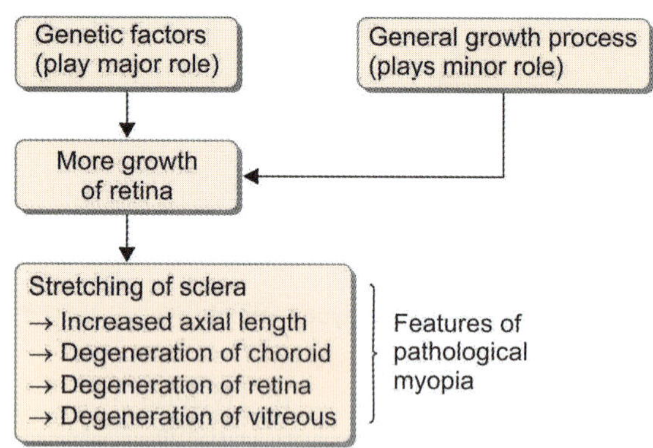

Etiological hypothesis for pathological myopia.

143. Type of squint, which can be corrected by spectacles:

a. Paralytic squint b. Convergence squint
c. Accommodation squint d. None of the above

In cases of accommodative esotropia, the eyes turn inward due to the effort of focussing far-sighted eyes, and the treatment of this type of strabismus necessarily involves refractive correction, which is usually done via corrective glasses or contact lenses, and in these cases surgical alignment is considered only if such correction does not resolve the eye turn.

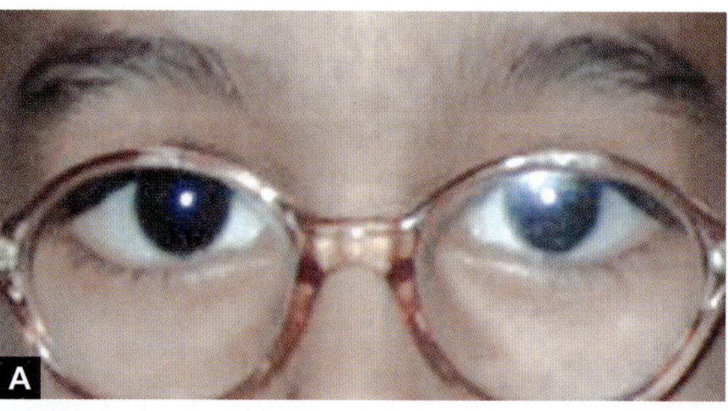

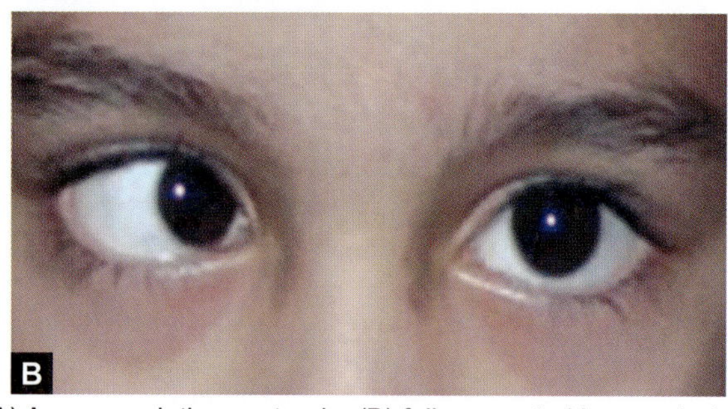

(A) Accommodative esotropia, (B) fully corrected by spectacles.

144. Radial keratotomy is best used in:

a. Hypermetropia b. Astigmatism
c. Anisometropia d. Myopia

Radial keratotomy (RK) is a refractive surgical procedure to correct myopia (nearsightedness) that was developed in 1974, by Svyatoslav Fyodorov, a Russian ophthalmologist.

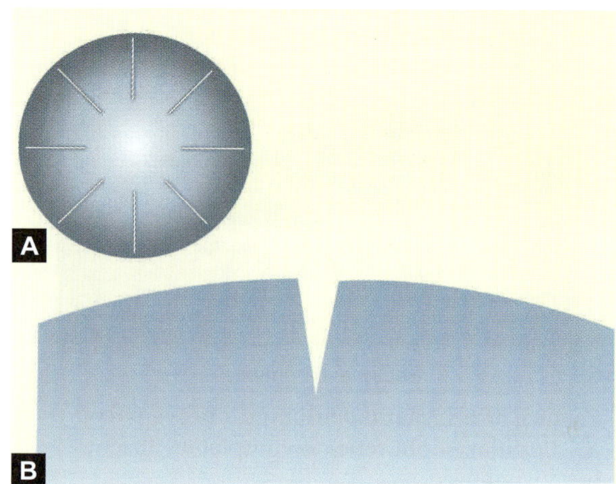

Radial keratotomy. (A) configuration of radial incisions; (B) depth of incision.

145. Lattice degeneration is seen in:

a. Myopia b. Hypermetropia
c. Presbyopia d. Astigmatism

Lattice degeneration is a disease of the human eye wherein the peripheral retina becomes atrophic in a lattice pattern and may develop tears, breaks, or holes, which may further progress to retinal detachment. It is an important cause of retinal detachment in young myopic individuals. The cause is unknown, but pathology reveals inadequate blood flow resulting in ischemia and fibrosis.

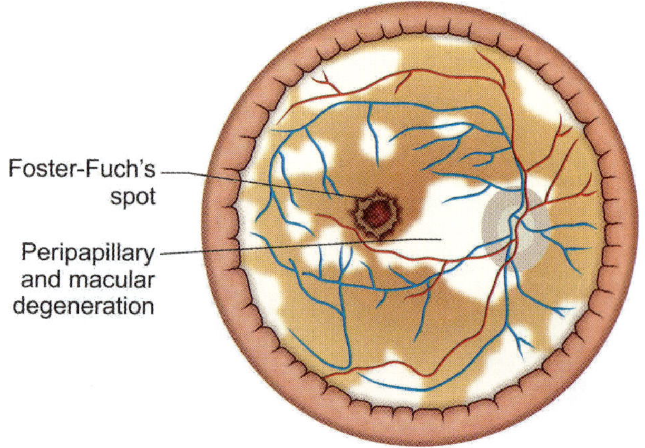

Fundus changes in pathological myopia.

146. True for chalazion:

a. Acute inflammation of Zeis gland
b. Acute inflammation of meibomian gland
c. Chronic inflammation of meibomian gland
d. Chronic inflammation of Zeis gland

A **chalazion**, also known as a **meibomian gland lipogranuloma**, is a cyst in the eyelid that is caused by inflammation of a blocked meibomian gland, usually on the upper eyelid. Chalazia differ from styes (hordeola) in that they are subacute and usually painless nodules. They may become acutely inflamed, but unlike a stye, chalazia usually sit inside the lid rather than on the lid margin.

Ans. **143. c.** Accommodat... **144. d.** Myopia **145. a.** Myopia **146. c.** Chronic inflammation...

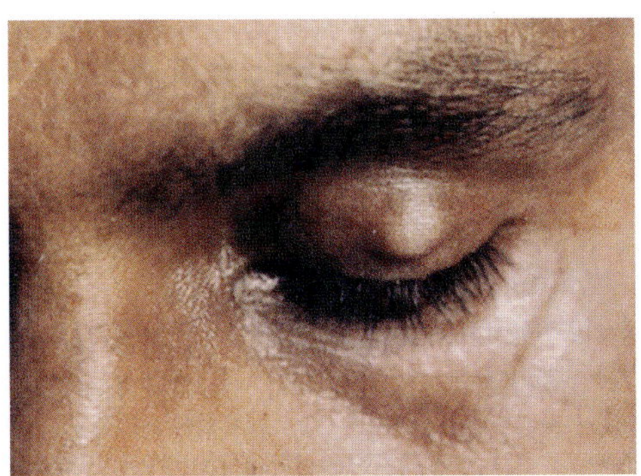

Chalazion upper eyelid.

147. A blow-out fracture of orbit refers to fracture involving:

a. Medial part of floor of orbit
b. Medial wall of orbit
c. Posterior wall of floor of orbit
d. Roof of the orbit

An orbital **blowout fracture** is a traumatic deformity of the orbital floor or medial wall, typically resulting from impact of a blunt object larger than the orbital aperture, or eye socket. There are two broad categories of blowout fractures: *open door*, which are large, displaced and comminuted, and *trapdoor*, which are linear, hinged, and minimally displaced. They are characterized by double vision, sunken ocular globes, and loss of sensation of the cheek and upper gums due to infraorbital nerve injury.

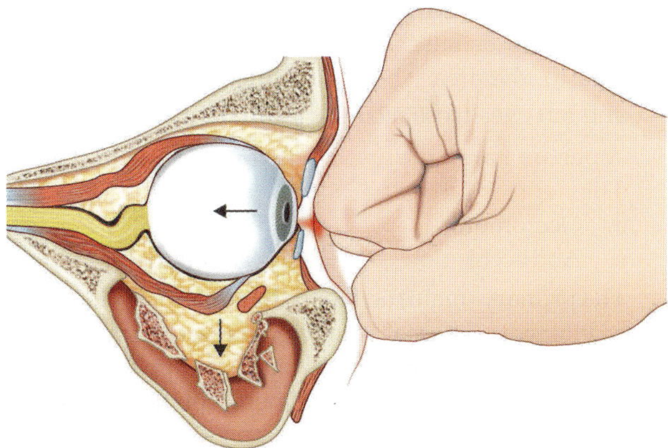

Mechanism of blow-out fracture of the orbital floor.

148. Visual field defect in pituitary tumour with suprascellular extension is:

a. Bitemporal hemianopia
b. Binasal hemianopia
c. Homonymous hemianopia
d. Pie in the sky vision

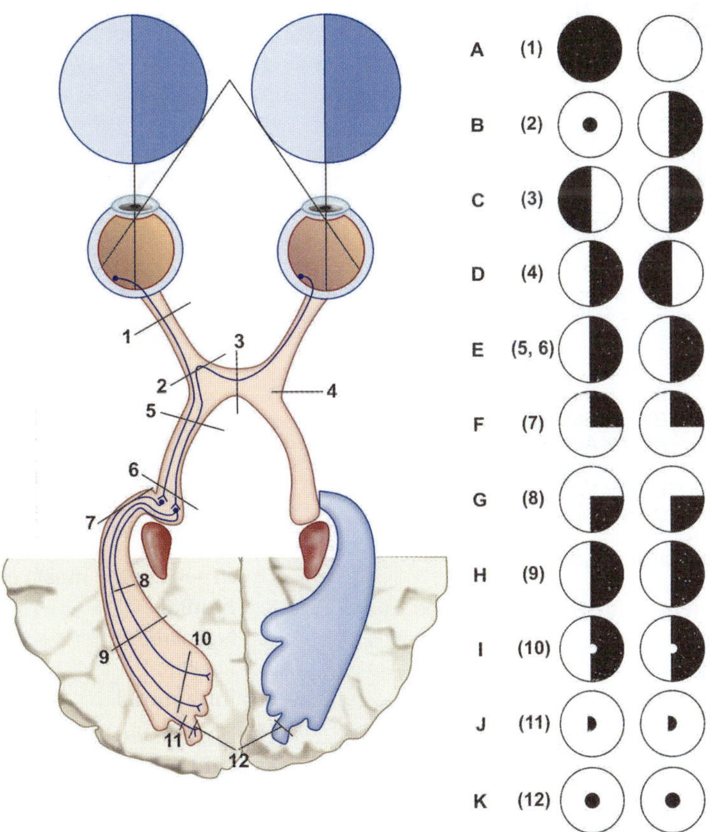

Lesions of the visual pathways at the level of: 1. optic nerve; 2. proximal part of optic nerve; 3. central chiasma; 4. lateral chiasma (both sides); 5. optic tract; 6. geniculate body; 7. part of optic radiations in temporal lobe; 8. part of optic radiations in parietal lobe; 9. optic radiations; 10. visual cortex sparing the macula; 11. visual cortex, only macula; 12. bilateral visual cortex only macula.

Ans. 147. a. Medial part... **148. a.** Bitemporal hemianopia

Bitemporal hemianopsia (**bitemporal heteronymous hemianopsia** or **bitemporal hemianopia**) is the medical description of a type of partial blindness where vision is missing in the outer half of both the right and left visual field. It is usually associated with lesions of the optic chiasm, the area where the optic nerves from the right and left eyes cross near the pituitary gland.

149. A person has inability to look downward and laterally. The nerve injured is:

a. Oculomotor
b. Trochlear
c. Abducent
d. Trigeminal

The primary (main) action of the superior oblique muscle is intorsion (internal rotation), the secondary action is depression (primarily in the adducted position) and the tertiary action is abduction (lateral rotation).

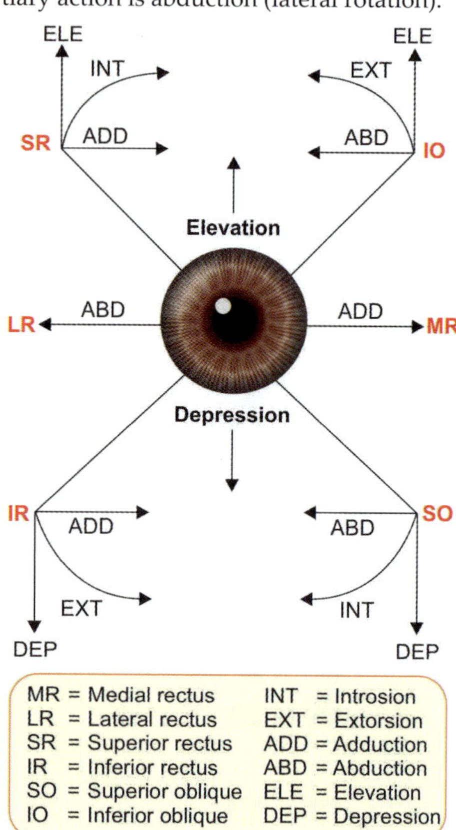

Action of the extraocular muscles.

150. Anterior ischemic optic neuropathy is characterized by:

a. Centrocecal scotoma
b. Altitudinal hemianopia
c. Ring scotoma
d. Increased blood supply

Altitudinal visual field defects describes a visual field defect in which either the upper or lower half of the visual field is selectively affected. The selective abnormality often creates a horizontal line across the visual field (known as "respecting the horizontal meridian"). Altitudinal defects occur in retinal vascular disease, glaucoma, and other disorders that affect the eye itself.

151. The operation of plication of inferior lid retractors is indicated in:

a. Senile ectropion
b. Senile entropion
c. Cicatricial entropion
d. Paralytic ectropion

Entropion often requires reinsertion of lower lid retractors. Augmentation of posterior lamellae (along with excision of any cicatrix) is required for cicatricial entropion and can be helpful in reoperations after simpler procedures have failed.

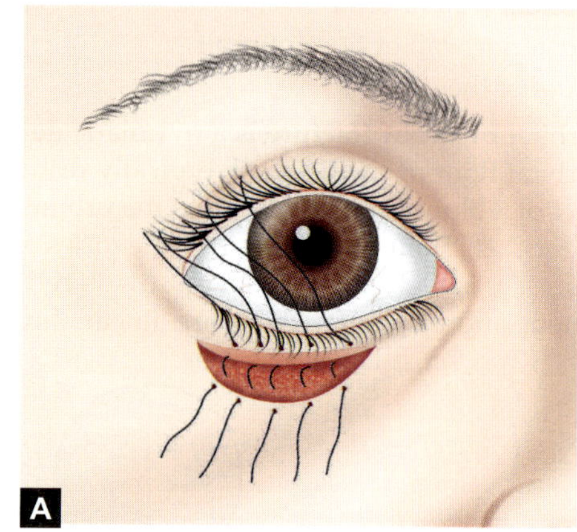

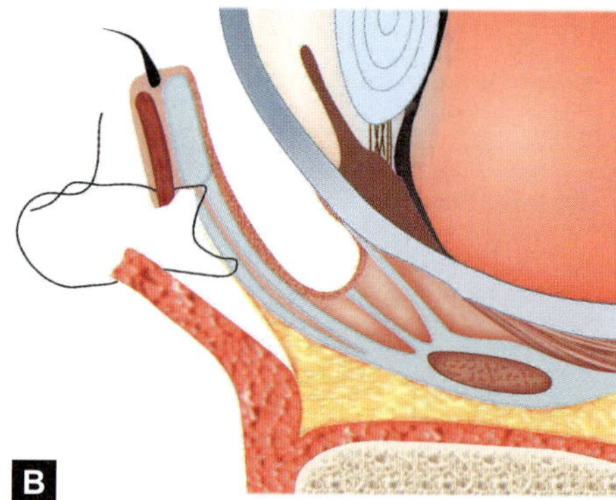

Plication of lower lid retractors: (A) front view; (B) cut section.

152. In herpes zoster, most commonly affected nerve is:

a. Frontal
b. Nasociliary
c. Lacrimal
d. Infraorbital

Herpes zoster ophthalmicus (**HZO**) and also known as **ophthalmic zoster** is a disease characterized by reactivation of dormant varicella zoster virus residing within the ophthalmic nerve (the first division of the trigeminal nerve). The frontal nerve is more commonly affected than the nasociliary nerve or lacrimal nerve.

Ans. 149. b. Trochlear **150. b.** Altitudinal hemian... **151. b.** Senile entropion **152. a.** Frontal

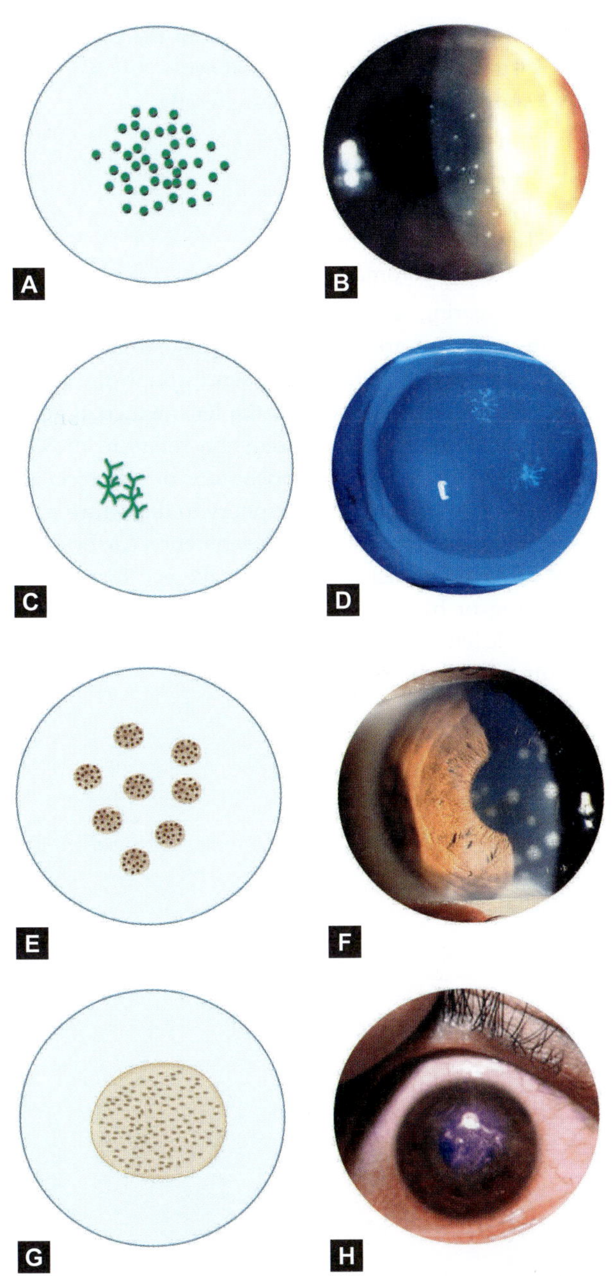

Types of zoster keratitis. Diagrammatic depictions and clinical photographs of: (A and B), Punctate epithelial keratitis; (C and D), Microdendritic epithelial ulcer; (E and F), Nummular keratitis; (G and H), Disciform keratitis.

153. Complication of lagophthalmos:

a. Refractive errors
b. Cataract
c. Exposure keratitis
d. Glaucoma

Lagophthalmos is defined as the inability to close the eyelids completely. Blinking covers the eye with a thin layer of tear fluid, thereby promoting a moist environment necessary for the cells of the exterior part of the eye. The tears also flush out foreign bodies and wash them away. This is crucial to maintain lubrication and proper eye health. If this process is impaired, as in lagophthalmos, the eye can suffer abrasions and infections. Lagophthalmos leads to corneal drying and ulceration.

154. Lesions of the visual cortex with homonymous hemianopia may be seen in occlusion of:

a. Basilar artery
b. Middle cerebral artery
c. Posterior cerebral artery
d. Anterior cerebral artery

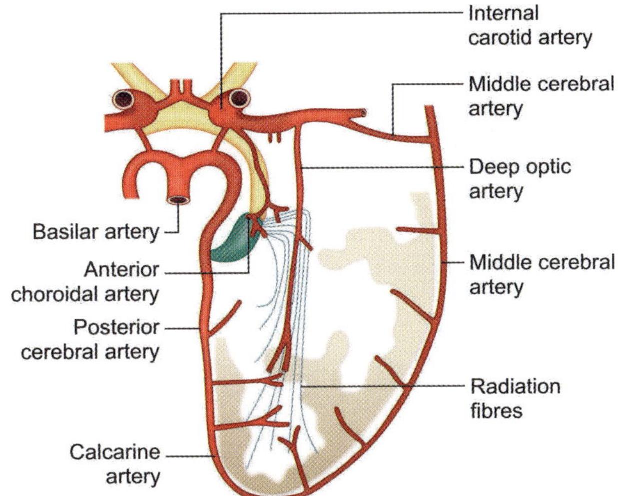

Blood supply of posterior visual pathway.

Vascular and neoplastic (malignant or benign tumours) lesions from the optic tract, to visual cortex can cause a contralateral homonymous hemianopsia. Injury to the right side of the brain will affect the left visual fields of each eye. The more posterior the cerebral lesion, the more symmetric (congruous) the homonymous hemianopsia will be. For example, a person who has a lesion of the right optic tract will no longer see objects. Homonymous hemianopsia secondary to posterior cerebral artery occlusion—may result in syndromes of memory impairment, opposite visual field loss (homonymous hemianopsia), and sometimes hemisensory deficits The PCA supplies the occipital lobe and the medial portion of the temporal lobe.

155. True statement for congenital dacryocystitis:

a. Uncommon condition
b. High grade acute inflammation
c. Involves lacrimal gland
d. Lower part of nasolacrimal duct occlusion is most common cause

Dacryocystitis is an infection of the lacrimal sac, secondary to obstruction of the nasolacrimal duct at the junction of lacrimal sac.

Ans. **153. c.** Exposure kerat... **154. c.** Posterior cerebral... **155. d.** Lower part of nasolacrimal duct occlusion is most...

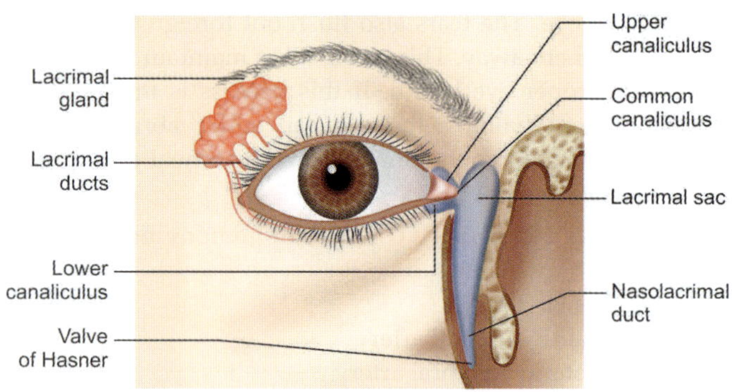

The lacrimal apparatus.

156. Feature of Foster Kennedy syndrome:

a. Optic atrophy
b. Contralateral papilloedema
c. Both of the above
d. None of the above

Foster Kennecly syndrome

- Optic atrophy in the ipsilateral eye
- Papilledema in the contralateral eye
- Central scotoma (loss of vision in the middle of the visual fields) in the ipsilateral eye
- Anosmia (loss of smell) ipsilaterally

157. Jack in the box phenomenon is:

a. Sickle cell scotoma
b. Bjerrum's scotoma
c. Roving ring scotoma
d. Arcuate scotoma

When wearing very high positive lenses (e.g. in aphakia) there exists an area in the periphery situated between the outer extent of the field seen through the lens and the field beyond the edge of the lens, which is not seen (**ring scotoma**). This phenomenon refers to the disappearance and sudden reappearance of an object when the eye moves from the periphery to the centre passing over the ring scotoma. This phenomenon can be avoided by turning the head rather than the eye for peripheral viewing or by correcting with contact lenses. Modern aspheric lenses minimize this phenomenon as they have reduced peripheral power.

Ans. **156. c.** Both of the above **157. c.** Roving ring scotoma

ANSWERS WITH REFERENCES

OPHTHALMOLOGY ANATOMY

1. **Ans. (d) Right superior rectus**
Ref: Nema's Ophthalmology, 4/e p307t

2. **Ans. (a) Superior oblique**
Ref: Nema's Ophthalmology, 4/e p

3. **Ans. (d) Endothelium**
Ref: Khurana's Ophthalmology 6/e p96

4. **Ans. (a) Aqueous humor**
Ref: Khurana's Ophthalmology 6/e p97

5. **Ans. (a) 2–3 mm**
Ref: Khurana's Ophthalmology 6/e p4

6. **Ans. (a) Fovea centralis**
Ref: Khurana's Ophthalmology 6/e 264

7. **Ans. (c) Carbonic anhydrase**
Ref: Khurana's Ophthalmology 6/e p223

8. **Ans. (b) Fovea centralis**
Ref: Khurana's Ophthalmology 6/e p266

9. **Ans. (c) Attachment of vitreous to posterior lens**
Ref: Khurana's Ophthalmology 6/e p258

10. **Ans. (b) Fourth cranial nerve**
Ref: Khurana's Ophthalmology 6/e p337

11. **Ans. (c) 24 mm**
Ref: Khurana's Ophthalmology 6/e p3

12. **Ans. (a) Endothelium**
Ref: Khurana's Ophthalmology 6/e p97

13. **Ans. (d) Peculiar arrangement of lamella**
Ref: Khurana's Ophthalmology 6/e p96

14. **Ans. (c) 3 mm**
Ref: Khurana's Ophthalmology 6/e p263

15. **Ans. (b) Sclera**
Ref: Khurana's Ophthalmology 6/e p10

16. **Ans. (b) Mesoderm**
Ref: Khurana's Ophthalmology 6/e p11

17. **Ans. (d) Ciliary body**
Ref: Khurana's Ophthalmology 6/e p437

18. **Ans. (a) Optic disc**
Ref: Khurana's Ophthalmology 6/e p263

19. **Ans. (a) Optic disc**
Ref: Khurana's Ophthalmology 6/e p263

20. **Ans. (b) Hypermetropic**
Ref: Khurana's Ophthalmology 6/e p13

21. **Ans. (a) Pupillary and the visual axis**
Ref: Khurana's Ophthalmology 6/e p31

22. **Ans. (b) Visual axis and optical axis**
Ref: Khurana's Ophthalmology 6/e p31

23. **Ans. (c) 45**
Ref: Khurana's Ophthalmology 6/e p95

24. **Ans. (d) 60 D**
Ref: Khurana's Ophthalmology 6/e p31

25. **Ans. (c) Behind the insertion of recti**
Ref: Khurana's Ophthalmology 6/e p141 (Figure 140)

26. **Ans. (d) Neural crest**
Ref: Khurana's Ophthalmology 6/e p12

OPHTHALMOLOGY PROCEDURES

27. **Ans. (d) Binocular vision**
Ref: Internet resources

28. **Ans. (a) Strabismus**
Ref: Nema's Ophthalmology, 4/e p314

29. **Ans. (b) 2–4% xylocaine**
Ref: Khurana's Ophthalmology 6/e p510

30. **Ans. (a) Field of charting**
Ref: Khurana's Ophthalmology 6/e p512

31. **Ans. (c) 15 times**
Ref: Khurana's Ophthalmology 6/e p589

32. **Ans. (c) Single mirror gonioscopes allows examination of 360 degrees of the angle**
Ref: Khurana's Ophthalmology 6/e p569

33. **Ans. (d) It has a large field of view.**
Ref: Khurana's Ophthalmology 6/e p587

34. **Ans. (b) Testing color vision**
Ref: Khurana's Ophthalmology 6/e p330

35. **Ans. (d) Hyperopes display an "against" movement**
Ref: Khurana's Ophthalmology 6/e p574

36. **Ans. (d) Color blindness**
Ref: Khurana's Ophthalmology 6/e p331

37. **Ans. (c) Acute congestive glaucoma and cataract**
Ref: Khurana's Ophthalmology 6/e p244

38. **Ans. (c)** **Specular microscope**
Ref: Khurana's Ophthalmology 6/e p502

39. **Ans. (c)** **Refractive errors**
Ref: Khurana's Ophthalmology 6/e p572

40. **Ans. (c)** **Corneal scars**
Ref: Khurana's Ophthalmology 6/e p502

41. **Ans. (d)** **Curvature of cornea**
Ref: Khurana's Ophthalmology 6/e p576

42. **Ans. (d)** **Ability to discriminate 2 points**
Ref: Khurana's Ophthalmology 6/e p17

OPHTHALMOLOGY PHARMACOLOGY

43. **Ans. (b)** **Red green**
Ref: Internet resources

44. **Ans. (b)** **Prednisolone**
Ref: Khurana's Ophthalmology 6/e p454

45. **Ans. (b)** **Ganciclovir**
Ref: Khurana's Ophthalmology 6/e p448

46. **Ans. (d)** **Tetracyclines**
Ref: Khurana's Ophthalmology 6/e p72

47. **Ans. (c)** **Cause mydriasis and prevent formation of posterior synechiae**
Ref: Khurana's Ophthalmology 6/e p159

48. **Ans. (d)** **Natamycin**
Ref: Khurana's Ophthalmology 6/e p448

49. **Ans. (a)** **Atropine ointment**
Ref: Khurana's Ophthalmology 6/e p573

50. **Ans. (b)** **Pilocarpine**
Ref: Khurana's Ophthalmology 6/e p449

51. **Ans. (d)** **Beta blockers**
Ref: Khurana's Ophthalmology 6/e p450

CONJUNCTIVA

52. **Ans. (d)** **Trachoma**
Ref: Nema's Ophthalmology, 4/e p113

53. **Ans. (b)** **Chlamydia**
Ref: Nema's Ophthalmology, 4/e p117

54. **Ans. (d)** **Spring catarrh**
Ref: Khurana's Ophthalmology 6/e p80

55. **Ans. (a)** **Vernal keratoconjunctivitis/VKC**
Ref: Khurana's Ophthalmology 6/e p80

56. **Ans. (d)** **Chlamydial conjunctivitis**
Ref: Khurana's Ophthalmology 6/e p68

57. **Ans. (a)** **Vitamin A deficiency**
Ref: Khurana's Ophthalmology 6/e p91

58. **Ans. (b)** **Trachoma**
Ref: Khurana's Ophthalmology 6/e p69

59. **Ans. (c)** **Phlyctenular**
Ref: Khurana's Ophthalmology 6/e p83

60. **Ans. (b)** **Trachoma**
Ref: Khurana's Ophthalmology 6/e p67

61. **Ans. (d)** **Sarcoidosis**
Ref: Khurana's Ophthalmology 6/e p91

62. **Ans. (d)** **All of the above**
Ref: Khurana's Ophthalmology 6/e p91

63. **Ans. (a)** **CMV**
Ref: Khurana's Ophthalmology 6/e p73

64. **Ans. (d)** **Corneal xerosis**
Ref: Khurana's Ophthalmology 6/e p468

65. **Ans. (a)** **Caterpillar hair in the eye**
Ref: Khurana's Ophthalmology 6/e p78

66. **Ans. (b)** **Allergic conjunctivitis**
Ref: Khurana's Ophthalmology 6/e p64

67. **Ans. (c)** **Moraxella**
Ref: Khurana's Ophthalmology 6/e p66

68. **Ans. (b)** **Spring catarrh**
Ref: Khurana's Ophthalmology 6/e p80

69. **Ans. (d)** **Ectropion**
Ref: Khurana's Ophthalmology 6/e p70

CORNEA

70. **Ans. (b)** **KF rings**
Ref: Nema's Ophthalmology, 4/e p154

71. **Ans. (c)** **HSV infection**
Ref: Nema's Ophthalmology, 4/e p142

72. **Ans. (a)** **Corneal dystrophy**
Ref: Khurana's Ophthalmology 6/e p126

73. **Ans. (c)** **Aspergillus**
Ref: Khurana's Ophthalmology 6/e p106

74. **Ans. (b)** **Affects cornea**
Ref: Khurana's Ophthalmology 6/e p117

75. **Ans. (a) Herpes simplex virus**
Ref: Khurana's Ophthalmology 6/e p109

76. **Ans. (c) Gonococcus**
Ref: Khurana's Ophthalmology 6/e p99

77. **Ans. (b) It manifests just after birth**
Ref: Khurana's Ophthalmology 6/e p132

78. **Ans. (b) Interstitial keratitis**
Ref: Khurana's Ophthalmology 6/e p121

79. **Ans. (b) Symmetrical and unilateral condition**
Ref: Khurana's Ophthalmology 6/e p130

80. **Ans. (c) Cornea verticillata**
Ref: Internet resources

81. **Ans. (d) All of the above**
Ref: Khurana's Ophthalmology 6/e p103

82. **Ans. (c) Fungus**
Ref: Khurana's Ophthalmology 6/e p106

83. **Ans. (b) Sodium fluorescein dye**
Ref: Khurana's Ophthalmology 6/e p104

84. **Ans. (b) Congenital syphilis**
Ref: Khurana's Ophthalmology 6/e p121

85. **Ans. (d) Purulent discharge**
Ref: Khurana's Ophthalmology 6/e p109

86. **Ans. (d) Acanthamoeba does NOT depend upon a human host for the completion of its life-cycle**
Ref: Khurana's Ophthalmology 6/e p113

87. **Ans. (c) Corneal epithelial damage**
Ref: Khurana's Ophthalmology 6/e p98

88. **Ans. (b) Seen in contact lenses users**
Ref: Khurana's Ophthalmology 6/e p113

UVEAL TRACT AND GLAUCOMA

89. **Ans. (b) Open angle glaucoma**
Ref: Nema's Ophthalmology, 4/e p208

90. **Ans. (b) Laser trabeculoplasty**
Ref: Nema's Ophthalmology, 4/e p205

91. **Ans. (c) Scotoma in Bjerrum's field**
Ref: Nema's Ophthalmology, 4/e p

92. **Ans. (c) CRAO**
Ref: Khurana's Ophthalmology 6/e p250, 272

93. **Ans. (d) Open angle glaucoma**
Ref: Khurana's Ophthalmology 6/e p237

94. **Ans. (a) Penetrating injury of ciliary body**
Ref: Khurana's Ophthalmology 6/e p437

95. **Ans. (a) Inferonasal**
Ref: Khurana's Ophthalmology 6/e p150

96. **Ans. (c) Angle closure glaucoma**
Ref: Khurana's Ophthalmology 6/e p247

97. **Ans. (d) Constricted**
Ref: Khurana's Ophthalmology 6/e p154

98. **Ans. (b) Decreased outflow**
Ref: Khurana's Ophthalmology 6/e p223

99. **Ans. (c) Unilateral**
Ref: Khurana's Ophthalmology 6/e p226

LENS

100. **Ans. (c) Vitreous detachment**
Ref: Nema's Ophthalmology, 4/e p228

101. **Ans. (b) Aphakia**
Ref: Nema's Ophthalmology, 4/e p234

102. **Ans. (c) Zonular**
Ref: Khurana's Ophthalmology 6/e p184

103. **Ans. (d) 6 weeks**
Ref: Internet resources

104. **Ans. (b) Diabetic cataract**
Ref: Khurana's Ophthalmology 6/e p193

105. **Ans. (d) Cataract**
Ref: Khurana's Ophthalmology 6/e p191

106. **Ans. (c) Alport's syndrome**
Ref: Khurana's Ophthalmology 6/e p218

107. **Ans. (c) Hallermann Streiff syndrome**
Ref: Internet resources

108. **Ans. (a) Chalcosis**
Ref: Khurana's Ophthalmology 6/e p194

109. **Ans. (a) Posterior cortex**
Ref: Khurana's Ophthalmology 6/e p182

110. **Ans. (d) Posterior capsule**
Ref: Khurana's Ophthalmology 6/e p194

111. **Ans. (b) Intraocular lens**
Ref: Khurana's Ophthalmology 6/e p38

RETINA

112. **Ans. (d) CRVO**
Ref: Nema's Ophthalmology, 4/e p248

113. **Ans. (a) Massive vitreous hemorrhage**
Ref: Nema's Ophthalmology, 4/e p241

114. **Ans. (b) Retinopathy of prematurity**
Ref: Khurana's Ophthalmology 6/e p270

115. **Ans. (c) Vitreous hemorrhage**
Ref: Khurana's Ophthalmology 6/e p278

116. **Ans. (d) Retinal edema**
Ref: Khurana's Ophthalmology 6/e p279

117. **Ans. (c) Hypertensive retinopathy**
Ref: Khurana's Ophthalmology 6/e p275

118. **Ans. (d) Retinitis pigmentosa**
Ref: Khurana's Ophthalmology 6/e p288

119. **Ans. (c) Retinal artery**
Ref: Khurana's Ophthalmology 6/e p331

120. **Ans. (c) Diabetes**
Ref: Khurana's Ophthalmology 6/e p303

121. **Ans. (a) Dot and blot hemorrhages**
Ref: Khurana's Ophthalmology 6/e p287

122. **Ans. (d) Neovascularization**
Ref: Khurana's Ophthalmology 6/e p278

123. **Ans. (c) Fellow eye is never involved**
Ref: Khurana's Ophthalmology 6/e p299

124. **Ans. (a) Consecutive optic atrophy**
Ref: Khurana's Ophthalmology 6/e p288

125. **Ans. (d) All of the above**
Ref: Khurana's Ophthalmology 6/e p291

OPHTHALMIC ONCOLOGY

126. **Ans. (b) Reduced intraocular pressure**
Ref: Nema's Ophthalmology, 4/e p290

127. **Ans. (b) Retinoblastoma**
Ref: Khurana's Ophthalmology 6/e p306

128. **Ans. (b) Always unilateral**
Ref: Khurana's Ophthalmology 6/e p304

129. **Ans. (b) Rhabdomyosarcoma**
Ref: Khurana's Ophthalmology 6/e p419

130. **Ans. (b) Intracerebral calcification**
Ref: Khurana's Ophthalmology 6/e p305

131. **Ans. (c) Retinoblastoma**
Ref: Khurana's Ophthalmology 6/e p304

132. **Ans. (d) Chromosome 13**
Ref: Khurana's Ophthalmology 6/e

133. **Ans. (b) Malignant melanoma of choroid**
Ref: Khurana's Ophthalmology 6/e p176

MISCELLANEOUS

134. **Ans. (d) Normal vision**
Ref: Nema's Ophthalmology, 4/e p298

135. **Ans. (d) Dacryo-cysto-rhinostomy**
Ref: Nema's Ophthalmology, 4/e p345

136. **Ans. (b) Lateral rectus**
Ref: Internet resources

137. **Ans. (d) Poliosis**
Ref: Khurana's Ophthalmology 6/e p365

138. **Ans. (d) Drooping of eyelid**
Ref: Khurana's Ophthalmology 6/e p355

139. **Ans. (a) Uncorrected hypermetropia**
Ref: Khurana's Ophthalmology 6/e p34

140. **Ans. (a) High anisometropia**
Ref: Khurana's Ophthalmology 6/e p342

141. **Ans. (c) Giant cell arteritis**
Ref: Khurana's Ophthalmology 6/e p322

142. **Ans. (c) 3D**
Ref: Khurana's Ophthalmology 6/e p40

143. **Ans. (c) Accommodation squint**
Ref: Khurana's Ophthalmology 6/e p349

144. **Ans. (d) Myopia**
Ref: Khurana's Ophthalmology 6/e p52

145. **Ans. (a) Myopia**
Ref: Khurana's Ophthalmology 6/e p41

146. **Ans. (c) Chronic inflammation of meibomian gland**
Ref: Khurana's Ophthalmology 6/e p369

147. **Ans. (a) Medial part of floor of orbit**
Ref: Khurana's Ophthalmology 6/e p423

148. **Ans. (a) Bitemporal hemianopia**
Ref: Khurana's Ophthalmology 6/e p314

149. **Ans. (b) Trochlear**
Ref: Khurana's Ophthalmology 6/e p338

150. **Ans. (b) Altitudinal hemianopia**
Ref: Khurana's Ophthalmology 6/e p322

151. **Ans. (b) Senile entropion**
Ref: Khurana's Ophthalmology 6/e p374

152. **Ans. (a) Frontal**
Ref: Khurana's Ophthalmology 6/e p111

153. **Ans. (c) Exposure keratitis**
Ref: Khurana's Ophthalmology 6/e p378

154. **Ans. (c) Posterior cerebral artery**
Ref: Khurana's Ophthalmology 6/e p311

155. **Ans. (d) Lower part of nasolacrimal duct occlusion is most common cause**
Ref: Khurana's Ophthalmology 6/e p386

156. **Ans. (c) Both of the above**
Ref: Internet resources

157. **Ans. (c) Roving ring scotoma**
Ref: Khurana's Ophthalmology 6/e p38

PRACTICE QUESTIONS

OPHTHAL ANATOMY

1. Posterior chamber contains:
a. Vitreous humour
b. Aqueous humour
c. Retinal vessels
d. All

OPHTHAL PROCEDURES

2. Schirmer test is done to detect:
a. Epiphora
b. Dacryocystitis
c. Keratitis
d. Dry eye

3. Which of the following clinical procedure is best to evaluate cystoid macular edema:
a. Indirect ophthalmoscopy
b. Direct ophthalmoscopy
c. Slit lam examination
d. Distant direct ophthalmoscopy

4. Image formed by plane mirror:
a. Decreased size, virtual
b. Same size, virtual
c. Increased size, virtual
d. Erect, virtual

5. Field of vision is maximum on which quadrant:
a. Superior
b. Inferior
c. Temporal
d. Nasal

6. Pi-hole test is used for:
a. Astigmatism
b. Refractive error
c. Presbyopia
d. Keratoconus

OPHTHAL PHARMACOLOGY

7. Which beta blocker is commonly used in open angle glaucoma:
a. Propranolol
b. Timolol
c. Atenolol
d. Labetalol

8. Duration of cycloplegic effect of atropine lasts for:
a. 1–3 days
b. 3–6 days
c. 6–9 days
d. 9–12 days

9. True regarding phenylephrine:
a. Cycloplegic
b. Mydriatic
c. Cycloplegic and mydriatic both
d. None

CONJUNCTIVA

10. Location of Herberts pits in trachoma:
a. Limbus
b. Margin of lids
c. Palpebral conjunctiva
d. Lens

11. True for pterygium:
a. Inflammatory process
b. Elastotic degeneration
c. Seen in young population
d. Occurs anywhere

12. Deficiency of which of the following layer of tear leads to Keratoconjunctivitis Sicca:
a. Mucin
b. Lipid
c. Aqueous
d. All of the above

CORNEA

13. Neurotrophic keratopathy is seen in:
a. Trigeminal nerve injury
b. Facial nerve injury
c. Both
d. None

14. Prognosis of chemical acid injury to eye is determined by:
a. Concentration of acid
b. Duration of contact
c. Corneal penetration
d. All of the above

15. Location of Krukenberg's spindles:
a. Anterior surface of cornea
b. Posterior surface of cornea
c. Anterior surface of lens
d. Posterior surface of lens

16. Which of the following is a true statement for Bowmans membrane of cornea:
a. A true elastic membrane
b. It is having maximum regenerative power
c. More capable of preventing infection than Descemets membrane
d. It is a cellular layer

Ans.
1. **b.** Aqueous...
2. **d.** Dry eye
3. **c.** Slit lam examination
4. **b.** Same size, virtual
5. **c.** Temporal
6. **b.** Refractive error
7. **b.** Timolol
8. **d.** 9–12 days
9. **b.** Mydriatic
10. **a.** Limbus
11. **b.** Elastotic...
12. **c.** Aqueous
13. **a.** Trigeminal...
14. **d.** All of the above
15. **b.** Posterior surface...
16. **c.** More capable

UVEAL TRACT

17. Mid-dilated fixed pupil is seen in:
- a. Subacute primary angle closure
- b. Acute primary angle closure
- c. Chronic primary angle closure glaucoma
- d. Open angle glaucoma

18. A child presented with enlarged eyes with lacrimation and photophobia. Intra-ocular tension was found to be elevated. Next step:
- a. Gonioscopy
- b. Conservative management
- c. Surgical procedure/Goniotomy
- d. Wait and watch

19. Which of the following condition is associated with iridodonesis:
- a. Anterior uveitis
- b. Subluxation of lens
- c. Posterior uveitis
- d. Intumescent cataract

20. Which is an important pathology in angle closure glaucoma:
- a. Increased aqueous production
- b. Pupillary block
- c. Phacomorphic mechanisms
- d. Genetic factors

LENS

21. Physiological insufficiency of accommodation leads to:
- a. Myopia
- b. Hypermetropia
- c. Presbyopia
- d. Anisometropia

22. Index myopia results from:
- a. Increase in anteroposterior length of eyeball
- b. Nuclear cataract
- c. Increased curvature of cornea
- d. Excessive accommodation

23. Phacomorphic glaucoma with shallow anterior chamber may be seen in:
- a. Acute anterior uveitis
- b. Intumescent cataract
- c. Steroid induced
- d. Traumatic

RETINA

24. Number of burns made in pan-retinal photocoagulation:
- a. 800–1200
- b. 1200–1600
- c. 1600–2000
- d. 2000–3000

25. Neuroretinal rim is broadest in which location:
- a. Temporal
- b. Inferior
- c. Superior
- d. Nasal

26. Which of the following condition presents as yellowish waxy spots on posterior pole of retina with microvascular spasm:
- a. Diabetic retinopathy
- b. Retinitis pigmentosa
- c. Hypertensive retinitis
- d. Sickle cell retinitis

OPHTHAL ONCOLOGY

27. Which of the following eyelid tumour does NOT have a lymphatic spread:
- a. Squamous cell carcinoma
- b. Malignant melanoma
- c. Basal cell carcinoma
- d. None

MISCELLANEOUS

28. See-saw nystagmus is seen in:
- a. Disease of retina
- b. Labyrinthitis
- c. Brainstem lesions
- d. CNS depression

29. All of the following are suggestive of hypervitaminosis A EXCEPT:
- a. Xerophthalmia
- b. Pseudotumor cerebri
- c. Dryness of skin
- d. Emesis

Ans. 17. **b.** Acute primary... 18. **c.** Surgical 19. **b.** Subluxation of lens 20. **b.** Pupillary block 21. **c.** Presbyopia 22. **b.** Nuclear cataract 23. **b.** Intumescent cataract 24. **b.** 1200–1600 25. **b.** Inferior 26. **c.** Hypertensive retinitis 27. **c.** Basal cell carcinoma 28. **c.** Brainstem lesions 29. **a.** Xerophthalmia

IMAGE-BASED QUESTIONS

1. Which substance is accumulated in this type of cataract:

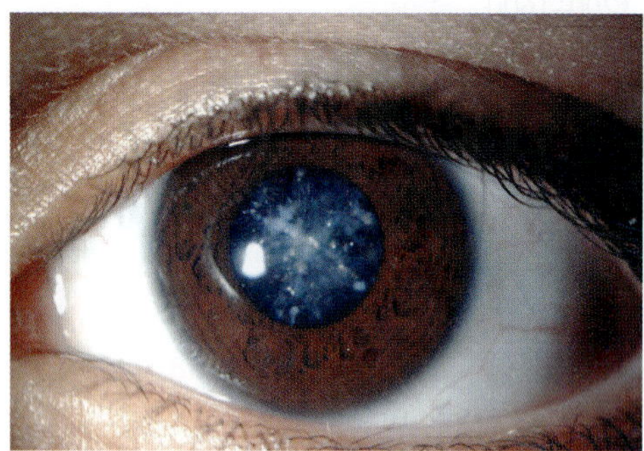

a. Galactitol b. Dulcitol
c. Homogentisate d. Sorbitol

This is a typical snowflake/snowstorm cataract suggestive of classical diabetic cataract. It is a rare condition, usually occurring in young adults due to osmotic over hydration of lens. Osmotic over hydration of the lens occurs due to accumulation of sorbitol, when glucose is metabolized by NADPH+ dependent aldose reducatse.

2. Such type of cataract is seen in:

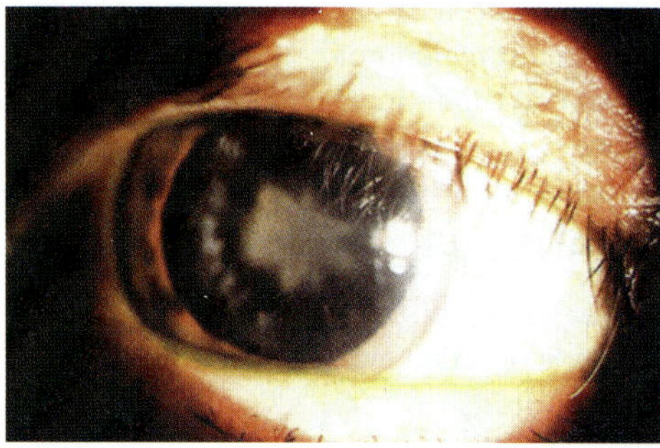

a. Diabetes b. Hypertension
c. Blunt trauma d. Penetrating trauma

Rosette cataract is seen in blunt trauma to lens.

3. Such type of cataract is typically seen in:

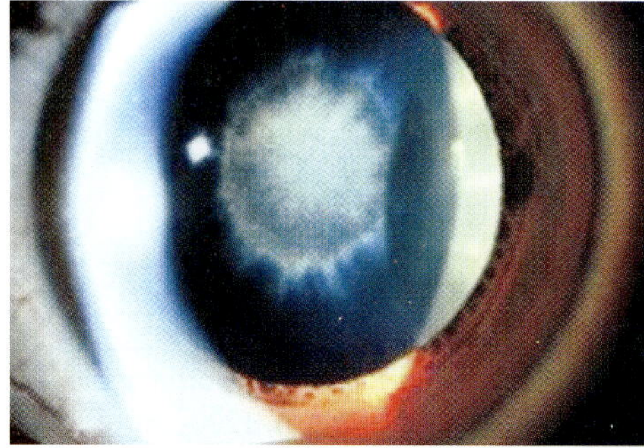

a. Diabetes b. Blunt trauma
c. Galactosemia
d. Hepatolenticular degeneration

Sunflower cataract characterized by yellowish brown dots may be observed rarely in patients with Wilson disease/chalcosis/hepatolenticular degeneration, due to the deposition of cuprous oxide in the anterior lens capsule and subcapsular cortex in a stellate pattern.

4. Action of which extraocular muscle:

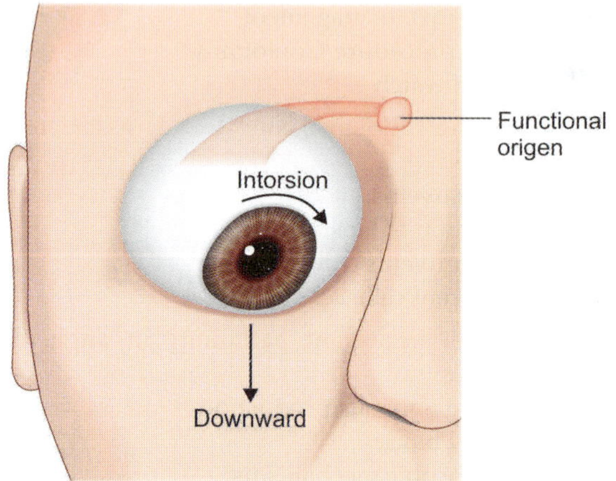

a. Inferior oblique b. Inferior rectus
c. Superior oblique d. Superior rectus

For superior oblique, primary action is intorsiWon, secondary action is depression and tertiary action is abduction.

5. What is being measured:

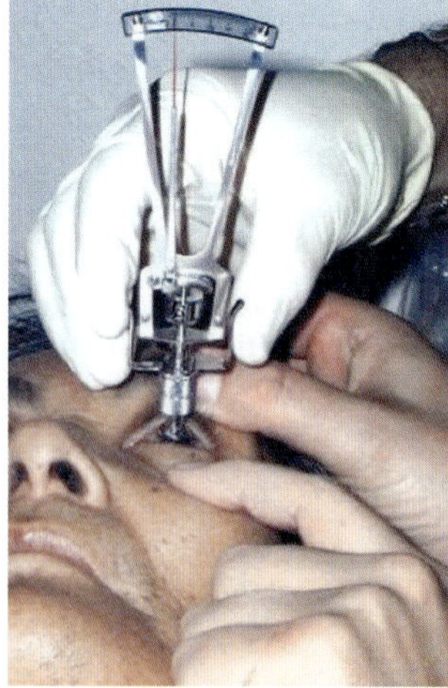

a. Curvature of cornea b. Thickness of cornea
c. Angle of anterior chamber
d. Intraocular pressure

The intraocular pressure is being measured with the help of an instrument called tonometer (Schiotz tonometer in figure)

6. **Injury to which part of the visual pathway will give this kind of lesion:**

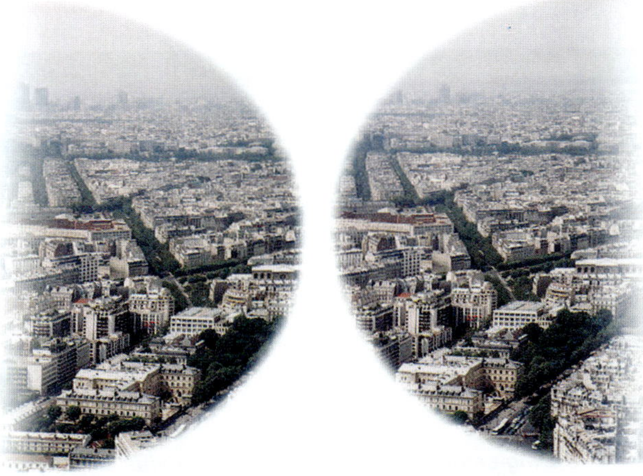

a. Optic nerve
b. Optic chiasm
c. Optic tract
d. Optic radiation

The lesion is bitemporal hemianopia, suggestive of lesion in optic chiasm

7. **Which reflex is being shown:**

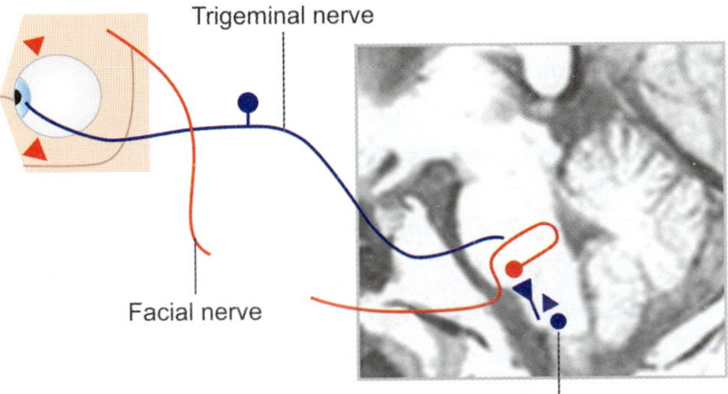

a. Corneal reflex
b. Light reflex
c. Gag reflex
d. Pupillary reflex

Corneal reflex: Light touching of conjunctiva with a wisp of cotton leads to blinking of eye

8. **Appearance of right eye suggests the paralysis of which cranial nerve:**

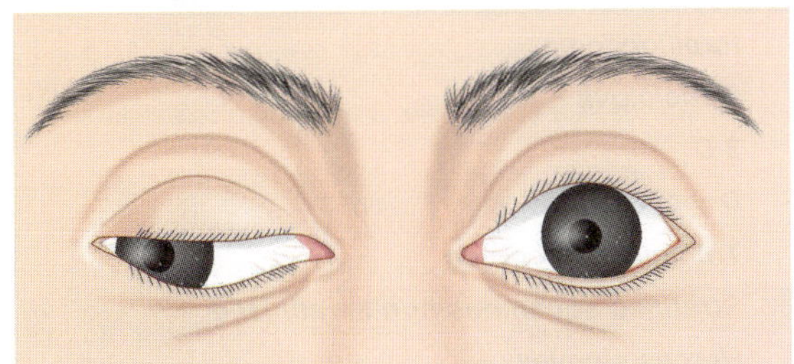

a. 2nd
b. 3rd
c. 4th
d. 6th

Ptosis and mydriasis suggest the paralysis of 3rd cranial nerve.

9. **Following procedure is done for which condition:**

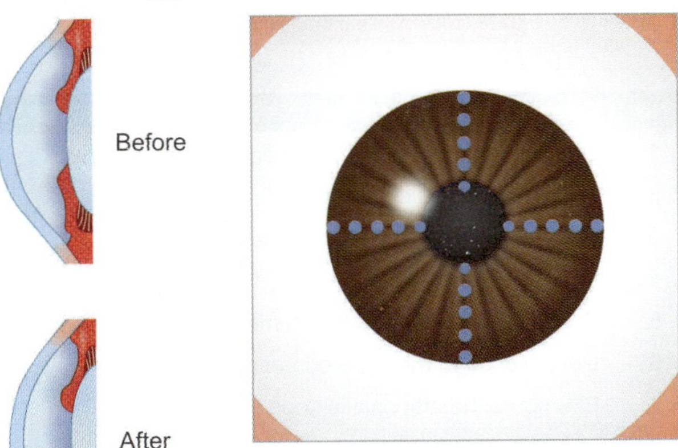

a. Hypermetropia
b. Myopia
c. Presbyopia
d. Astigmatism

Radial keratotomy/RK refer to making deep (90% of corneal thickness) radial incisions in the peripheral part of cornea leaving the central 4 mm optical zone. These incisions on healing ; flatten the central cornea thereby reducing its refractive power. This procedure gives good correction in low to moderate myopia (2 to 6 D)

10. **Name the procedure:**

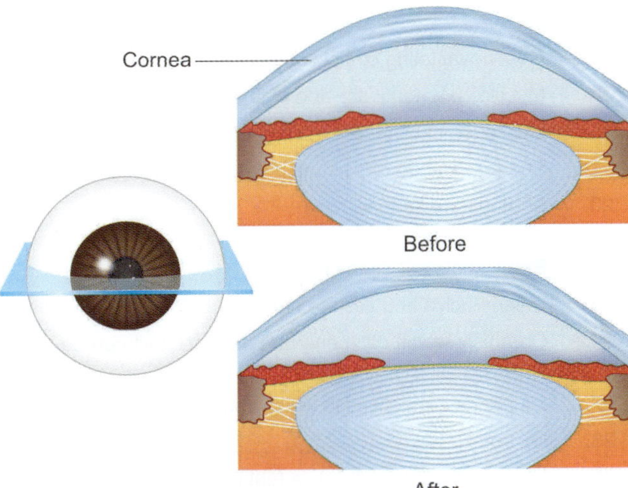

a. Laser trabeculotomy
b. Peripheral iridectomy
c. Laser-in-situ keratomileusis
d. Refractive lenticule extraction

In LASIK (laser-in-situ keratomileusis), a flap of 130-160 micron thickness of anterior corneal tissue is raised with the help of an automated microkeratome. After creating a corneal flap midtsromal tissue is ablated directly with an excimer laser beam, ultimately flattening the cornea. Currently, this procedure is being considered the refractive surgery of choice for myopia upto -8D

MCQ POINTS

S. No.	Question statements	Answers
1.	Drug of choice (DOC) for corneal herpes zoster is	***Acyclovir***
2.	Antero-posterior length of eyeball	***24 mm***
3.	Nerve supply of superior oblique muscle	***Trochlear***
4.	Epithelium of cornea	***Stratified squamous non-keratinized***
5.	Sphincter and dilator pupillae muscles are derived from	***Neuroectoderm***
6.	Device used to measure curvature of cornea	***Keratometer***
7.	Bitemporal hemianopia is seen in lesion of	***Optic chiasm***
8.	Most sensitive part of retina	***Fovea***
9.	Angular conjunctivitis is caused by	***Moraxella***
10.	Ropy discharge is suggestive of	***Spring catarrh/vernal keratoconjunctivitis***
11.	Herberts pits are seen in	***Trachoma***
12.	Pupil in angle closure glaucoma is	***Vertically oval, mid dilated and fixed***
13.	Maximum refractive power is within the ... of lens	***Centre***
14.	Laser used in after cataract	***Nd: YAG***
15.	Relative afferent pupillary defect is seen in	***Optic neuritis***
16.	Drug of choice for acute anterior uveitis	***Steroids***
17.	Most common intraocular malignancy in children	***Retinoblastoma***
18.	Irregular black deposits of clumped pigment in the peripheral retina is seen in	***Retinitis pigmentosa***
19.	Most devastating complication of HIV infection of eye	***Cytomegalovirus infection***
20.	Muscle commonly affected in thyroid ophthalmopathy	***Inferior rectus***
21.	MC cause of blindness in children in India:	***Vitamin A deficiency***
22.	Shortest and quickly acting mydriatic	***Tropicamide***
23.	KF rings are seen in	***Wilson disease/chalcosis/hepatolenticular degeneration***
24.	Roths spots are seen in	***Subacute bacterial endocarditis/septicemia***
25.	Dalen Fuch's nodules are seen in	***Sympathetic ophthalmitis***
26.	Organism which can penetrate normal intact cornea	***Neisseria gonorrhoeae, Neisseria meningitidis, Corynebacterium diphtheria***
27.	Iris pearls are noticed in which condition	***Leprosy***
28.	Iris bombe is a feature of	***Ring synechiae (complication of anterior uveitis)***
29.	Mushroom shaped disc is a feature of	***Papilloedema***
30.	Drug of choice (DOC) for CMV retinitis	***Ganciclovir***
31.	If length of eyeball changes by 1 mm, refractive index changes by	***3 D***
32.	Schirmer test is done for	***Dry eyes***
33.	Pachymeter measures	***Thickness of cornea***
34.	Epithelial lining of conjunctiva	***Stratified squamous non-keratinized***
35.	Dendritic ulcer is commonly seen in	***Herpes simplex***
36.	Neurotrophic keratitis involves	***Trigeminal nerve***
37.	Recurrent corneal erosions are seen in	***Corneal dystrophy***
38.	Acanthamoeba keratitis is usually associated with	***Contact lens***

S. No.	Question statements	Answers
39.	HLA associated with anterior uveitis	***HLA B27***
40.	Most serious complication seen in one eye after traumatic injury to other eye	***Sympathetic ophthalmitis***
41.	Vertically oval, mid dilated and shallow anterior chamber is seen in	***Acute congestive glaucoma***
42.	Posterior staphyloma is commonly associated with	***High myopia***
43.	Ideal site of implantation of intraocular lens	***Posterior chamber in capsular bag***
44.	Cataract in diabetes is due to accumulation of	***Sorbitol***
45.	Characteristic feature of diabetic retinopathy	***Microaneurysm***
46.	Visual field defect seen in pituitary tumour with suprasellar extension	***Bitemporal hemianopia***
47.	Flexner Wintersteiner rosettes on microscopy are seen in	***Retinoblastoma***
48.	Initial manoeuvre done in congenital dacryocystitis:	***Massaging***
49.	MC cause of vitreous hemorrhage in young individuals	***Trauma***
50.	Afferent limb of light reflex is mediated by which cranial nerve	***2nd***
51.	Lens used to correct astigmatism	***Cylindrical***
52.	A pupil responds to accommodation but light reflex is absent. This is	***Argyll Robertson pupil***
53.	Excessive accommodation may result in	***Pseudomyopia***
54.	Inability to completely close the palpebral aperture is known as	***Lagophthalmos***
55.	Chronic, sterile inflammation of the meibomian gland is known as	***Chalazion***
56.	As per WHO, definition of blindness is visual acuity less than	***3/60 (with best possible correction)***
57.	Thinnest part of lens	***Posterior***
58.	Operation of plication of lower lid retractors is done for	***Senile entropion***
59.	Satellite lesions are seen in which corneal ulcer	***Fungal***
60.	MC intraocular malignancy in adults	***Malignant melanoma of choroid***
61.	Iris pearls are seen in	***Leprosy***
62.	Homonymous hemianopia is caused by lesion of	***Optic tract***
63.	Recurrent vitreous hemorrhage is a feature of	***Eales disease***
64.	Epidemic keratoconjuctivitis is caused by	***Adenovirus***
65.	Coloboma of the lid is commonest in which part of lid	***Upper eyelid, medial half***
66.	Chalcosis is caused by which metal	***Copper***
67.	Edema of retina following blunt trauma is known as	***Berlin's edema***
68.	Vossius ring affects which part of eye	***Lens***
69.	Enlargement of blind spot is a feature of	***Papilloedema***
70.	Cause of sudden loss of vision in diabetic patient	***Massive vitreous hemorrhage***
71.	Earliest change of diabetic retinopathy	***Microaneurysm***
72.	MC used drug in open angle glaucoma is	***Timolol***
73.	Fincham's test is done to differentiate between	***Colored halos of acute congestive glaucoma and cataract***
74.	Typical appearance of true diabetic cataract is	***Snowflake***
75.	MC parasitic cause of uveitis is	***Toxoplasmosis***

CHAPTER

3

GENERAL MEDICINE

KEY POINTS

ECG Changes in Hyper- and Hypokalemia

Hypokalemia	Hyperkalemia
ST segment depressed	Peaked tall T waves
Flat or inverted T waves	Sine- wave, P wave decreased
U waves	Widening of QRs complex
PR prolonged	PR interval prolonged Ventricular asystole/ventricular fibrillation

Classic Triad of Myeloma

- Marrow plasmacytosis > 10 Per cent
- Lytic bone lesions
- Serum and /or urine M component

Remember

- Thiazides are used for treating hypercalciuria
- Tumour lysis causes hypocalcemia (NOT hypercalcemia)

Acute Respiratory Failure

- Type 1:
  - Severe hypoxemia refractory to oxygen
  - Due to airspace filling: Intrapulmonary shunting
- Type 2:
  - Alveolar hypoventilation
  - Increased $PaCO_2$
- Type 3: Perioperative
- Type 4:
  - Circulatory shock,
  - Acute respiratory failure

Pneumocystis Carinii Pneumoniae

- Prophylaxis is given in HIV positive patients with CD4 count of less than 200
- Single double: Strength tablet of sulphamethoxazole-trimethoprim is given daily.

Mycobacterium Avium Intracellulare

- Treatment of choice: Clarithromycin + ethambutol + rifabutin

Bronchial Asthma

Creola boides Desquamated epithelial cells
Curschman's spirals Bronchial mucous casts

Sarcoidosis

- Pseudo tuberculosis/Osteitis tuberculosa/Multiplex cystoids/Jungling disease/Schaumann's disease
- Biopsy evidence of mononuclear cell granulomatous inflammatory process is mandatory for definitive diagnosis of sarcoidosis
- Lung is the most common site to biopsied

Shrinking Lung Syndrome

- Seen in SLE
- Diaphragmatic dysfunction with loss of lung volume

Paraneoplastic Syndromes in Lung Cancer

Small cell Ca	Adenocarcinoma	Squamous cell Ca
Eaton-Lambert	Clubbing	Hypercalcemia
Syndrome		
Cushing's syndrome		
Acromegaly		
SIADH		

Management of Lung Carcinoma

- Treatment of small cell carcinoma: Chemotherapy
- Treatment of squamous cell Carcinoma and adenocarcinoma: Radiotherapy and surgery
- Best response to chemotherapy and radiotherapy is shown by small cell carcinoma, but it has worst prognosis.

Bronchial Carcinoids

- No known relationship to cigarette smoking
- Neuroendocrine differentiation of Kulchitsky cells of bronchial mucosa
- Carcinoid syndrome:
  - Episodic flushing, diarrhea, bonchospasm, cyanosis
  - Due to release of vasoactive amines like serotonin, from carcinoid tumors
- Pancoast tumor is a type of squamous cell carcinoma.
- Clara cell are seen in broncho-alveolar carcinoma.
- Most common site of metastasis from lung carcinoma is adrenal glands

Pulse	Description	Seen in	
Anacrotic	Slow rising, twice	AS	
	Beating, both in systole		
Pulsus bisferiens	Rapid rising, twice	Idiopathic Beating, both in systole subaortic stenosis with mild AR	Hypertrophic
Dicrotic pulse	Twice beating, 1in Systoe, 1 in diastole	Decreased peripheral resistance and diastolic pressure like typhoid CCF, cardiac tamponade, open heart surgery	
Pulsus parvus et tardus	Slow rising	AS	
Pulsus alternans	Strong and weak Beats alternately	Left ventricular failure, toxic myocarditis, Paroxysmal tachycardia, Following a premature beat	
Pulsus paradoxus	Systemic blood Pressure falls more Pericarditis	Superior vena cava obstruction, than 10 mm Hg effusion, severe on inspiration	COPD, pericardial CCF, constrictive
Pulsus bigeminus	Coupling of pulses	Alternate premature beat, AV block, SA node block with ventricular escape	
Water hammer Pulse	Increased stroke volume	Fever, pregnancy, alcoholism, anemia, Beriberi, Cor-pulmonale, cirrhosis, Paget's disease, AV fistula, thyrotoxicosis, AR, PDA, rupture sinus of Valsalva , bradycardia, systolic hypertension	

Jugular Venous Pulsation

Normal waves with their causes

Waves	Causes
A	**A**trial contraction
C	Ventricular **C**ontraction
V	Inflow from **V**enacavae
X	Atrial rela**X**ation
Y	Atrial empt**X**ing

Abnormal Waves with Causes

Waves	Causes
Large 'a'	Tricuspid stenosis/Pulmonay stenosis/pulmonary hypertension
Absent 'a'	Atrial fibrillation
Cannon 'a'	Complete heart block
c-v waves	Tricuspid regurgitation
Deep y descent	Chronic constrictive pericarditis
Raised JVP	Right ventricular failure
Kussmaul's sign	Constrictive pericarditis, Constrictive Cardiomyopathy, Pericardial effusion, Severe right heartfailure.
Deep x descent	Acute cardiac tamponade
Prominent v ware	Tricuspid regurgitation
Accentuated x descent	Constrictive pericarditis
Reversed x descent	Tricuspid regurgitation

Heart Sounds

Loud S1	Mitral stenosis
Soft S1	Mitral regurgitation, mitral stenosis
Reversed splitting of S2	LBBB

A-V Block

- 1st degree: PR interval > 200 msec, every P is followed by QRS
- 2nd degree: Progressive increase in PR till P is not
- Mobitz's type I: Transmitted. Block is usually in the His-Purkinje system
- 3rd degree: Atria and ventricles beat independently.

Arrhythmias	Drug of choice
Atrial extrasystole	Quinidine
PSVT	Adenosine/Verapamil
Atrial flutter	Cardioversion/Verapamil
Ventricular extrasystole	Lidocaine
Ventricular tachycardia	Lidocaine/cardioversion
Ventricular fibrillation	Defibrillation, Lidocaine
Wolff-Parkinson: White syndrome	Cardioversion/Amiodarone

Torsades De Pointes

- Ventricular tachycardia characterized by polymorphic QRS complexes that change in amplitude and cycle length
- Magnesium sulfate is the drug of choice.

Jone's Criteria for Rheumatic Fever

Major criteria	Minor criteria
Carditis	Fever
Sydenham's	Arthralgia
Subcutaneous nodules	Prolonged PR interval
Erythema marginatum	Elevated acute phase reactants
Migratory polyarthritis	

Essential Criteria

- Evidence of recent group A streptococcal infection
- Positive throat culture of rapid antigen detection test
- Elevated or increasing streptococcal antibody test.

Gamna-Gandy bodies

- Are foci of fibrosis containing iron and calcium
- Seen in sickle cell anemia, CML, cirrhosis with portal hypertension.

Signs in Aortic Regurgitation

Sign	Explanation
Watson's sign	Bounding peripheral pulses
Waterhammer pulse	
Corrigan's pulse	Rapid upstroke and collapse of the carotid artery pulse
de Musset's sign	Head nodding in time with the heart beat
Quincke's sign	Pulsation of the capillary bed in the nail
Duroziez's sign	Systolic and diastolic murmurs described as 'pistol shots' heard over the femoral artery when it is gradually compressed
Traube's sign	A double sound heard over the femoral artery when it is compressed distally
Lighthouse sign	Blanching and flushing of forehead
Landolfi's sign	Alternating constriction and dilatation of pupil
Becker's sign	Pulsations of retinal vessels
Muller's sign	Pulsations of uvula
Mayen's sign	Diastolic drop of BP > mm Hg with arm raised
Rosenbach's sign	Pulsatile liver
Gerhardt's sign	Enlarged spleen
Hill'sign	A ≥ 20 mm Hg difference in popliteal and brachial systolic cuff pressures, seen in chronic severe AI
Lincoln sign	Pulsatile popliteal
Sherman sigh	Dorsalis pedis pulse is quickly located and unexpectedly prominent in age > 75 year

Mitral Valve Prolapse/Barlow's Syndrome/ Floppy Valve Syndrome

- Commoner in females
- Mostly asymptomatic
- Non-ejection systolic click
- Echocardiography is the investigation of choice

Murmur	Characteristics
Murmur of AR	High pitched, blowing, decrescendo, diastolic, best heard in third intercostals space along left sternal border.
Austin Flint murmur	Soft, low pitched ejection murmur (seen in AR)
Mill wheel murmur	Air embolism
Lerman scratch	Grating systolic sound, heard over sternum in second space seen in thyrotoxicosis
Graham Steel murmur	Pulmonary regurgitation
Seagull murmur	Seen in rheumatic fever, due to turbulence of low around swollen valves.

Continuous Murmurs

- Patent ductus arteriosus
- Coronary fistula
- Ruptured aneurysm of sinus of Valsalva
- Aortic septal defect
- Anomalous left coronary artery
- Mammary soufflé
- Intercostal arteriovenous fistula
- Cervical venous hum
- Bronchial collateral circulation

Conditions and their Effects on Murmur

- Standing increases murmur of MVP, HOCM
- Sustained handgrip accentuates murmur of MR, AR, HOCM

Lesion Seen in Infective Endocarditis

- Osler's nodes: Painful tender pea-sized erythomatous nodules in the pulp of fingers and soles in patients of infective endocarditis
- Janeway lesions: Small maculopapular erythematous or hemorrhagic emboli to distal digital arteries, commonly seen in palm and soles
- Roth's spots: Oval, retinal hemorrhages with a clear pale center
- Splinter hemorrhages: Linear, subungual dark red streaks commonly seen in fingers.

CK

- Rises at 4-8 hours,
- Peaks at 16-24 hours
- Returns to normal at 3-4 days

Troponin T

- Begins to rise at 4-6 hours
- Peaks at 12-24 hours
- Returns to normal at 7-10 days

Contraindication to Thrombolytic Therapy

Absolute	Relative
Past history of cerebrovascular hemorrhage	Current use of anticoagulants
Any cerebrovascular event in the past one year	Recent invasive or surgical procedure or prolonged cardiopulmonary resuscitation
Suspicion of aortic dissection	Active peptic ulcer disease
Active internal bleeding	Adequately controlled severe hypertension.
	Known bleeding diasthesis
	Pregnancy
	A hemorrhagic ophthalmic condition

Enzyme Markers in MI

Creatinine phosphokinase	Appears within 2-4 hours, peaks by 24 hours, returns to normal by 3 days.	Very sensitive, less specific
Lactate dehydrogenase	Seen within 24 hours, peaks by 4-5 days, returns to normal in days.	Not specific
Troponin T/ I	Rises within 4-8 hours, Peaks in 10 days	MC used Very sensitive and specific

Troponin is Elevated in

- Myocardial infarction
- Pulmonary embolism
- Congestive heart failure

Principle Features of Cardiac Tamponade

- Elevation of intracardiac pressure
- Limitation of ventricular
- Limitation of ventricular filling
- Reduction of cardiac output

Conditions Associated with Hypochromic Microcytic Anemia/HcMcA are:

- Thalassemia (normal level of free erythrocyte protoporphyrin)
- Iron deficiency anemia
  - Increased TIBC
  - Increased red cell distribution width
  - Decreased ferritin
  - Decreased MCV
  - Decreased MCH
- Sideroblastic anemia
- Lead toxicity
- Anemia of chronic diseases
  - HcMcA may or may not be seen
  - Increased serum ferritin
  - Decreased serum iron levels
  - Decreased total iron binding capacity/ TIBC
- HcMcA with decreased serum iron and increased TIBC suggests: Iron deficiency anemia
- HcMcA with decreased serum iron and decreased TIBC suggests: Anemia of chronic diseases
- Conditions associated with normocytic, normochromic anemia are:
  - Sickle cell anemia
  - Fanconi anemia
  - Hereditary spherocytosis
- Haemochromatosis: Elevated serum ferritin, elevated serum iron and elevated percent tarnsferrin saturation

Hyperbaric Oxygen is Used in the Treatment of

- CO poisoning
- Gas gangrene
- Radiation induced tissue injury
- Diabetic leg ulcers
- Very severe blood loss, anemia
- Decompression sickness.

Hemolytic Transfusion Reactions

- Most common symptom is sensation of heat and pain along the vein into which the blood is being transfused, flushing on face, lumbar pain
- Oliguria and hemoglobinuria is seen
- In anesthetized patients: Abnormal bleeding and continued hypertension despite adequate replacement are seen

Concentrations of Abnormal Hemoglobin Complexes Producing Cyanosis

- Sulph Hb: 0.5 per cent
- Meth Hb: 1.5 per cent
- Deoxy Hb: 5 per cent

Age at Diagnosis is the Most Important Prognostic Factor in AML

- ALL: Peak incidence is before 10 years
- AML: After 65 years

Bernard-Soulier Syndrome

- Platelet function disorder characterized by deficiency of glycoprotein Ib (von Willebrand's factor receptor)
- Thromobocytopenia with giant platelets

Glanzmann's Thrombasthenia

- Deficiency of glycoprotein IIb and III a (fibrinogen receptor Platelet count is nomals

Hodgkin's Disease

Most common type	Nodular sclerosis
Best prognosis	Lymphocytic predominance
Popcorn cells are seen in	Lymphocytic predominance
Lacunar cells seen in	Noddlar sclerosis
Reed-Sternberg cells	Seen in all varieties, maximum in mixed cellularity

Order of Involvement Nodes in Hodgkin's Disease

Cervical, mediastinal, para-aortic

Epstein-Barr Virus (Associated with)

- Infectious mononucleosis
- Thymoma
- Burkitt's lymphoma
- CNS lymphoma
- Hodgkin's disease
- NHL
- B cell lymphoma
- T cell lymphoma
- Oral hairy leukoplakia
- Tonsillar carcinoma
- Angioimmunoblastic lymphoma

Cold AIHA	Warm AIHA
IgM	IgG
Mycoplasma infection	Lymphomas
Mononucleosis	SLE
Idiopathic Paroxysmal	Methyldopa
cold hemoglobinuria (IgG)	

Therapeutic Nuclear Magnetic Resonance

- I 131: Thyroid cancer, Graves disease
- I 131MIBI: Pheochromocytomas, Neuroblastomas
- Yttrium-90 – Octreotide: Carcinoma with Somatostatin receptors
- P- 32, Sr- 87: Bone metastasis, pain palliation, Rheumatoid arthritis
- I 131, I 125 lipoidol: Hepatic carcinoma
- Au-198: Pleural/Pericardial effusion

HLA Association of Diseases

- HLA A3: Hemochromatosis
- HLA B5/ B51: Behcets's syndrome
- HLA B27: Ankylosing spondylitis, Reiter's syndrome, Reactive arthritis, Psoriatic arthritis, JRA.
- HLA DR2: Narcolepsy, Multiple Sclerosis
- HLA DR3: Celiac disease, Sjogren's syndrome, Dermatitis herpetiformis, Chronic active hepatitis, Adrenal insufficiency.
- HLA B8/HLA DR3: Grave's disease , Myasthenia gravis.
- HLA DR4/ DW4: Rheumatoid arthritis
- HLA DR2/DR3/DR4: IDDM
- HLA DQ2/ HLA B8: Gluten sensitive enteropathy.
- HLA BW47: Inherited error of metabolism

Immune Thrombocytopenic Purpura

- Therapy includes steroids, intravenous immunoglobulins, anti D immunoglobulin and splenectomy.

Polymyositis

- Ocular muscles are not involved

Dermatomyositis

- Classical rash: Helkiotreope rash in butterfly distribution
- Gottron rash
- Erythema of the knuckles with a rasied violaceous scaly eruption seen in dermatomyositis

Pyrexia of Unknown Origin

- In 1961, Petersdorf and Beeson suggested the following criteria
- Fever higher than 38.3°C (101°F) on several occasions, persisting without diagnosis for at least 3 weeks.
- At least 1 week's investigation in hospital
- Tuberculosis is the commonest cause of PUO

Hereditary Angioedema

- Deficiency of C1 inhibitor
- Autosomal dominant

Myasthenia Gravis

- Extraocular muscles are most commonly affected first
- Pupils are never affected
- Associated with thymoma
- Edrophomium, a quick and short acting anticholinersterase is used for diagnosis.

Lambert-Eaton Neuromuscular Syndrome

- Associated with malignancy in only 50 per cent
- Most commonly associated with small cell carcinoma

- Neoplasm induced IgG antibody against the voltage gated calcium channels in the terminus of the motor neuron

Ulcerative colitis	Crohn's disease
Cigarette smoking is protective	Cigarette smoking causes disease
Commonest symptom is bloody	Commonest symptom is non
Diarrhea and abdominal pain	Bloody diarrhea, abdominal pain
No cobblestoning of mucosa	Cobblestoning of mucosa +
Rectum is always involved	Rectum is spared
Continuous lesions	Skip lesions
No recurrence after surgery	Recurs after surgery
Antibiotics not effective	Antibiotics are effective
Toxic megacolon is seen	Not seen
Lead pipe appearance on barium meal	String sign on barium meal
pANCA present	ASCA present

Causes of Pseudomembranous Colitis

- Clostridium difficile
- Ischemic colitis
- Volvulus
- Staphylococcus
- Shigella
- Candida

Liver

- 5′ nucleotidase-determines whether rasied alkaline phosphatese is hepatic in origin.
- Gamma glutary1 transpeptidase/GGT: Increased in cholestasis, Increased in patients of alcohol abuse.
- Auxilliary liver transplant: Transplanted liver provides temporary support till the native liver recovers.

Purtscher's Retinopathy

- Complication of acute pancreatitis
- Sudden and severe loss of vision
- Due to occlusion of posterior retinal artery with aggregated granulocytes
- Fundoscopic appearance of cotton wool spots and hemorrhages confined to an area of optic disc and macula.

Grading of Hepatic Encephalopathy

Grade	Clinical features
Subclinic	Impaired psychomotor testing
1	Asterixis
2	Disorientation
3	Stupor
4	Deep coma

Terms

- Somogyi effect: Overnight hyperglycemia after hypoglycemia due to counter regulatory hormones. Management – decrease insulin dose
- Dawn phenomenon: Early morning hyperglycemia. Management – increase dose or delay it
- Honeymoon period: Seen in type I diabetes, Drastic decrease in insulin requirement followed by rise due to temporary recovery of beta cells
- Brittle diabetes: Seen in type I diabetes, Rapid changes in blood glucose level, from hypoglycemia to ketoacidosis

Classical Triad of Pyonephrosis

- Anemia
- Fever
- Loin swelling

Causes of Papillary Necrosis

- Analgesic abuse
- Diabetes mellitus
- Infant in shock
- Pyelonephritis
- Obstruction
- Sickle cell disease
- Ethanol

Dietl's Crisis

- Intermittent unilateral hydronephrosis after an attack of renal colic,
- Followed hours later by passage of urine,
- Disappearance of swelling and relief of pain.

Bartter's Syndrome

- Hypertrophy and hyperplasia of Juxtaglomerular cell
- Hypokalemic alkalosis and hyperaldosteronism

Diagnostic Nuclear Magnetic Resonance

- I-131, I-123: Thyroid
- Tc- 99m DTPA: Kidney glomerular function. Mucociliary clearance of lungs in pneumocystis carinii pneumoniae infection in AIDS
- HIDA: Liver function and biliary clearance
- Tc- 99m MAA: Lung perfusion
- Tc- 99m DMSA: Kidney cortical scarring
- Tc- 99m MIBI: Thyroid carcinoma
- Cr-51: RBC scan
- Thallium: Myocardial infarction
- Tc- 99m pertechnate: Hot spots
- I 131 hippuran: Kidney
- Xe- 133: Lung ventilation scan

- Tc 99 m MDP: Bone tumors and infections
- Gallium- 67, Iridium – 111: Leucocyte scan Strontium: Fracture neck femur
- Gallium 67: Sarcoidosis

MEA/MEN

MEA I	Parathyroid gland- chief cell hyperplasia
(Werner's)	hyperparathyroidism, Pancreas – islet cell tumour, Zollinger- Ellison syndrome, Pituitary- anterior acromegaly, Cushing's syndrome
MEA II a	Parathyroid gland- pheochromocytoma
	Thyroid- medullar carcinoma
MEA II b	Parathyroid gland – chief cell hyperplasia – Hyperparathyroidism, Adernal gland-Pheochromocytoma, Neurofibromatosis Thyroid – Medullary carcinoma

Thyroid

- Jod Basedow thyrotoxicosis: Large doses of iodine given to hyperplastic endemic goiter which is iodine-avid may produce temporary hyperthyroidism and occasionally persistent hyperthyroidism
- Wolf- Chaikoff effect: In normal individuals large doses of iodine act directly on the thyroid to produce a mild and transient inhibition of organic binding of iodide and hence of hormone synthesis

Primary Hyperparathyroidism

- Bones, groans, stones and psychic moans.

Landry-Guillain-Barre Syndrome

- Acute inflammartory demyelinating polyradiculopathy
- History of preceding viral infection
- Ascending weakness
- Albumino-cytological dissociation present
- Treatment includes steroids, plasma exchange, intravenous immunoglobulin.

Miller-Fisher Variant of Guillain-Barre Syndrome

- External ophthalmoplegia
- Ataxia
- Areflexia

Wallenberg's Syndrome/Lateral Medullary Syndrome

- Due to PICA infarct
- Ipsilateral loss of pain and temperature over the face
- Ipsilateral 9th, 10th, and 11th cranial nerve palsy
- Ipsilateral Horner's syndrome
- Ipsilateral cerebellar signs
- Ipsilateral vestibular signs
- Contralateral loss of pain and temperature over the limbs

Jackson's Syndrome/Medial Medullary Syndrome

- Ipsilateral twelfth nerve palsy
- Contralateral hemiplegic
- Contralateral loss of joint position sense and vibration

Millard-Gubler Syndrome/Ventral Pontine Syndrome

- Ipsilateral seventh nerve palsy
- Contralateral hemiplegia

Raymond-Foville Syndrome

- Ipsilateral facial palsy
- Ipsilateral abducens palsy
- Contralateral hemiparesis

Weber's Syndrome

- Ipsilateral third nerve palsy
- Contralateral hemiplegia

Benedikt's Syndrome

- Ipsilateral rubral tumor
- Contralateral hemiparesis

CNS Causes of Hemiplegia

- Thrombosis of unpaired anterior cerebral artery
- Superior sagittal sinus
- Parasagittal meningioma
- Cortical venous sinus thrombosis

Similar Sounding Terms

- Tabes dorsalis: Neurosyphilis affecting posterior column of spinal cord
- Tabes mesenterica: Tuberculous affection of mesenteric lymph nodes
- Tabes ergotica: A condition similar to Tabes dorsalis due to ergotism
- Friedrich's tabes: Friedrich's ataxia
- Lupus vulgaris: Skin TB
- Lupus pernio: A form of Sarcoidosis.

Syphilitic Aneurysm

- Most common ste of syphilitic aneurysm is ascending and transverse portion of the arch of aorta
- It also leads to ventricular dilatation (Cor bovinum)

Brown-Sequard Syndrome

- Ipsilateral lower motor neuron paralysis in the segment.
- Ipsilateral spastic paralysis below the level
- Ipsilateral band of cutaneous anesthesia at the level
- Ipsilateral band of posterior column sensation loss below the level
- Contralateral loss of pain and temperature sensation below the level
- Contralateral impaired tactile sensation below the level.

Thalamic Pain Syndrome (Dejerine-Roussy Syndrome)

- Affects contralateral side of the body
- Due to thalamic infarct in ventral posterolateral nucleus

Frontal Disinhibition Syndrome

- Loss of initiative, creativity and curiosity
- Pervasive emotional apathy
- Anomic aphasia is the single most common language disturbance seen in head trauma, metabolic encephalopathy and Alzheimer's disease
- Prolactin is increased after an episode of seizures.

Déjà vu

- Déjà vu and Jamais vu phenomenon are seen in partial seizures
- Déjà vu is seen in temporal lobe epilepsy, normal people, psychosis, hysteria
- Déjà vu feeling of familiarity with unfamiliar situations
- Jamais vu: Felling of unfamiliarity with familiar situations.

West Syndrome

- Epileptic encephalopathy
- Onset between 4–8 months of age
- Salaam attacks
- Hypoarrhythmia on EEG
- Treatment with ACTH or vigabatrin

Gait	Condition
Circumduction	Hemiplegia
Scissoring gait	Spastic paraplegia
Festinating gait	Parkinson's disease
Wadding gait	Muscular dystrophies
Stamping gait	Sensory ataxia
Broad based gait	Cerebellar disorders
Broad based high stepping gait	Posterior column disorders
Charlie Chaplin gait	Tibial torsion, Homocystinuria
Lurching gait	Cerebellar ataxia

Intracranial Aneurysm

- Most common site is between anterior cerebral and anterior communicating artery
- Intracranial aneurysms: Rupture is likely if >7 mm in diameter
- Progressively enlarging unruptured aneurysm most commonly involve occulomotor nerve
- Most common nerve to be involved with raised intracranial tension is the abducent nerve
- Most common site of hypertensive hemorrhage in brain is putamen
- Marchiafava: Bignami syndrome: Widespread demyelination of cerebral hemispheres due to chronic alcoholism.

Craniopharyngioma

- It is called 90 per cent tumor
- 90 per cent are calcified
- 90 per cent are cystic
- 90 per cent show enhancement

Brain Secondaries

- Most common secondaries to brain are from:
- Carcinoma lung
  - Carcinoma breast
  - Carcinoma kidney

Cluster Headache

- 1-3 short lived daily attacks, of unilateral, orbital or temporal pain of 4-8 weeks interval followed by pain free interval often of 1 year
- Associated with red, tearful eye, nasal stuffiness
- Commonly in males

Epilepsy

- Twilight sleep is seen in epilepsy
- Twilight sleep is the state of narrowing of field of consciousness for short duration followed by amnesia.
- Jacksonian march: Seen in simple partial seizures, the abnormal motor activity begins in a limited area and then gradually spreads to involve larger areas.
- Todd's paralysis: Type of postictal focal neurological deficit seen in partial motor seizures.
- Absence seizures: Typically, 3 Hz spike and wave pattern discharge is seen.

Clinical Triad of Tuberous Sclerosis

- Adenoma sebaceum
- Epilepsy
- Mental retardation

Wilms' Tumor is Assoiated with

- WAGR syndrome (Wilm's tumor, Aniridia, Genital abnormalities, mental retardation)
- Denys- Drash syndorome
- Beckwith- Weidemann syndrome

Charcot's Triad (Seen in Ascending Cholangitis)

- Jaundice
- Abdominal pain
- Fever

Saint's Triad

- Diverticulosis
- Gallstones
- Hiatus hernia

Reynold's Pentad

- Jaundice
- Abdominal pain
- Fever
- Shock
- Confusion

Diseases Associated with Massive Splenomegaly

- Chronic myelogenous leukemia
- Lymphomas
- Hairy cell leukemia
- Myelofibrosis with myeloid metaplasia
- Polycythemia vera
- Gaucher's disease
- Chronic lymphocytic leukemia
- Sarcoidosis
- Autoimmune hemolytic anemia
- Splenic hemangiomatosis
- Malaria
- Kala azar

Strawberry Tongue

- Scarlet fever
- Kawasaki's disease
- Toxic shock syndrome

Diseases with their Specific Antibodies

- SLE: Anti ds DNA (specific) Anti Sm {Smith}
- Drug induced SLE: Anti Histone
- Systemic sclerosis: Anti DNA Topoisomerase {Scl 70}
- Scleroderma {CREST}: Anticentromere
- Sjogren's syndrome: SSA (Ro) SSB (La)
- Primary biliary cirrhosis: Antimitochondrial
- Inflammatory myopathy : Histidyl t- RNA synthetase
- Mixed connective tissue disorders: Antiribonucleoprotein
- Churg Strauss: Antiribonucleoprotein ANCA
- Multifocal motor neuropathy: Anti GM1
- Wegener's granulmatosis, Henoch-Schonlein purpura: c-ANCA
- Idiopathic crescentric nephritis , Ulcerative colitis, Microspcopic polyangitis, Polyarteritis nodosa: p-ANCA
- Crohn's disease: Anti-saccharomyces crevisiae (ASCA)
- Celiac sprue: Antiendomysial and Antigliadin
- Psychosis/Depression due To CNS SLE: Antiribosomal –P.

Vaccines Recommended in HIV Positive Patients

- Pneumococcal vaccine: Consider revaccination five years after initial dose.
- Hepatitis B vaccine: Administer to patients without serologic evidence of past or present Hepatitis B infection. Vaccinated patients after the third dose; nonresponders should receive booster injections
- Hemophilus influenzae type B vaccine: Administer to asplenic patients and those with history of recurrent hemophilus infection.
- Influenza vaccine: Administer to patients at high-risk for exposure to or morbidity from influenza. There is evidence that the vaccine may transiently promote HIV replication.
- Tetanus toxoid: Td booster is recommended every 10 years.
- Polio vaccine: IPV is administered.

CRITERIA FOR AIDS—If Two of the Major with at Least One of the Minor Signs are Present

Major signs	Minor signs
Weight loss of more than 10 per cent of body weight	Persistent cough for more than 1 month
Chronic diarrhea for more than 1 month	Generalized pruritic dermatitis
Prolonged fever for more than 1 month	History of herpes zoster oro-pharyngeal candidiasis
	Chronic progressive or disseminated herpes simplex infection. Generalized lymphadenopathy

POEMS Syndrome

- Polyneuropathy
- Organomegaly
- Endocrinopathy
- M protein band on electrophoresis with less than 5 percent plasma cells in bone marrow
- Skin hyperpigmentation.

Glasgow Coma Scale

Remember EVM- 4-5-6

Eye Opening

4. Spontaneous
3. On verbal stimuli
2. On pain stimuli
1. No response

Verbal Response

5. Oriented
4. Confused
3. Inappropriate
2. Nonspecific sounds
1. No response

Motor Activity

6. Follows command
5. Localizes pain
4. Withdraws to pain (pressure on nail bed, words If no response supraorbital pressure or suprasternal pressure)
3. Flexion to pain
2. Extension to pain
1. None

   Maximum score – 15
   Minimum score – 3

Neurological derangement	Score
Severe	8 or less
Moderate	9 – 12
Minor	13 – more

Other Scales Used in ICU

- SOFA-Sequential Organ Failure Assessment Score
- SAPS II- Simplified Acute Physiology Score
- APACHE II/III – Acute Physiology and Chronic Health Evaluation
- Rancho Los Amigos cognitive scale.

MCQs WITH SHORT EXPLANATIONS

HEMATOLOGY

1. **Which is NOT true regarding haemochromatosis:**
   a. Hepatic cirrhosis b. CNS manifestations
   c. Heart failure d. Impotence

Features of Haemochromatosis
- Cirrhosis of the liver
- Diabetes due to pancreatic islet cell failure
- Cardiomyopathy
- Arthritis (calcium pyrophosphate deposition in joints)
- Testicular failure
- Slate grey discoloration of the skin

2. **Which of the following is NOT a feature of vitamin K deficiency:**
   a. Associated thrombocytopenia with prolonged bleeding
   b. Deficiency is rarely seen, except in infants
   c. Factor X is first to be affected
   d. Warfarin causes vitamin K deficiency

Vitamin K is required for the synthesis of clotting factors and hence deficiency leads to prolonged coagulation and bleeding (NOT because of thrombocytopenia)

3. **All of the following are true for thalassemia major EXCEPT:**
   a. Target cells b. Hepatosplenomegaly
   c. Need of transfusion d. Macrocytic anemia

Thalassemia major shows microcytic hypochromic anemia

4. **FALSE regarding sickle cell anemia:**
   a. Autosomal recessive b. Painful crisis
   c. Raised ESR
   d. Increased target cells seen

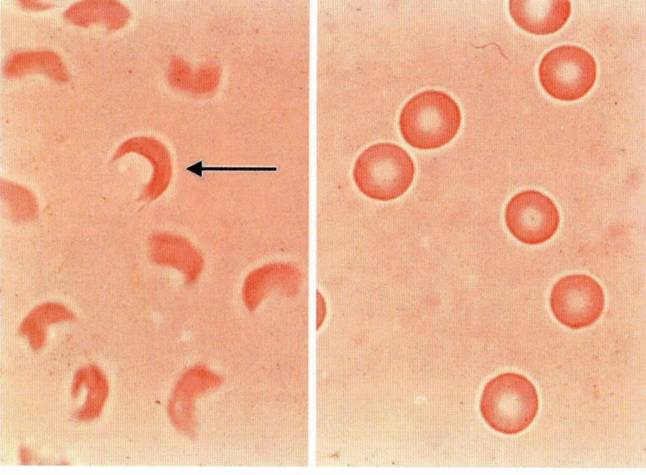

Sickle cell anemia (HbS)
Note: (A) sickling-arrow (B) oxygenated blood

The ESR is decreased in polycythemia, hyperviscosity, sickle cell anemia, leukemia, low plasma protein (due to liver or kidney disease) and congestive heart failure.

5. **NOT a cause of microcytic hypochromic anemia:**
   a. Lead poisoning
   b. Thalassemia
   c. Iron deficiency anemia
   d. Fanconi anemia

Fanconi anemia/ congenital pancytopenia (special form of aplastic anemia) is an autosomal recessive disorder characterized by developmental abnormalities, bone marrow failure and cancer predisposition; especially squamous cell carcinoma and acute myeloid leukemia.

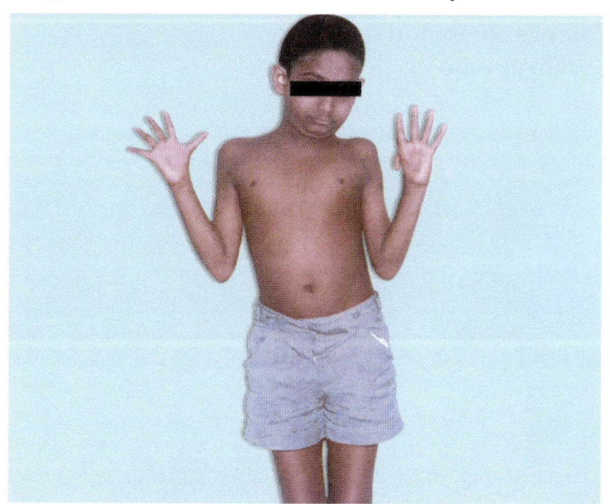

Fanconi's anemia, boy aged 12 years
Note hypoplastic thumb left hand

6. **A patient presents with microcytic hypochromic anemia. Serum iron levels and TIBC are decreased and serum ferritin is increased. Likely diagnosis is:**
   a. Iron deficiency anemia
   b. Anemia of chronic diseases/ ACD
   c. Thalassemia
   d. Sideroblastic anemia

Ferritin levels are higher in ACD due to an increase in storage iron in reticuloendothelial/ RE cells and also the acute inflammatory reaction raising ferritin levels.

Shows the clinical parameters to distinguish between IDA and ACD

Parameter	ACD	IDA	Combined ACD+IDA
Iron	Reduced	Reduced	Reduced
Transferrin	Reduced	Increased	Reduced

Contd...

Ans. 1. **b.** CNS mani... 2. **a.** Associated... 3. **d.** Macrocytic anemia 4. **c.** Raised ESR 5. **d.** Fanconi anemia 6. **b.** Anemia of chronic diseases/ACD

Contd...

Parameter	*ACD*	*IDA*	*Combined ACD+IDA*
Transferrin saturation	Reduced	Reduced	Reduced
Ferritin	Normal	Reduced	Reduced or normal
STR	Normal	Increased	Normal or increased
STR/log ferritin	<1	>2 High	> 2
Cytokine levels	Increased	Normal	Increased

7. Which of the findings are consistent with the diagnosis of iron deficiency anemia:

a. Increased TIBC, decreased serum ferritin
b. Decreased TIBC, decreased serum ferritin
c. Increased TIBC, increased serum ferritin
d. Decreased TIBC, increased serum ferritin

Total Iron Binding Capacity/TIBC in both males and females is 340 mg/dL, with the range of 250-450 mg/dL. Estimation of serum ferritin is helpful to assess the iron stores in the body, and therefore, wherever facilities permit, this should be done. Values below 15 microg/L, suggest depletion of stores.

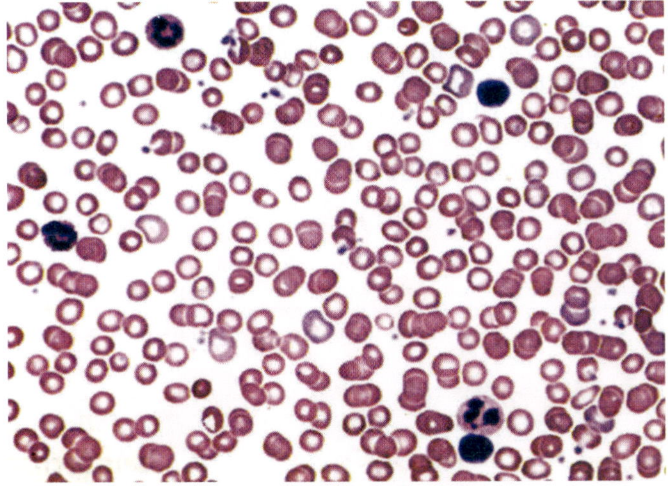

PB iron deficiency anemia

8. Most sensitive and specific test to diagnose iron deficiency anemia is:

a. Serum iron levels
b. Serum ferritin levels
c. Serum transferrin receptor population
d. Transferrin saturation

Ferritin contains two types of monomers – the light (L-monomer) and the heavy (H-monomer). The L-monomer which is basic, binds very readily and tightly to the iron. This property makes it suitable for storing iron.

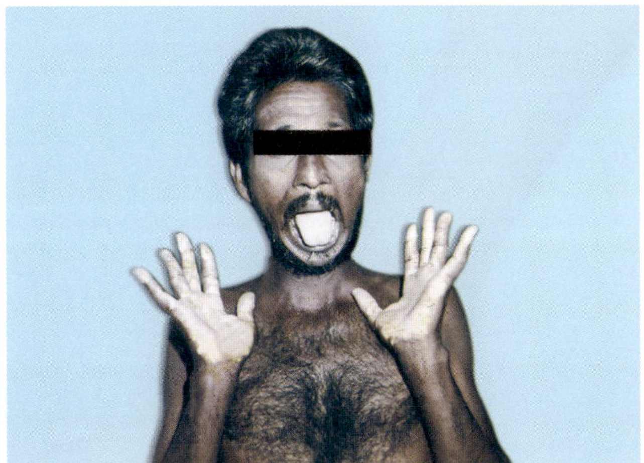

Male iron deficiency anemia. Note: Pallor: small pale tongue

9. NOT a feature of iron deficiency anemia:

a. Hypersegmented neutrophils
b. Microcytosis preceeds hypochromia
c. MCHC < 50%
d. MC cause of anemia in India

In megaloblastic anemia, granulocytes are larger than normal, showing increased lobulation with the average lobe count higher than 5 (macropolycytes). This change in leukocytes is very helpful in diagnosis when the morphology of erythrocytes is equivocal.

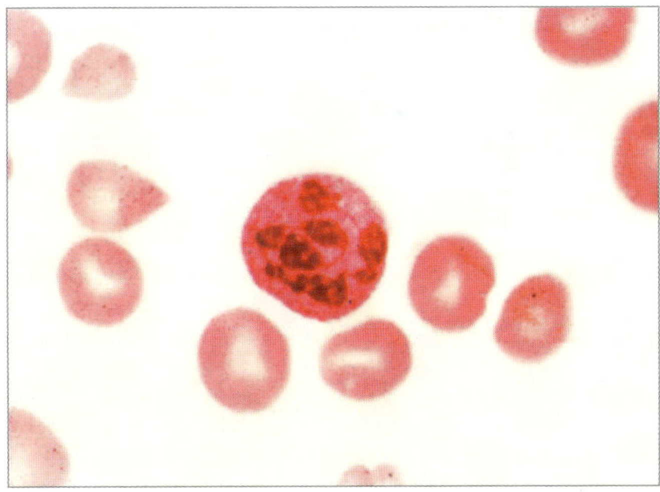

PB megaloblastic anemia with hypersegmented neutrophil

10. FALSE regarding Henoch-Schonlein purpura:

a. IgM antibodies are foundb. Palpable purpura
c. Self limiting
d. Ig antibodies are involved

Although the cause of anaphylactoid purpura/Henoch-Schonlein purpura (HSP)/hypersensitivity angitis/ rheumatic purpura is unknown, IgA has a pivotal role in the pathogenesis of HSP. Among the two subclasses of IgA – (IgA1 and IgA2) only IgA1 is involved in HSP. IgA1 is deposited in blood vessel walls and renal mesangium.

Ans. 7. **a.** Increased TIBC... 8. **b.** Serum ferritin levels 9. **a.** Hypersegmented... 10. **a.** IgM antibodies are found

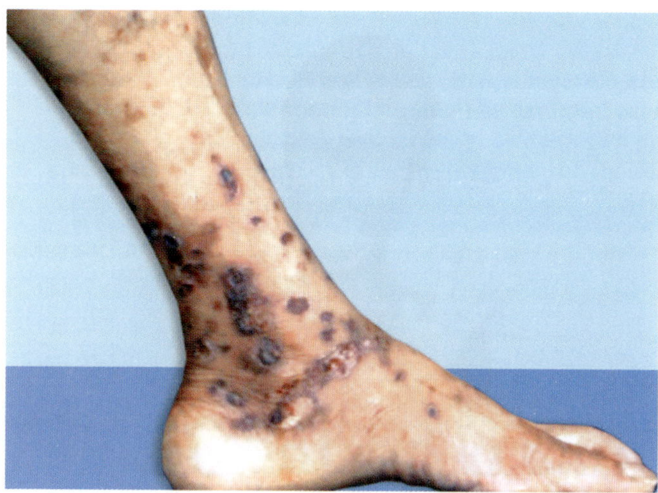

Pitted lesions persisting after relief of anaphylactoid purpura

11. Hemolytic anemia as a result of intrinsic red cell defect is a feature of:

a. Auto-immune hemolytic anemia
b. Hereditary spherocytosis
c. Pyruvate kinase deficiency
d. G-6PD deficiency

HS is the MC inherited disorder of erythrocyte membrane. It is an autosomal dominant disorder presenting as a chronic hemolytic anemia with the presence of spherocytes in peripheral blood, intermittent jaundice, and splenomegaly.

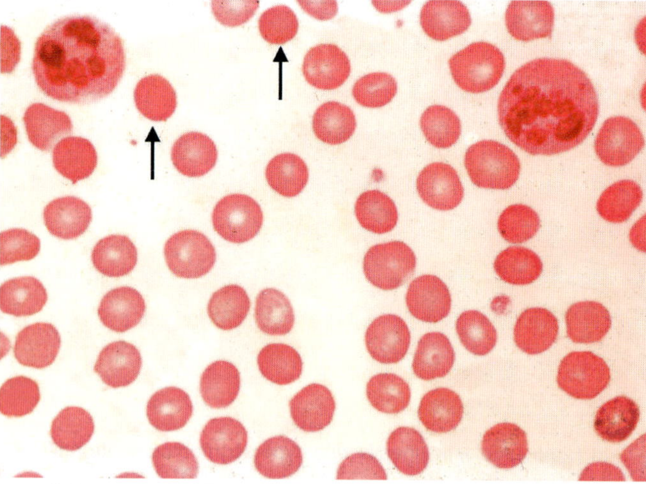

Spherocytosis-PB: Note: The small densely stained RBCs-(spherocytes)-arrows

12. In hemolytic anemia, all of the following are true EXCEPT:

a. Bone marrow hyperplasia
b. Reticulocytosis
c. Increased unconjugated bilirubin
d. Increased haptoglobin

Haptoglobin combine with hemoglobin liberated from red cells to form comlexes which are rapidly destroyed. Consequently, haptoglobin level in serum is lowered in active hemolysis.

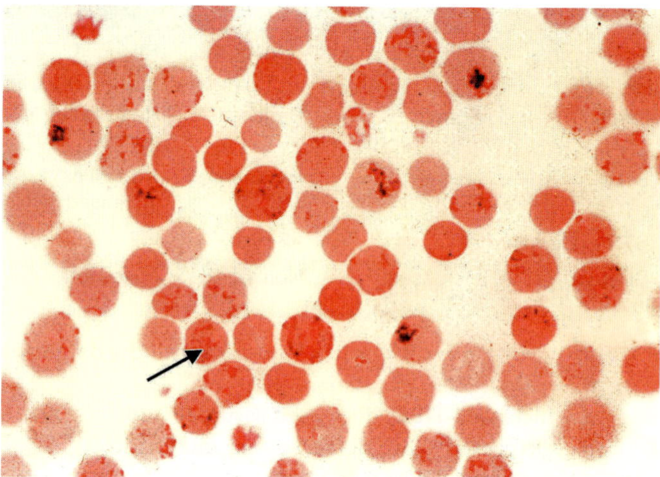

Hemolytic anemia peripheral blood x 1000 reticulocytes increased-note reticulum within erythrocytes-arrow

13. Microangiopathic hemolytic anemia is associated with:

a. Diabetes Mellitus
b. Vitamin B12 deficiency
c. Hemolytic uremic syndrome
d. All of the above

Microangiopathic hemolytic anemia (MHA) comprises thrombotic thrombocytopenic purpura (TTP), hemolytic uremic syndrome (HUS), chemotherapy induced microangiopathic hemolytic anemia, malignant hypertension and the HELPP syndrome (hemolysis, elevated liver enzyme levels and a low platelet count occurring in association with pre-eclampsia).

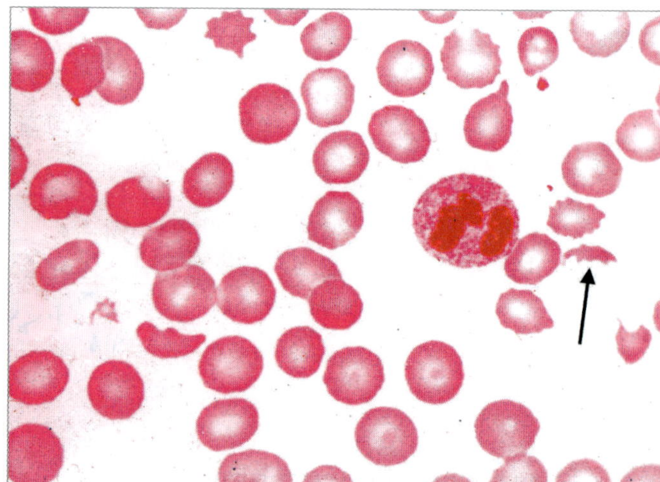

Blood smear–schistocytes in microangiopathic hemolytic anemia (arrow)

14. In alpha-thalassemia trait, electrophoresis shows:

a. Increased HbF and normal HbA2
b. Normal HbF and normal HbA2
c. Normal HbF and decreased HbA2
d. Decreased HbF and normal HbA2

Ans. **11. b.** Hereditary... **12. d.** Increased haptoglobin **13. c.** Hemolytic uremic... **14. b.** Normal HbF and...

Alpha-thalassemia trait result from deletion or inactivation of two alpha-globin genes (--/αα in cis configuration or –α/-α in trans configuration). Carriers of α^o- thalassemia show microcytosis (low MCV), hypochromia (low MCH), normal percentages of HbA2 and HbF, and RBC inclusion bodies.

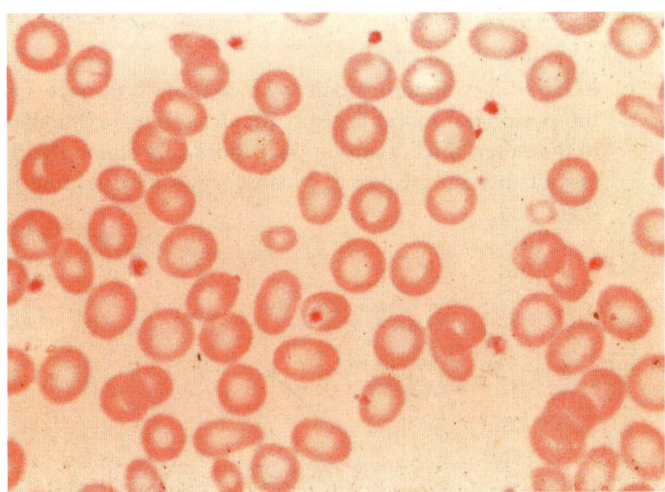

PB thalassemia minor. Note: Mild hypochromia

15. A patient presents with increased serum iron, decreased TIBC, increased % saturation and increased serum ferritin. Most likely diagnosis is:

a. Anemia of chronic disease
b. Sideroblastic anemia
c. Iron deficiency anemia
d. Thalassemia major

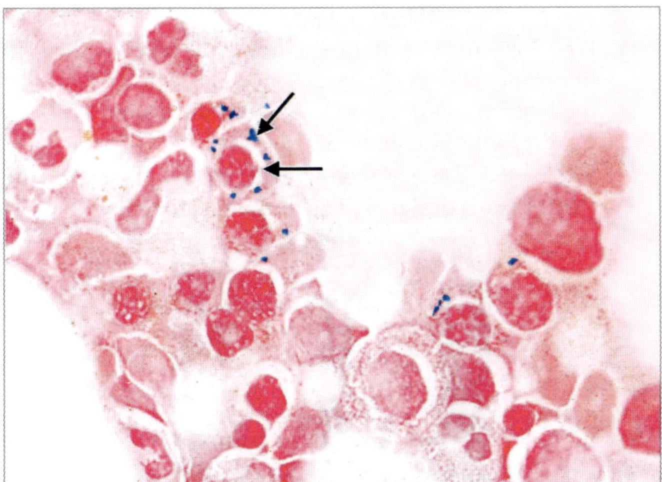

Sideroblastic anemia bone marrow. Note: Ringed sideroblast stained by Prussian blue method arrows

Lab features of sideroblastic anemia

- Anemia is moderate to severe and dimorphic
- Basophilic stippling
- Target cells
- Pappenheimer bodies
- MCV decreased
- RDW (red blood cell distribution width) is increased
- Increased serum iron, percentage saturation and ferritin
- TIBC of the cells is normal to decreased

16. NOT a cause of macrocytic anemia:

a. Liver disease
b. Copper deficiency
c. Thiamine deficiency
d. Orotic aciduria

Copper deficiency leads to hypochromic, microcytic anemia in experimental animals. Copper deficiency may occur in infanys fed solely on milk or due to severe malnutrition.

Classification of anemia based on erythrocyte morphology	
Microcytic hypochromic anemia	Iron deficiency, thalassemias, hemoglobinopathies, and hemolytic anemia
Normocytic normochromic anemia	Aplastic anemia
Macrocytic normochromic anemia	Folate deficiency, vitamin B12 deficiency, hypothyroidism
Macrocytic hypochromic anemia (dimorphic)	This picture is due to combined deficiency of iron and folate or B12

17. A patient presented with macroglossia and loss of tongue papilla. His Hb is 8.5 and MCV is 100. Next step in investigation:

a. Vitamin B12 estimation
b. Brush biopsy of the lesion
c. Fluconazole lesion
d. Incision biopsy

Features of megaloblastic anemia

- Large beefy tongue
- Hemoglobin level may vary from 5 to 8 g/dL
- MCHC is within normal range (28-32%)
- MCV is increased and may be as high as 120 ft

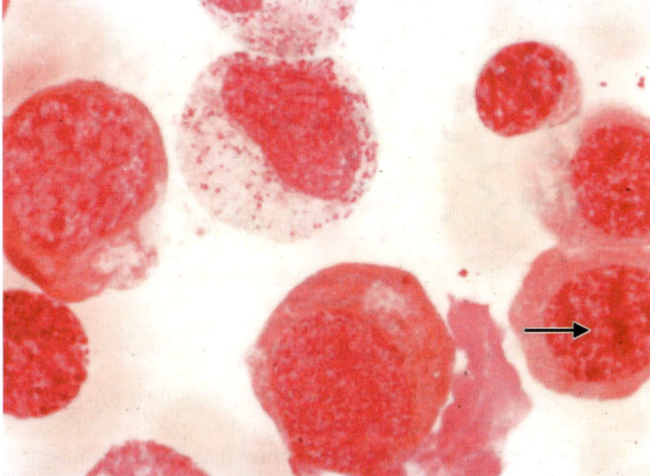

Megaloblastic bone marrow. Note: Megaloblast: nuclear chromatin is loose—arrow

Ans. 15. **b.** Sideroblastic... 16. **b.** Copper deficiency 17. **a.** Vitamin B12

18. Megaloblastic anemia should be treated with both folic acid and vitamin B12 because:

a. Folic acid alone causes improvement of hematologic but worsening of neurological symptoms
b. It is a cofactor
c. It is an enzyme
d. None of the above

Oral administration of 1 mg or more of folic acid daily is adequate to correct the folate deficiency. Supplementation of folic acid will improve the anemia due to deficiency of vitamin B12 also, but not the neurological complications.

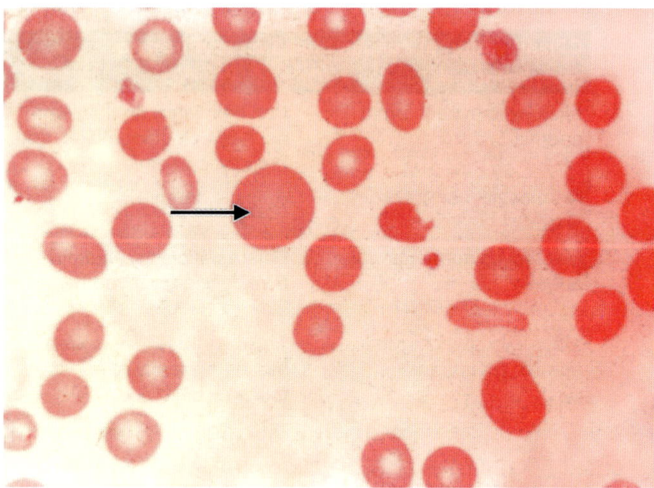

PB megaloblastic anemia. Note: Macrocyte—arrow

19. Philadelphia chromosome is NOT involved in:

a. ALL
b. CLL
c. AML
d. CML

Ph[1]

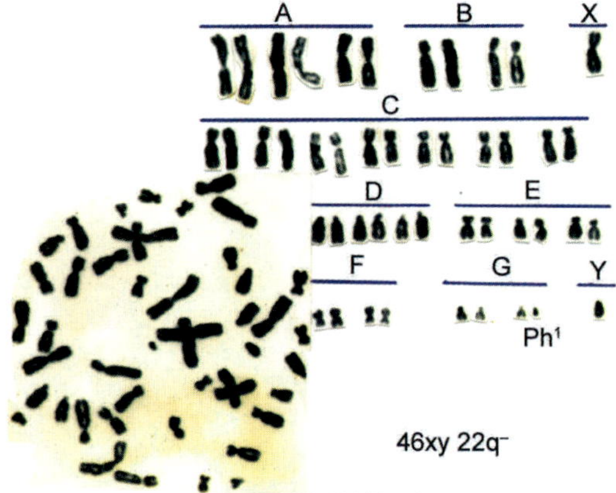

Chronic Myeloid Leukemia
Karyotyping
Note: Ph Chromosome

CML karyotype showing Ph[1] chromosome

Over 95% of CML shows a constant chromosomal abnormality in the myeloid, erythrid and megakaryocytic cells. This abnormal chromosome known as Philadephia chromosome (Ph[1]) is formed by the reciprocal translocation of the long arms of chromosome 22 and chromosome 9.

A subgroup of ALL, especially in adults shows Ph[1] chromosome positivity on karotyping

Occasionally seen in acute myelogenous leukemia

20. NOT a feature of hereditary Spherocytosis:

a. Autosomal dominant
b. Increased RBC surface area
c. Increased MCHC
d. Normal or increased MCV

In hereditary spherocytosis, over 30% of erythrocytes is the peripheral blood are spherocytes. They are smaller in diameter, thicker and appear uniformly stained with loss of the central pallor. Mean corpuscular volume is increased.

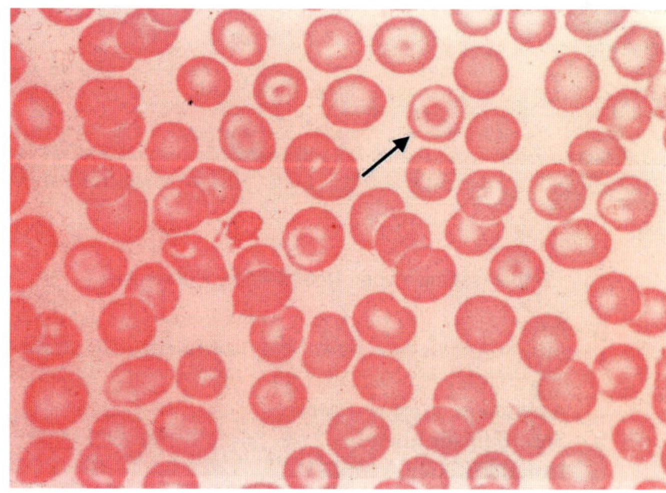

Peripheral blood-post splenectomy
Note:Target cells-arrow

21. First investigation to be done in a patient with thrombocytopenia:

a. Platelet count
b. Bleeding time
c. Prothrombin time
d. aPTT

When the platelet count falls below 1,00,000/cmm (1010/L), it is designated as thrombocytopenia.

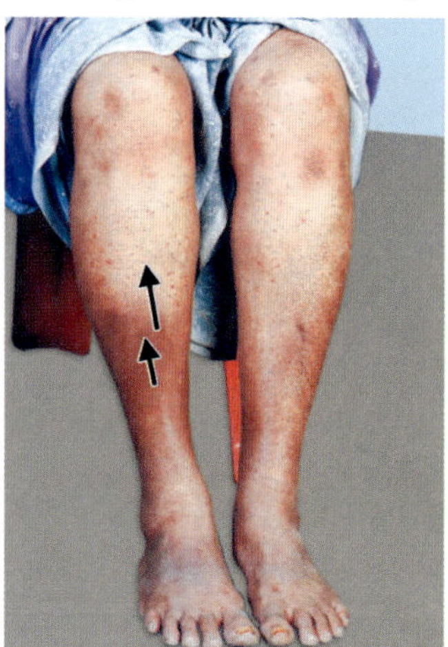

Female purpura over legs

Ans. **18. a.** Folic acid alone... **19. b.** CLL **20. b.** Increased RBC... **21. a.** Platelet count

22. Gum hyperplasia is seen in:

a. CLL b. CML
c. ALL d. AML

Some people with AML may experience swelling of the gums because of infiltraion of leukemic cells into the gum tissues.

Classification of neoplasia involving leukocytes

1. Acute leukemias
Acute myeloid leukemia (AML) French, American, British (FAB) Classification. Differentiation of the immature cells forms the main criteria.

Subclass	Type of cell
M_0	Undifferentiated by light microscopy
M_1	Poorly differentiated
M_2	More differentiated
M_3	Dysplastic promyelocytes
(acute promyelocytic leukemia)	M_3h-hyper granular PML
	M_3v-inapparent or fine granules
	M_3a-less hypergranular blasts
M_4	Both granulocytic and Monocytic
M_4	Eo-Myelodysplastic eosinophils
M_5	Monocytic differentiation M_5a-predominantly blasts M_5b-differentiation into promonocytes and monocytes
M_6	Myeloblasts with dysplastic erythroid precursors
M_7	Megakaryoblastic

Acute lymphatic leukemia (FAB):
When stained with Wright's stain three types—L1, L2 and L3 can be distinguished morphologically

L1 The blast cells are small and there is no appreciable variation in size and shape. The nuclear chromatin is smooth and the nucleoli are indistinct.

L2 The blast cells vary in size with prominent nucleoli and a variable amount of cytoplasm.

L3 The cells are deeply basophilic with vacuolated cytoplasm.Immunological markers and other cytochemical markers help to identify the cell precisely.

Different hematological cancers can be distinct at the molecular level even though they may appear similar morphologically. This is true for acute and chronic leukemias and lymphomas. Acute lymphatic leukemias can be broadly grouped into three

1. Precursor B lymphoblastic leukemia
2. Precursor T lymphoblastic leukemia
3. Burkitt lymphoma or leukemia

In addition there are acute leukemias of ambiguous lineage. These are:

1. Biphenotypic acute leukemias
2. Undifferentiated acute leukemias

The availability of immunological probes like monoclonal antibodies, techniques like flow cytometry and DNA microarray analysis have enabled the sub-typing of acute leukemias and lymphomas based on immunological markers such as CD positivity (cluster group of differentiation). This has helped to devise specifically effective therapy with less of side effects.

Classification of neoplasia involving leukocytes

2. Chronic leukemias
Chronic myeloid leukemia (CML)
Chronic lymphatic leukemia (CLL)
Hairy cell leukemia (variant of CLL)
Prolymphocytic leukemia (variant of CLL)
Plasma cell leukemia
Chronic myelomonocytic leukemia
Sézary syndrome: (leukemic phase of mycosis fungoides)

23. NOT a side effect of blood transfusion:

a. Hypokalemia b. Hypomagnesemia
c. Hypocalcemia d. Iron overload

Metabolic complications may develop due to citrate toxicity, potassium toxicity, toxic substances eluted from synthetic containers, and vasoactive substances, especially after massive transfusion.

The storage requirements and shelf- life of blood products

Blood product	*Storage specification*	*Shelf-life*
1. Red cells	2–6°C	35 days
2. Frozen red cells	2–6°C	24 hours (reconstituted)
3. Washed red cells	2–6°C	6 hours
4. Granulocyte	Room temperature	24 hours concentrates
5. Platelet concentrates	Room temperature with agitation	5 days
6. Fresh frozen plasma	–20–40°C	12 months
7. Cryoprecipitate	–20–40°C	12 months

24. Osmotic fragility is increased in:

a. Sickle cell anemia b. Thalassemia
c. Hereditary spherocytosis
d. Chronic lead poisoning

Osmotic fragility of erythrocytes is determined by estimating the hemolysis when a standard volume of erythrocytes is added to increasing dilutions of sodium chloride. Osmotic fragility is increased in spherocytosis and decreased in thalassemia.

APPENDIX
Normal hematological values

1. Hemoglobin		
	Infants	16–18 g/dL
	Men	13–16 g/dL
	Women	11–14.5 g/dL
2. Red cells		
	Infants	$5–6 \times 10^{12}$/L
	Men	$4–6.6 \times 10^{12}$/L
	Women	$3.5–4.5 \times 10^{12}$/L
3. PCV		
	Men	40–54%
	Women	35–47%
4. MCV		76–94 fl

Contd...

Ans. 22. d. AML 23. a. Hypokalemia 24. c. Hereditary spherocytosis

Contd...

APPENDIX Normal hematological values		
5. MCH		27–32 picogram (pg)
6. MCHC	32–36 g/dL	
7. Reticulocytes	0.2–2.5%	
8. ESR		
	Males	0–10 mm 1st hour (Westergren)
	Females	0–20 mm 1st hour (Westergren)
9. White cells		
	Infants	15-16 × 10^9/L
	Adults	5-10 × 10^9/L
10. Differential leukocyte count		
Adults:		
Neutrophils		40–75%
Lymphocytes		20–45%
Monocytes		2–9%
Eosinophils		1–5%
Basophils		0.0–1%
11. Platelets	150,000-400,000 per mm^3 (1.5–4 × 10^{11}/L)	
12. Bleeding time	(Ivy's method) upto 10 min	
13. Coagulation time	(Lee and White method at 37°C) 5–11 min	
14. Prothrombin time	12–14 sec	
15. Plasma fibrinogen	150–400 mg/dL	
16. Serum iron	60–160 μg/dL	
17. Total iron binding capacity (TIBC) (Transferrin)	280–400 μg/dL	
18. Serum ferritin		
	Males	40–340 μg/dL
	Females	14–148 μg/dL
19. Serum folate	6–20 ng/mL	
20. RBC folate	160–640 ng/mL	
21. Serum vitamin B_{12}	100–1000 pg/mL	

25. FALSE regarding sickle cell anemia:

a. Mutations in alpha chain
b. Symptoms ameliorated by HbF
c. Veno-occlusive crisis is cause of morbidity
d. Bone pain is presenting feature

Hemoglobin S is formed by the substitution of valine in place of glutamic acid in the sixth residue of the beta chain of adult hemoglobin and it is a slow-moving hemoglobin.

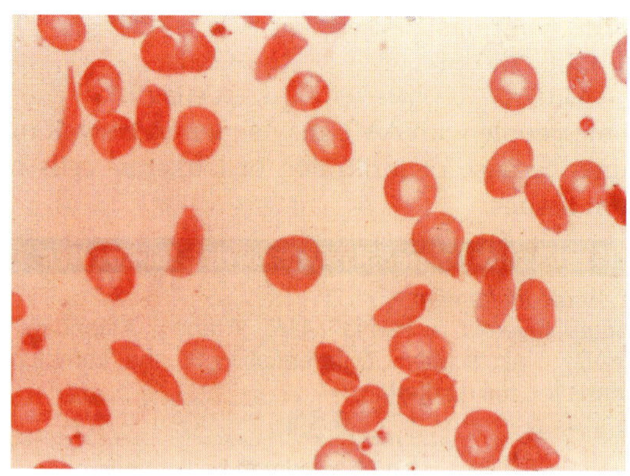

PB sickle cell anemia.
Note: The sickle showed erythrocytes

26. FALSE regarding beta thalassemia trait:

a. Raised HbF b. Raised HbA2
c. Microcytosis d. Severe anemia

Thalassemia minor/ trait is seen in parents of children with thalassemia major who have genetic abnormalities and morphological abnormalities in erythrocytes but no anemia.

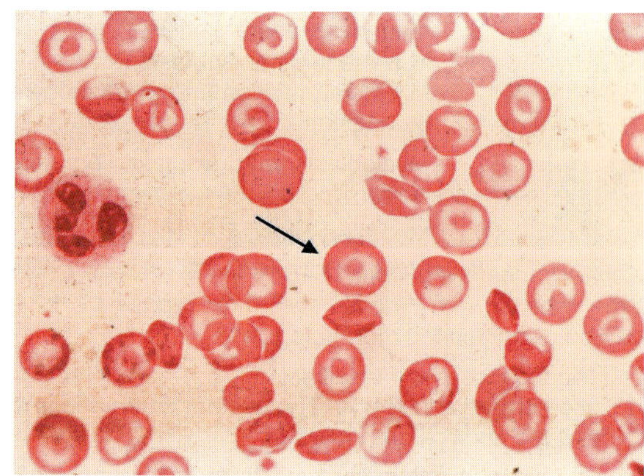

PB target cells in thalassemia—arrow

27. Hair on end appearance on skull radiograph is seen in:

a. Thalassemia b. Hydrocephalus
c. Chronic malaria d. Aplastic anemia

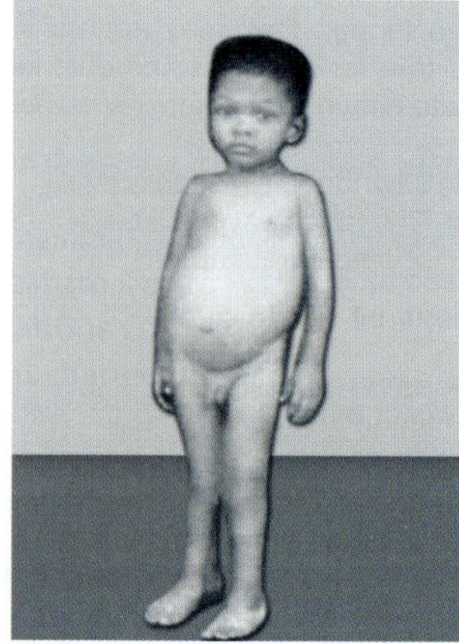

Boy aged 4 years. Thalassemia major Note the gross splenomegaly

Ans. **25. a.** Mutations... **26. b.** Raised HbA2 **27. a.** Thalassemia...

In thalassemia, "Hair-on-end" appearance on skull X-ray and thinning and widening of metacarpal shafts indicate enlargement of bone marrow tissue.

28. FALSE regarding paroxysmal nocturnal hemoglobinuria:

a. Hemosiderinuria
b. Pancytopenia
c. Increased leucocyte alkaline phosphatase score
d. Cellular marrow

Lower levels of LAP are found in pathologies that involve undeveloped leukocytes, such as chronic myelogenous leukemia (CML), paroxysmal nocturnal hemoglobinuria (PNH) and acute myelogenous leukemia (AML).

29. Polycythemia may be associated with:

a. Carcinoma breast
b. Hepatic hemangioma
c. Renal cell carcinoma
d. Mesothelioma

Malignant tumors producing excessive erythropoietin (causing secondary polycythemia)

- Hepatocellular carcinoma
- Renal cell cancer
- Cerebellar hemangioblastoma

30. True for von-Willebrand disease:

a. Normal partial thromboplastin time
b. Decreased platelets
c. Normal prothrombin time
d. Normal bleeding time

Laboratory tests for VW disease show prolonged bleeding time, reduced levels of factor VIII, reduced levels of vWF antigen and reduction of ristocetin cofactor.

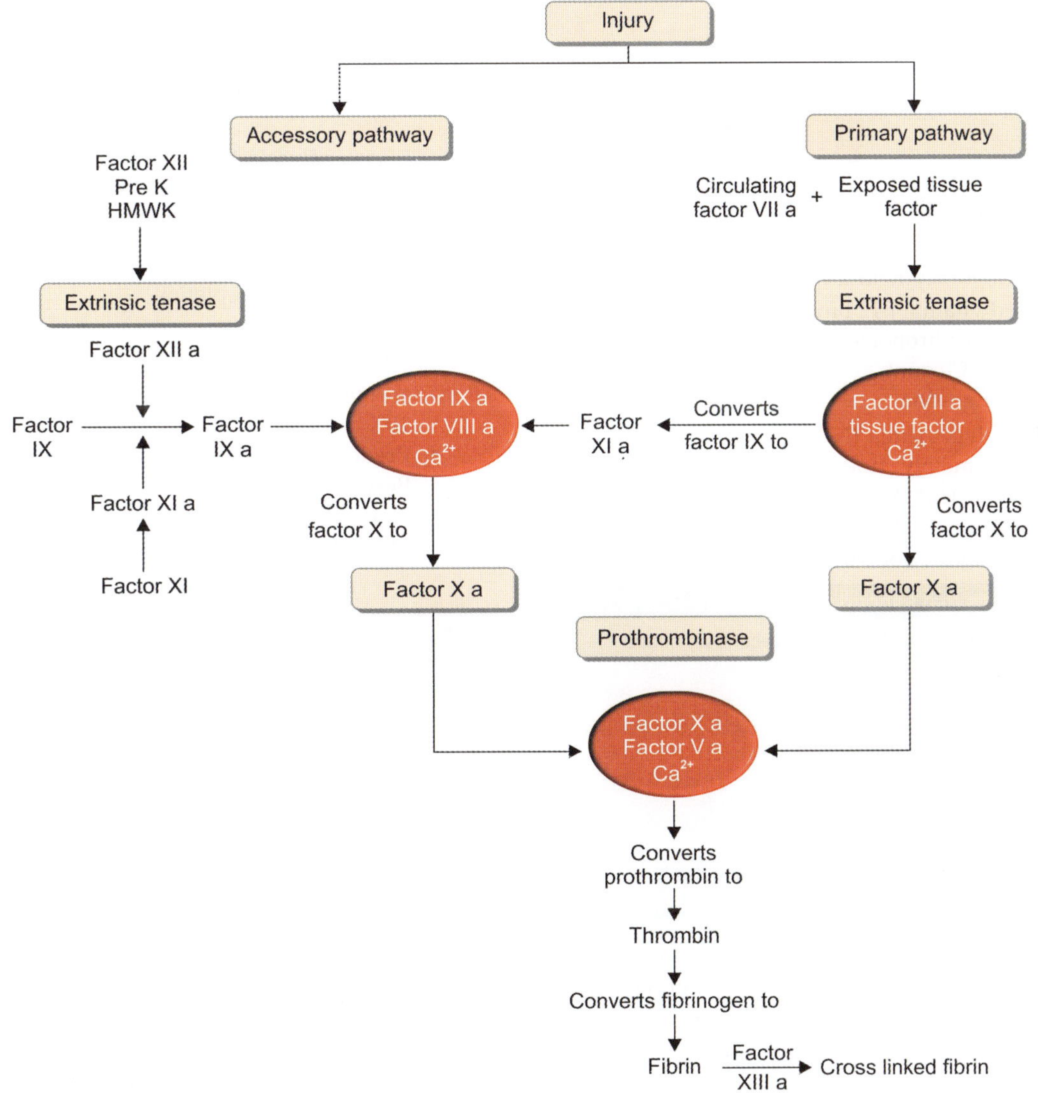

Overview of hemostasis. Note: The term extrinsic and intrinsic 'tenase' indicate their enzymic activity

Ans. **28. c.** Increased... **29. c.** Renal cell carcinoma **30. c.** Normal prothrombin time

31. FALSE regarding aplastic anemia:

a. Splenomegaly b. Reticulocytopenia
c. Thrombocytopenia d. Neutropenia

The picture of peripheral pancytopenia with aplastic bone marrow confirms the diagnosis of aplastic anemia. Acute myeloid leukemia may be mistaken for aplastic anemia in the initial stages, but presence of splenomegaly is suggestive of AML.

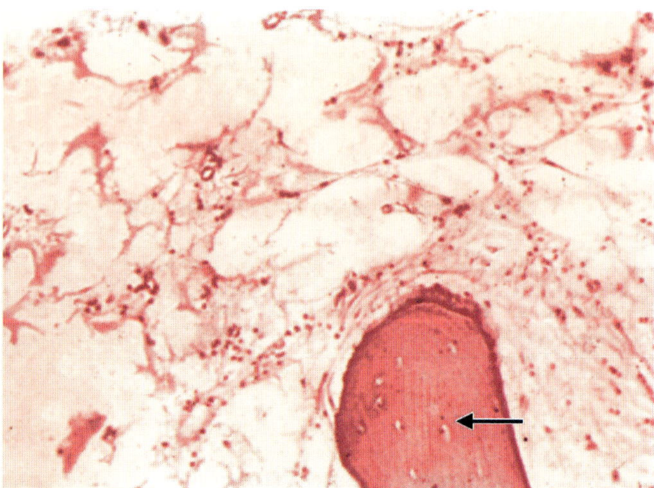

Aplastic anemia – Bone marrow. Note: (1) Reduction in cellularity (2) Increase in fat spaces and (3) arrow points to a spicule of bone

32. NOT seen in polycythemia rubra vera/ PRV:

a. Increased vitamin B12 binding capacity
b. Increased erythropoietin level
c. Increase RBC count
d. Ocular congestion

Secondary polycythemia (NOT primary polycythemia/ PRV) occurs mainly due to increased amounts of erythropoietin (EPO) secreted as a physiological response to hypoxic stimulus, or abnormal secretion of EPO from the kidney or from ectopic foci.

Features that support the diagnosis of PRV
1. Polycythemia without any known secondary cause
2. Splenomegaly
3. Elevated white blood cell count > 12 × 10^9/L
4. Increased basophil count
5. Thrombocytosis > 400 × 10^9/L
6. Elevated serum uric acid levels
7. Elevated leukocyte alkaline phosphatase levels
8. Elevated serum vitamin B_{12} and vitamin B_{12}-binding protein levels.

33. A patient is being evaluated for anemia. Bone marrow tap is 'dry'. Peripheral smear showed tear drop cells. Most likely diagnosis is:

a. Leukemia
b. Lymphoma
c. Myelofibrosis
d. Polycythemia rubra vera

The erythrocytes in myelofibrosis shows marked aniso and poikilocytosis with polychromasia and characteristic 'tear drop' cells. Bone marrow aspiration often results in dry tap.

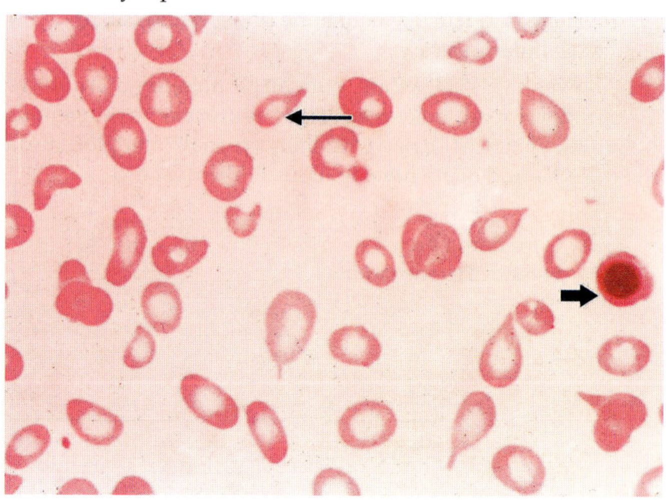

PB myelofibrosis. Note: The teardrop cell (arrow). Normoblast (arrow head)

34. Type of Hodgkin's disease with best prognosis:

a. Lymphocytic predominant
b. Lymphocytic depletion
c. Mixed cellularity
d. Nodular sclerosis

Lymphocyte predominant type of HD

- 10%
- Predominance of lymphocytes with a few RS cells
- Best prognosis
- Nodular variety of lymphocyte predominant HD is of B-cell origin

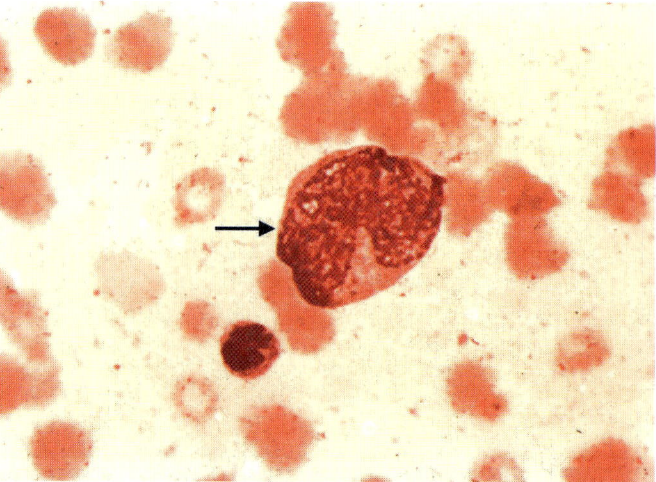

Bone marrow Hodgkin's disease. Note: The Reed-Sternberg's cell (arrow)

Ans. 31. **a.** Splenomegaly 32. **b.** Increased erythro... 33. **c.** Myelofibrosis 34. **a.** Lymphocyctic...

35. Hemophilia A is characterized by all EXCEPT:

a. Bleeding into soft tissues, muscles and joints
b. Reduced VIII levels
c. Prolonged partial thromboplastin time
d. Prolonged prothrombin time

Clinical hallmark of hemophilia A are joint and muscle hemorrhages, easy bruising and prolonged potentially fatal hemorrhage following trauma or surgery, but no excessive bleeding after abrasions or minor cuts. Bleeding time, platelet count, and prothrombin time are normal but PTTK (APTT) is prolonged. Assay of factor VIII helps to establish the diagnosis and assess the severity. Factor VIII assay also helps to monitor replacement therapy.

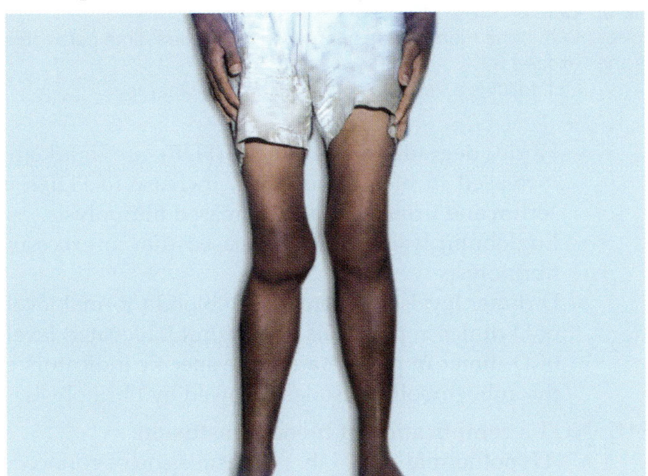

Male: Hemophilial arthritis knees

36. Bleeding time is prolonged in:

a. Hemolytic telangiectasia
b. Henoch Schonlein purpura
c. von Willebrand's disease
d. Hemophilia

Prolongation of bleeding time (Ivy) beyond 12 minutes is definitely abnormal. In dysfunction of platelets and capillaries, BT is prolonged. Common causes of the prolongation of BT are thrombocytopenia (platelet count below 1,00,000/cmm), thrombopathies, von Willebrand's diseases and scurvy.

Coagulation: Nomenclature of the coagulation proteins has been accepted internationally.	
Factor I	Fibrinogen
Factor II	Prothrombin
Factor III	Tissue thromboplastin
Factor IV	Calcium ions
Factor V	Proaccelerin-labile factor
Factor VII	Stable factor-Proconvertin
Factor VIII	Antihemophilic globulin (AHG, AHF)
Factor IX	Plasma thromboplastin component (PTC), Christmas factor
Factor X	Stuart-Prower factor
Factor XI	Plasma thromboplastin antecedent-PTA
Factor XII	Hageman's factor
Factor XIII	Fibrin stabilising factor.

37. Methemoglobinemia may result from exposure to:

a. Sodium chlorate
b. Aniline
c. Isopropyl alcohol
d. Carbon monoxide

Methemoglobinemia is a disorder characterized by the presence of a higher than normal level of methemoglobin (metHb, i.e., ferric/ Fe^{3+} rather than ferrous/ fe^{2+} hemoglobin) in the blood. Classical drug causers of methemoglobinemia include antibiotics (trimethoprim, sulfonamides, and dapsone), local anesthetics (especially articaine, benzocaine, and prilocaine), aniline dyes, metocolopramide etc.

38. NOT a cause of massive splenomegaly:

a. AML
b. CML
c. Hairy cell leukemia
d. Malaria

Liver, spleen and lymph nodes are moderately enlarged in 70-80% of cases in acute leukemia.

Differences between acute and chronic leukemias

	Acute leukemia	*Chronic leukemia*
Age group	More in the first and second decades but can occur in all age groups	Mostly in the 4th, 5th and 6th decades but even young children may be affected rarely
Sex ratio	M:F is 2:1	M:F is 1:1
Duration of symptoms	Weeks to months	Several months to one year
Presenting complaints	Anemia, fever, infections, hemorrhagic tendencies or complications, especially neurological	Vague symptoms, loss of weight, mass in the abdomen, or lymph nodular masses
Organomegaly	Liver, spleen and lymph nodes are moderately enlarged in 70-80% of cases	Moderate to gross splenomegaly is the rule in CML. Moderate to gross lymphadenopathy occurs in CLL.

Contd...

Ans. 35. **d.** Prolonged... 36. **c.** von Willebrand's... 37. **b.** Aniline 38. **a.** AML

Contd...

	Acute leukemia	*Chronic leukemia*
Blood picture	Total leukocyte count is moderately elevated (15-30 × 10_9/litre = 15-30,000/cmm), Blast cells form 10-90% of the total. Platelets are often reduced	Total leukocyte count is grossly elevated, 15-25 × 10^{10}/L (150-250,000/cmm)
Bone marrow	Shows depression of erythroid cells, myeloid cells and megakaryocytes, and infiltration by the abnormal cells. Blast cells form more than 30% and may be even up to 90%	CML shows increase in myeloid cells, especially myelocytes, metamyelocytes, and neurtrophils, infiltration by small lymphocytes is seen in CLL Erythroid and megakaryocytic precursors show variable cellularity.
Chromosomal studies	Different patterns in different subtypes	Ph chromosome is demonstrable in over 95% cases of CML.
Course and prognosis	Untreated, fatal within weeks to six months due to infections, hemorrhage, anemia or other complications	Untreated, CML has a median survival of 18–24 months, CLL has a generally more prolonged course
Response to treatment	Spontaneous remissions have rarely been reported. With modern treatment, over proportion of 90% of cases go into remission and 60–70% get complete cure. Acute lymphatic leukemia in children gives the best results	With modern chemotherapy a small CML is cured With bone marrow transplantation at the ideal-time cure rates exceed 50%. CLL follows a variable course with chemotherapy

39. NOT a cause of palpable purpura:

a. Acute meningococcemia
b. Disseminated gonococcal infection
c. Small vessel vasculitis d. Thrombocytopenia

Causes of palpable purpura

- Rocky mountain spotted fever
- Acute meningococcemia
- Disseminated gonoccal infection
- Ecthyma gangrenosum
- Henoch-Schonlein purpura
- Microscopic polyangitis

40. Most specific investigation in disseminated intravascular coagulation:

a. D-dimer assay b. Bleeding time
c. Clotting time d. Fibrinogen level

Common causes of disseminated intravascular coagulation (DIC)
1. Obstetric: Abruptio placentae, intra-uterine fetal death, septic abortion, and amniotic fluid embolism.
2. Infections: Falciparum malaria, gram-negative septicemia, meningococcemia, septic shock, rickettsial infections, viral infections and several others.
3. Malignant disease: Diseases of prostate, breast, lung, pancreas and others.
4. Hematological malignancies: Acute promyelocytic leukemia.
5. Mismatched blood transfusion with hemolytic transfusion reaction.
6. Cavernous hemangioma.
7. Miscellaneous: Trauma, fat embolism, burns, hypothermia, viper bites, and scorpion bite.

Diagnostic findings in DIC

- Reduction in platelets, fibrinogen (normal fibrinogen in plasma as 150-400 mg/dL), and factors II, V and VIII.
- Prolonged PT and partial thromboplastin time
- Fibrin degradation products (FDP) are markedly increased in blood and urine. Increase in FDP's in serum and urine indicates increased fibrinolysis.
- Euglobulin lysis time is increased due to excessive fibrinolysis
- D-dimer levels are increased in blood (normal levels of D-dimer in plasma is <500 ng/mL). Elevated levels of D-dimer in plasma are more specific indicators of thromboembolic episodes followed by fibrinolysis.

41. NOT a complication of blood transfusion:

a. Hypothermia b. Transmission of gonococci
c. Citrate toxicity d. Hyperkalemia

Transfusion transmitted diseases
1. *Viral infections* a. Human immunodeficiency virus HIV I and HIV II. Data from Delhi gave seroprevalence for HIV rate as 0.71 to 0.77% for blood donors. In Trivandrum the seroprevalence of HIV is 0.2%. In Punjab it was 0.26%.
2. *Hepatitis viruses* All the hepatitis viruses HBV, HCV, delta virus, HAV, HGV and HEV can be transmitted. HBV and HCV are clinically the most important in this group. The approximate risk for transfusion associated hepatitis in India for HBV is 0.07% and for HCV is 0.04%.
Transfusion associated hepatitis (TAH) should be diagnosed if there is elevation of SGPT levels in the recipient to 1.5 times the normal value or more, on two occasions at 5 days interval when estimated at 14-180 days after the transfusion.
3. Other viruses: Human T-cell lymphotropic virus (HTLV) I and II, cytomegalovirus (CMV).
4. Parasitic infections: Malaria, trypanosomiasis, toxoplasmosis, babesiosis.
5. Bacterial infections: Yersinia enterocolitica, Staph. epidermidis, Bacillus cereus, syphilis and others. T. pallidium can remain viable in refrigerated blood for up to 5 days.

Ans. **39. d.** Thrombocy... **40. a.** D-dimer assay **41. b.** Transmission...

42. **Prolonged PT and normal aPTT is a feature of:**
    a. Factor VII deficiency b. Factor VIII deficiency
    c. Factor XII deficiency
    d. von-Willebrand's disease

Activated partial thromboplastin time (APTT)/ Partial thromboplastin time (PTT) measures the time required for the formation of thrombin and fibrin polymers by the intrinsic pathway. Normal APTT is 35 seconds. Value of APTT rises whenever the levels of one or more of the coagulation factors other than factor VII is reduced below 30% of the normal. When the common pathway is impaired, both PTT and APTT are prolonged.

43. **Changes of megaloblastic anemia which may NOT be corrected by administering folic acid:**
    a. Hyperplasia of bone marrow
    b. Neurological changes
    c. Megakaryocytic RBC d. Achlorhydria

Cyanocobalamin is required for the normal metabolism of myelin and other components of the nervous system. Therefore, deficiency of this factor leads to lesion in the nervous system as well (apart from megaloblastic anemia). Supplementation of folic acid will improve the anemia due to deficiency of vitamin B12, but not the neurological complications.

44. **A 50-year-old patient with abdominal discomfort since last 2 years, was found to have a large spleen of 3 kg. Bone marrow is difficult to aspirate. Most probable diagnosis is:**
    a. Sickle cell anemia b. Myelofibrosis
    c. Hemochromatosis d. Iron deficiency anemia

Most patients of myelofibrosis are over the age of 50 years, and they usually come to the medical attention for anemia and symptoms due to splenomegaly which is often massive even at presentation. Bone marrow aspiration often results in dry tap.

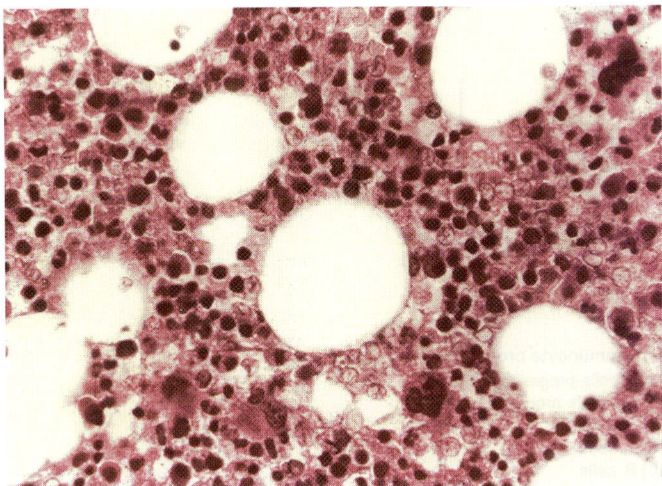

Normal bone marrow × 400

45. **FALSE statement regarding DIC is:**
    a. Thrombocytopenia b. Decreased fibrinogen
    c. Decreased PTT d. Increased PT

Lab diagnosis of DIC

- Platelet count below 1,00,000 and rapidly falling further
- Clotting time, prothrombin time and APTT are all prolonged
- Increase in FDP levels and D-dimer in plasma
- Coagulation inhibitor levels reduced

Differentiation between DIC and primary fibrinolysis

Tests	*Acute DIC*	*Primary fibrinolysis*
Platelet count	Decreased	Normal
Bleeding time	Prolonged	Normal
Clot retraction	Defective	Clot is dissolved
Red cell fragmentation	Present	Absent
Clotting time	Prolonged	Prolonged slightly
Prothrombin time Activated partial	Prolonged	Prolonged
Thromboplastin time	Prolonged	Slightly prolonged
Euglobulin lysis time	Shortened	Shortened
Fibrin split products (FDP) estimation	High titre	High titre
D-dimer levels	Raised	Raised
Thrombin time	Prolonged	Prolonged

46. **Fresh frozen plasma is used for:**
    a. Deficiency of coagulation factor
    b. Deficiency of RBC
    c. Deficiency of proteins
    d. Deficiency of WBC

Fresh frozen plasma (FFP) contains mainly factors V and VIII and is indicated in bleeding in multiple coagulopathies, liver disease, DIC, and bleeding due to massive blood transfusion as a first time therapy.

Blood components: Use and abuse

Component	*Indications*	*Abuse*
Red cells	To increase oxygen carrying capacity in anemic patients	a. As a volume expander b. To improve general "well-being"
Platelets	To control or prevent bleeding associated with deficiencies in platelet number or function	a. Routine treatment of immune thrombocytopenic purpura b. Prophylactically in other conditions
Fresh frozen plasma	As a replacement of clotting factors when specific deficiency is demonstrated	As a simple volume expander

47. **A young girl presents with repeated episodes of bleeding. BT and APTT is prolonged and PT is normal. What is the likely condition:**
    a. Hemophilia A b. Factor VII deficiency
    c. Von-Willebrand disease d. Factor XII deficiency

Ans. 42. **a.** Factor VII... 43. **b.** Neurological changes 44. **b.** Myelofibrosis 45. **c.** Decreased PTT
46. **a.** Deficiency of... 47. **c.** Von-Willebrand disease

Clinical features of vWD are similar to ITP, i.e. excessive post-traumatic bleeding, menorrhagia, and mucosal bleeding, especially from the nose, gums, gastrointestinal tract, and genitourinary tract. Bleeding time is prolonged.

Phenotype	Mechanism	Transmission
1 (1)	Partial quantitative deficiency of vWF and factor VIII	Autosomal dominant (AD)
2 (A)	Defect in platelet dependent vWF and lack of large multimers	AD
2 (B)	Heightened platelet dependent vWF functions associated with lack of large multimers	AD
2M	vWF functions and multimers reduced	AD
2N	Defective vWF binding to factor VIII	AD
3	Severe or complete deficiency pf vWF and moderately severe factor VIII deficiency	Autosomal recessive

48. Diagnostic test for Disseminated Intravascular coagulation is:

a. PT b. D-Dimer assay
c. APTT d. BT

Elevated levels of D-dimer in plasma are more specific indicators of thromboembolic episodes followed by fibrinolysis.

49. Stored blood as compared to fresh blood has:

a. More 2, 3 DPG b. High extracellular K^+
c. High extracellular hemoglobin
d. Increased platelets

Diagrammatic representation of Hematopoieses from a precursor stem cell

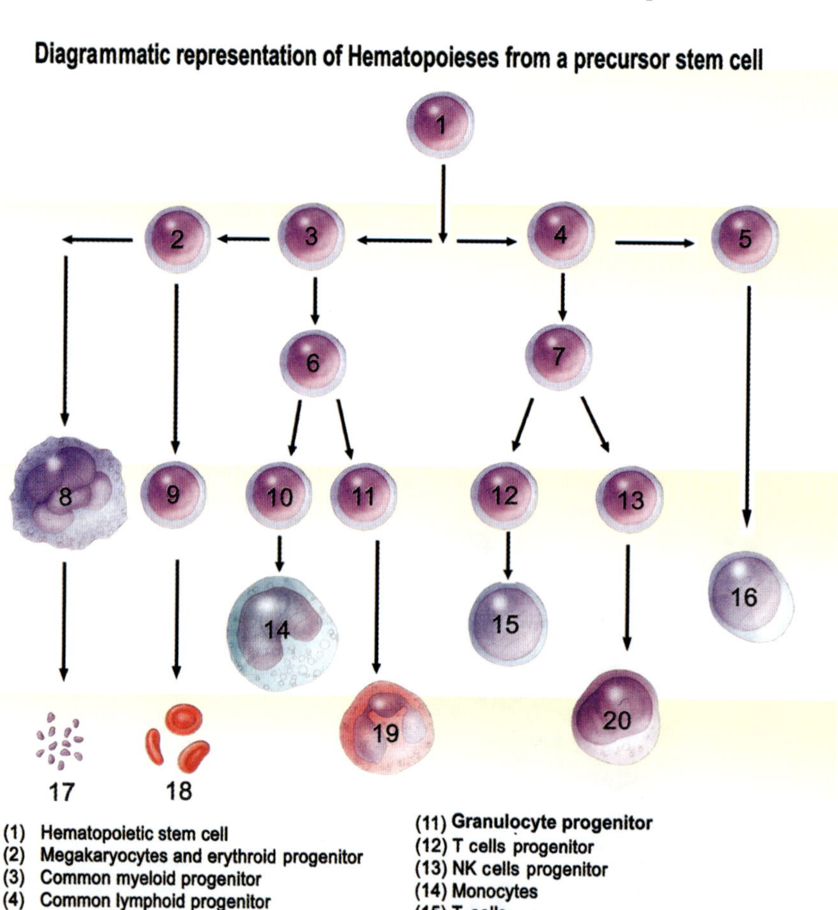

(1) Hematopoietic stem cell
(2) Megakaryocytes and erythroid progenitor
(3) Common myeloid progenitor
(4) Common lymphoid progenitor
(5) Unilineage committed progenitor for B cells
(6) Granulocytes and macrophages
(7) T cells and natural killer cells
(8) Megakaryocytes
(9) Erythrocytes
(10) Monocytes progenitor
(11) Granulocyte progenitor
(12) T cells progenitor
(13) NK cells progenitor
(14) Monocytes
(15) T cells
(16) B cells
(17) Platelets
(18) Erythrocytes
(19) Neutrophils, eosinophils, basophils
(20) NK cells

Scheme of hematopoiesis

Ans. 48. **b.** D-Dimer assay 49. **b.** High extracellular K^+

During blood storage, there is a slow but constant leakage of potassium from the cells into the surrounding plasma along a concentration gradient as a result of sodium potassium pump failure. The plasma level of potassium may increase by 0.5-1.0 mmol/L per day of refrigerator storage.

50. A peripheral smear with increased neutrophils, basophils, eosinophils and platelets is highly suggestive of:

a. Acute myeloid leukemia
b. Acute lymphoblastic leukemia
c. Chronic myelogenous leukemia
d. Myelodysplastic syndrome

CML should be considered in the diagnosis when there is moderate to massive splenomegaly in the presence of reasonably good general health. A very high total leukocyte count and the blood smear examination confirms the diagnosis. Presence of thrombocytosis and basophilia are supporting evidences. Low or absent leukocyte alkaline phosphatase score almost confirms the diagnosis.

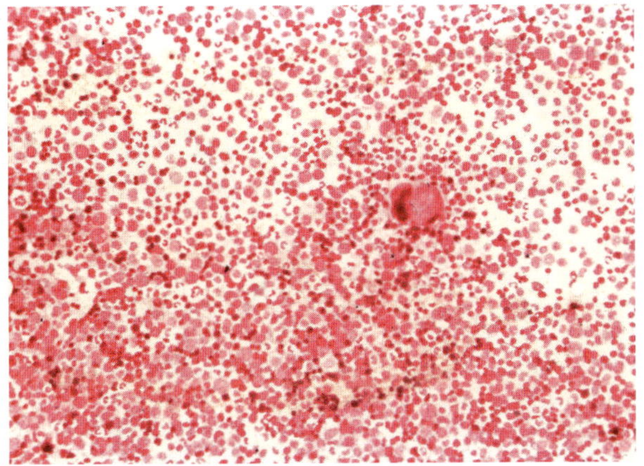

CML: Bone marrow × 400. Note myeloid hyperplasia. All the elements are present

51. In which leukemia, auto-immune hemolytic anemia is most common:

a. ALL
b. AML
c. CML
d. CLL

Causes of autoimmune hemolytic anemias	
Warm antibody type	*Cold antibody type*
1. Idiopathic (primary)	1. Idiopathic
2. Drugs, e.g. penicillin and methyldopa	2. Infections by viruses e.g. EB virus and mycoplasma infection
3. Systemic lupus erythematosus and other collagen disorders	3. Drugs, e.g. stibophen
4. Lymphomas and chronic lymphatic leukemia	4. Chronic lymphatic leukemia
5. Immune deficiency states	5. Paroxysmal cold hemoglobinuria

Autoimmune hemolytic anemia

- Autoantibodies develop against the erythrocytes.
- The antibody may agglutinate the red cells at 37 degree C (warm antibody) or at lower temperatures (cold antibody).
- Warm antibodies generally belong to IgG class whereas cold antibodies are IgM.
- In the warm antibody type hemolysis takes place extravascularly in the spleen, while in the cold antibody type hemolysis occurs intravascularly or in the liver.

52. Which is NOT seen in iron deficiency anemia:

a. Hyper-segmented neutrophils
b. Microcytosis preceeds hypochromia
c. MCHC < 50%
d. Commonest cause of anemia in India

Hypersegmented neutrophils are seen in peripheral smear of megaloblastic anemia.

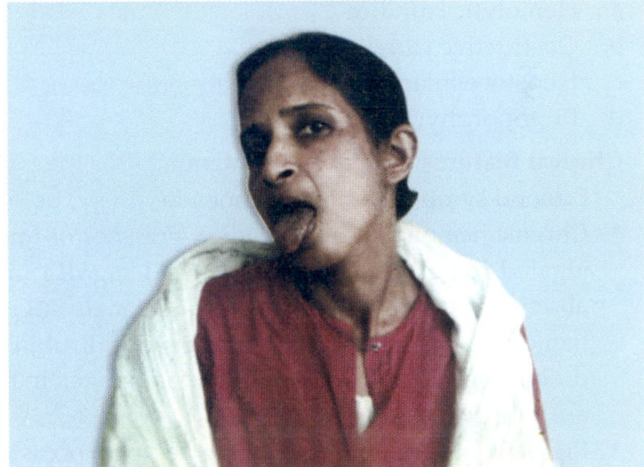

Female staining of tongue by oral iron therapy

53. An 80-year-old, asymptomatic man present with a total leucocyte count of 1 lakh, with 80% lymphocytes and 20% PMC's. What is the most probable diagnosis:

a. HIV
b. CML
c. CLL
d. TB

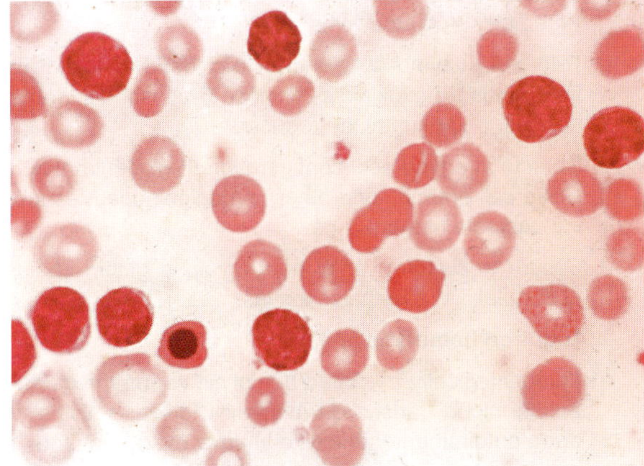

Peripheral blood film chronic lymphatic leukemia. Note: Mature looking lymphocytes

Ans. **50. c.** Chronic myelog... **51. d.** CLL **52. a.** Hyper-segmented... **53. c.** CLL

Diagnostic finding of CLL in peripheral blood is the marked leucocytosis (50-200 × 10^9/L or 50,000-200,000/cmm) consisting almost totally of small mature lymphocytes. The cells are uniform in type and blasts are usually not seen except in the later stages.

54. The coagulation profile in a 13-year-old girl with menorrhagia having Von-Willebrand's disease is:

a. Isolated BT with a normal PT
b. Isolated prolonged PT with a normal BT
c. Prolongation of both PT and BT
d. Prolongation of thrombin time

Common causes of prolongation of the bleeding time are thrombocytopenia (platelet count below 100,000/cmm), thrombopathies, von Willebrand's disease and scurvy.

55. A young male with gallbladder stones shows following results: S. bilirubin – 2.5, Hb – 6 and urine test positive for urobilinogen. Diagnosis is:

a. Hemolytic jaundice
b. Obstructive jaundice
c. Hepatocellular jaundice
d. Protoporphyria

Clinical features of hemolytic anemia

- General symptomatology of anemia
- Chronic hemolysis leads jaundice. Presence of unconjugated hyperbilirubinemia (above 1 mg/dL) in the absence of primary hepatic disease strongly suggests hemolysis. The metabolic products of bilirubin like urobilinogen in the urine and stercobilinogen in feces are also increased.
- Pigment stones in the biliary tree are occasional complications seen in chronic hemolysis, caused by the excessive presence of bilirubin in bile

Classification of hemolytic disorders
1. Inherited hemolytic disorders
a. Red cell membrane defects, e.g. hereditary spherocytosis, hereditary elliptocytosis, hereditary acanthocytosis, hereditary stomatocytosis
b. Red cell enzyme deficiencies, e.g. deficiencies of pyruvate kinase, hexokinase, glucose-6-phosphate dehydrogenase, and glutathione reductase.
c. Defects in amino acid configuration of globin chains, e.g. sickle cell anemia, and other hemoglobinopathies including unstable hemoglobins
d. Failure to switch over of beta or alpha globin chains in post natal life, e.g. thalassemias
2. Acquired hemolytic anemia
a. Immunologically mediated hemolytic anemia, e.g. incompatible blood transfusion, hemolytic disease of the newborn, autoimmune hemolytic anemia (warm antibody and cold antibody types).
b. Microangiopathic hemolytic anemia, e.g. disseminated intravascular coagulation, hemolytic uremic syndrome, thrombotic thrombocytopenic purpura, mechanical causes like implantation of cardiac prosthesis and march hemoglobinuria
c. Caused by infections, e.g. malaria, Clostridium welchii infections, and bartonellosis
d. Caused by drugs, chemicals, and toxins, e.g. nitrofurantoin, sulphonamides, viper venom, and formic acid poisoning.
e. Paroxysmal nocturnal hemoglobinuria.

56. Coomb's positive hemolytic anemia is associated with:

a. TTP
b. PAN
c. SLE
d. HUS

Most of the cases of SLE show normocytic normochromic anemia. Other abnormalities include Coomb's positive autoimmune hemolytic anemia, leucopenia, and thrombocytopenia.

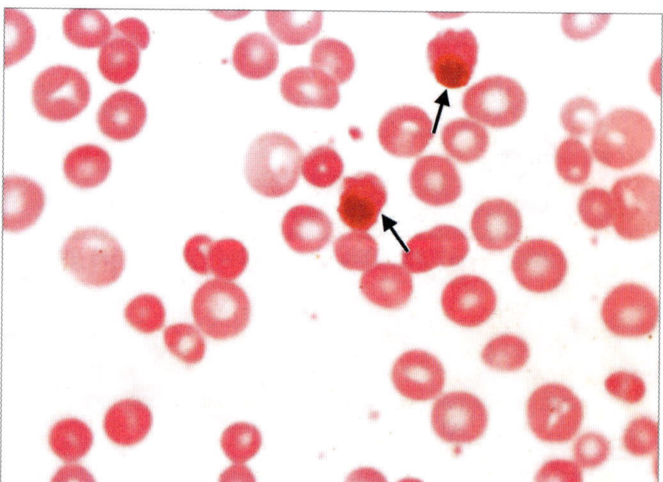

Hemolytic crisis: PB: Note: Anisopoikilocytosis, and presence of normoblasts-arrows

CARDIOVASCULAR SYSTEM

57. ECG features of Extrasystole are all EXCEPT:

a. Absent p wave
b. Wide QRS complex
c. ST segment elevation
d. Opposite T waves to QRS

ST segment elevation

- Myocardial infarction (see also ECG in myocardial infarction). ST elevation in select leads is more common with MI. ST elevation only occurs in full thickness infarction
- Prinzmetal's angina
- Acute pericarditis: ST elevation in all leads is more common with acute pericarditis.
- Left ventricular aneurysm
- Hyperkalemia

Ans. 54. a. Isolated BT with... 55. a. Hemolytic jaundice 56. c. SLE 57. c. ST segment elevation

58. 'a' wave on jugular venous pulse, is ABSENT in:
a. Complete heart block b. Tricuspid regurgitation
c. Atrial fibrillation d. Mitral stenosis

AF/ A Fibrillation
- JVP: a waves absent (no unifocal atrial depolarization)
- ECG: p waves absent

59. Severe mitral stenosis is reflected by:
a. Loud first heart sound
b. Loud opening snap
c. Intensity of mid-diastolic murmur
d. Duration of mid-diastolic murmur

A mid-diastolic rumbling murmur with presystolic accentuation will be heard after the opening snap. The murmur is best heard at the apical region and is not radiated. Since it is a low-pitch sound, it is heard best with the bell of the stethoscope. Its duration increases with worsening disease

60. A-55-year old male presented with history of angina and dyspnea for the past few days. Appearance of blood is thick red-brownish color. Findings are consistent with the diagnosis of:
a. G-6-PD deficiency b. Methemoglobinemia
c. Hemolytic anemia d. Sickle cell anemia

Arterial blood with elevated methemoglobin levels has a characteristic chocolate-brown color as compared to normal bright red oxygen-containing arterial blood.

61. All of the following are included in major criteria for Rheumatic fever EXCEPT:
a. Carditis b. Migratory polyarthritis
c. ASO titre d. St. Vitu's dance

According to revised Jones criteria, the diagnosis of rheumatic fever can be made when two of the major criteria, or one major criterion plus two minor criteria, are present along with evidence of streptococcal infection: elevated or rising anti-streptolysin O titre or DNAase.

62. Transesophageal echocardiography/ TEE is better than transthoracic echocardiography as:
a. Better evaluation of left ventricle
b. Better evaluation of left atria & left atrial appendage thrombus
c. Better evaluation of commissural fusion
d. Better evaluation of valve cusps

TEE is used to assess cardiac disorders when transthoracic study is technically difficult, as in obese patients and in patients with COPD. It reveals better detail of small abnormal structures (e.g., endocarditic vegetations or patent foramen ovale) and posterior cardiac structures (e.g., left atrium, left atrial appendage, interatrial septum, pulmonary vein anatomy) because they are closer to the esophagus than to the anterior chest wall. TEE can also produce images of the ascending aorta, which arises behind the 3rd costal cartilage; of structures < 3 mm (e.g., thrombi, vegetations); and of prosthetic valves.

63. In stable angina:
a. CK-MB is elevated
b. Troponin I is elevated
c. Myoglobin is elevated
d. Levels of cardiac markers remain unchanged

Diagnosis of stable angina pectoris
- Should be diagnosed by history
- Resting ECG may be normal in approximately half of patients with chronic stable angina
- Depression/ elevation of the S-T segment during exercise (treadmill) are diagnostic of angina
- Myocardial perfusion imaging using radioactive isotopes and stress echocardiography are useful in diagnosis of myocardial ischemia.

Showing the details of common biochemical markers diagnostic of myocardial infarction

Marker and normal level	*Time to show rise in serum levels hours after onset*	*Peak level*	*Time to return to normal*	*Time for collection of blood*
SGOT 5–40 IU/L	8–12	18–36 hours	3–4 days	Once in 12 hours
LDH 20–220 IU/L	10	24–48 hours	10–14 day	24 hours
CK MB	3–12	24 hours	48–72 hours	Every 12 hours for 3 days
C TnT	3–12	12 hours to 2 days	5–14 days	Once at least every 12 hours
C Tn1	3–12	24 hours	5–10 days	Once at least every 12 hours

64. FALSE for infective endocarditis:
a. May cause embolic complications
b. Splinter hemorrhages seen
c. Rose spots may be seen
d. May lead to acute regurgitant valvular lesions

Rose spots are seen in typhoid/enteric fever. In IE, Roth's spots (circular hemorrhages with central white spots) are seen on the retina.

Ans. 58. **c.** Atrial fibrillation 59. **d.** Duration of mid... 60. **b.** Methemoglobinemia 61. **c.** ASO titre
62. **b.** Better evaluation... 63. **d.** Levels of cardiac... 64. **c.** Rose spots may be seen

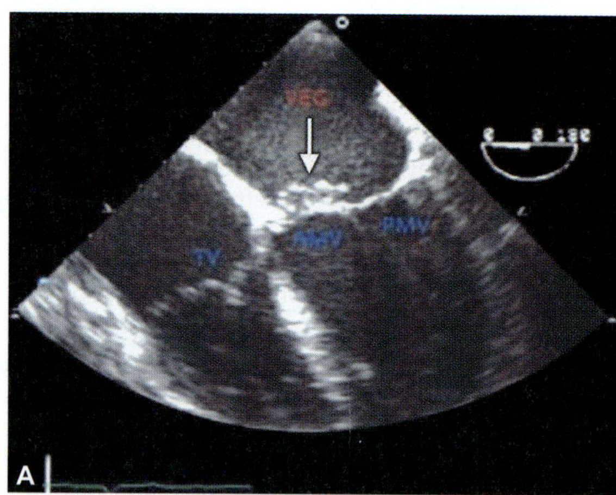

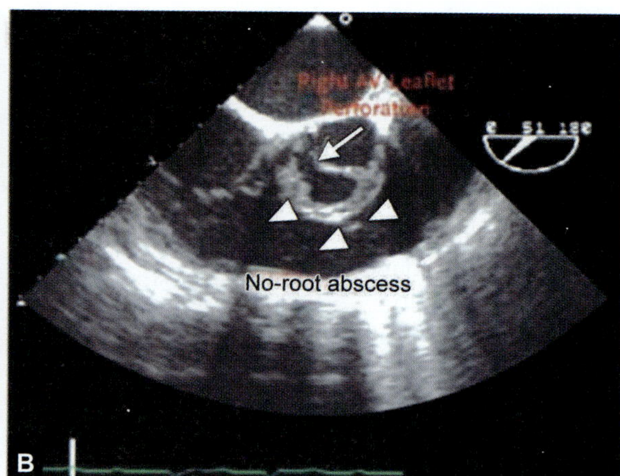

Transesophageal echocardiogram picture of a (A). Vegetation attached to mitral valve (B) Aortic root abscess on right side - arrow

65. Severe hemorrhagic shock is said to be present, when blood loss is:

a. Less than 20% b. 20-40%
c. 40–60% d. More than 60%

In stage 4 hypovolemia shock, over 40% of blood is lost (over 2000 mL).

Classification of Shock
1. Hypovolemic
2. Traumatic
3. Cardiogenic Intrinsic Compressive
4. Septic Hyperdynamic Hypodynamic
5. Neurogenic
6. Hypoadrenal

66. Murmur heard in aortic regurgitation is:

a. Continuous murmur b. Austin flint murmur
c. Crescendo-decrescendo d. Graham Steele's Murmur

Regurgitation
Aorta
IV

Colour Doppler echocardiograph showing aortic regurgitation

A mid-diastolic, or presystolic murmur or a combination of both may be heard well over the apex beat (Austin Flint murmur) in AR. This is produced because of the premature closure of the mitral valve caused by the regurgitant stream of blood.

67. Pericardial effusion is best diagnosed by:

a. Chest X-ray b. Echocardiography
c. ECG d. Angiography

Echocardiography is the procedure of choice for the diagnosis of pericardial effusion. Pericardial effusion appears as an 'echo-free' space between the visceral and parietal pericardium. Early diastolic collapse of right atrium and right ventricle seen in echo indicate presence of tamponade.

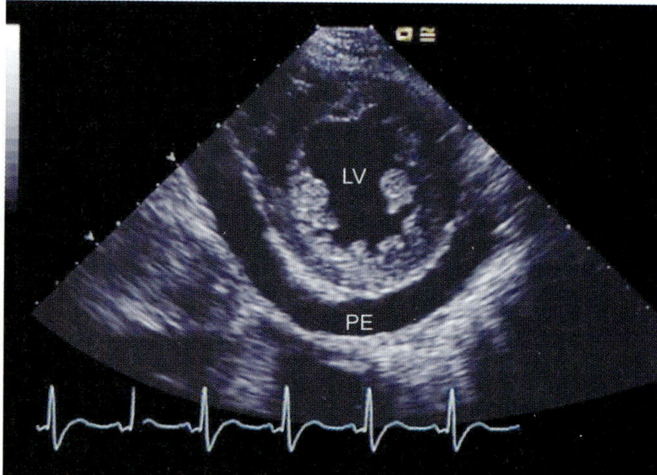

2D –Echocardiographic picture of pericardial effusion which is seen as echo free space behind the left ventricle. LV – left ventricle, PE – pericardial effusion

68. Treatment of orthostatic hypotension includes all EXCEPT:

a. High salt and fluid intake b. Physical maneuvers
c. Dobutamine d. Fludricortisone

Ans. **65. c.** 40–60% **66. b.** Austin flint murmur **67. b.** Echocardiography **68. c.** Dobutamine

Management of orthostatic hypotension

- Put the patient supine and elevate the legs or press thighs against the abdomen to improve venous retrun
- Stimulating drinks such as coffee or lime juice containing 20 g sugar and 6 g salt help to raise the blood pressure within a short time
- Intravenous drip of 10% glucose saline
- Pressor agents such as ephedrine 30 mg oral or intravenous infusion of dopamine may be required
- Fludricortisone in doses of 0.01 to 0.02 mg/ day is the best treatment on a long term basis

Various neurological disorders that can lead to orthostatic hypotension	
1. Afferent lesions	Neuropathies
2. Central lesions	Multiple system atrophy, Parkinson's disease
3. Spinal lesions	Lesions of cervical and dorsal regions of the spinal cord
4. Ganglionic lesions	Progressive autonomic failure
5. Post-ganglionic lesions	Neuropathies

69. Drug of choice for variant angina is:

a. CCB
b. Sodium nitroprusside
c. Aspirin
d. Propranolol

Management of variant/ Prinzmetal's angina

- Nitrates are beneficial, the action being exclusively direct vasodilating effect on spastic coronaries
- Calcium antagonists are very effective in preventing the corornary artery spasm of variant angina and they should be used in maximally tolerated doses. Caclium antagonists along with long and short acting nitrates are the mainstay of therapy.

Calcium antagonists		
Dihydropyridine group	*Dosage*	*Side effects*
1. Amlodipine	2.5–10 mg/d	Headache, edema of the legs and feet
2. Felodipine	2.5–10 mg/d	Headache, edema
3. Nicardipine	20–40 mg t.i.d	Headache, dizziness, flushing, edema
Other groups of drugs		
Diltiazem		
Immediate release	30-90 mg t.i.d	Hypotension
Slow release	60-180 mg b.i.d	Myocardial depression Bradycardia
Verapamil		
Immediate release	80-120 mg t.i.d	Myocardial depression
Slow release	120-480 mg/d	Bradycardia

70. Best indicator of MI after 3 days:

a. CPK
b. Cardiac specifc troponin T
c. Aspartate amino-transkinase
d. All of the above

Troponin I and troponin T are released into the plasma so that reliable diagnostic sensitivity is reached by 12 to 16 h and maximal activity is reached by 24 to 36 h. The levels return to normal within 10-12 days.

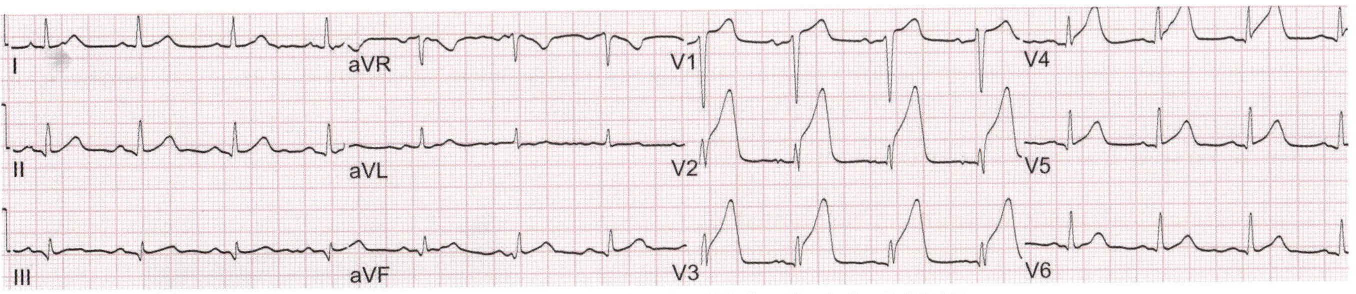

ECG of anterior wall MI showing ST elevation in leads V1-V5

71. Most common form of shock is:

A. Hypovolemic shock
b. Cardiogenic shock
c. Neurogenic shock
d. Septicemic shock

Shock is a clinical syndrome resulting from gross impairment of tissue perfusion and widespread cellular dysfunction caused by diminution in oxygen delivery.

72. Angina pectoris occurs commonly in:

a. AR
b. MR
c. AS
d. MS

The three most important presentations of significant aortic stenosis are angina pectoris, syncope, and left ventricular failure.

Ans. 69. **a.** CCB 70. **b.** Cardiac specifc... 71. **a.** Hypovolemic shock 72. **c.** AS

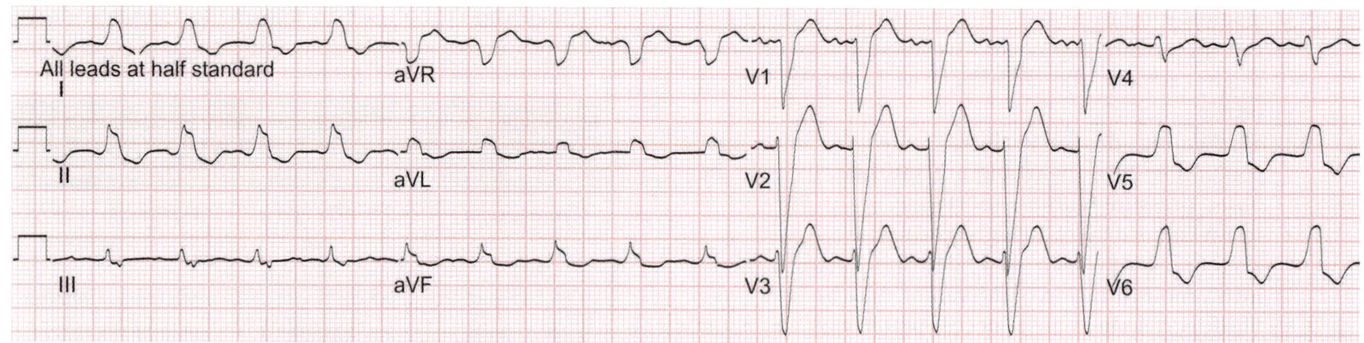

ECG showing left ventricular hypertrophy in aortic stenosis. Note: 1. Deep S waves in V1 and V2 and tall broad R waves in V5, V6. ST depression in leads V5, V6. The amplitude of SV2 + RV5 or V6 is above 35 mm

73. 'p' waves are ABSENT in:

a. Atrial fibrillation
b. Atrial flutter
c. Complete heart block
d. All of the above

Atrial fibrillation is a very frequent complication of mitral stenosis. ECG shows absence of p waves.

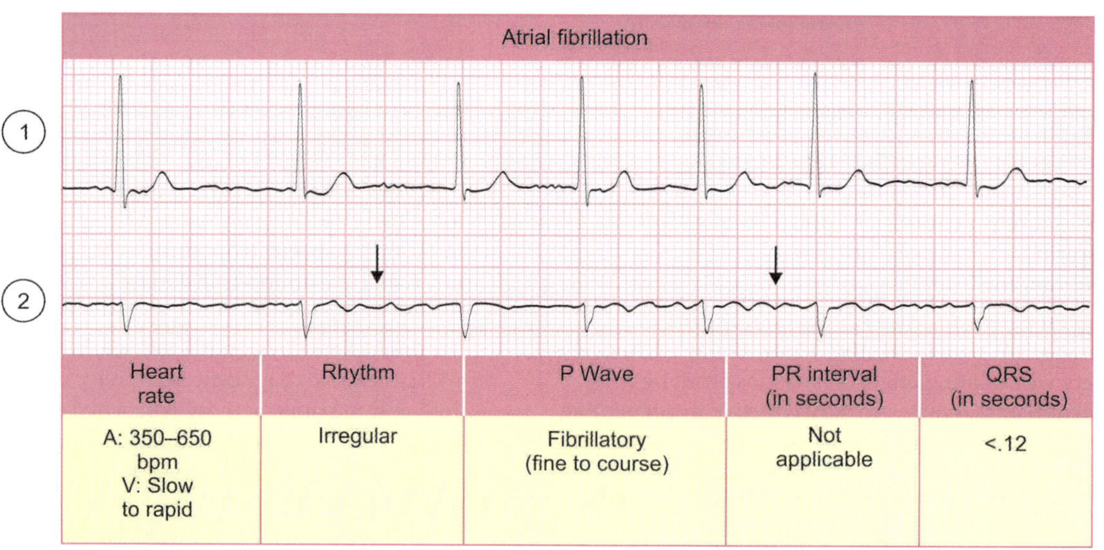

Heart rate	Rhythm	P Wave	PR interval (in seconds)	QRS (in seconds)
A: 350–650 bpm V: Slow to rapid	Irregular	Fibrillatory (fine to course)	Not applicable	<.12

Atrial fibrillation: Note: 1. Totally irregular RR intervals 2. Absence of –P waves 3. Fibrillary waves marked by arrows. Usually the QRS rate is fast in untreated atrial fibrillation. This record is made after starting treatment and showing of the heart rate
(1) Upper tracing lead 2
(2) Lower tracing shows the fibrillary waves best brought out in lead V1

74. Most important factor determining myocardial O_2 consumption:

a. Myocardial fibre tension
b. Cardiac output
c. Blood volume
d. Heart rate

Heart receives its oxygen supply and nutrition from the coronary arterial blood flow which is 72-85 mL/100 g of cardiac muscle/min in resting phase. The heart utilizes 8-10 mL of oxygen/100 g every time. The oxygen demand during systole is thrice that during diastole.

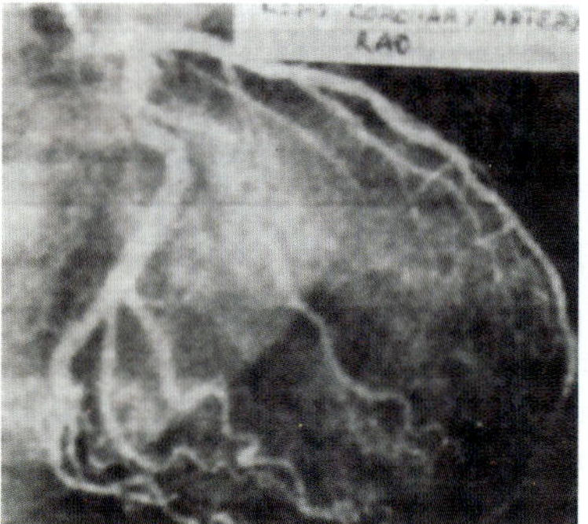
Normal coronary angiogram showing the various branches filling normally

Ans. **73. a.** Atrial fibrillation **74. a.** Myocardial fibre...

75. NOT a cause of asymmetrical pulse:

a. Coarctation of aorta
b. Aorta arteritis
c. Dissection of aorta
d. Supravalvular aortic stenosis

A discrepant or unequal pulse between left and right radial artery is observed in anomalous or aberrant course of artery, coarctation of aorta, aortitis, dissecting aneurysm, peripheral embolism etc.

76. NOT a major criteria for diagnosing acute rheumatic fever:

a. Erythema marginatum
b. Erythema nodusum
c. Carditis
d. Rheumatic chorea

Erythema marginatum are erythematous, non-pruritic annular lesions with serpiginous borders, usually seen over the anterior aspects of the chest and abdomen and over the thighs. They spread peripherally like ripples with central clearing.

Jones' criteria (revised)*

Major manifestations	*Minor manifestations*
Carditis	Previous rheumatic fever or History of rheumatic heart disease
Polyarthritis	Fever
Chorea	Acute phase reactants
Erythema marginatum Subcutaneous nodules and evidence of preceding streptococcal infection, i.e., ASO titer	Prolongation of PR interval in the ECG
*Duckett Jones	

77. Atherosclerosis is inversely related to:

a. Chylomicrons
b. Triglycerides
c. LDL
d. HDL

The role of HDL is probably to transport cholesterol and remove lipids from the arterial walls. The HDL reduces uptake of LDL by cells. Increase in the levels of LDL and VLDL and decrease of HDL are associated with higher incidence of atheroma and its complications.

Properties of the major lipoprotein fractions

Lipoprotein	*Major lipid*	*Major apoproteins*	*Sp. gr.*	*Electrophoretic mobility*
Chylomicron	Dietary triglyceride	AI, AII,BI, CI, CII,CIII	Below 1.006	No movement
VLDL	Endogenous triglyceride	B, CI, CII, CIII, E	Below 1.006	Pre-beta
LDL	Cholesterol esters	B	1.019 to 1.063	Beta
HDL	Cholesterol esters	AI, AII	1.063 to 1.210	Alpha
Remnants and triglyceride	Cholesterol esters	B, CIII, E	Less than 1.019	Slow pre-beta

78. MC cause of paroxysmal hypertension:

a. Cushing's syndrome
b. Hyperthyroidism
c. Acromegaly
d. Phaeochromocytoma

The most prominent feature of pheochromocytoma is hypertension, which is pparoxysmal in the initial stages, but later becomes persistent. Headache, flushing, excessive sweating, tachycardia, fever, glycosuria, and postural hypotension accompany hypertensive paroxysms.

JNC VII classification of blood pressure for adults (>18 years) (Joint national committee on prevention, detection, evaluation and treatment of high blood pressure)

BP classification	*SBP (mm Hg)*		*DBP (mm Hg)*
Normal	< 120	and	< 80
Prehypertension	120-139	or	80-89
Stage 1 Hypertension	140-159	or	90-99
Stage 2 Hypertension	> 160	or	> 100
When SBP and DBP fall in different categories, higher category should be selected to classify the individual's BP status.			

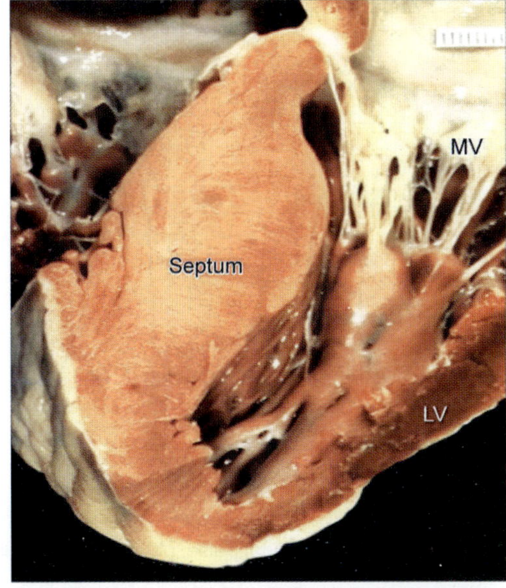

Pathological specimen of hypertrophic cardiomyopathy showing asymmetric hypertrophy of IVS (ASH) and normal thickness LV free wall. *Septum – interventricular septum, LV-LV free wall, MV-mitral valve*
Ref: J.P. Veinot: Cardiomyopathy and Pericardial diseases

79. Valsalva manouevere increases murmur of:

a. AR
b. MS
c. HOCM
d. All of the above

Ans. 75. **d.** Supravalvular... 76. **b.** Erythema nodusum 77. **d.** HDL 78. **d.** Phaeochromocytoma 79. **c.** HOCM

The murmur of HOCM increases in intensity by reducing preload (valsalva manoeuvre, nitrates) or reducing afterload (vasodilators).

80. Dressler's syndrome is due to:

a. Cor pulmonale b. Mitral stenosis
c. Myocardial infarction d. Pulmonary embolism

One of the delayed complication of MI is Dressler's syndrome, which is probably an immune-mediated reaction in which pericarditis, pleurisy, fever, arthritis, and elevation of ESR, develop 1-6 weeks after the infarction.

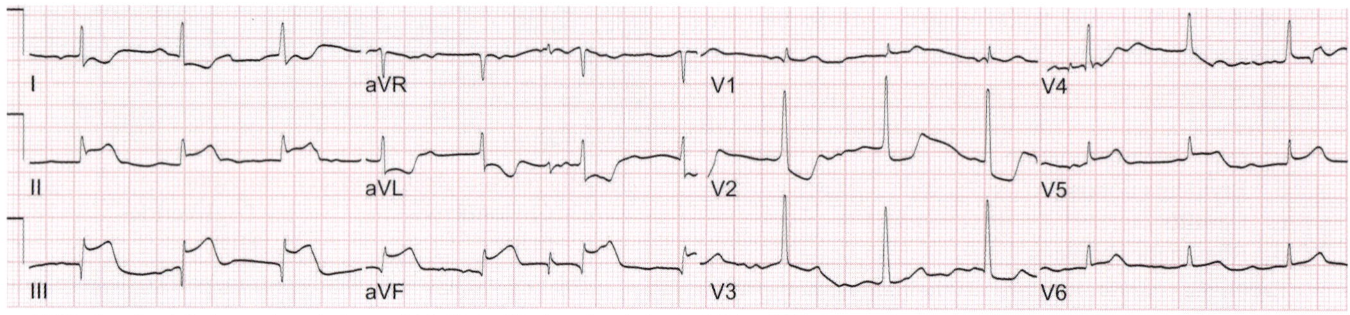

ECG showing inferior and posterior wall MI. Note ST elevation in 2, 3, aVF and ST depression in 1, aVL. Also tall R waves with upright T waves in V1 and V2

81. 'a' wave in JVP indicates:

a. Atrial relaxation
b. Atrial contraction
c. Bulging of tricuspid valve into right atrium
d. Ventricular contraction

'a'–wave of JVP is caused by atrial contraction and is presystolic. It is more prominent when the right atrium is contracting against increased resistance. It disappears in atrial fibrillation.

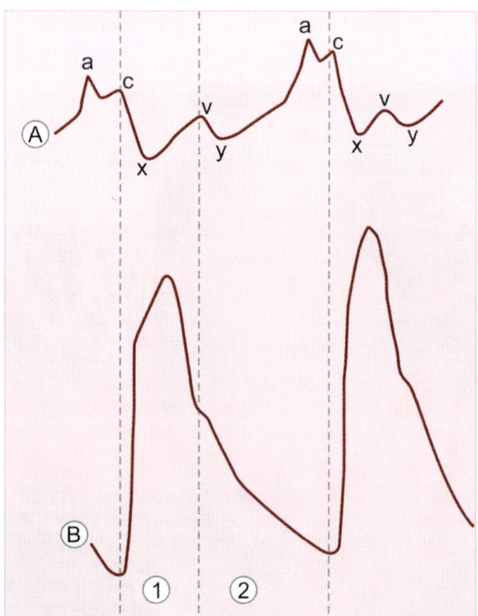

Jugular venous tracing and arterial pulse: (A) Jugular venous pulse (B) Carotid arterial pulse (1) Systole (2) Diastole

82. Wide split fixed 2nd heart sound is heard in:

a. Normal individuals b. Left bundle branch block
c. ASD d. VSD

In ASD, during inspiration more venacaval blood flows into the right side of the heart and during expiration more of the left atrial blood flows through the shunt. These phenomenon account for the ejection of the same quantity of blood across the pulmonary valve during inspiration and expiration. Therefore, the split of the pulmonary second sound remains fixed. The ausculatatory hallmark of ASD is wide, fixed split of the second heart sound.

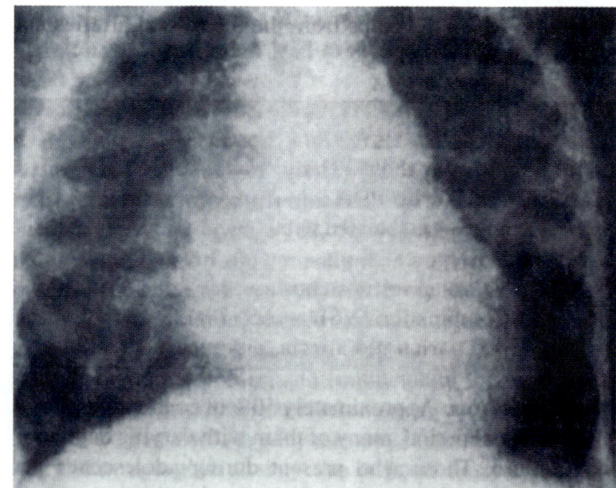

Atrial septal defects Note: Cardiac enlargements, prominents main pulmonary artery and plethoric lung fields

83. Most important in aetiology of coronary artery disease is:

a. VLDL b. LDL
c. HDL d. All of the above

HDL is protective against atheroma, whereas LDL favors atherogenesis. Lipoproteins abnormalities are particularly marked in the metabolic syndrome (syndrome X) in which the HDL level is reduced.

Ans. **80. c.** Myocardial infa... **81. b.** Atrial contraction **82. c.** ASD **83. b.** LDL

84. Pulsus alterans is a feature of:

a. Severe AS + AR b. Severe AR
c. Bronchial asthma d. Left ventricular failure

In LVF, pulse becomes rapid as a result of compensatory adrenergic activity. Pulsus alterans is suggestive of left ventricular failure.

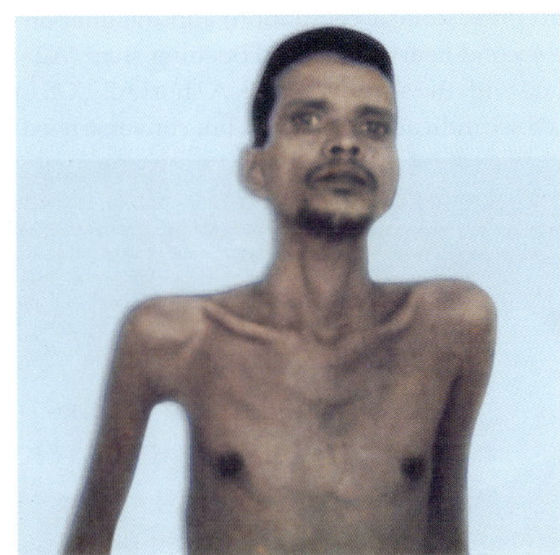

Cardiac cachexia
Note: Feature of cardiac failure and emaciation

85. Earliest diagnosis of MI is by:

a. AST b. LDH
c. CK d. CK-MB

CK-MB shows two isoforms: CKMB1 and CKMB2. Elevation of CKMB2 is more suggestive of cardiac infarction in the absence of other obvious reasons. Levels of CKMB isoform >1.0 U/L, or a ratio of CKMB2/CKMB1 >1.5 is diagnostic of acute MI. The level of CK rises within 4-8 hours of infarction, reaches its peak in 24 hours and falls to normal level within 2-3 days.

ECG leads showing changes	Location of infarct
V1 to V3	Anteroseptal
V4 to V6, L1 and aVL	Anterolateral
aVF, L2 and L3	Inferior wall
ST depression in V1 and V2	
Presence of tall R-waves and upright T-waves in lead V1 and V2	True posterior infarct
ST elevation in Rt sided chest leads and Q waves (V3R, V4R)	Right ventricular infarct

Note:
1. In true posterior infarct. V1 will show upright R and T waves, unlike as in right ventricular hypertrophy in which T is inverted.
2. Right ventricular infarction has to be suspected when there is jugular venous changes resembling constrictive pericarditis and shock without hypovolemia. In such circumstances right sided leads should be taken to demonstrate RV infarction. Presence of right ventricular infarction calls for special management.

86. Mitral regurgitation is NOT a feature of:

a. Ostium primum ASD b. Marfan's syndrome
c. Down's syndrome
d. Endomyocardial fibroelastosis

Patient with left ventricular involvement in endomyocardial fibrosis, present very early with varying grades of dyspnea and palpitations – clinically they may resemble mitral incompetence. Physical examination reveals cardiomegaly, loud apical third heart sound and pansystolic murmur in the mitral area.

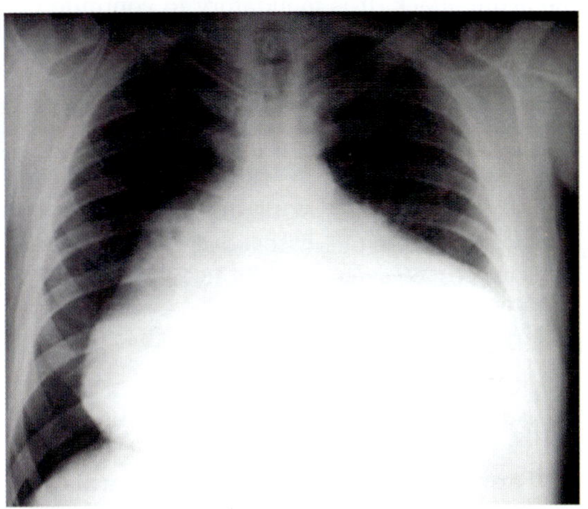

X-ray chest in right ventricular EMF showing gross cardiomegaly and enlarged right atrium

87. 100% Oxygen is NOT effective in:

a. Pulmonary edema b. MI
c. Tetralogy of Fallot d. COPD

The right ventricular outflow tract (RVOT) obstruction in TOF causes reduction in pulmonary blood flow. Arterial desaturation occurs because of right to left shunt across the VSD. Both right and left ventricular blood enters the aorta.

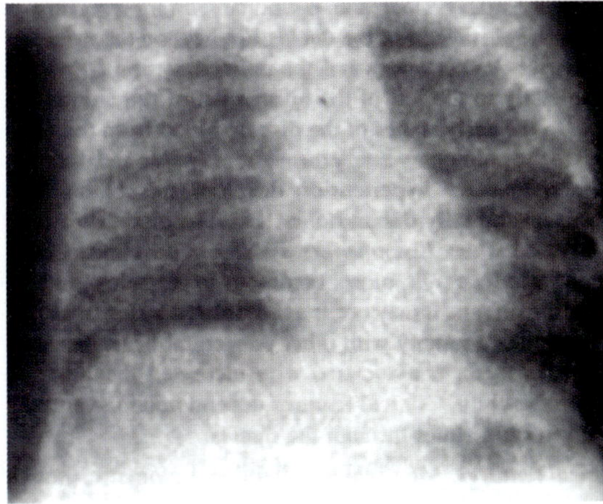

Tetralogy of Fallot
Note: Normal heart size with upturned apex. Concavity at the site of the pulmonary artery. Lung vascularity is reduced. Aorta is left sided in the majority

Ans. 84. d. Left ventricular... 85. d. CK-MB 86. d. Endomyocardial... 87. c. Tetralogy of Fallot

88. True regarding secondary prophylaxis of a 6-year-old child with carditis is:

a. Duration of prophylaxis is life long
b. Duration of prophylaxis is till 18 years
c. Duration of prophylaxis is at least 5 years after onset
d. Duration of prophylaxis is till 25 years of age

It is desirable to continue rheumatic prophylaxis (benzathine penicillin 1.2 mega units once every three weeks) lifelong but the chance of recurrence comes down with increasing age and the passage of time after the acute attack. It is mandatory to continue penicillin prophylaxis at least till the age of 25 years or for 5 years after the initial attack, whichever is later.

Comparison to the streptococcal lesion in acute rheumatic fever (ARF) and glomerulonephritis (GN)

	ARF	*GN*
1. Site of lesion	Mostly throat	Throat or skin
2. Prior sensitization	Essential	Not necessary
3. Serotypes of streptococci	3,5,6,14,18,19	12,44,2,52,55, 57,4
4. Immune response	Marked	Moderate

89. Carotid massage is effective in:

a. Atrial flutter
b. Atrial fibrillation
c. Ventricular tachycardia
d. Paroxysmal supraventricular tachycardia

Carotid sinus massage in the recumbent posture may serve to abolish PAT (paroxysmal atrial tachycardia/ PAT). Only one side should be massaged at a time. PSVT includes PAT.

90. Severity of mitral stenosis is determined by:

a. Intensity of S1 heart sound
b. Diastolic murmur duration
c. Opening snap
d. Intensity of diastolic murmur

The duration of the murmur (mid-diastolic murmur with presystolic accentuation) and the interval between the second heart sound and opening snap (A2 - OS) correlate with the severity of MS. A short A2 – OS interval of <0.08 sec indicates severe MS, but converse need not true.

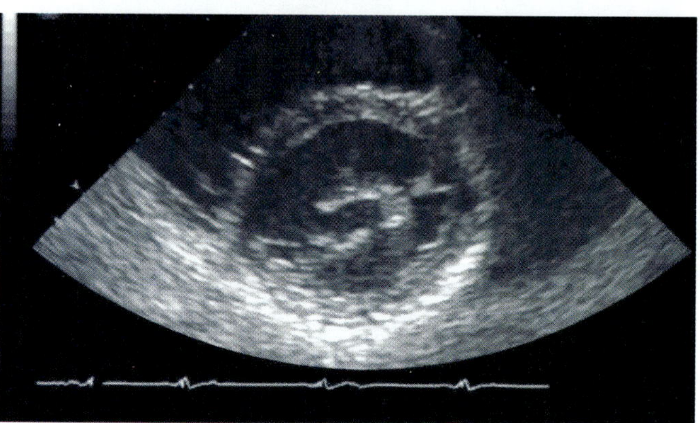

Echocardiogram in mitral stenosis: Short axis view
Note: The stenotic mitral valve orifice. Valve aperture below 1 cm² indicates severe stenos

91. ST segment elevation is seen in:

a. Prinzmetal's angina
b. Acute pericarditis
c. Acute MI
d. All of the above

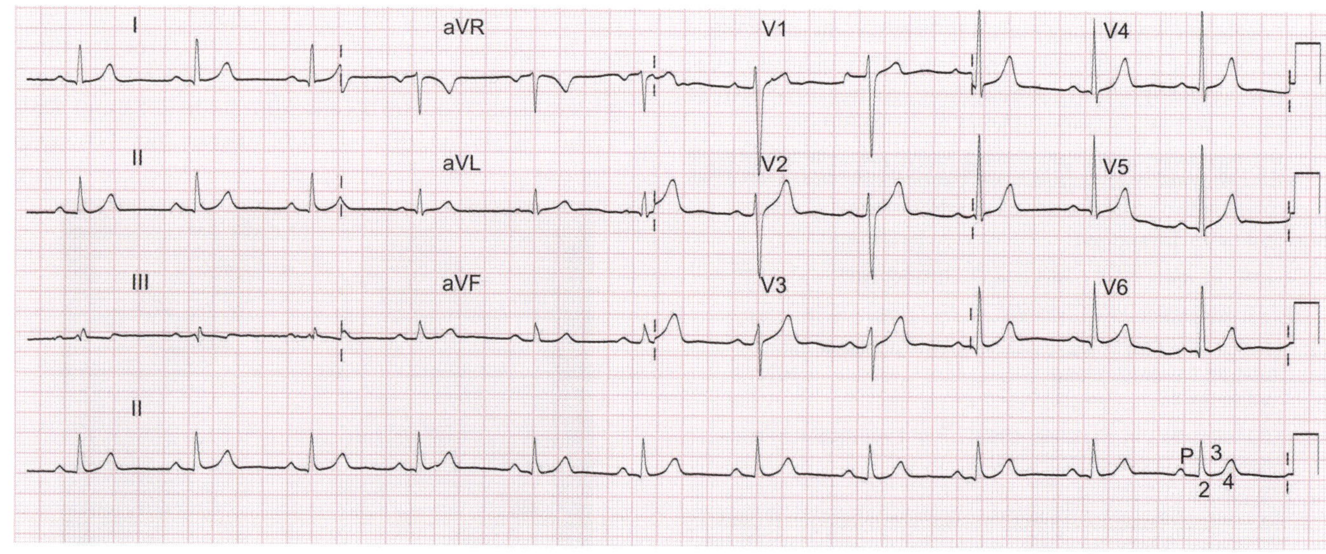

Normal ECG. ECG shows sinus rhythm. Each QRS complex is preceded by a P wave. PR interval in this ECG is 0.16 sec. (Normal PR interval is up to 0.21 sec). QRS duration is also normal, i.e. 0.08 sec (Normal up to 0.1 sec). No ST segment of T wave changes
I, II, III, limb leads
aVR, aVL, aVF augmented unipolar leads
V1-V6 unipolar chest leads
2. QRS segment 5. Position of U wave, 3. ST segment, 4. T wave

Ans. 88. **d.** Duration of... 89. **d.** Paroxysmal... 90. **b.** Diastolic murmur... 91. **d.** All of the above

ST segment elevation

- MI
- Prinzmetal's angina
- Acute pericarditis
- Left ventricular aneurysm
- Blunt trauma to chest
- Hyperkalemia
- Early repolarization
- Pulmonary embolism

92. Congenital long QT syndrome can result in:

a. Recurrent supraventricular tachycardia
b. Acute MI
c. Polymorphic ventricular tachycardia
d. Complete heart block

Torsades-de-pointesisanacquiredorcongenitalpolymorphic ventricular tachycardia in the range of 180-250/min characterized by QRS complexes of progressively changing amplitude and contour, that seem to revolve around the isoelectric line. The ECG shows proloned QT interval.

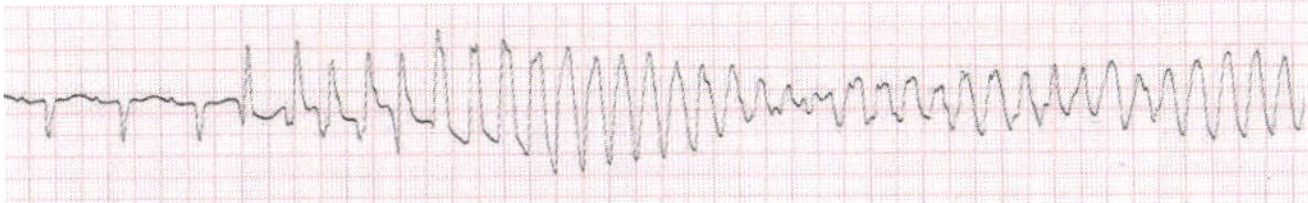

Torsades de pointes: Note: 1. Torsades is a form of malignant ventricular tachycardia 2. The QRS is polymorphic 3. The axis of the QRS shifts across the baseline around a point 4. Often this occurs in the setting of prolonged QT interval

93. ST segment elevation of EKG is NOT seen in:

a. Prinzmetal angina
b. Ventricular aneurysm
c. Unstable angina
d. Early repolarization variant

In unstable angina, ST segment depression (or transient ST segment elevation) and T-wave changes occur in up to 50% of patients. New ST segment deviation, even of 0.05 mV, is a specific and important measure of ischemia and prognosis.

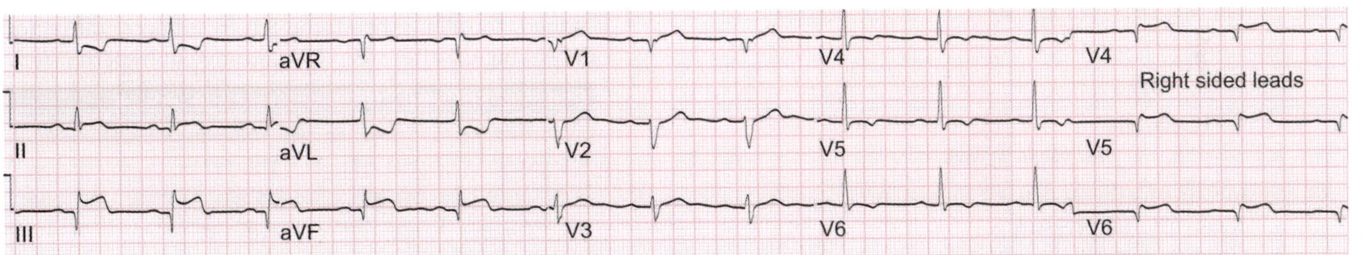

ECG showing inferior MI with right ventricular MI. Note ST elevation in 2, 3, aVF, V1 and right chest leads. ST depression in I, aVL

94. Acute asymptomatic sinus bradycardia usually responds to:

a. Norepinephrine
b. Atropine
c. Dopamine
d. Adrenaline

Sinus bradycardia implies a sinus rate below 60/min. Often this is seen normally in athletes and heavy manual labourers. Drugs like digoxin, verapamil and propranolol may produce sinus bradycardia. Atropine causes sinus tachycardia.

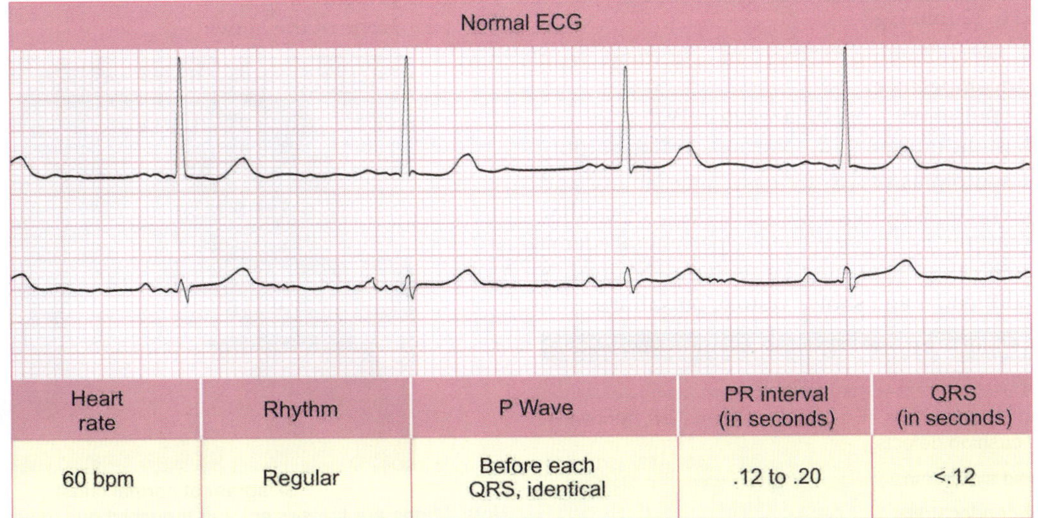

Heart rate	Rhythm	P Wave	PR interval (in seconds)	QRS (in seconds)
60 bpm	Regular	Before each QRS, identical	.12 to .20	<.12

Normal ECG with sinus bradycardia. Note: The QRS rate is around 60/minute. The rhythm is regular with normal P and other complexes. QRS duration is less than 0.12 seconds

Ans. 92. c. Polymorphic... 93. c. Unstable angina 94. b. Atropine

95. Continuous murmur is a feature of:

a. Atherosclerosis
b. Dissecting aortic aneurysm
c. Arteriovenous fistula
d. Thromboangitis obliterans

The mature fistula in hemodialysis patient should course conspicuously in the subcutaneous tissue and have a prominent thrill and continuous medium-pitched bruit similar to the continuous murmur of a patent ductus arteriosus. Disappearance of the thrill and bruit is diagnostic of hemodialysis-access thrombosis.

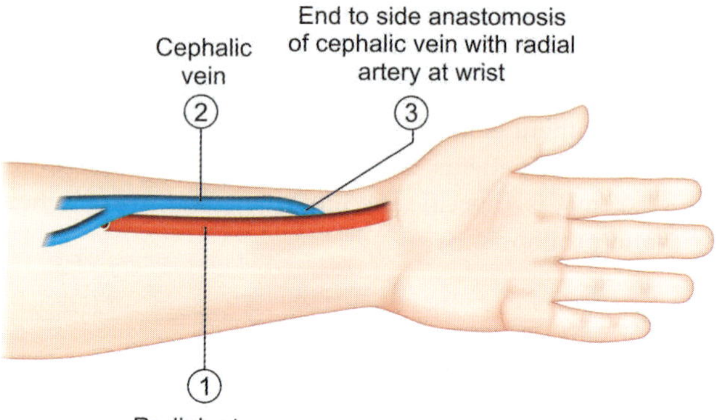

AV fistula at wrist

96. Swan Ganz Catheter is used to measure:

a. Mean arterial pressure
b. Cardiac output
c. Blood volume
d. Pulmonary capillary wedge pressure

Pulmonary arterial wedge pressure/PCWP is the pressure measured by wedging a pulmonary catheter/ Swan Ganz catheter with an inflated balloon into a small pulmonary arterial branch. Because of the large compliance of the pulmonary circulation, it provides an indirect measure of the left atrial pressure. Physiological pressure is 6–12 mm Hg.

97. Which of the following is seen in a patient with tricuspid Incompetence:

a. Hepatic pulsation
b. a wave in JVP
c. Mid diastolic murmur
d. Normal cardiac output

The usual symptoms of TR are easy fatiguability and effort intolerance resulting from reduction of cardiac output. In severe cases there is usually peripheral edema and in some cases there may be ascites. The liver is enlarged and tender and shows systolic pulsations.

Causes of primary TR
1. Rheumatic valvulitis,
2. Congenital anomalies (Ebstein's malformation, atrioventricular cushion defects)
3. Carcinoid syndrome
4. Infective endocarditis
5. Trauma.

98. Pulsus bisferiens occurs in:

a. HOCM
b. AR
c. AS and AR
d. All of the above

The term "bisferiens pulse" is used, when the pulse wave shows two upstrokes (both in systole). This is seen when there is a combination of aortic stenosis and incompetence or sometimes even in pure aortic incompetence. Pulsus bisferiens may be more clearly identified over the carotid artery.

99. Most common feature of essential hypertension:

a. Visual disturbances
b. Headache
c. Palpitations
d. Dizziness

When the blood pressure is elevated without an evident organic cause, it is called essential hypertension. The condition is asymptomatic and over 50% of the patients are unaware of the condition. In symptomatic, the symptoms are vague and non-specific. These symptoms include fatigue, dizziness, palpitations, headache and anxiety. Though many types of headache have been described, throbbing headache felt in suboccipital region on waking up after sleep is suggestive of hypertension.

Showing SBP and DBP in different age groups		
Age	*Normal*	*Significant hypertension*
< 2 years	104–111	112–117
	70–73	74–81
10–12 years	122–125	126–133
	78–81	82–89

Note: BP in a one day old infant is ± 70 mm Hg. It rises to ± 85 mm Hg at 1 year.
Boys have a slightly higher BP than girls.

100. Opening of the aortic valve is initiated by:

a. Contraction of atria
b. Contraction of ventricle
c. When ventricular pressure is more than aortic pressure
d. None of the above

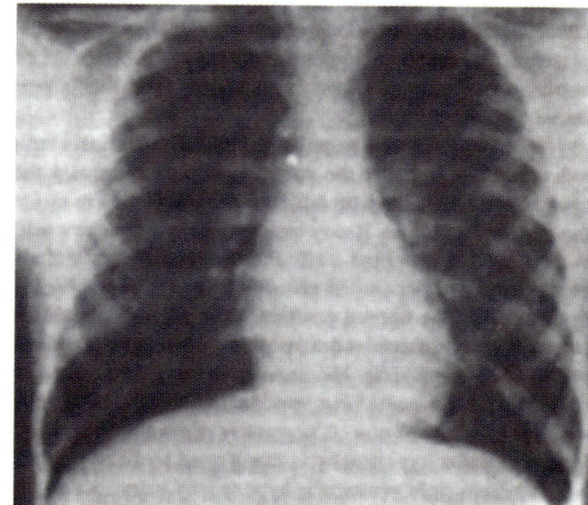
Skiagram of normal chest

Note: Lungs are translucent and bronchial and vascular markings are traceable to the chest wall. The cardiothoracic ratio is less than 50%. The blood vessels at the hilum and major bronchi are visible.

Ans. **95. c.** Arteriovenous... **96. d.** Pulmonary capillary... **97. a.** Hepatic pulsation **98. d.** All of the above **99. b.** Headache **100. c.** When ventricular...

With the onset of the ventricular systole, A-V valves close and the A-V valve apparatus bulges towards the atria giving rise to the c-wave in the jugular veins. As the ventricular pressure increases rapidly, the semilunar valves open and blood is ejected into the aorta and the pulmonary artery.

101. A Carey Coomb's murmur in a child with multiple joints pain is suggestive of:
a. Infective endocarditis
b. Rheumatoid arthritis
c. Rheumatic fever
d. Libman-Sack's endocarditis

In RF, sometimes a low pitched mid-diastolic murmur may be heard in the mitral area due to acute mitral valvulitis (Carey-Coombs murmur). It is transient and disappears as the valvulitis subsides. As the valvulitis heals, fibrosis occurs and this distorts the valve apparatus resulting in stenotic and regurgitant lesions.

102. False regarding jugular venous pulse:
a. Pressure typically raises in right ventricular failure
b. Pressure typically raised in partial obstruction of superior vena cava
c. Commonly not visible with normal heart
d. Pulsations exaggerated in tricuspid incompetence

In health, at 45 degree incline the upper limit of the venous column lies just behind the right sternoclavicular joint, which is at the same horizontal level as the sternal angle. When the right atrial pressure is increased, as in right sided heart failure, the venous column is seen above the right sternoclavicular joint and the vertical height of this condition is measured to express the increase in venous pressure.

Differences between the jugular venous pulse and carotid artery pulse

Jugular vein	*Carotid artery*
1. Better seen then felt	Seen and felt well
2. Wavy column with 2-3 waves	Jerky, only one wave
3. During inspiration the vein becomes empty	Not much change with the phase of respiration
4. Vein becomes more promi-nent when the patient lies flat	No change
5. Hepatojugular reflux present	No change

103. Pulmonary wedge pressure corresponds to:
a. Right atrial pressure
b. Right ventricular pressure
c. Left atrial pressure
d. Left ventricular pressure

A suitable catheter can be passed into the right side of the heart and manipulated into the pulmonary artery and advanced till it gets impacted into a small branch. Measurement of the pressure at this site (pulmonary wedge pressure) reflects the left atrial pressure.

104. Left ventricular hypertrophy is caused by all EXCEPT:
a. Aortic stenosis
b. Chronic cor pulmonale
c. Chronic kidney disease
d. Essential hypertension

Cor pulmonale is the enlargement of the right ventricle secondary to diseases of the lung parenchyma, pulmonary circulation, thoracic cage or the mechanics of ventilation. Right sided heart dysfunction secondary to the left-sided heart failure, valvular dysfunction, or congenital heart disease is excluded in the definition of cor pulmonale.

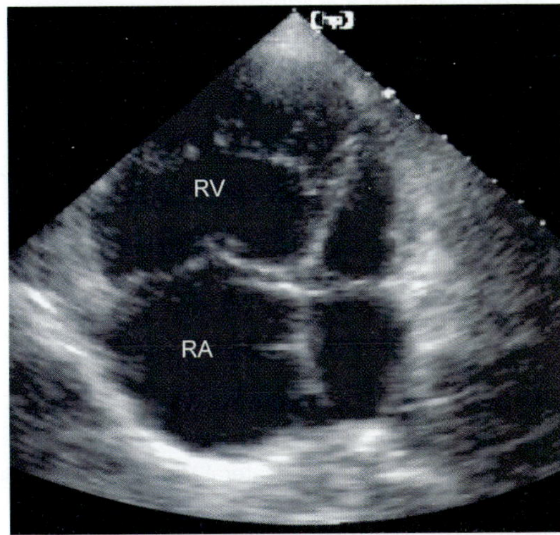

2D Echocardiogram in cor pulmonale showing dilated right ventricle and right atrium
RV – right ventricle, RA – right atrium

105. Malignant hypertension can lead to all of the following EXCEPT:
a. Hypertensive retinopathy
b. Respiratory failure
c. Renal failure
d. Stroke

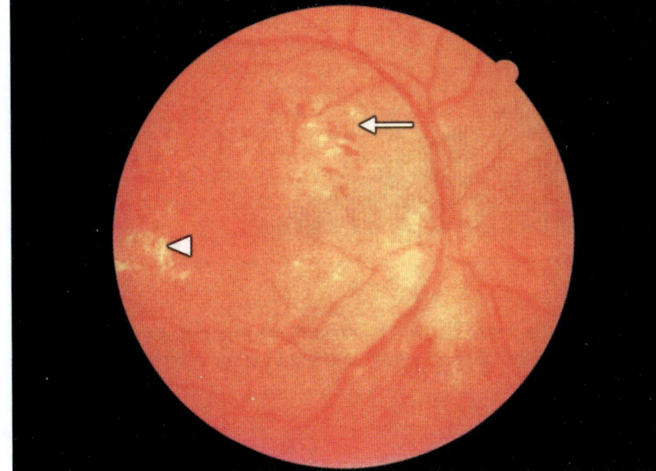
Hypertensive retinopathy in malignant hypertension.
Note: Papilledema, hemorrhages (arrow and soft exudates—arrowhead)

Ans. 101. c. Rheumatic fever 102. c. Commonly not... 103. c. Left atrial pressure 104. b. Chronic cor pulmonale 105. b. Respiratory...

Complications of hypertension

- Retinal arteriole undergoes changes. The retinal changes give an indication of the progress of hypertension and help to determine the prognosis.
- Atheroma of the retinal arteries results in reduction of blood supply to the kidney and progressive loss of renal function
- Strokes are among the most common complications in hypertension

106. ECG changes in atrial fibrillation do NOT include:

a. Irregular QRS complex
b. Irregularity of R-R interval
c. Tall P waves
d. None of the above

Confirmation of the diagnosis of AF is made by ECG which shows absence of P-waves and the presence of fibrillary waves instead. The QRS complexes are irregular in rhythm but may be normal in pattern.

107. Rupture of myocardium takes place in what duration after myocardial infarction:

a. First week
b. Second week
c. Third week
d. Fourth week

Cardiac rupture may develop by the third to the fifth day of MI. The infracted area gives way giving rise to hemopericardium, cardiac tamponade, and death in majority of cases.

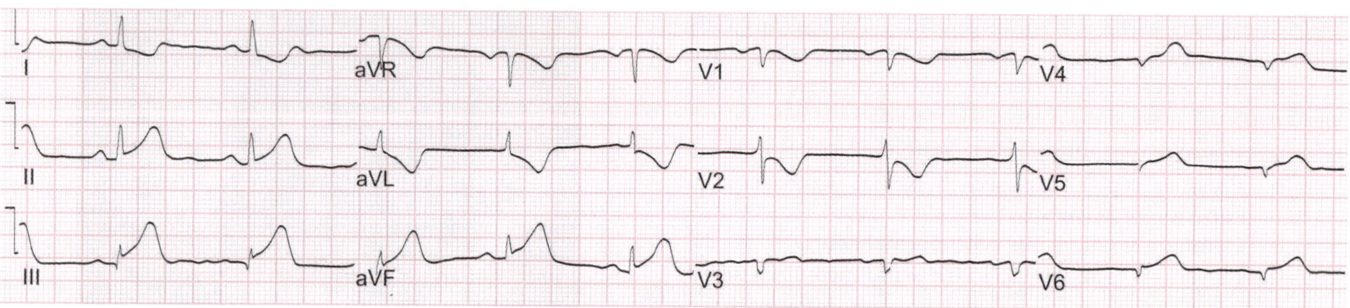

ECG showing inferior and lateral MI. Note ST elevation in leads 2, 3, aVF, V5,V6 and ST depression in leads I, aVL, V1,V2

108. Austin Flint Murmur is commonly mistaken for the murmur of:

a. Mitral regurgitation
b. Pulmonary regurgitation
c. Tricuspid stenosis
d. Mitral stenosis

Austin Flint murmur of aortic regurgitation is a mid-diastolic, or presystolic murmur, may be heard well over the apex. Murmur is mitral stenosis is a mid-diastolic murmur with presystolic accentuation.

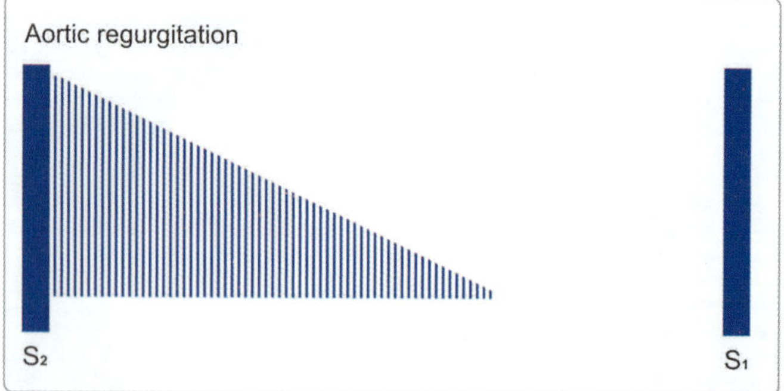

The timing of murmur of AR: The diastolic murmur starts with the aortic component of the second sound and extends for variable duration into diastole

109. Pansystolic murmur at the apex with soft first heart sound is the key sign of:

a. Aortic regurgitation
b. Mitral regurgitation
c. Ventricular septal defect
d. Atrial septal defect

The characteristic murmur of MR is medium to high-pitched pansystolic murmur heard best over the apex beat. In cases, where the anterior mitral leaflet is damaged, the murmur is conducted to the axilla because the direction of the regurgitant stream from the left ventricle is towards the body of the left atrium.

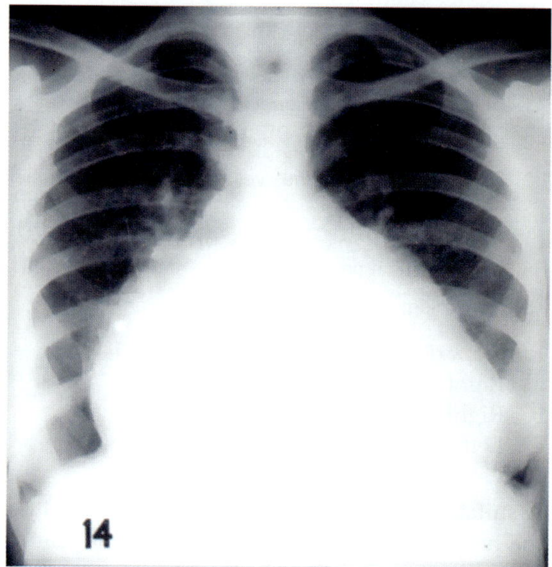

X-ray chest showing cardiac enlargement of left ventricular type. Note: The convex left border with the apex reaching down. Note also left atrial enlargement

Ans. **106. c.** Tall P waves **107. a.** First week **108. d.** Mitral stenosis **109. b.** Mitral regurgitation

110. WRONG match is:

a. 'c' wave – onset of atrial systole
b. 'a-x' descent – atrial relaxation
c. 'v-y' descent – emptying of blood from right atrium into right ventricle
d. 'y-a' ascent – filling of the right atrium from the vena cava

c wave of JVP is recordable but not actually visible as a separate wave. It reflects the bulging motion of the closed tricuspid valve during isovolumic systole.

111. Continuous murmur is found in all EXCEPT:

a. Mitral regurgitation with mitral stenosis
b. Patent ductus arteriosus
c. Rupture of sinus of vasalva
d. Systemic arteriovenous fistula

In a large number of cases of rheumatic fever affection of the mitral valve there is a combination of mitral stenosis and incompetence. The clinical findings are modified depending upon the severity of each lesion. Continuous murmur is neither heard in MS (heard is a mid-diastolic murmur) nor in MR (heard is a pansystolic murmur).

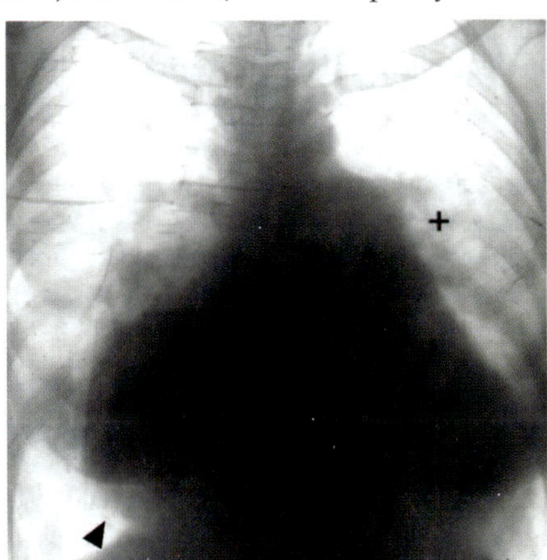

X-ray chest advanced mitral stenosis. Note: 1. Prominence of pulmonary artery segment (+) (previously referred to as pulmonary conus) 2. left arterial shadow within the right atrial border—arrowhead 3. cardiomegaly

112. Pulsus paradoxus is seen in all EXCEPT:

a. IPPV
b. COPD
c. Cardiac tamponade
d. Constrictive pericarditis

In normal subjects, during inspiration, the pulse volume falls slightly, but this is often not noticeable. Marked fall of pulse volume and pulse pressure during inspiration is called "pulsus paradoxus". This is seen in pericardial effusion, constrictive pericarditis and COPD.

113. Hypercalcemia on ECG tracing shows:

a. Increased QT interval
b. Decreased QT interval
c. Greatly increased PR interval
d. Tall T waves

Electrocardiogram in hypercalcemia shows shortened QT interval and other non-specific changes.

114. Torsades de pointes lead to:

a. Short QT
b. Wide QT
c. Short QRS
d. Wide QRS

Torsades-de-pointes shows prolonged Q-T interval on ECG.

115. Systolic ejection murmur of HOCM diminishes when patient:

a. Stands up
b. Inhale amyl-nitrite
c. Lies down
d. Performs vasalva manouevre

Lying down results in increase in preload, which decreases the intensity of murmur of HOCM.

Gene	Chromosome	Frequency (%)
B-Myosin heavy chain	14q1	35-45
Cardiac Troponin T	1q31	15
∞ - tropomyosin	15q2	5
Myosin binding protein C	11p 13-q 13	10

116. Drug used to perform stress ECHO:

a. Noradrenaline
b. Adrenaline
c. Dobutamine
d. Thallium

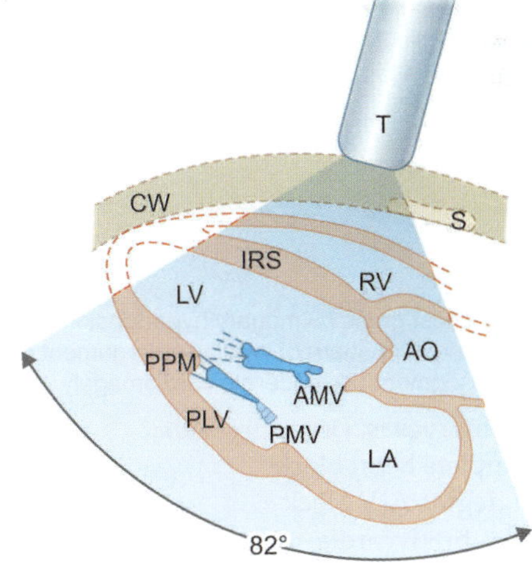

Schematic drawing showing a sagittal section of the heart through the long axis of the left ventricle. The path of the ultrasound beam emitted by the transducer (T) placed over the chest wall, as it is swept through an arc of 82° is illustrated.
T—Transducer; CW—Chest wall; S—Sternum; RV—Right ventricle; IVS—Intraventricular septum, RV—Right ventricular wall; AMV—Anterior leaflet of mitral valve; PMV—Posterior leaflet of mitral valve; LV—Left ventricle; PPM—Papillary muscle; PLV—Posterior left ventricular wall; AO—Aorta; LA— Left atrium

Ans. **110. a.** 'c' wave... **111. a.** Mitral regurgitation... **112. a.** IPPV **113. b.** Decreased QT interval **114. b.** Wide QT **115. c.** Lies down **116. c.** Dobutamine

Stress echocardiography is a very useful technique in the evaluation of coronary artery disease and valvular heart disease. This is done by evaluating the cardiac chambers by echocardiography at rest and during and immediately after applying some forms of stress. Commonly used modalities of stress are exercise, atrial pacing and pharmacologic methods (dobutamine, adenosine).

117. NOT a cause of left ventricular hypertrophy:

a. AR
b. AS
c. MR
d. MS

In MS, obstruction to the left atrial blood entering the left ventricle leads to elevation of intra-atrial pressure. The left atrial pressure is reflected back in the pulmonary veins leading to pulmonary venous hypertension. Subsequently pulmonary arterial hypertension sets in. Chronic pulmonary hypertension leads to right ventricular hypertrophy and eventually right ventricular failure and tricuspid regurgitation.

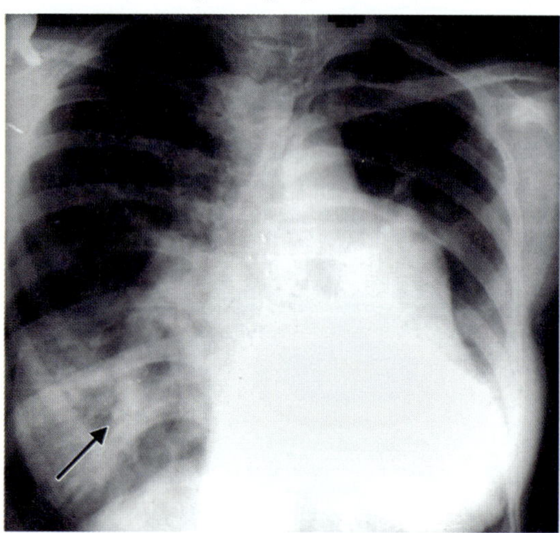

X-ray chest gross pulmonary hypertension etc.
Note: (1) right ventricular pattern of cardiac enlargement (2) prominent pulmonary artery segment (3) moderate cardiomegaly

118. Large 'a' waves in JVP represents:

a. Complete heart block
b. 1st degree A-V block
c. Sinus bradycardia
d. Tachycardia

Complete heart block should be suspected when the heart rate is 30-40/min or less, not increasing with exercise. Physical examination reveals slow, high volume pulse, forceful apex beat (due to diastolic overdistension), presence of irregular cannon waves in jugular veins, widened pulse pressure (high systolic and normal or low diastolic), and varying intensity of the first heart sound.

Etiology of Heart Block
1. Primary degeneration of the conducting tissues. (Lev's disease, Lenegre's disease)
2. Diseases affecting the myocardium: myocardial infarction, chronic coronary artery disease and myocarditis.
3. Drugs and toxins: digoxin, quinidine, procainamide, beta adrenergic blocking drugs, cerbera thevetia and cerbera odollam.
4. Trauma to the conducting tissue during surgery.
5. Congenital abnormality of the conducting tissue (congenital heart block).
6. Infections: Tertiary syphilis, South American trypanosomiasis (Chagas' disease) and cysticercosis.
7. Sick-sinus syndrome.

119. Acute anginal attack can be terminated by:

a. Nitroglycerin
b. Digoxin
c. Lignocaine
d. Verapamil

Nitrates form the mainstay of therapy for unstable angina pectoris. Intravenous nitroglycerine controls the angina and prevents recurrence. Nitrates can be given sublingually, orally, topically or intravenously.

Commonly used nitrates		
1. Nitroglycerine	Sublingual tablets	0.3 to 0.6 mg up to 1,5 mg
	Buccal spray	400 μg as needed
	Transdermal	15 × 15 cm patch containing 7.5-40 mg
	Oral sustained release	2.5 mg-13 mg
	Buccal	1-3 mg 3 times daily
	Intravenous	5-20 μg/min
2. Isosorbide dinitrate	Sublingual Oral	2.5-15 mg 5-80 mg, 2-3 times daily
	Buccal spray	1.25 mg metered doses
	Chewable tablets	5 mg
	Oral slow release	40 mg o.d or b.i.d
	Intravenous ointment	1.25-5 mg/h 100 mg/24 h 20 mg twice daily
3 Isosorbide mononitrate oral		60-240 mg once daily

Ans. 117. d. MS **118. a.** Complete heart bloc **119. a.** Nitroglycerin

120. Carotid sinus massage will terminate-:
a. Atrial flutter
b. Atrial fibrillation
c. Supraventricular arryhthmia
d. Supraventicular tachycardia

If there is no hemodynamic compromise, vagal pressure can be applied initially to reduce the rate in SVT. This is followed up with adenosine (6-12 mg I/V rapid bolus) and later intravenous verapamil or diltiazem.

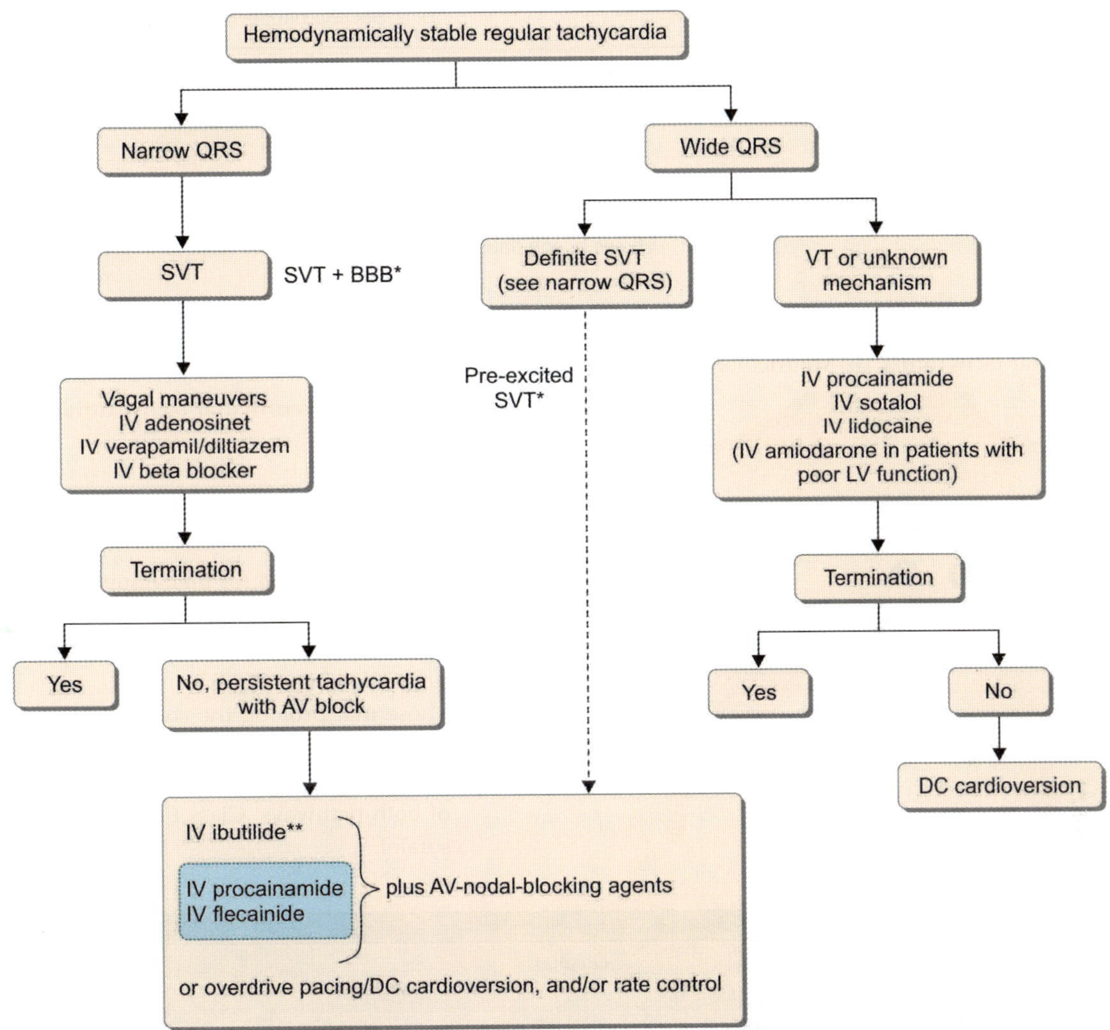

Guidelines for the management of tachyarrhythmias. Acute management of patients with hemodynamically stable and regular tachycardia. *A 12-lead ECG during sinus rhythm must be available for diagnosis. Adenosine should be used with caution in patients with severe coronary artery disease and may produce AF, which may result in rapid ventricular rates for patients with pre-excitation. **Ibutilide is especially effective for patients with artrial flutter but should not be used in patients with EF less than 30% due to increased risk of polymorphic VT. AF indicates atrial fibrillation; AV, artrioventricular, BBB, bundle-branch block; DC, direct current; IV, intravenous; LV, left ventricular; QRS, ventricular activation on ECG; SVT, supraventricular tachycardia; VT, ventricular tachycardia
Modified from ACC/AHA/ESC guidelines for the management of tachyarrhythmias. *Ref:* Circulation 2003;108:1871-1909.

121. Most common arrhythmia:
a. Inappropriate sinus tachycardia
b. Junctional Premature complexes
c. Atrial fibrillation
d. Atrial flutter

Atrial fibrillation is the condition in which the coordinated contractions of the atrium is abolished and the atrial muscle fibrillates. Abnormality of atrial activation is caused by impulses arising from different foci at the rate of 400-600/min. Since coordinated contraction at this rate is not possible, fibrillation sets in. This is the most common sustained arrhythmia in clinical practice.

122. Pacemaker is indicated in:
a. Acute myocardial infarction with first degree AV block
b. Acute myocardial infarction with fascicular block

Ans. **120. d.** Supraventicular...**121. c.** Atrial fibrillation **122. c.** Sick sinus syndrome

c. Sick sinus syndrome
d. All of the above

Once the diagnosis of SSS is established, in symptomatic patients, implantation of suitable permanent pacemaker is the treatment of choice particularly in those with symptomatic bradycardias. It helps to relieve the symptoms and improve the quality of life.

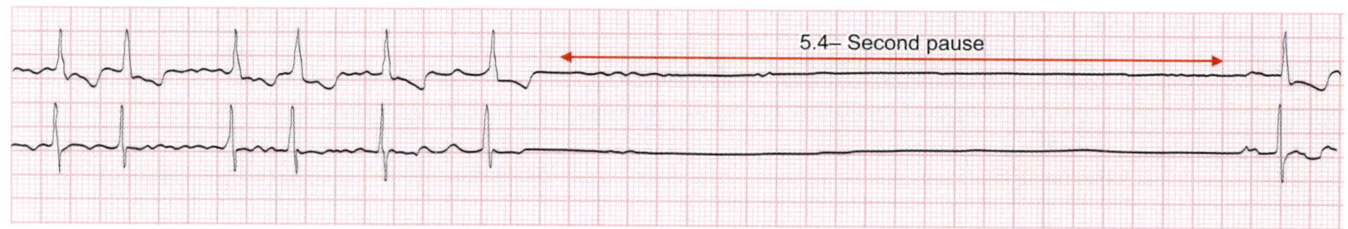

Sick sinus syndrome: note the tachy and bradyarrhythmias 1. The first half shows atrial fibrillation with fast heart rate 2. The latter half shows a long pause

123. On ECG, p wave is absent in:

a. WPW syndrome
b. Atrial fibrillation
c. Ventricular tachycardia
d. Ventricular fibrillation

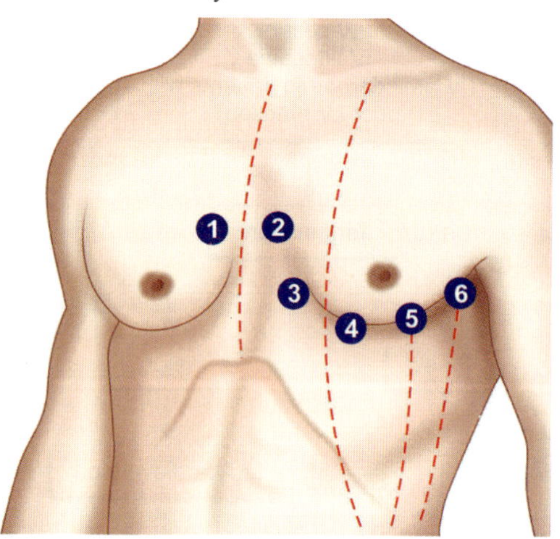

Position of chest leads—V1-V6

Confirmation of the diagnosis on AF is made by ECG which shows absence of P-waves and the presence of fibrillary waves instead.

124. DOC for supraventricular tachycardia:

a. Adenosine
b. Propranolol
c. Verapamil
d. Digoxin

Drugs are employed for managing SVT

- Those that prolong the conduction time or refractoriness in the AV node, e.g. Adenosine, propranolol and digoxin
- Those that prolong the conduction or refractoriness of the accessory pathway, e.g. Class IA and Class IC drugs.
- Prolongation of conduction time and refractoriness of both pathways, Class III drugs, e.g. Amiodarone, sotalol.

Anti-arrhythmic Drugs – Dosage and Indications

Sl.No.	Anti arrhythmic drugs	Dosage		Indications
		Oral	Parenteral	
1.	Quinidine	200-400 mg 3-4 times a day (up to 600 mg Q 6 H)	IM-600 mg followed by 400 mg every 2 hours or IV-800 mg in 50 mL 5% Dextrose @ 1mL/mt infusion	Atrial flutter, atrial fibrillation AVNRT
2.	Procainamide	2-4 g/day in 3-4 divided doses (max daily dose 6 gm)	IM or IV 25-50 mg over 1 mt to rpt at 5 mts interval till arrhythmia is controlled. Or IV infusion 2-6 mg/mt	Atrial fibrillation SVT (AVNRT, AVRT)
3.	Disopyramide	100-200 mg Q 6H Max 1200 mg/day	IV – 1 -2 mg/kg bolus followed by 1 mg/kg/hr	SVT (AVNRT, AVRT), atrial flutter, atrial fibrillation, VT
4.	Lignocaine	N A	IV 1-2 mg/kg bolus max 5 mg/kg then infusion at 1-4 mg/mt	Rapid termination of VT refractory VT/VF
5.	Mexiletine	200 mg tid	100-250 mg I V bolus followed by 250 mg infusion over 1-2 hrs	Ventricular tachycardia
6.	Phenytoin	1 g loading dose day 1 followed by 500 mg on D2 and D3 and 300-400 mg daily thereafter	IV 100 mg, repeated, up to max 1 g	Digoxin related atrial and ventricular arrhythmias

Contd...

Ans. 123. b. Atrial fibrillation **124. a.** Adenosine

Contd...

Sl.No.	Anti arrhythmic drugs	Dosage		Indications
		Oral	Parenteral	
7.	Flecainide	100 mg every 12 H max 400 mg/day	I V – 2 mg/kg then 100-200 mg Q 12 H	Paroxysmal AF, SVT, VT
8.	Esmolol	N A	I V 500 mcg/kg loading followed by 50–200 mcg/kg/mt	Rapid rate control in SVT
9.	Amiodarone	200 mg tid × 1 week then 200 mg bd for a week, maintenance 100-200 mg/d	150-300 mg IV bolus then 1 mg/kg/mt for 6 hrs and 0.5 mg/kg/mt for 18 hrs	Atrial flutter fibrillation AVNRT refractory VT/VF and VF
10.	Sotalol	80 mg/d in 1-2 divided doses, max of 640 mg/d	I V 100 mg over 1-2 mt	Atrial flutter atrial fibrillation, VT
11.	Bretylium	4 mg/kg/daily	I V 5-10 mg/kg bolus followed by 0.5-2 mg/mt infusion	Refractory VT and VF
12.	Ibutilide	N A	I V 1 mg over 10 mts to repeat if needed	Termination of a/c episode of atrial flutter/ atrial fibrillation
13.	Dofetilide	0.1-0.5 mg BD	IV 2.5 mcg/kg, to repeat if needed	Acute and chronic AF
14.	Verapamil	120-480 mg/day in 3-4 divided doses	I V 5-10 mg over 2-3 mts	SVT
15.	Adenosine	N A	6-12 mg I V as rapid bolus	Termination of PSVT
16.	Digoxin	0.5-1 mg loading followed by 0.125 mg 0.25 mg daily	I V 0.5-1 mg	Atrial flutter fibrillation control of heart rate

Key: SVT – Supraventricular tachycardia
VT – Ventricular – do –
AVNRT – AV nodal re-entrant – do –
VF – Ventricular fibrillation
AF –Atrial fibrillation
PSVT – Paroxysmal SVT

125. In pericardial effusion, all are seen EXCEPT:

a. Raised JVP
b. Hepatomegaly
c. Pedal edema
d. Loud heart sounds

Physical examination of pericardial effusion reveals reduced force or absence of apical impulse, enlargement of the area of cardiac dullness, muffled heart sounds and pericardial rub.

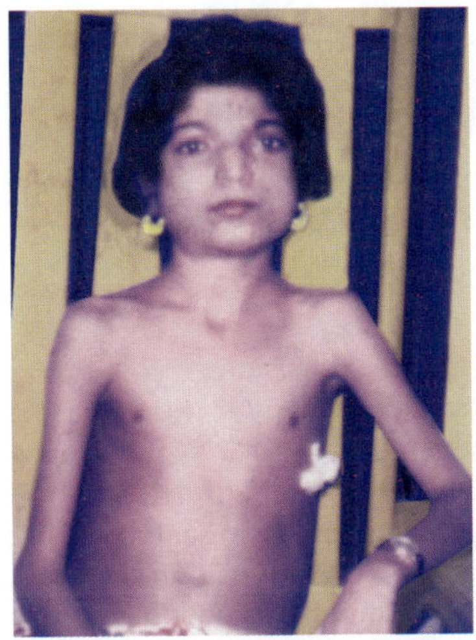

14 years female with chronic pericardial effusion. The cotton seal is over the site of aspiration

126. Kussmaul's sign is seen in all EXCEPT:

a. Constrictive pericarditis
b. Right ventricular infarct
c. Restrictive cardiomyopathy
d. Cardiac tamponade

In pericardial effusion/cardiac tamponade, normal decrease in venous pressure on inspiration is maintained.

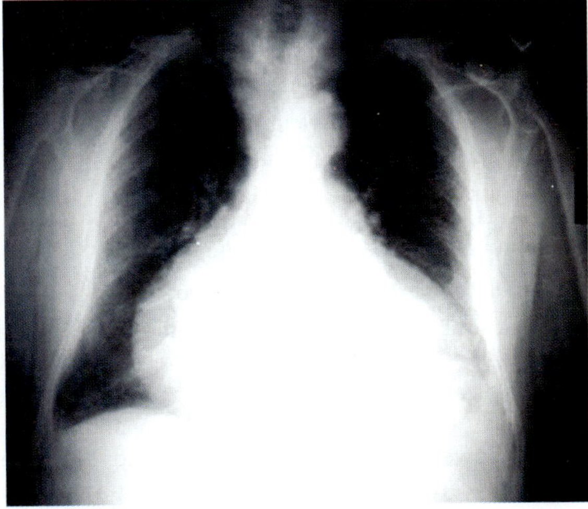

Chest X-ray in pericardial effusion showing flask shaped enlargement of heart and stenciled appearance of cardiac borders

MCQs with Short Explanations

Ans. **125. d.** Loud heart... **126. d.** Cardiac tamponade

127. NOT seen in cardiac tamponade:

a. Pulsus paradoxus
b. Diastolic collapse of right ventricle on echocardiogram
c. Electrical alterans
d. Kussmaul's sign

Clinical features of cardiac tamponade

- A paradoxical pulse is present. Paradoxical pulse is the exaggerated inspiratory fall in systolic blood pressure, often exceeding 10 mm Hg.
- Early diastolic collapse of the right atrium and right ventricle seen in echo indicates presence of cardiac tamponade
- ECG usually shows sinus tachycardia, reduced voltage and sometimes, electrical laterans of the QRS complex.

128. In post-ductal coarctation of aorta, collaterals to lower limb are NOT formed by:

a. Intercostal artery
b. Vertebral artery
c. Suprascapular artery
d. Internal thoracic artery

When coarctation is severe, arterial blood from the proximal part is taken to the distal part through collateral circulation which develops from intercostal arteries and the subclavian system.

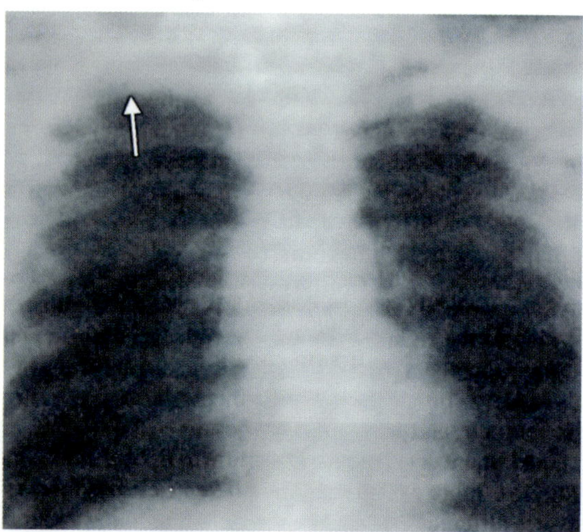

Coarctation of the aorta. Note 3 sign on the aorta—'x', and rib notching (arrows)

129. Best marker for dyslipidemia:

a. Triglyceride and cholesterol
b. LDL/ HDL ratio
c. LDL/ cholesterol ratio
d. Apo-A1

The desirable level of total cholesterol for Indians is ideally 150-200 mg/dL. Decreased level of HDL below 35 mg/dL is an independent risk factor for atherosclerosis. Presence of low HDL levels is an indication for active lowering of total cholesterol and LDL. Levels of triglycerides above 200 mg/dL especially when accompanied by a low HDL/LDL ratio increases the risk of coronary atheroma six fold.

Frederickson's classification

Types	*Lipoproteins*	*Groups*
Type 1	Chylomicron	Group III
Type 2a	LDL	Group I
Type 2b	LDL and VLDL	
Type 3	Remnants	Group II
Type 4	VLDL	
Type 5	VLDL and chylomicrons	

130. NOT true for VSD:

a. Defect is usually in membranous part
b. Endocarditis is commonest complication
c. Large VSD causes infundibular stenosis
d. Small holes close spontaneously

Large VSDs lead to congestive cardiac failure in infancy. Recurrent respiratory infection and failure to thrive may also be noticed. Those who survive develop varying degrees of pulmonary hypertension. Small VSDs are asymptomatic and they are detected on routine examination. Moderate VSDs present with palpitation and recurrent respiratory infections.

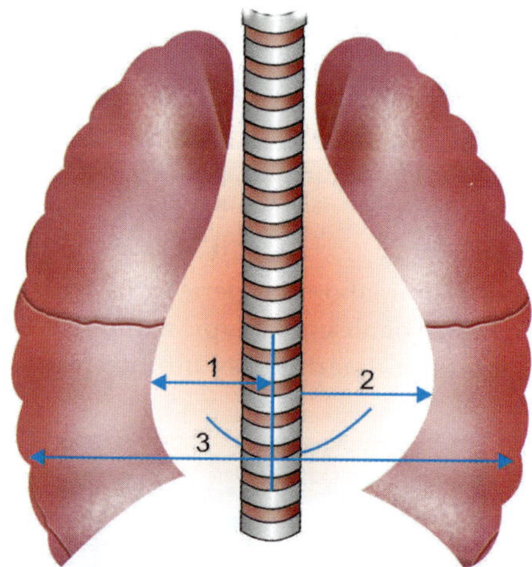

Line drawing of chest X-ray Note: Transverse diameter of the heart is 1 + 2 Cardiothoracic ratio (CTR) $\frac{1+2}{3}$

131. Which condition present as severe chest pain radiating to back:

a Acute aortic occlusion
b. Aortic dissection
c. Rheumatic aortitis
d. Tetralogy of fallot

The symptoms of dissecting aneurysm of aorta start with sudden onset of severe pain in the chest, interscapular region, neck, mid-back, abdomen, sacral region, and lower limbs. The pain may be mistaken for myocardial infarction.

Ans. **127. d.** Kussmaul's sign **128. a.** Intercostal artery **129. b.** LDL/ HDL ratio **130. c.** Large VSD causes... **131. b.** Aortic dissection

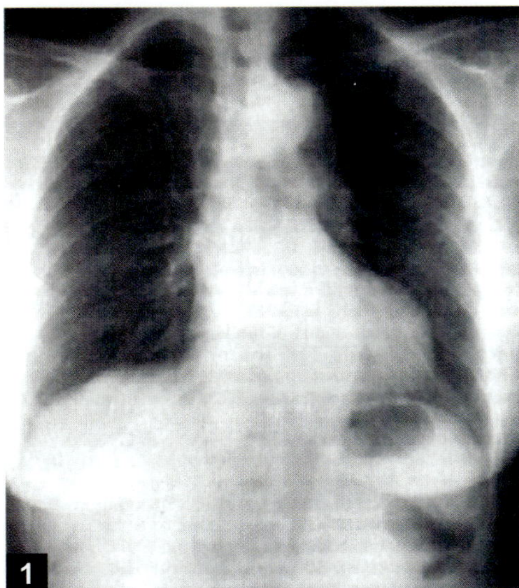

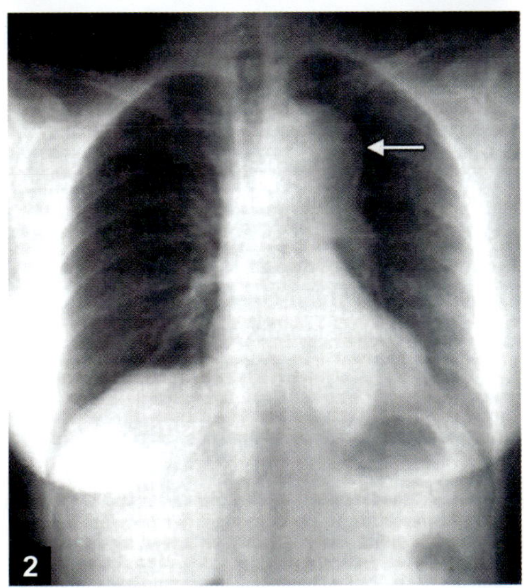

Chest X-ray of patient with dissection of the aorta (1) Original X-ray taken 2 years previously (2) Note the widening of the aortic knuckle—arrow

132. Advantages of stenting over balloon angioplasty are:

a. Improved efficacy in bifurcation lesions
b. Control over elastic recoil
c. Lesser incidence of restenosis
d. All of the above

PTCA (percutaneous transluminal coronary angioplasty) is a radiological intervention procedure undertaken by cardiologists in which the stenotic segment of the arteries are dilated by suitable balloons passed through catheters, percutaneously through the femoral artery, retrograde into the aorta and then into the coronary arteries. By inflating the balloon the atheroma is crushed and the arterial lumen is restored. The lumen is maintained patent by the use of different types of stents.

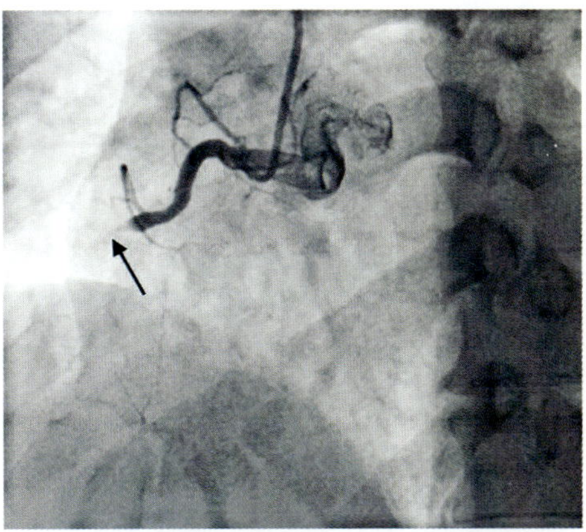

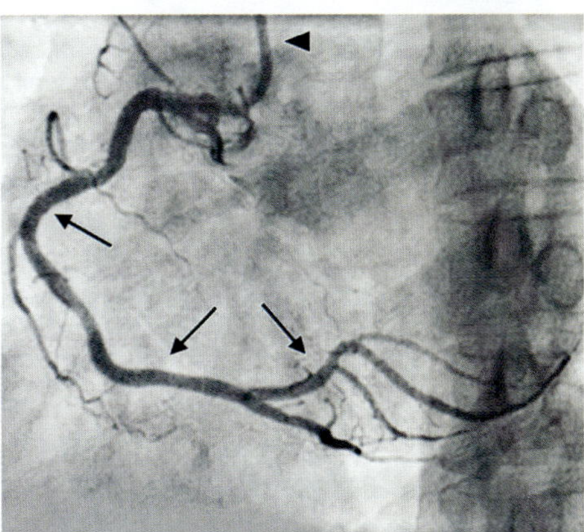

Coronary angiogram in a patient with acute inferior wall myocardial infarction showing RCA. First picture: Before primary PTCA, RCA was totally occluded with thrombus.(arrow). Second picture: After primary PTCA, showing RCA with good flow and the branches (arrows)

133. One of the main disadvantage of stenting is:

a. Elastic recoil
b. Late stent thrombosis
c. Restenosis
d. Lesser efficacy in bifurcation lesions

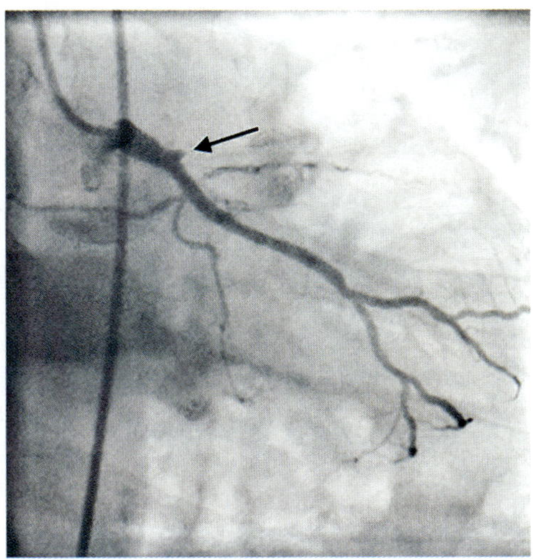

Ans. **132. d.** All of the above **133. b.** Late stent thrombosis

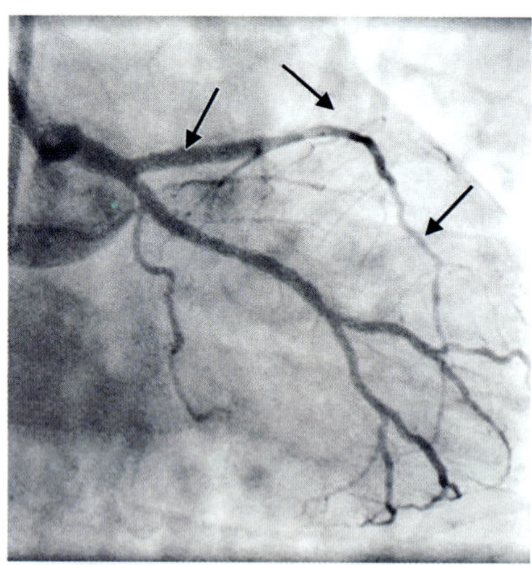

Coronary angiogram in a patient with acute anterior wall myocardial infarction showing LAD. First picture: Before primary PTCA, LAD was totally occluded from ostium with thrombus and is not seen (arrow). Second picture: After primary PTCA, showing LAD with good flow and the branches (arrows)

The original stents introduced in 1987 were simple metallic stents. In them the re-occlusion rate was 30% and above within 1 year. Subsequently drug eluting stents were introduced. These elute drugs such as sirolimus, paclitaxel and others which serve to inhibit re-occlusion. Drug eluting stents are considerably more expensive than the plain stents.

134. Preferred biochemical markers in patients presenting with myocardial infarction:

a. Myoglobin
b. Cardiac specific Troponins
c. CK-MB
d. All of the above

Myocardial injury leads to a rapid rise in cardiac troponin in plasma. Troponin I and troponin T are released into the plasma so that reliable diagnostic sensitivity is reached by 12 to 16 h and maximal activity is reached by 24 to 36 h. The levels return to normal within 10-12 days.

The location of infarct depends upon the vessel occluded
❑ Left anterior descending branch: Anterior and apical portions of left ventricle.
❑ Left circumflex branch: Lateral and inferoposterior walls of the left ventricle.
❑ Right coronary artery: Inferoposterior wall and inferior portion of the interventricular septum.

135. Split second heart sound is heard in:

a. Mitral stenosis
b. Left bundle branch block
c. Complete right bundle branch block
d. Pulmonary hypertension

The second heart sound in the pulmonary area shows two components – the aortic and the pulmonary (A2 and P2). Right bundle branch block and pulmonary stenosis would lead to delayed closure of pulmonary valve and wide splitting of second heart sound.

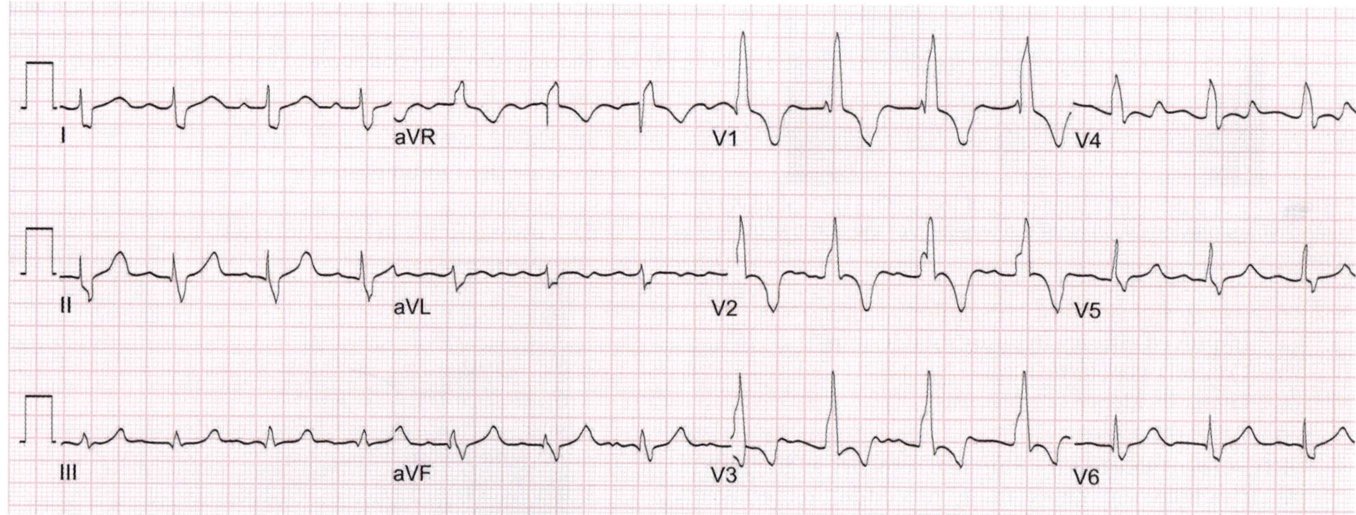

RBBB: complete right bundle branch block Note: 1. Prolongation of QRS duration above 0.12 seconds 2. Slurred R'waves in V1 and V2 3. Wide S waves in L1, aVL and V5 and V6

136. Which of the following is a high pitched sound:

a. 1st heart sound
b. Tumor plop
c. Opening Snap
d. 4th heart sound

In MS, an opening snap is heard which is a sharp sound (high-pitched) and best heard over the apex beat, but conducted widely over the precordium, especially towards the sternum.

Ans. 134. b. Cardiac specific...**135. c.** Complete right bundle **136. c.** Opening Snap

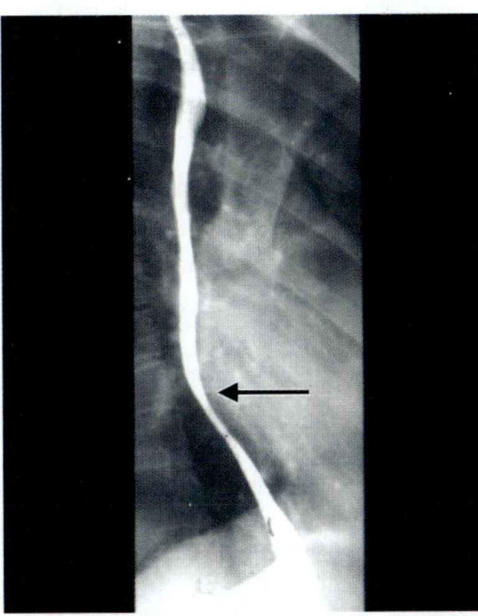

X-ray chest with barium swallow – mitral stenosis. Note: The indentation caused by the left atrium on the barium filled esophagus—arrow

137. Which of the following is characterized by hampered diastolic filling of ventricles, a positive Kussmaul's sign and pericardial calcification:

a. Constrictive pericarditis
b. Right ventricular infarct
c. Restrictive Cardiomyopathy
d. Cardiac tamponade

Constrictive pericarditis is a condition in which a thickened, scarred, and often, calcified pericardium forms a tough cover around the heart limiting diastolic filling of the ventricles.

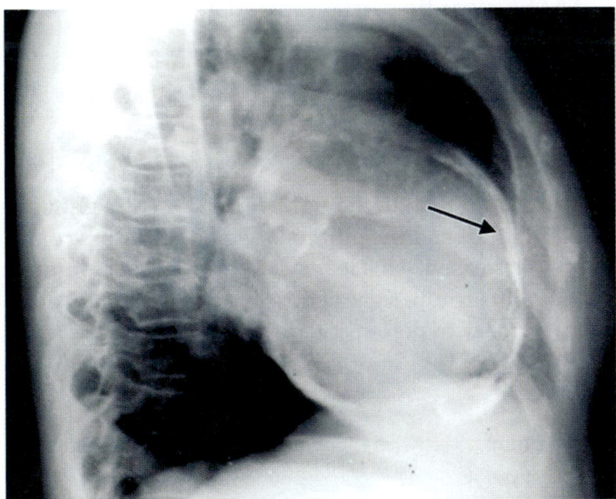

X- ray chest lateral view in constrictive pericarditis showing calcification around the cardiac silhouette (arrow)

138. Following acute failure of left ventricle in man, pulmonary edema generally begins to appear when left atrial pressure approaches:

a. 5 mm Hg
b. 15 mm Hg
c. 25 mm Hg
d. 35 mm Hg

When directly or indirectly caused by increased left ventricular pressure, pulmonary edema may form when mean pulmonary pressure rises from the normal of 15 mm Hg to above 25 mm Hg.

Framingham criteria for diagnosis of congestive heart failure (CHF)
Major criteria 1. Paroxysmal nocturnal dyspnea 2. Neck veins distension 3. Rales (crackles) over the lower portions of the lung 4. Cardiomegaly 5. Acute pulmonary edema 6. S3 gallop 7. Increased venous pressure > 16 mm Hg 8. Circulation time >25 sec 9. Hepatojugular reflux
Minor criteria 1. Ankle edema 2. Night cough 3. Dyspnea on exertion 4. Hepatomegaly 5. Pleural effusion 6. Decrease of vital capacity exceeding 1/3 7. Tachycardia > 120/mt
Major or minor criteria 1. Weight loss > 4.5 kg in 5 days in response to treatment. 2. Major +2 minor criteria if present concurrently establishes the diagnosis of CHF
Note: Framingham is a township in the USA where a cohort of persons have been followed up meticulously over a long period of time and several biological parameters have been recorded continuously. This study has become a classic prospective study, for several disorders, especially for cardiovascular disorders. The follow up and observation are still continuing.

139. Drug used for prophylaxis of rheumatic heart disease:

a. Sulfadiazine
b. Phenoxy-methyl penicillin
c. Benzathine penicillin
d. All of the above

Since rheumatic recurrence is invariably precipitated by streptococcal reinfection, benzathine penicillin 1.2 mega units is given once every three weeks to prevent streptococcal reinfection and rheumatic recurrence. As an alternative, oral penicillin 200,000 units twice daily must be given. Penicillin-sensitive individuals may be treated with erythromycin 250 mg/day.

Effects of streptococcal products on the host	
Erythrogenic toxins—	3 types: Pyrogenic, cytotoxic, suppression of reticuloendothelial activity, immunosuppression and inducing susceptibility to endotoxin
Streptolysin O	Lysis of erythrocytes, cytotoxic action on neutrophils, platelets and cardiac tissue

Contd...

Ans. **137. a.** Constrictive... **138. c.** 25 mm Hg **139. d.** All of the above

Contd...

Effects of streptococcal products on the host	
Streptokinase	Fibrinolysis
Deoxyribonucleases	Hydrolyse nucleic acids and nucleoproteins. These are antigenic
Hyaluronidase	Spreading factor, helps the organism to spread in tissues
Nicotinamide adenine dinucleotidase (NADase)	Antigenic

140. Drug contraindicated in HOCM is:

a. Verapamil b. Propranolol
c. Digoxin d. Amiadarone

Contraindications to Digoxin

- AV blocks – second degree, complete heart block and unstable AV blocks
- Pure diastolic dysfunction
- Wolff-Parkinson-White syndrome
- Suspected digitoxicity
- Hypertrophic obstructive cardiomyopathy

141. Wolff-Parkinson-White disease may be associated with which of the congenital heart defect:

a. Tetralogy of Fallot b. PDA
c. Ebstein's anomaly d. All of the above

Ebstein's anomaly is a congenital heart defect in which the septal and posterior leaflets of the tricuspid valve are displaced towards the apex of the right ventricle of the heart. About 50% of individuals with Ebstein's anomaly have evidence of Wolff-Parkinson-White syndrome, secondary to the atrialized right ventricular tissue.

Prenatal teratogens	
Agent	*Cardiac defect*
Ethanol	VSD
Phenytoin	VSD
Lithium	Ebstein's anomaly
Retinoic acid	TGA
Rubella	PDA, PS
Valproic acid	Coarctation of aorta
Vitamin D	Supravalvular PS
Warfarin	PDA, PS

142. Best time to administer long term nitrates for nocturnal angina:

a. Early morning b. Noon
c. Evening d. Late night

Most expert recommend that people not take the long acting nitrate for an 8-12 hour period each day, usually at night unless that is when angina occurs. This approach helps maintain the long-term effectiveness of the drug. Unlike beta-blockers, nitrates do not reduce the risk of heart attacks and suden death, but they greatly reduce symptoms in people with coronary artery disease.

143. Left ventricular hypertrophy is NOT a feature of:

a. Mitral regurgitation b. Isolated mitral stenosis
c. Isolated ventricular septal defect
d. Aortic stenosis

Chronic pulmonary hypertension in MS leads to right ventricular hypertrophy and eventually right ventricular failure and tricuspid regurgitation.

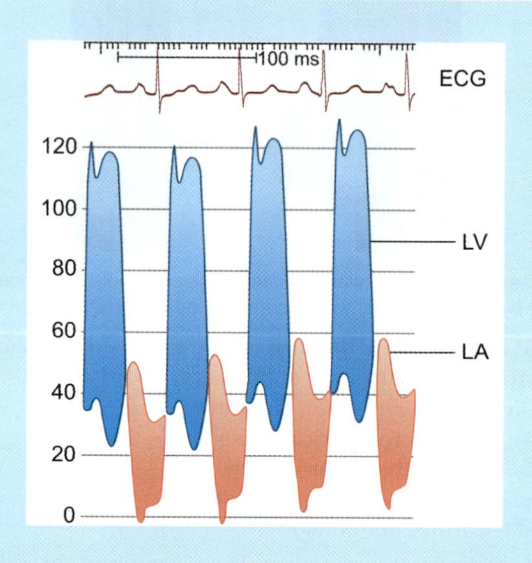

Mitral stenosis: cardiac catheterization; LV and LA pressures are superimposed, showing the gradient in diastole between LA and LV indicating high pressure in the atrium in mitral stenosis

144. FALSE regarding atrial septal defect:

a. Right atrial hypertrophy
b. Left atrial hypertrophy
c. Right ventricular hypertrophy
d. Pulmonary hypertension

In ASD the blood is shunted from left atrium to right atrium and then to the right ventricle. The right ventricular output and the pulmonary blood flow are considerably increased. This leads to progressive enlargment of the right atrium, right ventricle, and pulmonary arteries. Pulmonary hypertension develops.

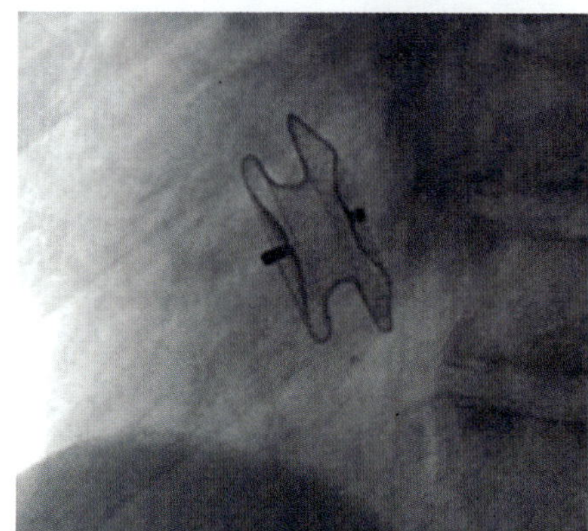

Amplatzer ASD occluder deployed to close an ASD

Ans. **140. c.** Digoxin **141. c.** Ebstein's anomaly **142. c.** Evening **143. b.** Isolated mitral stenosis **144. b.** Left atrial...

145. FALSE about ventricular septal defect:
a. Small hole closes spontaneously
b. Defect is usually in membranous part
c. Endocarditis is commonest complication
d. Pulmonary oligemia in chest X-ray

X-ray findings of VSD
- With small defects, heart size and pulmonary blood flow are normal
- With large defects, moderate to marked enlargement of heart, prominent main pulmonary artery and pulmonary plethora are seen
- There is no right atrial enlragement unlike ASD and unlike PDA, the aorta is not prominent

Acyanotic
Left to right shunt
1. Atrial septal defect (ASD)
2. Ventricular septal defect (VSD)
3. Patent ductus arteriosus (PDA)

Obstructive lesions
1. Aortic stenosis (AS)
2. Pulmonary stensois (PS)
3. Coarctation of aorta (CoA)

Cyanotic
Reduced pulmonary blood flow
1. Tetralogy of Fallot (TOF)
2. Transposition of great arteries (TGA), VSD, PS
3. Corrected TGA (c-TGA)-VSD—PS
4. Tricuspid atresia-VSD—PS

146. A 65-year-old man presents with triad of angina, syncope and congestive heart failure. Which of the following valvular lesion can be suspected:
a. Mitral stenosis b. Tricuspid regurgitation
c. Aortic stenosis d. Aortic regurgitation

The three most important presentations of significant aortic stenosis are angina pectoris, syncope and left ventricular failure.

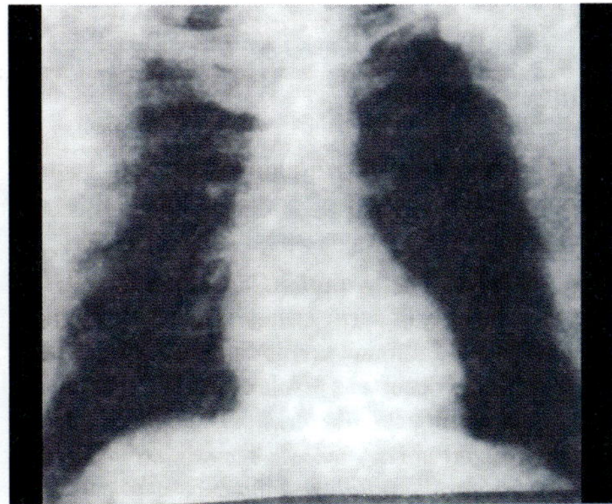

X-ray chest – Aortic stenosis
Note: Left ventricular type cardiac contour. Muscle hypertrophy is more prominent than dilatation

147. NOT a feature of tetralogy of fallot:
a. Ejection systolic murmur in 2nd intercostals space
b. Single 2nd heart sound
c. Predominantly left to right shunt
d. Normal JVP

In TOF, there is pulmonary stenosis, ventricular septal defect, overriding of the aorta, and right ventricular hypertrophy. The right ventricular outflow tract (RVOT) obstruction causes reduction in pulmonary blood flow. Arterial desaturation occurs because of right to left shunt across the VSD. Both right and left ventricular blood enters the aorta.

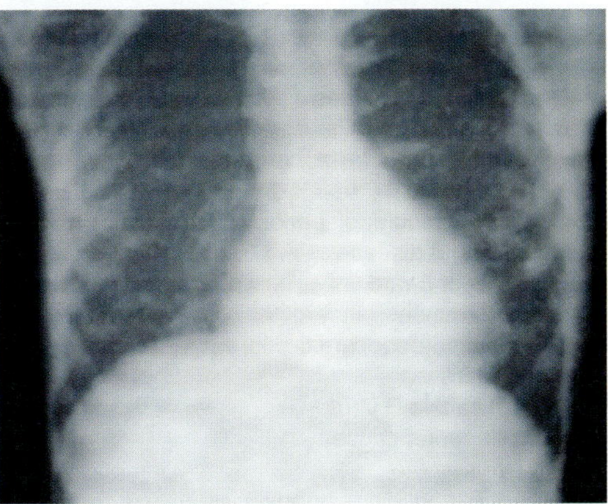

Tetralogy of Fallot with right sided aortic arch Note: Concave pulmonary artery segment, decreased lung vascularity and right sided aortic arch. This occurs in 20% of subjects

148. In MI, correct sequence of increase in enzyme levels is:
a. LDH, CPK, AST b. AST, CPK, LDH
c. CK, LDH, AST d. CK, AST, LDH

CK-MB begins to rise at 3-12 hours, AST at 8-12 hours and LDH, after 10 hours.

149. Coarctation of aorta may be associated with:
a. Marfan's syndrome b. Down's syndrome
c. Turner's syndrome d. Klinefelter's syndrome

In Turner's syndrome, coarctation is a typical manifestation. Coarctation is uncommon with cyanotic congenital heart diseases like tetralogy of Fallot and pulmonary atresia since these conditions lead to dilatation of the aortic root and good growth of the isthmus.

CHD in selected chromosomal aberrations

Condition	*Common defects*
1. Trisomy 21 (Down's syndrome)	Endocardial cushion defects
2. Turner's syndrome	Coarctation of aorta, AS, ASD
3. Klinefelter's syndrome	PDA
4. Cri Du Chat syndrome	VSD, PDA, ASD
5. Trisomy 13 (Patau's syndrome)	VSD, PDA
6. Trisomy 18 (Edward's syndrome)	VSD, PDA, PS

150. A 20-year-old female patient has non-exertional chest pain. On auscultation, she had non-ejection click. Investigation of choice would be:
a. Serum markers b. Chest X-ray
c. Electrocardiography d. Echocardiography

Ans. **145. d.** Pulmonary... **146. c.** Aortic stenosis **147. c.** Predominantly... **148. d.** CK, AST, LDH
149. c. Turner's... **150. d.** Echocardiography

Diagnosis of mitral valve prolapse/MVP/midsystolic click syndrome/floppy valave syndrome/Barlow's syndrome is made on the presence of a non-ejection systolic click with or without late systolic murmur, best made out over the apex on auscultation. Diagnosis can be confirmed by echocardiography which is the investigation of choice.

Chronic valvular heart disease—etiology

- ❑ Congenital
- ❑ Ischemic heart disease
- ❑ Degenerative changes
- ❑ Infiltrative and storage diseases
- ❑ Heritable disorders of connective tissue, e.g.: Marfan's syndrome
- ❑ Collagen vascular diseases
- ❑ Rheumatoid disease
- ❑ Tumours of heart
- ❑ Infective causes
  - Infective endocarditis
  - Syphilis
  - Coxsackie B virus
- ❑ Miscellaneous causes
  - Trauma
  - Anticardiolipin antibody
  - Hypereosinophilic syndrome

151. False regarding Austin-Flint murmur is:

a. Systolic murmur
b. Severe aortic regurgitation
c. Originates at anterior mitral valve leaflet
d. May be confused with murmur of mitral stenosis

In AR, a mid-diastolic, or presystolic murmur or a combination of both may be heard well over the apex beat (Austin-Flint murmur).

Peripheral signs of AR	
Alfred de Musset's sign	Head nodding with heart beat
Landolfi's sign	Change in pupil size with heart beat
Muller's sign	Uvula pulsation
Rosenbach's sign	Liver pulsations
Gerhardt's sign	Spleen pulsations
Quincke's sign	Digital capillary pulsations
Pistol shot sound	Systolic booming sound over femoral artery
Traube's sign	Systolic and diastolic booming sound over femoral artery
Duroziez's sign	Systolic sounds on proximal compression and diastolic sounds on distal compression over femoral arteries
Hill's sign	Lower limb systolic BP exceeding Upper limb systolic BP by > 60 mm Hg
Corrigan's pulse	High volume collapsing pulse
Becker's sign	Retinal artery pulsations
Corrigan's sign	Prominent carotid pulsation

152. Austin flint murmur is a:

a. Pansystolic murmur b. Midsystolic murmur
c. Mid-diastolic murmur d. Continuous murmur

Austin-Flint murmur of AR, is a mid-diastolic murmur.

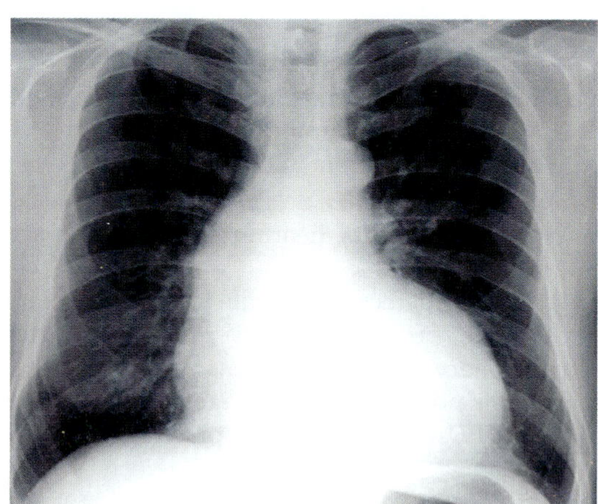

X-ray chest AR showing cardiac dilatation (LV type) and dilated aorta

153. Dyspnea at rest is which grade:

a. 1 b. 2
c. 3 d. 4

Grade IV (gross) dyspnea is total incapacity and dyspnea at rest and recumbency.

154. Where pulsatile liver and ascites is found:

a. Critical pulmonary stenosis
b. MR
c. TR d. MS

In TR, the liver is enlarged and tender and shows systolic pulsation. In severe cases there is usually peripheral edema and is some cases there may be ascites.

155. All are true regarding hypertrophic cardiomyopathy EXCEPT:

a. Digoxin is helpful
b. Irregular thickness of septa
c. Dynamic obstruction d. Double apical impulse

Digoxin is contraindicated in HOCM.

156. Site of vegetations in endocarditis of RHD is:

a. Along the line of closure of valves
b. Both sides of valves
c. Valve cusps d. Free margin of valves

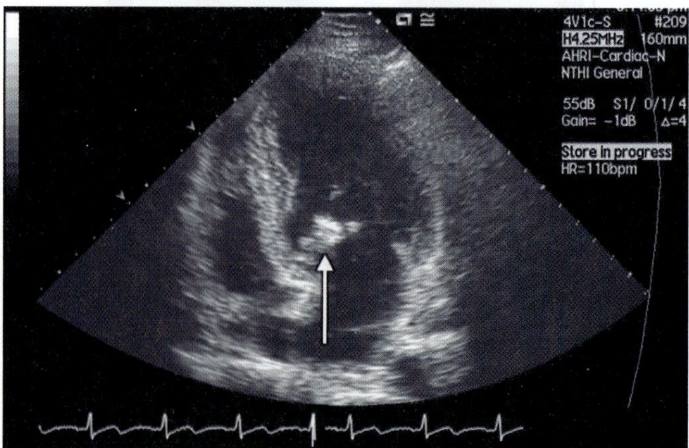

Transthoracic echocardiogram shows vegetation attached to anterior mitral leaflet—arrow

Ans. **151. a.** Systolic murmur **152. c.** Mid-diastolic murmur **153. d.** 4 **154. c.** TR
155. a. Digoxin is... **156. a.** Along the line...

Volume II Clinical Subjects

The small verrucous vegetations seen along the line of closure line of the mitral valve are associated with acute rheumatic fever. The warty vegetations average only a few millimeters and form along the line of closure over areas of endocardial inflammation.

157. Asynchronous cardioversion is given in:

a. AF b. Ventricular fibrillation
c. Atrial flutter d. Ventricular tachycardia

In VF, the heart is defibrillated by direct current (DC) shock of 300-400 joules.

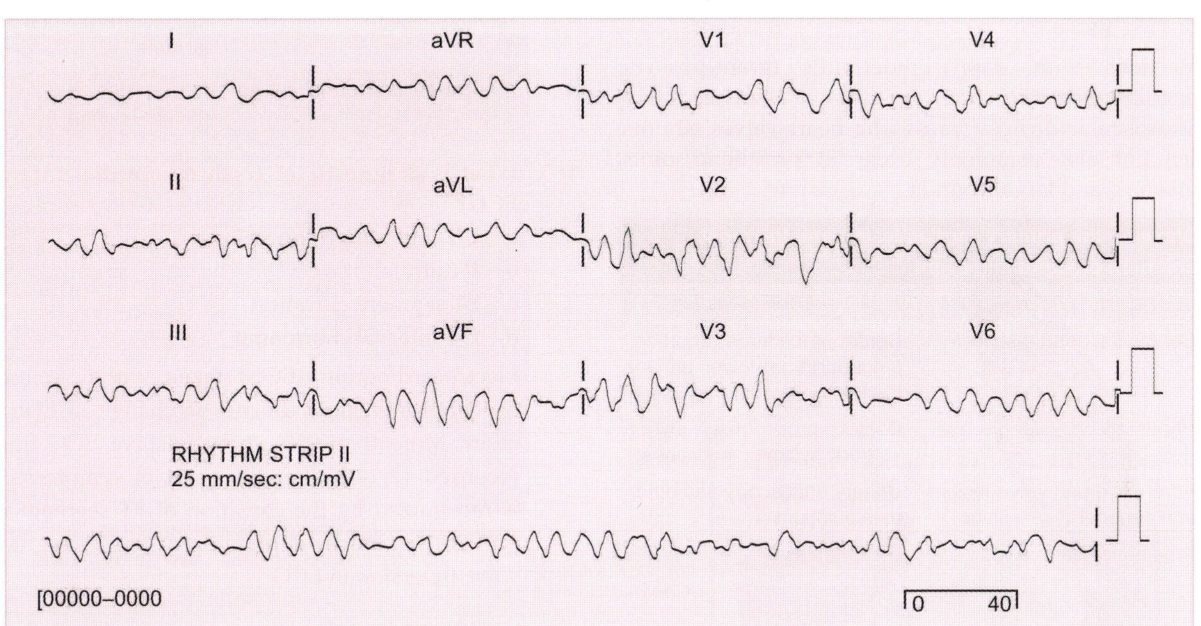

Ventricular fibrillation: Note: 1. Totally irregular QRS activity with undulating base line. 2. Absence of normal QRS and T waves

158. All are ECG findings in Wolff-Parkinson-White syndrome EXCEPT:

a. Narrow QRS complexes b. Normal QT interval
c. Slurred and tall QRS d. Short PR interval

In WPW syndrome, the ECG shows shortening of the PR interval and slurring of the ascending limb of the QRS complex, termed the delta wave, in addition to widening of the QRS complex.

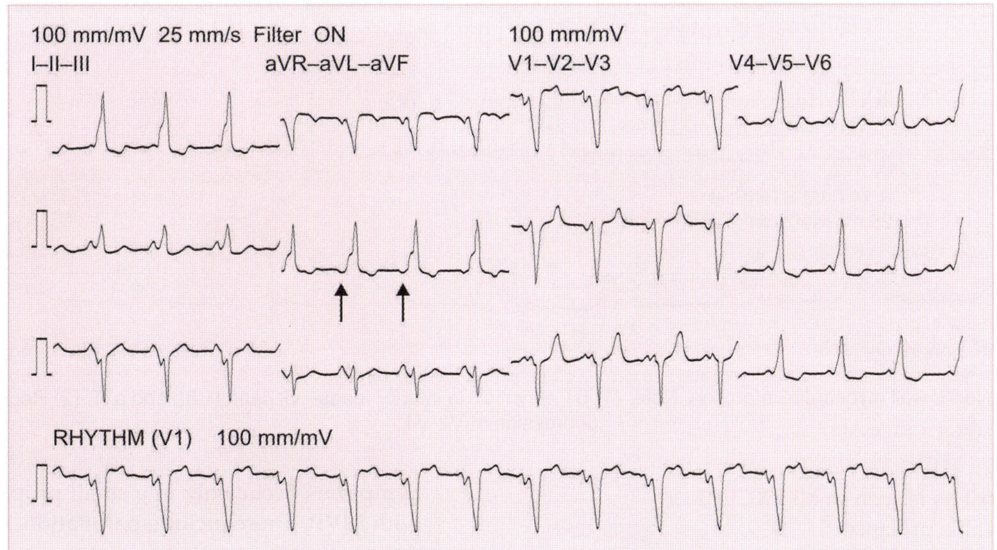

Wolff-Parkinson-White (WPW) syndrome: Note: The classic triad of WPW syndrome include: 1. short PR interval 2. delta wave (arrows) and 3. QRS widening. The delta wave represents the conduction through the aberrant bypass tract

Ans. 157. **b.** Ventricular... 158. **a.** Narrow QRS...

159. A patient has prosthetic valve replacement and he developed endocarditis 8 months later. Organism responsible is:

a. Staphylococcus aureus
b. Streptococcus viridans
c. Staphylococcus epidermidis
d. HACEK

Infections with staph epidermidis (gram-positive, coagulase-negative cocci) are usually associated with intravascular devices (prosthetic heart valves, shunts, etc.) but also commonly occur in prosthetic joints, catheters, and large wounds.

Showing the primary cardiac lesion and the most common precipitating event

Pre-existing heart disease	*Precipitating factors*
Congenital heart disease	Dental procedures, abortion, procedures on lower urinary tract, intravenous drug use
Rheumatic valvular disease	Dental procedures, minor surgery, systemic infections.
Atherosclerotic valve lesions and degenerative lesions	Urinary endoscopy and other manipulations
Prosthetic heart valves	Bacteremias
Cardiac surgery	Intravenous cannulae and shunts, foreign materials
Normal valves in immuno-compromised	Emergency room procedures including IV catheter and injections
Drug addicts: Normal valves	Intravenous drug injection, needle-sharing

160. What is diagnostic of fresh myocardial infarction in ECG?

a. QT interval prolongation
b. P mitrale
c. ST segment elevation
d. QT interval shortening

Electrocardiogram (ECG) taken within a few hours of symptoms show diagnostic change in over 80% of cases. More than 95% show positive ECG findings if recorded 12-24 h after the onset of symptoms. STEMI is recognized by the elevation of ST segment in ECG. NSTEMI produces depression of the ST segment or T wave inversion in ECG.

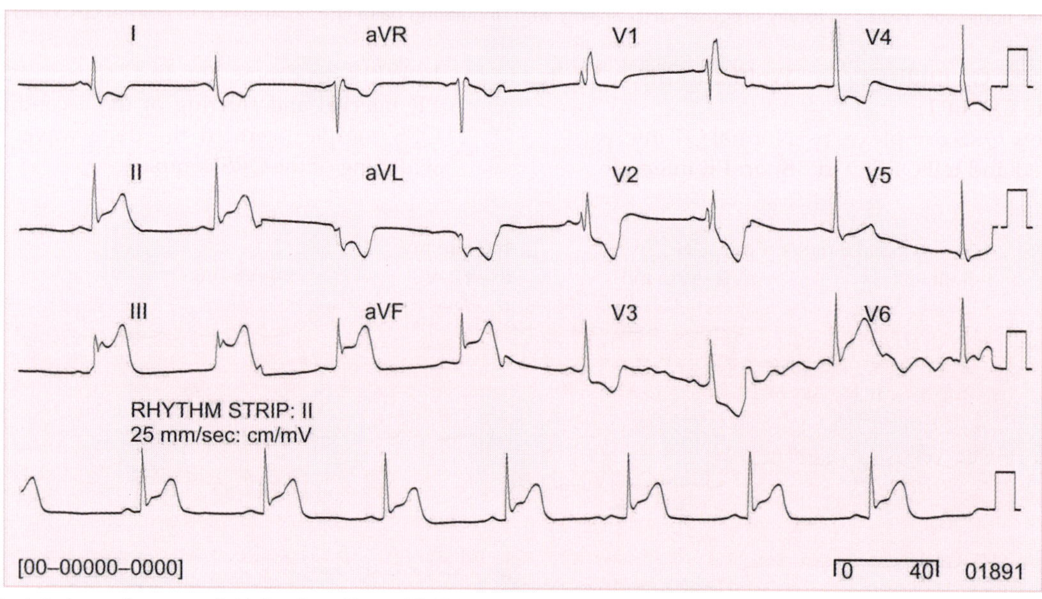

ECG: Hyperacute inferior wall myocardial infarction. Note: (1) ST elevation in inferior leads– viz lead II, III, and aVF (2) Reciprocal ST segment depression in V2-V4

161. Pulsus bisfriens is seen in all EXCEPT:

a. Mitral valve prolapse
b. Aortic stenosis with aortic regurgitation
c. Severe aortic regurgitation
d. HOCM

Symptoms occur only in a small proportion of patients with MVP. These include palpitation, vague chest pain, dyspnea, and non-cardiac symptoms such as vascular headache and anxiety state. In most cases chest pain is non-cardiac.

Ans. **159. c.** Staphylococcus... **160. c.** ST segment elevation **161. a.** Mitral valve prolapse

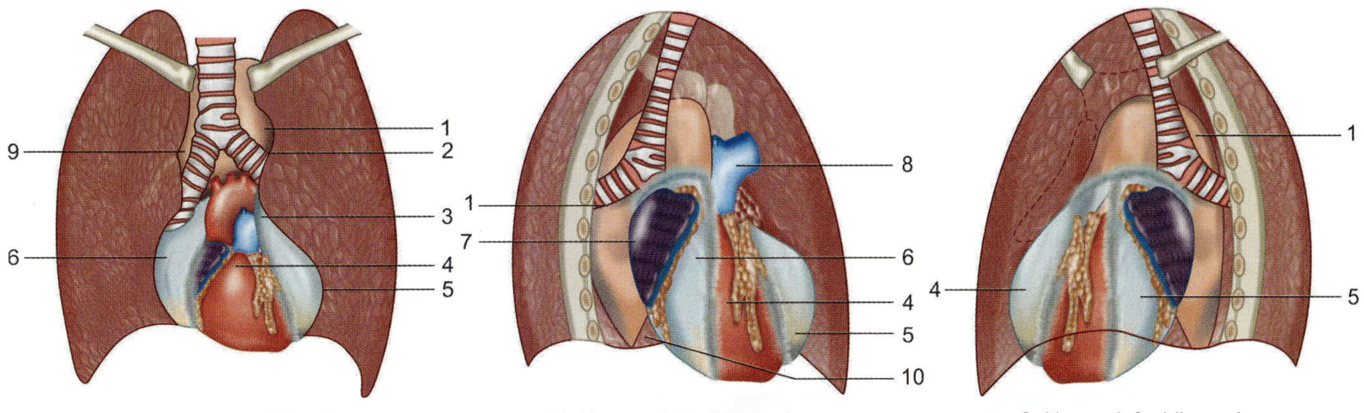

A: X-ray—PA view of the chest B: X-ray—right oblique view C: X-ray—left oblique view

162. On ECG, ST segment elevation is seen in all of the following conditions EXCEPT:
a. Left ventricular aneurysm
b. Acute pericarditis
c. Myocardial infarction
d. Hypocalcemia

The ECG signs of hypocalcemia include prolongation of the QT interval, flat or inverted T waves in severe hypocalcemia, slight decrease in QRS duration and ST segment lengthening.

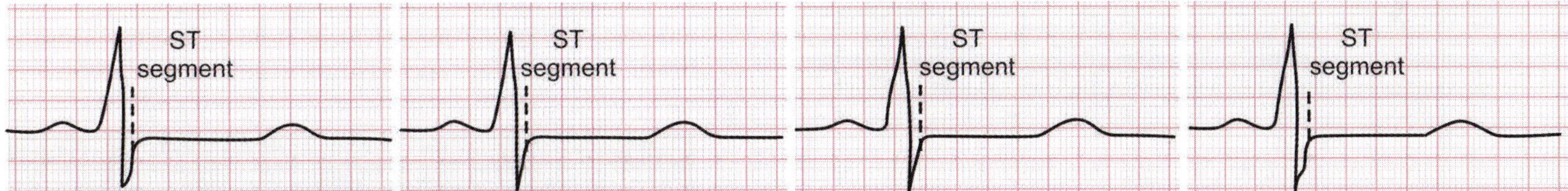

Hypocalcemia—ECG. Note: (1) prolongation of the QT interval, (2) flat or inverted T waves in severe hypocalcemia, (3) slight decrease in QRS duration, (4) ST segment lengthening

EXCRETORY SYSTEM

163. Acute renal failure lead to:
a. Hypokalemic acidosis b. Hyperkalemic alkalosis
c. Hypokalemic alkalosis d. Hyperkalemic acidosis

In all cases of acute kidney injury (AKI), creatinine and urea build up in the blood over several days, and fluid and electrolyte disorders develop. The most serious of these disorders are hyperkalemia and fluid overload (possibly causing pulmonary edema). Phosphate retention leads to hyperphosphatemia. Hypocalcemia is thought to occur because the impaired kidney no longer produces calcitriol and because hyperphosphatemia causes Ca phosphate precipitation in the tissues. Acidosis develops because hydrogen ions cannot be excreted.

164. All are features of nephrotic syndrome EXCEPT:
a. Lipiduria b. Hyperlipidemia
c. Thromboembolism d. Hypertension

Hypertension is a feature of nephritic syndrome (NOT nephrotic)

165. Which of the following is the most common cause of chronic renal failure in adults:
a. TB b. Multiple myeloma
c. DM d. HTN

Chronic Kidney Disease may result from any cause of renal dysfunction of sufficient magnitude. The most common cause is diabetic nephropathy, followed by hypertensive nephroangiosclerosis and various primary and secondary glomerulopathies.

166. NOT a feature of acute glomerulonephritis:
a. Bence Jones proteins b. Hematuria
c. Edema d. Hypertension

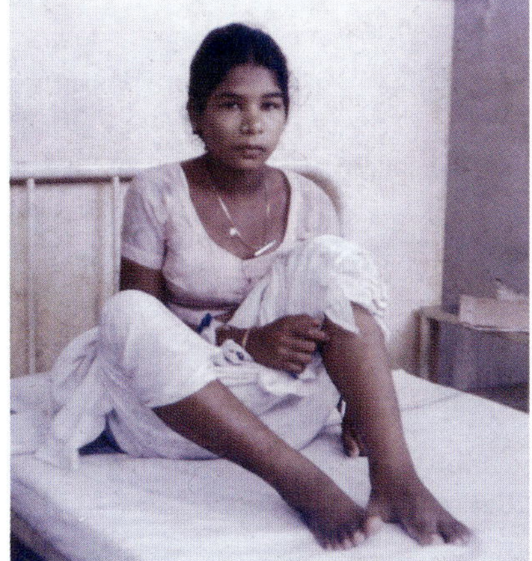
Acute glomerulonephritis: woman 30 years Note: Puffiness of face and moderate edema

Ans. **162. d.** Hypocalcemia **163. d.** Hyperkalemic acidosis **164. d.** Hypertension **165. c.** DM
166. a. Bence Jones proteins

In about 50% patients with multiple myeloma, light chains of immunogloulins called Bence Jones protein is detected in urine. It may also be seen in other condition like macroglobulinemia, lymphoma, leukemia, amyloidosis and other malignancies.

167. Syndrome characterized by proteinuria, hematuria and hypertension:

a. Nephrotic syndrome b. Acute nephritis
c. Renal cell carcinoma d. Nephrocalcinosis

Acute nephritic syndrome is characterized by hematuria, red blood casts, proteinuria, oliguria, hypertension, fluid retention and sometimes, renal failure.

Common Causes
1. Post-streptococcal acute glomerulonephritis
2. Other post-infective acute nephritic syndromes following staphylococcal, pneumococcal, and viral infections.
3. Focal glomerulonephritis and membranoproliferative glomerulonephritis.
4. Collagen disorders, especially systemic lupus erythematosus and polyarteritis nodosa.
5. Miscellaneous group: Henoch-Schönlein syndrome, infective endocarditis, hypersensitivity angiitis, hemolytic uremic syndrome and early stages of Goodpasture's syndrome.

168. Nephrogenic diabetes insipidus is caused by all of the following EXCEPT:

a. Toxicity of lithium
b. Diabetes mellitus
c. Hypocalcemia
d. Hypokalemia

Nephrogenic diabetes inspidus/ NDI

- The renal tubules are refractory to the action of normal levels of circulating ADH
- This may be congenital as in primary NDI or secondary to diseases such as chronic renal failure, diabetes mellitus, hypercalcemia, hypokalemia and sickle cell anemia or due to drugs such as lithium or demeclocycline

Polypeptides	GHRH, GHRIH, TRH, ADH, Oxytocin, GH, IGF-1
Single chain peptide	CRH, ACTH, prolactin
Glycoproteins	LH, FSH, TSH, hCG
Steroids	Cortisol, estrogen and androgens
Amines	Dopamine
Iodinated tyrosine	T3, T4

169. Kimmelstiel-Wilson bodies are characteristic of:

a. Malignant hypertension
b. SLE
c. Diabetic nephropathy
d. Amyloidosis

The MC lesion in diabetic nephropathy is diffuse glomerulosclerosis, but nodular glomerulosclerosis (Kimmelstiel-Wilson nodules) is pathognomonic.

Criteria for diagnosis of prediabetes		
Category	*Fasting plasma glucose*	*2-hr post-prandial*
1. Normal	< 100 mg/dL	< 140 mg/dL
2. Impaired fasting glucose (IFG)	100-125 mg/dL	<140 mg/dL
3. Impaired glucose tolerance (IGT)	<100 mg/dL	140-200 mg/dL

170. Hemodialysis is NOT effective in:

a. Salicylate poisoning
b. Digoxin poisoning
c. Barbiturate poisoning
d. Methanol poisoning

Drugs that can be effectively dialysed inlcudes barbiturates, phenytoin, primidone, paraldehyde, chloral hydrate, amphetamine, alcohol, methanol, ethylene glycol, salicylates, paracetamol, several antibiotics, isoniazid, quinine, quinidine, metallic salts including lithium, bromide, iodide and potassium, ergotamine, carbon tetrachloride, toxic principles of mushroom and others.

Types of elimination procedure ideal for specific toxic agents	
Salicylates	1,2,3
Phenobarbitone	1,2-3
Barbitone	1-2-3
Methanol/ethanol	1-2-3
Lithium	1-2
Isopropanol	1-2
Short and Medium acting barbiturates	3-
Glutethimide	3-
Meprobamate	3-
Methaqualone	3-
Disopyramide	3-
Theophylline	3-
Key: 1. Peritoneal dialysis 2. Hemodialysis 3. Hemoperfusion	

171. MC cause of nephrotic syndrome in adults:

a. Goodpasture syndrome
b. Membranous GN
c. Minimal change disease
d. RPGN

Membranous nephropathy (MN) is the most common cause of adult-onset NS accounting for about 50% of the cases. In children the frequency is 5-7%. The peak incidence is in 4th to 5th decades of life. Male to female ratio is 2:1>

Ans. **167. b.** Acute nephritis **168. c.** Hypocalcemia **169. c.** Diabetic nephropathy **170. b.** Digoxin poisoning **171. b.** Membranous GN

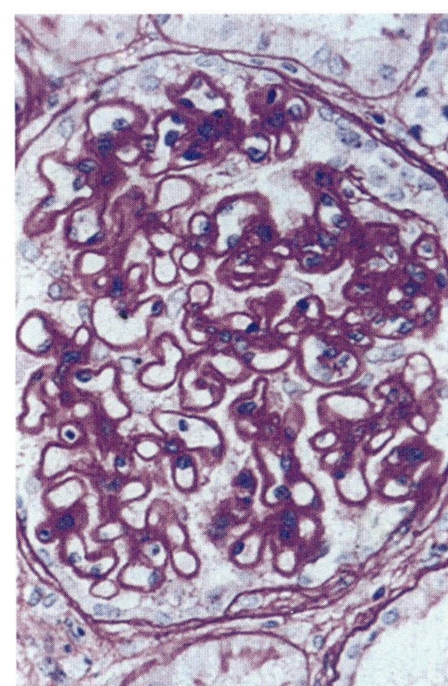

Membranous nephropathy. Note thickened capillary wall due to immune deposits on the subepithelial side of the BM. Over growth of BM between the deposits as spikes

172. In Fanconi syndrome, failure of tubular resorption leads to excessive excretion of all EXCEPT:

a. Uric acid b. Amino acid
c. Chloride d. Glucose

Fanconi syndrome is a rare disorder of kidney tubule function that results in excess amounts of glucose, bicarbonate, phosphates (phosphorous salts), uric acid. Potassium, and certain amino acids being excreted in the urine. Fanconi syndrome is unrelated to – and should not be confused with – Fanconi anemia (a type of aplastic anemia).

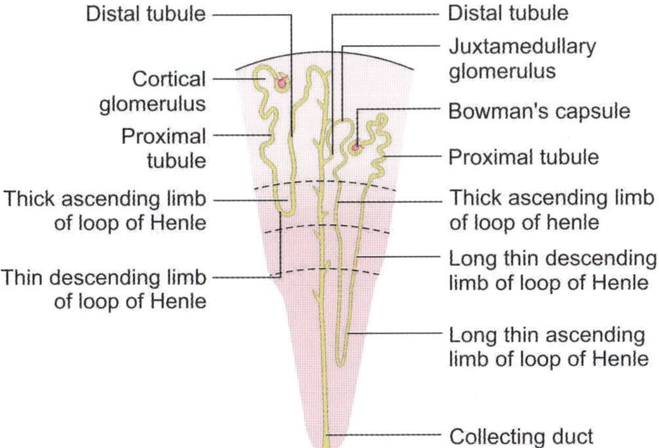

Arrangement of cortical and juxtamedullary nephrons

173. HIV nephropathy is:

a. Fibrillary glomerulopathy
b. Collapsing glomerulopathy
c. Immunotactoid glomerulopathy
d. Membranous glomerulonephritis

HIV associated nephropathy is one of the subtypes of FSGS, which accounts for 30% of nephrotic syndrome in adults and 50% of all steroid resistant cases. Depending on histological variations, FSGS is subclassified as (a) classic (b) collapsing (c) cellular (d) tip lesion and (e) perihilar FSGS.

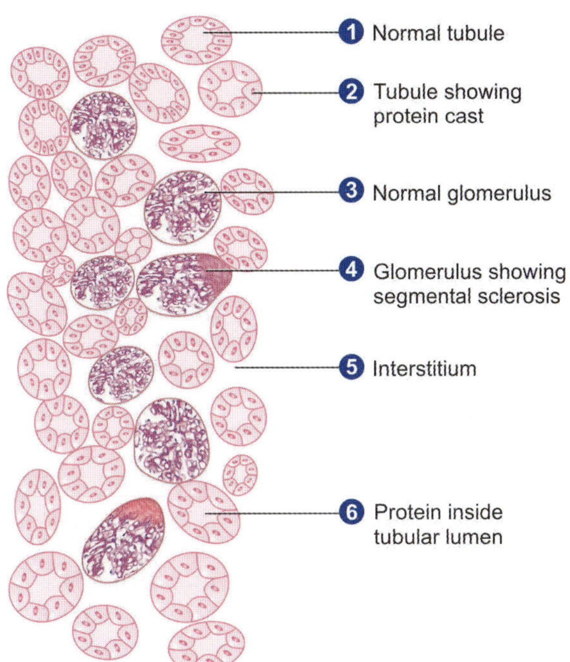

Diagram showing focal and segmental glomerular involvement
Note: 3 out of 7 glomeruli are affected. They show sclerosis involving < 50% of the glomerular capillary tuff

174. Cause of restless leg syndrome:

a. Hypophosphatemia
b. Hypercalcemia
c. Chronic renal failure
d. All of the above

RLS is a disorder that causes a strong urge to move one's legs. Risk factors for RLS include low iron levels, kidney failure, Parkinson disease, diabetes, rheumatoid arthritis, and pregnancy.

175. NOT a cause of skeletal abnormality in renal osteodystrophy:

a. Loss of vitamin D and calcium through dialysis
b. Hypophosphatemia
c. Hypocalcemia
d. Impaired synthesis of vitamin D_3

As renal failure progresses, hyperphosphatemia, hypokalemia and secondary hyperparathyroidism develop leading to skeletal abnormalities. Renal tubular defects and altered vitamin D metabolism also contributes to skeletal changes of renal osteodystrophy.

Ans. 172. b. Amino acid 173. b. Collapsing glome... 174. c. Chronic renal failure 175. b. Hypophosphatemia

Factor affecting the onset, progress and course of CKD	
Increased susceptibility to kidney damage ❑ Older age ❑ Family h/o CKD ❑ Reduced kidney mass ❑ Low birth weight ❑ Racial factors	**Directly initiate kidney damage** ❑ Diabetes mellitus ❑ Hypertension ❑ Autoimmune diseases ❑ Systemic infections ❑ Urinary tract infections ❑ Urinary stones ❑ Lower urinary tract obstruction ❑ Drug toxicity
Progression factors ❑ These cause worsening of kidney damage and faster decline in kidney function after initiation of kidney damage	**End stage factors** increase morbidity and mortality in kidney failure ❑ Late referral ❑ Lower dialysis dose
❑ Higher level of proteinuria ❑ Uncontrolled hypertension ❑ Poor glycemic control in diabetics ❑ Smoking ❑ Non-compliance with treatment	❑ Temporary vascular access ❑ Anemia ❑ Low serum albumin level

176. Sign and symptoms of CRF are seen when the renal function deteriorates by:

a. More than 40%
b. More than 50%
c. More than 60%
d. More than 70%

Chronic kidney disease is defined as either kidney damage or GFR <60 mL/min/1.73 m^2 for ≥3 months. The normal GFR of a young adult is around 120-130 mL/min/ 1.73 m^2.

Stages of Chronic Kidney Disease

Stage	*Description*	*GFR (mL/min/1.73 m^2)*
1.	Kidney damage with normal or increased GFR	≥ 90
2.	Kidney damage with mild decrease in GFR	60-89
3.	Moderate decrease in GFR	30-59
4.	Severe decrease in GFR	15-29
5.	Kidney failure	< 15 or dialysis

177. A patient has serum creatinine of 150-300 micromol/L. Which of the following require dosage reduction:

a. Cephalosporins
b. Enalapril
c. Gentamycin
d. Penicillin

Generally, it is better to be cautious in using ACEI (ACE inhibitors) in those with serum creatinine of >3.5 mg%. If ACEI are used, periodic monitoring of renal functions and serum potassium are needed. Withdrawal of the drug may be necessary if serum creatinine or potassium increases steadily.

Drug dose adjustment in renal failure

Drug	*Normal dose*	*In mild renal failure (SCr.2-4 mg%)*	*Moderate renal failure (4-8 mg%)*	*Severe renal failure (>8 mg%)*
Gentamicin	1.5 mg/kg q8h	1.5 mg/kg q12h	1 mg/kg q12h	1 mg/kg q24h
Amikacin	7.5 mg/kg q12h	7.5 mg/kg q24h	5 mg/kg q24h	5 mg/kg q24.4h
Cefazolin	1 g q6h	1 g q12h	1 g q24h	500 mg q24h
Cefotaxime	1-2 g q6h	1 g q8h	1 g q12h	500 mg-1 g q24h
Ceftazidime	1-2 g q6h	1 g q12h	1 g q24h	500 mg-1 g q24h
Crystalline penicillin	10-20 L q6h	10-20 L q6h	10-20 L q6h	10-20 L q8 h
Ampicillin	500 mg q6h	500 mg q6h	500 mg q6h	500 mg q12h
Ciprofloxacin	200 mg q12h	200 mg q12h	200 mg q12h	200 mg q24h
Vancomycin	500 mg q6h	500 mg once in	500 mg once in	500 mg once in 7 days
		3 days	5 days	
INH	300 mg OD	300 mg OD	200 mg OD	200 mg OD
Ethambutol	10 mg/kg OD	10 mg/kg OD	5 mg/kg OD	5 mg/kg OD
Rifampicin	450-600 mg OD	450-600 mg OD	450 mg OD	450 mg OD
Methyldopa	250-600 mg O8h	250-500 mg O8h	250-500 mg O12h	250-500 mg OD 12 h
Enalapril	2.5-10 mg OD	2.5-10 mg OD	2.5-10 mg OD	2.5-10 mg OD
Digoxin	0.25 mg OD	0.125 mg in 36 h	0.125 mg in 48 h	0.125 mg in 48 h

Ans. **176. b.** More than 50% **177. c.** Gentamycin

178. Which is NOT true for renal cell carcinoma:

a. Progesterone increases tumor size
b. Spreads through blood
c. Clear cell carcinoma is the common histological type
d. Commoner in males

RCC is associated with mutations in the short-arm of chromosome 3, with the implicated genes being either tumor suppressor genes (VHL and TSC) or oncogenes (like c-Met). It is not related to progesterone.

179. Renal vein thrombosis is associated with all of the following EXCEPT:

a. Trauma
b. Sickle cell anemia
c. Nephrotic syndrome
d. Dehydration

Vaso-occlusion by sickle cells is a two step process that begins with adhesion of red cells to endothelium, probably in the post-capillary venules. This is followed by a propagation phase caused by accumulation of poorly deformable red cells behind the site of adhesion.

180. Oliguric phase of renal failure, all are true EXCEPT:

a. Hypercalcemia
b. Hyponatremia
c. Anemia
d. Hyperkalemia

Early in the course of renal failure, loss of nephrons result in reduction of phosphate excretion and lead to hyperphosphatemia. This causes a fall in serum calcium due to its binding to the excess phosphorous.

Age (sex)	Mean GFR + SD (mL/min/1.73 m_2)
1 week (males and females)	40.6 ± 14.8
2-8 weeks (males and females)	65.8 ± 24.8
>8 weeks (males and females)	95.7 ± 21.7
2-12 years (males and females)	133.0 ± 27.0
13-21 years (males)	140.0 ± 30.0
13-21 years (females)	126.0 ± 22.0

181. Post-infective glomerulonephritis present as:

a. ARF
b. Nephrotic syndrome
c. Nephritic syndrome
d. Asymptomatic hematuria

PSGN starts about 2-3 weeks after streptococcal infection of the skin, throat or respiratory tract. In India, the most common precipitating cause was infected scabies or other skin infections.

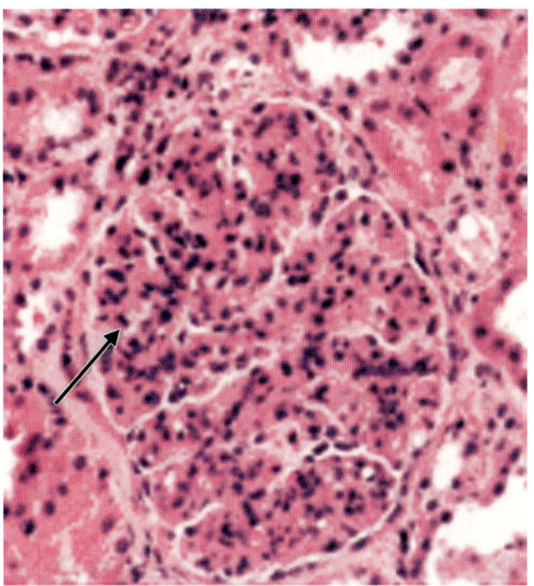

Renal biopsy poststreptococcal glomerulonephritis: Note enlargement of the glomeruli, increase in cellularity and occlusion of capillary lumen, polymorphonuclear infiltrates

182. First manifestation of Alport syndrome is:

a. Microscopic hematuria b. Proteinuria
c. Oliguria d. Sensorineural deafness

Alport syndrome is a genetic disorder characterized by glomerulonephritis, end stage kidney disease, and hearing loss. Blood in urine (hematuria) is an usual feature of Alport syndrome from early infancy, identifiable on urine dipsticks. In young children, episodes of visible (macroscopic) hematuria may occur.

183. In a child, non-functioning kidney is best diagnosed by:

a. USG b. IVU
c. DTPA renogram d. Creatinine clearance

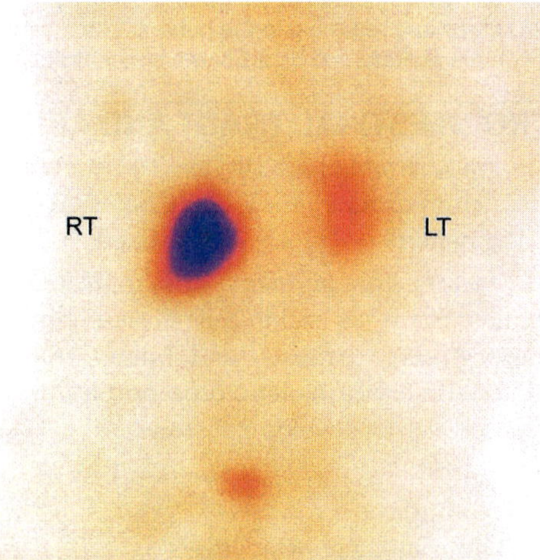

DTPA renogram showing retention of radiopharmaceutical in the renal pelvis of right kidney (From a case of congenital pelviureteric obstruction

Ans. **178. a.** Progesterone... **179. b.** Sickle cell anemia **180. a.** Hypercalcemia **181. c.** Nephritic syndrome
182. a. Microscopic... **183. c.** DTPA renogram

Isotope renography helps to assess renal perfusion and excretory function. It is particularly useful to diagnose renovascular hypertension, assess individual kidney function, renal scarring and to confirm pelvi-ureteric junction obstruction. The radiopharmaceutical agents include technetium labeled DTPA (diethylene triamine pentacetic acid).

184. Most common cause of death in patient on chronic hemodialysis:

a. Uremia b. Infection
c. Cardiovascular disease d. Malnutrition

Hypotension, pyrogen infections, first use syndrome and dialysis disequilibrium are the common acute complications of maintenance hemodialysis. Patients with cardiovascular disease may develop hemodynamic instability, angina, acute coronary events, arrhythmias and sudden death.

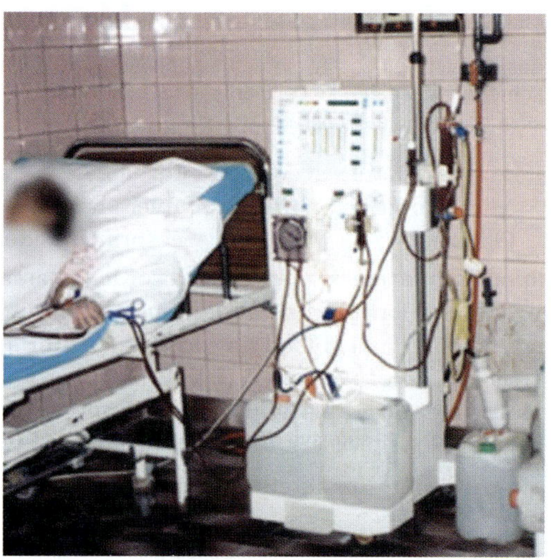

Hemodialysis machine

Note: Blood tubings connected to the patient circulating blood through the artificial kidney and returning to the patient. The 2 cans in the base of the unit contain acetate and bicarbonate concentrate

GASTROINTESTINAL TRACT AND ABDOMEN

185. Gallstones associated with hemolytic anemia:

a. Calcium oxalate b. Cholesterol
c. Pigmented d. Mixed

Risk factors for pigment stones include hemolytic anemias (such as sickle-cell disease and hereditary spherocytosis), cirrhosis, and biliary tract infections. People with erythropoietic protoporphyria (EPP) are at increased risk to develop gallstones.

186. Which of the following is the best test for diagnosing Carcinoid tumour:

a. 24 hour metanephrine levels
b. 24 hour Vanilylmandelic acid levels
c. 24 hour catecholamine
d. 24 hour urinary 5-HIAA

Since 5-HIAA is a metabolite of serotonin, testing is most frequently performed for the diagnosis of carcinoid tumors of the enterochromaffin (Kultschitzsky) cells of the small intestine, which release large amounts of serotonin. Values greater than 25 mg per 24 hours (higher if the patient has malabsorption) are strong evidence for carcinoid. The normal range is 2 to 6 mg per 24 hours.

187. All of the following are true for Plummer Vinson syndrome EXCEPT:

a. Premalignant b. Anemia
c. Lower esophageal web d. In females

Plummer–Vinson syndrome (**PVS**), also called **Paterson–Brown-kelly syndrome** or **sideropenic dysphagia**, is a rare disease characterized by difficulty in swallowing, iron deficiency anemia, and esophageal webs (postcricoid/ upper esophageal).

188. Crohn's disease is characterized by all EXCEPT:

a. Skip lesions b. Fistula
c. Toxic megacolon
d. Transmural involvement

Toxic megacolon is usually a complication of inflammatory bowel disease, such as ulcerative colitis (rarely with Crohn's disease) and of some infections of the colon, including Clostridium difficile infections, which have led to pseudomembranous colitis. Other forms of megacolon exist and can be congenital (present since birth, such as Hirschsprung's disease). Also, it can be caused by Entamoeba histolytica and Shigella.

189. Maternal to child transfer of hepatitis B virus is more if mother is:

a. HBsAg positive
b. IgG anti-HBcAg positive
c. HBeAg positive
d. IgM anti-HBcAg positive

Without intervention, a mother who is positive for HBsAg has a 20% risk of passing the infection to her offspring at the time of birth. This risk is as high as 90% if the mother is also positive for HBeAg (HBeAg correlates with active viral replication & high infectivity)

190. MC symptom of primary biliary cirrhosis:

a. Pruritus b. Vomiting
c. Diarrhea d. All of the above

PBC is characterized by chronic cholestasis, pigmentation, xanthomatous eruptions, and histological features of chronic non-suppurative, destructive cholangiohepatitis. Classically, the disease (PBC) affects middle-aged women and starts with fatigue, pruritus and jaundice.

191. Poor prognostic factor in acute pancreatitis:

a. Decreased PaO_2
b. Increased blood sugar
c. Decreased serum amylase
d. Decreased serum calcium

Ans. **184. c.** Cardiovascular... **185. c.** Pigmented **186. d.** 24 hour urinary... **187. c.** Lower esophageal web **188. c.** Toxic megacolon **189. c.** HBeAg **190. a.** Pruritus **191. d.** Decreased serum calcium

In general the mortality in acute pancreatitis is 10-20%. In hemorrhagic pancreatitis with profound shock, the mortality is high. Adverse factors include elderly age, severe shock, respiratory failure, fall of serum calcium below 8 mg/dL, azotemia and high fluid requirements.

192. Terry's nail is found in:

a. Pancreatitis b. Cirrhosis
c. Iron deficiency d. Vitamin C deficiency

Terry nails is a physical finding in which fingernails or toenails appear white with a characteristic 'ground glass' appearance, with no lunula. It frequently occurs in the setting of liver failure, cirrhosis, diabetes mellitus, hyperthyroidism, congestive heart failure or malnutrition.

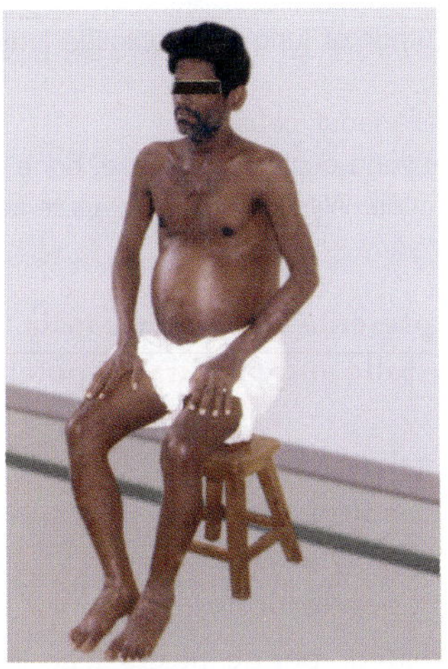

Male 60 years—cirrhosis liver with gross ascites and edema. Note: The pale nails and shiny abdomen

193. MC Cause of peritonitis in a patient with cirrhosis:

a. Corynebacterium b. Streptococcus
c. Staphylococcus aureus d. E. coli

In advanced liver cirrhosis, bacterial translocation of the gut microbes into the ascitic fluid occurs. This condition is known as spontaneous bacterial peritonitis which is seen in about 50% of patients with cirrhosis and ascites. Culture is positive for gram negative enterobacteriacae, usually a single type.

Etiological Factors in Cirrhosis	
1. Infections	Hepatitis B, C, D, *Schistosomiasis mansoni*, congenital syphilis
2. Drugs and toxins	Alcoholism, methotrexate, arsenic, methyldopa, isoniazid, and several others
3. Metabolic causes	Galactosemia, glycogen storage disease type IV, alpha-l-antitrypsin deficiency, hemochromatosis, Wilson's disease, urea cycle enzyme defects, tyrosinosis
4. Primary immunological disorders	Autoimmune hepatitis (lupoid) and primary biliary cirrhosis
5. Vascular causes	Hepatic venous obstruction, chronic congestive cardiac failure, constrictive pericarditis, veno-occlusive disease
6. Miscellaneous	Indian childhood cirrhosis
7. Biliary obstruction steatohepatitis	Gallstones, biliary atresia, biliary strictures, mucoviscidosis and non-alcoholic
8. Cryptogenic	No cause is detectable even after full investigations. The majority of cases are cryptogenic.

Contd...

Contd...

194. Gluten sensitive enteropathy is strongly associated with:

a. Blood group B b. HLA-DQ3
c. HLA-DR4 d. HLA-DQ2

HLA associations of celiac disease/gluten induced enteropathy include HLA-DQ$_2$ (DOA 1-*05/DOB$_1$/*0$_2$) or HLA D0$_8$ (DOA1*0301/DQBI*0302).

195. Raised sweat electrolytes is a feature of:

a. Malaria b. Whipple disease
c. Tropical sprue d. Cystic fibrosis

Diagnosis of cystic fibrosis of the pancreas/fibrocystic disease of the pancreas/ mucoviscoidosis is established by determining sweat electrolytes. Sweat is collected by stimulating diaphoresis with pilocarpine inotophoresis. Normal sweat chloride level is <40 mmol/L.

Criteria for diagnosis of cystic fibrosis
Major criteria 1. Sweat chloride exceeding 60 mmol/L in children and 80 mmol/L in adults. 2. Evidence of pulmonary involvement. 3. Obstructive azoospermia.
Minor criteria 1. Sweat chloride 40 mmol/L in children and 60 mmol/L in adults. 2. Family history of cystic fibrosis or azoospermia. Definite diagnosis is made if two major criteria, or a combination of one major and one minor criterion from two different organ systems are present.

196. Positive D-xylose test indicates all of the following EXCEPT:

a. Pancreatic insufficiency
b. Small intestinal mucosal disease
c. Impaired carbohydrate absorption in small intestine
d. Malabsorption

In xylose absorption test, 5 g of xylose is given orally and the urinary excretion over the next 5 h and the serum levels are determined. Normal persons excrete at least 1 g in urine in 5 hours and the blood levels reach 25 mg/dL 2 h after the oral dose. In malabsorption due to mucosal disease affecting the upper small intestine, urinary elimination is lowered.

Ans. 192. **b.** Cirrhosis 193. **d.** E. coli 194. **d.** HLA-DQ2 195. **d.** Cystic fibrosis
196. **a.** Pancreatic insufficiency

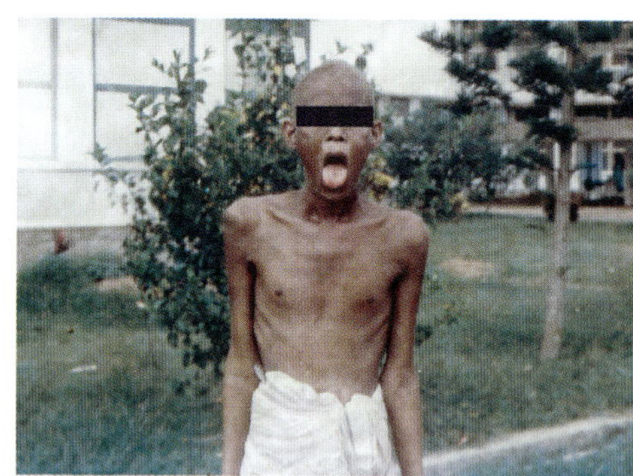

Malabsorption state—male 40—intestinal resection. Note: loss of weight and glossitis

197. Palmar erythema may be a manifestation of:

a. Liver failure
b. Adrenal failure
c. Heart failure
d. Renal failure

Finger clubbing, palmar erythema and spider naevi are common in chronic hepatic failure. Erythematous patches may occur over several parts of the body, especially the chest wall and supraclavicular regions.

Causes of Acute Hepatic Failure
1. *Viral hepatitis*—B, D, E and A and other viruses can cause AHF. Over 70% of cases of AHF are caused by viral infections. Overall incidence of AHF in viral hepatitis is around 1%. Frequency of AHF in different types of viral hepatitis is given below: HAV 0.35%. AHF is more common in the elderly and drug users. Prognosis is relatively better with survival over 60%. HBV 1%. HCV By itself, it is rare to produce AHF. In combination with HBV, it predisposes to AHF. HDV In combination with HBV it increases the frequency and severity of AHF. HEV This is likely to cause AHF, especially in pregnant women Other viruses such as CMV, EBV and herpes viruses 1, 2 and 6 cause AHF especially in immunocompromised subjects.
2. *Drugs*—halothane, monoamine oxidase-inhibitors such as iproniazid and phenelzin, isoniazid.
3. *Poisoning*—paracetamol, mushrooms, weedicides, copper sulfate, alcohol, organic solvents.
4. Shock—surgical shock or gram-negative toxic shock.
5. Occlusion of major hepatic veins (Budd-Chiari syndrome)
6. Acute fulminant biliary tract infection with obstruction.
7. *Other Causes* a. Disseminated malignant deposits obstructing sinusoidal blood flow, e.g., Cancer of stomach and breast, oat cell tumor of lung, myeloblastic leukemia, and carcinoids. b. Miscellaneous causes: Acute veno-occlusive disease, bone marrow transplantation, Wilson's disease, acute fatty liver of pregnancy.

198. A patient presents with tachycardia, BP of less than 100 mm systolic and postural hypotension. Diagnosis is:

a. Vasovagal attack
b. Diabetic neuropathy
c. Shy Drager syndrome
d. Bleeding peptic ulcer

If left untreated, peptic ulcers lead to complications. Acute complications include severe ulceration with intractable hematemesis. Hemorrhage leads to hypovolemic shock which depends on the extent and rate of hemorrhage and presence of other diseases. Loss of 20% of the blood volume results in postural hypotension and tachycardia. Shock supervenes if the bleeding continue or recurs.

Drugs used for peptic ulcer

Drugs	*Action*	*Dose for oral administration*	*Major side effects*
Antacids			
Aluminium hydroxide Magnesium hydroxide Magnesium trisilicate Magnesium carbonate	Neutralizes gastric acid	15-30 mL of suspension one and three hours after each meal and at bed time, for 6 weeks	Diarrhea or constipation, inhibition of absorption of iron, calcium and phosphates, and milk-alkali syndrome
Mucosal protecting agents			
Sodium alginate	Coats the mucosa	0.5-1 g after food and at bed time	Nil
Carbenoxolone sodium		100 mg tid for 4-8 weeks	Retention of sodium and loss of potassium
Sucralfate (aluminium salt of sucrose-octa sulfate).	Coats the mucosa	1 g four times a day	Nil
Antihelicobacter agents			

Contd...

Ans. **197. a.** Liver failure **198. d.** Bleeding peptic ulcer

Contd...

Drugs	*Action*	*Dose for oral administration*	*Major side effects*
Colloidal bismuth: tripotassium dicitrato-bismuthate (De-nol) Omeprazole, amoxycillin, clarithromycin preventing relapse	Eliminates *H. pylori,* thereby hastening ulcer-healing and	20 mL three or four times a day for 30 days	Unpleasant taste, staining of mouth and teeth
H2-receptor blocking agent	Suppression of acid secretion and favour ulcer-healing		Drowsiness, allergy, gynecomastia, impotence and inhibition of gastric intrinsic factor
Cimetidine		200 mg 6 h and 400 mg bed time	Reduction of gastric acidity may predispose to
Ranitidine		150 mg bid or 300 mg bed time	Salmonella infection
Famotidine		20 mg bid or 40 mg bed time	
Proton-pump inhibitor Omeprazole lansoprazole, pantoprazole, esmoprazole and rabiprazole	Inhibits H^+K^+ ATPase, and suppresses acid secretion,	10-20 mg twice a day and 20 mg bed time favours ulcer-healing	Very few, Diarrhea, skin rashes headache, impotence and gynecomastia 30 mg od
Prostaglandins Misoprostol	Cytoprotection and reduces acid production	200 mg four times a day	Diarrhea
Note: Antacids and acid inhibiting drugs are continued for 4-8 weeks in full doses and then maintenance treatment is given depending on the individual response.			

199. All are true regarding typhoid ulcer EXCEPT:

a. Ileum is the common site
b. Bleeding is common
c. Stricture is usual and causes obstruction
d. Perforation is common

The Peyer's patches in the terminal ileum becomes swollen and surface undergoes necrosis with formation of ulcers. Blood vessels here may be eroded leading to intestinal hemorrhage. Ulceration may extend to the muscularis mucosa and serosa and may result in intestinal perforation.

Gastrointestinal system: Performation of ileum with peritonitis, intestinal hemorrhage, paralytic ileus, cholecystitis
Respiratory: Pneumonia
Neuropsychiatric: Typhoid encephalopathy, typhoid meningitis, transverse myelitis, peripheral neuropathy
Hematological: Disseminated intravascular coagulation (DIC), thrombocytopenia
Genitourinary: Glomerulonephritis, pyelonephritis, urinary retention
Cardiovascular: Myocarditis, endocarditis, deep vein thrombosis, thrombophlebitis
Miscellaneous: Focal sepsis, abscess in liver, spleen, breast, typhoid osteomyelitis, parotitis, arthritis, bone abscess (Brodie's abscess)
Relapse

200. A patient gives chronic history of diarrhea and blood in stool, presents with multiple fistulae in the perineum and multiple strictures in small intestine. Most likely diagnosis is:

a. Crohn's disease
b. Radiation enteritis
c. Ulcerative colitis
d. Ischemic bowel disease

Crohn's disease affects persons aged 15-35 years or more, and it is characterized by remissions and relapses. Presenting symptoms include fatigue, weight loss, right lower quadrant pain, and diarrhea. The pain is continuous and localized but may be colicky. Moderate diarrhea follows. The feces is not visibly mixed with blood. Fistulous tracts, strictures, and fibrosis may be demonstrable in advanced cases.

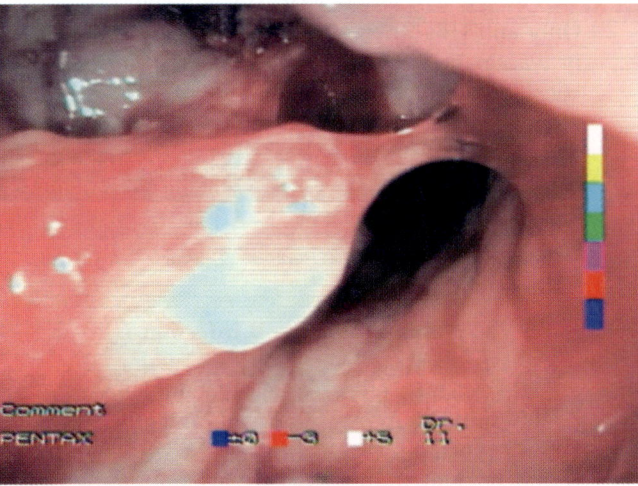

Crohn's disease—Fistulous track endoscopic view

201. Micronodular cirrhosis is seen in all EXCEPT:

a. Chronic hepatitis B
b. Alcoholic liver disease
c. Hemochromatosis
d. Chronic extrahepatic biliary obstruction

Ans. **199. c.** Stricture is usual...**200. a.** Crohn's disease **201. a.** Chronic hepatitis B

In micronodular cirrhosis, the nodules are less than 3 mm in diameter, uniform, and these are seen involving the whole liver. The fibrous bands are indistinct and fine. In macronodular cirrhosis the nodules are coarse, irregular, and may grow up to several centimeters. The liver surface is grossly disturbed. Chronic hepatitis B leads to macronodular cirrhosis.

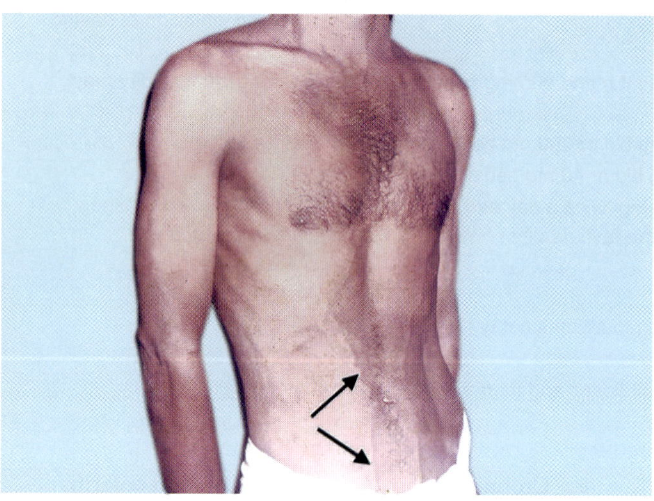

Cirrhosis liver abdomen showing caput medusae
Note: The prominent veins on the abdominal wall, arrows point to the direction a blood flow

202. A nurse having vaccinated with hepatitis B (no previous HBV infection). Which of the following will be seen in blood examination:

a. HBsAg
b. Anti HBs
c. Anti HBcAg
d. Anti HBsAg, anti HBcAg, core antigen

Only anti-HBs in blood indicate immunity as a result of vaccination. Values more than 10 microIU/L is considered protective.

	1st dose	2nd dose after one month	3rd dose after six months
Adults	1 mL	1 mL	1 mL
Infants and newborns	0.5 mL	0.5 mL	0.5 mL
Booster at 5 years			

203. Acute infection of hepatitis B infection is diagnosed by:

a. IgM anti HBsAg
b. IgM anti HBcAg
c. IgG anti HBsAg
d. IgG anti HBcAg

HBcAg (Hepatitis-B core antigen) is not detectable in serum, but with the onset of clinical illness anti-HBc IgM (IgM antibody to core antigen) appears and remains elevated throughout the course of the disease. Detection of anti-HBc IgM is diagnostic of HBV hepatitis. Initial antibody is IgM type later it is replaced by IgG type. Persistence of anti-HBc IgG in high titer indicates continuing infection.

Clinical feature	Replicating stage	Integrated stage
Infectivity	High	Low
HBsAg	Positive	Positive
HBeAg	Positive	Negative
Anti-HBe	Negative	Positive
HBV DNA	Positive	Negative

204. If only anti HBs is positive in serum and all others viral markers are negative, this indicates:

a. Acute hepatitis
b. Chronic active hepatitis
c. Persistent carrier
d. Immunized person with hepatitis B vaccine

Anti-HBs antibody (anti-HBs Ab) can be estimated to detect protective immunity. These are detectable in patients who recover from the disease and in those who are successfully vaccinated.

The four stages of hepatitis B infections				
	Replicative phase		*Integrative phase*	
Disease marker	Stage 1	Stage 2	Stage 1	Stage 2
HBsAg	Positive	Positive	Positive	Negative
Antibody to HBsAg	Negative	Negative	Negative	Positive
HBV DNA	Strongly positive	Positive	Negative	Negative
Antibody HBcAg	Positive	Positive	Positive	Positive
HBeAg	Positive	Positive	Negative	Negative
Antibody to HBeAg	Negative	Negative	Positive	Positive
Asparate and alanine aminotrans-ferase levels	Normal	Elevated	Normal	Normal

205. A person was screened for blood transfusion. Which of the following is safer for blood transfusion:

a. Anti HBs positive
b. Anti HBcAg positive (IgM)
c. HBsAg positive
d. HBeAg positive

Anti-HBs shows patient is immune to HBV and either the infection has resolved (and the patient is no more infective) or successful vaccination.

206. A 20-year-old male with massive hematemesis had history of fever for the past 14 days and H/O ingestion of some drug. He also has moderate splenomegaly. Most likely diagnosis is:

a. NSAID induced duodenal ulcer
b. Drug induced gastritis
c. Esophageal varices
d. None of the above

Ans. **202. b.** Anti HBs **203. b.** IgM anti HBcAg **204. d.** Immunized person... **205. a.** Anti HBs positive **206. c.** Esophageal varices

Signs of portal hypertension include asymptomatic splenomegaly, gradual development of portal systemic collateral veins and bouts of hematemesis or melena.

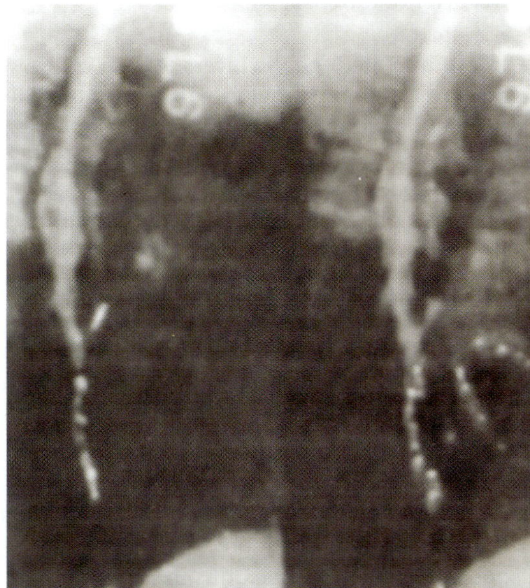

Portal hypertension—barium swallow X-ray showing esophageal varices. Note the longitudinal filling defects caused by the dilated veins

207. Which of the following has the best sensitivity and specificity for the diagnosis of celiac disease:

a. Anti-endomysial antibody/ EMA
b. Anti-tissue transglutaminase antibody/ tTG
c. Anti-gliadin antibody/ AGA
d. Anti-reticulin antibody

AGA has lower sensitivity. EMA are directed against the connective tissue surrounding the smooth muscles. It is sensitive and specific, but expensive. The epitope against which EMA is directed is identified as tTG. IgA tTG is more specific and sensitive. It is also cheaper. In low-prevalence areas a negative tTG test virtually rules out celiac disease.

208. In gastric outlet obstruction in a peptic ulcer patient, the site of obstruction is most likely to be:

a. Antrum
b. Duodenum
c. Pylorus
d. Fundus

Major chronic complication of peptic ulcer is the development of cicatricial stenosis of the pylorus resulting in pyloric obstruction.

209. NOT a premalignant condition of stomach:

a. Gastric ulcer
b. Pernicious anemia and achlorhydria
c. Hiatus hernia
d. Atrophic gastritis

Gastric carcinoma is common in Indians. Men are affected more than women. Atrophic gastritis and gastric polyps predispose to gastric carcinoma. It is more common in persons with blood group A.

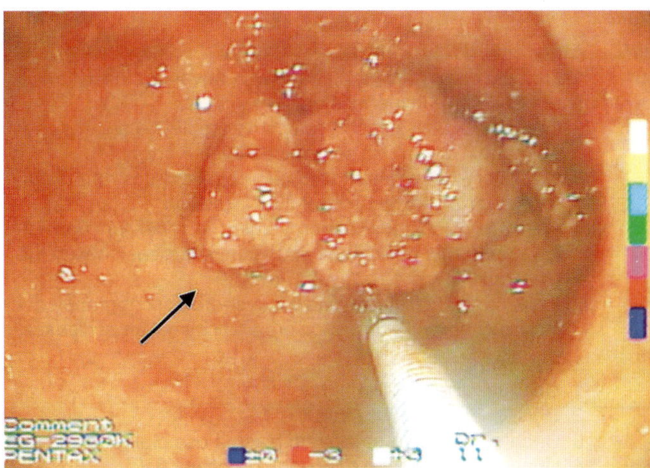

Carcinoma stomach. Note: the cauliflower growth (arrow)

210. Triad originally described for ZES is:

a. Peptic ulceration, gastric hypersecretion, non beta cell tumor
b. Peptic ulceration, gastric hypersecretion, beta cell tumor
c. Peptic ulceration, achlorhydria, non beta cell tumor
d. Peptic ulceration, achlorhydria, beta cell tumor

Zollinger-Ellison syndrome consists of recurrent ulceration of the stomach, duodenum and jejunum and marked increase in gastric acid secretion caused by a gastrin secreting tumor, commonly arising from the non-beta cells of the islets of Langerhans.

211. A patient was operated for colonic Carcinoma and later a solitary nodule was found in the liver. Treatment of choice is:

a. Surgery
b. Radiation
c. Chemotherapy
d. Conservative treatment

Even a few metastases in the liver are not a contraindication for surgery, since the liver metastases can also be removed.

212. Which of the following statements is INCORRECT with regard to hepatorenal syndrome/ HRS in a patient with cirrhosis:

a. The creatinine clearance is more than 40 ml/ min
b. The urinary sodium is less than 10 mmol/ L
c. The urine osmolality is lower than the plasma osmolality
d. There is poor response to volume expansion

Impairment of renal function, defined as a doubling of the initial serum creatinine to a level higher than 2.5 mg/dL, or a 50% reduction of the initial 24-hour creatinine clearance to a level lower than 20mL/min occurs in less than 2 weeks in type I HRS.

Diagnostic criteria

HRS should be suspected in any patient with acute or chronic liver disease and portal hypertension, when there is a rise in serum creatinine to above 1.5 mg/dL. The criteria are divided into major criteria, which must be present in all patients for diagnosis, and minor criteria, which provide support for diagnosis.

Contd...

Ans. 207. **b.** Anti-tissue... 208. **c.** Pylorus 209. **c.** Hiatus hernia 210. **a.** Peptic ulceration, gastric... 211. **a.** Surgery 212. **a.** The creatinine...

Contd...

Major criteria: 1. Chronic or acute liver disease with advanced hepatic failure and portal hypertension. 2. Low glomerular filtration rate, with creatinine clearance < 40 mL/min and blood serum creatinine > 1.5mg/dL 3. No history of treatment with nephrotoxic drugs, shock, infection, or significant recent fluid losses. 4. Absence of sustained improvement in renal function following diuretic withdrawal and volume expansion with 1.5 L isotonic saline. 5. Proteinuria < 500 mg/dL, and absence of ultrasonographic evidence of urinary obstruction or parenchymal renal disease.
Minor criteria: 1. Urine volume < 500 mL/day 2. Urine sodium < 10 mmol/L 3. Urine osmolality greater than plasma osmolality. 4. Urine red blood cells < 50 per high power field. 5. Serum sodium concentration < 130 mmol/L.

213. Which of the following statements about peptic ulcer disease is true:

a. Helicobacter pylori eradication increases the likelihood of occurrence of complications
b. The incidence of complications has remained unchanged
c. The incidence of Helicobacter pylori reinfection in India is very low
d. Helicobacter pylori eradication does NOT alter the recurrence ratio

Peptic ulcer

- If left untreated, peptic ulcers lead to complications. So eradication of H. pylori will reduce the likelihood of complications.
- Duodenal ulcer is more common in the rice-eating population of India
- There is a great tendency to recur after initial healing. It is seen even after surgery. The persistence of H. pylori infection is the most common cause of recurrence. So eradication of H. pylori reduces the recurrence.

214. The commonest hepatotropic virus causing increased chronic carrier state is:

a. HEV b. HAV
c. HBV d. HEV

Chronic hepatitis is defined as continuing inflammation the liver persisteing for more than six months. HBV is responsible for chronic hepatitis in 30-50%.

The important features of the viruses primarily causing hepatitis

	HAV	*HBV*	*HCV*	*HDV delta virus*	*HEV*	*HGV*
Type of virus	RNA	DNA	RNA	RNA	RNA	RNA
Source of infection	Feco-oral rarely parenteral	Parenteral, sexual and mother to baby	Parenteral, rarely sexual, and mother to baby	Parenteral	Feco-oral, rarely parenteral	Parenteral
Incubation period weeks	2-6	8-48	2-22	4-8	2-9	"
Onset of clinical illness	Acute	Insidious	Insidious	Acute	Acute	Clinical
Presence of jaundice	50%	33%	25%		20%	significance not established
Diagnostic markers	IgM HAV	HBsAg	Anti-HCV IgM	Anti-HDV IgM	Anti-HEV	HGV RNA
Establishment of chronic carrier state	Nil	5-10%	Up to 60%	Vast majority	Nil	"
Vertical transmission	—	+	+	+	—	"
Chronic hepatitis	Very rare	5%	30-50%	70%	Rare	"
Fulminant hepatitis	0.1%	Up to 1%	Not known	Up to 17%	Up to 10% in pregnant women	
Vaccination	Available	Available	No	—	No	No

215. All are features of hepatocellular carcinoma EXCEPT:

a. NOT common in Asians
b. Liver biopsy is diagnostic
c. Raised titre of HBV and HCV antibodies
d. Fibrolamellar type is having good prognosis

Primary carcinoma of the liver is a common neoplasm seen in India, South Africa, Malaysia and China. It is less common in Caucasians.

216. Minnesota tube used for control of variceal bleeding in portal hypertension has:

a. One lumen b. Two lumen
c. Three lumen d. Four lumen

Sengstaken Blackmore or Linten Nechlon tube may be useful for temporary tamponade while the patient is being transported to a higher centre. It is not as effective as somatostatin or endoscopic interventions. It

Ans. **213. b.** The incidence... **214. c.** HBV **215. a.** NOT common in... **216. d.** Four lumen is not used unless there are exceptional circumstances. Minnesota tubes are more modern models that have an opening near the upper esophagus. Blackmore tube (3 lumen) replaced by Minnesota tube (4 lumen) as it allows aspiration of both gastric and esophageal contents, not just gastric contents.

217. All of the following are components of Whipple's triad EXCEPT:

a. Symptoms of hypoglycemia
b. Increased insulin levels
c. Symptoms improve after glucose administration
d. Low blood glucose

Whipple triad is the clinical presentation of pancreatic insulinomas and consists of: fasting hypoglycemia (<50 mg/dl), symptoms of hypoglycemia and immediate relief of symptoms after the administration of I/V glucose.

218. Gold standard method of diagnosing celiac disease is:

a. Small bowel biopsy
b. Anti-endomysial antibodies
c. Blood picture
d. Biochemical tests

Diagnosis of celiac disease is made from the history, demonstration of malabsorption and characteristic histology. Histologically the mucosal atrophy, during the active stages of the disease and its clearance during abstinence from gluten containing diet can be demonstrated.

219. Most common cause of acute superior mesenteric arterial obstruction is:

a. Embolism
b. Thrombosis
c. Non occlusive ischemia
d. Atherosclerosis

Acute mesenteric ischemia refers to the sudden onset of small intestinal hypoperfusion, which can be due to acute embolic occlusion of the intestinal blood supply, most commonly the superior mesenteric artery (SMA).

220. Puddle sign is seen in:

a. Hydrothorax
b. Pneumothorax
c. Hydrocele
d. Ascites

When the quantity of fluid in ascites is less than 200 mL, it can be detected only by eliciting dullness to percussion around the umbilicus, the patient being examined in the knee elbow position – "puddle sign".

Causes of ascites	
Transudate Peritoneum is not actively involved	1. *Due to combination of hypoalbuminemia and rise in portal venous pressure, e.g. cirrhosis* 2. Hypoalbuminemia, e.g. protein malnutrition, nephrotic syndrome. 3. Increased flow of lymph from the hepatic surface. In hepatic venous obstruction, superficial hepatic veins distend and lymph transudes into the peritoneum, thus adding to the ascites and rise of portal pressure, e.g. Budd-Chiari syndrome. In this condition protein content of the fluid is high. 4. As part of generalized edema, e.g. congestive heart failure, myxedema.
Exudate Peritoneum is actively involved	1. Inflammations a. Infections-chronic peritonitis, e.g. tuberculosis and acute peritonitis. b. Dyscollagenosis, e.g. systemic lupus, polyarteritis nodosa. c. Acute pancreatitis, splenic infarct. 2. Malignancies a. Secondary carcinomatosis from liver, stomach, breast, colon, etc. b. Primary mesotheliomas of the peritoneum. c. Pseudomyxoma peritonei due to rupture of mucocele of appendix or ovarian cyst.
Miscellaneous	
Peritoneum may or may not be involved	a. Perforation of hollow viscus, e.g. stomach, appendix, small intestine. b. Fibroma of the ovary (Meig's syndrome). c. Lymphatic obstruction-filariasis, secondary carcinoma, lymphoma.

221. Investigation of choice for amoebic liver abscess:

a. Demonstration of parasites in stool
b. Serum Entamoeba antibodies
c. Aspiration of cyst fluid
d. X-ray abdomen

Serological tests are mainly used in extraintestinal amebiasis. Indirect hemagglutination antibody test is positive in 95% of extraintestinal and 70% of intestinal amebiasis.

Ans. **217. b.** Increased... **218. a.** Small bowel biopsy **219. a.** Embolism **220. d.** Ascites
221. b. Serum Entamoeba antibodies

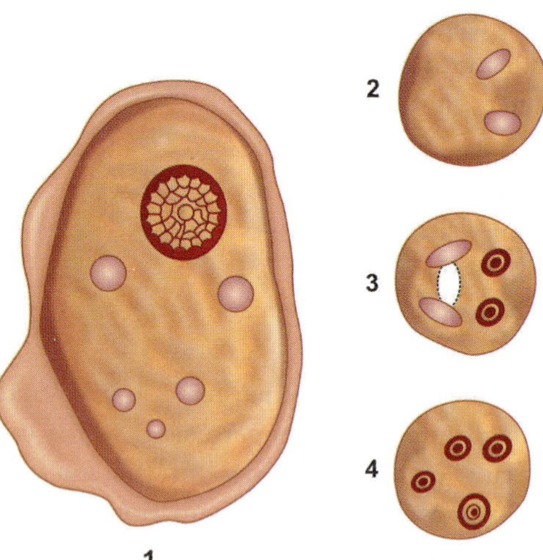

Entameba histolytica in stools (diagram)

INFECTIOUS DISEASE

222. Ebola virus is transmitted by:

a. Feco-oral
b. Inhalation
c. Contact with body fluids
d. Sexual

The Ebola virus spreads by direct contact with body fluids, such as blood, of an infected human or other animals. This may also occur through contact with an item recently contaminated with bodily fluids.

223. Vertical transfer of HIV is assessed by:

a. p24
b. Serum ELISA
c. Western blot
d. Immunoblot

The detection of HIV p24 antigen (by capture assay, an ELISA-t per assay) in serum or CSF is the key to early diagnosis, especially in window period (but it does not help in assessing mother-to-child transfer of HIV)

224. Post-splenectomy infections are common with:

a. Klebsiella
b. E. coli
c. Staph aureus
d. H. influenzae

As splenectomy causes an increased risk of sepsis due to encapsulated organisms (such as S. pneumoniae and Haemophilus influenzae) the patient should receive the pneumococcal conjugate vaccine, Hib vaccine, and the meningococcal vaccine

225. FALSE for leptospirosis:

a. Quinolones are the drug of choice
b. Jaundice and renal dysfunction is seen
c. Hemorrhagic diathesis may be seen
d. Negative dark field examination does not rule out the diagnosis

Leptospira are sensitive to several antibiotics such as penicillin, tetracyclines, erythromycin, quinolones, third generation cephalosporins, doxycyline and others. Penicillin is the drug of choice. Benzyl penicillin G in a dose of 1.5 mega units I/V every 6 hours produces dramatic improvement in 24-72 hours.

Points to remember
1. Leptospirosis has become a very common infection in many parts of India
2. Several serovars cause the disease
3. Brunt of the disease is borne by the liver and kidney,but several other organs may also be affected
4. Early diagnosis and treatment with penicillin or other antibiotics ensure cure in the vast majority.
5. Prompt dialysis therapy saves life in severe renal involvement

226. Drug of choice for Kala-azar is:

a. Dacarbazine
b. Stibogluconate sodium
c. Co-trimoxazole
d. Amphotericin-B

The specific drugs for kala-azar (visceral leishmaniasis) are the time-honoured pentavalent antimonials and aromatic diamidines, still used in areas where the parasite is sensitive. These drugs are effective and relatively cheap giving cure rates up to 95%. Pentavalent antimonial drugs in common use are sodium stibgluconate and methyl-1-glucamine antimoniate. Among the aromatic diamidine, pentamidine isethionate is more freely available and hence more commonly used in India. Other drugs include amphotericin-B, paromomycin and miltefosine which are all highly effective even against resistant organism.

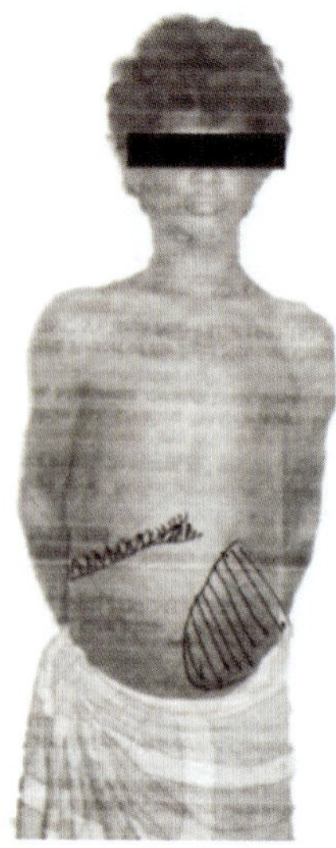
Patients with advance kala-azar—note the gross splenohepatomegaly and emaciation—adult 26 years

Ans. 222. **c.** Contact with... 223. **a.** p24 224. **d.** H. influenzae 225. **a.** Quinolones are the drug... 226. **b.** Stibogluconate...

227. Most common malignancy in AIDS is:

a. Kaposi sarcoma b. Hodgkins lymphoma
c. Leukemia d. Multiple myeloma

Kaposi's sarcoma/ KS was the first malignancy detected to be associated with HIV infection. The worldwide prevalence of KS in patients with AIDS may approach 34%.

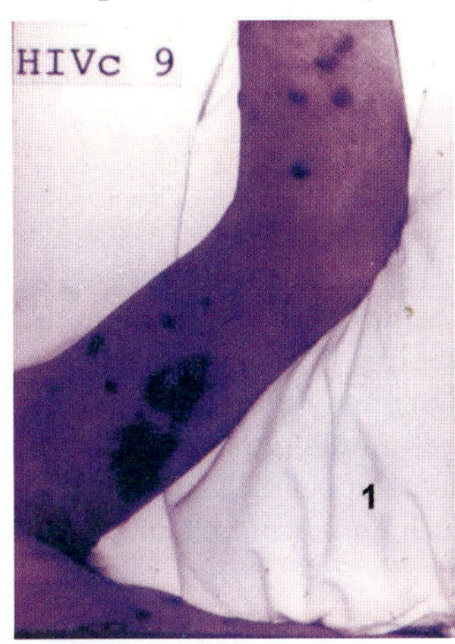

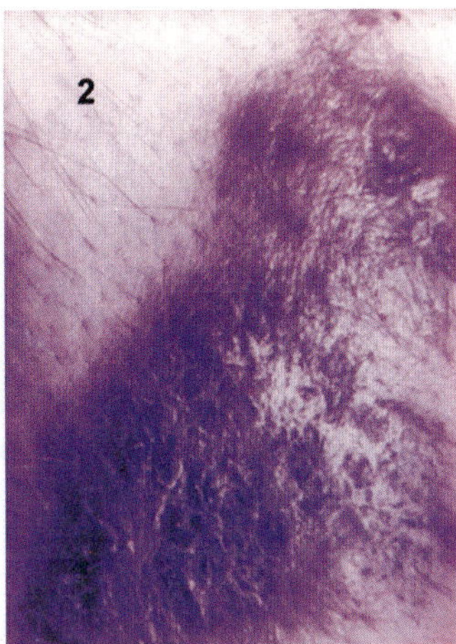

Kaposi's sarcoma. Note (1) General appearance—pigmented lesions (2) Enlarged view × 100

228. Average incubation period of AIDS is:

a. 1 year b. 3 years
c. 5 years d. 10 years

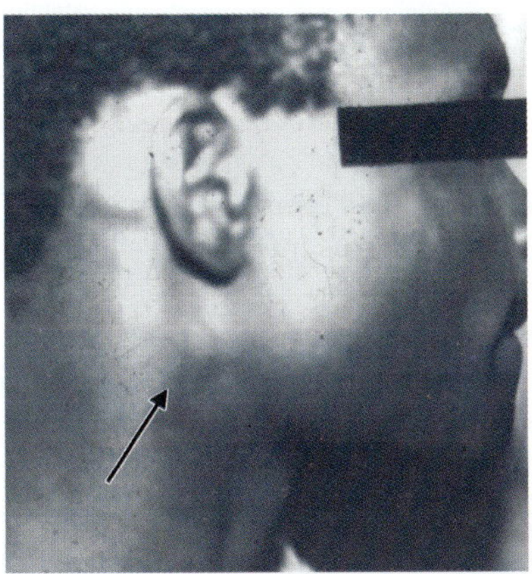

AIDS persistent lymphadenopathy neck

The median incubation period from HIV infection until development of AIDS is estimated at approximately 10 years for young adults.

229. Pathognomic lesion in HIV is:

a. Gingivitis b. Oral candidiasis
c. Herpes simplex d. Aphthous ulcers

Fungal infections occur extensively on the skin and mucous membranes in AIDS. Recurrent and persistent muco-cutaneous candidiasis is common.

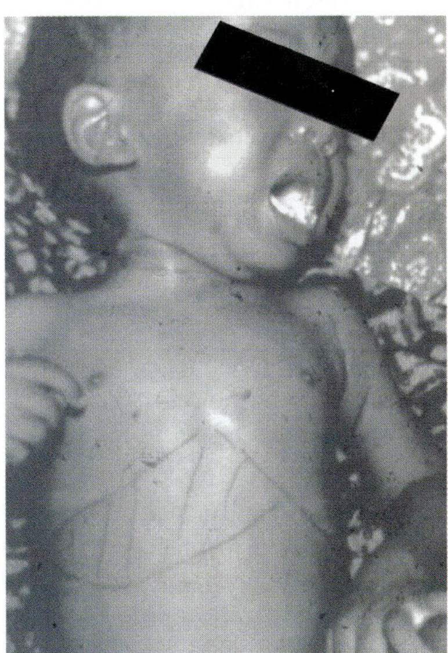

AIDS oral candidiasis

230. In plasmodium vivax malaria, relapse is caused by:

a. Sporozoite
b. Schizont
c. Hypnozoite
d. Gamteocyte

In the case of P. vivax, P. malariae and P. ovale many of the sporozoites can remain dormant in the liver cells for periods extending up to several months or years and get released into the circulation to start their erythrocytic phase. These dormant sporozoites are called hypnozoites. They lead to late relapses in case of P. vivax and P. ovale.

Morphological features of the different species of plasmodium

	P. vivax	*P. falciparum*	*P. malariae*	*P. ovale*
Size of parasitized erythrocyte	Larger	Not larger	Normal size	Variable, the erythrocyte is often oval
Common stages present in peripheral blood	All stages gametocytes	Only rings and	All stages	All stages
Pigmentary change in erythrocyte	Schuffner's dots seen in the erythrocyte outside the parasite	Maurer's clefts	Nil	Schuffner's dots
Number of merozoites in the schizont	8-16	12-24	6-12	8-12

Contd...

Ans. 227. **a.** Kaposi sarcoma 228. **d.** 10 years 229. **b.** Oral candidiasis 230. **c.** Hypnozoite

Contd...

	P. vivax	*P. falciparum*	*P. malariae*	*P. ovale*
Morphology of the rings	Thick and large	Fine rings-marginal forms (applique)*	Large coarse ring	Large ring
Multiple infection in erythrocyte	Nil	Present	Nil	Nil
Number of chromatin in the rings	One	One or two	One	One
Gametocyte	Oval or circular	Crescentic	Oval or circular	Oval or circular
* Applique forms of P. falciparum are the ring stages of the parasite attached along the margin of the erythrocyte.				

231. The most common cause of seizures in a patient of AIDS is:

a. Toxoplasmosis
b. Cryptococcal meningitis
c. Progressive multifocal leucoencephalopathy
d. CNS lymphoma

In AIDS, cerebral toxoplasmosis almost always result from the reactivation of a latent infection with Toxoplasma gondii. Patients may present with seizure, headache or focal neurological deficits.

AIDS Indicator Conditions
❑ Candidiasis, of esophagus, trachea, bronchi or lungs
❑ Cervical cancer, invasive*
❑ Coccidioidomycosis, extrapulmonary*
❑ Cryptococcosis, extrapulmonary
❑ Cryptosporidiosis with diarrhea longer than 1 month
❑ Cytomegalovirus of any organ other than liver, spleen, or lymph nodes
❑ Herpes simplex with mucocutaneous ulcer for more than 1 month duration or bronchitis, pneumonitis, esophagitis
❑ Histoplasmosis, extrapulmonary*
❑ HIV-associated dementia: disabling cognitive and/or motor dysfunction interfering with activities of daily living*
❑ HIV-associated wasting: involuntary weight loss >10% of baseline plus chronic diarrhea (2 loose stools/day 30 days) or chronic weakness and documented enigmatic fever 30 days*
❑ Isosporiasis with diarrhea greater than 1 month*
❑ Kaposi's sarcoma in patient under 60 years (or over 60 years*)
❑ Lymphoma of brain in patient under 60 years (or over 60 years*)
❑ Lymphoma, non-Hodgkin's of B-cell or unknown immunologic phenotype and histology showing small, noncleaved lymphoma or immunoblastic sarcoma
❑ Mycobacterium avium complex or M. kansasii disseminated tuberculosis*
❑ Nocardiosis*
❑ Pneumocystis carinii pneumonia
❑ Pneumonia, recurrent-bacterial (2 episodes in 12 months)*
❑ Progressive multifocal leukoencephalopathy
❑ Salmonella septicemia (non-typhoid), recurrent*
❑ Strongyloidiasis, extraintestinal
❑ Toxoplasmosis of internal organs
* Requires positive HIV serology Note: Criteria of Center for Disease Control (CDC) Atlanta

232. Opportunistic infections in HIV infected individual occur when CD4 cell count fall below:

a. 200/ mm^3
b. 400/ mm^3
c. 600/ mm^3
d. 800/ mm^3

As the CD4 count drops below 200 cells per cmm, the opportunistic infection appear. This is also the time when neoplasms like high grade B cell lymphoma, Kaposi's sarcoma, cervical intra-epithelial neoplasia and primary CNS lymphoma appear. Many infections which remain localized in immunocompetent subjects tend to become disseminated.

Route	*Percentage*	*Efficiency (%)*
Sexual	85.96	0.1-1
Perinatal transmission	3.64	14-45%
Blood and blood products	2.00	~100%
Injecting Drug users	2.39	0.5%
Others (not specified)	6.01	

233. In patients of acquired immunodeficiency syndrome, the commonest cause of space occupying lesion in brain is:

a. Non-Hodgkin's lymphoma
b. Cytomegalovirus infection
c. Cryptococcus
d. Toxoplasmosis

A CT or MRI scan of the head should be performed promptly in all cases of focal neurological deficit, suspected to be having cerebral toxoplasmosis. Ring enhancing lesions and solitary or multiple abscesses should suggest the toxoplasmosis infection.

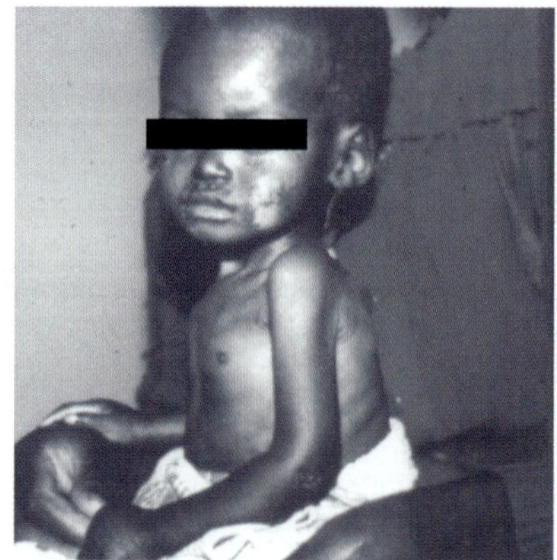

AIDS cachexia diarrhea

Ans. 231. a. Toxoplasmosis **232. a.** 200/ mm^3 **233. d.** Toxoplasmosis

234. True about dengue hemorrhagic fever are all EXCEPT:

a. Thrombocytopenia b. Thrombosis
c. Pleural effusion d. Fever

The minimum diagnostic criteria for DHF are a positive tourniquet test or spontaneous hemorrhages from multiple sites, thrombocytopenia (<1000,000/cmm), and evidence of plasma leakage as shown by increase in hematocrit by 20% or more from baseline, ascites or pleural effusion.

Points to remember

1. Dengue, which was considered to be a mild infection is emerging as a serious problem
2. Four distinct viruses can cause the disease. No cross protection is present. But may produce DHF and DSS in subsequent attacks.
3. Main cause of death: DHF and DSS –increased capillary permeability
4. Early fluid replacement and supportive measures save life.

235. XDR-TB is defined as:

a. Resistance to at least INH and rifampicin +/- other drugs
b. Resistance to any of the 3 first line drugs
c. Resistance to all 1st line drugs and any 3 second line injectable drugs
d. Resistance to at least INH and rifampicin + any quinolones + at least 1 injectable 2nd line drug

X-DR TB is newly coined term that denotes extensive resistance to drugs in the first and second line also. X-DR TB is classified as cases resistant to three or more of the second line drugs. The reason for developing X-DR TB is misuse and mismanagement of second line drugs.

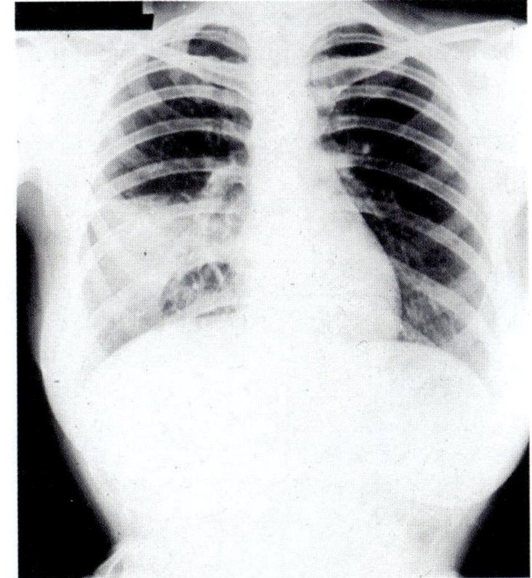

X-ray chest tuberculosis—middle lobe consolidation right

ENDOCRINOLOGY

236. Addison's disease is characterized by all EXCEPT:

a. Hypertension b. Hyponatremia
c. Hyperkalemia d. Hyperpigmentation

Characteristic symptoms are of Addison disease

- Severe vomiting and diarrhea, resulting in dehydration
- Low blood pressure (hypotension)
- Hypoglycemia (reduced level of blood glucose)
- Hyponatremia (low sodium level in the blood)
- Hyperkalemia (elevated potassium level in the blood)
- Hypercalcemia (elevated calcium level in the blood)

237. Hyperthyroid state is characterized by all EXCEPT:

a. Palpitations b. Increased BMR
c. Tachycardia d. Weight gain

Major clinical signs include weight loss (often accompanied by an increased appetite), anxiety, intolerance to heat, hair loss (especially of the outer third of the eyebrows), muscle aches, weakness, fatigue, hyperactivity, irritability, hyperglycemia, polyuria, polydipsia, delirium, tremor, pretibial myxedema (in Graves' disease), and sweating.

238. Regarding obesity, which is NOT true:

a. High risk of coronary artery disease
b. Associated with DM
c. Genetic predisposition
d. Smoking is a risk factor

The main active ingredient in cigarettes is nicotine. Nicotine acts by binding to a specific type of receptor on neurons (nerve cells) called the nicotinic acetylcholine receptor. Acetylcholine is one of the main signaling molecules (neurotransmitters) that neurons use to communicate with one another. Nicotine suppresses food intake, increases energy expenditure, and lowers body fatness. Smokers tend to be leaner than non-smokers. Infact giving up smoking causes weight gain

239. Primary hyperparathyroidism is characterized by all of the following EXCEPT:

a. Nephrocalcinosis b. High serum calcium
c. Low serum phosphate d. Diarrhoea

Primary hyperparathyroidism/HP may present as anorexia, nausea, vomiting and constipation. Peptic ulcer is rare (unless it occurs in the context of a MEN 1). Likewise, acute pancreatitis is rarely seen due to hypercalcemia associated with HP

240. Thyrotoxicosis is characterized by all EXCEPT:

a. Voracious appetite
b. Anxiety
c. Palpitation
d. Menorrhagia

Oligomenorrhoea (NOT menorrhagia) is a feature of Graves disease & menorrhagia is seen in hypothyroidism

241. All of the following are true for SIADH EXCEPT:

a. Normal KFT
b. Low uric acid
c. Relative hypernatremia
d. Normal BP with water retention

Ans. **234. b.** Thrombosis **235. d.** Resistance to at least... **236. a.** Hypertension **237. d.** Weight gain
238. d. Smoking is... **239. d.** Diarrhoea **240. d.** Menorrhagia **241. c.** Relative hypernatremia

The **syndrome of inappropriate antidiuretic hormone secretion** or **SIADH** (other names: Schwartz-Bartter syndrome, SIAD—syndrome of inappropriate antidiuresis) is characterized by excessive release of antidiuretic hormone from the posterior pituitary gland or another source. The result is often dilutional hyponatremia in which the plasma sodium levels are lowered and total body fluid is increased.

242. GH deficiency is characterized by all EXCEPT:

a. Stunting b. Delayed bone age
c. Hyperglycemia d. Delayed milestones

The effects of growth hormone deficiency vary depending on the age at which they occur. In children, growth failure and short stature are the major manifestations of GH deficiency, with common causes including genetic conditions and congenital malformations. It can also cause delayed sexual maturity. In adults, deficiency is rare (GH excess results in insulin resistance or even a rare form of type 2 diabetes i.e. hyperglycemia)

243. Secondary-hyperparathyroidism as a result of vitamin D deficiency is characterised by all EXCEPT:

a. Calciuria
b. Increased PTH
c. Increased serum alkaline phosphatase
d. Hypocalcemia

Secondary hyperparathyroidism/ HS with vitamin D deficiency:

- PTH: High
- Calcium: Low
- Urine Ca: Low
- Vitamin D: Low (<20)

244. Which of the following condition does NOT present with proptosis:

a. Grave's disease
b. Sarcoidosis
c. Pituitary adenoma
d. Myxoedema

Graves' ophthalmopathy due to Graves' disease (hyperthyroidism), usually causes bilateral proptosis (NOT myxoedema)

245. Hypothyroidism is associated with all of the following EXCEPT:

a. Hashimoto's thyroiditis
b. Struma ovarii
c. Lithium therapy
d. Iodine deficiency

A **struma ovarii** (literally: goitre of the ovary) is a rare form of monodermal teratoma that contains mostly thyroid tissue, which may cause hyperthyroidism

246. Hypocalcemia is characterized by all EXCEPT:

a. Tetany
b. Seizures
c. Osteoporosis
d. QT prolongation on ECG

Symptoms of hypocalcemia include neuromuscular irritability (including tetany as manifested by Chvostek's sign or Trousseau's sign, bronchospasm), electrocardiographic changes (prolonged QT interval), and seizures.

247. NOT a feature of Conn's syndrome:

a. Hyposecretion of renin b. Diastolic hypertension
c. Hyponatremia d. Hypokalemia

Conn's syndrome is a rare disorder caused by a primary increase in the production of aldosterone. The condition is characterized by hypertension, unprovoked hyperkalemia and low plasma renin activity.

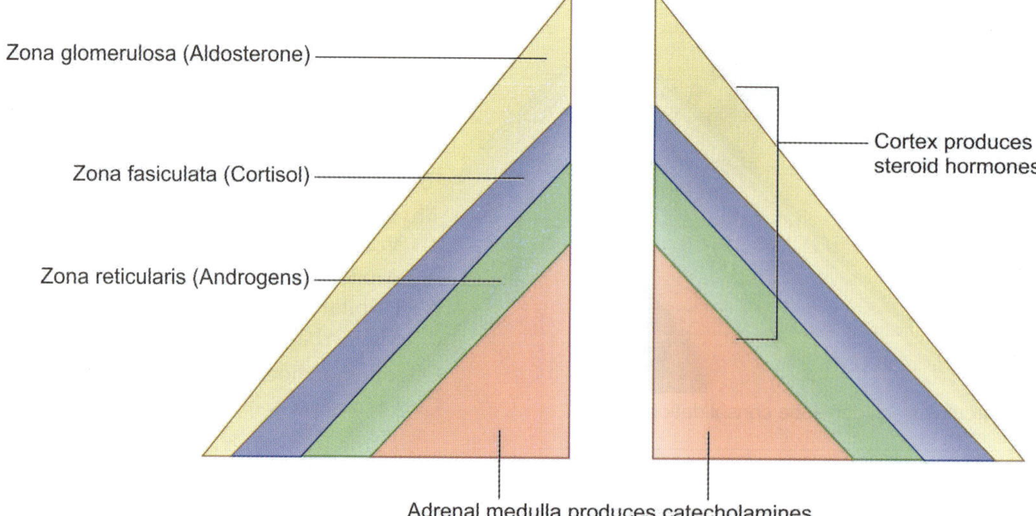

A diagrammatic representation of the layers of the adrenal gland

Ans. **242. c.** Hyperglycemia **243. a.** Calciuria **244. d.** Myxoedema **245. b.** Struma ovarii **246. c.** Osteoporosis **247. c.** Hyponatremia

248. GH secretion is inhibited by:

a. Stress b. Hyperglycemia

c. Exercise d. Hypoglycemia

Fasting level of GH in the plasma is below 4 ng/mL. Secretion occurs in burst lasting 1-2 h. Maximal secretion occurs during the stages III and IV of NREM sleep. Factors such as exercise, hypoglycemia, and rise in amino acid level enhances secretion.

Type of cells	Percentage	Secretion
Acidophils (eosinophils) Lactotrophs Somatotrophs	60-75% 15-20% 50%	 Prolactin GH
Basophils	25%	
Corticotrophs	10%	ACTH
Gonadotrophs	10%	FH, LH
Thyrotrophs	5%	TSH
Melanotrophs	—	MSH

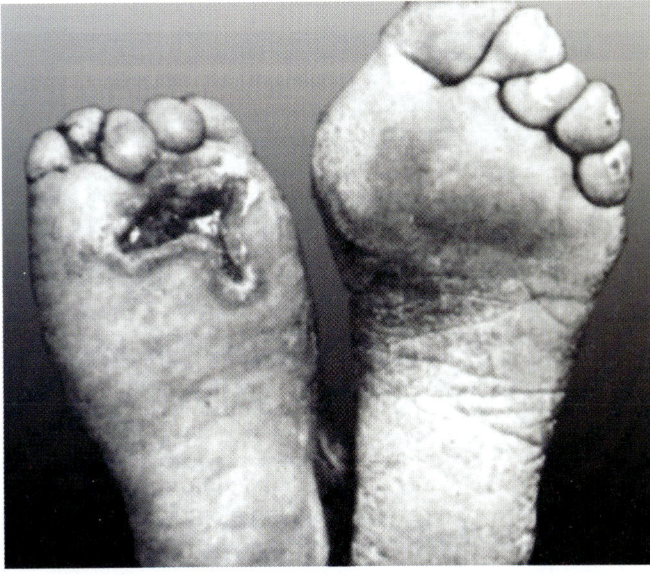

Trophic ulcer R foot— note the indolent deep ulcer

249. Most common form of diabetic neuropathy:

a. Distal symmetric polyneuropathy

b. Poly-radiculopathy

c. Autonomic neuropathy

d. Acute mononeuropathy

The most common neurological complication of DM is peripheral neuropathy. Clinical presentation may be varied. Symmetrical distal sensory neuropathy with pain, numbness, paresthesia, glove and stockings sensory loss and arreflexia is the common pattern seen in diabetics.

250. Adrenal insufficiency causes:

a. A rise in plasma sodium/ potassium ratio

b. Low blood pressure

c. Increase breakdown of protein

d. A fall in extra-cellular fluid volume

Cardiovascular abnormalities of Addison's disease/ primary adrenocortical insufficiency include low blood pressure especially postural hypotension, and diminution of heart size.

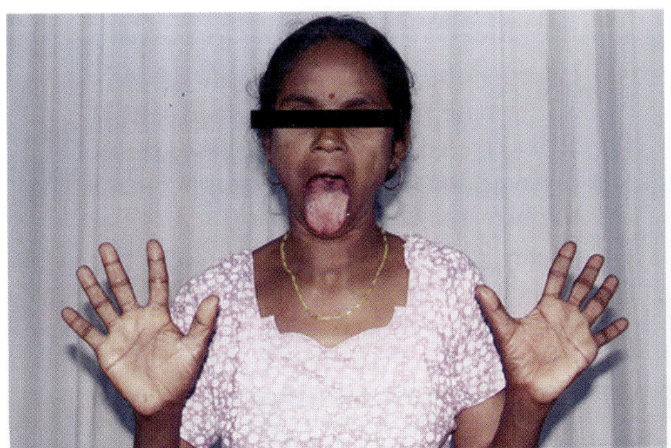

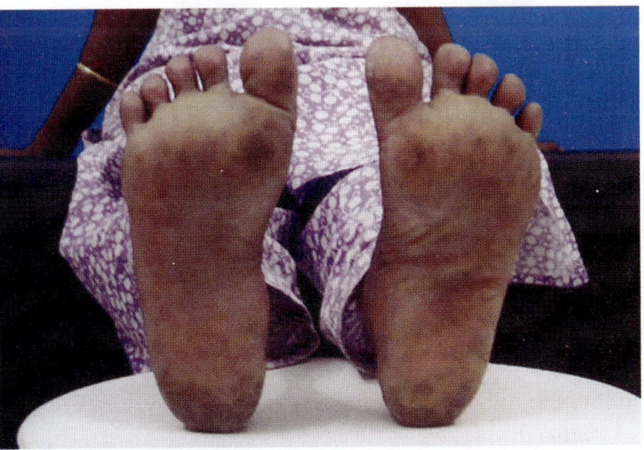

Female Addison's disease. Note pigmentation

251. Glycosylated hemoglobin %, indicating a good control of diabetes:

a. 7% b. 10%

c. 15% d. 20%

A diabetic is considered to be well controlled if the HbA1c is below 6.5%. As the life of a RBC is about 120 days, HbA1c is an index of the average sugar levels over the previous 3 months.

Clinical features	Type 1	Type 2
Usual age at onset (yrs)	5-30 years	35-65 years
Sex	M:F 1:1	F>M (in India)
Prevalence	15-18% in	95-98% of
Among diabetes	Caucasians 1% in Indians	Indians
Genetic	Heredity+	Heredity +++ No

Contd...

Ans. 248. b. Hyperglycemia 249. a. Distal symmetric... 250. b. Low blood pressure 251. a. 7%

Contd...

Clinical features	Type 1	Type 2
	Strong HLA association	HLA association
Nutrition	Lean	Often obese
Usual onset	Rapid with classic symptoms	Slow, insidious, often with only mild symptoms
Ketosis	Prone	Not prone
Islet cell antibodies	May be present within 1 year of onset	Absent
Treatment modality	Almost all require insulin for control of sugar	Majority can be controlled by oral hypoglycemic drugs (OHAs)

252. Ulcers in diabetes are precipitated by all EXCEPT:

a. Microangiopathic changes in blood vessels
b. Neuropathy
c. Position
d. Macroangiopathy

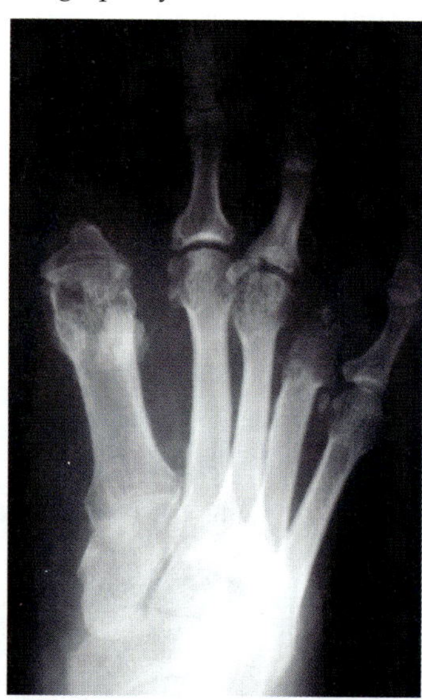

X-ray diabetic foot—note the resorption of the phalanges and distal parts of the metatarsals

Factors contributing to the foot problems

- Neuropathy – sensory, motor and autonomic
- Ischemia (Apart from major vascular occlusions, defect in microcirculation also contribute)
- Trauma – physical, mechanical, thermal, continuous mechanical stress, uneven weight bearing
- Infection

253. Medical adrenalectomy is done by:

a. Vincristine
b. Vinblastine
c. Mitotane
d. Methotrexate

Medical therapy for adrenal tumor is given if the primary cause is not corrected surgically. O, P'DDD (2, 2-bis – (2-chlorphenyl-4 chlorphenyl-1,1-dichlorethane - mitotane) given orally in divided doses to a total of 10-15 g/day causes atrophy and necrosis of the adrenal cortex and adrenal metastases. This drug may prolong life by a few months to years.

Important clinical features of Cushing's syndrome
❑ Truncal obesity
❑ Moon facies
❑ Hypertension
❑ Osteoporosis
❑ Protein depletion
❑ Glucose intolerance
❑ Purple striae
❑ Muscle wasting and weakness

254. Cushing's disease presents with:

a. Increased ACTH and increased cortisol
b. Decreased ACTH and decreased cortisol
c. Increased ACTH and decreased cortisol
d. Increased catecholamines

Cushing's disease refers specifically to the pituitary dependent hyperadrenal corticism. Cushing's syndrome is caused by persistent over secretion of glucocorticoids.

Interpretation of diagnostic tests in hyperadrenocortical states

Test	*Normal subjects*	*Pituitary cause (Cushing's disease)*	*Adrenal tumor and hyperplasia*	*Ectopic ACTH production*
Urinary 17 KGS	Normal	H	H	H
Plasma ACTH	Normal	H	L	H
Suppression by Dexamethasone 1 mg screening test	Suppression of plasma cortisol	No suppression	No suppression	Nil
2 mg/day × 3 days	Suppression	No suppression	Nil	Nil
8 mg/day × 2 days	Suppression	Suppression	No suppression (tumour) Suppression (hyperplasia)	No suppression

Ans. **252. c.** Position **253. c.** Mitotane **254. a.** Increased ACTH...

255. Syndrome of inappropriate ADH secretion is characterized by the following EXCEPT:
a. Hypo-osmolar urine
b. Water intoxication
c. Expanded fluid volume
d. Hyponatremia

SIADH is diagnosed by estimating serum sodium levels, which is below 125 mmol/L with high urine sodium levels above 20 mmol/L. Plasma osmolality must be less than 270 mOsm/kg with normal renal, adrenal and thyroid functions. Urine osmolality is more than 100 mOsm/kg.

Hypothalamic hormones, their action on the pituitary and the peripheral hormones liberated

Hypothalamic hormones	*Action on pituitary*	*Peripheral hormones released (or) Peripheral effect*
Thyrotropin releasing hormone (TRH) (1)	Thyroid stimulating hormone (TSH) (1)	T3,T4 and prolactin (1)
Gonadotropin releasing hormone (GnRH), (LHRH) (1)	Releases luteinising hormone (LH), and follicle stimulating hormone (FSH) (1)	Estrogens and androgenic steroids (2)
Growth hormone releasing hormone (GHRH)	Growth hormone (1) secreted	Somatomedin (IGH-1) (1)
Growth hormone releasing inhibiting hormone (GHRIH-somatostatin) (1)	G H inhibited TSH response to TRH reduced	
Prolactin inhibiting factor (PIF) (3)	Prolactin (PRL) (1) inhibited	Prolactin level kept at normal levels
Corticotropin releasing hormone (CRH) (1)	Adrenocorticotropic hormone (ACTH) (1)	Cortisol mainly (2)
Vasopressin (antidiuretic hormone ADH) (1)	-	Action on the renal tubules
Oxytocin (1)	-	Uterine contraction

Note: (1) peptide (2) steroids (3) amine

256. An obese NIDDM patient present with FBS=180 mg% and PPBS=260 mg%. Management include:
a. Glibencamide
b. Diet therapy + exercise + metformin
c. Insulin
d. Chlorpropamide

In type 2 DM, regular exercise forms an important component of therapy along with dietary regulation and oral hypoglycemic agents. Diet is the corner stone in the management of diabetes. The objective of dietary therapy is the optimization of glycemic control and to provide a nutritious and balanced diet.

Clinical differences between type 1 and type 2 DM

	Type 1 DM	*Type 2 DM*
Insulin deficiency	++++	+
Insulin resistance	Rare	+++ common
Insulin requirement	Low to moderate	Variable
Sulphonylurea drugs	Unresponsive	Responsive
Common cause of death	Nephropathy CHD, DKA	CHD, nephropathy, stroke and gangrene

CHD – coronary heart disease: DKA- diabetic ketoacidosis.

257. Hypertension with androgenisation of a female child is a feature of congenital adrenal hyperplasia due to deficiency of:
a. C-21 hydroxylase
b. C-11 hydroxylase
c. C-17 hydroxylase
d. Desmolase

11-beta hydroxylase deficient congenital adrenal hyperplasia (11-beta-OH CAH) is an uncommon form of congenital adrenal hyperplasia (CAH) resulting from a defect in the gene encoding the enzyme steroid 11-beta-hydroxylase which mediates the final step of cortisol synthesis in the adrenal. 11-beta-OH CAH results in hypertension due to excessive mineralocorticoid effects. It also causes excessive androgen production both before and after birth and can virilize a genetically female fetus or a child of either sex.

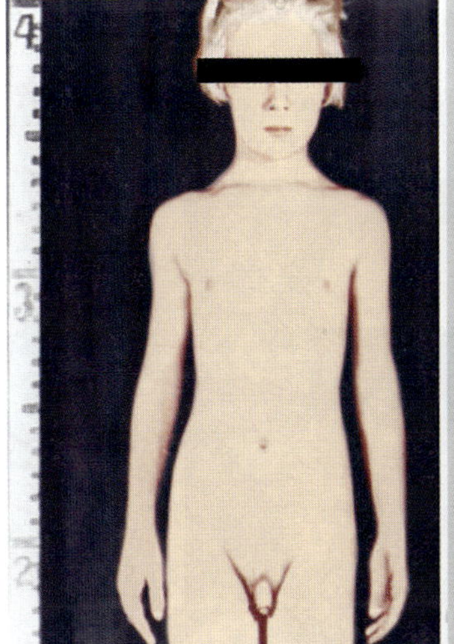
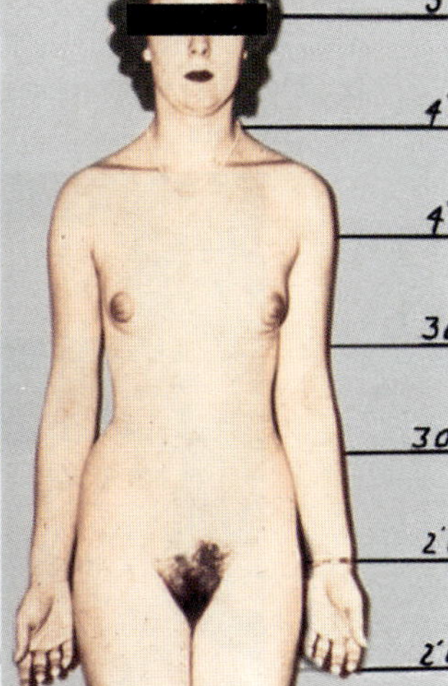

Virilizing adrenal hyperplasia. Note: Enlarged clitoris in the girl on the left. Normal girl of same

Ans. 255. **a.** Hypo-osmolar... 256. **b.** Diet therapy +... 257. **b.** C-11 hydroxylase

258. A patient is having random plasma glucose levels of 110 mg/dL and 113 mg/dL on two separate occasions. What you will advise him:

a. Declare him as having diabetes mellitus
b. Proceed for oral glucose tolerance test
c. Declare patient as normal
d. Check for glycosylated hemoglobin and if it is raised, declare him as having DM

The reference values for a 'normal' random glucose test in an average adult are 79-140 mg/dL (4.4 – 7.8 mmol/L), between 140-200 mg/dL is considered pre-diabetes, and >200 mg/dL is considered diabetes.

Criteria for diagnosis of diabetes mellitus (ADA 1997) – accepted all the world over
1. Symptoms of diabetes plus casual plasma glucose 200 mg/dl (Casual is defined as any part of the day without regard to time since the last meal. The classic symptoms of diabetes include polyuria, polydipsia and unexplained weight loss) OR
2. Fasting plasma glucose (FPG) 126 mg/dl (fasting is defined as no caloric intake for 8 hours) OR
3. A 2-hour post-glucose-load plasma glucose (2 hr PGBS) 200 mg/dL during oral glucose tolerance test (OGTT).
Note: The test should be performed as described by the WHO using a glucose load containing the equivalent of 75g of anhydrous glucose dissolved in water. In the absence of unequivocal hyperglycemia with acute metabolic decompensation, these criteria should be confirmed by repeat testing on a different day.
The expert committee on the diagnosis and classification of diabetes mellitus (American Medical Association) has defined normal plasma glucose as 100 mg/dL. Values between 100 and 126 are classified as impaired fasting plasma glucose (FPG).

259. A 21-year-old lady presented with history of tiredness, weight gain, depression and excessive somnolence. What will NOT be seen:

a. Hypertension
b. Delayed relaxation of tendon reflexes
c. Anemia
d. Tachycardia

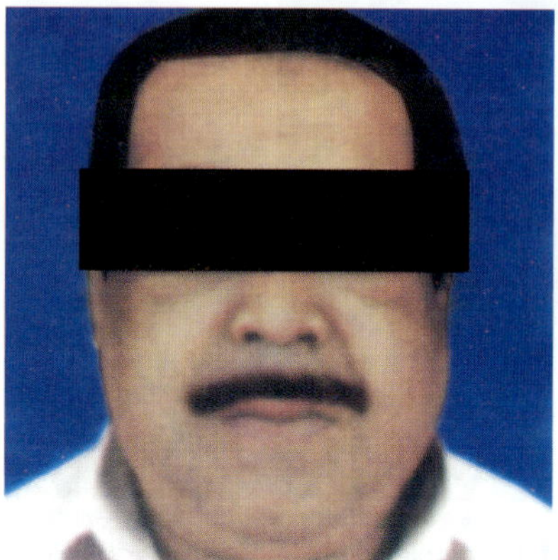

Myxedema: Male aged 50

Signs of hypothyroidism

- Dry coarse skin
- Cool extremities
- Myxedema
- Hair loss
- Bradycardia
- Delayed relaxation of tendon reflexes
- Carpal tunnel syndrome

260. Most common cause of spontaneous hypoglycemia in non-diabetic individual is:

a. Insulin
b. Oral hypoglycemic agents
c. Von Gierkes disease
d. Alcohol consumption

Hypoglycemia is the fall of blood glucose levels below 50-60 mg/dL at which symptoms occur in normal persons.

Precipitating factors for hypoglycemia
I. Meal-medicine mismatch: a. Decreased food intake, missing a meal or its delay, diarrhea, vomiting. b. Increased physical activity (unplanned, excessive strenuous physical activity) without reduction of the dose of drugs or adjustments in food intake. c. Increased dose of either insulin or oral hypoglycemic agents
II. Decrease in insulin requirements, which can occur when a juvenile diabetic goes into remission (honeymoon phase in type-1 diabetes), or soon after delivery in a pregnant woman (due to the drop in the placental hormones) or with the elimination of stress and control of infection.
III. Renal and hepatic insufficiency which decrease the insulin requirements.
IV. Drug interactions e.g. quinine, newer quinolones.
V. Excessive alcohol consumption

261. Acromegaly is associated with all of the following EXCEPT:

a. Nasal sinus enlargement
b. Increased heel pad thickness
c. Diabetes mellitus
d. Muscle hypotrophy

Though the muscles are hypertrophied in acromegaly, they may be weak due to proximal myopathy.

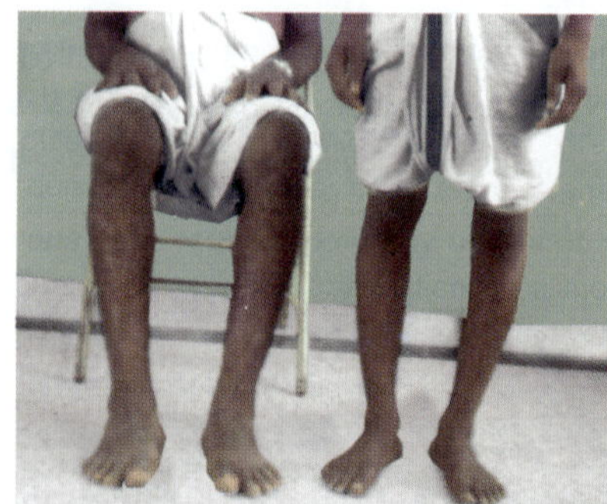

Acromegaly large legs and feet Note: Normal for comparison

Ans. **258. c.** Declare patient... **259. d.** Tachycardia **260. d.** Alcohol consump... **261. d.** Muscle hypotrophy

METABOLIC AND NUTRITIONAL DISORDERS

262. Wide anion gap metabolic acidosis is NOT a feature of:

a. Diarrhoea
b. Diabetic ketoacidosis
c. Methanol poisoning
d. Lactic acidosis

In patients with a normal anion gap the drop in HCO_3^- (diarrhea, Renal Tubular Acidosis type II) is the primary pathology. Since there is only one other major buffering anion, it must be compensated for almost completely by an increase in Cl^-. This is therefore also known as hyperchloremic acidosis.

263. Deficiency of which vitamin causes facial dyssebacea, angular stomatitis, cheilosis and normochromic-normocytic anemia:

a. Thiamine
b. Ascorbic acid
c. Riboflavin
d. Niacin

The classical syndrome of Riboflavin deficiency affects the mouth (sore throat, inflammation of the lining of mouth and tongue), angular cheilitis), the eyes (photophobia with bloodshot, itchy, watery eyes), the skin (moist, scaly skin particularly affecting the scrotum or labia majora and the nasolabial folds) and the blood (decreased red blood cell count with normal cell size and hemoglobin content i.e. normochromic normocytic anemia). In children it also results in reduced growth.

264. Associated with iodine deficiency are all EXCEPT:

a. Mental retardation
b. Wide open posterior fontanelle
c. Sclerema
d. Subnormal temperature

Sclerema neonatorum is a rare and severe skin condition that is characterized by diffuse hardening of the subcutaneous tissue with minimal inflammation. It usually affects premature, ill newborns.

265. Hypernatremia is characterized by all of the following EXCEPT:

a. Seizure
b. Thrombus
c. Brain hemorrhage
d. Central pontine myelinolysis

Central pontine myelinolysis presents most commonly as a complication of treatment of patients with profound, life-threatening chronic hyponatremia (low sodium). Hyponatremia should be corrected at a rate of no more than 12-20 mmol/L of sodium per day to prevent central pontine myelinolysis.

266. Presenting feature of a patient with deficiency of thiamine:

a. Gingival bleeding
b. Memory loss
c. Cardiac failure
d. Delayed wound healing

Wet beriberi is associated with mental confusion, muscular atrophy, edema, tachycardia, cardiomegaly, and congestive heart failure in addition to peripheral neuropathy

267. A 2-year-child is having a heart rate 40/ min and BP of 90/60 mm of Hg. Serum K+ is 6.5 mEq/ L. Management of such a case would be:

a. Ipratropium
b. Adrenaline
c. Sodium bicarbonate
d. Calcium gluconate

Calcium (calcium chloride or calcium gluconate) increases threshold potential through a mechanism that is still unclear, thus restoring normal gradient between threshold potential and resting membrane potential (improves myocardial contractility), which is elevated abnormally in hyperkalemia. The goal of treatment is to normalize the ECG and doses can be repeated if the ECG does not improve in 3 minutes.

268. Hypokalemia is associated with:

a. Respiratory alkalosis
b. Respiratory acidosis
c Metabolic alkalosis
d. Metabolic acidosis

In the kidney there is vacoulation of renal tubular cells in hypokalemia, leading to polyuria, polydypsia, metabolic alkalosis, increased ammonia synthesis and increased acid excretion in urine. The presence of acid urine in the setting of metabolic alkalosis is called paradoxical aciduria and it is a common feature in hypokalemic states.

Composition of intra and extracellular fluid compartments

Substance	*ICF*	*ECF*
1. Sodium Na^+	10 mmol/L	140 mmol/L
2. Potassium K^+	150 mmol/L	4 mmol/L
3. Chloride Cl^-	2 mmol/L	104 mmol/L
4. Bicarbonate HCO_3	6 mmol/L	24 mmol/L
5. Calcium Ca^{++}	50-100 nanomoles/L	2.25-2.65 mmol/L
6. Magnesium Mg^{++}	0.5 mmol/L	0.75-1 mmol/L
7. Phosphates,	1.4 mmol/L	0.8-1.5 mmol/L
Note: For univalent ions the mEq and mmol are the same		

269. NOT a cause of respiratory acidosis:

a. External intercostal muscle paralysis
b. Myasthenia gravis
c. Salicylate poisoning
d. Fibrosing alveolitis

Salicylate poisoning results in metabolic acidosis. Metabolic acidosis occurs when acid is added to the body or when alkali is lost from the body.

Ans. **262. a.** Diarrhoea **263. c.** Riboflavin **264. c.** Sclerema **265. d.** Central pontine...
266. c. Cardiac failure **267. d.** Calcium gluconate **268. c.** Metabolic alkalosis **269. c.** Salicylate poisoning

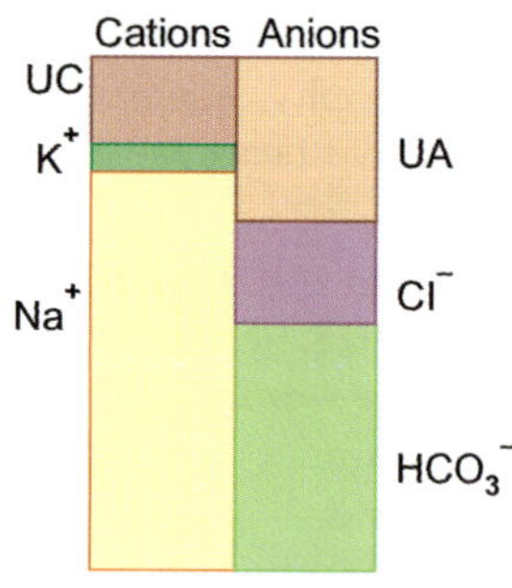

a) Normal cations include Na^+ K^+ and unmeasured cations (UC) Normal anions include HCO_3^-, Cl^- and unmeasured anions (UA)

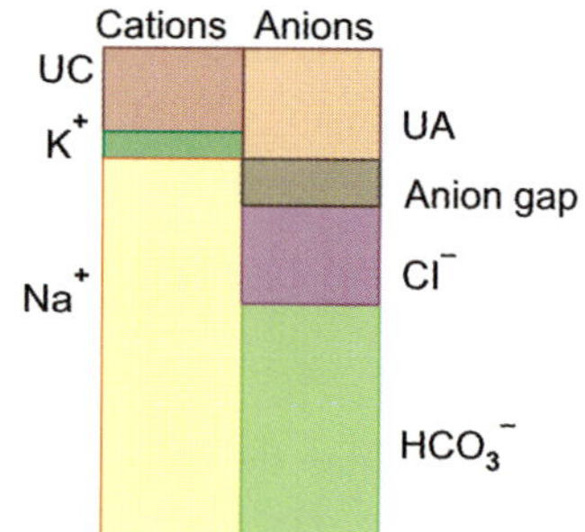

b) Anion gap = Sodium minus (bicarbonate + Chloride)

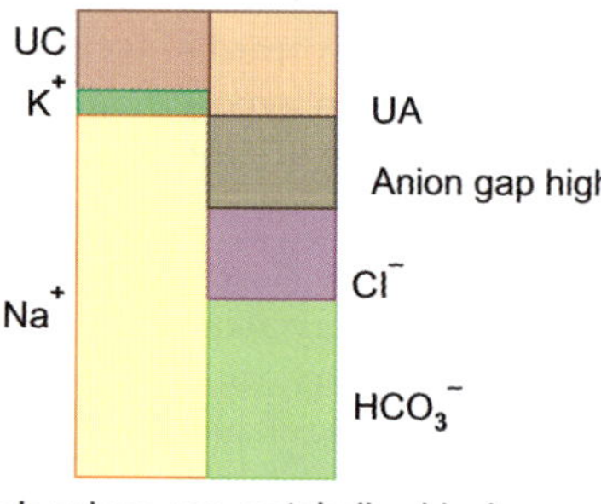

c) High anions gap metaboli acidosis Note: HCO_3 decreased, chloride normal anion gap increased

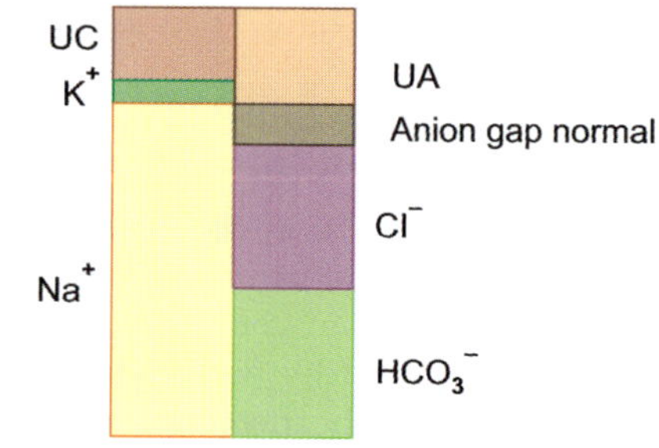

d) Normal anion gap metabolic acidosis Note: HCO decreased, chloride increased; anion gap–Normal

Showing anions, cations, anion gap and types of metabolic acidosis

270. Metal required for synthesis of retinol:

a. Molybdenum
b. Chromium
c. Zinc
d. Selenium

Zinc deficiency if often associated with low plasma vitamin A (retinol) concentrations. It has been suggested that the reduction in plasma retinol is secondary to reduced liver retinol binding protein (RBP) synthesis.

	Daily requirements
Man	750 µg
Woman	750 µg
Infants	300-400 µg
Children	400-600 µg
Adolescents	750 µg

271. Goat milk is deficient in which vitamin:

a. B12 b. B6
c. B1 d. Folate

Folic acid deficiency is commonly observed in children who are fed a severely restricted diet. This usually occurs with a diet restricted to goat's milk, which is deficient in folic acid.

272. Obesity is NOT associated with:

a. Arthritis b. Pancreatitis
c. Cholecystitis d. Hypertension

Complications of obesity

- Ill effect of increased weight: Slowness of movement, proneness to falls and accidents, osteoarthritis of weight bearing joints like knees, hips and spine
- Cardiovascular system: Atherosclerosis, hypercholesterolemia, angina, ischemic heart disease, hypertension, varicose veins, venous thrombosis, and recurrent embolism.
- Abdomen: Hernias develop owing to the increase in the intra-abdominal pressure. Gallbladder lesions are more common.

Shows the recommended values		
Weight class	*Global*	*Asians*
Normal	18.5–24.5	18.5–22.9
Over weight	25–29.9	23–24.9
Obese	> 30	>25
Severely obese	> 40	

273. Vitamin B_{12} deficiency can lead to all EXCEPT:

a. Myopathy b. Peripheral neuropathy
c. Optic atrophy d. Myelopathy

Ans. **270. c.** Zinc **271. d.** Folate **272. b.** Pancreatitis **273. a.** Myopathy

The neurological lesions of vitamin B12 deficiency include subacute combined degeneration of the spinal cord, optic neuritis, and demyelination of the cerebral white matter and peripheral nerves.

Neurological syndromes associated with nutrient deficiency	
Dementia/encephalopathy	Vitamin B_{12}, nicotinic acid, thiamine, folate
Seizures	Pyridoxine, biotin
Extrapyramidal syndrome	Nicotinic acid
Cerebellar ataxia	Vitamin E, vitamin B_{12},
Myelopathy	Vitamin B_{12}, folate, vitamin E
Optic neuropathy	Vitamin B_{12}, folate, vitamin E
Polyneuropathy	Thiamine, vitamin B_{12}, folate, pyridoxine, vitamin E, nicotinic acid
Myopathy	Vitamin B12, folate, vitamin E

274. Episodic weakness is associated with all EXCEPT:

a. Hyperglycemia b. Myotonia
c. Hyperkalemia d. Hypokalemia

The heterogenous group of muscle diseases known as periodic paralyses (PP) is characterized by episodes of flaccid muscle weakness occurring at irregular intervals. General characteristics of primary PP include the following: (1) they are hereditary; (2) most are associated with alteration in serum potassium levels; (3) myotonia sometimes coexists; and (4) both myotonia and PP result from defective ion channels.

275. Normal anion gap acidosis is a feature of:

a. Salicylate poisoning b. Renal tubular acidosis
c. Diabetic ketoacidosis d. All of the above

Metabolic acidosis with normal anion gap

- Renal causes
  - Proximal RTA (Type II RTA)
  - Distal RTA (Type I RTA)
  - Hyperkalemic distal RTA (Type IV RTA)
- Extrarenal causes
  - Diarrhea (loss of bicarbonate)
  - Pancreatic/ biliary fistula (loss of bicarbonate)
  - Uretero-sigmoidostomy leading to reabsorption of hydrogen ions and ammonia in exchange for bicarbonate in the gut.

276. Organ affected majorly in galactosemia:

a. Eyes, brain and kidney b. Liver, eyes and brain
c. Liver, eyes and kidney d. Lungs, liver and eyes

Galactosemia is transmitted as an autosomal recessive trait. In the fully developed form classical galactosemia presents with cataract, mental retardation, hepatic cirrhosis, and death in early life. The enzyme galactose-1-phosphate uridyl transferase is deficient.

277. Which of the following causes pseudotumor cerebrii:

a. Chronic subdural hematoma
b. Cerebellar tumors
c. Hypervitaminosis A
d. Cerebellar hemangiomas

Chronic toxicity of vitamin A is characterized by body aches, arthralgia, hair loss, anorexia, benign intracranial hypertension, weight loss and hepatomegaly.

Age	*Vitamin A dosage*
Infants < 6 months	50,000 IU/orally
Infants 6-12 months	100,000 IU/oral once in 4-6 months
Children >12 months	200,000 IU/orally once in 4-6/months
Mothers	200,000 IU orally within 8 weeks of delivery

NEUROLOGY

278. All of the following are commonly associated with seizures EXCEPT:

a. Hypocalcemia
b. Neurocysticercosis
c. Hypoglycemia
d. HIV encephalopathy

A number of disorders including: low blood sugar (hypoglycemia), low blood sodium, hyperosmolar nonketotic hyperglycemia, high blood sodium, low blood calcium (hypocalcemia) and high blood urea levels may cause seizures. As may hepatic encephalopathy and the genetic disorder porphyria

279. A comatose patient presented to the casuality. There was a history of road traffic accident. Pupil was dilated on one side. NCCT imaging of head showed peripheral lesion with concave border. Likely diagnosis:

a. Intraparenchymal bleed
b. Subdural hemorrhage
c. Subarachnoid hemorrhage
d. Normal

Unlike epidural hematomas, which cannot expand past the sutures of the skull, subdural hematomas can expand along the inside of the skull, creating a concave shape that follows the curve of the brain, stopping only at the dural reflections like the tentorium cerebelli and falx cerebri. On a CT scan, subdural hematomas are classically crescent-shaped, with a concave surface away from the skull.

280. Upper motor neuron lesion is characterized by all EXCEPT:

a. Hypotonia
b. Spasticity
c. Weakness of muscles
d. Absent superficial reflexes

Ans. **274. a.** Hyperglycemia **275. b.** Renal tubular... **276. b.** Liver, eyes and **277. c.** Hypervitaminosis A
278. d. HIV encephal... **279. b.** Subdural hemorrhage **280. a.** Hypotonia

Symptoms of upper motor neuron lesion include muscle weakness, decreased motor control including a loss of the ability to perform fine movements, increased vigor (and decreased threshold) of spinal reflexes including spasticity (hypertonia), and an extensor plantar response known as the Babinski sign

281. All of the following are features of CN VIII palsy EXCEPT:

a. Gag reflex b. Vertigo
c. Motion sickness d. Tinnitus

Gag/ Pharyngeal reflex

- The sensory limb is mediated predominantly by CN IX (glossopharyngeal nerve)
- The motor limb by CN X (vagus nerve).

282. Wernicke's aphasia is characterized by all EXCEPT:

a. Paraphasia
b. Poor repetition
c. Poor comprehension of spoken words
d. Non fluent but meaningful speech

In contrast to Expressive (motor aphasia) aphasia, damage to the temporal lobe may result in a fluent aphasia that is called receptive aphasia (also known as **Sensory aphasia** and **Wernicke's aphasia**). Patients suffering from receptive aphasia, unlike Broca's aphasia patients, produce speech without any grammatical problem. However, because the Wernicke's area, which is responsible for language comprehension, is damaged, receptive aphasia patients cannot convey the meaning.

283. A patient presented to the medicine OPD with complaints of headache. Physical examination revealed nuchal rigidity. Lumbar puncture was done and CSF showed normal glucose with clear CSF. Microscopic examination of CSF showed 50 lymphocytes/ mm 3 with lymphocytic pleiocytosis. Findings are consistent with the diagnosis of:

a. Fungal meningitis
b. Neoplastic meningitis
c. Viral meningitis
d. Bacterial meningitis

Normal glucose, normal protein & mild lymphocytic leukocytosis suggest viral meningitis

284. Which of the following is NOT a feature of Parkinsonism:

a. Chorea
b. Recurrent falls
c. Tremors
d. Freezing

Chorea is an abnormal involuntary movement disorder, one of a group of neurological disorders called dyskinesias. Dyskinesia can be anything from a slight tremor of the hands to an uncontrollable movement of the upper body or lower extremities. It is a disease of the caudate nucleus and putamen.

285. Unilateral ptosis is seen in all EXCEPT:

a. Pancoast tumour
b. Marfan syndrome
c. Thyroid ophthalmopathy
d. Myasthenia gravis

Exophthalmos can be either bilateral (as is often seen in Graves' disease)

286. Examples of proximal myopathy are all EXCEPT:

a. Thyroid myopathy
b. Drug induced myopathy
c. Duchenne muscular dystrophy
d. Myasthenia gravis

The hallmark of myasthenia gravis is fatigability. Muscles become progressively weaker during periods of activity, and improve after periods of rest. Muscles that control eye and eyelid movement, facial expressions, chewing, talking, and swallowing are especially susceptible.

287. All contribute to Circle of Willis EXCEPT:

a. Internal carotid artery b. Posterior cerebral artery
c. Anterior cerebral artery d. Middle cerebral artery

The basilar artery and middle cerebral arteries, supplying the brain, are not considered part of the circle.

288. A patient presented to the emergency room in an unconscious state. There was a history of road traffic accident. Physical examination revealed unilateral dilation of pupil. Likely cause could be:

a. Transcalvarial herniation
b. Cingulate herniation
c. Tonsillar herniation
d. Uncal herniation

In uncal herniation, a common subtype of transtentorial herniation, the innermost part of the temporal lobe, the uncus, can be squeezed so much that it moves towards the tentorium and puts pressure on the brainstem, most notably the midbrain. The uncus can squeeze the oculomotor nerve, which may affect the parasympathetic input to the eye on the side of the affected nerve, causing the pupil of the affected eye to dilate and fail to constrict in response to light as it should.

289. Lower motor neuron palsy is characterized by all EXCEPT:

a. Flaccid paralysis
b. Muscular hypertrophy
c. Hyporeflexia
d. Superficial reflexes present

Damage to lower motor neurons, lower motor neuron lesions (LMNL) cause muscle atrophy, decreased strength and decreased reflexes in affected areas. These findings are in contrast to findings in upper motor neuron lesions. LMNL is indicated by abnormal EMG potentials, fasciculations, paralysis, weakening of muscles, and neurogenicatrophy of skeletal muscle. Bell's Palsy, Bulbar palsy, Poliomyelitis and Amyotrophic lateral sclerosis (ALS) are all pathologies associated with lower motor neuron dysfunction.

Ans. 281. **a.** Gag reflex 282. **d.** Non fluent but... 283. **c.** Viral meningitis 284. **a.** Chorea
285. **c.** Thyroid ophth... 286. **d.** Myasthenia gravis 287. **d.** Middle cerebral... 288. **d.** Uncal herniation
289. **b.** Muscular hypertrophy

290. Features of tubercular meningitis are all EXCEPT:

a. Evidence of old pulmonary lesions or a miliary pattern is found on chest radiography
b. Culture of CSF is diagnostic in majority of cases and remains the gold standard
c. It is seen most often in young children but also develops in adults
d. CSF reveals a low WBC count

The CSF usually has a high protein, low glucose and a raised number of lymphocytes. Acid-fast bacilli are sometimes seen on a CSF smear, but more commonly, M. tuberculosis is grown in culture. A spiderweb clot in the collected CSF is characteristic of TB meningitis, but is a rare finding.

291. Neck rigidity WITHOUT fever is a feature of:

a. Space occupying lesion
b. Subarachnoid hemorrhage
c. Meningism
d. Meningitis

Bleeding into the subarachnoid space constitutes subarachnoid hemorrhage (SAH). The patient usually presents with excruciating pain of sudden onset followed by loss of consciousness. Signs of meningeal irritation like neck rigidity, Kernig's sign, and Brudzinski sign are usually present.

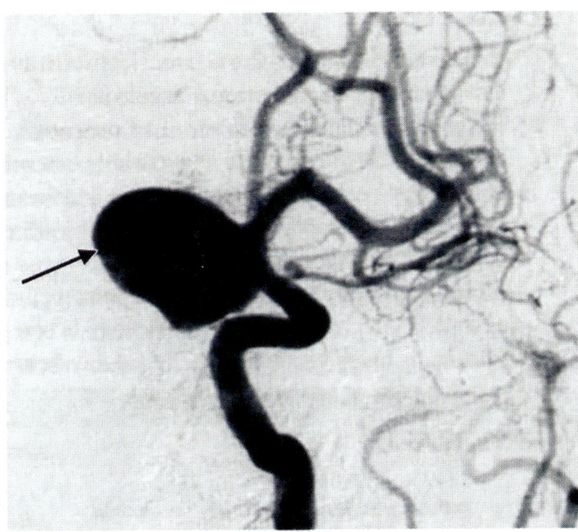
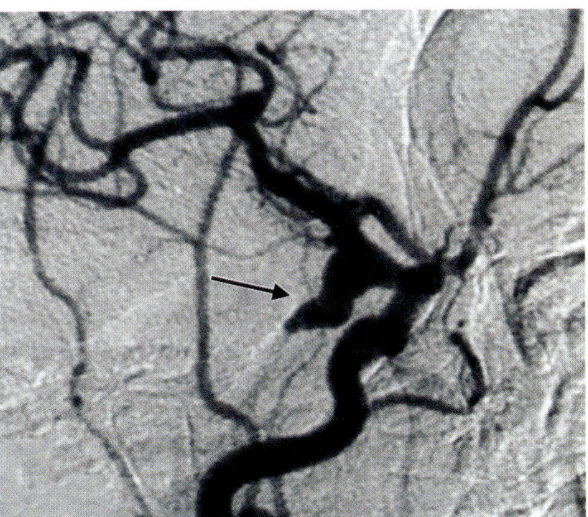

Carotid angiography. A and B show berry aneurysm—arrows

292. Albumino-cytological dissociation in CSF is a feature of:

a. Multiple sclerosis
b. GB syndrome
c. TB meningitis
d. Multiple myeloma

Cerebrospinal fluid characteristically shows albuminocytological dissociation if examined about a week after the onset of the disease in GBS. The term albuminocytological dissociation refers to the rise in proteins without a corresponding rise in cell count.

Salient features of the common types of peripheral neuropathy

Disease	Type of onset	Distribution	Pattern	Fiber affected	Pathology
Diabetes melitus	Acute or chronic	Proximal or distal	Polyneuropathy or mononeuropathy	Small and large	AD and SD
Porphyria	Acute	Proximal/diffuse	Polyneuropathy	-do-	AD
Vitamin B_{12} deficiency	Chronic	Distal	Polyneuropathy	-do-	AD
Lead poisoning	Subacute	Distal	Mononeuropathy	-do-	AD
Arsenic poisoning	Subacute	Distal	Polyneuropathy	-do-	AD
Leprosy	Subacute or chronic	Mononeuritic or distal symmetrical	Mono- or poly-neuropathy	Small	AD and SD
Diphtheria	Acute	Distal, proximal or diffuse	Poly- or mononeuropathy	Small and large	SD
Connective tissue disorders and vasculitis	Chronic or acute	Distal	Poly- or mono-neuropathy	-do-	SD
Guillain-Barré syndrome	Acute	Proximal or diffuse	Polyneuropathy	-do-	SD
Paraneoplastic	Chronic	Distal	Poly- or mononeuropathy	-do-	AD
Hereditary sensori-motor neuropathy	Chronic	Distal	Polyneuropathy	-do-	AD

Note: - AD – Axonal degeneration; SD – Segmental demyelination.

Ans. **290. d.** CSF reveals a... **291. b.** Subarachnoid... **292. b.** GB syndrome

293. When to declare a patient as brain dead:

a. Occassional shivering
b. Iso-electric EEG for 30 minutes
c. Heart rate absent
d. Hypothermia

The characteristic periodic EEG complexes in subacute sclerosing panencephalitis and Jocob-Creutzfeldt disease, the triphasic waves in hepatic coma and the electrocerebral silence in brain death are some of the diagnostic EEG patterns.

294. Lasegue's sign is seen in:

a. Transection of spinal cord
b. Myasthenia gravis
c. Intracranial lesions
d. Nerve root pressure

Straight leg raising test is positive in lumbar disc lesions – Lasegue's sign. This sign is elicited by passively lifting up the lower limb held straight by the examiner when the patient is in supine position. In normal subjects the limb can be brought to near-vertical position without discomfort. In lumbosacral root irritation due to disc prolapsed this movement is restricted by severe pain.

295. Coma and pin-point may be a manifestation of bleeding in:

a. Spinal cord b. Medulla
c. Thalamus d. Pons

In pontine hemorrhage the patient is deeply comatose with pin-point, but reacting pupil.

296. Hemiparesis is NOT a feature of:

a. Vertebral artery occlusion
b. Anterior cerebral artery occlusion
c. Middle cerebral artery occlusion
d. Carotid artery occlusion

In occlusion of the posterior inferior cerebellar artery supplying the lateral half of the medulla a characteristic syndrome called the lateral medullary syndrome (Wallenberg's syndrome) develops. This is perhaps the most common mode of presentation of vertebral artery occlusion. The resultant neurological features consist of sensory impairment over the face, Horner's syndrome and ataxia on the ipsilateral side, and impaired pain and temperature sensations on the contralateral side. In the pure form of this syndrome, there is no weakness or pyramidal tract dysfunction.

Pattern of clinical features in various vascular syndromes

Middle cerebral artery (MCA)	Anterior cerebral artery (ACA)	Common carotid artery (CCA)	Internal capsule (IC)	Vertebro-basilar artery (VBA)
Upper limbs weaker than lower	Lower limbs weaker than upper	Ipsilateral eye and contralateral hemiparesis resembling MCA, ACA or both	Equal weakness of upper and lower limbs	Bilateral affection
Aphasia if lesion is on the dominant side	Nil	±	Nil	Nil
Hemianopia often present	Absent	Present	Present	Present if PCA is affected
Hemianesthesia present	Cortical sensory loss in lower limbs	Hemianesthesia +	Present	Crossed anesthesia
Rarely cerebellar signs +	Absent	Absent	Rarely present	Cerebellar signs common
Recovery poor in patients with Wernicke's aphasia and hemianopia	Recovery poor due to frontal lobe infarct. Apathy and lack of drive	Variable	Variable	Recovery variable

297. NOT a cause of thick nerves:

a. Amyloidosis b. Leprosy
c. Alcoholic polyneuropathy
d. Refsum's disease

Peripheral nerves may be palpably hypertrophic in conditions such as leprosy, amyloidosis, acromegaly, neurofibromatosis, and Refsum's disease.

Causes of peripheral neuropathy

Hereditary	Hereditary sensory-motor neuropathies
Metabolic	Diabetes mellitus, hepatic failure, renal failure porphyria
Endocrine	Hypothyroidism
Toxic	Alcohol,organophosphates, arsenic, lead, gold, thallium, lithium
Drugs	Vincristine, INH
Immune mediated Chronic idiopathic demyelinating polyneuropathy (CIDP)	Guillain-Barré syndrome
Infections	Leprosy, diphtheria
Vasculitis	Polyarteritis nodosa, other forms of vasculitis in sarcoidosis, Wegener's granulomatosis, Behcet's syndrome
Nutritional	Vitamin deficiencies, e.g. Vit B_{12}, B_1, B_6
Miscellaneous	Lymphomas, paramalignant syndromes, critical illness neuropathy

Ans. 293. **b.** Iso-electric... 294. **d.** Nerve root pressure 295. **d.** Pons 296. **a.** Vertebral artery occlusion 297. **c.** Alcoholic polyn...

298. Raised protein WITHOUT pleocytosis is a feature of:

a. TB meningitis
b. Pyogenic meningitis
c. GB syndrome
d. Froin syndrome

Albuminocytological dissociation is a feature of GBS.

Alterations in CSF in health and CNS infections					
	Tension	*Colour*	*Cells*	*Protein*	*Sugar*
Normal	50-150 mm water	Clear	0-5 lymph/cm	30-40 mg/dL	60-80 mg/dl
Pyogenic meningitis	Raised	Turbid	>1000, mostly neutrophils	Increased considerably	Very low
Tuberculous meningitis	Raised	Cloudy (cob-web)	Up to 300-500, mostly lymphocytes	200-300 mg/dL or more	Very low
Viral meningitis	Raised	Clear	10-100, mostly lymphocytes	50-100 mg/dL	Normal
Syphilitic meningitis	Raised	Clear	Up to 20-500, mostly lymphocytes	100-200 mg/dL	Normal
General paralysis of the insane	Normal	Clear	up to 100, mostly lymphocytes	40-100 mg/dL	Normal
Tabes dorsalis	Normal	Clear	Up to 100, mostly lymphocytes	30-60 mg/dL	Normal
Encephalitis	Raised	Clear	Up to 100, mostly lymphocytes	Normal or marginally raised	Normal or raised

299. FALSE for prion's disease:

a. Myoclonus found only in 10% cases
b. Neurodegenerative disease
c. Biopsy of brain diagnostic
d. Caused by infectious protein

Transmissible spongiform encephalopathies refer to subacute, fatal, transmissible neurodegenerative disorders characterized by spongiform encephalopathy due to accumulation of abnormal proteins in the CNS.

Prion diseases in humans
Creutzfeldt-Jakob Disease (CJD)
Kuru
Fatal familial insomnia (rare)
Gerstmann-Straussler-Scheinker disease (rare)

300. A patient presented with sudden onset of thunderclap headache and dilated pupils. Findings are consistent with:

a. Meningitis
b. Brain stem encephalitis
c. Acute ischemia of midbrain
d. Acute aneurysmal hemorrhage

Rupture of an aneurysm results in subarachnoid hemorrhage. The patient usually presents with excruciating headache (thunderclap headache) of sudden onset followed by loss of consciousness.

Distinctive clinical features in stroke			
	Thrombosis	*Embolism*	*Hemorrhage*
Age group	Elderly	Young or old	Younger
Time of onset	Sleep	Activity	Activity
Waking the patient during sleep	No	No	Yes
Headache	Present due to vasodilation of extracranial vessels	Not much	Sudden bursting headache
Seizures	Occurs late, when gliosis develops	Solitary seizures at onset	Recurrent seizures
Disturbance of consciousness	Minor	Minor or nil	Often severe
Recovery	Slow, mortality less, morbidity more	Good recovery	Mortality more, but in survivors morbidity is less

301. Pathway involved in dissociative anesthesia in syringomyelia:

a. Cilio-retinal pathway
b. Anterior spinothalamic tract
c. Decussating branches of lateral spinothalamic tract
d. Dorsal column

Ans. **298. c.** GB syndrome **299. a.** Myoclonus found... **300. d.** Acute aneurysmal... **301. c.** Decussating branches...

Loss of pain and temperature sensation (carried in lateral spinothalamic tract) with preservation of touch (dissociative anesthesia) in an irregular distribution is the hallmark of syringomyelia. The patient may not appreciate burns and injuries.

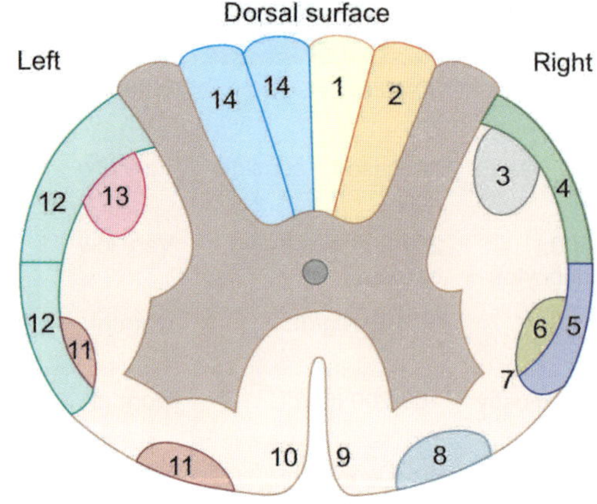

Spinal cord section—diagrammatic representation

Functional Representation	*Anatomy of tracts*
10. and 13. Voluntary movement	1. Fasciculus gracilis
11. Pain, temperature and touch	2. Fasciculus cuneatus
12. Equilibration	3. Lateral (crossed) pyramidal tract
14. Position sense, vibration sense, touch	4. Posterior spinocerebellar tract
	5. Anterior spinocerebellar tract
	6. Lateral spinothalamic tract
	7. Extrapyramidal tracts
	8. Anterior spinothalamic tract
	9. Anterior (uncrossed) pyramidal tract

302. Extensor plantar but ABSENT ankle jerk may be a feature of:

a. Syringomyelia
b. Tabes dorsalis
c. Friedreich's ataxia
d. Polio

Diagnosis of FA is entirely clinical. Insidious onset of ataxia with signs of cerebellar and posterior column dysfunction, absence of ankle jerks, and presence of Babinski's sign (extensor plantar) in the first two decades of life should suggest the diagnosis.

303. Scanning speech is seen in:

a. Pseudobulbar palsy
b. Motor neuron disease
c. Parkinsonism
d. Multiple sclerosis

Scanning speech, also known as explosive speech, is a type of ataxic dysarthria in which spoken words are broken up into separate syllables, often separated by a noticeable pause, and spoken with a varying force. It is a typical symptom of multiple sclerosis, and it constitutes one of the three symptoms of Charcoat's neurological triad.

Representation of various components of speech in anatomical areas of the cerebral cortex	
Components of speech	*Anatomical areas of cerebral cortex*
1. Ability to read and comprehend written speech	1. Visual cortex and its association areas
2. Ability to hear and comprehend	2. Heschl's gyrus (transverse temporal gyrus) and the superior temporal gyrus
3. Ability to comprehend symbols	3. Superior temporal gyrus and parieto-occipital areas
4. Ability to identify and name objects	4. Supra-marginal and angular gyrus
5. Genesis of motor engram of speech	5. Broca's area (posterior part of inferior frontal gyrus)
6. Genesis of motor engram for writing	6. Exner's area in the middle frontal gyrus
7. Execution of the expressive part through the motor system coordinated by the pyramidal, extrapyramidal and the cerebellar connections along with the emotional component executed by the prefrontal lobe and connections.	
8. The main white fibre tracts connecting the Broca's and Wernicke's areas constitute the arcuate fasciculus.	

304. Presence of hemiplegia with diminution of vision in the contralateral eye suggests occlusion of:

a. Middle cerebral artery
b. Basilar artery
c. Anterior cerebral artery
d. Internal carotid artery

The ICA supplies the eye as well as the anterior two-third of the cerebral hemisphere, via the anterior and middle cerebral arteries. Ipsilateral blindness occurring with contralateral hemiplegia is called carotid hemiplegia.

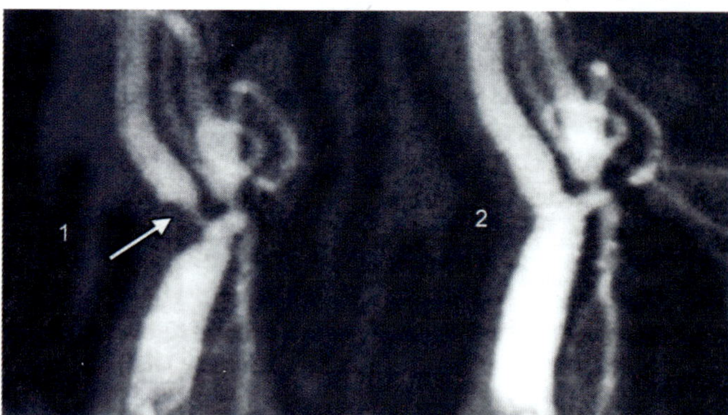

Internal carotid artery stenosis, arteriogram (1) Note the narrowing—arrow (2) after correction

305. Facial palsy is seen in:

a. Myasthenia gravis
b. Guillain Barre syndrome
c. Muscular dystrophy
d. Duchenne muscular dystrophy

The cranial nerves commonly involved in GBS are facial (40%), bulbar (30%) and ocular (10%).

Ans. 302. c. Friedreich's... **303. d.** Multiple sclerosis **304. d.** Internal carotid artery **305. b.** Guillain Barre syndrome

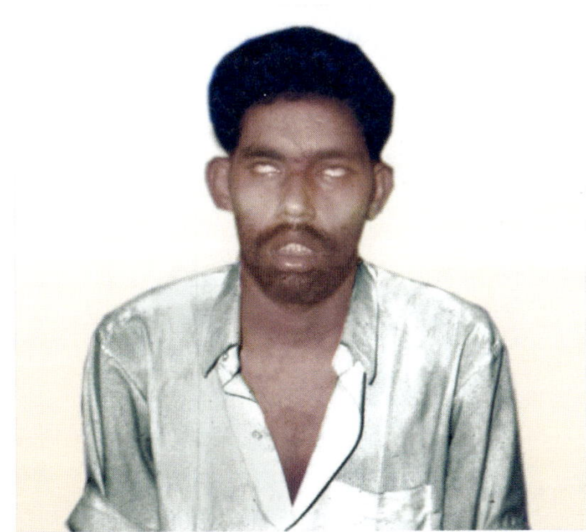

Bilateral facial palsy. Note inability to close the eyes and Bell's phenomenon

306. Cranial nerve most commonly involved in posterior communicating artery aneurysm is:

a. Oculomotor b. Facial
c. Optic d. Trigeminal

Posterior communicating artery aneurysms may press upon the ipsilateral oculomotor nerve.

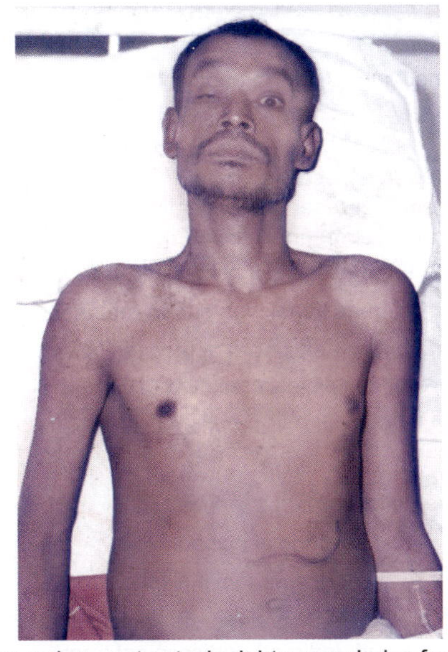

3rd nerve palsy—note ptosis right secondaries from abdominal tumor

307. Alzheimer's disease is associated with:

a. Delerium
b. Delusion
c. Dementia
d. All of the above

Alzheimer's disease is one of the more common causes of dementia in adults. This usually occurs in the elderly. The onset of mental symptoms is so insidious that neither the family nor the patient can dates its beginning.

Clinical importance of delusions

Types of delusion	*Characteristic false belief of*	*Typical mental disorder*
Paranoid		
Persecutory	Persecution – to kill or – to harm	Schizophrenia, Depression (when moved congruent)
Reference	Actions of others have special reference/meaning	-do
Grandiose	Oneself being high, big, rich	Mania
Poverty	Poverty or loss	Depression
Guilt	Sinful action	Depression
Nihilistic	Non-existence of part or whole of self or the world itself	Depression
Somatic/ hypochondriasis	Bodily disease	Depression
Jealousy	Illicit sexual relationship	Delusional disorder, Alcoholism
Love Primary Secondary delusions	Being loved	Delusional disorder Schizophrenia Mood disorder or any psychosis

308. For generalized tonic clonic Status epilepticus, treatment of choice is:

a. Ethosuximide b. Sodium valproate
c. Lamotrigine d. Lorazepam

Time is a critical factor in the management of status epilepticus. There are many therapeutic regimes but none of them is totally satisfactorily. Benzodiazepines such as diazepam, lorazepam, midazolam and clonazepam are all potent fast acting antiepileptic drugs, preferred for terminating the attack immediately. Lorazepam in doses of 0.1 mg/kg at 2 mg/minute is preferable to IV Diazepam as it has longer duration of action (>4 hrs) and lesser respiratory depression.

Type of epilepsy and choice of AED

Types of epilepsy	*Drugs of choice*
1. Generalized tonic-clonic seizures with partial onset	Phenytoin sodium Carbamazepine Phenobarbitone Sodium valproate
2. Simple partial seizures	Carbamazepine Phenytoin sodium Primidone Phenobarbitone Sodium valproate
3. Complex partial seizures	Carbamazepine Sodium valproate Primidone Phenytoin sodium Phenobarbitone

Contd...

Ans. **306. a.** Oculomotor **307. c.** Dementia **308. d.** Lorazepam

Contd...

Types of epilepsy	*Drugs of choice*
4. Absence seizures with 3/ sec spike and waves on EEG	Sodium valproate Ethosuximide Clonazepam
5. Myoclonic seizures	Sodium valproate Nitrazepam Clonazepam Ethosuximide
6. Infantile spasms	ACTH/ Corticosteroids Nitrazepam Clonazepam
7. Neonatal seizures, Febrile seizures	Phenobarbitone Sodium valproate
8. Status epilepticus	Diazepam Phenytoin sodium Phenobarbitone Lorazepam

309. True statement for primary cerebral lymphoma:

a. It is most commonly formed of T cells
b. It is usually solitary
c. It is seen in immunocompromised patient
d. Chemosensitive

Primary CNS lymphomas are late complications of HIV infection, occurring in up to 10% of AIDS patients. Almost all cases are EBV-associated.

310. The commonest cause of intracerebral bleed is:

a. Thrombocytopenia
b. Diabetes
c. Hypertension
d. Berry aneurysm

Intracerebral hemorrhage/spontaneous non-traumatic intracerebral hematoma is most common in the sixth and seventh decade of life. Among the known causes, hypertension was the most frequent. Rarely the blood pressure may be in the normal range when first examined after the stroke.

311. Upper motor neuron lesion is characterized by:

a. Weakness and spasticity
b. Fasciculations
c. Rigidity
d. Localized muscle atrophy

Signs of Upper Motor Neuron Lesions

- Loss of voluntary movements (paralysis)
- Increase in muscle tone (spasticity)
- Exaggerated stretch reflexes (hyper-reflexia)
- Alteration in superficial reflexes
- Absence of muscle atrophy (prolonged disuse of muscles in UMN lesions, give rise to disuse atrophy)
- Electrical reactions of the affected muscles are not altered.

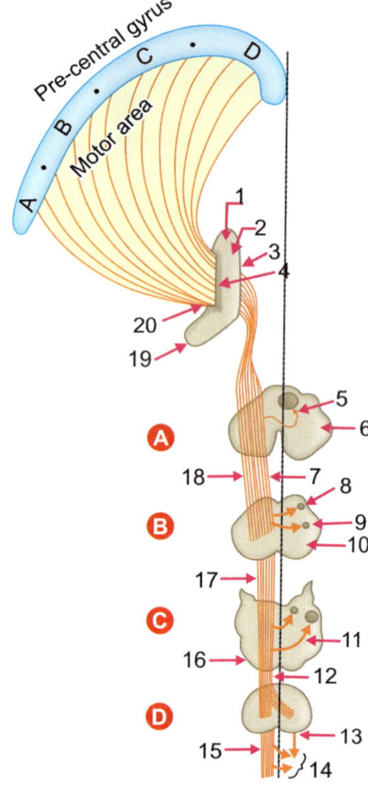

The motor pathways

(A) Midbrain (C) Medulla
(B) Pons (D) Spinal cord

A. Cortical area representing head
B. Cortical area representing upper limb
C. Cortical area representing trunk
D. Cortical area representing lower limb
1. Visual fibres
2. Sensory fibres
3. Posterior limb of internal capsule
Fibres for lower limb in internal capsule
5. Fibres to opposite midbrain nuclei
6. Cerebral peduncle (crus cerebri)
7. Fibres to opposite pontine nuclei
8. 6th nerve nucleus
9. 7th nerve nucleus
10. Ventral aspect of pons
11. Fibres to opposite medullary nuclei
12. Decussation of pyramidal tract
13. Lateral (crossed, indirect) corticospinal tract
14. Corticospinal fibres of direct tract crossing to supply opposite spinal nuclei
15. Anterior (direct) corticospinal tract
16. Medullary pyramid
17. Corticospinal (Pyramidal) tract
18. Fibres for lower limb in pons
19. Anterior limb of internal capsule
20. Fibres for head in internal capsule

312. CSF findings in a patient with tubercular meningitis:

a. Raised protein, normal glucose, increased WBC
b. Raised protein, normal glucose, normal lymphocytes

Ans. 309. c. It is seen in... **310. c.** Hypertension **311. a.** Weakness and... **312. c.** Raised protein...

c. Raised protein, decreased glucose, increased lymphocytes
d. Raised protein, decreased glucose, increased neutrophils

Rise in cells in CSF is called pleocytosis. Lymphocytic pleocytosis occurs in viral, tuberculous and syphilitic meningitis.

CSF findings in TBM
Appearance: Hazy or xanthochromic, presence of cob web formation
Routine analysis: Elevated protein, reduced sugar and lymphocytic pleocytosis
Microbiological techniques: Demonstration of acid-fast bacilli in CSF smears, isolation in solid media such as Lowenstein–Jensen medium
Molecular technique: Polymerase chain reaction (PCR) technique
Immunological techniques: Detection of mycobacterial antibodies, antigens, immune complexes
Radiometric technique: BACTEC technique
Biochemical techniques: Adenosine deaminase, detection of tuberculostearic acid by HPLC

313. All are true regarding cluster headache EXCEPT:
a. Most common in male
b. Periorbital in location
c. Bilateral
d. Symptoms seen in early hours of the morning

Cluster headache/histamine headache/Horton's headache is a migrainous variant. The name 'cluster headache' refers to its occurrence in bouts. The headache starts within 3 hours of falling asleep, it is non-throbbing, unilateral, and orbital in location.

Pain in the head may arise from different structures, which include:
1. The cranial vault consisting of skin, subcutaneous tissue, muscles, arteries, and periosteum of skull;
2. Intracranial venous sinuses and their tributaries;
3. Intracranial arteries before they penetrate brain parenchyma;
4. Meninges at the base of the brain;
5. Trigeminal, glossopharyngeal, vagal, and the first three cervical nerves; and
6. Structures of eye, ear, and nasal cavity.

RESPIRATORY SYSTEM

314. All of the following are true for obstructive lung disease EXCEPT:
a. Low FEV1
b. Increased RV
c. Low TLC
d. Low FEV1/ FVC

Two main components are measured to make the diagnosis: the forced expiratory volume in one second (FEV_1), which is the greatest volume of air that can be breathed out in the first second of a breath, and the forced vital capacity (FVC), which is the greatest volume of air that can be breathed out in a single large breath. Normally, 75–80% of the FVC comes out in the first second and a FEV_1/FVC ratio of less than 70% in someone with symptoms of COPD defines a person as having the disease. Lung volumes show an increase in TLC (total lung capacity) and residual volume/ RV due to gas trapping.

315. Typical pneumonia is associated with all EXCEPT:
a. Staph. aureus
b. Strept. pneumoniae
c. Chlamydia pneumoniae
d. H. influenzae

Atypical pneumonia can have a bacterial (mycoplasma, Chlamydia, coxiella), fungal, protozoan or viral cause

316. All of the following drugs are indicated in early management of chronic persistent asthma EXCEPT:
a. Inhaled high dose steroids
b. Long acting beta 2 agonist LABA
c. Oral corticosteroids
d. Short acting beta 2 agonist/ SABA

Management of chronic persistent asthma
- Step 1: Occasional use of inhaled SABA bronchodilators
- Regular inhaled anti-inflammatory agents
- High dose inhaled corticosteroids, or low dose inhaled corticosteroids plus a inhaled LABA
- High dose inhaled corticosteroids and regular bronchodilators
- Addition of regular oral corticosteroid therapy

317. A 65 year lady had a fall and sustained fracture shaft of femur. She was planned for operative intervention. But she collapsed after surgery. What could be the most probable cause:
a. Calf vein thrombosis
b. Pulmonary embolism
c. MI
d. Refracture

Symptoms of pulmonary embolism include difficulty breathing, chest pain on inspiration, and palpitations. Clinical signs include low blood oxygen saturation and cyanosis, rapid breathing, and a rapid heart rate. Severe cases of PE can lead to collapse, abnormally low blood pressure, and sudden death. Prolonged surgeries are a risk factor for development of DVT & subsequent PE.

318. A 60-year-old men was suffering from severe osteoarthritis in both the knees. He underwent total knee replacement surgery. After operation, he started complaining of calf pain & swelling in leg. 2 days later, she developed breathlessness & collapsed suddenly. Most likely cause of death:
a. Pulmonary embolism/ PE
b. MI
c. Stroke
d. ARDS

Ans. **313. c.** Bilateral **314. c.** Low TLC **315. c.** Chlamydia... **316. c.** Oral corticosteroids **317. b.** Pulmonary... **318. a.** Pulmonary embolism

Causes of PE (& deep venous thrombosis)

- Alterations in blood flow: immobilization (after surgery, injury, pregnancy (also procoagulant), obesity (also procoagulant), cancer (also procoagulant)
- Factors in the vessel wall: surgery, catheterizations causing direct injury ("endothelial injury")
- Factors affecting the properties of the blood (procoagulant state):
  - Estrogen-containing hormonal contraception
  - Genetic thrombophilia (factor V Leiden, prothrombin mutation G20210A, protein C deficiency, protein S deficiency, antithrombin deficiency, hyperhomocysteinemia and plasminogen/ fibrinolysis disorders)
  - Acquired thrombophilia (antiphospholipid syndrome, nephrotic syndrome, paroxysmal nocturnal hemoglobinuria)
  - Cancer (due to secretion of pro-coagulants)

319. What could be the most probable diagnosis of a 65-years-old patient with hemoptysis and stage III clubbing:

a. Sarcoidosis b. TB
c. Small cell Ca of lung/SCLC
d. Non small cell Ca of lung/NSCLC

Clubbing and hypertrophic pulmonary osteoarthropathy and Trousseau syndrome of hypercoagulability are caused more frequently by adenocarcinomas. Central tumors are generally squamous cell carcinomas (SCCs) and produce cough, dyspnea, atelectasis, postobstructive pneumonia, wheezing, and hemoptysis. (SCC & adenocarcinoma comes under NSCLC). None of the patients with clubbing and hypertrophic pulmonary osteoarthropathy had oat cell/ small cell Ca

320. Worst prognosis in lung cancer:

a. Small cell carcinoma b. Adenocarcinoma
c. Squamous cell carcinoma
d. All of the above

Two year survival rate is about 30% in cases with limited spread in small cell lung carcinoma/SCLC, whereas it is below 10% in more advanced cases. SCLC – the median survival without treatment is 6 to 8 weeks for limited disease. At presentation less than 30% have limited disease.

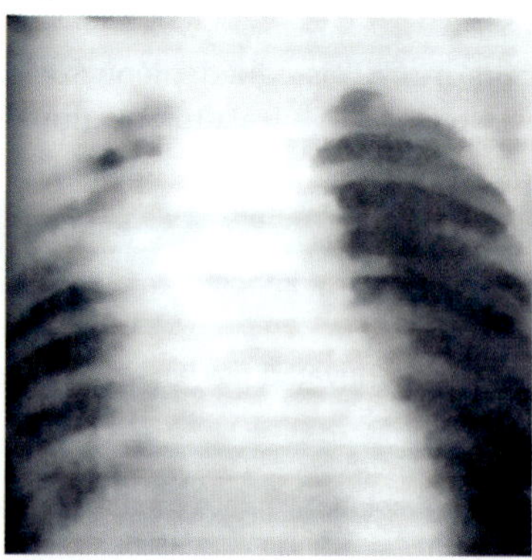

X-ray chest—carcinoma lung. Note: The mass with hazy margins extending outwards from the right border of the mediastinum

321. Cyanosis can NOT occur in severe anemia because:

a. Anemic blood has higher oxygen carrying capacity per gram of hemoglobin
b. It requires a critical concentration of reduced hemoglobin in blood
c. Patient improves his alveolar oxygen as a compensation for anemia
d. There is an increased blood flow through the skin

Bluish discoloration of the skin and mucous membranes due to the presence of excess of reduced hemoglobin in peripheral blood is called cyanosis.

322. In restrictive lung disease:

a. FVC is high b. FEV1 is high
c. FEV1/ FVC is high d. All of the above

Restrictive lung disease/restrictive ventilator defects are a category of extrapulmonary, pleural or parenchymal respiratory diseases that restrict lung expansion, result in a decreased lung volume, an increased work of breathing, and inadequate ventilation and/or oxygenation. Pulmonary function test demonstrates a decrease in the forced vital capacity.

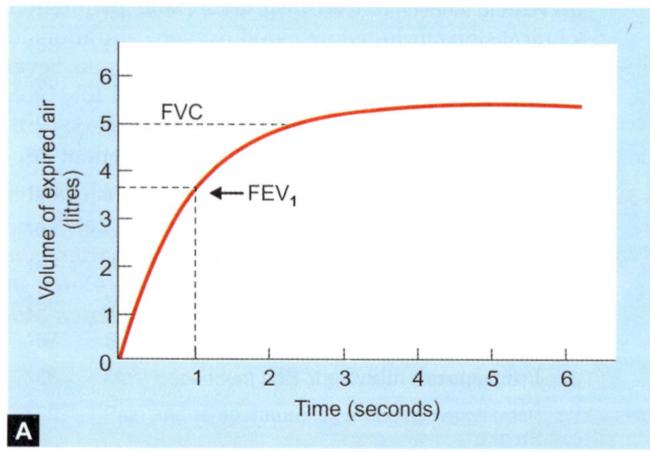

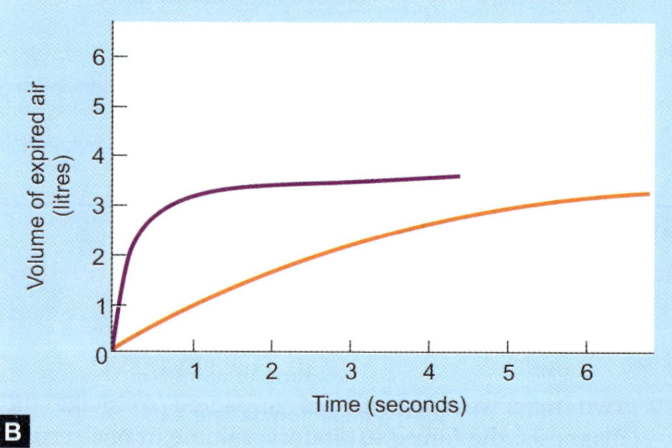

Volume-time curves obtained during forced expiration (A) Normal (B) Restrictive and obstructive lung diseases

Ans. **319. d.** Non small cell... **320. a.** Small cell carcinoma **321. b.** It requires a... **322. c.** FEV1/ FVC is high

323. Most likely cause of bihilar lymphadenopathy is:

a. Histoplasmosis b. TB
c. Sarcoidosis d. Aspergillosis

The commonest presentation of the sarcoidosis is as bilateral hilar lymphadenopathy with associated fever and erythema nodosum.

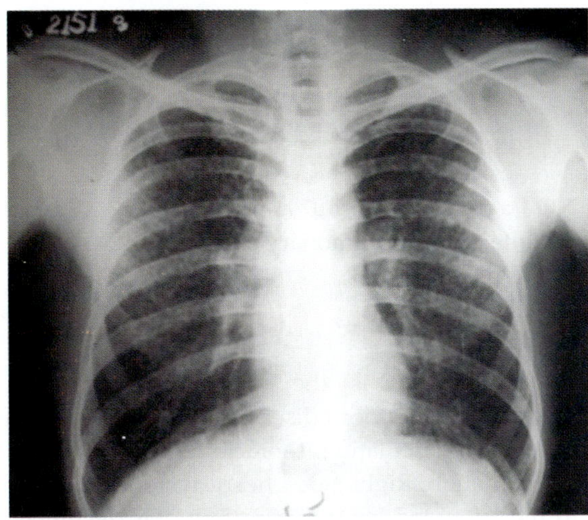

X-ray chest sarcoidosis. Note: Bilateral hilar adenopathy with miliary lesions

324. MC cause of hemoptysis:

a. Mitral stenosis b. Bronchiectasis
c. Pulmonary TB d. Bronchogenic Ca

Hemoptysis is present in many cases of bronchogenic carcinoma and the sputum is typically described as "currant jelly". Malignant cells may be detected in the sputum by examining a wet preparation with methylene blue staining and this can be confirmed by Papanicolaou's method.

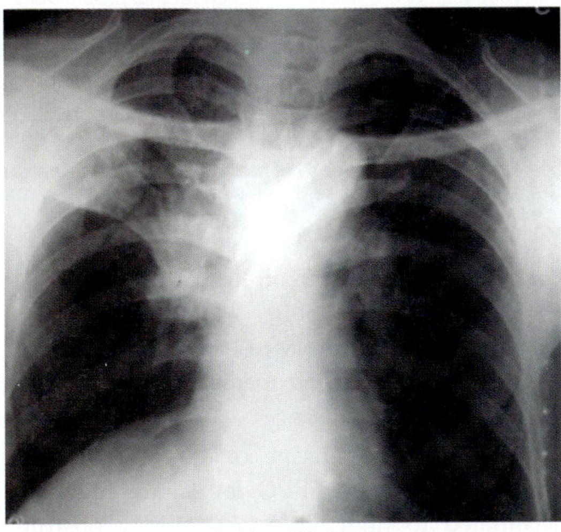

Golden 'S' sign

325. NOT a feature of pulmonary embolism:

a. Neck vein distension b. Hypertension
c. Tachypnea d. Dyspnea

Pulmonary Embolism

Symptoms	Sign
Dyspnea	Tachycardia
Cough	Tachypnea
Substernal chest pain	Crackles
Sweating	Wheezes
Syncope	JVP elevated
Hemoptysis	Right ventricular gallop
Later pleuritic chest pain	Loud pulmonic second sound

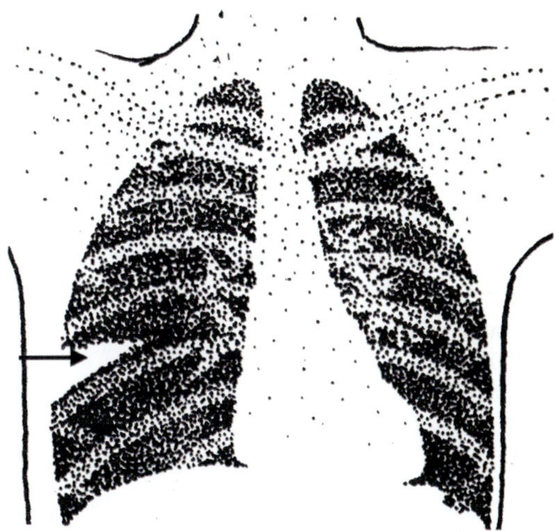

X-ray chest: Pulmonary infarct. Note: The triangular opacity with the base towards the pleura

326. NOT a cause of type-II respiratory failure:

a. Respiratory distress syndrome
b. COPD with emphysema
c. GB syndrome
d. Kyphoscoliosis

Type I respiratory failure is characterized by lowered PaO_2 and normal or low $PaCO_2$. This is usually the result of conditions in which ventilation is normal, but there is defective diffusion or ventilation-perfusion imbalance. Conditions like pulmonary edema, respiratory distress syndrome, extrinsic allergic alveolitis and interstitial pulmonary fibrosis lead to type I respiratory failure.

Causes of respiratory failure	
1. *Interference with the mechanics of the chest wall*	Severe kyphoscoliosis, obesity, flail chest injury with multiple rib fractures, paralysis of the chest wall muscles and diaphragm, immobility of the chest wall as in progressive systemic sclerosis
2. *Pleural disorders*	Large collection of pleural fluid, tension pneumothorax, gross thickening of the pleura and others
3. *Diseases of the airways*	Severe asthma, advanced chronic bronchitis and emphysema, laryngeal edema, mechanical obstruction of air passages

Contd...

Ans. 323. **c.** Sarcoidosis 324. **d.** Bronchogenic Ca 325. **b.** Hypertension 326. **a.** Respiratory distress...

Contd...

Causes of respiratory failure	
4. *Pulmonary diseases*	Pulmonary interstitial fibrosis, neonatal and adult respiratory distress syndrome, allergic alveolitis, extensive malignancy, bilateral pneumonia
5. *Diseases of pulmonary vasculature*	Primary pulmonary hypertension, polyarteritis nodosa, repeated pulmonary embolism
6. *Metabolic*	Metabolic alkalosis
7. Depression of the respiratory centre	Injury to brainstem, raised intracranial tension and narcotic poisoning lead to central respiratory failure

327. Minimum air required to produce air embolism:
a. 50 mL
b. 100 mL
c. 150 mL
d. 200 mL

Human case reports suggest that injecting more than 100 mL of air into the venous system at rates greater than 100 mL/s can be fatal.

328. Caplan's syndrome is a manifestation of:
a. RA b. SLE
c. Both d. None

Caplan's syndrome is a special phenomenon occurring in subjects with rheumatoid disease who develop pneumoconiosis. Large coalescing nodules develop in the lungs. These are demonstrable by X-rays.

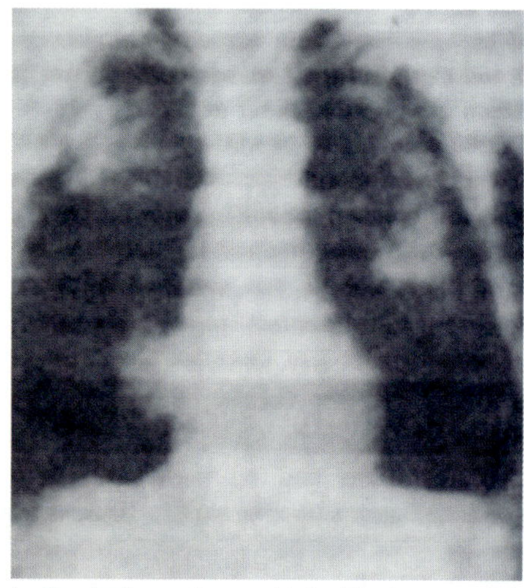

X-ray chest—Caplan's syndrome. Note: The large nodular shadows

329. NOT an indication for ICU admission of a bronchial asthma patient:
a. $PaCO_2$ more than 40 mm Hg
b. PaO_2 less than 60 mm Hg
c. Prolonged wheeze
d. Confusion

If the condition in an asthmatic patient does not respond to treatment or the respiratory embarrassment is increasing, ventilation should be assisted.

1. Pulses paradoxus
2. Central cyanosis despite O_2 inhalation
3. Deterioration of arterial blood gases despite treatment a. PaO_2 < 60 mm Hg (8 kPa) and falling b. $PaCO_2$ > 40 mm Hg (6 kPa) and rising c. pH of 7.3 and falling
4. Extreme physical exhaustion
5. Clouding of consciousness, confusion, drowsiness
6. Coma, and
7. Respiratory arrest

330. NOT a cause of Cor pulmonale:
a. Intermittent pulmonary embolism
b. Kyphoscoliosis
c. COPD
d. Mitral stenosis

Cor pulmonale is the enlargement of the right ventricle secondary to disease of the lung parenchyma, pulmonary circulation, thoracic cage or the mechanics of ventilation. Right-sided heart dysfunction secondary to the left-sided heart failure, valvular dysfunction, or congenital heart disease is excluded in the definition of cor pulmonale.

Causes
1. *Diseases of the lung parenchyma:* a. Chronic obstructive pulmonary diseases—emphysema, chronic bronchitis, bronchial asthma. b. Restrictive lung diseases—diffuse interstitial fibrosis, pulmonary hemosiderosis, radiation fibrosis, scleroderma. c. Pneumoconiosis. d. Bronchiectasis and cystic disease of the lungs.
2. *Diseases of the chest wall which restrict proper ventilation.* 3. *Diseases affecting the pulmonary arteries or veins:* Primary pulmonary hypertension, pulmonary arteritis, veno-occlusive disease, schistosomiasis, recurrent thromboembolism, sickle cell anemia. For example kyphoscoliosis, myopathies, myasthenia gravis, and extreme obesity.
4. *Diseases which depress the respiratory center resulting in diminution of the respiratory drive.*
5. *Chronic mountain sickness.*

331. Earliest change noticed on high altitude:
a. Increased hemoglobin
b. Increased inspiratory reserve
c. Increased diffusion capacity
d. Increased 2,3 DPG

Conditions of low tissue oxygen concentration such as high altitude (2,3-BPG levels are higher in those acclimated to high altitudes), airway obstruction, or congestive heart failure will tend to cause RBCs to generate more 2,3-BPG in their effort to generate energy by allowing more oxygen to be released in tissues, deprived of oxygen.

Ans. **327. b.** 100 mL **328. a.** RA **329. c.** Prolonged wheeze **330. d.** Mitral stenosis **331. d.** Increased 2,3 DPG

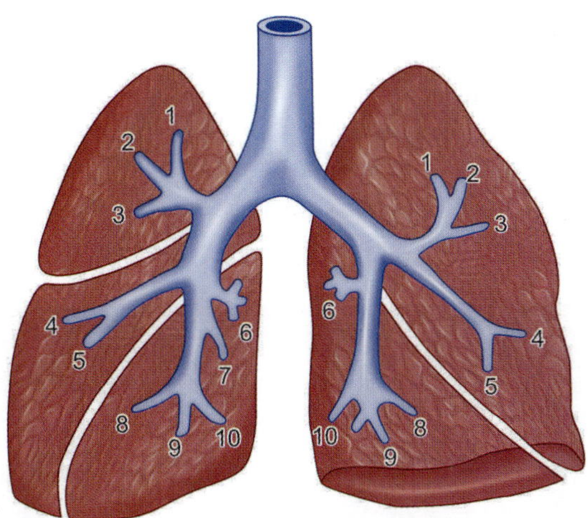

Divisions of bronchi

Right upper lobe	Left upper lobe
1. Apical	1. Apical
2. Posterior	2. Posterior
3. Anterior	3. Anterior
Right middle lobe	Lingular lobe
4. Lateral	4. Superior
5. Medial	5. Inferior
Right lower lobe	Left lower lobe
6. Apical lower lobe	6. Apical lower lobe
7. Medial basal	——
8. Anterior basal	8. Anterior basal
9. Lateral basal	9. Lateral basal
10. Posterior basal	10. Posterior basal

332. In type-II respiratory failure, there is:

a. Low PO_2, low PCO_2 b. Low PO_2, high PCO_2
c. Normal PO_2, high PCO_2 d. Low PO_2, normal PCO_2

In type-II respiratory failure, PaO_2 is reduced and $PaCO_2$ is elevated. Hypoxia is the more prominent feature. This results from conditions characterized by defective ventilation occurring along with ventilation-perfusion imbalance. Alveolar hypoventilation occurs in chronic bronchitis, emphysema, asthma and respiratory paralysis.

333. A patient presents with acute respiratory distress, stridor and unability to speak. Likely diagnosis is:

a. Asthma b. Aspiration pneumonia
c. Foreign body aspiration d. Pleural effusion

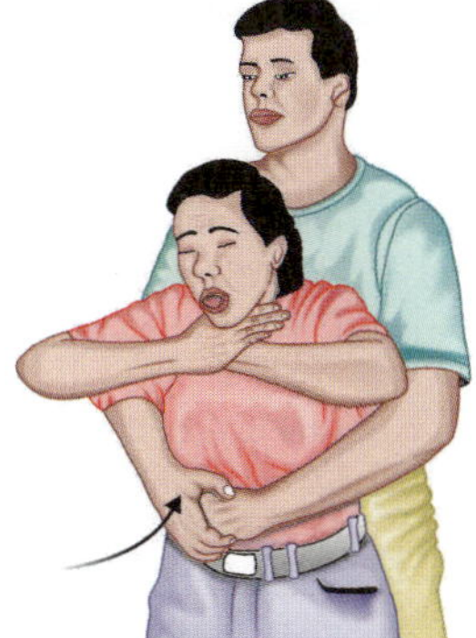

Heimlich maneuver. Application of sudden pressure over the abdomino-thoracic region may dislodge the laryngeal foreign body

Stridor, aphonia, and dyspnea are the hallmarks of laryngeal obstruction.

334. A 60-year-old patient, who has been on bed rest for the past 10 days, complains of breathlessness and chest pain. Chest X-ray is normal. Next investigation would be:

a. Lung ventilation – perfusion scan
b. Pulmonary arteriography
c. Pulmonary venous angiography
d. Echocardiography

Acute massive pulmonary embolism manifests with sudden dyspnea, angina pain, hemoptysis and circulatory collapse in a patient who is apparently well and progressing from other underlying disorders. Isotope lung scan is a useful investigation to demonstrate segmental perfusion defects.

Scintiscan pulmonary embolism. Note: The isotope does not reach the affected side (left side)

335. MC causative agent for lobar pneumonia is:

a. Staphylococcus aureus b. Streptococcus pyogenes
c. Streptococcus pneumonia
d. Haemophilus influenza

50-80% of cases of community acquired pneumonia are caused by pneumococcus.

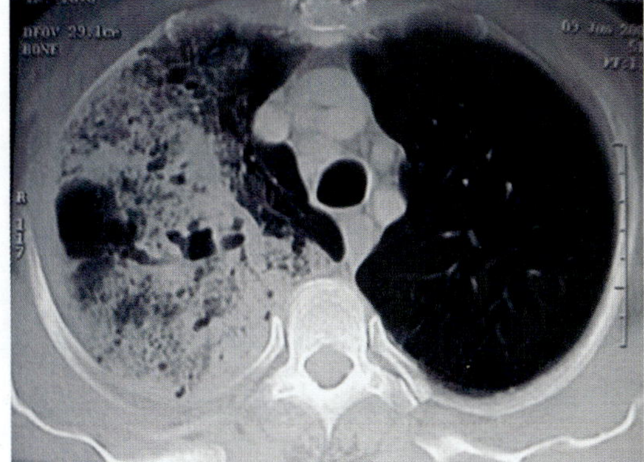

HRCT Pneumococcal Pneumonia Note the dense consolidation and air spaces in between

Ans. 332. **b.** Low pO_2, high... 333. **c.** Foreign body... 334. **a.** Lung ventilation... 335. **c.** Streptococcus pneumonia

336. **NOT a pulmonary function test abnormality of interstitial lung disease:**
a. Reduced total lung capacity
b. Reduced diffusion capacity
c. Reduced FEV1/ FVC ratio
d. Reduced vital capacity

Interstitial fibrosis is the end result of interstitial lung diseases. Pulmonary function test will show restrictive pattern, usually decreased vital capacity.

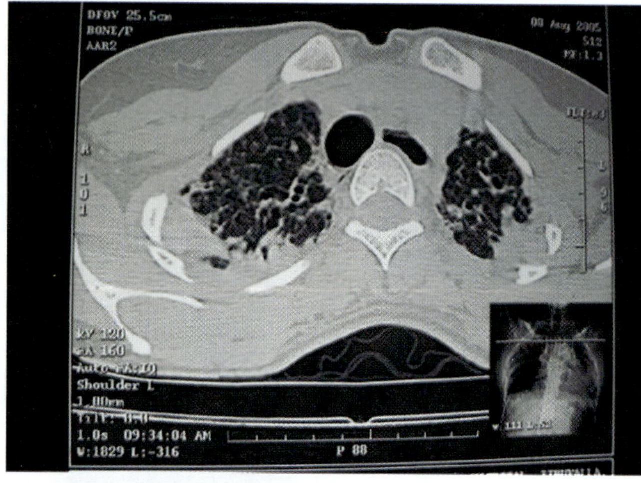

HRCT of pulmonary interstitial fibrosis. Note: The thickening of interalveolar septa

337. **Which organ should be imaged in suspected cases of bronchogenic carcinoma:**
a. Pancreas
b. Spleen
c. Kidneys
d. Adrenals

Widespread secondaries may occur in cases of bronchogenic carcinoma in the liver, bone, adrenal glands, brain, kidney, spleen, peritoneum, skin, and other organ.

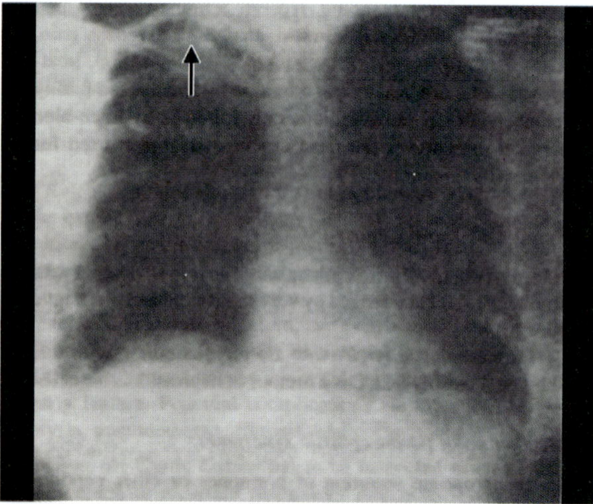

Pancoast's tumor. Note: The rounded opacity in the right upper region—arrowhead

338. **Lung carcinoma, associated with SIADH:**
a. Oat cell carcinoma
b. Transitional cell carcinoma
c. Adenocarcinoma
d. Squamous carcinoma

Paraneoplastic syndromes are more common with Small Cell Lung Ca/ Oat-cell Ca. Possibly SCLC is a tumor of neuroendocrine cells.

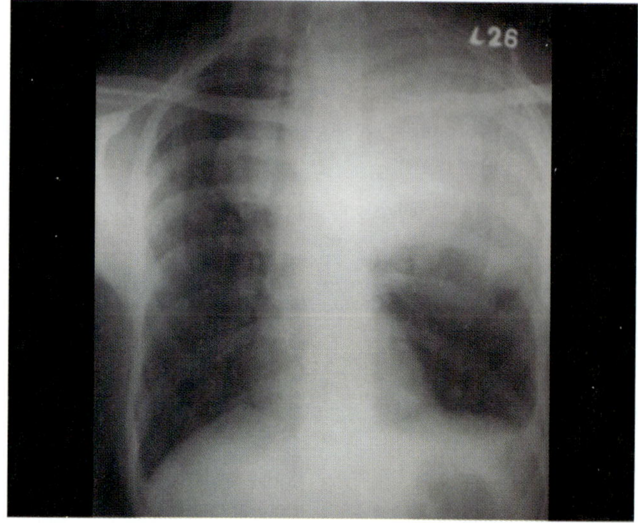

X-ray chest. Bronchogenic carcinoma. Note: Tumor with bilateral massive lymph node metastases

339. **In an asthmatic patient, inhaling a bronchodilator will show a greatest improvement in:**
a. FVC
b. FEF
c. FEV1
d. Tidal volume

Objective assessment of the severity of airways obstruction and response to bronchodilator therapy can be made by use of bedside peak flow meter. Respiratory function tests reveal gross reduction in FEV1, FEV1/FVC ratio and peak expiratory flow rate (PEFR) and increase in the time taken for forced expiration.

Levels of severity of acute asthma exacerbations	
Brittle asthma	Wide PEF variability despite intense therapy. Sudden severe attacks on a background of well controlled asthma
Moderate asthma exacerbation	Increasing symptoms PEF >50-75% of best predicted value None of the features of acute severe asthma
Acute severe asthma	Any one of the following: ❑ PEF 33-50% of best/predicted ❑ Respiratory rate > 25/min ❑ Heart rate > 110/min ❑ Inability to complete sentences in one breath

Contd...

Ans. **336. c.** Reduced FEV1... **337. d.** Adrenals **338. a.** Oat cell carcinoma **339. d.** Tidal volume

Contd...

Levels of severity of acute asthma exacerbations	
Life-threatening asthma	Any of the following in a patient with acute severe asthma ❑ PEF < 33% of best/predicted, PEF not recordable ❑ SPO_2 < 92%
	❑ Central cyanosis ❑ PaO_2 < 8 kPa (60 mm Hg), especially on oxygen ❑ $PaCO_2$ Normal (4.6-6.0 kPa) ❑ Low pH Silent chest, bradycardia, feeble respiratory efforts, dysrhythmia, hypotension, exhaustion, confusion and coma
Near fatal asthma	Raised $PaCO_2$ and/or requiring mechanical ventilation

340. True regarding asthma:

a. Increased FRC, increased residual volume
b. Increased FRC, decreased residual volume
c. Decreased FRC, decreased residual volume
d. Decreased FRC, increased residual volume

Lung volume and capacities

- Residual volume: Volume of gas still remaining in the lungs after maximal expiration.
- Functional residual capacity: Volume of gas remaining in the lung at the end of tidal expiration.

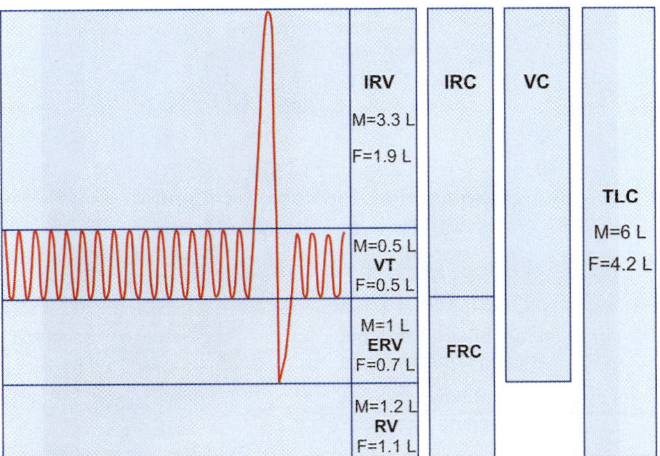

Static lung volumes. IRV, inspiratory reserve volume; VT, tidal volume; ERV, expiratory reserve volume; RV, residual volume; IRC, inspiratory reserve capacity; FRC, functional reserve capacity; VC vital capacity; RLC, total lung capacity

341. FEV1/ FVC value below 70 is suggestive of:

a. Pulmonary edema
b. Acute interstitial pneumonia
c. Severe pectus excavatum d. Pulmonary emphysema

Chronic bronchitis emphysema syndrome which is mainly due to narrowing of the airways is diagnosed when: FEV1 is <80% of the predicted value and the FEV1/FVC or FEV1/vital capacity is <70%.

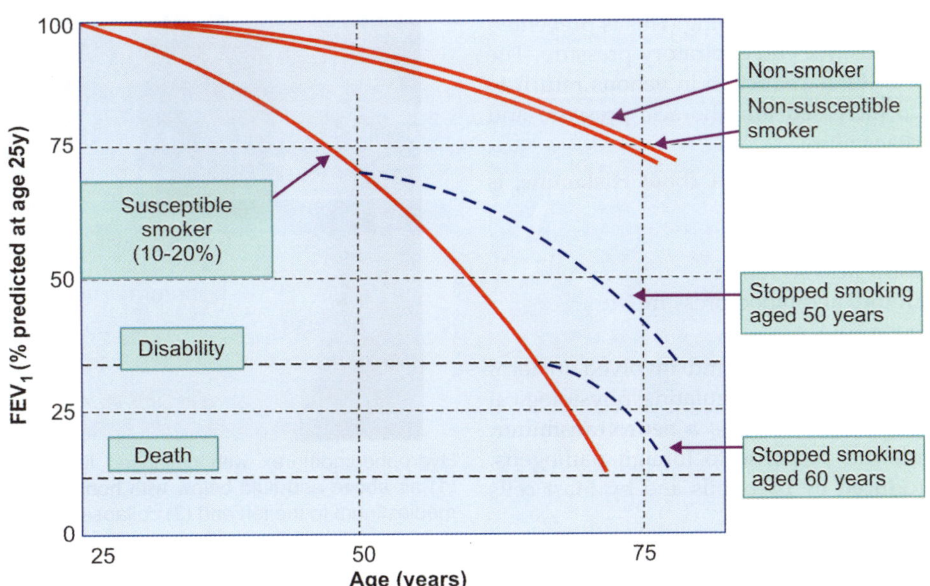

Annual decline in lung function. Note the relation between decline in FEV_1 in the normals (non-smokers) and smokers. Rate of decline in FEV_1 is many times higher in smokers. Note also the improvement in FEV1 on stopping smoking

342. NOT a cause of clubbing of fingers:

a. Congenital
b. Cirrhosis
c. Chronic interstitial lung disease
d. Acute pneumonia

Digital clubbing (Syn: Hippocratic fingers) is caused by increase in the volume of soft tissues in and around the distal phalanges of the fingers and toes, especially the nailbeds. This leads to increased curvature of the nails.

Ans. 340. a. Increased FRC... **341. d.** Pulmonary... **342. d.** Acute pneumonia

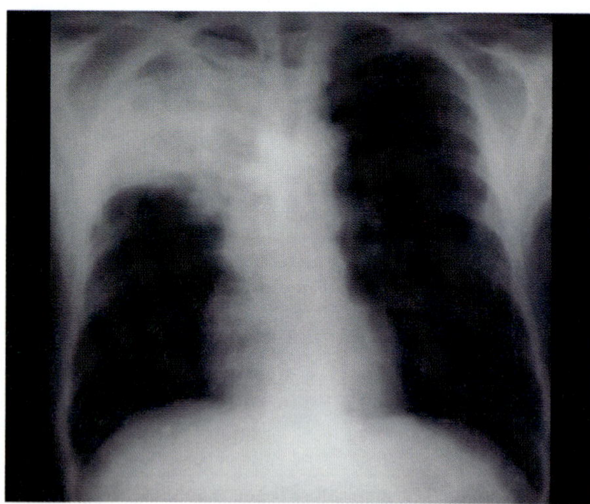

X-ray chest showing lobar pneumonia Note: the consolidation of the upper zone right lung uniform opacity with clearcut margins, midline structures not shifted

343. All are true about PEEP (positive end-expiratory pressure) EXCEPT:

a. Useful in situations where PO_2 is low
b. Increased venous return
c. Improved tidal respiration
d. Reopens bronchioles

One of the problems encountered in patients with respiratory failure maintained on assisted respiration is premature closure of the terminal airways during expiration, giving rise to air trapping. This is prevented by maintaining a positive end expiratory pressure. The disadvantage of PEEP is reduction in venous return to the heart due to increased intrathoracic pressure and consequent cardiac failure.

344. Which of the following statement about Histamine, is true:

a. Is found in Mast cells
b. Increases gastric acid secretion
c. Related to arousal and blood pressure
d. All of the above

Histamine is an organic compound involved in local immune responses as well as regulating physiological function in the gut and acting as a neurotransmitter. As a part of immune response to foreign pathogens, histamine is produced by basophils and by mast cells found in nearby connective tissue.

345. The following drugs can be used for the management of status asthmaticus EXCEPT:

a. Magnesium sulphate b. Montelukast
c. Corticosteroid d. Adrenaline

Leukotriene receptor antagonist (Monteleukast) is indicated as add-on therapy in mild to moderate asthma, which is not adequately controlled with an inhaled corticosteroid and a short acting beta-2 stimulant used as required. It reduces the dose of inhaled steroids in moderate to severe asthma. It may also be used to prevent exercise or drug induced asthma (e.g. aspirin-sensitive asthma).

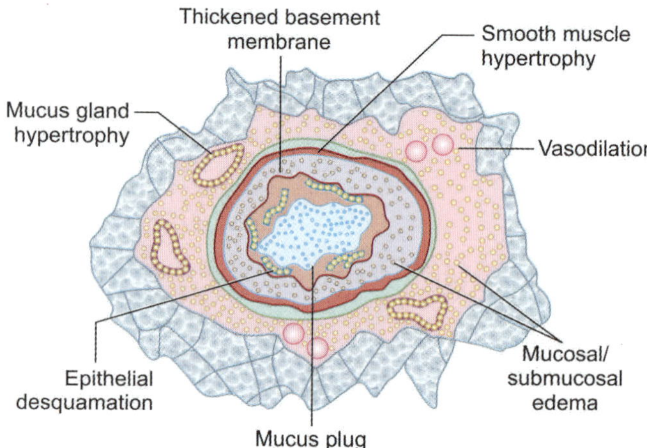

Pathological features of asthma

346. NOT a feature of pleural effusion:

a. Horizontal fluid level
b. Low lung volume
c. Muffled heart sounds
d. Decreased chest movements

Chest radiograph of a case of hydropenumothorax reveals a horizontal upper level of fluid with the findings of pneumothorax above it.

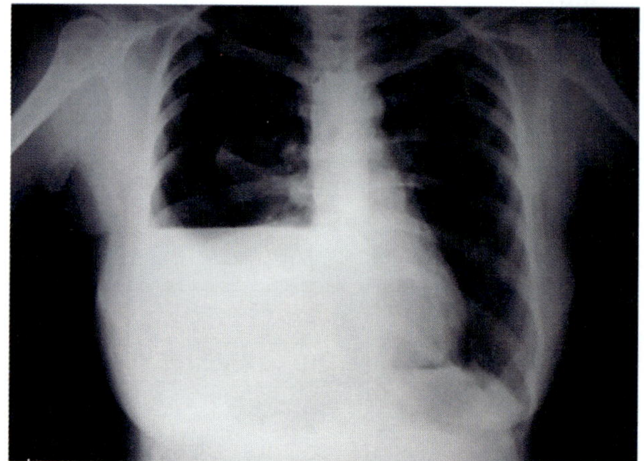

Hydropneumothorax with collapsed lung. Note: On the right side (1) air above and fluid below with horizontal level of fluid (2) shift of mediastinum to the left and (3) collapsed lung on the right hilum

347. Criteria for acute respiratory distress syndrome inlcude:

a. PaO_2/FiO_2 ratio is </= 100
b. PaO_2/FiO_2 ratio is </= 200
c. PaO_2/FiO_2 ratio is </= 300
d. PaO_2/FiO_2 ratio is </= 400

Diagnostic criteria for ARDS

- Acute onset of respiratory failure
- PaO_2/FiO_2: <300 mm Hg = acute lung injury (ALI)

Ans. 343. **b.** Increased venous 344. **d.** All of the above 345. **b.** Montelukast 346. **a.** Horizontal fluid level
347. **b.** PaO_2/FiO_2 ratio...

- PaO_2/FiO_2: <200 mm Hg = acute respiratory distress syndrome (ARDS)
- Chest radiograph: Bilateral alveolar infiltrates consistent with pulmonary edema
- Pulmonary capillary wedge pressure <18 mm Hg

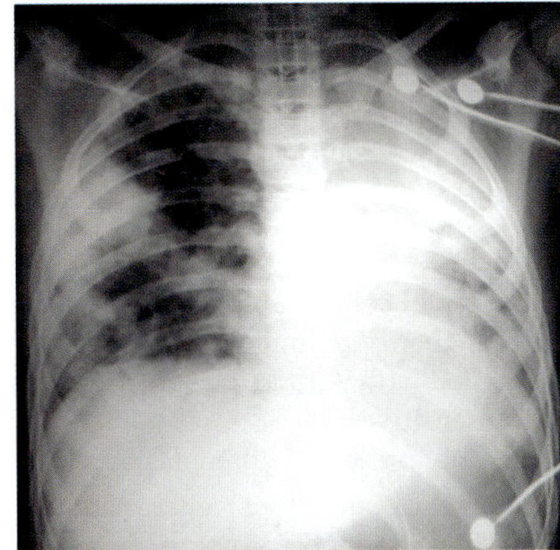

X-ray chest shows bilateral alveolar infiltrate consistent with pulmonary edema

348. Fever persisting even after treatment of pneumonia is most likely due to:

a. Empyema b. Fungal lesion
c. Hydrothorax d. All of the above

Collection of pus in the pleural cavity is called empyema. Empyema may result from the extension of infection from the underlying lung, or it may complicate chest injuries, thoracocentesis, or generalized pyemia. Pneumonia, lung abscess, bronchiectasis, tuberculous cavities, hepatopulmonary amebiasis, bronchogenic carcinoma, osteomyelitis of the ribs, fungal infections and actinomycosis are all important causes. Onset is marked by high fever, pleuritic or dull chest pain and dry cough.

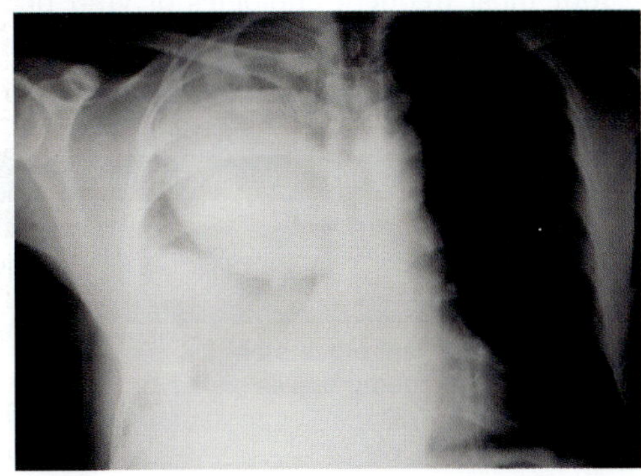

X-ray chest multiple encysted empyema right. Note: Multiple well defined rounded shadows

349. The most predictive and dangerous side effect of propranolol that makes it to be avoided in a patient of COPD is induction of:

a. Respiratory failure b. Acute asthmatic attack
c. Glaucoma d. Pleural effusion

Contraindications of beta-blockers

- Bronchospasm, asthma
- Symptomatic bradycardia with heart rate below 60/minute
- Higher grade of blocks in patients who have no implanted pacemakers
- Patients on IV inotropic support
- Acutely ill patients

350. Alpha 1 antitrypsin deficiency is associated with:

a. Centriacinar emphysema b. Panacinar emphysema
c. Irregular emphysema d. Paraseptal emphysema

Persons who have alpha-1 antitrypsin/AAT deficiency develop panacinar emphysema by the third or fourth decade of life. AAT deficiency can be treated by replacing AAT by IV infusion weekly or monthly to individuals whose serum AAT levels are below 1 mmol/L and who have abnormal lung function.

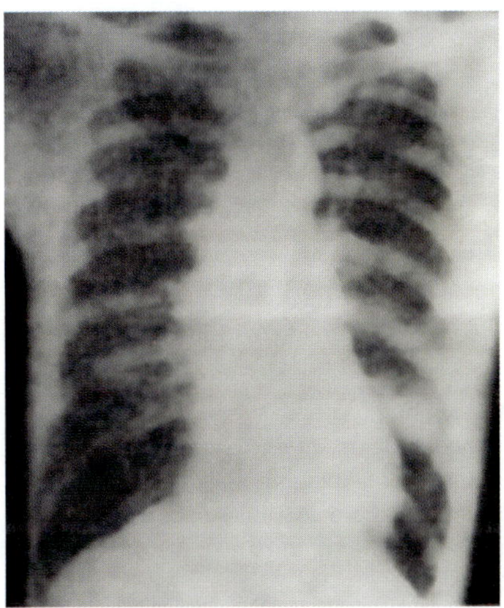

X-ray chest—Emphysema. Note: The inflated position of the rib cage, lower level of the diaphragm and hypertranslucent lung fields

351. NOT a cause of transudative pleural effusion:

a. Nephrotic syndrome
b. Rheumatoid arthritis
c. Constrictive pericarditis
d. Pulmonary embolism

Recurrent pleural effusion (exudative) may occur in RA, which is usually unilateral.

Types of Pleural Effusion – Transudate and Exudate

Cause of Transudate Pleural Effusion	*Cause of Exudate Pleural Effusion*
LVF	Tuberculosis
Cirrhosis	Parapneumonic
Nephrotic syndrome	Malignancy (primary and metastatic)
Hypoalbuminemia	Collagen vascular diseases
Hypothyroidism	RHD disease, SLE, Churg-Strauss syndrome

Contd...

Ans. 348. a. Empyema 349. b. Acute asthmatic... 350. b. Panacinar... 351. b. Rheumatoid arthritis

Contd...

Cause of Transudate Pleural Effusion	*Cause of Exudate Pleural Effusion*
Pulmonary embolism	Post-myocardial infarction syndrome
Meig's syndrome	Pulmonary infarction
Peritoneal dialysis	Pancreatitis Pseudopancreatic cyst Esophageal rupture Drugs Chylothorax, Pseudochylothorax

352. Rasmussen aneurysm involves:

a. Posterior intercostal artery
b. Vertebral artery
c. Pulmonary artery
d. Bronchial artery

Rasmussen aneurysm is an uncommon complication of pulmonary tuberculosis and represents a pulmonary artery aneurysm adjacent or within a tuberculous cavity.

Early: **Occurring within months**
1. Mild hemoptysis 2. Pneumothorax 3. Pleural effusion 4. Poncet's syndrome
Intermediate: **Occurring within several months or a** few years
1. Massive hemoptysis 2. Secondary infection of cavities 3. Pneumothorax, pleural effusion, empyema 4. Progressive fibrosis with dyspnea 5. Spread to other organs such as larynx, pericardium and others 6. Non-healing of lesion due to drug resistance of organisms.
Late: **Occurring after several years.**
1. Pulmonary fibrosis with compensatory emphysema, cor pulmonale, pleuropulmonary fibrosis. 2. Bronchiectasis 3. Persistence of open cavities without healing 4. Aspergilloma i.e., growth of *Aspergillus fumigatus* in the cavities in the form of a fungus ball 5. *Coexistence of apical tuberculosis with carcinoma* 6 Secondary amyloidosis.

353. Farmers lung is due to:

a. Cryptostroma corticale
b. Aspergillus
c. Thermophilic actinomycetes
d. Grain duct

While inhaled allergens often provoke the creation of IgE antibodies (in farmer's lung) that circulate in the blood stream, these types of immune responses are most often initiated by exposure to thermophilic actinomycetes (most commonly Saccharopolyspora rectivirgula), which generates IgG-type antibodies.

Some common types of bronchioloalveolitis

Condition	*Source*
Farmer's lung	Mouldy hay, straw, grain dust
Bagassosis	Sugarcane dust
Byssinosis	Cotton dust
Mushroom worker's lung	Mushroom compost
Malt-worker's lung	Mouldy barley, malt dust
Maple bark stripper's lung	Mouldy bark
Bird fanciers' lung	Bird's droppings
Cheese worker's lung	Mouldy cheese

354. FALSE for small cell Ca of lung:

a. MC malignancy of lung
b. Associated with paraneoplastic syndromes
c. Chemosensitive
d. Commonly presents with metastasis to bone

The incidence of squamous cell carcinoma is coming down and that of adenocarcinoma is going up.

World Health Organisation (WHO) classification of malignant tumors of the lungs

Type	*Frequency*
Squamous cell (epidermoid)	30%
Small cell carcinoma	20
Adenocarcinoma	25
Large cell carcinoma (anaplastic)	10-15
Adenosquamous carcinoma Carcinoid tumor	
Bronchial gland tumors *Others*	

355. Virus causing pneumonia are all EXCEPT:

a. RSV
b. Adenovirus
c. Influenza virus
d. None

The four most frequent etiologies of viral pneumonia in children and immunocompetent adults are influenza virus, respiratory syncytial virus (RSV), adenovirus, and parainfluenza virus (PIV).

Causes of community acquired pneumonia

Organism	*Frequency %*
1. Pneumococcus	50-80
2. Aerobic gram-negative bacilli	3-11
3. *Kl. pneumoniae*	2-6
4. *Staph.aureus*	1-10
5. Mixed anaerobes	2-12
6. *Mycoplasma pneumoniae*	3-44
	(in young adults)
7. *Hemophilus influenzae*	2.5-15
8. Viral-influenza A and B, parainfluenza, adenovirus,	1-16
9. *Strep. pyogenes*	1

Ans. **352. c.** Pulmonary... **353. c.** Thermophilic... **354. a.** MC malignancy... **355. d.** None

356. **Shrinking lung is seen in:**
a. Scleroderma b. Rheumatoid arthritis
c. SLE d. Dermatomyositis

A syndrome of shrinking lung is uncommon but virtually pathognomonic of SLE. It is characterized by progressive reduction in lung volume with evidence of diaphragmatic weakness.

Presentation of SLE	Frequency (%)
Arthralgia/arthritis	70-90%
Fever	50%
Cutaneous rashes	50-80%
Malar rash	40%
Lymph node involvement	40%
Renal lesions	45-65%
Neuropsychiatric symptoms	35-40%
Cardiac lesions	30%
Pleuropulmonary lesions	20-25%
Hepatosplenomegaly	20-25%
Discoid lupus	10%
Ocular lesions	10%

357. **All of the following conditions are associated with clubbing EXCEPT:**
a. Bronchogenic carcinoma
b. Chronic bronchitis
c. Empyema
d. Bronchiectasis

Suppurative lesions like bronchiectasis, lung abscess, empyema, and infected cysts; advanced tuberculosis with bronchiectatic changes, bronchogenic carcinoma, pneumoconiosis, fibrosing alveolitis, and pleural fibroma, all are respiratory causes of clubbing.

358. **Paradoxical breathing is seen in:**
a. Severe left ventricular failure
b. Flail chest
c. Metabolic acidosis
d. COPD

Flail chest results when ribs are fractured in two places. The fractured segment of the thoracic wall floats independently of the rest of the chest wall and moves paradoxically.

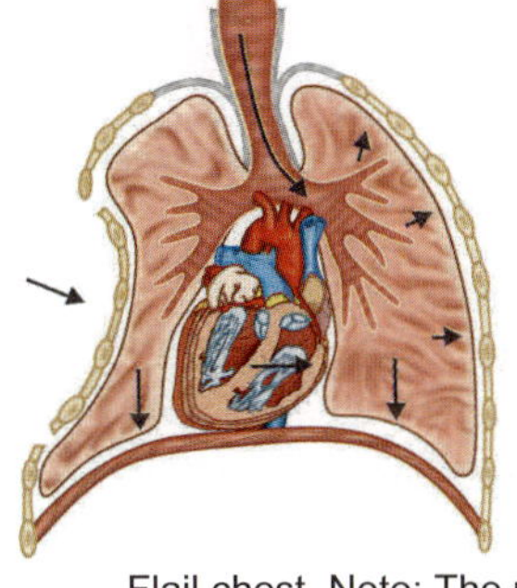
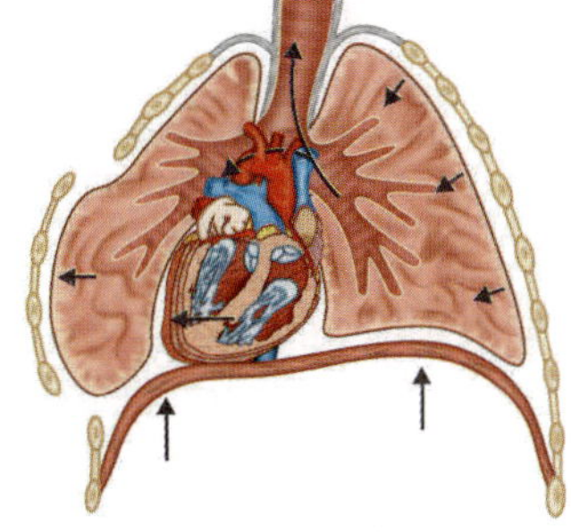

Flail chest. Note: The paradoxical movements of lung

359. **Ascent to high altitude may cause all of the following EXCEPT:**
a. Cerebral edema b. Pulmonary edema
c. Cerebral palsy d. Venous thrombosis

Cerebral palsy (CP) is a group of permanent movement disorders that appear in early childhood. Signs and symptoms vary among people. Often, symptoms include poor coordination, stiff muscles, weak muscles, and tremors. There may be problems with sensation, vision, hearing, swallowing, and speaking.

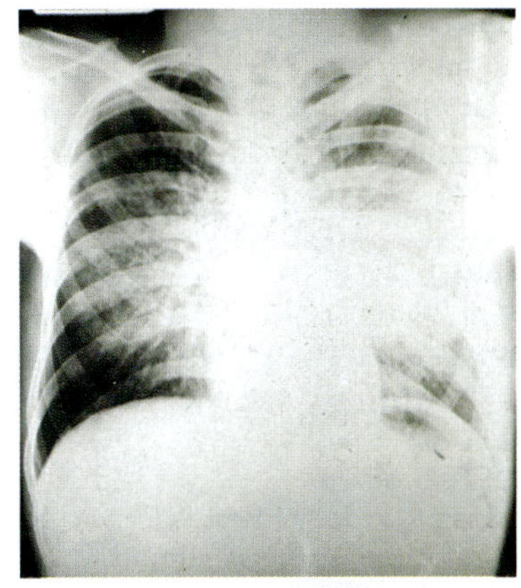

X-ray chest: High altitude pulmonary edema Note the bat-wing like opacities arising from the hilum

ONCOLOGY

360. **Smoking is associated with carcinoma of all the organs EXCEPT:**
a. Oral cavity b. Kidney
c. Bladder d. Liver

Most cases of HCC are secondary to either a viral hepatitis infection (hepatitis B or C), cirrhosis (alcoholism being the most common cause of liver cirrhosis), aflatoxin, hemachromatosis or Wilson disease.

361. **Thymoma can be associated with all EXCEPT:**
a. Superior mediastinum syndrome
b. Myasthenia gravis
c. Hypergammaglobulinemia
d. Pure red cell aplasia

10–15% of patients with MG have a thymoma and, conversely, 30–45% of patients with thymomas have MG. Additional associated autoimmune conditions include pure red cell aplasia and Good syndrome (thymoma with combined immunodeficiency and hypogammaglobulinemia).

MISCELLANEOUS

362. **All of the following conditions are related to defective DNA repair EXCEPT:**
a. Herediatry nonpolyposis colon cancer
b. Xeroderma pigmentosa
c. Friedrich ataxia
d. None of the above

Ans. 356. c. SLE 357. b. Chronic bronchitis 358. b. Flail chest 359. c. Cerebral palsy
360. d. Liver 361. c. Hypergammag... 362. c. Friedrich ataxia

Friedreich's ataxia is an autosomal recessive disorder that occurs when the FXN gene contains amplified intronic GAA repeats. The FXN gene encodes the protein frataxin. GAA repeat expansion causes frataxin levels to be reduced. Frataxin is an iron-binding protein responsible for forming iron–sulphur clusters. One result of frataxin deficiency is mitochondrial iron overload which can cause damage to many proteins.

363. All of the following are true for Duchenne muscular dystrophy EXCEPT:

a. Cause of death is pneumonia
b. Positive Gower sign
c. Symptomatic females
d. Pseudohypertrophy of calf muscles

Duchenne muscular dystrophy (DMD) is a recessive X-linked form of muscular dystrophy, affecting around 1 in 3,600 males, which results in muscle degeneration and eventual death. The disorder is caused by a mutation in the dystrophin gene, located on the human X chromosome, which codes for the protein dystrophin.

364. True statements for Wegener's granulomatosis are all EXCEPT:

a. p-ANCA positive
b. Both lung & kidney involved
c. Non-granulomatous vasculitis
d. Associated with inflammatory bowel disease

Granulomatosis with polyangiitis (GPA), the disease formerly known as Wegener's granulomatosis (WG), is a systemic disorder that involves both granulomatosis and polyangiitis. It is a form of vasculitis (inflammation of blood vessels) that affects small- and medium-size vessels in many organs. Damage to the lungs and kidneys can be fatal. It requires long-term immunosuppression

365. NOT a feature of Hurler syndrome:

a. X-linked b. MR
c. Joint stiffness d. Coarse facial features

Hurler syndrome is often classified as a lysosomal storage disease, and is clinically related to Hunter Syndrome. Hunter syndrome is X-linked while Hurler syndrome is autosomal recessive.

366. Which of the following immunoglobulin & complement are involved in Henoch Schonlein purpura:

a. IgG, C3 b. IgA, C3
c. IgA, C1 d. IgG, C1

Immunofluorescence demonstrates IgA and C3 (a protein of the complement system) in the blood vessel wall. However, overall serum complement levels are normal.

367. Which of the following is used in management of Wilson disease:

a. Copper b. Phosphorus
c. Zinc d. Aluminium

Generally, penicillamine is the first treatment used for Wilson disease. Those intolerant to penicillamine may instead be commenced on trientine hydrochloride, which also has chelating properties. Once all results have returned to normal, zinc (usually in the form of a zinc acetate prescription called Galzin) may be used instead of chelators to maintain stable copper levels in the body. Zinc stimulates metallothionein, a protein in gut cells that binds copper and prevents their absorption and transport to the liver.

368. NOT true for X-linked recessive diseases:

a. Unaffected males do not transmit the trait to any offspring
b. Females are frequently carriers
c. Males are commonly affected
d. Male to male transmission only

In XLR, only males are affected, females are only carrier. Among offsprings of an affected male, none of the sons will carry the trait, while all the daughters will be carriers.

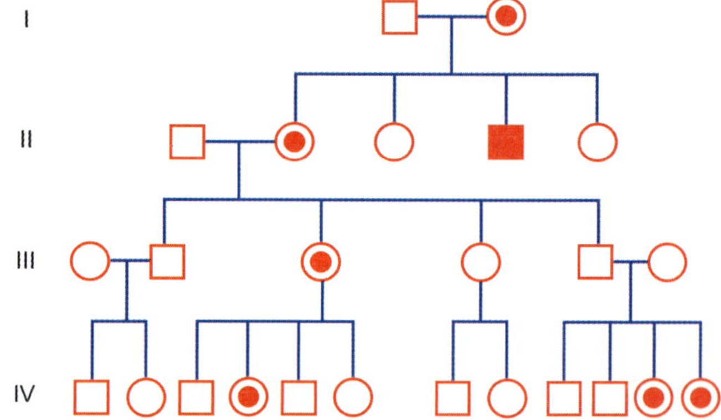

Pedigree of a disorder with X-linked recessive inheritance (oblique transmission). Circles with dots in the centre represent carrier females

369. Does NOT have autosomal recessive inheritance:

a. Wilson disease b. Cystic fibrosis
c. Hemophilia-A d. None of the above

Hemophilia (also christmas disease and pseudohypertrophic muscular dystrophy) has XLR inheritance.

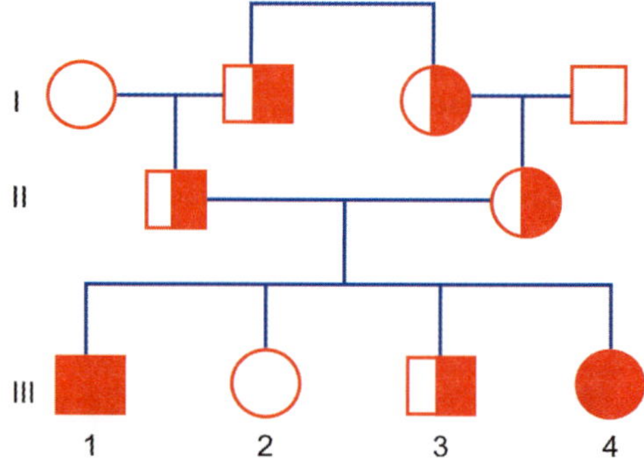

Pedigree of a disorder with autosomal recessive inheritance (horizontal transmission). Roman numerals I-III indicate generations. The nos. 1-4 indicate siblings. Blacked out symbol means an affected individual. Those with one-half blackened indicate carriers

370. Dystrophin gene is of great diagnostic value in:

a. Oculopharyngeal dystrophy
b. Duchenne's muscular dystrophy
c. Myotonic dystrophy
d. Limb girdle dystrophy

Ans. 363. c. Symptomatic... 364. c. Non-granulomatous... 365. a. X-linked 366. b. IgA, C3
367. c. Zinc 368. d. Male to male... 369. c. Hemophilia-A 370. b. Duchenne's muscular...

Summary of the features of common myopathies					
Muscle disorder	*Age of onset*	*Pattern of involvement*	*Muscle enzymes*	*EMG*	*Prognosis*
1. Duchenne muscular dystrophy (DMD)	Before 4 years	Proximal muscles	Markedly elevated	Myopathic	Gross disability in 10 years
2. Congenital myopathy	Infancy	Proximal muscles	Normal or marginally elevated	Myopathic	Insidious course
3. Limb-girdle dystrophy	2nd or 3rd decade	Proximal muscles	Mild to moderate elevation	Myopathic by middle age	Severe disability
4. Facioscapulohumeral dystrophy	Childhood to adult life	Facial and shoulder girdle muscles	Mild to moderate	Myopathic	Normal life expectancy
5. Dystrophia myotonica	20-30 years	Facial muscles, temporalis, masseter, quadriceps and distal limb muscles	Mild elevation	Myotonic pattern "dive-bomber phenomenon"	Severely disabled in 15-20 years
6. Polymyositis	20-60 years	Proximal limb muscles, trunk muscles, neck pharyngeal and laryngeal muscles	Markedly elevated	Myopathic, spontaneous activity in the form of fibrillations	Responds to corticosteroids and immuno-suppresants

Duchenne and Becker type dystrophies are due to defects in the same gene locus and its product "dystrophin" is probably required for maintaining the stability of muscle membrane. Mutations of dystrophin gene, usually deletion or gene inversion; lead to total or near total loss of dystrophin protein from skeletal muscle causing early and progressive loss of muscle function.

371. True regarding Foster Kennedy syndrome:
a. Associated with cerebral abscess
b. Tumor is in subfrontal area
c. Papilledema is on the side of tumor
d. Optic atrophy is on the opposite side of tumor

Foster Kennedy syndrome
- Optic atrophy in the ipsilateral eye
- Disc edema in the contralateral eye
- Central scotoma (loss of vision in the middle of the visual fields) in the ipsilateral eye
- Anosmia (loss of smell) ipsilaterally

372. C-reactive protein is NOT raised in:
a. Non-allergic asthma
b. Sickle cell anemia
c. Active rheumatoid arthritis
d. Rheumatic fever

C-reactive protein is a beta globulin which is absent in normal plasma but appears in the presence of different types of inflammatory arthritis. The CRP levels rise up to 100 folds during infection, tissue injury and inflammation.

The advantages of CRP over ESR
1. More rapid procedure; only a few minutes.
2. CRP is positive even before ESR starts rising.
3. CRP can be quantified by serial dilution.
4. It helps to distinguish between rheumatoid arthritis (RA) and systemic lupus erythematosus (SLE). In RA it is elevated, whereas in uncomplicated SLE it is not.

373. NOT an autosomal dominant disorder:
a. Sickle cell anemia
b. Familial hypercholesterolemia
c. Huntington's chorea
d. Hereditary spherocytosis

Sickle-cell conditions have an autosomal recessive pattern of inheritance from parents.

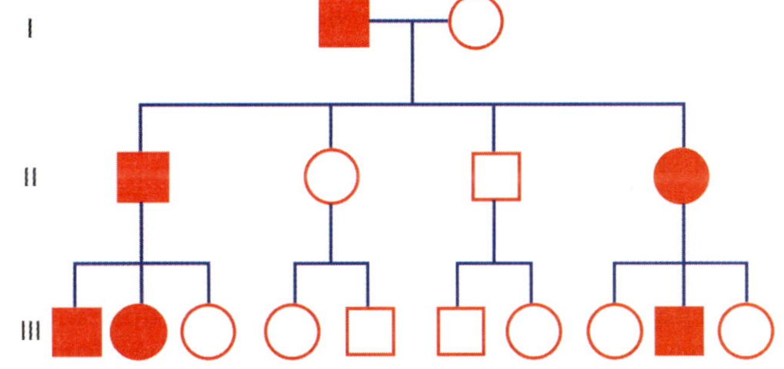

Pedigree of a disorder with autosomal dominant inheritance (vertical transmission). Normal persons do not pass on the trait to their offspring

374. Correct sequence of cell cycle:
a. G0-G1-S-G2-M
b. G0-G1-G2-S-M
c. G0-M-G2-S-G1
d. G0-G1-S-M-G2

Interphase proceeds in three stages, G1, S, and G2, followed by the cycle of mitosis and cytokinesis. The cell's nuclear chromosomes are duplicated during S phase.

375. Hematoxylin bodies are a feature of:
a. Amyloidosis
b. SLE
c. Silicosis
d. Sarcoidosis

A hematoxylin body, or LE body, is a dense, homogeneous, basophilic particle, easily stainable with hematoxylin. It consists of degraded nuclear material from an injured cell, along with autoantibodies and a limited amount of cytoplasm.

Ans. 371. b. Tumor is in... 372. b. Sickle cell anemia 373. a. Sickle cell anemia 374. a. G0-G1-S-G2-M 375. b. SLE

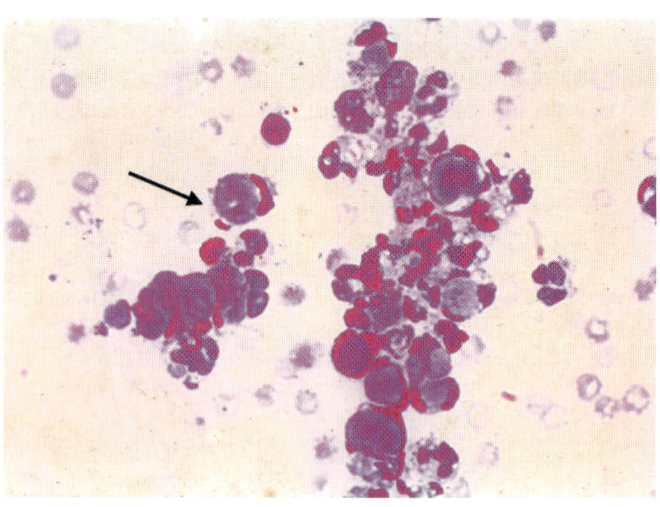

LE cell—a neutrophic leukocyte engulfing amorphous eosinophilic material—its own nucleus pushed to the periphery—arrow)

376. Drug of choice for refractory histiocytosis:

a. Cytosine arabinoside b. Fluadarbine
c. Cladarabine d. Methotrexate

Patients with refractory histiocytosis with high-risk organ (liver, spleen, or bone marrow) involvement and resistant multisystem low-risk organ involvement have been treated with an intensive acute myeloid leukemia-like protocol. Prompt change of therapy to cladribine and cytosine arabinoside appeared to provide an improvement in overall survival (OS).

377. Mucin clot test is employed for:

a. Protein in pleural fluid
b. Hyaluronate in synovial fluid
c. Proteins in CSF
d. Mucin in stool

Mucin clot test reflects the polymerization of synovial fluid hyaluronate; a few drops of synovial fluid added to acetic acid form a clot; poor clot formation occurs in a variety of inflammatory conditions including septic arthritis, gouty arthritis, and rheumatoid arthritis.

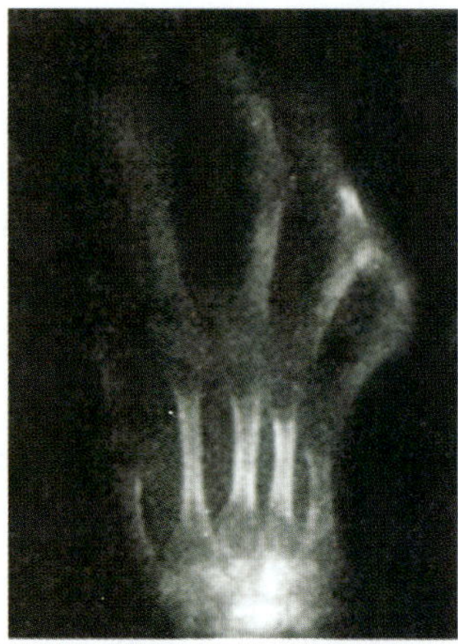

X-ray of rheumatoid hand. Note the juxta-articular rarefaction of bone

378. HLA-B27 is NOT associated with:

a. Myasthenia gravis b. Acute anterior uveitis
c. Reiter's syndrome d. Ankylosing spondylitis

MG is a disease characterized by weakness and easy fatiguability of skeletal muscles with predilection for cranial and limb muscles.

The positivity rates for HLA B27 in the different forms of arthritis.
Ankylosing spondylitis—above 90%
Reiter's syndrome—75%
Psoriatic arthropathy—50-75%
Enteropathic arthritis—30-70%

379. Antibody seen in myositis:

a. Anti-ku b. Anti-Sm
c. Anti-scl 70 d. Anti-Jo 1

Anti-Jo-1 antibody is a myositis specific autoantibody most commonly found in patients with idiopathic inflammatory myopathies (IIM). This antibody is directed against the histidyl-tRNA synthetase which catalyses the binding of the histidine to its cognate tRNA during protein synthesis.

Clinical features of the different types of myositis			
	DM	*PM*	*IBM*
Age	All	Second decade	Above 50 yrs
Sex	Females more	Females more	Males more
	DM	*PM*	*IBM*
Distribution of	Proximal	Proximal	Distal
Muscle weakness	Symmetrical	Symmetrical	Symmetrical
DM—Dermatomyositis; PM—Polmyositis; IBM—Inclusion body myositis			

380. Gene therapy is given in:

a. Severe combined immune-deficiency syndrome
b. Sickle cell anemia
c. Thalassemia
d. Cystic fibrosis

Though gene therapy is largely beneficial, insertion of a defective gene may lead to adverse effects in future, e.g. lymphatic leukemia in children treated with single gene therapy for severe combined immunodeficiency.

381. Treatment of choice for long term therapy of Kawasaki disease:

a. Azathioprine b. Steroid
c. Immunoglobulin d. Antibiotics

Treatment during the acute febrile phase of Kawasaki disease consists of aspirin given in a dose of 80-100 mg/kg bw/day to be tapered off later and IVIG given as IV infusion in a dose of 2 g/kg bw over 10 hours.

Ans. 376. **c.** Cladarabine 377. **b.** Hyaluronate in... 378. **a.** Myasthenia gravis 379. **d.** Anti-Jo 1
380. **a.** Severe comb... 381. **c.** Immunoglobulin

Classification of the primary vasculitis		
Size of vessel	*Sites*	*Clinical entity*
Large vessels	1. Temporal arteritis	Giant cell arteritis syn: temporal arteritis polymyalgia rheumatica
	2. Aorta and main arteries to head and limbs. Occasionally pulmonary arteries	Takayasu's arteritis
Medium size vessel	1. Diffuse lesions in several arteries 2. Coronary arteries	Polyarteritis nodosa Kawasaki disease
Small vessels—arterioles capillaries or venules	Kidneys, lungs	Microscopic polyangiitis, Goodpasture's syndrome
	Upper and lower respiratory tract	Wegener's granulomatosis, Churg-Strauss syndrome
	Skin, mucous membrane, genitalia, joints	Behcet's syndrome
	Skin, joints, abdominal viscera, kidneys	Henoch-Schönlein purpura
Cutaneous vessels	Isolated angiitis without systemic lesion	Isolated cutaneous leucoclastic vasculitis

382. Most useful test in a patient with generalized restriction of eye movements in all directions, intermittent ptosis, proximal muscle weakness and fatiguability is:

a. Muscle biopsy b. EMG
c. Edrophonium test d. CPK

Tensilon (Edrophonium chloride) is given IV in a dose of 2 mg initially in a test dose followed by 8 mg slowly, improves myasthenic weakness dramatically within 60 seconds.

383. HLA associated with myasthenia gravis:

a. B8 b. DR4
c. DW3 d. B27

MG is associated with HLA B21 and B8.

HLA association with diseases commonly seen in India	
Ankylosing spondylitis	HLA B-27
Reiter's disease	HLA B-27
Acute anterior uveitis	HLA B-27
Rheumatoid arthritis	HLA DR4
Juvenile	RA HLA DR5, DR8
Insulin dependent diabetes	HLA B-8, B-21, DR3
Graves' disease	HLA DR2, DQ2
Rheumatic heart disease	HLA DR3
Myasthenia gravis	HLA B-21, B-8
Tuberculoid leprosy	HLA DR2, DR6
Lepromatous leprosy	HLA DQW1
Pulmonary tuberculosis	HLA DR2, DR6

Contd...

Contd...

384. NOT a feature of Neurofibromatosis-1:

a. Ash leaf spots b. Family history
c. Optic glioma d. Axillary freckle

Ash leaf spots are seen in tuberous sclerosis.

Diagnostic criteria in neurofibromatosis	
Type I *Two or more of the following must be present*	*Type II* *At least one criterion must be present for diagnosis*
1. Cafe-au-lait macules with the greatest diameter 5 mm in prepubertal and 15 mm in postpubertal patients, atleast six in number.	1. Bilateral eighth nerve tumors seen by imaging techniques.
2. Two or more neuro-fibromas of any type or one plexiform neuroma	2. Parent, sibling or child with neurofibromatosis-2 showing neurologica tumours or juvenile posterior lenticular opacity.
3. Presence of optic glioma	
4. Two or more Lisch nodules	
5. Bony lesion in sphenoid or long bones	
6. Parent, sibling or child with neurofibromatosis	

385. What is the indication of using systemic steroids in a case of rheumatoid arthritis:

a. Carpal tunnel syndrome
b. Presence of deformities
c. Mononeuritis multiplex
d. Involvement of articular cartilage

Multiple mononeuropathy (mononeuritis multiplex) is the simultaneous malfunction of two or more peripheral nerves in separate areas of the body.

Diagnostic criteria for rheumatoid arthritis (RA)
1. Morning stiffness extending for 1 hour or more.
2. Arthritis of three or more joints.
3. Arthritis of hand joints.
4. Symmetrical arthritis.
5. Rheumatoid nodules.
6. Positive rheumatoid factor test: significant titer in India is >20 μU/mL
7. Radiological abnormalities. Four or more of these criteria occurring for more than six weeks should make the diagnosis probable.

Ans. 382. c. Edrophonium... **383. a.** B8 **384. a.** Ash leaf spots **385. c.** Mononeuritis multiplex

386. Characteristics of SIRS (systemic inflammatory response syndrome) include the following EXCEPT:

a. Leucocytosis
b. Thrombocytopenia
c. Infectious or non-infectious cause
d. Oral temperature more than 38°C

Manifestations of SIRS

- Body temperature less than 36°C (96.8 °F) or greater than 38 °C (100.4 °F)
- Heart rate greater than 90 beats per minute
- Tachypnea (high respiratory rate), with greater than 20 breaths per minute; or, an arterial partial pressure of carbon dioxide less than 4.3 kPa (32 mm Hg)
- White blood cell count less than 4000 cells/mm^3 (4×10^9 cells/L) or greater than 12,000 cells/mm^3 (12×10^9 cells/L); or the presence of greater than 10% immature neutrophils (band forms). Band forms greater than 3% is called bandemia or a "left-shift."
- Hyperglycemia (blood glucose >6.66 mmol/L [120 mg/dL]) in absence of diabetes mellitus
- Altered mental state

387. All of the following are autosomal dominant disorders EXCEPT:

a. Tuberous sclerosis
b. Polyposis coli
c. Cystic fibrosis
d. Myotonic dystrophy

CF is an autosomal recessive disease. The defective gene is located in the long arm of chromosome 7.

388. All are seen in hemochromatosis EXCEPT:

a. Hypogonadism
b. Arthropathy
c. Bronze diabetes
d. Desferrioxamine is the treatment of choice

In hemochromatosis/bronzed diabetes, simple venesection to remove 500 mL blood once in two weeks or at shorter intervals help to prolong life by a mean of 8.2 years and improves hepatic function. The iron chelating agent desferrioxamine has been used when venesection is contraindicated by the presence of anemia, but the drug is less effective. In secondary hemochromatosis desferrioxamine is effective.

389. Best indicator for beneficial effect of atropine in a patient with organophosphorous poisoning is:

a. Heart rate
b. Pupil
c. Blood pressure
d. Ventilation

A dose of 2 mg atropine is given initially in organophosphorous compounds poisoning, and 1 mg or more is repeated every 10 minutes (or even at shorter intervals) till the pupil are dilated to normal size and pulmonary edema and bronchorrhea is cleared.

Effects of AChE inhibition on cholinergic nervous system functions

Muscarinic effects	*Nicotinic effects*	*CNS effects*
Excessive salivation	Muscle cramping	Restlessness
Lacrimation	Weakness	Headache
Urination	Respiratory failure	Emotional lability
Diarrhea		Drowsiness
G I distress		Tremor
Emesis		Slurred speech
Miosis		Confusion
Bronchitis		Delirium
Bronchospasm		General weakness
Bradycardia		Ataxia
Sweating		Seizures

Ans. 386. b. Thrombocy... 387. c. Cystic fibrosis 388. d. Desferrioxamine... 389. b. Pupil

ANSWERS WITH REFERENCES

HEMATOLOGY

1. **Ans. (b)** CNS manifestations
Ref: Davidson's Medicine, 19/e p871

2. **Ans. (a)** Associated thrombocytopenia with prolonged bleeding
Ref: Davidson's Medicine, 19/e p321

3. **Ans. (d)** Macrocytic anemia
Ref: Davidson's Medicine, 19/e p928t

4. **Ans. (c)** Raised ESR
Ref: KV Krishna Das's Medicine 5/e p1008

5. **Ans. (d)** Fanconi anemia
Ref: KV Krishna Das's Medicine 5/e p1020

6. **Ans. (b)** Anemia of chronic diseases/ACD
Ref: KV Krishna Das's Medicine 5/e p997

7. **Ans. (a)** Increased TIBC, decreased serum ferritin
Ref: KV Krishna Das's Medicine 5/e p986

8. **Ans. (b)** Serum ferritin levels
Ref: KV Krishna Das's Medicine 5/e p991

9. **Ans. (a)** Hypersegmented neutrophils
Ref: KV Krishna Das's Medicine 5/e p987

10. **Ans. (a)** IgM antibodies are found
Ref: KV Krishna Das's Medicine 5/e p1090

11. **Ans. (b)** Herediatry spherocytosis
Ref: KV Krishna Das's Medicine 5/e p1004

12. **Ans. (d)** Increased haptoglobin
Ref: KV Krishna Das's Medicine 5/e p1000

13. **Ans. (c)** Hemolytic uremic syndrome
Ref: KV Krishna Das's Medicine 5/e p1103

14. **Ans. (b)** Normal HbF and normal HbA2
Ref: KV Krishna Das's Medicine 5/e p988

15. **Ans. (b)** Sideroblastic anemia
Ref: KV Krishna Das's Medicine 5/e p989

16. **Ans. (b)** Copper deficiency
Ref: KV Krishna Das's Medicine 5/e p984

17. **Ans. (a)** Vitamin B12 estimation
Ref: KV Krishna Das's Medicine 5/e p994

18. **Ans. (a)** Folic acid alone causes improvement of hematologic but worsening of neurological symptoms
Ref: KV Krishna Das's Medicine 5/e p987

19. **Ans. (b)** CLL
Ref: KV Krishna Das's Medicine 5/e p1043

20. **Ans. (b)** Increased RBC surface area
Ref: KV Krishna Das's Medicine 5/e p1005

21. **Ans. (a)** Platelet count
Ref: KV Krishna Das's Medicine 5/e p1084

22. **Ans. (d)** AML
Ref: KV Krishna Das's Medicine 5/e p1029

23. **Ans. (a)** Hypokalemia
Ref: KV Krishna Das's Medicine 5/e p1025

24. **Ans. (c)** Hereditary spherocytosis
Ref: KV Krishna Das's Medicine 5/e p983

25. **Ans. (a)** Mutations in alpha chain
Ref: KV Krishna Das's Medicine 5/e p987

26. **Ans. (b)** Raised HbA2
Ref: KV Krishna Das's Medicine 5/e p988

27. **Ans. (a)** Thalassemia
Ref: KV Krishna Das's Medicine 5/e p1012

28. **Ans. (c)** Increased leucocyte alkaline phosphatase score
Ref: KV Krishna Das's Medicine 5/e p

29. **Ans. (c)** Renal cell carcinoma
Ref: KV Krishna Das's Medicine 5/e p1072

30. **Ans. (c)** Normal prothrombin time
Ref: KV Krishna Das's Medicine 5/e p1080

31. **Ans. (a)** Splenomegaly
Ref: KV Krishna Das's Medicine 5/e p1018

32. **Ans. (b)** Increased erythropoietin level
Ref: KV Krishna Das's Medicine 5/e p1073

33. **Ans. (c)** Myelofibrosis
Ref: KV Krishna Das's Medicine 5/e p1071

34. **Ans. (a)** Lymphocytic predominant
Ref: KV Krishna Das's Medicine 5/e p1064

35. **Ans. (d)** Prolonged prothrombin time
Ref: KV Krishna Das's Medicine 5/e p1093

36. **Ans. (c)** von Willebrand's disease
Ref: KV Krishna Das's Medicine 5/e p1078

37. **Ans. (b)** Aniline
Ref: Internet resources

38. **Ans. (a)** AML
Ref: KV Krishna Das's Medicine 5/e p1031

39. **Ans. (d)** Thrombocytopenia
Ref: Internet resources

40. **Ans. (a)** D-dimer assay
Ref: KV Krishna Das's Medicine 5/e p1102

41. **Ans. (b)** Transmission of gonococci
Ref: KV Krishna Das's Medicine 5/e p1026

42. **Ans. (a)** Factor VII deficiency
Ref: KV Krishna Das's Medicine 5/e

43. **Ans. (b)** Neurological changes
Ref: KV Krishna Das's Medicine 5/e p995

44. **Ans. (b)** Myelofibrosis
Ref: KV Krishna Das's Medicine 5/e p971

45. **Ans. (c)** Decreased PTT
Ref: KV Krishna Das's Medicine 5/e p1097

46. **Ans. (a)** Deficiency of coagulation factor
Ref: KV Krishna Das's Medicine 5/e p1024

47. **Ans. (c)** Von-Willebrand disease
Ref: KV Krishna Das's Medicine 5/e p1095

48. **Ans. (b)** D-Dimer assay
Ref: KV Krishna Das's Medicine 5/e p1102

49. **Ans. (b)** High extracellular K+
Ref: KV Krishna Das's Medicine 5/e p971

50. **Ans. (c)** Chronic myelogenous leukemia
Ref: KV Krishna Das's Medicine 5/e p1043

51. **Ans. (d)** CLL
Ref: KV Krishna Das's Medicine 5/e p1001

52. **Ans. (a)** Hyper-segmented neutrophils
Ref: KV Krishna Das's Medicine 5/e p992

53. **Ans. (c)** CLL
Ref: KV Krishna Das's Medicine 5/e p1048

54. **Ans. (a)** Isolated BT with a normal PT
Ref: KV Krishna Das's Medicine 5/e p1081

55. **Ans. (a)** Hemolytic jaundice
Ref: KV Krishna Das's Medicine 5/e p999

56. **Ans. (c)** SLE
Ref: KV Krishna Das's Medicine 5/e p999

CARDIOVASCULAR SYSTEM

57. **Ans. (c)** ST segment elevation
Ref: PJ Mehta's Practical Medicine, 17/e p329

58. **Ans. (c)** Atrial fibrillation
Ref: Davidson's Medicine, 19/e p359

59. **Ans. (d)** Duration of mid-diastolic murmur
Ref: PJ Mehta's Practical Medicine, 17/e p168

60. **Ans. (b)** Methemogobinemia
Ref: Internet resources

61. **Ans. (c)** ASO titre
Ref: Davidson's Medicine, 19/e p451

62. **Ans. (b)** Better evaluation of left atria & left atrial appendage thrombus
Ref: Davidson's Medicine, 19/e p370

63. **Ans. (d)** Levels of cardiac markers remain unchanged
Ref: KV Krishna Das's Medicine 5/e p847

64. **Ans. (c)** Rose spots may be seen
Ref: KV Krishna Das's Medicine 5/e p804

65. **Ans. (c)** 40-60%
Ref: KV Krishna Das's Medicine 5/e p765

66. **Ans. (b)** Austin flint murmur
Ref: KV Krishna Das's Medicine 5/e p795

67. **Ans. (b)** Echocardiography
Ref: KV Krishna Das's Medicine 5/e p872

68. **Ans. (c)** Dobutamine
Ref: KV Krishna Das's Medicine 5/e p841

69. **Ans. (a)** CCB
Ref: KV Krishna Das's Medicine 5/e p859

70. **Ans. (b)** Cardiac specifc troponin T
Ref: KV Krishna Das's Medicine 5/e p846

71. **Ans. (a)** Hypovolemic shock
Ref: KV Krishna Das's Medicine 5/e p765

72. **Ans. (c)** AS
Ref: KV Krishna Das's Medicine 5/e p793

73. **Ans. (a)** Atrial fibrillation
Ref: KV Krishna Das's Medicine 5/e p812

74. **Ans. (a)** Myocardial fibre tension
Ref: KV Krishna Das's Medicine 5/e p752

75. **Ans. (d)** Supravalvular aortic stenosis
Ref: Internet resources

76. **Ans. (b)** Erythema nodusum
Ref: KV Krishna Das's Medicine 5/e p194

77. **Ans. (d)** HDL
Ref: KV Krishna Das's Medicine 5/e p588

78. **Ans. (d) Pheochromocytoma**
Ref: KV Krishna Das's Medicine 5/e p829

79. **Ans. (c) HOCM**
Ref: KV Krishna Das's Medicine 5/e p867

80. **Ans. (c) Myocardial infarction**
Ref: KV Krishna Das's Medicine 5/e p846

81. **Ans. (b) Atrial contraction**
Ref: KV Krishna Das's Medicine 5/e p745

82. **Ans. (c) ASD**
Ref: KV Krishna Das's Medicine 5/e p775

83. **Ans. (b) LDL**
Ref: KV Krishna Das's Medicine 5/e p588

84. **Ans. (d) Left ventricular failure**
Ref: KV Krishna Das's Medicine 5/e p757

85. **Ans. (d) CK-MB**
Ref: KV Krishna Das's Medicine 5/e p847

86. **Ans. (d) Endomyocardial fibroelastosis**
Ref: KV Krishna Das's Medicine 5/e p869

87. **Ans. (c) Tetralogy of Fallot**
Ref: KV Krishna Das's Medicine 5/e p (Figure 118.11A)

88. **Ans. (d) Duration of prophylaxis is till 25 years of age**
Ref: KV Krishna Das's Medicine 5/e p191

89. **Ans. (d) Paroxysmal supraventricular tachycardia**
Ref: KV Krishna Das's Medicine 5/e p817

90. **Ans. (b) Diastolic murmur duration**
Ref: KV Krishna Das's Medicine 5/e p787

91. **Ans. (d) All of the above**
Ref: KV Krishna Das's Medicine 5/e p749

92. **Ans. (c) Polymorphic ventricular tachycardia**
Ref: KV Krishna Das's Medicine 5/e p811

93. **Ans. (c) Unstable angina**
Ref: KV Krishna Das's Medicine 5/e p857

94. **Ans. (b) Atropine**
Ref: KV Krishna Das's Medicine 5/e p808

95. **Ans. (c) Arteriovenous Fistula**
Ref: KV Krishna Das's Medicine 5/e p1170

96. **Ans. (d) Pulmonary capillary wedge pressure**
Ref: Internet resources

97. **Ans. (a) Hepatic pulsation**
Ref: KV Krishna Das's Medicine 5/e p797

98. **Ans. (d) All of the above**
Ref: KV Krishna Das's Medicine 5/e p745

99. **Ans. (b) Headache**
Ref: KV Krishna Das's Medicine 5/e p829

100. **Ans. (c) When ventricular pressure is more than aortic pressure**
Ref: KV Krishna Das's Medicine 5/e p747

101. **Ans. (c) Rheumatic fever**
Ref: KV Krishna Das's Medicine 5/e p192

102. **Ans. (c) Commonly not visible with normal heart**
Ref: KV Krishna Das's Medicine 5/e p746

103. **Ans. (c) Left atrial pressure**
Ref: KV Krishna Das's Medicine 5/e p752

104. **Ans. (b) Chronic cor pulmonale**
Ref: KV Krishna Das's Medicine 5/e p875

105. **Ans. (b) Respiratory failure**
Ref: KV Krishna Das's Medicine 5/e p832

106. **Ans. (c) Tall P waves**
Ref: KV Krishna Das's Medicine 5/e p821

107. **Ans. (a) First week**
Ref: KV Krishna Das's Medicine 5/e p846

108. **Ans. (d) Mitral stenosis**
Ref: KV Krishna Das's Medicine 5/e p794

109. **Ans. (b) Mitral regurgitation**
Ref: KV Krishna Das's Medicine 5/e p789

110. **Ans. (a) 'c' wave – onset of atrial systole**
Ref: KV Krishna Das's Medicine 5/e p745

111. **Ans. (a) Mitral regurgitation with mitral stenosis**
Ref: KV Krishna Das's Medicine 5/e p784

112. **Ans. (a) IPPV**
Ref: KV Krishna Das's Medicine 5/e p745

113. **Ans. (b) Decreased QT interval**
Ref: KV Krishna Das's Medicine 5/e p645

114. **Ans. (b) Wide QT**
Ref: KV Krishna Das's Medicine 5/e p820

115. **Ans. (c) Lies down**
Ref: KV Krishna Das's Medicine 5/e p866

116. **Ans. (c) Dobutamine**
Ref: KV Krishna Das's Medicine 5/e p750

117. **Ans. (d) MS**
Ref: KV Krishna Das's Medicine 5/e p784

118. **Ans. (a) Complete heart bloc**
Ref: KV Krishna Das's Medicine 5/e p823

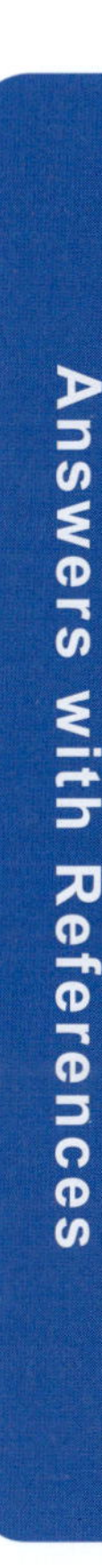

119. **Ans. (a)** Nitroglycerin
Ref: KV Krishna Das's Medicine 5/e p659

120. **Ans. (d)** Supraventicular tachycardia
Ref: KV Krishna Das's Medicine 5/e p819

121. **Ans. (c)** Atrial fibrillation
Ref: KV Krishna Das's Medicine 5/e p820

122. **Ans. (c)** Sick sinus syndrome
Ref: KV Krishna Das's Medicine 5/e p815

123. **Ans. (b)** Atrial fibrillation
Ref: KV Krishna Das's Medicine 5/e p749

124. **Ans. (a)** Adenosine
Ref: KV Krishna Das's Medicine 5/e p827

125. **Ans. (d)** Loud heart sounds
Ref: KV Krishna Das's Medicine 5/e p871

126. **Ans. (d)** Cardiac tamponade
Ref: KV Krishna Das's Medicine 5/e p872

127. **Ans. (d)** Kussamaul's sign
Ref: KV Krishna Das's Medicine 5/e p871

128. **Ans. (a)** Intercostal artery
Ref: KV Krishna Das's Medicine 5/e p772

129. **Ans. (b)** LDL/HDL ratio
Ref: KV Krishna Das's Medicine 5/e p589

130. **Ans. (c)** Large VSD causes infundibular stenosis
Ref: KV Krishna Das's Medicine 5/e p748

131. **Ans. (b)** Aortic dissection
Ref: KV Krishna Das's Medicine 5/e p878

132. **Ans. (d)** All of the above
Ref: KV Krishna Das's Medicine 5/e p856

133. **Ans. (b)** Late stent thrombosis
Ref: KV Krishna Das's Medicine 5/e p856

134. **Ans. (b)** Cardiac specific Troponins
Ref: KV Krishna Das's Medicine 5/e p844

135. **Ans. (c)** Complete right bundle branch block
Ref: KV Krishna Das's Medicine 5/e p815

136. **Ans. (c)** Opening Snap
Ref: KV Krishna Das's Medicine 5/e p784

137. **Ans. (a)** Constrictive pericarditis
Ref: KV Krishna Das's Medicine 5/e p872

138. **Ans. (c)** 25 mm Hg
Ref: KV Krishna Das's Medicine 5/e p758

139. **Ans. (d)** All of the above
Ref: KV Krishna Das's Medicine 5/e p189

140. **Ans. (c)** Digoxin
Ref: KV Krishna Das's Medicine 5/e p762

141. **Ans. (c)** Ebstein's anomaly
Ref: KV Krishna Das's Medicine 5/e p769

142. **Ans. (c)** Evening
Ref: Internet resources

143. **Ans. (b)** Isolated mitral stenosis
Ref: KV Krishna Das's Medicine 5/e p787

144. **Ans. (b)** Left atrial hypertrophy
Ref: KV Krishna Das's Medicine 5/e p776

145. **Ans. (d)** Pulmonary oligemia in chest X-ray
Ref: KV Krishna Das's Medicine 5/e p769

146. **Ans. (c)** Aortic stenosis
Ref: KV Krishna Das's Medicine 5/e p793

147. **Ans. (c)** Predominantly left to right shunt
Ref: KV Krishna Das's Medicine 5/e p780

148. **Ans. (d)** CK, AST, LDH
Ref: KV Krishna Das's Medicine 5/e p848

149. **Ans. (c)** Turner's syndrome
Ref: KV Krishna Das's Medicine 5/e p769

150. **Ans. (d)** Echocardiography
Ref: KV Krishna Das's Medicine 5/e p782

151. **Ans. (a)** Systolic murmur
Ref: KV Krishna Das's Medicine 5/e p795

152. **Ans. (c)** Middiastolic murmur
Ref: KV Krishna Das's Medicine 5/e p795

153. **Ans. (d)** 4
Ref: KV Krishna Das's Medicine 5/e p743

154. **Ans. (c)** TR
Ref: KV Krishna Das's Medicine 5/e p797

155. **Ans. (a)** Digoxin is helpful
Ref: KV Krishna Das's Medicine 5/e p762

156. **Ans. (a)** Along the line of closure of valves
Ref: KV Krishna Das's Medicine 5/e p803

157. **Ans. (b)** Ventricular fibrillation
Ref: KV Krishna Das's Medicine 5/e p812

158. **Ans. (a)** Narrow QRS complexes
Ref: KV Krishna Das's Medicine 5/e p810

159. **Ans. (c)** Staphylococcus epidermidis
Ref: KV Krishna Das's Medicine 5/e p801

160. **Ans. (c)** ST segment elevation
Ref: KV Krishna Das's Medicine 5/e p846

161. **Ans. (a)** Mitral valve prolapse
Ref: KV Krishna Das's Medicine 5/e p748

162. **Ans. (d)** Hypocalcemia
Ref: KV Krishna Das's Medicine 5/e p432

EXCRETORY SYSTEM

163. **Ans. (d)** Hyperkalemic acidosis
Ref: Davidson's Medicine, 19/e p598

164. **Ans. (d)** Hypertension
Ref: Davidson's Medicine, 19/e p587t

165. **Ans. (c)** DM
Ref: Davidson's Medicine, 19/e p600t

166. **Ans. (a)** Bence Jones proteins
Ref: KV Krishna Das's Medicine 5/e p1113

167. **Ans. (b)** Acute nephritis
Ref: KV Krishna Das's Medicine 5/e p1122

168. **Ans. (c)** Hypocalcemia
Ref: KV Krishna Das's Medicine 5/e p606

169. **Ans. (c)** Diabetic nephropathy
Ref: KV Krishna Das's Medicine 5/e p545

170. **Ans. (b)** Digoxin poisoning
Ref: KV Krishna Das's Medicine 5/e p115

171. **Ans. (b)** Membranous GN
Ref: KV Krishna Das's Medicine 5/e p1129

172. **Ans. (b)** Amino acid
Ref: KV Krishna Das's Medicine 5/e p1109

173. **Ans. (b)** Collapsing glomerulopathy
Ref: KV Krishna Das's Medicine 5/e p1128

174. **Ans. (c)** Chronic renal failure
Ref: Internet resources

175. **Ans. (b)** Hypophosphatemia
Ref: KV Krishna Das's Medicine 5/e p1164

176. **Ans. (b)** More than 50%
Ref: KV Krishna Das's Medicine 5/e p1162

177. **Ans. (c)** Gentamycin
Ref: KV Krishna Das's Medicine 5/e p1176

178. **Ans. (a)** Progesterone increases tumor size
Ref: Internet resources

179. **Ans. (b)** Sickle cell anemia
Ref: KV Krishna Das's Medicine 5/e p1009

180. **Ans. (a)** Hypercalcemia
Ref: KV Krishna Das's Medicine 5/e p1162

181. **Ans. (c)** Nephritic syndrome
Ref: KV Krishna Das's Medicine 5/e p1123

182. **Ans. (a)** Microscopic hematuria
Ref: Internet resources

183. **Ans. (c)** DTPA renogram
Ref: KV Krishna Das's Medicine 5/e p1121

184. **Ans. (c)** Cardiovascular disease
Ref: KV Krishna Das's Medicine 5/e p1169

GASTROINTESTINAL TRACT AND ABDOMEN

185. **Ans. (c)** Pigmented
Ref: Davidson's Medicine, 19/e p883

186. **Ans. (d)** 24 hour urinary 5-HIAA
Ref: Davidson's Medicine, 19/e p801t

187. **Ans. (c)** Lower esophageal web
Ref: Davidson's Medicine, 19/e p780

188. **Ans. (c)** Toxic megacolon
Ref: Davidson's Medicine, 19/e p811

189. **Ans. (c)** HBeAg
Ref: PJ Mehta's Practical Medicine, 17/e p65t

190. **Ans. (a)** Pruritis
Ref: KV Krishna Das's Medicine 5/e p508

191. **Ans. (d)** Decreased serum calcium
Ref: KV Krishna Das's Medicine 5/e p536

192. **Ans. (b)** Cirrhosis
Ref: KV Krishna Das's Medicine 5/e p505

193. **Ans. (d)** E. coli
Ref: KV Krishna Das's Medicine 5/e p505

194. **Ans. (d)** HLA-DQ2
Ref: KV Krishna Das's Medicine 5/e p476

195. **Ans. (d)** Cystic fibrosis
Ref: KV Krishna Das's Medicine 5/e p540

196. **Ans. (a)** Pancreatic insufficiency
Ref: KV Krishna Das's Medicine 5/e p474

197. **Ans. (a)** Liver failure
Ref: KV Krishna Das's Medicine 5/e p515

198. **Ans. (d)** Bleeding peptic ulcer
Ref: KV Krishna Das's Medicine 5/e p468

199. **Ans. (c)** Stricture is usual and causes obstruction
Ref: KV Krishna Das's Medicine 5/e p211

200. **Ans. (a)** Crohn's disease
Ref: KV Krishna Das's Medicine 5/e p480

201. Ans. (a) Chronic hepatitis B
Ref: KV Krishna Das's Medicine 5/e p506

202. Ans. (b) Anti HBs
Ref: KV Krishna Das's Medicine 5/e p327

203. Ans. (c) IgG anti HBsAg
Ref: KV Krishna Das's Medicine 5/e p526

204. Ans. (d) Immunized person with hepatitis B vaccine
Ref: KV Krishna Das's Medicine 5/e p319

205. Ans. (a) Anti HBs positive
Ref: KV Krishna Das's Medicine 5/e p318

206. Ans. (c) Esophageal varices
Ref: KV Krishna Das's Medicine 5/e p519

207. Ans. (b) Anti-tissue transglutaminase antibody/tTG
Ref: KV Krishna Das's Medicine 5/e p476

208. Ans. (c) Pylorus
Ref: KV Krishna Das's Medicine 5/e p469

209. Ans. (c) Hiatus hernia
Ref: KV Krishna Das's Medicine 5/e p470

210. Ans. (a) Peptic ulceration, gastric hypersecretion, non beta cell tumour
Ref: KV Krishna Das's Medicine 5/e p470

211. Ans. (a) Surgery
Ref: KV Krishna Das's Medicine 5/e p490

212. Ans. (a) The creatinine clearance is more than 40 ml/min
Ref: KV Krishna Das's Medicine 5/e p523

213. Ans. (b) The incidence of complications has remained unchanged
Ref: KV Krishna Das's Medicine 5/e p466

214. Ans. (c) HBV
Ref: KV Krishna Das's Medicine 5/e p317

215. Ans. (a) NOT common in Asians
Ref: KV Krishna Das's Medicine 5/e p529

216. Ans. (d) Four lumen
Ref: KV Krishna Das's Medicine 5/e p521

217. Ans. (b) Increased insulin levels
Ref: Internet resources

218. Ans. (a) Small bowel biopsy
Ref: KV Krishna Das's Medicine 5/e p476

219. Ans. (a) Embolism
Ref: Internet resources

220. Ans. (d) Ascites
Ref: KV Krishna Das's Medicine 5/e p492

221. Ans. (b) Serum Entamoeba antibodies
Ref: KV Krishna Das's Medicine 5/e p383

INFECTIOUS DISEASE

222. Ans. (c) Contact with body fluids
Ref: Davidson's Medicine, 19/e p62t

223. Ans. (a) p24
Ref: PJ Mehta's Practical Medicine, 17/e p95

224. Ans. (d) H. influenzae
Ref: Davidson's Medicine, 19/e p923t

225. Ans. (a) Quinolones are the drug of choice
Ref: KV Krishna Das's Medicine 5/e p242

226. Ans. (b) Stibogluconate sodium
Ref: KV Krishna Das's Medicine 5/e p372

227. Ans. (a) Kaposi sarcoma
Ref: KV Krishna Das's Medicine 5/e p270

228. Ans. (d) 10 years
Ref: KV Krishna Das's Medicine 5/e p268

229. Ans. (b) Oral candidiasis
Ref: KV Krishna Das's Medicine 5/e p268

230. Ans. (c) Hypnozoite
Ref: KV Krishna Das's Medicine 5/e p365

231. Ans. (a) Toxoplasmosis
Ref: KV Krishna Das's Medicine 5/e p267

232. Ans. (a) 200/mm3
Ref: KV Krishna Das's Medicine 5/e p267

233. Ans. (d) Toxoplasmosis
Ref: KV Krishna Das's Medicine 5/e p268

234. Ans. (b) Thrombosis
Ref: KV Krishna Das's Medicine 5/e p342

235. Ans. (d) Resistance to at least INH and rifampicin + any quinolones + at least 1 injectable 2nd line drug
Ref: KV Krishna Das's Medicine 5/e p277

ENDOCRINOLOGY

236. Ans. (a) Hypertension
Ref: Davidson's Medicine, 19/e p684, 726t

237. Ans. (d) Weight gain
Ref: Davidson's Medicine, 19/e p691t

238. **Ans. (d) Smoking is a risk factor**
Ref: Davidson's Medicine, 19/e p302

239. **Ans. (d) Diarrhoea**
Ref: Internet resources

240. **Ans. (d) Menorrhagia**
Ref: Davidson's Medicine, 19/e p692t

241. **Ans. (c) Relative hypernatremia**
Ref: Davidson's Medicine, 19/e p282

242. **Ans. (c) Hyperglycemia**
Ref: Davidson's Medicine, 19/e p743t

243. **Ans. (a) Calciuria**
Ref: Davidson's Medicine, 19/e p717t, 718t

244. **Ans. (d) Myxoedema**
Ref: Davidson's Medicine, 19/e p694

245. **Ans. (b) Struma ovarii**
Ref: Davidson's Medicine, 19/e p701

246. **Ans. (c) Osteoporosis**
Ref: Davidson's Medicine, 19/e p717

247. **Ans. (c) Hyponatremia**
Ref: KV Krishna Das's Medicine 5/e p651

248. **Ans. (b) Hyperglycemia**
Ref: KV Krishna Das's Medicine 5/e p608 (Unnumbered table left upper side)

249. **Ans. (a) Distal symmetric polyneuropathy**
Ref: KV Krishna Das's Medicine 5/e p579

250. **Ans. (b) Low blood pressure**
Ref: KV Krishna Das's Medicine 5/e p658

251. **Ans. (a) 7%**
Ref: KV Krishna Das's Medicine 5/e p550

252. **Ans. (c) Position**
Ref: KV Krishna Das's Medicine 5/e p580

253. **Ans. (d) Methotrexate**
Ref: KV Krishna Das's Medicine 5/e p655

254. **Ans. (a) Increased ACTH and increased cortisol**
Ref: KV Krishna Das's Medicine 5/e p653

255. **Ans. (a) Hypo-osmolar urine**
Ref: KV Krishna Das's Medicine 5/e p608

256. **Ans. (b) Diet therapy + exercise + metformin**
Ref: KV Krishna Das's Medicine 5/e p552

257. **Ans. (b) C-11 hydroxylase**
Ref: KV Krishna Das's Medicine 5/e p656

258. **Ans. (c) Declare patient as normal**
Ref: KV Krishna Das's Medicine 5/e p547

259. **Ans. (d) Tachycardia**
Ref: KV Krishna Das's Medicine 5/e p637

260. **Ans. (d) Alcohol consumption**
Ref: KV Krishna Das's Medicine 5/e p568

261. **Ans. (d) Muscle hypotrophy**
Ref: KV Krishna Das's Medicine 5/e p618

METABOLIC AND NUTRITIONAL DISORDERS

262. **Ans. (a) Diarrhoea**
Ref: Davidson's Medicine, 19/e p290

263. **Ans. (c) Riboflavin**
Ref: Davidson's Medicine, 19/e p321

264. **Ans. (c) Sclerema**
Ref: Davidson's Medicine, 19/e p324

265. **Ans. (d) Central pontine myelinolysis**
Ref: Davidson's Medicine, 19/e p281

266. **Ans. (c) Cardiac failure**
Ref: Davidson's Medicine, 19/e p321

267. **Ans. (d) Calcium gluconate**
Ref: Davidson's Medicine, 19/e p286t

268. **Ans. (c) Metabolic alkalosis**
Ref: KV Krishna Das's Medicine 5/e p424

269. **Ans. (c) Salicylate poisoning**
Ref: KV Krishna Das's Medicine 5/e p435

270. **Ans. (c) Zinc**
Ref: KV Krishna Das's Medicine 5/e p150

271. **Ans. (d) Folate**
Ref: Internet resources

272. **Ans. (b) Pancreatitis**
Ref: KV Krishna Das's Medicine 5/e p168

273. **Ans. (a) Myopathy**
Ref: KV Krishna Das's Medicine 5/e p1225

274. **Ans. (a) Hyperglycemia**
Ref: Internet resources

275. **Ans. (b) Renal tubular acidosis**
Ref: KV Krishna Das's Medicine 5/e p436

276. **Ans. (b) Liver, eyes and brain**
Ref: KV Krishna Das's Medicine 5/e p584

277. **Ans. (c) Hypervitaminosis A**
Ref: KV Krishna Das's Medicine 5/e p151

NEUROLOGY

278. **Ans. (d)** HIV encephalopathy
Ref: Davidson's Medicine, 19/e p1126t

279. **Ans. (b)** Subdural hemorrhage
Ref: Sumer Sethi's Radiology, 5/e p6

280. **Ans. (a)** Hypotonia
Ref: PJ Mehta's Practical Medicine, 17/e p242

281. **Ans. (a)** Gag reflex
Ref: PJ Mehta's Practical Medicine, 17/e p237

282. **Ans. (d)** Nonfluent but meaningful speech
Ref: Davidson's Medicine, 19/e p1149

283. **Ans. (c)** Viral meningitis
Ref: Davidson's Medicine, 19/e p1193t

284. **Ans. (a)** Chorea
Ref: PJ Mehta's Practical Medicine, 17/e p209

285. **Ans. (c)** Thyroid ophthalmopathy
Ref: Davidson's Medicine, 19/e p694f

286. **Ans. (d)** Myasthenia gravis
Ref: Davidson's Medicine, 19/e p1184

287. **Ans. (d)** Middle cerebral artery
Ref: Davidson's Medicine, 19/e p262f

288. **Ans. (d)** Uncal herniation
Ref: PJ Mehta's Practical Medicine, 17/e p277t

289. **Ans. (b)** Muscular hypertrophy
Ref: PJ Mehta's Practical Medicine, 17/e p242t

290. **Ans. (d)** CSF reveals a low WBC count
Ref: Davidson's Medicine, 19/e p1193t

291. **Ans. (b)** Subarachnoid hemorrhage
Ref: KV Krishna Das's Medicine 5/e p1278

292. **Ans. (b)** GB syndrome
Ref: KV Krishna Das's Medicine 5/e p1326

293. **Ans. (b)** Iso-electric EEG for 30 minutes
Ref: KV Krishna Das's Medicine 5/e p1195

294. **Ans. (d)** Nerve root pressure
Ref: KV Krishna Das's Medicine 5/e p1319

295. **Ans. (d)** Pons
Ref: KV Krishna Das's Medicine 5/e p1276

296. **Ans. (a)** Vertebral artery occlusion
Ref: KV Krishna Das's Medicine 5/e p1271

297. **Ans. (c)** Alcoholic polyneuropathy
Ref: KV Krishna Das's Medicine 5/e p1323

298. **Ans. (c)** GB syndrome
Ref: KV Krishna Das's Medicine 5/e p1194

299. **Ans. (a)** Myoclonus found only in 10% cases
Ref: KV Krishna Das's Medicine 5/e p1236

300. **Ans. (d)** Acute aneurysmal hemorrhage
Ref: KV Krishna Das's Medicine 5/e p1269

301. **Ans. (c)** Decussating branches of lateral spinothalamic tract
Ref: KV Krishna Das's Medicine 5/e p1304

302. **Ans. (c)** Friedreich's ataxia
Ref: KV Krishna Das's Medicine 5/e p1300

303. **Ans. (d)** Multiple sclerosis
Ref: KV Krishna Das's Medicine 5/e p1188

304. **Ans. (d)** Internal carotid artery
Ref: KV Krishna Das's Medicine 5/e p1273

305. **Ans. (b)** Guillain Barre syndrome
Ref: KV Krishna Das's Medicine 5/e p1209

306. **Ans. (a)** Oculomotor
Ref: KV Krishna Das's Medicine 5/e p1205

307. **Ans. (c)** Dementia
Ref: KV Krishna Das's Medicine 5/e p1400

308. **Ans. (d)** Lorazepam
Ref: KV Krishna Das's Medicine 5/e p1252

309. **Ans. (c)** It is seen in immunocompromised patient
Ref: KV Krishna Das's Medicine 5/e p271

310. **Ans. (c)** Hypertension
Ref: KV Krishna Das's Medicine 5/e p1275

311. **Ans. (a)** Weakness and spasticity
Ref: KV Krishna Das's Medicine 5/e p1180

312. **Ans. (c)** Raised protein, decreased glucose, increased lymphocytes
Ref: KV Krishna Das's Medicine 5/e p1234

313. **Ans. (c)** Bilateral
Ref: KV Krishna Das's Medicine 5/e p1220

RESPIRATORY SYSTEM

314. **Ans. (c)** TLC
Ref: Davidson's Medicine, 19/e p510

315. **Ans. (c)** Chlamydia pneumoniae
Ref: Davidson's Medicine, 19/e p102

316. **Ans. (c)** Oral corticosteroids
Ref: Davidson's Medicine, 19/e p518

317. **Ans. (b) Pulmonary embolism**
Ref: Davidson's Medicine, 19/e p953t, 956t

318. **Ans. (a) Pulmonary embolism**
Ref: Davidson's Medicine, 19/e p953t

319. **Ans. (d) Non small cell Ca of lung/ NSCLC**
Ref: S. Das Surgery, 4/e p763

320. **Ans. (a) Small cell carcinoma**
Ref: KV Krishna Das's Medicine 5/e p 949

321. **Ans. (b) It requires a critical concentration of reduced hemoglobin in blood**
Ref: KV Krishna Das's Medicine 5/e p896

322. **Ans. (c) FEV1/FVC is high**
Ref: KV Krishna Das's Medicine 5/e p892

323. **Ans. (c) Sarcoidosis**
Ref: KV Krishna Das's Medicine 5/e p953

324. **Ans. (d) Bronchogenic Ca**
Ref: KV Krishna Das's Medicine 5/e p948

325. **Ans. (b) Hypertension**
Ref: KV Krishna Das's Medicine 5/e p941

326. **Ans. (a) Respiratory distress syndrome**
Ref: KV Krishna Das's Medicine 5/e p901

327. **Ans. (b) 100 ml**
Ref: Internet resources

328. **Ans. (a) RA**
Ref: KV Krishna Das's Medicine 5/e p936

329. **Ans. (c) Prolonged wheeze**
Ref: KV Krishna Das's Medicine 5/e p924

330. **Ans. (d) Mitral stenosis**
Ref: KV Krishna Das's Medicine 5/e p874

331. **Ans. (d) Increased 2,3 DPG**
Ref: KV Krishna Das's Medicine 5/e p886

332. **Ans. (b) Low PO2, high PCO2**
Ref: KV Krishna Das's Medicine 5/e p901

333. **Ans. (c) Foreign body aspiration**
Ref: KV Krishna Das's Medicine 5/e p909

334. **Ans. (a) Lung ventilation – perfusion scan**
Ref: KV Krishna Das's Medicine 5/e p942

335. **Ans. (c) Streptococcus pneumonia**
Ref: KV Krishna Das's Medicine 5/e p911

336. **Ans. (c) Reduced FEV1/FVC ratio**
Ref: KV Krishna Das's Medicine 5/e p939

337. **Ans. (d) Adrenals**
Ref: KV Krishna Das's Medicine 5/e p949

338. **Ans. (a) Oat cell carcinoma**
Ref: KV Krishna Das's Medicine 5/e p948

339. **Ans. (d) Tidal volume**
Ref: KV Krishna Das's Medicine 5/e p923

340. **Ans. (a) Increased FRC, increased residual volume**
Ref: KV Krishna Das's Medicine 5/e p891

341. **Ans. (d) Pulmonary emphysema**
Ref: KV Krishna Das's Medicine 5/e p893

342. **Ans. (d) Acute pneumonia**
Ref: KV Krishna Das's Medicine 5/e p910

343. **Ans. (b) Increased venous return**
Ref: KV Krishna Das's Medicine 5/e p903

344. **Ans. (d) All of the above**
Ref: Internet resources

345. **Ans. (b) Montelukast**
Ref: KV Krishna Das's Medicine 5/e p919

346. **Ans. (a) Horizontal fluid level**
Ref: KV Krishna Das's Medicine 5/e p961

347. **Ans. (b) PaO_2/FiO_2 ratio is </= 200**
Ref: KV Krishna Das's Medicine 5/e p904

348. **Ans. (a) Empyema**
Ref: KV Krishna Das's Medicine 5/e p958

349. **Ans. (b) Acute asthmatic attack**
Ref: KV Krishna Das's Medicine 5/e p762

350. **Ans. (b) Panacinar emphysema**
Ref: KV Krishna Das's Medicine 5/e p933

351. **Ans. (b) Rheumatoid arthritis**
Ref: KV Krishna Das's Medicine 5/e p957

352. **Ans. (c) Pulmonary artery**
Ref: KV Krishna Das's Medicine 5/e p278

353. **Ans. (c) Thermophilic actinomycetes**
Ref: KV Krishna Das's Medicine 5/e p918

354. **Ans. (a) MC malignancy of lung**
Ref: KV Krishna Das's Medicine 5/e p946

355. **Ans. (d) None**
Ref: KV Krishna Das's Medicine 5/e p911

356. **Ans. (c) SLE**
Ref: KV Krishna Das's Medicine 5/e p704

357. **Ans. (b) Chronic bronchitis**
Ref: KV Krishna Das's Medicine 5/e p895

358. Ans. (b) Flail chest
Ref: KV Krishna Das's Medicine 5/e p963

359. Ans. (c) Cerebral palsy
Ref: KV Krishna Das's Medicine 5/e p97

ONCOLOGY

360. Ans. (d) Liver
Ref: Davidson's Medicine, 19/e p876

361. Ans. (c) Hypergammaglobulinemia
Ref: Internet resources

MISCELLANEOUS

362. Ans. (c) Friedrich ataxia
Ref: Satyanarayana's Biochemistry, 3/e p538, 539

363. Ans. (c) Symptomatic females
Ref: Robbin's Basic Pathology, 7/e p780

364. Ans. (c) Non-granulomatous vasculitis
Ref: Robbin's Basic Pathology, 7/e p351

365. Ans. (a) X-linked
Ref: Robbin's Basic Pathology, 7/e p224

366. Ans. (b) IgA, C3
Ref: Robbin's Basic Pathology, 7/e p525

367. Ans. (c) Zinc
Ref: Davidson's Medicine, 19/e p872

368. Ans. (d) Male to male transmission only
Ref: KV Krishna Das's Medicine 5/e p9

369. Ans. (c) Hemophilia-A
Ref: KV Krishna Das's Medicine 5/e p8

370. Ans. (b) Duchenne's muscular dystrophy
Ref: KV Krishna Das's Medicine 5/e p1341

371. Ans. (b) Tumour is in subfrontal area
Ref: Internet resources

372. Ans. (b) Sickle cell anemia
Ref: KV Krishna Das's Medicine 5/e p689

373. Ans. (a) Sickle cell anemia
Ref: KV Krishna Das's Medicine 5/e p8

374. Ans. (a) G0-G1-S-G2-M
Ref: Internet resources

375. Ans. (b) SLE
Ref: KV Krishna Das's Medicine 5/e p706

376. Ans. (c) Cladarabine
Ref: Internet resources

377. Ans. (b) Hyaluronate in synovial fluid
Ref: KV Krishna Das's Medicine 5/e p696

378. Ans. (a) Myasthenia gravis
Ref: KV Krishna Das's Medicine 5/e p721

379. Ans. (d) Anti-Jo 1
Ref: KV Krishna Das's Medicine 5/e p1340

380. Ans. (a) Severe combined immune-deficiency syndrome
Ref: KV Krishna Das's Medicine 5/e p14

381. Ans. (c) Immunoglobulin
Ref: KV Krishna Das's Medicine 5/e p714

382. Ans. (c) Edrophonium test
Ref: KV Krishna Das's Medicine 5/e p1333

383. Ans. (a) B8
Ref: KV Krishna Das's Medicine 5/e p26

384. Ans. (a) Ash leaf spots
Ref: KV Krishna Das's Medicine 5/e p1328

385. Ans. (c) Mononeuritis multiplex
Ref: KV Krishna Das's Medicine 5/e p696

386. Ans. (b) Thrombocytopenia
Ref: KV Krishna Das's Medicine 5/e p

387. Ans. (c) Cystic fibrosis
Ref: KV Krishna Das's Medicine 5/e p539

388. Ans. (d) Desferrioxamine is the treatment of choice
Ref: KV Krishna Das's Medicine 5/e p591

389. Ans. (b) Pupil
Ref: KV Krishna Das's Medicine 5/e p117

PRACTICE QUESTIONS

HEMATOLOGY

1. Increase in which of the following shows satisfactory response to iron therapy for iron deficiency anemia:
   a. Serum ferritin
   b. Serum transferrin
   c. Erythrocyte count
   d. Hemoglobin

2. Which of the following indicates best prognosis in leukemia:
   a. Age between 1-10 years
   b. Total lymphocyte count > 1 lakh
   c. Petechiae
   d. Philadelphia chromosome

3. Which of the following is NOT a feature of cobalamin deficiency:
   a. Microcytosis b. Long tract signs
   c. Loss of proprioception d. Rhomberg sign

4. A strict vegetarian diet consumer developed progressive pallor. Peripheral smear showed hypersegmented neutrophils. MCV was found to be more than 100. Most likely diagnosis:
   a. Herediatry spherocytosis
   b. Megaloblastic anemia
   c. Dimorphic anemia
   d. Thalassemia

CARDIOVASCULAR SYSTEM

5. Postural hypotension is defined as a drop of:
   a. Systolic BP of more than 10 mm Hg on standing for 5 minutes
   b. Systolic BP of more than 20 mm Hg on standing for 5 minutes
   c. Diastolic BP of more than 10 mm Hg on standing for 5 minutes
   d. Diastolic BP of more than 20 mm Hg on standing for 5 minutes

6. ST segment depression in lead V1 and V2 suggests:
   a. Anterolateral infarct b. Anteroseptal infarct
   c. True posterior infarct d. Right ventricular infarct

7. What is the indication of using Digitalis in a patient with mitral stenosis:
   a. Atrial fibrillation
   b. Right ventricular failure
   c. Acute pulmonary edema
   d. Myocarditis

8. What is the best line of management of a young lady with diastolic blood pressure of 100 mm Hg:
   a. Rest
   b. Sedative
   c. Anti-hypertensive agent
   d. Diuretic

9. Which of the following is included in American Rheumatic Heart Association criteria for diagnosing rheumatic fever:
   a. Oral ulcer
   b. Malar rash
   c. Erythema marginatum
   d. Telangiectasia of nail

10. Duroziez sign is associated with which of the following valvular lesion:
   a. Aortic regurgitation
   b. Aortic stenosis
   c. Mitral regurgitation
   d. Mitral stenosis

11. Best method to differentiate between non-ST segment elevated MI/ NSTEMI and stable angina:
   a. Electrocardiography
   b. Cardiac markers
   c. Transthoracic Echocardiography
   d. Multi-uptake gated acquisition scan

12. Which of the following cardiac marker is last to rise and peak:
   a. CPK-myocardial bound
   b. LDH
   c. AST
   d. Troponin I

13. In which of the following condition, Y descent is absent and X wave is prominent:
   a. Restrictive cardiomyopathy
   b. Cardiac tamponade
   c. Constrictive pericarditis
   d. Right ventricular failure

Ans. 1. **d.** Hemoglobin 2. **a.** Age between 1-10 years 3. **a.** Microcytosis 4. **b.** Megaloblastic anemia
5. **b.** Systolic BP of... 6. **c.** True posterior infarct 7. **a.** Atrial fibrillation 8. **c.** Anti-hypertensive agent
9. **c.** Erythema marg... 10. **a.** Aortic regurgitation 11. **b.** Cardiac markers 12. **b.** LDH
13. **b.** Cardiac tamponade

14. Drug of choice for supraventricular tachycardia/ SVT:
a. Adenosine
b. Propranolol
c. Amiodarone
d. Lidocaine

15. Location and nature of murmur in aortic stenosis:
a. Right 2nd intercostal; low pitch murmur
b. Apex; low pitch mumur
c. Left sternal area; low pitch murmur
d. Pansystolic murmur; high pitch murmur

16. In mitral stenosis, a high pitched heart sound heard on auscultation:
a. Mid-diastolic murmur
b. Opening snap
c. Both
d. None

17. Rheumatic heart disease, prophylactic treatment should be given with:
a. 1.2 mega units of Benzathine penicillin once weekly
b. 1.2 mega units of Benzathine penicillin once every three weeks
c. 2.4 mega units of Benzathine penicillin once weekly
d. 2.4 mega units of Benzathine penicillin once every three weeks

18. Central venous pressure is measured to assess:
a. Total amount of blood
b. Urinary output
c. Adequacy of fluid replacement
d. Acid base disturbance

19. A male developed giddiness and syncope on sitting up from lying down position. This is indicative of:
a. Hypertension
b. Essential hypertension
c. Orthostatic hypotension
d. Paroxysmal hypertension

20. Wide fixed split second heart sound:
a. Vnetricular septal defect
b. Atrial septal defect
c. Patent ductus arteriosus
d. Pulmonary stenosis

21. Quincke's sign is seen in:
a. Aortic stenosis
b. Aortic regurgitation
c. Mitral regurgitation
d. Mitral stenosis

22. Which of the following is NOT associated with ST segment elevation on ECG:
a. Myocardial infarction
b. Coronary artery spasm
c. Constrictive pericarditis
d. Ventricular aneurysm

23. Balloon angioplasty is done through which artery:
a. Carotid artery
b. Femoral artery
c. Brachial artery
d. Popliteal artery

24. Dilated cardiomyopathy is characterised by:
a. Diastolic dysfunction
b. Restricted filling of ventricles
c. Systolic dysfunction
d. Reduced diastolic volume

25. Isolated systolic hypertension is seen in all EXCEPT:
a. Atherosclerosis
b. Coarctation of aorta
c. Severe aortic regurgitation
d. Hypothyroidism

26. MC cardiac lesion in a child with rheumatic fever:
a. Mitral regurgitation
b. Mitral stenosis
c. Aortic stenosis
d. Aortic regurgitation

EXCRETORY SYSTEM

27. Which of the following is NOT true regarding minimal change disease/ MCD in children:
a. Not associated with hypertension
b. Common in children less than 10 years
c. Massive proteinuria >3.5 gm/ day
d. Immune deposits

28. Earliest manifestation of diabetic nephropathy:
a. End stage renal disease
b. Isolated Hypertension
c. Macroscopic albuminuria
d. Microscopic albuminuria

29. All of the following are steroid resistant EXCEPT:
a. Post-streptococcal glomerulonephritis
b. RPGN
c. Minimal change disease
d. Recurrent hematuria

Ans. **14. a.** Adenosine **15. a.** Right 2nd intercostal... **16. b.** Opening snap **17. b.** 1.2 mega units...
18. c. Adequacy of fluid... **19. c.** Orthostatic hypotension **20. b.** Atrial septal defect **21. b.** Aortic regurgitation
22. c. Constrictive per... **23. b.** Femoral artery **24. c.** Systolic dysfunction **25. d.** Hypothyroidism
26. b. Mitral stenosis **27. d.** Immune deposits **28. d.** Microscopic album... **29. c.** Minimal change disease

30. Symptoms of chronic kidney disease will manifest if the GFR falls below:
a. 20 b. 40
c. 60 d. 80

31. Which of the following is useful in chronic kidney disease:
a. Beta blocker b. Amlodipine
c. ACE inhibitors d. All of the above

32. In a case of nephrolithiais, which will you prefer:
a. Low sodium diet b. Low calcium diet
c. High sodium diet d. Low citrate diet

33. Among the following, which is an indication for performing dialysis in acute renal failure:
a. Hypertension b. Hyperkalemia
c. Hypernatremia d. Metabolic alkalosis

34. Which of the following is the MC cause of glomerulonephritis:
a. Post-streptococcal glomerulonephritis
b. Diabetes mellitus
c. Autosomal recessive polycystic kidney disease
d. Crescentic glomerulonpehritis

35. Which of the following condition is associated with membranous glomerulopathy:
a. Diabetes mellitus b. Hypertension
c. Acute renal failure d. Solid organ carcinoma

GASTROINTESTINAL TRACT AND ABDOMEN

36. Which of the following cause of jaundice presents with markedly raised alkaline phsphatase:
a. Biliary cirrhosis
b. Spirochaetal jaundice
c. Carcinoma head of pancreas
d. Acute viral hepatitis

37. DOC for pseudomembranous colitis:
a. Penicillin b. Erythromycin
c. Metronidazole d. Albendazole

38. A young adult is brought to the emergency department with complains of epigastric region pain which radiates to back and vomiting. He had a party last night. On examination fever and tachycardia was noted. Which of the following is best to make a diagnosis:
a. Serum lipase
b. CPK-myocardial bound
c. Alkaline phosphatase
d. Serum amylase

39. Australia antigen is related to:
a. HBcAg b. HBsAg
c. HBeAg d. IgM Anti-HBc

40. Which of the following is specific antibody in Celiac disease:
a. Anti-tissue transglutaminase antibody/ tTG
b. Anti-gliadin antibody/ AGA
c. Anti-endomysial antibody/ EMA
d. All of the above

41. Which of the following correlate with active viral replication of hepatitis B virus:
a. HBsAg b. Anti-HBs
c. IgM Anti-HBc d. HBV DNA

INFECTIOUS DISEASES

42. Quadrivalent meningococcal vaccine is NOT against which serotype:
a. Type A b. Type B
c. Type C d. Type Y

43. All of the following are true for mumps EXCEPT:
a. Recurrent attacks b. Parotitis
c. Generalized infection d. Orchitis in males

44. MC site of hydatid cyst:
a. Lung b. Liver
c. Spleen d. Kidney

45. MC carcinoma associated with AIDS is caused by:
a. HPV-16 b. Retrovirus
c. HHV-8 d. HIV

46. SSPE is a complication of:
a. Mumps b. Measles
c. Rubella d. Vitamin B_{12} deficiency

47. MC complication of measles:
a. Otitis media b. Encephalitis
c. SSPE d. Diarrhoea

48. HIV principally affects which of the following:
a. B cells
b. Neutrophils
c. CD4+ cells (T lymphocytes)
d. RBC

Ans. 30. **c.** 60 31. **c.** ACE inhibitors 32. **a.** Low sodium diet 33. **b.** Hyperkalemia
34. **a.** Post-streptoc... 35. **d.** Solid organ carcinoma 36. **c.** Carcinoma head... 37. **c.** Metronidazole
38. **a.** Serum lipase 39. **b.** HBsAg 40. **a.** Anti-tissue transglut... 41. **d.** HBV DNA
42. **b.** Type B 43. **a.** Recurrent attacks 44. **b.** Liver 45. **c.** HHV-8
46. **b.** Measles 47. **a.** Otitis media 48. **c.** CD4+ cells (T lymphocytes)

49. A 42 year old patient with previous respiratory problem presented with fever, weight loss and loss of appetite. He is having a lump in right iliac fossa. On examination signs of ileal stenosis can be elicited. Most likely diagnosis:

a. Typhoid b. TB
c. Crohn's disease d. Ulcerative colitis

50. A know case of HIV infection presented with acute watery diarrhoea associated with fever and general malaise. Organism responsible for this presentation is:

a. Cryptococcus b. Cryptosporodium
c. Salmonella d. Vibrio cholerae

ENDOCRINOLOGY

51. Which of the following is true for SIADH:

a. Hyponatremia with increased plasma osmolality
b. Hyperatremia with decreased plasma osmolality
c. Hyponatremia with decreased plasma osmolality
d. Hyperatremia with increased plasma osmolality

52. In Bartter's syndrome, pathology is in which part of kidney:

a. Collecting duct
b. PCT
c. Thick ascending loop of Henle
d. DCT

53. Which type of neuropathy is seen in diabetes mellitus:

a. Sensory polyneuropathy
b. Autonomic neuropathy
c. Radiculopathy
d. Myelopathy

54. A young lady was having a random blood sugar level of 600 mg/ dL and sodium concentration of 110 mEq/ L. What will happen to sodium levels if Insulin is given to her:

a. Increase in sodium levels
b. Decrease in sodium levels
c. Unchanged sodium levels
d. Variable

METABOLIC AND NUTRITIONAL DISORDERS

55. Schiling's test is done to detect:

a. Vitamin B_{12} malabsorption
b. Pancreatic insufficiency
c. Pernicious anemia
d. Iron deficiency anemia

56. Which of the following is NOT an ECG finding of hypokalemia:

a. U wave b. Tall T wave
c. ST depression d. Prolonged QT interval

57. Hormone used for managing hyperkalemia:

a. Glucagon b. Insulin
c. Growth hormone d. Adrenaline

NEUROLOGY

58. A young man cannot speak fluently, but can inform the things in writing. Which brain area is affected:

a. Broaca area b. Wernickes area
c. Paracentral lobule d. Insula

59. Cerebral bleeding in a hypertensive is commonly seen at:

a. Cerebellum b. Cerebrum
c. Thalamus d. Putamen

RESPIRATORY SYSTEM

60. A 60 year old patient got pneumonia. He is apparently normal and oriented. Respiratory rate is >50/ minute. Management:

a. Chest physiotherapy
b. Symptomatic and supportive
c. Wait and watch
d. Primary treatment and referral to hospital

61. Lower lobes of the lung are damaged in which pneumoconiosis:

a. Silicosis
b. Coal worker's pneumoconiosis
c. Byssinosis
d. Asbestosis

62. NOT a feature of ARDS:

a. Reduced surfactant
b. Exudate in alveoli
c. Reduced lung compliance
d. $paO_2/ FiO_2 >200$

63. Biot breathing is a feature of:

a. Flail chest b. Uremia
c. High altitude d. Meningitis

64. Effect of hyperventilation:

a. Increased carbon dioxide
b. Decreased carbon dioxide
c. Increased pO_2
d. Decreased pO_2

65. A patient was diagnosed to have chronic obstructive pulmonary disease. Which of the following is important in management:

a. Quit smoking b. Bronchodilators
c. Low flow oxygen d. Mucolytics

Ans. **49. b.** TB **50. b.** Cryptosporodium **51. c.** Hyponatremia **52. c.** Thick ascending...
53. a. Sensory polyn... **54. a.** Increase in sodium... **55. a.** Vitamin B_{12} malab... **56. b.** Tall T wave
57. b. Insulin **58. a.** Broaca area **59. d.** Putamen **60. d.** Primary treatment...
61. d. Asbestosis **62. d.** $paO_2/ FiO_2 >200$ **63. d.** Meningitis **64. b.** Decreased carbon...
65. a. Quit smoking

66. **A patient is a heavy smoker. Now while considering ill-effects of smoking, what is most important:**
   a. Duration of smoking
   b. Number of times smoking in a day
   c. Brand of cigarette
   d. Filter of cigarette

67. **All of the following cases will respond to raised level of CO_2 EXCEPT:**
   a. Narcotic overdosage
   b. Obesity
   c. Pulmonary edema
   d. Type I respiratory failure

68. **Which of the following is NOT a feature of Aspirin sensitive asthma:**
   a. Nasal polyps
   b. Treatment with inhaled steroids
   c. Rhinosinusitis
   d. Involves Immunoglobulin E

ONCOLOGY

69. **Smoking causes which tumour:**
   a. Vaginal carcinoma b. Laryngeal carcinoma
   c. Liver carcinoma d. Tongue carcinoma

70. **Raised level of catecholamines, vanillylmandelic acid and homovanillic acid in urine suggest:**
   a. Neuroblastoma b. Retinonblastoma
   c. Wilms tumour d. Phaeochromocytoma

MISCELLANEOUS

71. **Micronutrient used in Wilson disease:**
   a. Copper b. Aluminium
   c. Iron d. Zinc

72. **A patient having intermittent ptosis, diplopia, proximal muscle weakness and fatiguability after sustained exercise. Which of the following is an useful test:**
   a. Short ACTH test b. Edrophonium test
   c. Schilling test d. Creatine kinase

73. **True regarding toxic epidermal necrolysis:**
   a. >10% body area involved
   b. >20% body area involved
   c. >30% body area involved
   d. >40% body area involved

74. **What could be the most probable diagnosis of a young lady presenting with bilateral hilar lymphadenopathy and joint pain. ACE levels are also found to be elevated:**
   a. Sarcoidosis b. Silicosis
   c. Hodgkins lymphoma d. Non-Hodgkins lymphoma

75. **What could be the most probable diagnosis of a young female who developed rashes on sun exposed parts. She also had pain in both the knees and low grade fever:**
   a. Systemic lupus erythematosis
   b. Rheumatoid arthritis
   c. Photodermatitis
   d. Porphyria

76. **Which of the following complication can be seen in patient with long standing Rheumatoid arthritis:**
   a. Milk alkali syndrome b. Nephrolithiasis
   c. Paradoxical aciduria d. Secondary amyloidosis

77. **A 40 year old female presents with hip pain, pericarditis, hematuria and muscle pains. Laboratory investigation showed raised ESR, moderate to severe proteinuria. and anti-nuclear antibody positivity. Most likely diagnosis:**
   a. Rheumatoid arthritis b. SLE
   c. Scleroderma d. Sjogren's syndrome

78. **Drug of choice for tetanus:**
   a. Metronidazole b. Penicillin
   c. Ampicillin d. Amooxycillin

79. **Which is seen in anorexia nervosa:**
   a. Arrhythmia b. Menorrhagia
   c. Intolerance to heat d. All of the above

Ans. **66. a.** Duration of... **67. a.** Narcotic... **68. d.** Involves Immuno... **69. b.** Laryngeal carcinoma **70. d.** Phaeochromocy... **71. d.** Zinc **72. b.** Edrophonium test **73. c.** >30% body area involved **74. a.** Sarcoidosis **75. a.** Systemic lupus eryth... **76. d.** Secondary amyloid... **77. b.** SLE **78. b.** Penicillin **79. a.** Arrhythmia

IMAGE-BASED QUESTIONS

1. Following image represents the deficiency signs of:

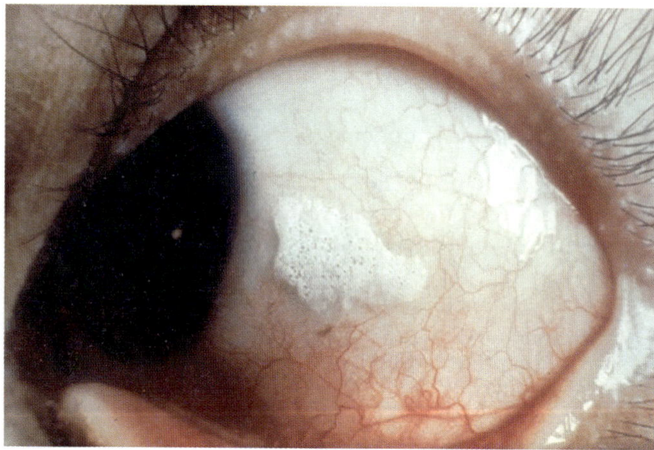

a. Vitamin A b. Vitamin B
c. Vitamin C d. Vitamin D

In vitamin A deficiency, the bulbar conjunctiva becomes dry, and rough greyish triangular foamy raised patches appear (Bitot's spots).

2. ECG changes are suggestive of:

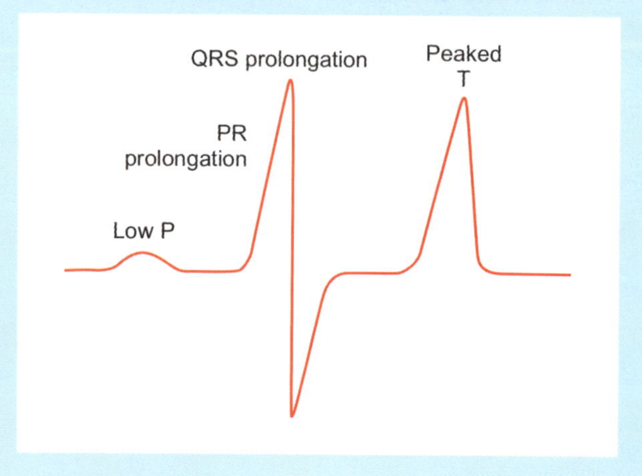

a. Hypercalcemia
b. Hypernatremia
c. Hyperkalemia
d. Hypermagnesemia

The ECG changes in hyperkalemia are: (i) tall peaked T waves (serum K^+ 6-7 mmol/L) (ii) prolongation of PR interval and absent p waves (serum K^+ 7-8 mmol/L) (iii) widening of QRS (serum K^+ 7-8 mmol/L) (iv) sine wave, ventricular tachycardia, ventricular fibrillation (serum K^+ 8-9 mmol/L) (v) cardiac arrest (serum K^+ >9 mmol/L)

3. Spot diagnosis:

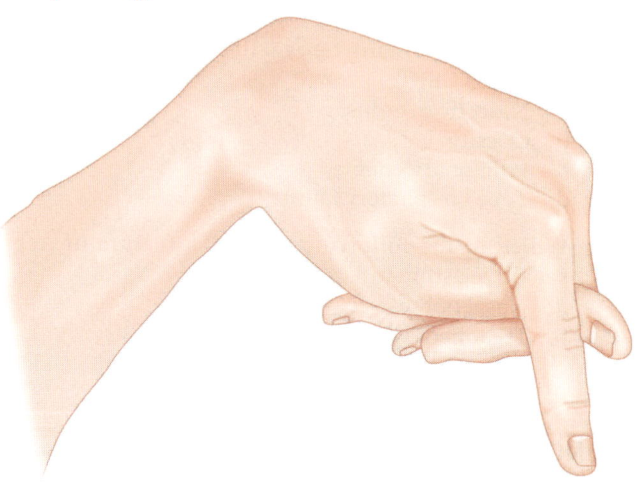

a. Hyponatremia
b. Hypernatremia
c. Hypocalcemia
d. Hypercalcemia

Tetany occurs due to hypocalcemia. It manifests as muscle cramps, paresthesia of the hands, feet and mouth, spasmophilia (carpopedal spasm, bronchospasm and laryngospasm) and severe neuromuscular irritability.

4. Spot diagnosis:

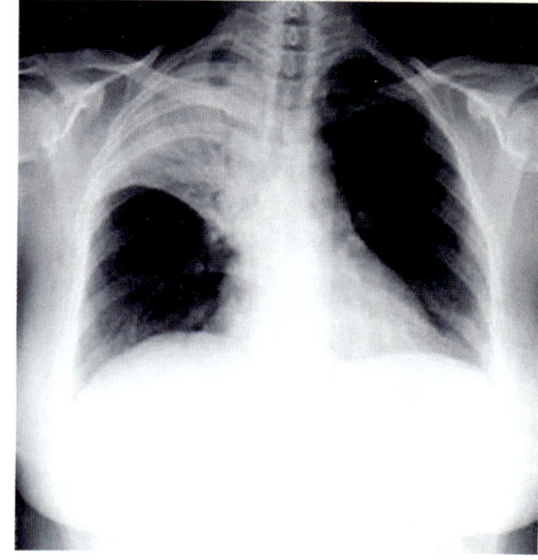

a. Pleural effusion b. Pneumothorax
c. Consolidation d. Empyema

Presence of homogenous opacities with well defined margins indicate pulmonary consolidation. Since there is no change in the volume of the lung the trachea and mediastinum are not shifted.

5. **Sputum microscopy of a patinet with asthma showed the following image. Diagnosis:**

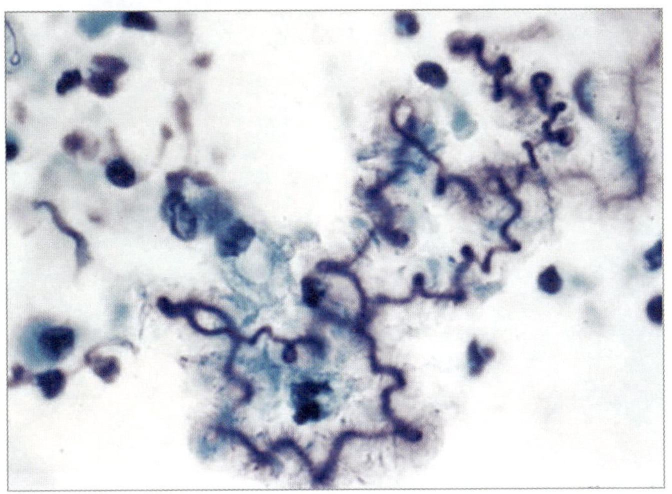

a. Anitschkov cells
b. Curschmann's spiral
c. Reid's index
d. Caterpillar cells

Sputum of a patient with asthma may reveal numerous eosinophils, mucus plugs and Curschmann's spirals (cast of smaller airways)

6. **Spot diagnosis:**

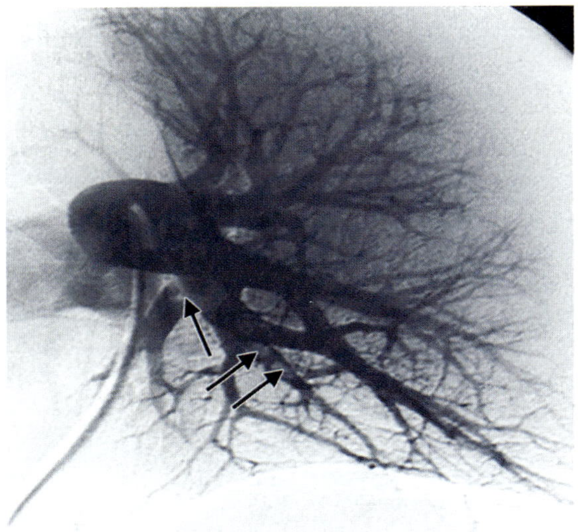

a. Fungal alveolitis
b. Interstitial lung disease
c. Chronic bronchitis
d. Pulmonary embolism

Pulmonary angiography is the most specific method for pulmonary embolism which unequivocally demonstrates pulmonary arterial obstruction. The common findings include abrupt "cut-off" or amputation of lobar or segmental arteries and intraluminal filling defects (arrows)

7. **Spot diagnosis:**

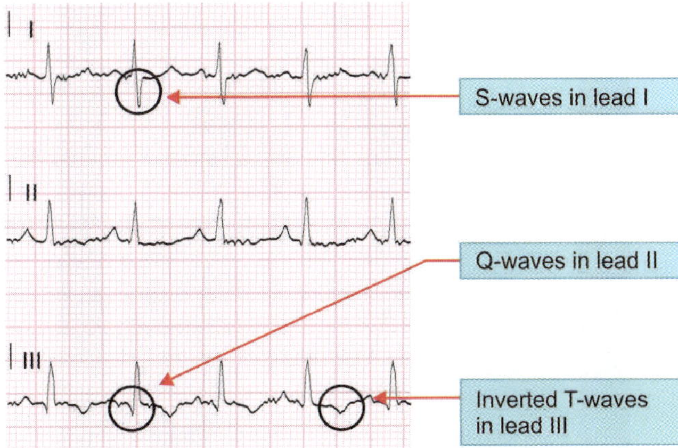

a. Myocardial infarction
b. Pulmonary edema
c. Pulmonary infarction
d. Pulmonary embolism

Classic ECG abnormalities develop only in few cases of pulmonary embolism, which shows prominent S-wave in leads I and II with the development of Q wave and T-wave inversion in lead III.

8. **Spot diagnosis (pathology on right side):**

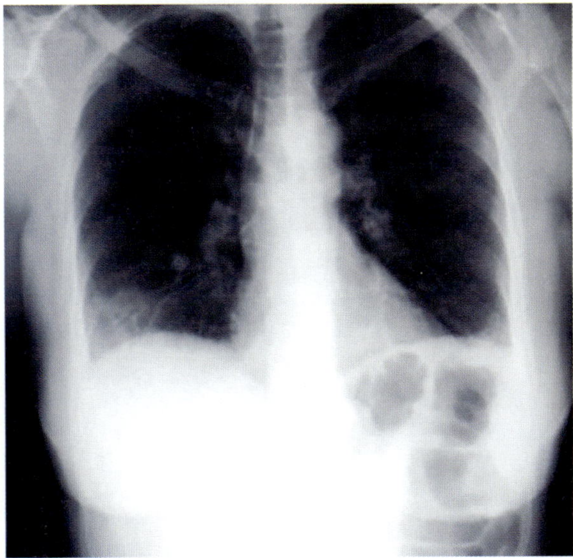

a. Pneumothorax
b. Lung collapse
c. Pulmonary embolism
d. Pneumonia

Pulmonary infarct (in pulmonary embolism) produces a trainagular opacity with the base of the triangle towards the pleura and its apex towards the hilum (Hampton's hump)

9. Spot diagnosis:

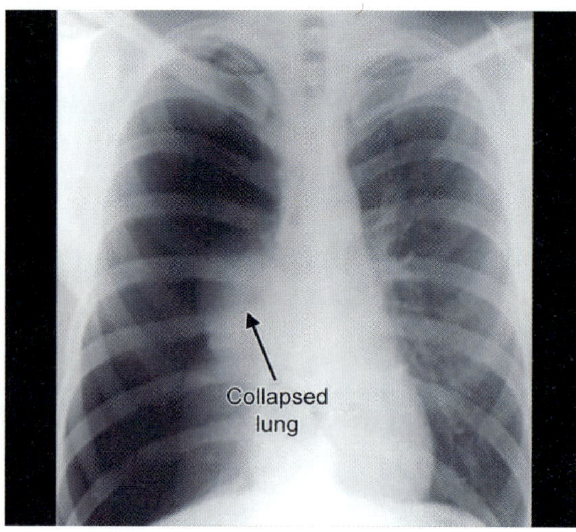

a. Pulmonary arterial hypertension
b. Pulmonary embolism
c. Coarctation of aorta
d. Pneumothorax

The radiological features of pneumothorax are diagnostic in a well developed case of pneumothorax. The affected side is hypertranslucent due to collection of free air in the pleural cavity and absence of normal lung markings. The outer margin of the collpased lung is seen as a sharp margin against the background of air. There is shift of the trachea and mediastinum to the opposite side.

10. Spot diagnosis:

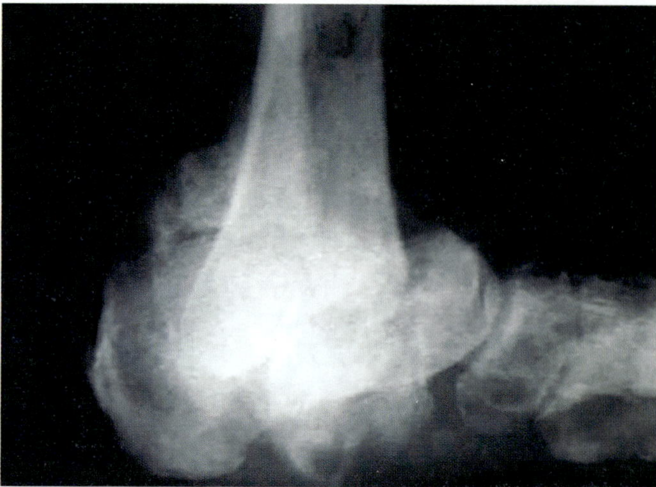

a. Cluttons joint
b. CTEV
c. Charcot's joint
d. Rheumatoid arthritis

Destructive changes in joints induced by denervation was described by Jean Martin Charcot (French physician) in 1868. The affected joints undergo denegrative changes due to hypermobility and laxity of the capsule and ligaments, and the articular surfaces may disintegrate.

MCQ POINTS

S. No.	Question statements	Answers
1.	MC type of cardiomyopathy	***Hypertrophic***
2.	Minimal change disease is managed by	***Steroids***
3.	IOC for interstitial lung disease	***High resolution CT scan***
4.	Loeffler's syndrome is caused by	***Ascarias***
5.	2 conditions where Paradoxical breathing is seen	***Unilateral diaphragmatic palsy, Flail chest***
6.	Charcot leyden crystals are seen in sputum of	***Asthma***
7.	MC type of emphysema	***Centri-acinar***
8.	Signs seen on HRCT in bronchiectasis	***Tram track, signet ring***
9.	C/I to use of digoxin:	***HOCM***
10.	Pneumoconiosis associated with cotton dust	***Byssinosis***
11.	Acid fastness of mycobacterium TB is due to	***Mycolic acid in cell wall***
12.	DOC for pneumocystis carinii	***Co-trimoxazole***
13.	MC carcinoma causing superior vena cava syndrome	***Small cell Ca***
14.	MC manifestation of pulmonary embolism	***Dyspnea***
15.	Ground glass appearance on chest X-ray is seen in	***ARDS***
16.	In JVP, c wave is due to	***Tricuspid valve closure***
17.	In ECG, p wave is due to	***Atrial depolarization***
18.	DOC for PSVT	***Adenosine***
19.	MacCallum patch is seen in which condition	***Rheumatic heart disease***
20.	IOC for mitral stenosis	***ECHO***
21.	Austin flint murmur is heard in	***Severe aortic regurgitation***
22.	Drug contraindicated in HOCM	***Digoxin***
23.	Enzyme which rises earliest in MI	***Myoglobin***
24.	Becks triad is associated with	***Cardiac tamponade***
25.	Earliest feature of iron deficiency anemia	***Reduced serum ferritin***
26.	SACD of spinal cord is associated with deficiency of	***Vitamin B12 deficiency***
27.	Erythropoietin levels are … in polycythemia rubra vera	***Normal/ low***
28.	Raised osmotic fragility of RBC is seen in	***Hereditary spherocytosis***
29.	Haptoglobin levels are …. in hemolytic anemia	***Low***
30.	Basic defect in hereditary spherocytosis	***Ankyrin***
31.	Malignant cell of Hodgkin lymphoma	***Reed Sternberg***
32.	MC type of Hodgkin lymphoma in India	***Mixed cellularity***
33.	Wire-loop lesions are seen in	***SLE***
34.	Shrinking lung syndrome is seen in	***SLE***
35.	Pseudo-hypertrophy of muscles is a feature of	***Duchenne muscular dystrophy***
36.	Surgical procedure done in myasthenia gravis	***Thymectomy***
37.	MC site of peptic ulcer	***Duodenum-first part***
38.	Specific test for diagnosing Whipple's disease	***Biopsy***
39.	Mainstay of therapy for inflammatory bowel disease	***5-Amino salicylic acid***
40.	First viral marker to appear after HBV infection	***HBsAg***
41.	IgM anti-HBc indicates	***Recent infection***
42.	Hepatitis virus carrying worst prognosis in pregnancy	***HEV***
43.	KF rings in Descemet membrane of cornea is seen in	***Wilson disease***

S. No.	Question statements	Answers
44.	Skip lesions are seen in	***Crohn's disease***
45.	MC complication of peptic ulcer	***Hemorrhage***
46.	Anti-centromere antibody is associated with	***Scleroderma***
47.	Standard treatment of Kawasaki disease	***I/V immunoglobulins***
48.	Necrotizing vasculitis of small and medium sized muscular arteries is a feature of	***Polyarteritis nodosa***
49.	Lab findings of von-Willebrand disease include .. BT and … PT	***Raised BT, normal PT***
50.	Hemophilia A is low levels of factor….	***VIII***
51.	Pretibial myxedema is seen in which condition	***Thyrotoxicosis***
52.	MC cause of sudden death in MI	***Ventricular fibrillation***
53.	Bite cells are seen in	***G-6PD deficiency***
54.	Uncompensated metabolic alkalosis is characterized by ….pH, ….. HCO_3 and …… pCO_2	***High pH, High bicarbonate and normal CO_2***
55.	Granulomatous condition associated with hypercalcemia	***Sarcoidosis***
56.	Displacement of cardiac apex to left and downward indicates hypertrophy of which chamber	***Left ventricle***
57.	Caplan syndrome is combination of	***Pneumoconiosis + RA***
58.	Osler's nodes are seen in	***SABE***
59.	Sipple's syndrome is also known as	***MEN-IIA***
60.	Pneumocystis prophylaxis is started when CD4 count is below	***200***
61.	Hemiballismus is seen in lesions of which nuclei	***Subthalamic nuclei***
62.	Value of TSH in hypothyroidism	***Increased***
63.	Mask like facies is a feature of	***Parkinsonism***
64.	Defective osteoid formation is a feature of which disease	***Scurvy***
65.	DOC for toxoplasmosis	***Sulfadiazine + pyrimethamine***
66.	Anti-gliadin antibodies and villous atrophy suggest the diagnosis of	***Celiac disease***
67.	MC site of hypertensive intracerebral bleed	***Putamen***
68.	Antibodies seen in primary biliary cirrhosis	***Anti-mitochondrial***
69.	HLA associated with IDDM	***DR3 (mainly)***
70.	Inferior notching of ribs is seen in	***Coarctation of aorta***
71.	A patient presented with proteinuria, hematuria and hypertension. Diagnosis is	***Nephritic syndrome***
72.	Auto-splenectomy is a feature of	***Sickle cell anemia***
73.	Anti-HBs presence signifies	***Immunity to HBV***
74.	Best measure of iron status of body	***Serum ferritin***
75.	MC symptom of primary biliary cirrhosis	***Pruritus***
76.	Gastric MALT lymphoma is caused by which organism	***H. pylori***
77.	Pretibial myxedema is seen in	***Hyperthyroidism***
78.	Tremors at rest occurs in lesions of	***Basal ganglia***
79.	Maltworker's lung is caused by	***Aspergillus fumigates***
80.	Uncompensated metabolic alkalosis is characterized by ….. pH, …… HCO_3 and …… Pco_2	***High, high, normal***
81.	Dietary fibres decreases serum cholesterol by	***Reduces absorption***
82.	Sinus bradycardia is defined as heart rate less than	***60***
83.	MC cause of infective endocarditis	***Staph. Aureus***
84.	Which chlyamydial infection is associated with atherosclerosis	***Chlamydia pneumonia***

S. No.	Question statements	Answers
85.	Anemia in CRF is due to	***Decreased erythropoietin***
86.	MC cause of secondary hypertension	***Renal parenchymal disease***
87.	Prominent U waves on ECG are seen in	***Hypokalemia***
88.	Loud P2 is heard in	***Pulmonary hypertension***
89.	Fainting attacks are more common in which valvular condition	***Aortic stenosis***
90.	Angina pectoris is more common in which valvular condition	***Aortic stenosis***
91.	Effect of hypoxia on pulmonary circulation	***Vasoconstriction***
92.	Which artery is involved in lateral medullary syndrome	***Vertebral artery (posterior inferior cerebellar artery)***
93.	Glycosylated hemoglobin value, which indicates good control of sugar	***7%***
94.	Spike and dome pattern of EEG is seen in which epilepsy	***Petit mal/ absence seizures***
95.	Keratoderma blenorrhagica is seen in	***Reiter's syndrome***
96.	Treatment of hyperviscosity in Waldenstorm's hypergammaglobulinemia	***Plasmapheresis***
97.	Size of spleen in hairy cell leukemia	***Massive splenomegaly***
98.	Prothrombin time in von Willebrand's disease	***Normal***
99.	HLA association of myasthenia gravis	***B8***
100.	Pseudomembranous colitis is caused by which bacteria	***Clostridium difficile***
101.	Bleeding into which part of CNS can cause pin point pupil	***Pons***
102.	Karyotype of Klinefelter's syndrome	***47XXY***
103.	Stibgluconate sodium is DOC for	***Kala-azar***
104.	Shagreen patch is seen in	***Tuberous sclerosis***
105.	HIV virus primarily affects which cells	***CD4***
106.	Philadelphia chromosome is seen in which leukemia	***Adult CML***
107.	Drug used for amoebiasis and giardiasis	***Metronidazole***
108.	Correct sequence of increase in enzymes in MI	***Myoglobin – CPK – AST- LDH***
109.	Earliest diagnosis of MI is by which enzyme	***CPK-MB***
110.	Best indicator of MI after 72 hours is	***Troponin***
111.	Electrolytes are increased in sweat in which condition	***Cystic fibrosis***
112.	Co-arctation of aorta is associated which syndrome	***Turner syndrome***
113.	Blue sclera is a feature of	***Osteogenesis imperfect***
114.	Steroid induced myopathy mainly involves which muscles	***Pelvis***
115.	Emergency peri-cardiocentesis is done for	***Acute cardiac tamponade***
116.	Sensation first lost in syringomyelia	***Pain and temperature***
117.	Dystrophin gene is of most value in diagnosing which condition	***Duchenne muscular dystrophy***
118.	Angular stomatitis is associated with deficiency of which vitamiin	***Riboflavin***
119.	Mode of inheritance of cystic fibrosis	***Autosomal recessive***
120.	Mycosis fungoides is a tumor of which cell	***T cell***
121.	Anticholinergic commonly used in management of asthma	***Ipratropium***
122.	Western blot test is used for which disease	***HIV***
123.	Early manifestation of hyponatremia	***Altered sensorium***
124.	DOC for status epilepticus	***Lorazepam***
125.	Blindness in temporal arteritis is due to involvement of which artery	***Posterior ciliary artery***
126.	Pseudo-tumor cerebri is caused by	***Hypervitaminosis A***
127.	Type of anemia associated with SACD of spinal cord	***Megaloblastic***

S. No.	Question statements	Answers
128.	Which Hepatitis infection commonly progresses to chronicity	***HCV***
129.	DOC for trigeminal neuralgia	***Carbamazepine***
130.	Anti-Jo1 antibodies are seen in	***Polymyositis***
131.	MC cause of subacute bacterial endocarditis is	***Strept viridians***
132.	Lung carcinoma with worst prognosis	***Small cell***
133.	Most serious complication of onchocerciasis	***Blindness***
134.	Pupil in datura poisoning	***Dilated***
135.	Hyaline cast in urine suggest	***Normal***
136.	Increase in number of component cells of a tissue resulting in increase in size is known as	***Hyperplasia***
137.	Festinating gait is seen in	***Parkinsonism***
138.	Defective mineralization of osteoid is a feature of which disease	***Rickets***
139.	Management of congenital hydrocoele	***Herniotomy***
140.	Drug induced SLE is related to	***Anti-histone antibodies***
141.	Salt losing nephropathy is also known as	***Interstitial nephritis***
142.	DOC for ventricular tachycardia (due to digitalis)	***Lidocaine***
143.	MOA of zileuton	***5-lipoxygenase***
144.	Differential cyanosis is seen in	***PDA (with reversal of shunts)***
145.	Cranial MC involved in raised intracranial pressure	***6th***
146.	DOC for HOCM	***Propranolol***
147.	HBeAg presence signifies	***Infectivity***
148.	Feature of JVP in atrial fibrillation	***Absent***
149.	Thrombotic occlusion of hepatic vein is a feature of	***Budd Chiari syndrome***
150.	WBC cast in urine suggest	***Pyelonephritis***
151.	Multiple punched out lesion on skull X-ray is a feature of	***Multiple myeloma***
152.	Histological feature of malignant hypertension	***Hyperplastic arteriosclerosis***
153.	DOC for hairy cell leukemia	***Cladribine***
154.	Changes seen on electron microscopy in minimal change disease	***Loss of foot process***
155.	Hyaline arteriosclerosis is associated with	***Benign hypertension***
156.	Graham steel murmur is heard in	***Severe pulmonary regurgitation***
157.	Diagnosis of phaeochromocytoma is done by	***Urinary Vaniyl Mandelic Acid***
158.	Medullary Ca of thyroid is a component of MEN type	***II***
159.	Color changes of Raynauds phenomenon	***White – blue – red***
160.	Bronze diabetes is related to	***Hemochromatosis***
161.	Appearance of gallbladder in starvation	***Distended***
162.	Hereditary fructose intolerance is because of deficiency of which enzyme	***Aldolase B***
163.	MC cause of meningitis in infants	***E. coli, Group B streptococcus***
164.	Clutton's joint is related to	***Late congenital syphilis***
165.	Waddling gait is seen in	***Bilateral CDH/ DDH***
166.	MC heart tumor	***Secondaries***
167.	Specific antibodies associated with SLE	***Anti-ds DNA***
168.	Most dependent part of pelvis in standing position	***Pouch of douglas***
169.	Pain and temperature is carried by which tract	***Lateral spinothalamic tract***
170.	Hyper-translucency on chest X-ray with hyper-resonant percussion suggest	***Pneumothorax***

S. No.	Question statements	Answers
171.	Albumino-cytological dissociation on CSF examination suggests	***Guillain Barre syndrome***
172.	Gold standard for diagnosing interstitial lung disease	***High Resolution CT scan***
173.	Diabetic keto-acidosis is commoner in which type of DM	***Type I***
174.	MC inherited bleeding disorder	***von-Willebrand disease***
175.	RBC cast in urine suggest	***Glomerular pathology***
176.	Parameter used to monitor short term DM control	***Serum fructosamine***
177.	Characteristic histological feature of DM nephropathy	***Nodular glomerulosclerosis***
178.	DOC for minimal change disease	***Steroids***
179.	Changes seen on light microscopy in minimal change disease	***Normal***
180.	Kimmelstein Wilson nodule is associated with	***Diabetic nephropathy***
181.	Mode of inheritance of adult polycystic kidney	***Autosomal dominant***
182.	IOC for chronic SAH	***MRI***
183.	MC cause of primary hyperparathyroidism	***Parathyroid adenoma***
184.	MC cause of dementia in elderly	***Alzheimer's***
185.	Creutzfeldt Jacobson disease is caused by	***Prions***
186.	Earliest feature of Friedreich's ataxia	***Ataxia***
187.	Intention tremor are seen in .... lesion	***Cerebellar***
188.	MC cause of meningitis in children	***H. influenza***
189.	MC cause of neuropathic joint disease	***Diabetes***
190.	High stepping gait is seen in	***Foot drop***
191.	MC posterior fossa tumor	***Cerebellar astrocytoma***
192.	Antibodies associated with drug induced SLE	***Anti-histone***
193.	Ascending motor paralysis is a feature of	***Guillain Barre syndrome***
194.	Tract involved in neuro-syphilis	***Dorsal column***
195.	In CSF examination, cob web appearance of CSF is a feature of ..... meningitis	***TB***
196.	Cloudy appearance of CSF is observed in.... meningitis	***Pyogenic***
197.	Gold standard for diagnosing pulmonary embolism	***Pulmonary angiography***
198.	Leading cause of end stage renal disease	***Diabetes***
199.	A 8-year-old girl with recurrent episodes of bleeding. BT is prolonged but PT is normal. Condition is	***von-Willebrand disease***

CHAPTER

4

GENERAL SURGERY

KEY POINTS

Vascular Entities

Port-wine stain	Vascular malformation present at birth
	Does not regress
Strawberry angioma	Capillary hemangioma not present at birth appear at 1–3 weeks slowly regresses
Salmon patch	Present at birth

Hemorrhage

Primary hemorrhage	Immediately postoperative
Secondary hemorrhage	Within 7–14 days postoperative due to infection
Reactionary hemorrhage	Within 24 hours of surgery, due to slippage of ligature or hypertension.

Buerger's Disease

- Thromboangitis obliterans
- Inflammatory reaction in the arterial wall, and neighboring veins and nerves
- More common in middle-aged men
- Associated with smoking
- Segmental, small and medium-sized arteries are affected
- Both distal extremities are affected.

Arterial Occlusion Syndrome

- Leriche's syndrome: Occlusion in the region of bifurcation of aorta and internal iliac arteries, leading to intermittent claudication
- Most common vessel to be involved in embolism is femoral.

Stages Seen in Raynaud's Phenomenon

- Stage of local syncope /stage of blanching: Pallor
- Stage of local asphyxia/ stage of dusky anoxia: Cyanosis
- Stage of recovery /stage of red engorgement: Redness.

Signs/Symptoms of Ischemia

- Pain
- Pulse—absent
- Pallor
- Paraesthesia
- Paralysis

Storage of Blood

CPD	Weeks
CPDA-I	5 Weeks

Conditions Indicating Significant Ischemia

- Ischemic ulceration
- Neuropathy
- Rest pain
- Gangrene
- Claudication is due to mild ischemia.

Amputation level	Stump length
Arm	8 inches
Forearm	8 inches
Leg	5.5 inches
Thigh	10–12 inches

Amputation eponym	Description
Lisfranc's	Disarticulation through tarsometatarsal joint
Chopart's	Disarticulation through midtarsal joint
Syme's	Removal of foot anterior to medial malleolus
Burger's	Below knee
Gittistoke's	Supracondylar

Cranial Hematomas with their Causes

Type	Causes
Epidural hematoma	Rupture of middle meningeal artery
Subdural heamatoma	Torn bridging veins (superior cerebral vein)
Subarachnoid haematoma	Aneurysm rupture
Intracerebral hemorrhage	Rupture of lenticulostriate arteries.

Shape of Hematomas on CT-Scan

Acute subdural haematoma	Concavo-convex
Extradural haematoma	Biconvex

Signs of DVT

Homan's sign	Pain in the calf on dorsiflexion of the foot
Moses's sign	Pain is caused by squeezing of the calf muscle from side to side

Fistula and Sinus

Fistula	Communicating track between two epithelial surfaces. One connecting hollow viscus with surface is called external fistula. One connecting two hollow viscera
Sinus	Bind track lined by granulomatous tissue, leading from the surface down to the tissues, which may contain cavity.

Aneurysms

True aneurysm	Contains all the three layers of arterial wall
False aneurysm	Single layer of fibrous tissue as the wall of sac
Mycotic aneurysm	Produced by the growth of microorganisms in the wall of the vessel.
Cirsoid aneurysm	Mass of dilated pulsating serpiginous vessels, found in congenital arteriovenous aneurysms
Aneurismal varix	Artery and vein are communicating directly with a short wide channel
Varicose aneurysm	Anastomosis between artery and vein is indirect through an intermediate sac.

Remember

- Atherosclerotic aneurysms are the commonest.
- Cimino fistula—for renal dialysis temporary iatrogenic A—V fistula is made in the wrist or ankle.
- Branham's sign:
  - If a finger is pressed on the artery proximal to A-V fistula, there will be slowing of pulse rate and rise in the diastolic pressure.
- Marjolin's ulcer:
  - Squamous cell carcinoma which arises in a chronic benign ulcer or scar.
  - Most commonly seen in long standing venous ulcer.

Wallace's Rule of Nine

To estimate the total body surface area in burn patient

In adult	In children
Head–9	Head–18
Chest front–9	Chest front–9
Abdomen front–9	Abdomen front–9
Chest back–9	Chest back–9
Lower back–9	Lower back–9
Each upper limb–9	Each upper limb–9
Each thigh–9	Each lower limb–13.5
Each leg–9	Perineum–1
Perineum–1	
Hand–1 per cent	

Infections in Burns

- Most common nonbacterial opportunistic organism form burn wounds is candidiasis
- Most common bacterial infection in burn wounds is pseudomonas.

Healing

Healing by primary intention	Clean, surgically closed wounds
Healing by secondary intention	Unsutured, infected wounds healing by granulation tissue formation
Healing by tertiary intention	Delayed closure for infected surgical wounds, in which skin was kept open in initial operation

Classification of Wounds

Clean	Viscus not opened
Clean contaminated	Viscus opened without spillage
Contaminated	Viscus opened with spillage
Dirty	Infected wounds, like abscesses
Absorbable sutures	**Nonabsorbable**
Catgut	Polyster
Vicry 1	Polyamide
Homopolymer of glycolide	Polypropylene
Homopolymer of polydioxanone	Polyethylene skin cotton

Skin Grafts

- Partial thickness graft
  - Thin graft/thiersch graft: Through the tips of papillae.
  - Thick graft/split skin grafts: All of epidermis and variable part of dermis.
- Whole thickness skin graft/Wolfe's graft: Includes entire epidermis and dermis.

Partial thickness graft	Full thickness graft
Includes whole of dermis	Includes whole of epidermis and part of epidermis and dermis.
Wound contraction is more	Wound contraction is minimal
Skin on the donor site can regenerate on its own	Skin on the donor site cannot regenerate and hence needs to be closed.
Used for resurfacing large areas	Used for resurfacing small areas, as they match color and texture.
Donor sites include upper thighs, buttocks and abdominal walls	Donor site includes post-auricular area and upper eyelids.

Skin Graft

Skin graft can be stored in refrigerator for 2 weeks at 4 degress centigrade

Skin Graft Survives in Recipient Bed by

- Imbibition: Absorption of nutrients into the graft which serves to feed the graft for the first 24 hours to 48 hours
- Inoculation: Process whereby donor and recipient capillaries become aligned
- Revascularization: Differentiation of connecting vessels into the arterioles and venules.

Graft type	Characteristic
Autograft	Received from self
Allograft	Received from same species
Isograft	Received from different individual who is genetically identical
Xenograft	Received from different species.

Rodent Ulcer/Basal Cell Carcinoma

- 90 per cent of basal cell carcinomas are seen in the face.
- Majority occur above the line connecting angle of mouth with lobule of the ear.
- Commonest site is around the inner canthus of eye (Tear cancer).
- Typical rolled edge.
- Spreads by local spread.
- Geographical or 'field fire' basal cell carcinoma has irregular raised edge around the flat white scar.
- Regional lymph node metastasis is characteristic.
- Superficial radiotherapy is the treatment of choice.

Melanomas

- Lymphatic spread is the commonest route of spread
- Radioresistant
- Best treated by surgery and local regional and perfusion with high doses cytotoxic agents.

Melanoma

Most common type	Superficial spreading
Least common type	Lentigo maligna melanoma
Least malignant	Lentigo maligna/Hutchinson's freckle
Most malignant	Nodular variety
Most common site in males	Lower back
Most common site in females	Legs
Salivary gland	Histological type
Parotid	Serous
Submandibular	Mixed
Sublingual	Mucous

Pleomorphic Adenoma

- Commonest benign tumor of salivary glands
- Radioresistant
- Patey's operation/superficial parotidectomy is done.

Warthin's Tumor

- Benign tumor
- Only involves parotid and usually lower portion
- Shows hot spot on Tc 99 m pertechnetate scan
- Superficial parotidectomy is done.
- Hemangioma is the most common benign tumors of parotid in children.

Indications of Radiotherapy in Parotid Tumors

- Recurrent disease
- Residual disease left at surgery
- High grade lesion
- Those who refuse surgery
- Unfit for surgery
- Unresectable local lesion

Triad of Mikulicz's Disease

- Enlargement of salivary glands
- Narrow palpebral fissure
- Parchment like dryness of mouth.

Carcinoma Breast

Carcinoma breast is more common on	Left side
Most common sit	Upper outer quadrant
Most common histological variant	Ductal carcinoma
Histological variant with good prognosis even in presence of axillary lymph node metastasi carcinoma	Medullary

Lymphoedema Grading

Grade	Characteristic
0	Sublinical
1	Pits on pressure, disappears on elevation /rest
2	Non-pitting; does not disappear on elevation and rest
3	Irreversible skin changes like fibrosis and papillae.

Cystic Hygroma

- Cystic swelling containing clear lymph
- It is caused due to sequestration of apportion of a jugular sac from the lymphatic system, which fails to join and regular lymphatic system
- Commonest site is posterior triangle of neck
- Manifests in early infancy
- Brilliantly translucent
- Excision is the treatment of choice.

Branchial Cyst

- MC site: Upper part of neck
- Wall is made of: Lymphoid tissue

Ranula

- Retention cyst of sublingual glands.

Tongue Carcinoma

- Most common site is anterior 2/3rd
- Near the lateral margin.

Thyroglossal Cyst

- Cystic swelling developing from the remnant of thyroglossal tract
- Subhyoid position is the commonest
- Moves with deglutition
- Excision is treatment.

Thyroglossal Fistula

- Never congenital
- Caused by the external opening of an infected thyroglossal cyst.

Sternomastoid Tumor/Congenital Torticollis

- Caused by the infarction of the central portion of one of the sternomastoid muscle at the time of birth.

The thyroid moves with deglutition due to its attachment with the larynx and trachea by

- Ligament of berry
- Posterior lamina of the pretracheal fascia
- Levator glandulae thyroidae.

Thyroid Lymphoma

- Rapidly growing
- Diffuse large type is variant.

Thyroidectomy

- Neck swelling immediately following thyroid surgery is due to: Tension hematoma (so open immediately).

Thyroid Surgeries

Superior thyroid artery	Ligated close to superior pole to avoid external laryngeal nerve.
Inferior thyroid artery	Ligated away from pole to avoid recurrent laryngeal nerve.

Zenker's Diverticulum

- Most common complication of esophageal atresia
- Seen in elderly
- Characteristic site is within inferior pharyngeal constrictor, between the oblique fibers and horizontal fibers, at Killian's triangle
- Lung abscess due to aspiration is the most common complication.

Plummer–Vinson Syndrome/Brown-Kelly-Paterson Syndrome/Sideropenic Dysphagia

- Esophageal web with iron deficiency anemia
- Premalignant: Precricoid carcinoma
- Palmar and solar keratosis is seen in esophageal cancer.

Sclerosing Agents for Endoscopic Sclerotherapy

- Polidocanol/polydochy1
- N-buty1- cyanonacrylate (glue injection)
- Absolute alcohol, phenol
- Ethanolamine maleate /oleate
- Sodium teradecy1 sulfhate
- Stomach is the conduit of choice after esophagectomy.

Congenital Hypertrophic Pyloric Stenosis

- Shows hypochloremic alkalosis
- Congenital pyloric stenosis is best diagnosed by USG
- Hypertrophied pyloric muscle mass > 4 mm or pyloric length >14 mm.

Dumping Syndrome

Early dumping syndrome	Late dumping syndrome
Immediately after meals	Second hour after meals
Relief by lying down	Relief by exercise
Symptoms of epigastric fullness, sweating, light headedness, tachycardia, colic	Symptoms of tremor, fainting prostration

Site of Duodenal Ulcer Perforation and Effect

Posterior duodenal ulcer perforation	Intense hemorrhage due to rupture of gastro-duodenal artery
Anterior duodenal ulcer perforation	Pneumoperitoneum and peritonitis

Vagotomy

Truncal vagotomy/vagectomy	Both the trunk of vagus nerves are resected
Selective vagotomy	Removal of all gastric fibers of the vagus nerves, leaving the hepatic and celiac branches.
Highly selective vagotomy	Denervation of acid secreting part of stomach, keeping supply to the alkali secreting part of the stomach and other abdominal viscera intact.

Typhoid

- Typhoid ulcers are placed longitudinally along the ileum
- Perforation of typhoid ulcer usually occurs in the 3rd week
- Most common complication of typhoid: Paralytic ileus
- Most common presentation: Intestinal bleeding
- Most common site involved: Ileum.

Remember

- Tubercular ulcer are place transversely along the ileum
- Acute mesenteric lymphadenitis is the disease with symptoms and signs most similar to those of acute appendicitis
- Strawberry lesion of recto-sigmoid is due to infection by spirochete vincenti and bacillus fusiformis. Carcinoid tumor is most frequently found in distal third of appendix
- Most common position of appendix: Retrocecal
- Bleeding is the earliest complication of rectal carcinoma followed by alteration of bowel movements
- Treatment of duodenal atresia is duodeno-jejunostomy or duodeno-duodenostomy
- Red currant jelly stool is seen in intussusception
- Most serious complication of end colostomies is parastomal hernia
- Bishop koop's operation is done in meconium ileus.

Type of edge	Ulcer
Undermined edge	Tuberculous ulcer
Punched out edge	Gummatous ulcer, deep trophic ulcer
Sloping edge	Healing traumatic ulcer
Raised beaded edge	Rodent ulcer
Rolled out edge	Squamous cell carcinoma

Ulcer with Eponyms

Bazin's ulcer	Small multiple in ankle region. Associated with erythrocyanosis frigida; seen exclusively in young women. Low grade ischemia of ankle, due to abnormally small or absent perforating arteries, arising from the posterior tibial or peroneal arteries.
Footballer's ulcer	Non-healing ulcer over shin due to direct trauma by football
Phagedenic ulcer	Tropical ulcers seen in malnourished, poorly immunized with history of trauma or insect bite. Infection is caused by Vincent's organisms
Hunner's ulcer	Interstitial cystitis. Bladder capacity is reduced to 30–50 mL

Blind Loop Syndrome

- Stagnation of small intestinal contents by strictures, stenosis, blind- pouch syndrome, or diverticula
- The bacterial flora in the stagnant area is increased in number
- Leading to anemia, hypoproteinemia, steatorhhea
- In distal small intestine, the abnormal bacterial flora compete for vitamin B_{12}, leading to deficiency
- In proximal small intestine, they deconjugate bile salts, leading to steatorhhea
- Also leads to hypoproteinemia and avitaminosis.

Polyposis Coli

Not premalignant	Premalignant
Juvenile polyposis	Tubular adenoma
Peutz-Jegher's	Villous adenoma
Syndrome	Familial adenomatous polyposis coli-100 per cent Malignancy risk, autosomal dominant. Gardner's syndrome, Turcot's syndrome – 100 Perc ent progression to malignancy

Meckel's Diverticulum

- Meckel's diverticulum is a true diverticulum, situated on antimesenteric border
- Present in 2 per cent population 2 inches long
- 2 feet proximal to ileocolic valve
- Most common complication of Meckel's diverticulum is intestinal obstruction followed by bleeding and diverticulitis.

Remember

Meckel's diverticulum	Result of partial obliteration of vitelline duct
Persistent vitelline fistula	Result of failure of closure of vitelline duct.

Classic Quartet of Intestinal Obstruction

- Pain
- Abdominal distention
- Vomiting
- Constipation

Remember

Aspirin/NSAID are protective against colorectal Ca.

Carcinoma Colon

Carcinoma colon left	Carcinoma colon right
Obstructive syndromes	Anemia is more common predominate

Duke's Classification of Colon Carcinoma

Stage A Growth is limited to the bowel
Stage B Spread into adjoining structures, without lymphatic metastasis
Stage C Lymphatic metastases

Duke's Classification of Rectal Carcinoma

Stage A Growth limited to rectal wall
Stage B Beyond rectal wall, but no involvement of lymph nodes.
Stage C Growth beyond rectal wall, with involvement of regional lymph nodes.

Tumor Markers

Tumour marker	Associated tumours
HCG	Trophoblastic tumors, nonseminomatous testicular tumors
Calcitonin	Medullary carcinoma of thyroid
Alpha fetoprotein	Liver cell cancer, nonseminomatous germ cell tumors of testis
CEA	Carcinoma colon, pancreas, lung, stomach, breast.
Acid phosphatase	Prostate cancer
PSA	Prostate cancer
Neuron specific enolase	Small cell lung cancer, neuroblastoma
Immunoglobulins	Multiple myeloma
CA 125	Ovarian cancer, pancreatic cancer
Ca 19-9	Colon cancer, pancreatic cancer
Ca 15-3	Breast cancer
5-HIA	Carcinoid tumors
S. alkaline phosphatase	Osteosarcoma
Homovanillic acid, VMA	Neuroblastoma, pheochromocytoma
Ca 50 / Ca 242	Colorectal, pancreatic, gastric.
Neuron specific Enolase	Neuroendocrine tumors, small cell lung carcinomas, Medullary thyroid carcinomas

Remember

- Characteristic of AML: Auer rods
- Philadelphia chromosome: CML
- Kaposi's sarcoma is the most common neoplasm in patients with AIDS.
- Commonest malignancy in women in developing countries is cervical cancer
- Commonest malignancy in women in developed countries is breast cancer
- Commonest cancer in elderly is prostate cancer
- Burkitt's lymphoma: Most rapidly progressive tumor.
- Most common inherited malignancy is retinoblastoma.

Short Bowel Syndrome

- Massive bowel resection.
- Minimum amount of small bowel required to prevent short bowel syndrome is 100 cm
- Absorption of fat, water, electrolytes, and vitamin B_{12} is affected.
- Associated with hypergastrinemia.

Causes

- Massive intestinal resection
- Regional enteritis with multiple bowel reactions
- A jejuno-ileal bypass for morbid obesity.

Grading of Piles

First degree	Contained within the anal canal
Second degree	Extruded on defecation, but return at the end or act
Third degree	Prolapse on defecation and then need to be manually reduced
Fourth degree	Prolapse on defecation and then cannot be reduced

Treatment of Piles

First degree	Sclerosants
Second degree	Sclerosants, rubber banding
Third degree	Sclerosants, rubber banding
Fourth degree	Rubber banding, hemorrhoidectomy.

Goodsall's Rule

- Anal fistulae with an external opening in relation to anterior half of anus tends to have a straight path, whereas those related to posterior half, usually have curving tracks and may be of the horseshoe variety.

Hernia	Description
Hernia through foramen of Moragni	Herniation through the retrosternal defect between sternal and costal attachment of diaphragm

Contd...

Key Points

Contd...

Hernia	Description
Hernia through foramen of Bochdalek	Herniation posterolaterally through pleuro-parietal opening
Spigelian	Interparietal and subumbilical herniation, lateral to rectus muscle at the level of arcuate line
Richter's hernia	Herniation of circumference of intestine
Littre's hernia	Herniation of Meckel's diverticulum
Maydl's hernia	Hernia en W

Remember

- Landmark for differentiating femoral hernia from inguinal hernia is the pubic tubercle
  - Neck of the sac of inguinal hernia is above and medial to it, while that of femoral hernia is below and lateral to it.
- Landmark for differentiating direct from indirect inguinal hernia is inferior epigastric vessels.
  - Neck of direct is medial to it, while that of indirect is lateral to it.

Hernia Surgeries

Herniotomy	Neck of the sac is transfixed and ligated and then the hernial sac is excised, no repair is done
Herniorrhaphy	Herniotomy with repair of posterior wall of the inguinal canal
Hernioplasty	Herniorrhaphy with reinforced repair of the posterior wall of the inguinal canal by filling the gap between the conjoined tendon and inguinal ligament.

Trousseau's Sign of Malignancy/Trousseau's Syndrome

- Some malignancies, especially adenocarcinomas of the pancreas and lung, are associated with hypercoagulability
- In patients with malignancy—associated hypercoagulable states, the blood may spontaneously form clots in the portal vessels, the deep veins of the extremities, or the superficial veins anywhere on the body.
- When recurrent clots form in different superficial veins around the body, this is described as migratory thrombophlebitis.
- Armand Trousseau first described this finding in himself; he was subsequently found to have pancreatic cancer.

Mesna–Sodium 2–Mercapto Ethane Sulfate

- Protective agent in cancer chemotherapy (Cyclophosphamide) to prevent hemorrhagic cystitis
- Acrolein is thought to be responsible for its action.

Insulinoma

- MC endocrine tumors of pancreas (from beta cells)
- Usually single
- Whipple's triad is seen
- Distributed equally throughout pancreas
- Total capsule removal is ensured to prevent tumor recurrence.

Somatostatinoma

- Endocrine tumors that secrete excessive amount of somatostatin
- Characterized by
  - DM
  - Gallbladder disease
  - Diarrhea
  - Steatorrhea.

VIPoma

- VIP is secreted
- Characterized by:
  - Large volume watery diarrhea
  - Dehydration
  - Hypokalemia.

Pancreatic Duct

Duct of Wirsung	Major pancreatic duct
Duct of Santorini	Minor pancreatic duct

Pancreatitis

Most commonly elevated and tested enzyme	Serum amylase
Low serum amylase is seen	Serum protein loss in congestive heart failure
Single best enzyme for pancreatitis	Serum lipase
Pancreases the only source of	Serum trypsinogen
Drugs inducing pancreatitis	L - asparginase, thiazides, steroids
Organism causing pancreatitis	Mumps
Best prognosis	Gall stone pancreatitis

Pancreatitis

- Grey Turner's sign: In hemorrhagic pancreatitis, bluish discoloration in the flank is seen .
- Cullen' s sing: In hemorrhagic pancreatitis, bluish discoloration in the periumbilical area is seen
- Most common site of pseudo pancreatic cyst is body and tail pancreas
- Pseudo cyst >5 cm in diameter is an indication of drainage
- Pseudo cyst <5 cm and <6 weeks duration should be observed only.

Pancreatic Tumors

Gastrinoma	Arises from G-cells, secretes gastrin, Produces Zollinger-Ellison syndrome Malignant tumor.
Insulinoma	Most common, arises from beta cells, Hypoglycemia
Glucagonoma	Arises from alpha cells. Causes diabetes, anemia, thrombosis, skin rashes
Somatostatinoma	Arises from delta cells. Causes diabetes, gallstone, steatorrhea, hypochlorhydria, malignant
VIPoma	Verner-Morrison syndrome, D1 tumor, diarrhea with hypokalemia, hypochlorhydria (pancreatic cholera).

Whipple's Criteria for Diagnosis of Hypoglycemia

- Symptoms of hypoglycemia
- Serum glucose < 2.8 mmoles/L
- Prompt relief of symptoms after glucose administration.

OPSI/Opportunistic Postsplenectomy Infection

- Streptococcus pneumoniae
- N. meningitides
- H. influenza
- Babesia microti

Blood Disorders Treatable by Splenectomy

- Hereditary spherocytosis
- Hereditary elliptocysis
- Thalassemia major
- Acquired hemolytic anemia
- ITP
- Idiopathic myelofibrosis
- Opitz's disease.

Kehr's Sign

- Splenic rupture
- Peritoneal hemorrhage irritates diaphragm, causes referred pain to the left shoulder
- Balance sign: Rupture spleen shows non- shifting dullness in the left flank.

Hypersplenism

- Splenomegaly
- Anemia ,leucopenia, and thrombocytopenia
- Compensatory bone marrow—hyperplasia
- Improvement after splenectomy
- Banti's syndrome
- Congestive splenomegaly with hypersplenism associated with cirrhosis and portal hypertension.

Couinaud's Segments

- Based on hepatic vein and portal vein division
- Segment I is caudate lobe
- Segment I has independent vascular supply
- Segment IV is quadrate lobe

Portal Circulation

Normal portal pressure	6–12 mm of Hg. 10–15 mm of water
Portal hypertension	> 40 mm of water

Portosystemic Venous Shunts

- Anastomoses between veins of falciform ligament and superior and inferior epigastric veins: Caput medusae
- Anastomoses between gastric vein and esophageal veins: Esophageal varices
- Anastomoses between superior hemorrhoidal vein and middle and inferior rectal veins: Hemorrhoids
- Anastomoses between veins of retroperitoneal structures and the body wall (veins of Retzius).

Amoebic Liver Abscess

- MC site: Right lobe (postero-superior surface)
- Anchovy sauce pus (choclate colored pus due to RBC lysis)
- Complication of amoebic liver abscess:
  - Pleuro-pulmonary involvement
  - Rupture into pleural space etc.

Pyogenic Liver Abscess

- Usually single and large
- MC route of infection: Infection through bile duct (hematogenous route is 2nd MC route).

Hepatocellular Ca

- Predisposing factors:
  - HBV,
  - HCV
  - Alcoholic liver disease etc.
- Commonest marker for HCC: Alpha Fetoprotein
- Other markers:
  - Neurotensin
  - PIVKA 2
- Imaging modality for screening HCC: USG
- Percutaneous biopsy (USG/ CT guided) can be diagnostic.

Fibrolamellar Ca

- Not associated with cirrhosis
- Slow growing
- Good prognosis, if treated.

Child–Pugh Grading

Features	1 point	2 points	3 points
Encephalopathy	-	Grade1/2	Grade 3,4
Ascites	Absent	Sight	Moderate
Serum bilirubin	1–2 mg	2–3 mg	> 3 mg
Serum albumin	> 3.5 mg	2.8–3.5 mg	<2.8 mg
Prothrombin time (seconds prolonged)	1–4	4–6	>6

Most Common Indications for Liver Transplantation

- Adults: Chronic liver failure
- In children: Biliary atresia is the most common indication.

Metabolic Diseases which can be Cured by Liver Transplantation

- Wilson's disease
- Alpha 1 antitrypsin deficiency
- Oxalosis

Hogarth Pringle Maneuver

- Hepatic artery is compressed between fingers and thumb in lesser omentum through foramen, to stop bleeding from injured cystic artery, when it cannot be controlled by packing, suction and ligation of bleeding artery.

Gallstone Ileus

- MC site of obstruction is: Ileum
- Management: Enterotomy and removal of stone.

Charcot's Triad is Seen in Cholangitis and Bile Duct Stones

- Pain
- Jaundice
- Fever

Hemobilia–Triad

- Biliary colic
- Jaundice
- Melaena

Emphysematous Cholecystitis

- Associated with presence of gas in the gallbladder
- Seen in diabetics, due to infection with gas forming bacilli
- Ultrasound shows gas in the gallbladder
- Needs to be operated immediately.

Structures in Free Border of Lesser Peritoneum from Anterior to Posterior

- Common bile duct
- Hepatic artery
- Portal vein

Saint's Triad

- Gallstones
- Diverticulosis coli
- Hiatus hernia

Calot's Triangle

- Cystic artery superiorly
- Cystic duct inferiorly
- Common hepatic duct medially
- Contents: Lymph node of Lund

Remember

- Blood supply to the liver is derived 80 per cent from portal vein and 20 per cent from hepatic artery
- CAROLI's disease: Congenital dilatation of intrahepatic biliary tree
- Caterpillar turn or Moynihan's hump: Tortuous right hepatic artery
- Most common route of infection of liver is along the bile ducts followed by via the hepatic artery.
- Commonest cause of liver abscess is pyogenic 80 per cent
- Honey comb liver is found in actinomycosis
- In Budd-Chiari syndrome, obstruction occurs at hepatic vein
- Hemangioma is the commonest benign tumor of the liver
- Commonest primary lesion causing metastasis to liver is colon carcinoma, pancreas, and breast
- Gold standard for liver imaging is triple phase spiral CT scan
- Up to 80 per cent of liver resection may be tolerated
- Acute cholecystitis: Most commonly caused by E. coli.

Indications of Percutaneous Nephrolithotomy

- Stones bigger than 3 cm
- Staghorn calculus
- Hard stones
- Anatomic abnormality like scoliosis or obesity
- Stones unresponsive to ESWL
- Coexisting obstructive uropathy.

Contraindications to ESWL

- Pregnant women
- Abdominal aortic aneurysm
- Uncorrectable coagulation disorders

- Hard stones
- Stones in poorly draining hydronephrotic kidney.

Management of Ureteric Stones

Upper third	ESWL
Middle third	ESWL/Ureteroscopic removal
Lower third	Ureteroscopic extraction

Triple Phosphate Stones

- Consists of calcium-ammonium—magnesium phosphate
- Usually formed as a result of inflammation
- Form Staghorn calculus.

Chemical	Associated cancer
Benzene	Leukemias
Vinyl chloride	Angiosarcoma of liver
Beta- naphthylamine	Urinary bladder carcinoma
Azo dyes	Hepatoma
Aflatoxin	Hepatoma

Tumors Associated with Absolute Erythrocytosis

- Hypernephroma (renal cell carcinoma)
- Cerebellar hemangioblastoma
- Hepatoma
- Adrenal adenoma
- Pheochromocytoma
- Meningioma
- Uterine fibromyoma.

Renal TB

- Sterile pyuria is a consistent feature
- Most sensitive technique for early detection: IVU

Thimble Bladder

- Seen in late stages of tuberculosis
- Fibrosis leads to reduced capacity.

TB Urinary System

- Sterile pyuria is seen in tuberculosis
- Golf hole ureteric orifice is seen in late stages of tuberculosis of urinary system as the ureter is pulled upward.

Remember

- Duplication of renal pelvis is the commonest congenital abnormality of the upper tract
- Commonest cause of lower urinary tract infection in boys is posterior urethral valve
- Meatal ulcer with scabbing is the most common cause of acute retention in boys.

Highly radiosensitive tumors	Highly radioresistant
Seminoma	Hepatoma
Ewing's tumor	Melanoma
Lymphoma	Osteosarcoma
Wilm's tumor	Pancreatic cancer
Multiple myeloma	
Dysgerminoma	

Remember

- Most radiocurable tumor is Hodgkin's disease.

Locations of Ectopic Testis

- Superficial inguinal pouch (commonest)
- In front of the pubis
- Superficial perineal pouch
- Near the saphenous opening.

Undescended testis	Ectopic testis
The testis is arrested in its normal path of descent	Testis deviates from its normal path of descent
Usually undeveloped	Fully developed
Scrotum is not well developed	Scrotum is well developed
Spermatogernesis is poor	Spermatogenesis is perfect
May be associated with indirect inguinal hernia	Never associated with indirect inguinal hernia

Seminoma

- Radiosensitive,
- Corresponds to dysgerminoma of ovary
- Treatment of choice is: Surgery.

Hypospadias

- Hooded prepuce
- Meatal stenosis
- Bifid scrotum
- Best time of surgery: 6–10 months of age.

Paraphimosis

- Complication: Gangrene (due to hampering of venous and lymphatic return from glans)
- May require circumcision (if manipulation fails).

Peyronie's Disease

- Hard plaques of fibrosis can be felt in the tunica
- Usually idiopathic
- May be associated with:
  - Trauma
  - Dupuytrens contracture
- Histologically similar to keloid or Dupuytren's contracture
- Self limiting.

Incomplete Descent of Testes

- Complication: Malignant change (even if the testes have been brought down surgically)
- Best time to operate: 9–15 months of age.

Spermatocele

- Diverticulum of epididymis, which:
  - Contains fluid (with spermatozoa) resembliing barley fluid and
  - Can be transilluminated.

Varicocele

- MC on: Left side
- Negative tranillumination test
- MC cause of male infertility, which is surgically treated.

Testicular Torsion

- Urine analysis is negative
- Elevation will not decrease the pain (negative Phen's sign)
- Roche's sign
- In torsion of testis, the epitidymis cannot be distinguished from the body of the testis, whereas in epididymitis, the body of the testis can be felt in the enlarged crescent of the epididymis.
- Operation should not be delayed for more than 4 hours from the time of onset of symptoms.

Indications for Operative Treatment of Penetrating Thoracic Injuries

- Caked hemothorax
- Large air leaks with inadequate ventilation or persistent collapse of lung
- Drainage of more than 1500 mL of blood when chest tube is first inserted
- Continuous hemorrhage of more than 200 mL per hour for > 3 consecutive hours
- Esophageal perforation
- Pericardial tamponade.

Timings of Operation

Cleft lip operation	Done at 3-6 months.
Cleft palate operation	Done between 6 months to 1.5 years.

Remember

- Suture removal after cleft lip operation is done on fifth day.

Conditions Related to Dental Tissue

Epulis	A swelling situated on the gum arising from the alveolar margin.
Dental cyst	Associated with chronically infected pulpless tooth. Always associated with a normally erupted tooth.
Dentigerous cyst	Associated with non-erupted permanent tooth.
	Cyst contains molar tooth.
Adamantinoma	True neoplasm of odontogenic epithelium
	Epithelial tumor arising from ameloblasts.

Coagulation System

Vitamin K dependent factor are 2, 7, 9, 10 proteins C and S.	
Extrinsic system of coagulation	Factor 7
Common system of coagulation	Factors 1, 2, 5, 10
Intrinsic system of coagulation	Factors 8, 9, 11,12
PT	Detects deficiency of common and extrinsic system of coagulation. Elevated in deficiency of factors 1, 2, 5, 7, 10.
	Also elevated in liver disease and early vitamin K Deficiency.
PTT (aPTT/ PPTk)	Detects deficiency of intrinsic and common system of coagulation. Elevated in deficiency of factors 1, 2, 5, 8, 9,10, 11, 12. Also elevated in liver disease and late vitamin K deficiency, Von Willebrand's disease, lupus anticoagulants.
Clot solubility in urea	Detects factor 13.

Frey's Syndrome

- Damage to the auriculotemporal nerve and greater auricular nerve
- On healing there is cross joining, go that when the patient eats, there is sweating in the parotid region.

Crocodile Tears

- Following facial nerve paralysis, due to inaccurate regrowth of fibers.
- So on eating, there is lacrimation.

Beck's Triad of Cardiac Tamponade

- Muffled heart sounds
- Distended neck veins
- Hypotension

Biological Fractionation of Radiotherapy is Explained by

- Repair of sublethal damage
- Repopulation between fractions
- Redistribution of cells in the cell cycle
- Reoxygenation of tumor
- Inherent rediosensitivity
- Recruitment of cells into the proliferating fraction.

Remember

- Most radiosensitive portion of cell cycle G2-M phase
- Thimble chamber: Used for detection and measurement of radiation.

Penetrating Power

- Neutron > Gamma >X-ray >Beta > Alpha (Helium)

Ionizing Power and Damaging Power

- Alpha (Helium) > Beta >X-ray > Gamma

Translocations

Cancer	Translocation
CML	t (9, 22)
Burkitt's lymphoma	t (8, 14)
Ewing's tumor	t (11, 22)
Acute promyelocytic leukemia	t (15, 17)

Tumor suppressor genes

Rb	Retinoblastoma and osteogenic sarcoma
p53	Many tumors and Li Fraumeni syndrome
Wt 1	Wilms' tumors and aniridia
Nf1	Neurofibromatosis

p53

- p53 is the guardian of genome
- p53 mutation is the most common genetic alteration seen in human cancer
- It is the causative in Li-Fraumeni familial cancer syndrome.

Ann Arbor staging for Hodgkin's disease

Stage I Involvement of single lymph node region
Stage II Involvement of 2 or more lymph node regions on same side of diaphragm
Stage III Involvement of lymph node region on both sides of diaphragm
Stage IV Disseminated involvement of one or more extra lymphatic organs with or without.

Half Lives

Tc-99 m	6 hours
I-131	8 days
I-125	60 days
Co-60	5.2 years
Ra 226	1699 years

Terms

- Pott's puffy tumor is seen in chronic frontal osteomyelitis, it is subperiosteal swelling with edema of scalp
- Dercum's disease/Adiposis dolorosa: Variant of lipoma in which there are tender lipomatosis on the trunk
- Teitze disease: Painful and non-suppurative swelling of 2nd and 3rd costal cartilage
- Fournier's gangrene: Idiopathic gangrene of scrotum, mostly by hemolytic streptococci.

Proctalgia Fugax

- Intermittent
- Levator muscle spasm
- Painful spasm of anal sphincter which awakens the patient at night.

Felon

- Infection of the distal pulp space, usually secondary to a puncture wound
- Late osteomyelitis may develop.

Remember

- Enlargement of Krause's nodes (located at jugular foramen) leads to jugular foramen syndrome (compression of 9th, 10th , 11th cranial nerve)
- PSA over 4 ng/mL is abnormal
- Superior vena cava syndrome is most commonly caused by lung cancer
- TURP syndrome is seen due to glycine absorption
- Thymoma is the most common mediastinal tumor
- Most common malignant tumor of the mediastinum is Seminoma
- Honeymoon pyelitis: Acute pyelitis occurring in females soon after marriage.
- Seminoma is the most common testicular tumor
- Thrombosis of splenic veins leading to thormbophlebitic splenomegaly
- Hypospadias: Commonest type Glandular
- Champagne urine: Fistula into urinary tract by diverticulosis gives rise to pneumaturia.
- Intussusception is the most common cause of intestinal obstruction in children under 2 years of age.

Raspberry Tumor

- A small part of vitello-intestinal duct remains patent near the umbilicus
- Giving to rise to a mucus discharging sinus, with its epithelium everted.

MCQs WITH SHORT EXPLANATIONS

BURNS

1. Which of the following is NOT a feature of burns:

a. Sepsis
b. Shock
c. Acute kidney injury
d. Hyperproteinemia

Hypoproteinemia is obvious in burns due to excessive loss of plasma proteins as a result of increase in the capillary permeability and infection.

2. All of the following are true regarding fluid resuscitation in burn patients EXCEPT:

a. Consider intravenous resuscitation in children with burns greater than 15% TBSA
b. Oral fluids must contain salts
c. Most preferred fluid is Ringer's lactate
d. Half of the calculated volume of fluid should be given in first 8 hours

Fluid resuscitation in burns

- Fluid used are normal saline, ringer lactate, Hartmann fluid, plasma. Ringer lactate is the fluid of choice
- Parkland regime is commonly used
  - 4 mL/ % burn/ body weight/ 24 hours
  - Maximum percentage considered is 50%
  - Half the volume is given in first 8 hours, rest given in 16 hours.

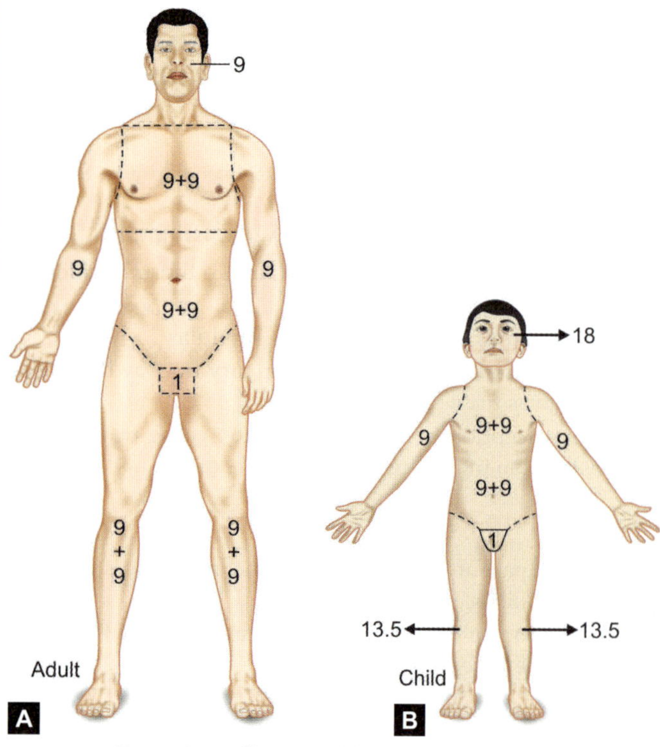

Percentage of burns in (A) Adults; (B) Children

3. According to rule of nines, burns involving perineum are:

a. 1%
b. 9%
c. 18%
d. 27%

Perineum constitutes 1% of burns in children and adults.

Types of burns
❑ Thermal injury
– Scald—spillage of hot liquids
– Flame burns
– Flash burns due to exposure of natural gas, alcohol, combustible liquids
– Contact burns—contact with hot metals/objects/materials
❑ Electrical injury
❑ Chemical burns—acid/alkali
❑ Cold injury—frost bite
❑ Ionising radiation
❑ Sun burns

4. NOT seen in 3rd degree burns:

a. Loss of skin appendages
b. No vesicles
c. Red color
d. Extremely painful

Third degree burns

- In third degree burns, the affected area is charred, parchment like, painless and insensitive, with thrombosis of superficial vessels.
- It requires grafting
- Charred, denatured, insensitive, contracted full thickness burn is called eschar.
- These wound must hel by re-epithelialization from wound edge.

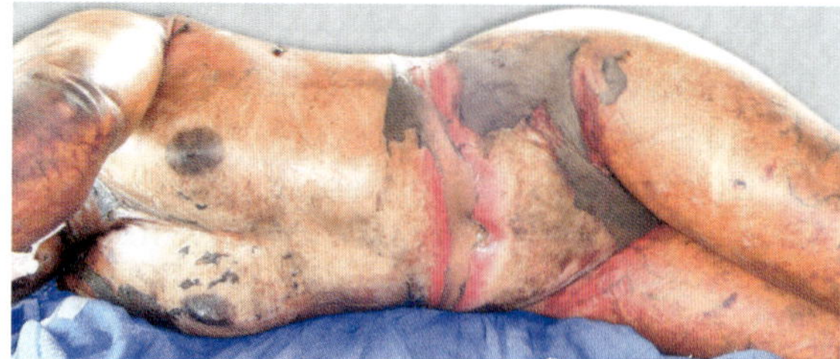

Extensive third degree burns with eschar

5. In second degree burns, re-epithelialization occurs by:

a. 1 week
b. 2 weeks
c. 3 weeks
d. 4 weeks

Second degree burns

- Affected area is mottled, red, painful, with blisters, heals by epithelialization in 14–21 days
- Superficial second degree burn heals, causing pigmentation

Ans. 1. **d.** Hyperthermia 2. **a.** Consider intravenous... 3. **a.** 1% 4. **d.** Extremely painful 5. **c.** 3 weeks

- Deep second degree burn heals, causing scarring, and pigmentation. Sensation is present but no blanching.

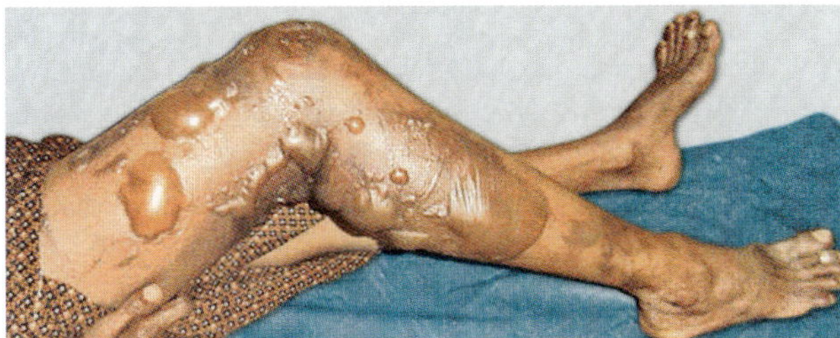

Second degree burns with blisters

6. FALSE regarding deep 2nd degree burns:

a. Heal by scar deposition
b. Painless
c. Damage to deeper dermis
d. Less blanching

Second degree burns are red, painful with blisters.

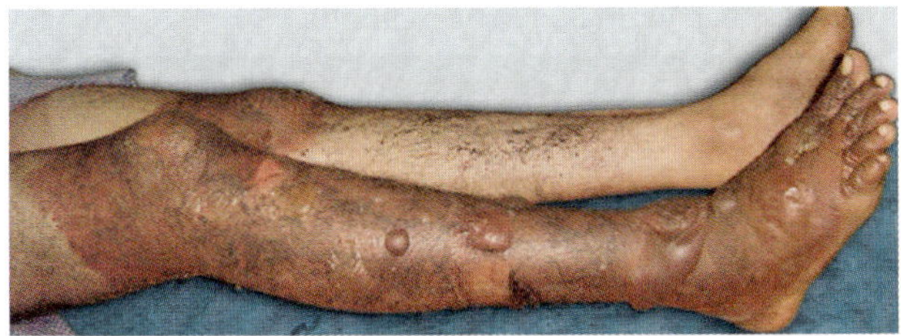

Second degree burns in the leg with blebs

7. NOT seen in severe burns:

a. Hypovolemia b. Sepsis
c. Duodenal ulcer d. Hyperthermia

Effects of burn injury

- Shock due to hypovolemia
- Infection by staphylococcus aureus, beta hemolytic Streptococcus, Pseudomonas, Klebsiella leads to becteremia, septicemia
- GIT: Hypovolemic, ischemia of mucosa, erosive gastritis – Curling's ulcer (seen in burns >35%).

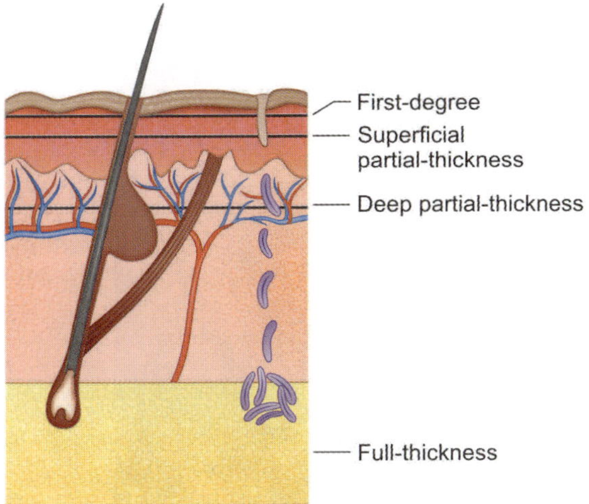

Degrees of burns

8. NOT true for 3rd degree burns:

a. Vesicles are absent b. Painful
c. Leathery skin
d. Reddish due to hemoglobin infiltration

Area with third degree burns is charred, parchment like, painless and insensitive.

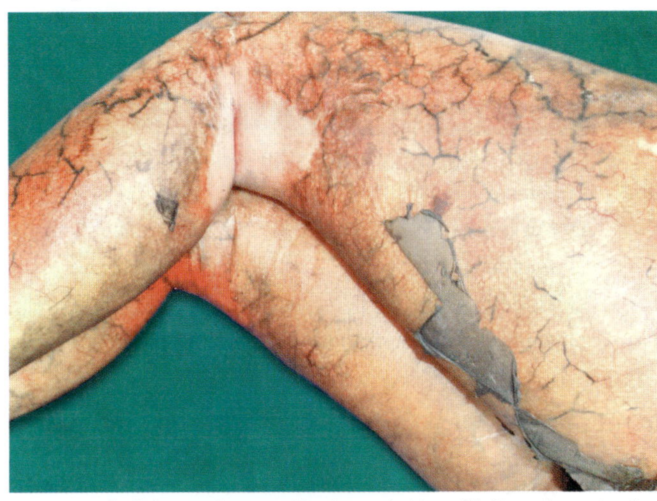

3rd degree burns with charred skin, with thrombosed veins and eschar

9. Most important aspect of management of burn injury in the first 24 hours:

a. Fluid resuscitation b. Dressing
c. Escharatomy d. Antibiotics

Fluid therapy in burns

- In first 24 hours, only crystalloids should be given (Crystalloids are one which can pass through capillary wall like saline either hypo, iso or hypertonic, dextrose saline, Ringer lactate).
- After 24 hours and up to 30–38 hours, colloids should be given to compensate plasma loss (colloids are one which are retained in intravascular compartment). Plasma, hemaccel (gelatin), dextran, hetastarch are used.

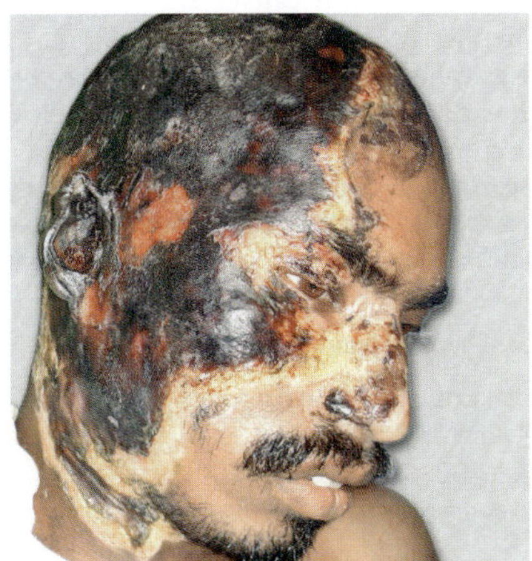

Face burns in an adult—severe 3rd degree

Ans. 6. **b.** Painless 7. **d.** Hyperthermia 8. **b.** Painful 9. **a.** Fluid resuscitation

10. MC cause of death due to burns in early period is:

a. Sepsis
b. Hypovolumic shock
c. Both
d. None of the above

Heat causes coagulation necrosis of skin and subcutaneous tissue → release of vasoactive peptides → altered capillary permeability → loss of fluid → severe hypovolemia.

Causes of death in burns
❑ Hypovolemia (refractory and uncontrolled) and shock
❑ Renal failure
❑ Pulmonary edema and ARDS
❑ Septicemia
❑ Multiorgan failure
❑ Acute airway block in head and neck burns

11. In burns management (within 24 hours), which of the following is the medium of choice:

a. Dextrose 5%
b. Normal saline
c. Ringer lactate
d. Isolyte-M

Ringer lactate is the fluid of choice for fluid resuscitation in burns.

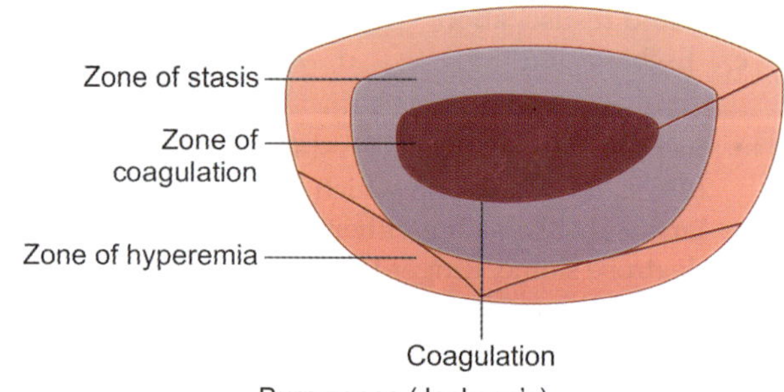

Burn zones (Jackson's)

12. A patient with burns died within 24 hours. What could be the most probable cause?

a. Circulatory shock
b. Physical burn injury to the airways above the larynx
c. Physical burn injury to the airways below the larynx
d. Circumferential burn

Assessment of airway injury is important in burns
❑ Occurs in burns around face and neck, or trapped in burning room
❑ Presents with hoarseness or stridor
❑ Inhaled burning gases can cause upper airway burns and laryngeal edema
❑ Smoke inhalation can cause chemical alveolitis, pulmonary edema, ARDS and respiratory failure
❑ Steam inhalation can cause damage to respiratory epithelium and subglottic edema
❑ Carbon monoxide inhalation more than 10% is dangerous as it forms carboxyhemoglobin (CO has got 240 times more affinity to hemoglobin than oxygen) which blocks oxygen transport completely causing respiratory arrest, hypoxia and metabolic acidosis
❑ Chest wall burn causes mechanical block of ventilation—needs escharotomy in chest wall and procedure is painless
❑ Airway burn may require early elective intubation or tracheostomy or emergency cricothyroidotomy as a life-saving method

13. Initial method to prevent infection in burn patients:

a. Physiotherapy
b. Intravenous antibiotics
c. Handwashing
d. Topical antibiotics

Burn patient should be managed in burn unit (ideally air-conditioned) with barrier nursing, sterile clothes, bed sheets with all septic methods.

Initial management
Clothing should be removed
Cooling of the part by running water for 20 minutes
Cleaning the part to remove dust, mud, etc.
Chemoprophylaxis—tetanus toxoid; antibiotics; local antiseptics
Covering with dressings by different methods
Comforting with sedation and pain killer

14. True for superficial burns:

a. Always require skin grafting
b. Dry and inelastic
c. Blister formation
d. Painless

Partial thickness burn is either first or second degree burn which is red and painful, often with blisters.

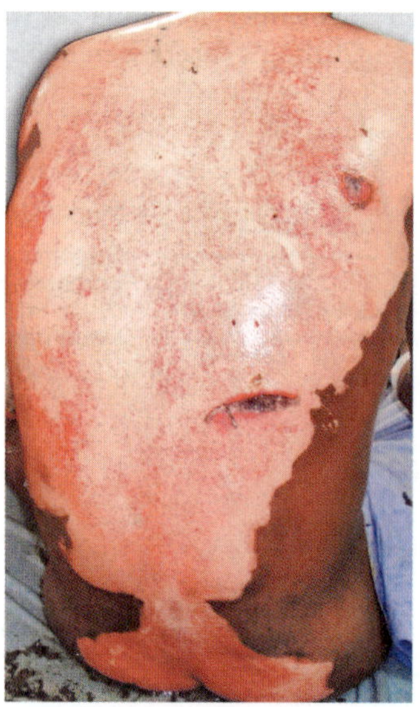

First degree burn

Ans. 10. b. Hypovolumic... 11. c. Ringer lactate 12. b. Physical burn injury... 13. c. Handwashing 14. c. Blister formation

15. A third degree circumferential burn in the arm and forearm region, which of the following is the most important for monitoring:

a. Blood gasses
b. Carboxy-oxygen levels
c. Macroglobinuria and cryoglobinuria
d. Peripheral pulse and circulation

Circumferential eschar in the upper limb, lower limb, neck, thorax can cause more edema which initially causes venous compression and later arterial compression causing ischemia, gangrene of the distal part. So distal area should be monitored for circulation.

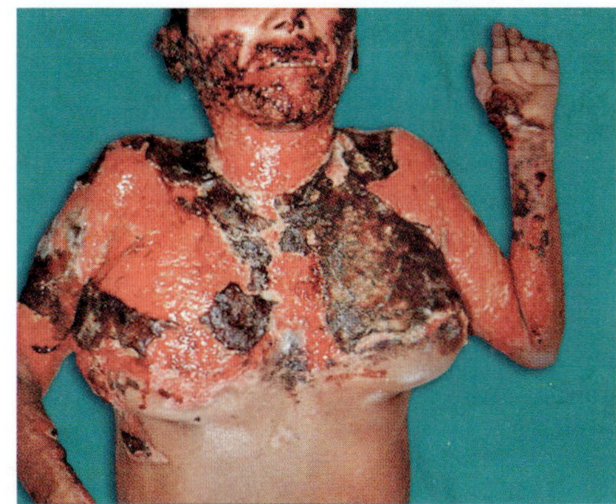

Burns over chest wall with eschar. Note the extent of involvement

16. Whole hand burns represent what percentage of total body surface area:

a. 1%
b. 9%
c. 18%
d. 27%

Patient's entire hand is 1%. Clean piece of paper is cut to the size of hand and through that percentage of burns is assessed.

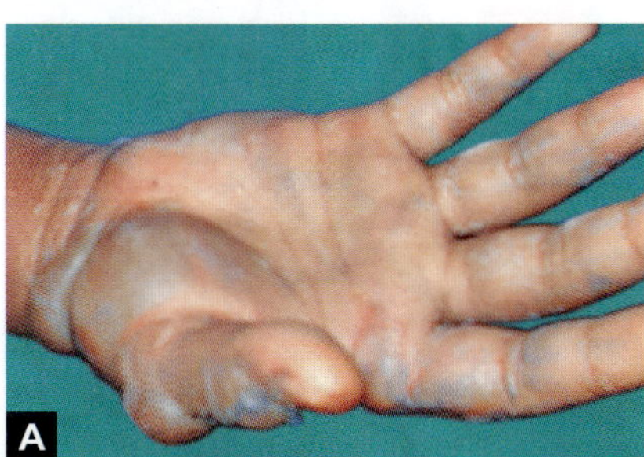

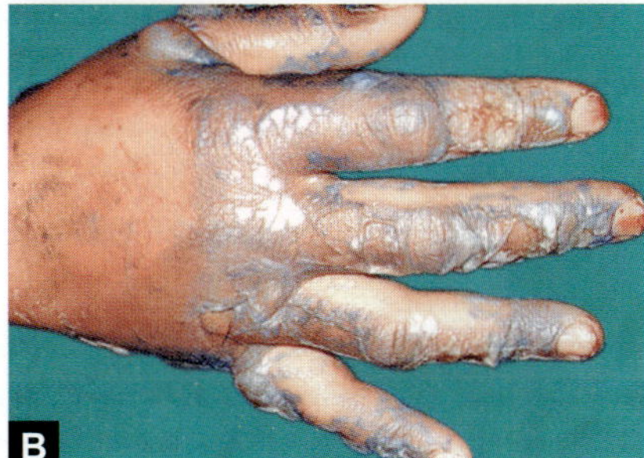

A and B: Burns hand both palmar and dorsal aspect

17. I/V fluid resuscitation rule for burns:

a. (% body surface area) × (weight in pounds) × 4 = Volume in mL
b. (% body surface area) × (weight in Kgs) × 4 = Volume in Lts
c. (% body surface area) × (weight in Kgs) × 5 = Volume in mL
d. (% body surface area) × (weight in Kgs) × 4 = Volume in mL

Parkland regime: 4 mL/% burn/ kg body weight/ 24 hours

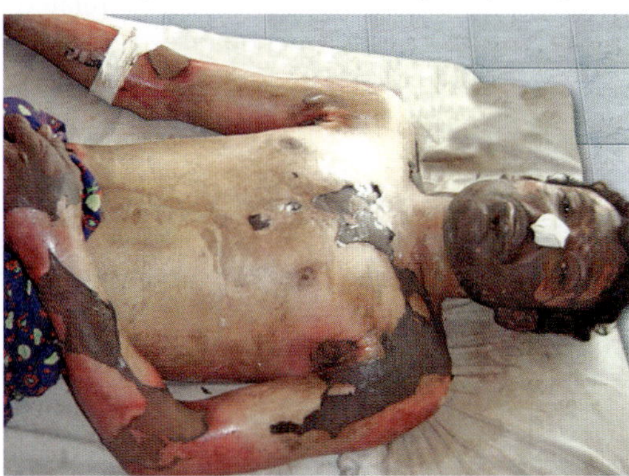

Extensive burns more than 50%

18. Escharotomy is done in:

a. Superficial burns
b. Deep burns
c. Circumferential full thickness burns
d. Burns in childrens

If required, deep longitudinal full thickness incisions are made in different areas so as to prevent collection of edema fluid and also to prevent compression over the vessels. This is called escharotomy.

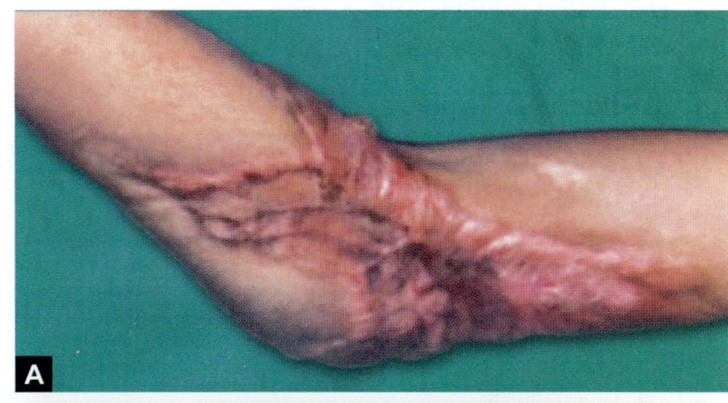

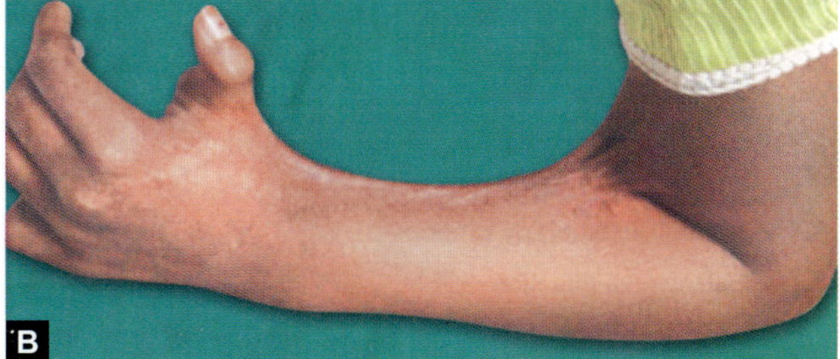

A and B: Elbow contracture due to burns

Ans. **15. d.** Peripheral pulse... **16. a.** 1% **17. d.** (% body surface... **18. c.** Circumferential

VASCULAR SYSTEM

19. Complications of chronic lower limb edema are all EXCEPT:

a. Infection of soft tissue
b. Thickening of skin
c. Ulceration
d. Varicose vein

Varicose veins (due to incompetent valves of veins of lower limb) are more common in women than in men, and are linked with heredity. Other related factors are pregnancy, obesity, menopause, aging, prolonged standing, leg injury, and abdominal straining.

20. FALSE for Thromboangiitis oblliterans/Berger disease:

a. Phlebitis migrans b. Nerves may be involved
c. Involvement of ulnar artery & peroneal arteries
d. Small acral vessels of limb are involved which result in hypohydrosis

Thromboangiitis obliterans (TAO), an inflammatory vasculopathy also known as Buerger disease, is characterized by an inflammatory endarteritis that causes a prothrombotic state and subsequent vaso-occlusive phenomena (NO hypohydrosis).

21. Initial fluid of choice in hypovolemic shock is:

a. Hartman solution b. Dextrose normal saline
c. Normal saline d. Dextran

NS is typically the first fluid used when hypovolemia is severe enough to threaten the adequacy of blood circulation, and has long been believed to be the safest fluid to give quickly in large volumes.

22. MC cause of unilateral lymphoedema of lower limb:

a. Lymphoedema tarda
b. Ca penis with metastasis
c. Filariasis
d. Tubercular lymphadenopathy

Causes of secondary lymphoedema
❑ Trauma
❑ Surgery—inguinal block or axillary block dissection/post-mastectomy with axillary clearance
❑ Filarial lymphoedema due to *Wuchereria bancrofti*—common cause in coastal region
❑ Tuberculosis
❑ Syphilis
❑ Fungal infection
❑ Advanced malignancy—hard, fixed lymph nodes in axilla or in inguinal region
❑ Postradiotherapy lymphoedema
❑ Bacterial infection
❑ Rare causes: Rheumatoid arthritis, snake and insect bites, DVT, chronic venous insufficiency

23. Hemostasis in scalp wounds is best achieved by:

a. Direct pressure over the wound
b. Catching and crushing the bleeders by hemostats
c. Eversion of galea aponeurotica
d. Coagulation of bleeders

Pressure or packing is done at the earliest.

Signs of significant blood loss
Pulse > 100/minute
Systolic BP< 100 mm Hg
Diastolic BP drop on sitting or standing > 10 mm Hg
Pallor/sweating
Shock index (ratio of pulse rate to blood pressure) > 1 (cardiac index)

24. Blood loss during major surgery is best assessed by:

a. Visual assessment
b. Swabs/suction bottles
c. Transesophageal USG doppler
d. Cardiac output by thermodilution

Weighing the swab before and after use is an important method of on-table assessment of blood loss.

Total amount of blood loss = Total difference in swab weight × 1.5

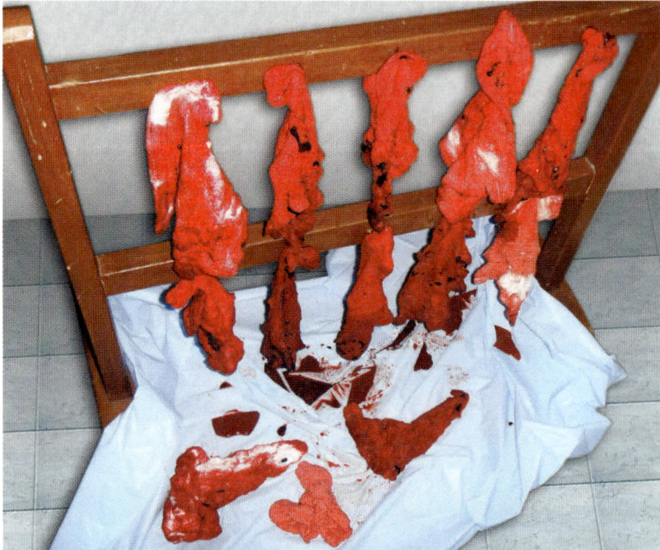

Mops used during major surgery should be kept in a rack so that quantity of bleeding during surgery can be assessed approximately.

25. NOT seen in massive blood transfusion:

a. DIC b. Hypothermia
c. Hypercalcemia d. Thrombocytopenia

Hypocalcemia is seen in massive blood transfusion.

It is defined as replacement or transfusion of blood equivalent to patient's blood volume in < 24 hours corresponding to that particular age (In adult it is 5-6 litres, in infants it is 85 mL/kg body weight.) Or single transfusion of blood more than 2,500 mL continuously

Ans. 19. d. Varicose veins 20. d. Small acral vessels... 21. c. Normal saline 22. c. Filariasis
23. a. Direct pressure... 24. b. Swabs/suction bottles 25. c. Hypercalcemia

Massive transfusion is used in severe trauma associated with liver, vessel, cardiac, pulmonary, pelvic injuries. Often it is required during surgical bleeding (primary hemorrhage on table) of major surgeries
Adverse effects of massive transfusion
a. Severe electrolyte imbalance (hypocalcemia, hyperkalemia, acidosis)
b. Coagulopathy—altered platelet and coagulation factors. – Dilutional thrombocytopenia
c. Citrate toxicity
d. Hypothermia
e. Poor oxygen delivery—due to reduced 2,3 DPG
f. Infections
g. Incompatibility and transfusion reactions
h. ARDS, DIC

26. Superficial thrombophlebitis is seen in:
a. AV fistula
b. Raynaud's disease
c. Buerger's disease
d. Aneurysm

Buerger's disease/thromboangitis obliterans/TAO is segmental, progressive, occlusive, inflammatory disease of small and medium sized vessels with superficial thrombophlebitis, often may present as Raynaud's phenomenon with microabscesses, along with neutrophil and giant cell infiltration, with skip lesions.

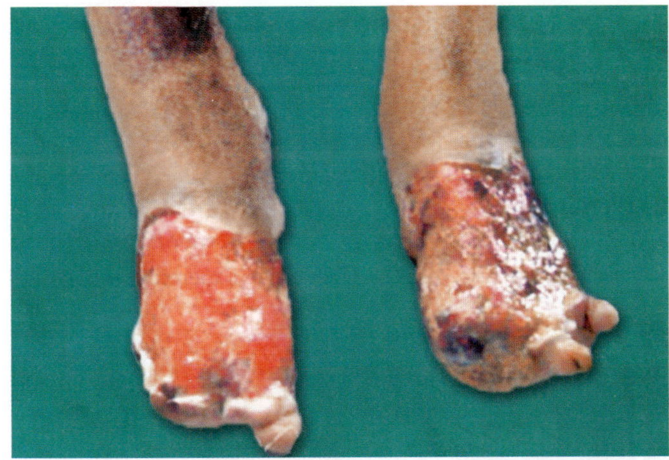

Bilateral TAO in a young male with large ischemic ulcers. Patient underwent amputation of both limbs (Below-knee)

27. Which of the following is associated with Virchow's triad:
a. Hypercoagulability
b. Disseminated malignancy
c. DVT
d. All of the above

Virchow's triad include stasis, hypercoagulability and vein wall injury. It predisposes for DVT. Spontaneous thrombosis is common in visceral neoplasm like carcinoma pancreas or carcinoma stomach. It is often migrating type.

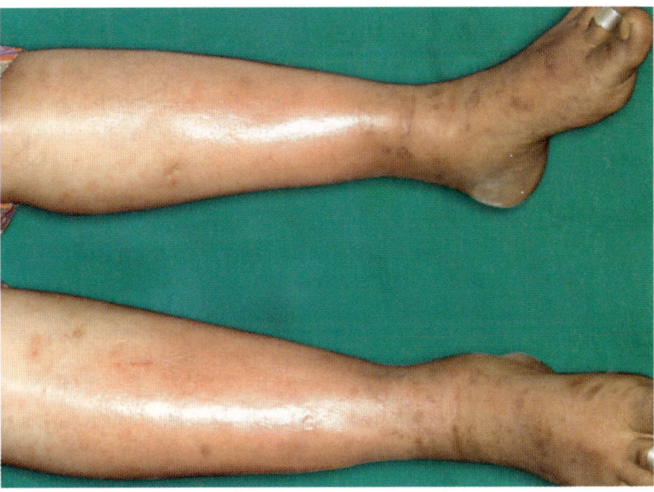

Deep vein thrombosis (DVT) in both legs.
30% cases of DVT are bilateral

28. Hemorrhage leads to:
a. Septicemic shock
b. Neurogenic shock
c. Hypovolemic shock
d. Cardiogenic shock

Classification of hemorrhagic shock (circulatory failure)

Class	*Blood loss*	*Features*
I	Up to 15% (< 750 mL)	Normal
II	Blood loss 15-30% (750–1500 mL)	Palor, thirsty, tachycardia
III	Blood loss 30-40% (1500-2000 mL)	Hypotension, tachycardia, oliguria, confusion
IV	Blood loss > 40% (> 2000 mL)	Rapid pulse, low BP, anuria, unconsciousness, MODS

29. True for shock:
a. Hypotension
b. Hypoperfusion to tissues
c. Hypoxia
d. All of the above

Effects of shock on heart: Low perfusion → low venous return → decreased cardiac output → hypotension → tachycardia. Persistent shock causes hypoxia and release of myocardial depressants leading to further cardiac damage.

Causes of shock
1. Hypovolemic shock—due to reduction in total blood volume. It may be due to: a. Hemorrhage External from wounds, open fractures Internal from injury to spleen, liver, mesentery or pelvis b. *Severe burns*, which results in loss of plasma c. Peritonitis, intestinal obstruction d. Vomiting and diarrhea of any cause

Cond...

Ans. 26. c. Buerger's disease 27. d. All of the above 28. c. Hypovolemic shock 29. d. All of the above

Cond...

2. Cardiac causes
  a. Acute myocardial infarction, acute carditis
  b. Acute pulmonary embolism wherein embolus blocks the pulmonary artery at bifurcation or one of the major branches
  c. Drug induced
  d. Toxemia of any causes
  e. Cardiac surgical conditions like valvular diseases, congenital heart diseases
  f. Cardiac compression causes
    i. Cardiac tamponade due to collection of blood, pus, fluid in the pericardial space which prevents the heart to expand leading to shock.
    ii. Trauma to heart

3. Septic shock—is due to bacterial infections which release toxins leading to shock

4. Neurogenic shock—due to sudden anxious or painful stimuli causing severe splanchnic vessel vasodilatation. Here, patient either goes for cardiac arrest and dies or recovers fully spontaneously—spinal cord injury/anesthesia can cause neurogenic shock

5. Anaphylactic shock—is due to Type 1 hypersensitivity reaction

6. Respiratory causes
  a. Atelectasis (collapse) of lung
  b. Thoracic injuries
  c. Tension pneumothorax
  d. Anesthetic complications

7. Other causes
  a. Acute adrenal insufficiency (Addison's disease)
  b. Myxoedema

30. Most common vessels to be affected in Buerger's disease:
a. Femoral artery b. Iliac artery
c. Popliteal artery
d. Anterior and posterior tibial artery

Buerger's disease is non-atherosclerotic inflammatory disorder involving medium sized and distal vessels with cell mediated sensitivity to type I and type III collagen.

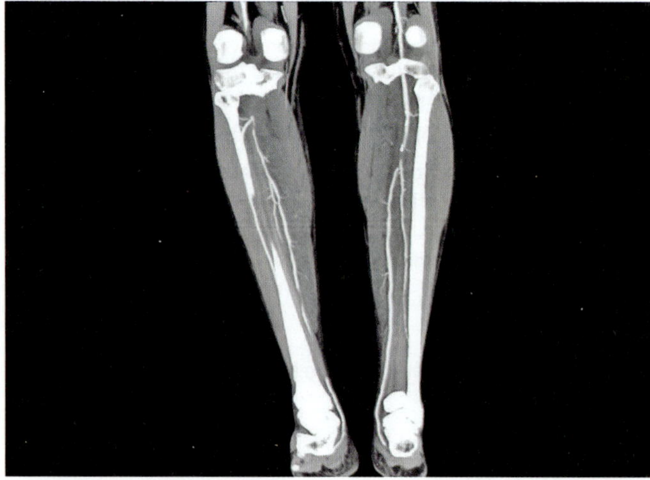
CT angiogram of lower limb (leg area) showing segmental block

31. Earliest and MC feature of deep venous thrombosis:
a. Calf tenderness
b. Rise in temperature
c. Swelling of calf muscle
d. Homan's sign

Features of DVT
Commonly it is asymptomatic—60%
Fever—most common
Tense, tender, warm, pale/bluish, shiny swelling calf
Positive Homan's, Mose's or Neuhof's signs
Inverted champagne bottle sign
Features of pulmonary embolism

32. All may predispose to DVT EXCEPT:
a. OCP b. Nephrotic syndrome
c. Sickle cell anemia d. Thrombocytosis

Polycythemia vera (NOT sickle cell anemia) predisposes to DVT.

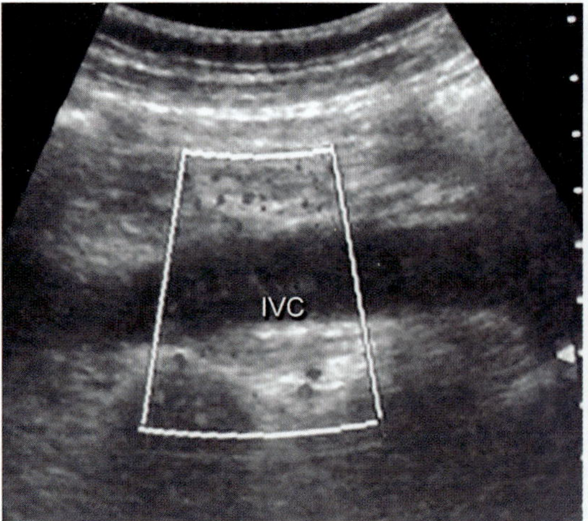

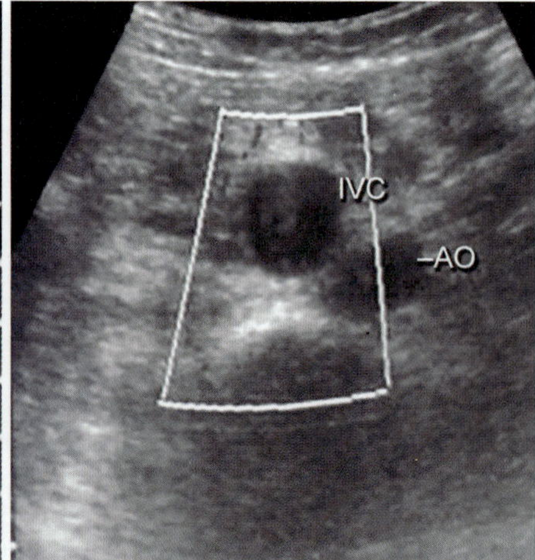

U/S showing thrombosis of the IVC

Ans. 30. **d.** Anterior and... 31. **b.** Rise in temperature 32. **c.** Sickle cell anemia

33. An obese patient developed acute edematous lower limb following a pelvic surgery. DVT is suspected. Most useful investigation is:

a. Duplex scanning   b. Fibrinogen uptake
c. Venography   d. Plethysmography

Duplex scanning in DVT shows non-compressible vein which is wider than normal. On compression over calf muscles, it does not show any augmentation of flow. Normal venous sound at the area of femoral vein which disappears during inspiration is conspicuously absent in DVT.

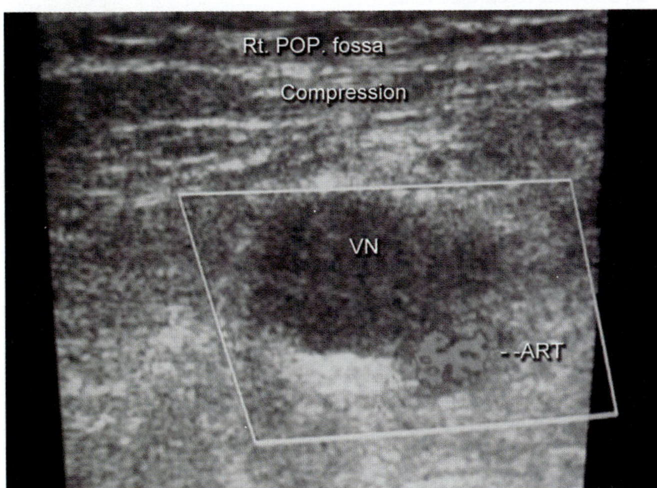

Doppler study showing DVT

34. Hunterian ligature is employed for:

a. Dislocation of TM joint   b. Lymphangitis
c. Aneurysm   d. A-V fistula

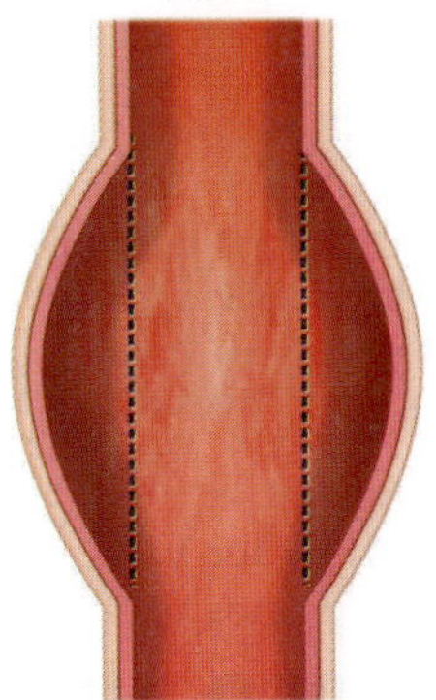

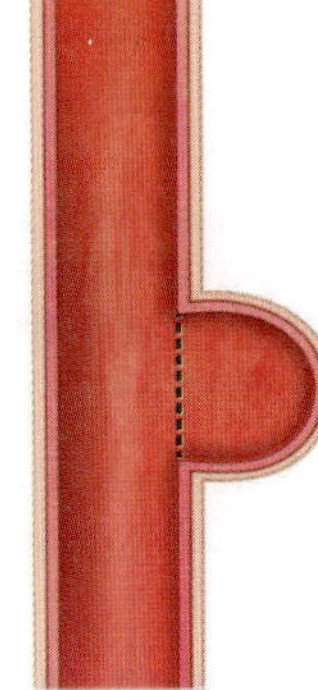

Fusiform type   Saccular type

Fusiform and saccular types of aneurysms

Older methods for managing aneurysms by putting ligatures

Level of ligature	Method
Ligation just proximal to aneurysmal sac	Anel's
Ligation proximally proximal to an arterial branch	Hunter's
Ligation just distal to aneurysmal sac	Brasdor's
Ligation distally distal to an arterial branch	Wardrop's
Ligation one proximal and another distal to aneurysmal sac	Antylus's

35. Drug used for sclerotherapy of varicose veins are all of the following EXCEPT:

a. Ethanolamine Oleate   b. Polidocanol
c. Ethanol   d. Sodium tetradecyl sulfate

Sclerosants used are:
❑ Sodium tetradecyl sulphate 3% (STDS)—commonly used
❑ Sodium morrhuate
❑ Ethanolamine oleate
❑ Polidocanol —3% or 1%

36. Raynaud's syndrome occurs in all of the following EXCEPT:

a. SLE   b. Rheumatoid arthritis
c. Osteoarthritis   d. Cryoglobulinemia

One of the common causes of Raynaud's phenomenon is collagen vascular diseases like scleroderma, rheumatoid disease causing vasculitis (all autoimmune diseases).

Raynaud's syndrome
Sequence of clinical features due to arteriolar spasm.
❑ Local syncope: It is due to vasospasm, causing white cold palm and digits along with tingling and numbness
❑ Local asphyxia: It is due to accumulation of deoxygenated blood as the result of vasospasm causing bluish discoloration of palm and digits with burning sensation (due to accumulated metabolites)

37. In traumatic cases, shock is most likely due to:

a. Injury to intra abdominal solid organ
b. Head injury
c. Septicemia   d. Cardiac failure

General clinical features of abdominal trauma include features of shock—pallor, tachycardia, hypotension, cold periphery, sweating and oliguria.

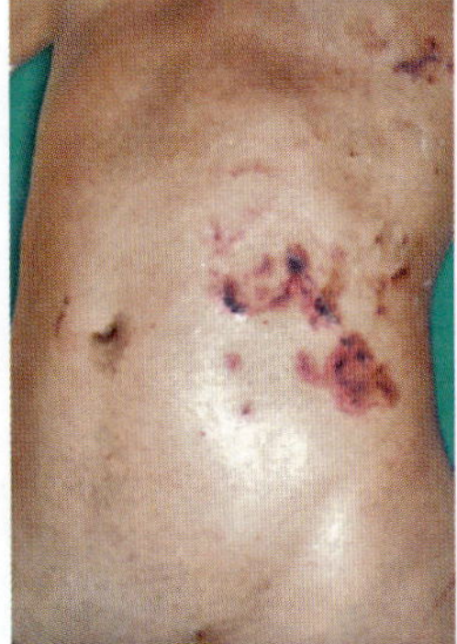

Blunt injury abdomen. Note the bruising over abdominal skin—*London's sign*

MCQs with Short Explanations

Ans. 33. a. Duplex scanning 34. c. Aneurysm 35. c. Ethanol 36. c. Osteoarthritis 37. a. Injury to intra abdominal solid organ

38. All of the following are true regarding DVT EXCEPT:

a. Pulmonary emboli is the immediate risk
b. May lead to lung infarction
c. Associated with deficiency of protein C
d. Prior history of DVT is an important risk factor

Most of the DVT is asymptomatic and presents suddenly with features of pulmonary embolism like chest pain, breathlessness and hemoptysis.

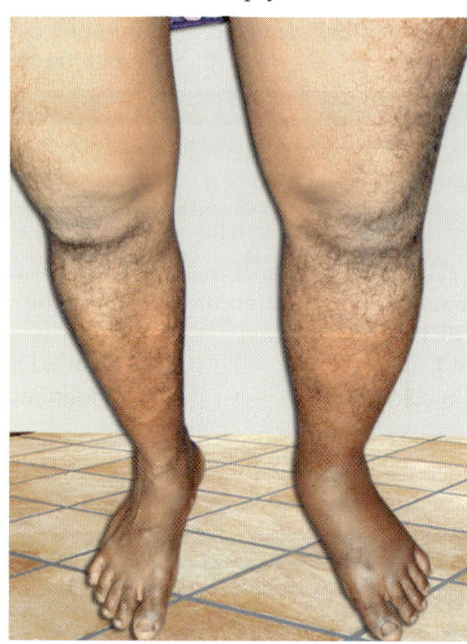

Unilateral left leg DVT. Note the edema and color changes

39. Sequence of color changes observed in Raynaud's disease:

a. Red, blue, white   b. White, blue, red
c. Blue, red, white   d. White, red, blue

Features of pallor/ blanching (syncope), dusky cyanosis (asphyxia), rubor/ painful red engorgement (recovery) are the presentation of Raynaud's phenomenon.

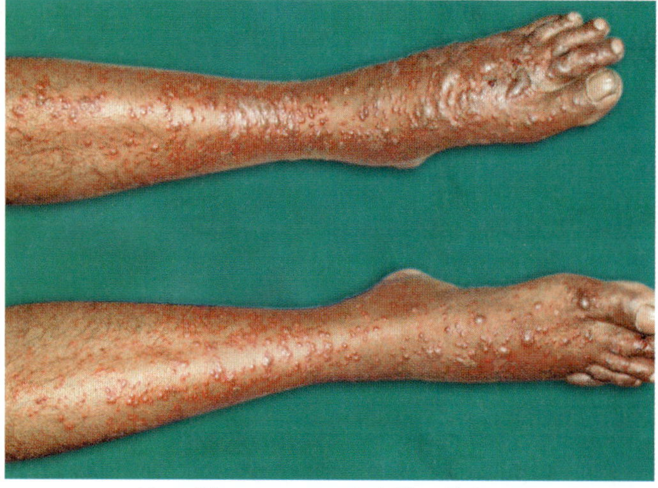

Vasculitis can cause arterial insufficiency

40. Which of the following is better indicator of need for blood transfusion:

a. Urine output   b. Hematocrit
c. Skin color   d. Clinical examination

The hematocrit measures the volume of red blood cells compared to the total blood volume (red blood cells and plasma). Hematocrit is also sometimes called packed cell volume (PCV), volume of packed red cells (VPRC), or erythrocyte volume fraction (EVF).

Complications of blood transfusion
❑ Congestive cardiac failure
❑ Transfusion reactions HBV, HCV – Incompatibility. Major and minor reactions with fever, rigors, pain, hypotension – Pyrexial reactions due to pyrogenic ingredients in the blood – Allergic reactions – Sensitization to leukocytes and platelets – Immunological sensitization
❑ Infections – Serum hepatitis – HIV infection – Bacterial infection – Malaria transmission – Epstein-Barr virus infection – Cytomegalovirus infection – Syphilis, Yersinia – *Babesia microti* infection – *Trypanosoma cruzi* infection
❑ Air embolism
❑ Thrombophlebitis
❑ Coagulation failure – Dilution of clotting factors – DIC – Dilutional thrombocytopenia occurs in patients with massive blood transfusion
❑ Circulatory overload causing heart failure
❑ Hemochromatosis in patients with CRF receiving repeated blood transfusions
❑ Citrate intoxication causes bradycardia and hypocalcemia. For every four units of blood 10 mL of 10% calcium chloride or gluconate should be infused intravenously
❑ Iron overload

41. Cryoprecipitate is a rich source of:

a. Thromboplastin   b. Factor VIII
c. Factor X   d. Factor VII

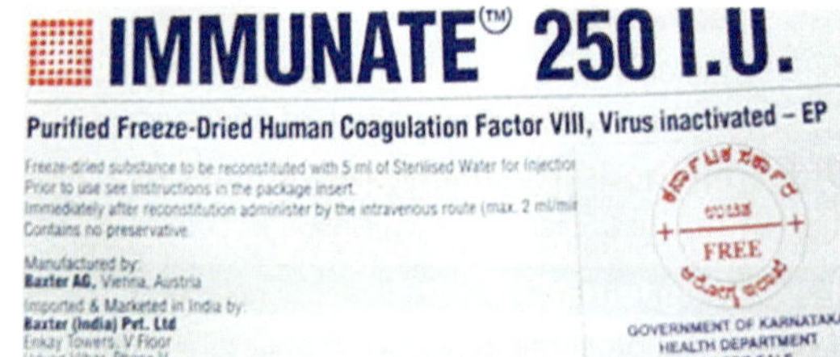

Purified freeze dried human coagulation factor VIII is available for use in hemophilia patients

Ans. 38. **b.** May lead to... 39. **b.** White, blue, red 40. **b.** Hematocrit 41. **b.** Factor VIII

When fresh frozen plasma is allowed to thaw at 4 °C, visible white supernatant layer develops and is called as cryoprecipitate which is rich in Factor VIII and fibrinogen.

42. Platelets can be stored at:

a. 20–24 °C for 5 days b. 20–24 °C for 8 days
c. 4–8 °C for 5 days d. 4–8 °C for 8 days

Storage at ambient, room temperature (22 °C) preserved a normal platelet life-span. Platelets stored at this higher temperature should be adequate for transfusion purposes for as long as 96 hours.

43. Massive transfusion in previous healthy adult male can cause hemorrhage due to:

a. Increased tPA
b. Dilutional thrombocytopenia
c. Vitamin K deficiency
d. Decreased fibrinogen

Coagulopathy is noticed in massive blood transfusion—altered platelet and coagulation factors—dilutional thrombocytopenia.

44. Blood platelets in stored blood do NOT remain functional after:

a. 24 hours b. 48 hours
c. 72 hours d. 96 hours

In stored blood
❑ RBCs last for 3 weeks
❑ WBCs are destroyed rapidly
❑ Platelets also get reduced in 24 hours
❑ Clotting factors are labile and so their levels fall quickly

45. Migratory thrombophlebitis is a feature of:

a. Buerger's disease b. Varicose veins
c. Pancreatic carcinoma d. Pancreatitis

Thrombophlebitis migrans (Trousseau's sign) is spontaneous migrating thrombophelibitis seen in visceral malignancy like pancreas, stomach.

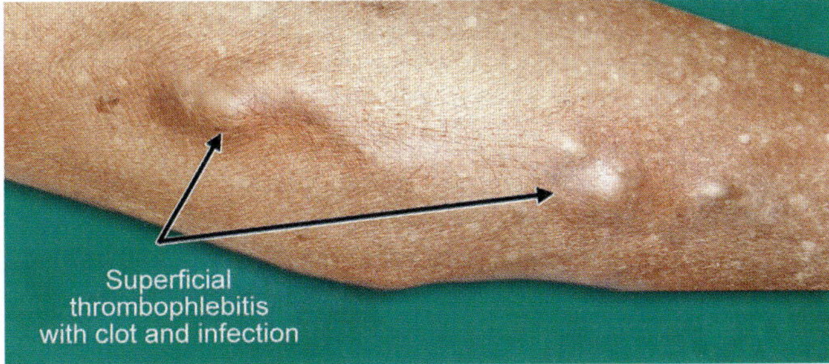

Superficial thrombophlebitis with clot and infection

46. On arteriogram, 'string of beads sign' is suggestive of:

a. Mural hyperplasia
b. Subadventitial fibroplasia
c. Renal embolism
d. Fibromuscular hyperplasia

The 'string of beads' feature in medial fibromuscular dysplasia. The sign is caused by areas of relative stenoses alternating with small aneurysms. FMD is a non-atherosclerotic, non-inflammatory disease of the blood vessels that causes abnormal growth within the wall of an artery.

47. Buerger's disease usually affects all of the following EXCEPT:

a. Small sized arteries
b. Medium sized arteries
c. Large arteries
d. Deep vein

There is vasospasms → intimal hyperplasia → thrombosis (commonly medium sized vessels are involved) → panarteritis → obliteration; tender, cord like veins with superficial migrataory thrombophlebitis (30%); with the nerve involvement due to vasa nervorum block// spasm. Arterial lumen is blcoked but not thickened like atherosclerosis.

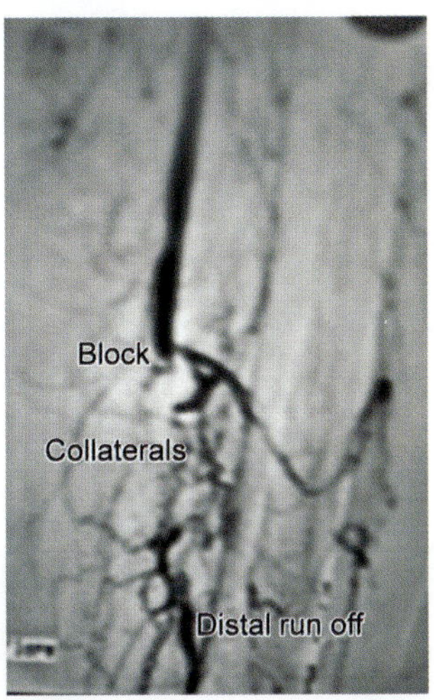

Angiogram showing block in main vessel with opened up collaterals and adequate distal run off

48. Features of hypovolumic shock are all EXCEPT:

a. Oliguria b. Bradycardia
c. Low BP d. Acidosis

Tachycardia (and NOT bradycardia) is seen in shock

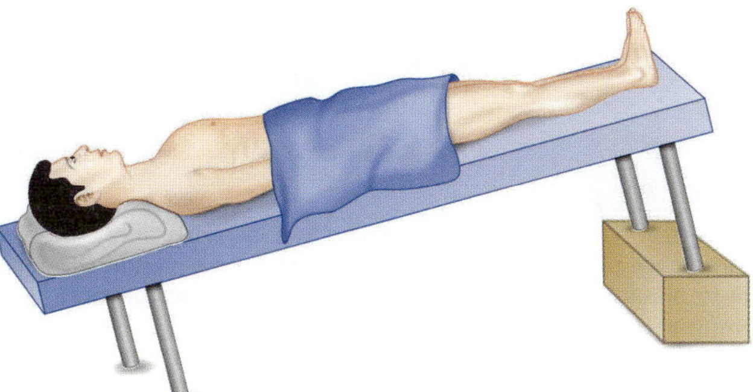

Trendelenburg position—head down position, used in patient in shock

Ans. 42. **a.** 20–24 deg... 43. **b.** Dilutional... 44. **a.** 24 hours 45. **c.** Pancreatic carcinoma 46. **d.** Fibromuscular... 47. **c.** Large arteries 48. **b.** Bradycardia

49. Adson's test is positive in:

a. Follicular cyst b. Radicular cyst
c. Cervical spondylosis d. Cervical rib

Adson's test is done for cervical rib. The hand is raised above after feeling the radial pulse. The patient is asked to take a deep breath and turn the head to the same side. Any change in pulse, i.e. either becoming feeble or absent, is noted.

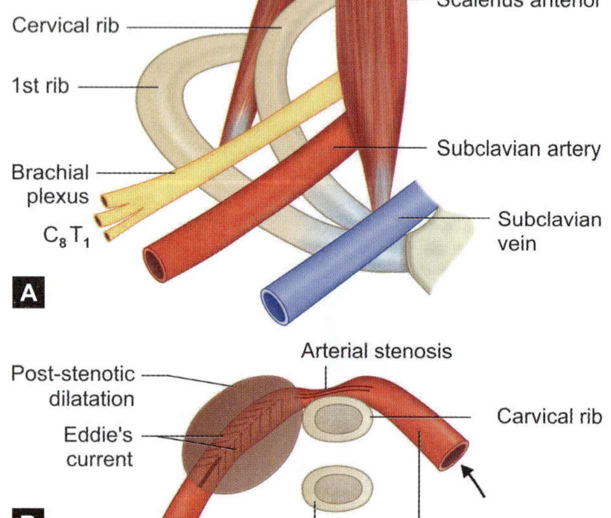

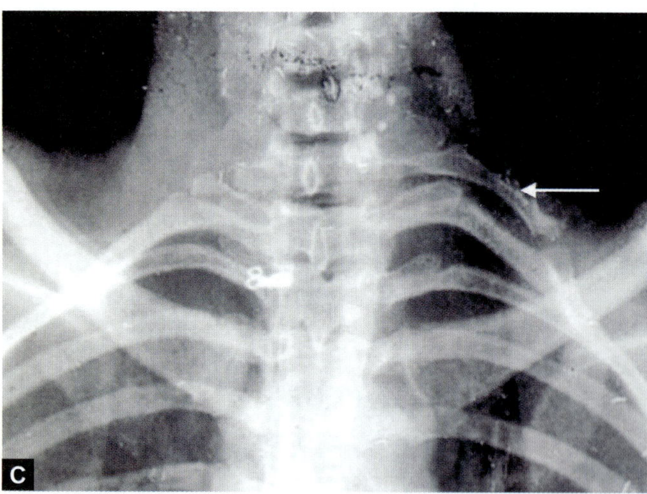

Anatomy of cervical rib and its relation to subclavian artery and vein and brachial plexus. Note the Eddie's current, post-stenotic dilatation due to arterial compression by cervical rib. **X-ray shows left sided complete cervical rib.**

50. Commonest cause of A-V fistula:

a. Traumatic b. Surgical creation
c. Tumor erosion d. Congenital

Congenital arteriovenous malformation/fistula

During development period, AV communication occurs.
It is high flow type of vascular malformation.
It is 30% of all vascular malformations.

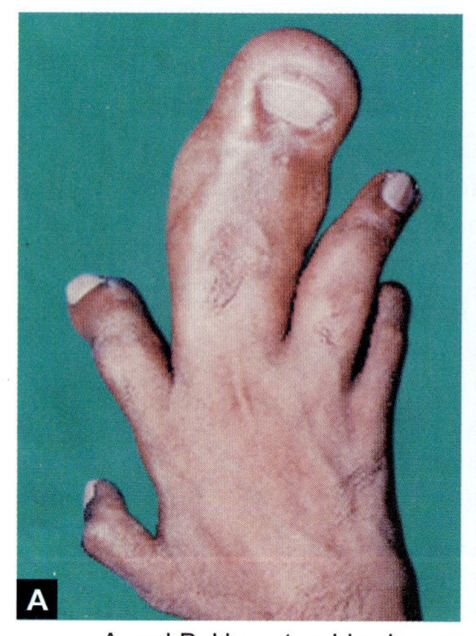

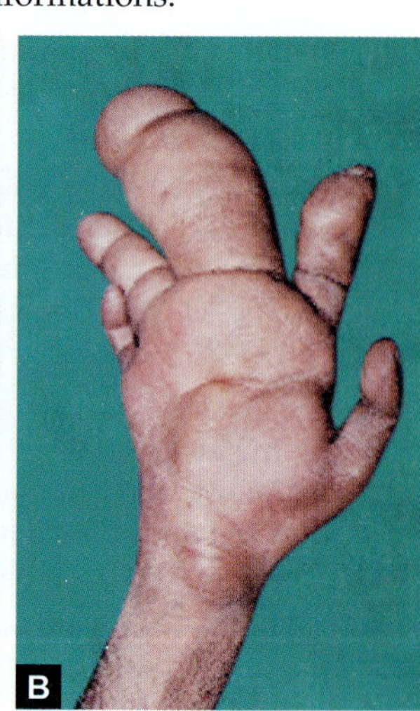

A and B: Hypertrophic changes due to AV malformation

51. Harvey's sign is:

a. Loss of hair from eyebrow
b. Seen in DVT
c. Related to venous refilling after emptying a length of vein
d. Transmitted pressure wave on coughing in a varicose vein

If two index fingers are placed firmly side by side on avein and the finger nearer the heart is moved so as to empty a short length of vein, the release of the distal finger will allow the speed of venous refilling to be observed.

52. Intermittent claudication means:

a. Cyanosis of leg
b. Pain in the leg only on exercise
c. Pain in leg on rest
d. Pain in leg

Claudication
❑ *Arterial*—typically develops after walking for certain distance and resolves rapidly within 5 minutes once walking is stopped
❑ *Neurogenic*—pain develops in standing or walking and disappears immediately after stopping walk; normal feeling pulses without ischemic changes are present. It is usually due to narrow lumbar canal (spinal canal stenosis)
❑ *Venous*—it is rare but definitely occurs. It is observed in chronic pelvic venous obstruction as a mechanical high venous pressure. It is usually due to iliac vein thrombosis. Peripheral pulses are normal.

53. MC site of subclavian artery obstruction:

a. 1st part b. 2nd part
c. 3rd part d. 4th part

Ans. 49. **d.** Cervical rib 50. **d.** Congenital 51. **c.** Related to venous... 52. **b.** Pain in the leg only... 53. **a.** 1st part

Stenosis of subclavian artery typically occurs in first part. Within this subset, the majority of stenoses occur proximal to the origin of the vertebral artery.

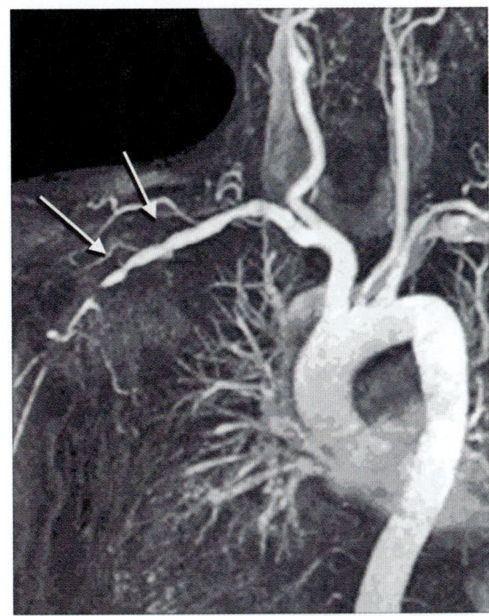

Upper limb angiogram showing blocks in subclavian artery

54. MC site of peripheral aneurysm:

a. Brachial artery b. Popliteal artery
c. Radial artery d. Femoral artery

Peripheral aneurysms are less common compared to aneurysms in the cavity. Popliteal type is the MC one.

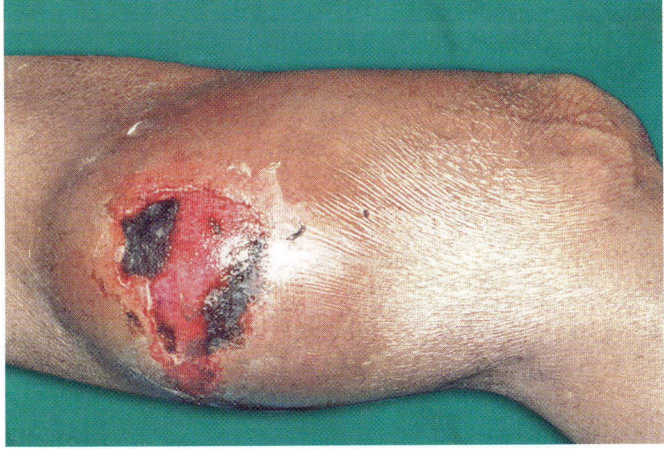

Popliteal aneurysm about to rupture. It is the most common peripheral aneurysm

55. Artery commonly involved in cirsoid aneurysm:

a. Occipital b. Superficial temporal
c. Internal carotid d. External carotid

Cirsoid aneurysm is a rare variant of capillary hemangioma occurring in the skin, beneath which abnormal artery communicates with distended veins. It is commonly seen in superficial temporal artery and its branches.

56. MC cause of aneurysm of abdominal aorta is:

a. Trauma b. Atherosclerosis
c. Syphilis d. Cystic medial necrosis

Acquired causes of abdominal aorta aneurysm include degenerative condition like atherosclerosis (most common cause), mucoid degeneration of intima and media (in South African young Negroes).

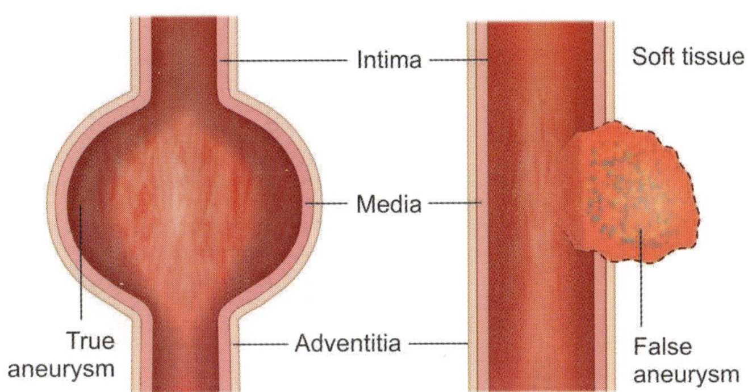

True and false aneurysms. In true type, all layers are intact. **In false type all layers breached with hematoma having a false capsule**

57. Ganglion spared in lumbar sympathectomy is:

a. L1 b. L2
c. L3 d. L4

L1 is retained on one side in bilateral cases. If both sides are removed, it will lead to failure of ejaculation and so sterility (Dry ejaculation).

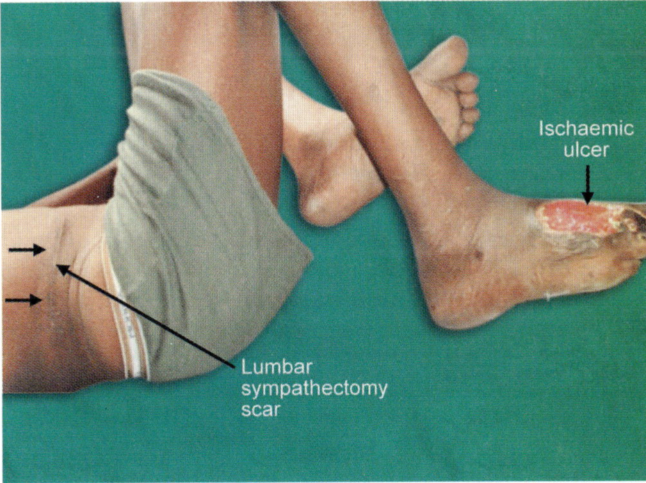

Lumbar sympathectomy scar with ischemic ulcer foot showing healing sign

58. Arterio-Venous fistula can lead to all EXCEPT:

a. Sinus tachycardia b. Increased preload
c. Cardiac arrhythmias d. Increased cardiac output

In AV fistula, shunting of blood with thrill and bruit with hyperdynamic circulation is common. Because of hyperdynamic circulation, there is increased cardiac output and so often congestive cardiac failure.

Ans. **54. b.** Popliteal artery **55. b.** Superficial temporal **56. b.** Atherosclerosis **57. a.** L1 **58. c.** Cardiac arrhythmias

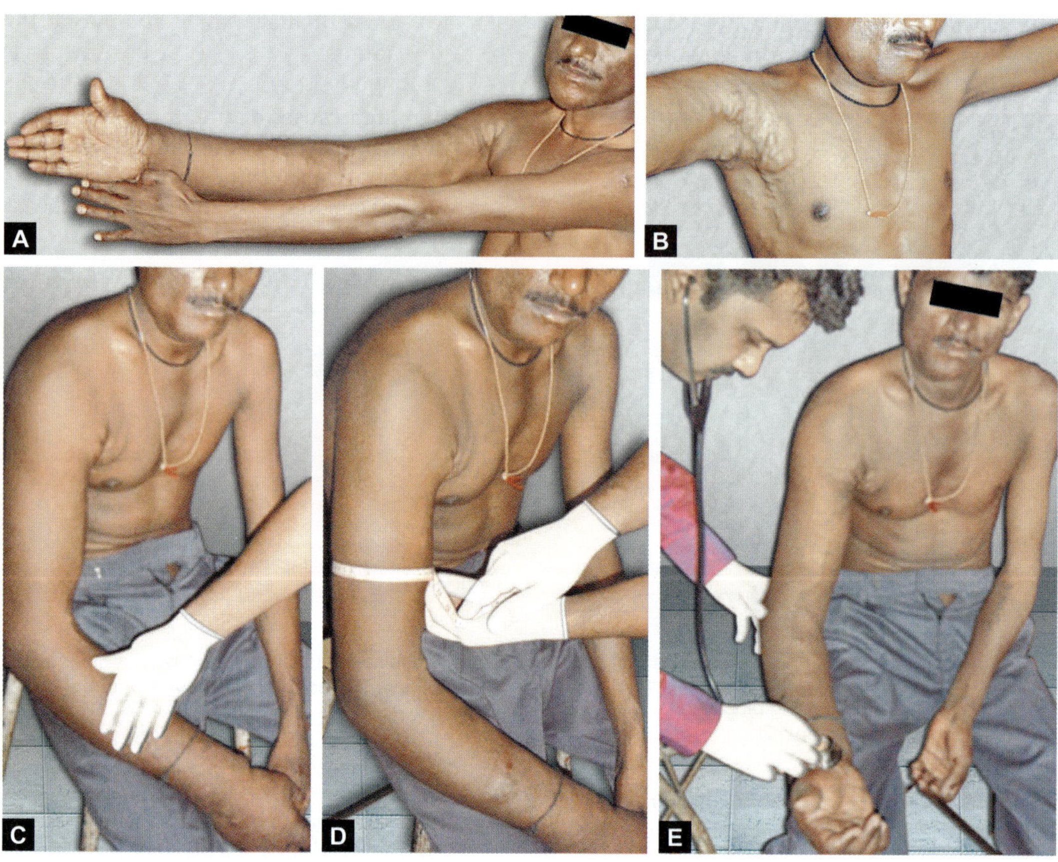

Congenital arteriovenous malformation involving right upper limb, axillary region and part of right half of neck and face. Note the limb lengthening and widened girth. Limb is warmer. Limb should be measured at each level. Auscultation reveals continuous bruit over the limb. Note the dilated tortuous veins due to hyperdynamic circulation.

59. Cryoprecipitate is NOT helpful in treating:

a. DIC
b. von Willebrand's disease
c. Christmas disease
d. Hemophilia A

Cryoprecipitate is used in inherited deficiency of factor VIII (classical hemophilia/ hemophilia A), fibrinogen, Factor XIII, von Willebrand's disease and DIC.

Blood clotting factors

Factor No.	Common name
I	Fibrinogen
II	Prothrombin
III	Thromboplastin
IV	Ionic calcium
V	Hereditary labile factor, activator (AC) globulin, proaccelerin
VI	Accelerin, supposed to be active form of Factor V
VII	Proconvertin; serum prothrombin—conversion accelerator (SPCA)
VIII	Antihemophilic factor (AHF)
IX	Plasma thromboplastin component (PTC; Christmas factor)
X	Stuart-Prower factor
XI	Plasma thromboplastin antecedent (PTA)
XII	Hageman factor
XIII	Fibrin stabilizing factor, fibrinase
XIV	Prekallikrein
XV	Kallikrein
XVI	Platelet factor

60. Test which is not done for varicose veins:

a. Perthe's test
b. Tourniquet test
c. Trendelenberg test
d. Adson's test

Adson's test is done for cervical rib.

Ans. **59. c.** Christmas disease **60. d.** Adson's test

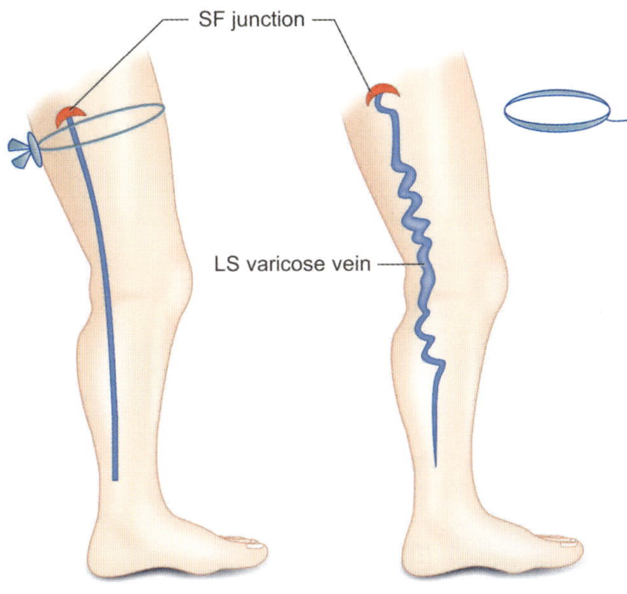

Brodie-Trendelenburg test. Note the reversal of blood flow while releasing the tourniquet

61. Modified Allen's test is done for:

a. Brachial artery b. Popliteal artery
c. Dorsalis pedis artery d. Radial artery

Allen's test is used in hand to test the patency of radial and ulnar arteries. Both radial and ulnar arteries of the patient is felt and pressed firmly at the wrist. Patient clinches his hand firmly (often repeated clinchning) and holds it tightly. After 1 minute clinch is released to open the palm of the hand which looks pale. Pressure on the radial artery in the wrist is released to see area of distribution of radial artery. Normally, it becomes flushed with pink color. If there is block in radial artery, the area will remain white. Test is repeated again for ulnar artery.

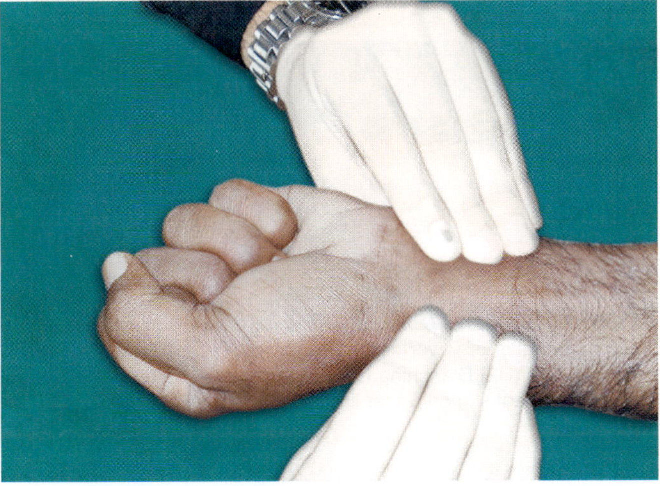
Allen's test done upper limb ischemia to look for perfusion of hand

62. A 60-year-old-male has been operated for carcinoma of cecum and right hemicolectomy has been done. On the 4th postoperative day, the patient develops fever, swelling and pain in the legs. The most important clinical entity one should look for is:

a. Urinary tract infection b. Intravenous line infection
c. Chest infection d. Deep vein thrombosis

Postoperative thrombosis is the MC cause of DVT. It is common after the age of 40 years. Incidence following surgeries is 30%. In 30% of cases, both legs are affected.

Effects and sequelae of DVT
❑ Pulmonary *embolism*—15%
❑ Infection; venous gangrene
❑ Partial recanalization, chronic venous hypertension around the ankle region causing venous ulcers—*chronic venous insufficiency*—CVI
❑ Recurrent DVT—30%
❑ Propagation of thrombus proximally—20-30%

63. Sympathectomy is done for all EXCEPT:

a. Causalgia
b. Intermittent claudication
c. Rest pain d. Raynaud's disease

Indications
❑ Cervical rib with vascular manifestations—useful
❑ Raynaud's phenomenon—useful
❑ Hyperhidrosis—very useful
❑ Upper limb vasospasm due to other causes—useful
❑ Acrocyanosis—useful
❑ Causalgia—very useful
❑ Sudeck's osteodystrophy

64. The most common cause of peripheral limb ischemia in India is:

a. Trauma b. Atherosclerosis
c. Buerger's disease d. Takayasu's disease

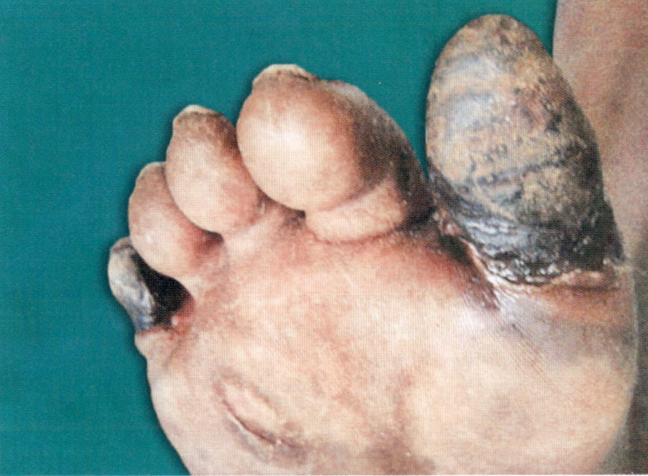
Gangrene of great and little toes in a patient with vascular compromise

Ans. **61. d.** Radial artery **62. d.** Deep vein thrombosis **63. b.** Intermittent... **64. b.** Atherosclerosis

Causes of limb ischemia

- Atherosclerosis
- Embolism (acute)
- Arteriopathies – Buerger's disease, Raynaud's disease, Takayasu's disease
- Diabetes
- Scleroderma
- Physical agents – trauma, tourniquet, radiation injury

65. Milroy's disease is lymphedema which:

a. Is due to malignant disease
b. Follows erysipelas
c. Is familial
d. Follows filariasis

Primary type	
It affects commonly females.	
❑ It is common in lower limb and left side.	
It can be:	
❑ Familial	
❑ Syndromic (Turner's / Klinefelter's / Down's / Klipple Trenauny Weber)	
It can be:	
❑ Lymphoedema congenital (10%)	Present at birth—< 2 years Familial type is called as *Nonne-Milroy's disease.* It is type I familial, autosomal dominant—chromosome 5 related; bilateral upper and lower limbs, genitalia and face may be involved. Incidence is 1:6000 of live births.
❑ Lymphoedema praecox	Present at puberty—up to 2–35 years (80%). Familial type is called as *Letessier-Meige's syndrome.* It is type II familial. It occurs between puberty and middle age.
❑ Lymphoedema tarda	Present in adult life—after 35 years
❑ *It can be radiologically (lymphangiography):*	
❑ Hypoplasia 70%	
❑ Aplasia 15%	
❑ Hyperplasia (varicose lymphatics) 15%	

66. Treatment of acute lymphangitis:

a. Antibiotic and rest
b. Immediate lymphangiography
c. Immediate multiple incisions
d. All of the above

Management of acute lymphangitis

- Antibiotics like penicillin and cloxacillin
- Elevation, rest, glycerine magnesium sulfa dressing
- Management of toxemia or septicemia with critical care.

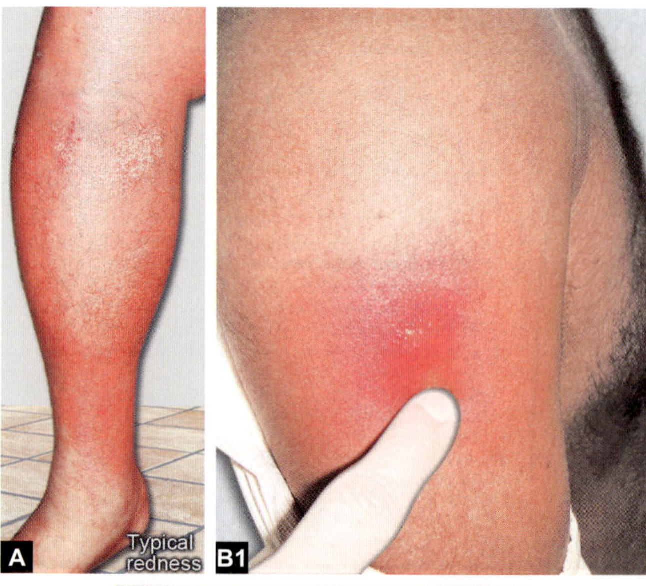

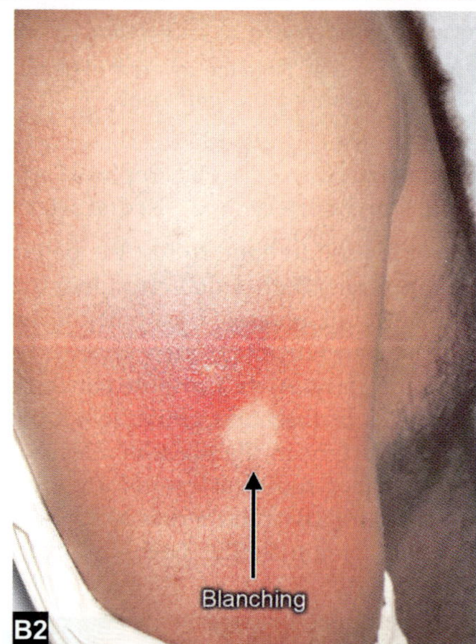

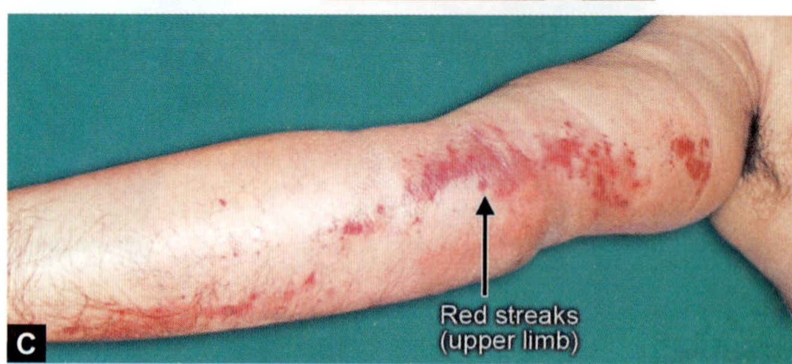

(A) Lymphangitis of lower limb showing redness. (B1) Lymphangitis of upper limb; (B2) Blanching is seen immediately after pressure; (C) Typical red streaks in an upper limb lymphangitis

67. When a patient suffers from critical limb ischemia, the ankle-brachial index (ABPI) is less than:

a. 1.0
b. 0.9
c. 0.7
d. 0.3

Ans. **65. c.** Is familial **66. a.** Antibiotic and rest **67. d.** 0.3

Critical limb ischemia is persistently recurring ischemic rest pain for 2 weeks, which requires regular analgesics for >2 weeks or ulceration or gangrene of the foot or toes with an ankle systolic pressure <50 mm Hg or toe systolic pressure <30 mm Hg. Ankle brachial pressure index (ABPI) will be less than 0.3.

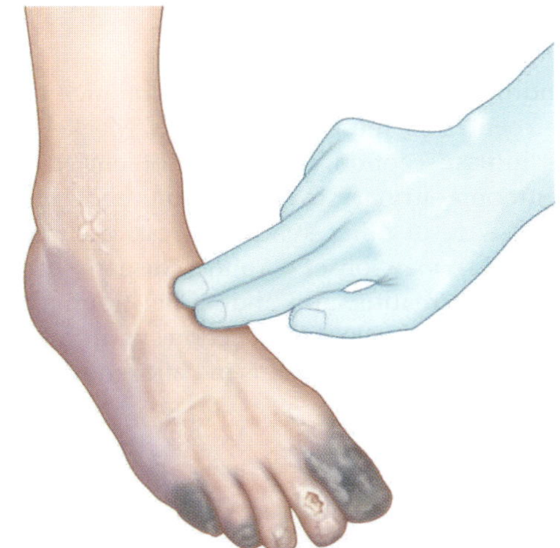

Gangrene of great and little toes in a patient with vascular compromise

68. Investigation of choice for varicose veins:

a. Duplex ultrasound imaging
b. Standard Doppler examination
c. Varicography
d. Venography

Duplex scan is a highly reliable ultrasound Doppler imaging technique (here high resolution B mode ultrasound imaging and Doppler ultrasound is used) which along with direct visualization of veins, gives the functional and anatomical information, and also color map.

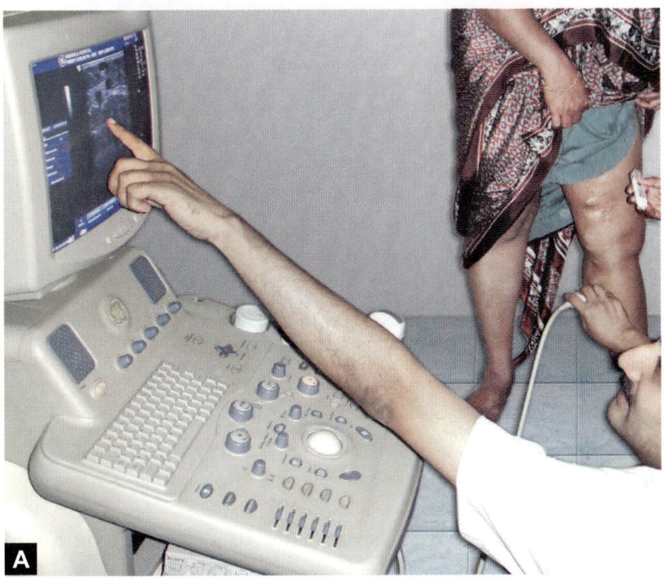

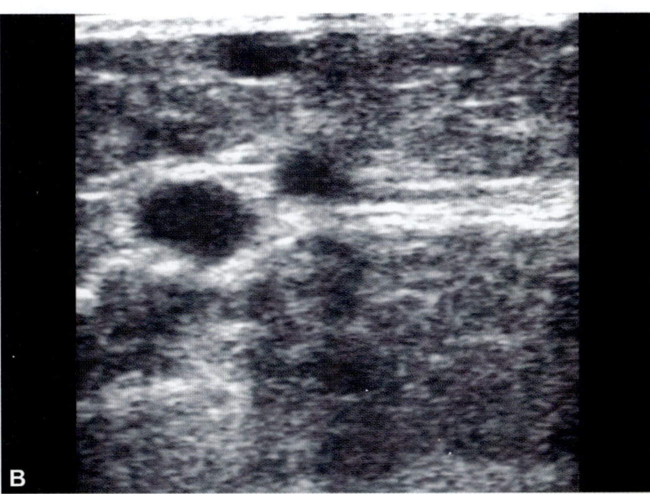

Duplex scan for venous diseases of lower limb should also be done in standing position

69. Triad following massive blood transfusion includes:

a. Acidosis, hyperthermia, hyperkalemia
b. Acidosis, hypothermia, hyperkalemia
c. Alkalosis, hypothermia, hyperkalemia
d. Alkalosis, hyperthermia, hyperkalemia

After 2 weeks of storage, PRBCs/ packed RBCs have a pH below 7.0, and each unit has an acid load of approximately 6 mEq. One of these mEq of acid comes from the fact that PRBCs are made from venous blood with a starting pH of 7.35, a second mEq is acquired in buffering the citric acid in the anticoagulant, and 4 mEqs are generated by glycolysis during the PRBC storage.

70. True statement about arterial occlusion in the leg are all EXCEPT:

a. Rest pain in limbs
b. Pain in limbs on taking very first step
c. Pain relieved by standing still
d. Pain in limbs on walking

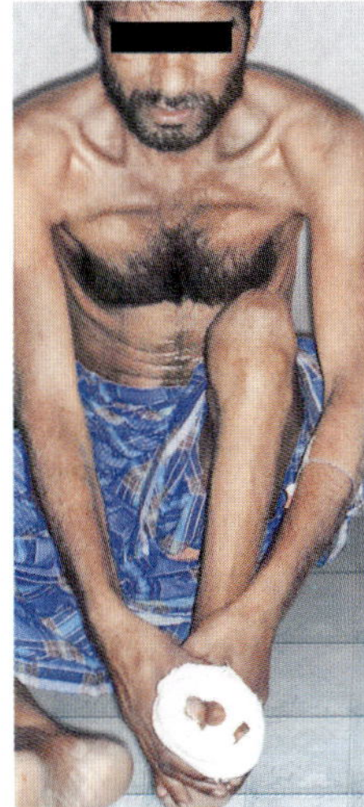

Rest pain in a patient suffering from TAO. Holding the foot reduces the pain slightly

Ans. 68. **a.** Duplex ultra... 69. **b.** Acidosis, hypothermia... 70. **b.** Pain in limbs on taking very first step

Intermittent claudication (pain) in the lower limbs develops when the muscles are exercising. Cause for pain is accumulation of substance P and metabolites, because of arterial occlusion. During exercise increased perfusion and increased opening of collaterals wash the metabolites.

ABDOMEN

71. Anchovy sauce pus is seen in:
a. Hydatid cyst
b. Hepatocellular carcinoma
c. Amoebic liver abscess
d. Pyogenic liver abscess

When Entamoeba histolytica spreads outside a patient's gut, it usually involves the liver. Here it can cause an ''abscess' filled with liquid necrotic liver. To start with this is yellow or yellow-green, later it becomes a syrupy dark reddish-yellow (''anchovy sauce'). The central area of necrosis is surrounded by zones of progressively less damaged tissue and amoebae.

72. Parameter used to assess severity of pancreatitis:
a. Serum amylase levels
b. Faecal trypsin levels
c. ARDS development
d. Ranson criteria

Ranson criteria
- It form a clinical prediction rule for predicting the severity of acute pancreatitis.
- Alternatively, pancreatitis severity can be assessed by any of the following:
  - APACHE II score ≥ 8
  - Organ failure
  - Substantial pancreatic necrosis (at least 30% glandular necrosis according to contrast-enhanced CT)

73. APACHE score considers all EXCEPT:
a. pH of blood
b. Heart rate
c. Serum bilirubin
d. Respiratory rate

APACHE II ("Acute Physiology and Chronic Health Evaluation II") is a severity-of-disease classification system (Knaus et al., 1985), one of several ICU scoring systems. . The point score is calculated from a patient's age and 12 routine physiological measurements:
- $AaDO_2$ or PaO_2 (depending on FiO_2)
- Temperature (rectal)
- Mean arterial pressure
- pH arterial
- Heart rate
- Respiratory rate
- Sodium (serum)
- Potassium (serum)
- Creatinine
- Hematocrit
- White blood cell count
- Glasgow Coma Scale

74. Differential diagnosis of appendicitis in children:
a. Intussusception
b. Lymphadenitis
c. Gastroenteritis
d. All of the above

Condition in children which may mimick appendictis: Gastroenteritis, mesenteric adenitis, Meckel's diverticulitis, intussusception, Henoch-Schönlein purpura, lobar pneumonia, urinary tract infection (abdominal pain in the absence of other symptoms can occur in children with UTI), new-onset Crohn's disease or ulcerative colitis, pancreatitis, and abdominal trauma from child abuse; distal intestinal obstruction syndrome in children with cystic fibrosis; typhlitis in children with leukemia.

75. MC abdominal organ involved in blunt injury to abdomen is:
a. Spleen
b. Liver
c. Pancreas
d. Stomach

Abdominal trauma can be blunt or stab/penetrating or abdominal wall injuries. Spleen is the MC organ involved in blunt trauma. Liver is the MC organ involved in penetrating injuries.

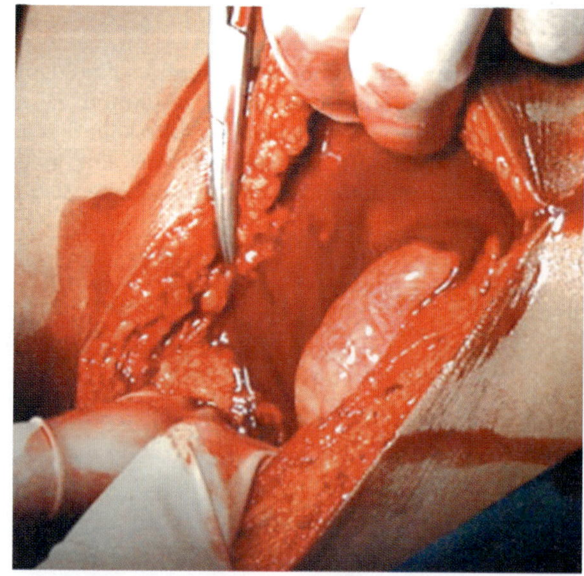

Traumatic hemoperitoneum

76. Diameter of common bile duct:
a. 2.5 cm
b. 3.5 cm
c. 5.5 cm
d. 7.5 cm

Common bile duct is normally 10–12 cm in length and 6–8 mm in diameter.

Ans. 71. **c.** Amoebic liver... 72. **d.** Ranson criteria 73. **c.** Serum bilirubin 74. **d.** All of the above 75. **a.** Spleen 76. **d.** 7.5 cm

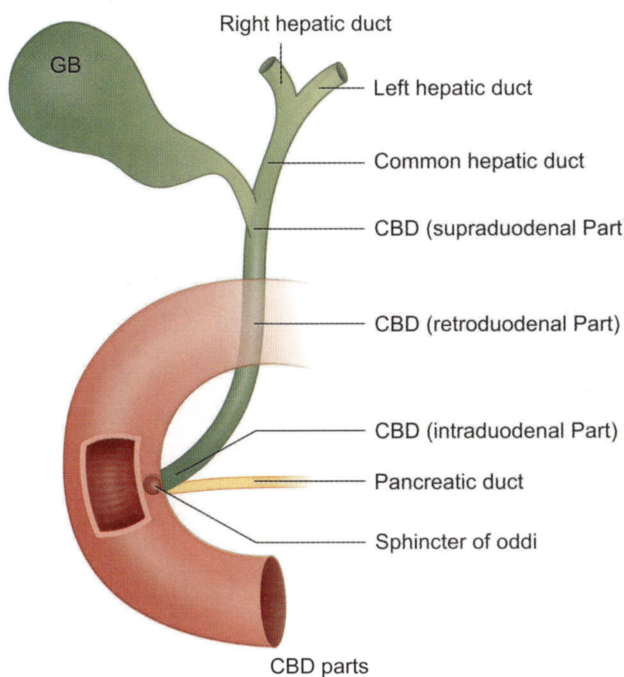

CBD parts

77. Best way to localize extra-adrenal pheochromocytoma:
a. X-ray b. Nucelotide scan
c. VMA excretion d. Clinical examination

Iodine labeled meta-iodo-benzyl-guanidine (I, MIBG) is useful to find out extra-adrenal involvement—SPECT scan is very useful. I^{131} MIBG scan is safe, noninvasive with 100% sensitivity and 95% specificity.

Tumor is
❑ 10% malignant
❑ 10% extra-adrenal
❑ 10% bilateral
❑ 10% familial
❑ 10% childhood
❑ 10% multiple
❑ 10% not associated with hypertension
❑ 10% calcified

78. NOT an indication for liver transplantation:
a. Primary hyperoxaluria
b. Wilson's disease
c. Hepatocellular carcinoma
d. Fatty liver

Treatment of fatty liver disease is to decrease the potential risk exposures to the liver. For those with alcoholic liver disease, abstaining from alcohol is a must. For those with NAFLD (non-alcoholic fatty liver disease) or NASH (non-alcoholic related steatohepatitis), appropriate diet, weight loss, diabetes control, and cholesterol/ triglyceride control are important both for treatment, and to prevent progression of the disease from NAFLD to NASH, and from NASH to cirrhosis.

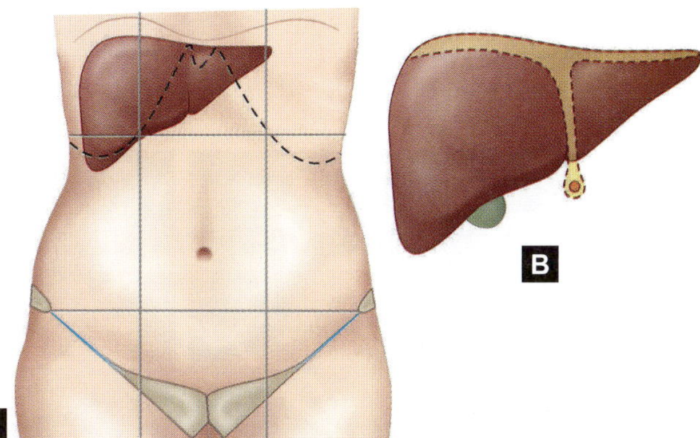

A and B: Anatomical location of liver and its lobes

79. Cirrhosis may be seen secondary to:
a. Hepatocellular carcinoma
b. Pancreatitis
c. Bile duct obstruction d. Gallbladder calculi

Primary sclerosing cholangitis is one important cause of cirrhosis. Diagnosis of PSC is best established with contrast cholangiography showing diffuse, multifocal strictures and focal dilatation of bile ducts, leading to a beaded appearance.

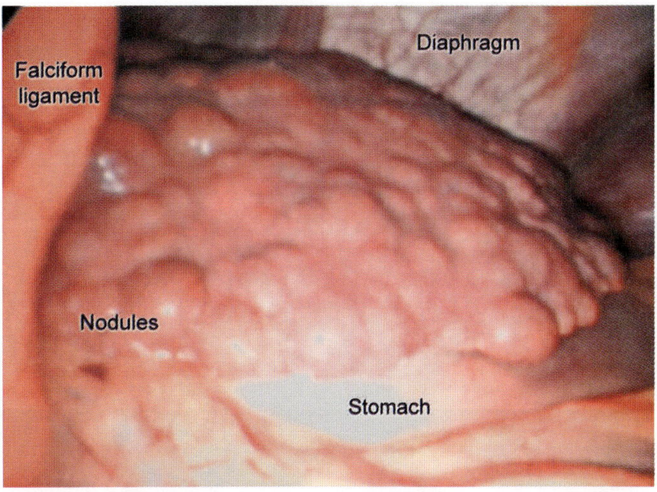

Laparoscopic view of cirrhosis with nodules on the surface

80. A patient is having 2 months old 2 × 2 cm cyst in pancreatic tail. Preferred management for such a case:
a. Observation b. Percutaneous aspiration
c. External drainage d. Cystogastrotomy

Indications for surgery/intervention
❑ Size more than 6 cm
❑ Formed pseudocyst
❑ Infected pseudocyst
❑ Cyst persisting after 6 weeks/progressive cyst
❑ Multiple cysts/cyst due to trauma
❑ Communicating cysts/cyst with severe pain
❑ Thick-walled pseudocyst

Ans. 77. **b.** Nucleotide scan 78. **d.** Fatty liver 79. **c.** Bile duct obstruction 80. **a.** Observation

81. Commonest pancreatic tumor is:

a. Non-islet cell tumor
b. Insulinoma
c. Cystadenoma
d. Ductal adenocarcinoma

Insulinomas are the commonest endocrine pancreatic tumour (60%) arising from B/ beta cells of pancreas.

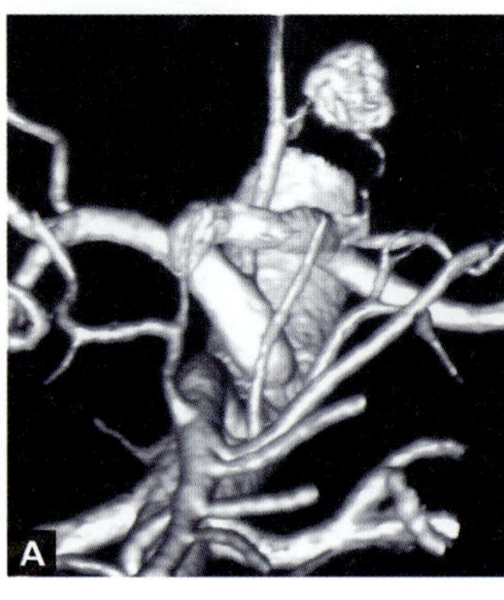
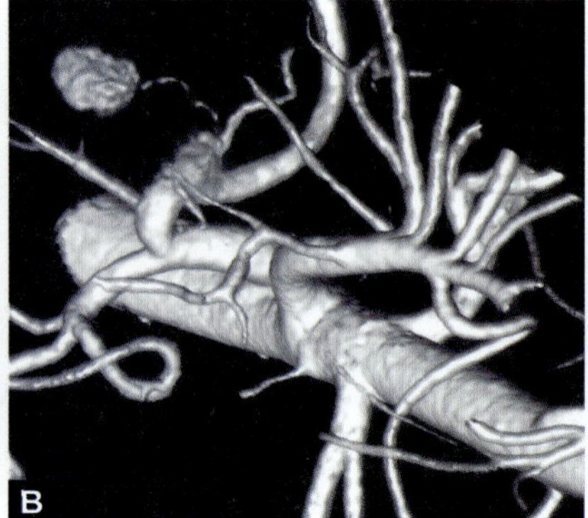
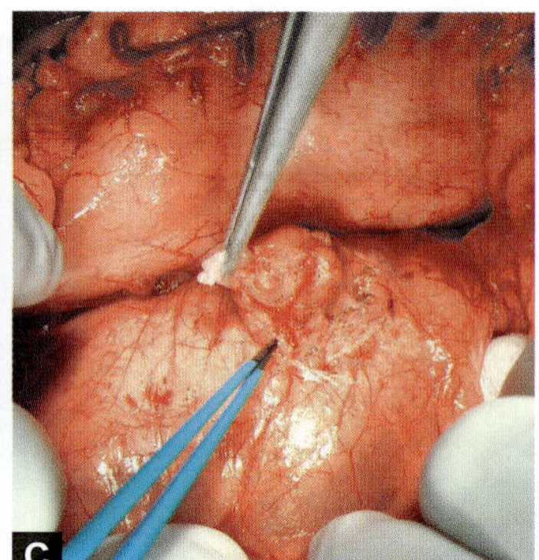

Insulinoma imaging picture and on table look (*Courtesy:* Dr Arunkumar, MCh).

82. Most important sign in acute pancreatitis:

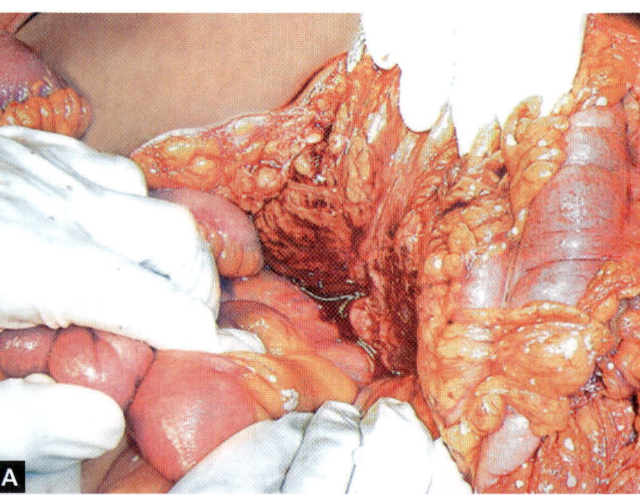
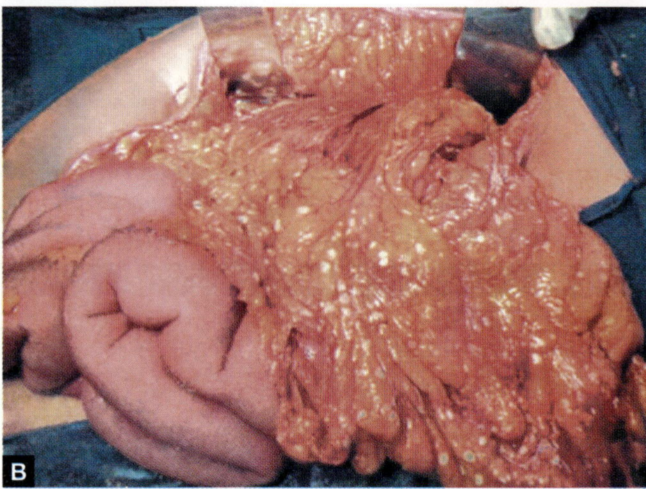

A and B: Features of acute pancreatitis with necrosis in the omentum and over pancreas; with hemorrhage.

a. Fever
b. Vomiting
c. Hyperesthesia in lower abdomen
d. Pain in upper abdomen

In acute pancreatitis, there is sudden onset of upper abdominal pain which is referred to back. Pain is severe, agonizing and refractory. Pain may be relieved or reduced by leaning forward.

83. MC nodule seen in liver:

a. Cholangioadenoma
b. Hemangioma
c. Hamartoma
d. Single adenoma

Hemangiomas are the commonest benign tumor of the liver.

Benign tumors of the liver
❑ It is two times common than malignant liver tumor
❑ It is seen in 20% of population
❑ Hemangioma is the most common benign tumor
❑ CT and MRI are the essential investigations
❑ MRI shows 95% accuracy
❑ Diagnostic accuracy of liver biopsy is low—40%
❑ Hepatic adenoma is potentially malignant
❑ FNH and hemangiomas are not premalignant
❑ Primary (HCC) tumor or secondaries are differential diagnosis; AFP and CEA are helpful to differentiate

84. Number of lobes in liver as per Couinaud's classification:

a. 3
b. 4
c. 6
d. 8

Ans. 81. **b.** Insulinoma 82. **d.** Pain in upper abdomen 83. **b.** Hemangioma 84. **d.** 8

Liver is divided into functional right and left lobes by a line passing from the left of the gallbladder fossa to the left of IVC—Cantlie's line creating Couniaud's segments. There are eight segments.

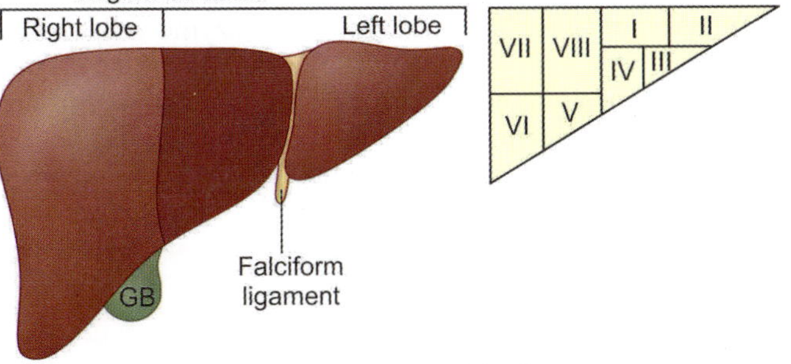

Segmental anatomy of the liver

85. NOT a complication of pseudopancreatic cyst:

a. Malignancy
b. Rupture
c. Hemorrhage into cyst
d. Infection

Complications of pseudocyst
❑ Rupture—3%—into bowel or peritoneum
❑ Infection, commonest—20%
❑ Bleeding from the splenic vessels—7%
❑ Cholangitis
❑ Duodenal obstruction
❑ Portal/splenic vein thrombosis and segmental portal hypertension
❑ Cholestasis due to CBD block

86. All of the following are associated with the gallstones EXCEPT:

a. Acute pancreatitis
b. Acute cholecystitis
c. Acute appendicitis
d. Acute cholangitis

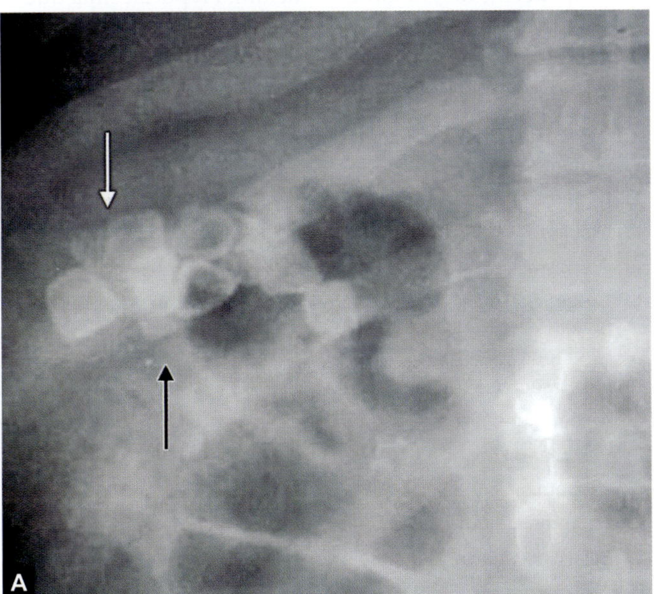

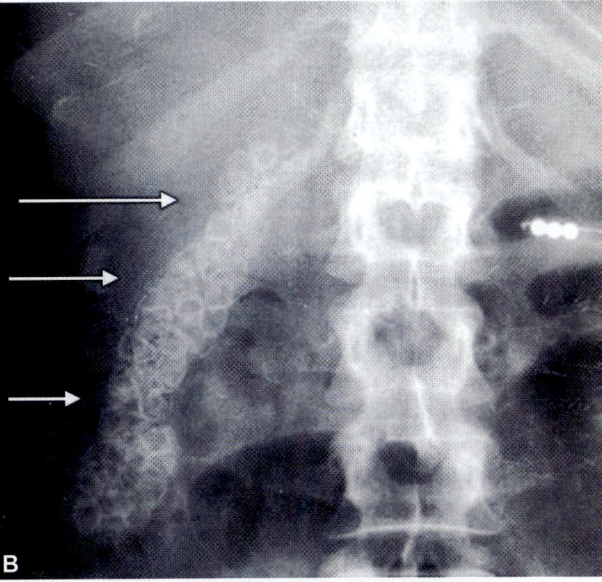

Multiple gallstones in a plain X-ray. Only 10% gallstones are radio-opaque. Often they are faceted because of compactness and equal pressure exerted by each stone. Center of the gallstone is often found radiolucent and is called as *Mercedes Benz sign/Seagull sign*

Effects of gallstones

In the gallbladder	In the CBD	In the intestine
❑ Biliary colic with periodicity ❑ Acute cholecystitis ❑ Chronic cholecystitis ❑ Empyema gall bladder ❑ Perforation causing biliary peritonitis or pericholecystitic abscess ❑ Mucocele of gall bladder ❑ Limely gallbladder ❑ Carcinoma gall- bladder	❑ Secondary CBD stones ❑ Cholangitis ❑ Pancreatitis ❑ Mirizzi syndrome	❑ Cholecystoduodenal fistula causing gallstone ileus and so intestinal obstruction

87. Investigation of choice for acute cholecystitis:

a. Plain radiography
b. USG
c. CT scan
d. Barium studies

Ultrasound abdomen is very useful in acute cholecystitis, reveals presence or absence of gallstones; and thickening of gallbladder wall.

Ans. 85. **a.** Malignancy 86. **c.** Acute appendicitis 87. **b.** USG

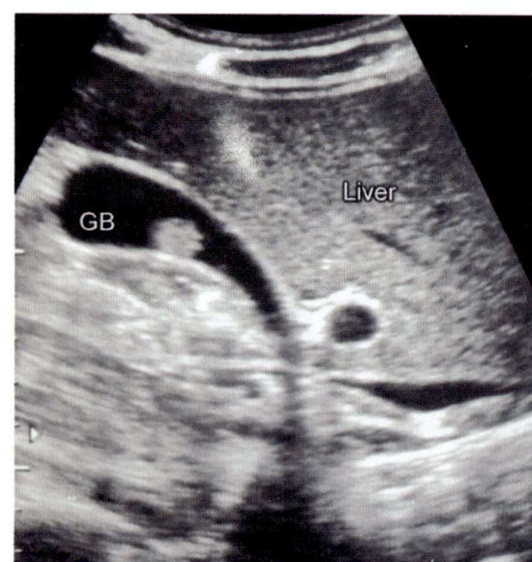

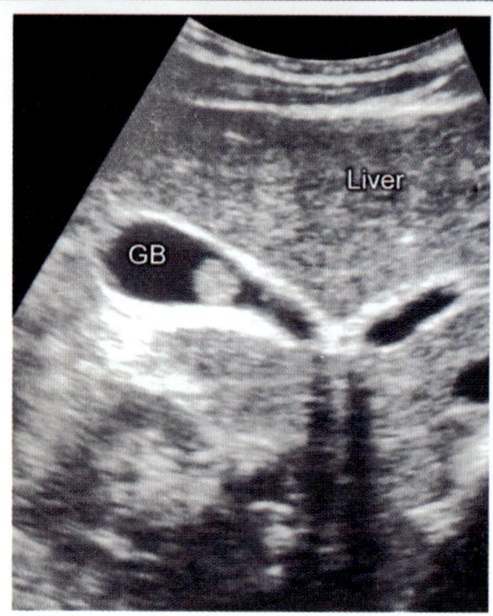

Ultrasound gallbladder showing echogenic lesion. US should be done with change of position to find out movement of the lesion with posterior acoustic shadow to say it as gallstone. Otherwise it will be gallbladder polyp or sludge ball

88. Most common cause of hemobilia is:

a. Cholangitis
b. Gallstone
c. Liver abscess
d. Trauma

Causes of hemobilia

- Accidental trauma, iatrogenic trauma (50%). In accidents hemobilia is more commonly caused by blunt trauma than by penetrating one.
- Percutaneous diagnostic and therapeutic procedures.
- Vascular disease of the hepatic system – 10%
- Malignant liver diseases > common (5%) than benign.

Triad of Sandblom in hemobilia
❑ Jaundice—60%
❑ Pain—70%
❑ Upper GI bleed with melaena (90%), hematemesis (60%)

89. Grey Turner's sign in seen in:

a. Acute appendicitis   b. Acute pancreatitis
c. Acute cholecystitis   d. Acute hepatitis

In severe cases of acute pancreatitis, extensive necrosis with hemorrhage occurs causing acute hemorrhagic necrotizing pancreatitis (Fulminant pancreatitis), which has got a high mortality. Here enzyme seep across the retroperitoneum causing hemorrhagic spots and ecchymosis in the flanks (Grey Turner's sign) or through falciform ligament causing discoloration around the umbilicus (Cullen's sign), umbilical black eye or below the inguinal ligament (Fox sign).

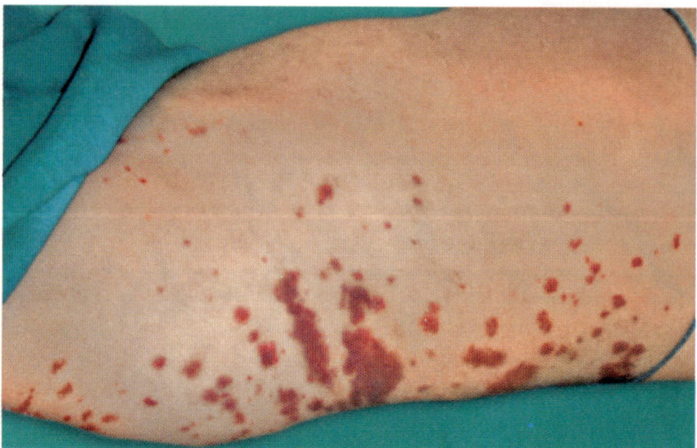

Grey-Turner's sign in a patient with acute pancreatitis

90. Acute pancreatitis results in all of the following EXCEPT:

a. Hypercalcemia   b. Increased amylase level
c. Subcutaneous fat necrosis
d. Hyperlipidemia

One of complication of acute pancreatitis is hypocalcemia. Hypocalcemia is either due to decreased albumin level or specific loss of ionized calcium. Hypocalcemia due to reduced ionized calcium carries poor prognosis.

Other causes
❑ Trauma
❑ After biliary, gastric, splenic surgery, ERCP
❑ Hyperparathyroidism
❑ Hypercalcemia, hyperlipidemia
❑ Diabetes
❑ Porphyria
❑ Drugs: Steroids(?), INH, diuretics (thiazides), septran, azathioprine, 5-amino salicylic acid, estrogens, tetracycline, valproic acid, petamidine – 5%
❑ Viral infections (mumps, coxsackie)
❑ Autoimmune diseases
❑ Vascular diseases
❑ Idiopathic
❑ Scorpion venom—Common in Trinidad
❑ Biliary ascariasis, Clonorchis sinensis

Contd...

Ans. 88. **d.** Trauma   89. **b.** Acute pancreatitis   90. **a.** Hypercalcemia

Contd...

Other causes
❑ Mycoplasma pneumoniae
❑ Infectious mononucleosis
❑ Pancreatic divisum

91. Acute pancreatitis is associated with:

a. Elevated serum amylase b. Alcohol
c. Gallbladder stones d. All of the above

Serum amylase levels is very high (>1000 Somogyi units) or shows rising titer in acute pancreatitis.

Major causes
❑ Biliary tract disease 50%—stones—common cause
❑ Alcoholism 25%

92. Trauma to spleen is best diagnosed by:

a. X-ray abdomen
b. USG
c. CT scan
d. Diagnostic peritoneal lavage

CT scan, in cases of splenic injury, will show type of splenic injury and its class.

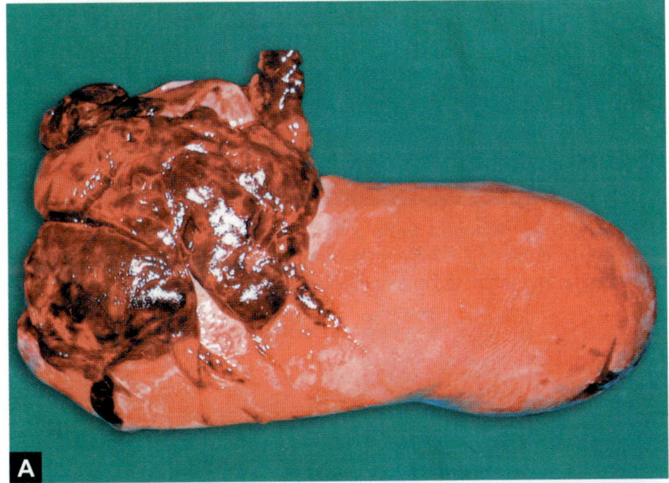

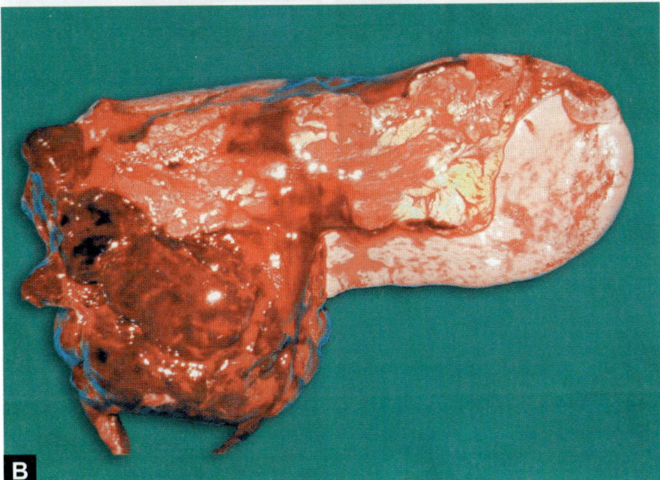

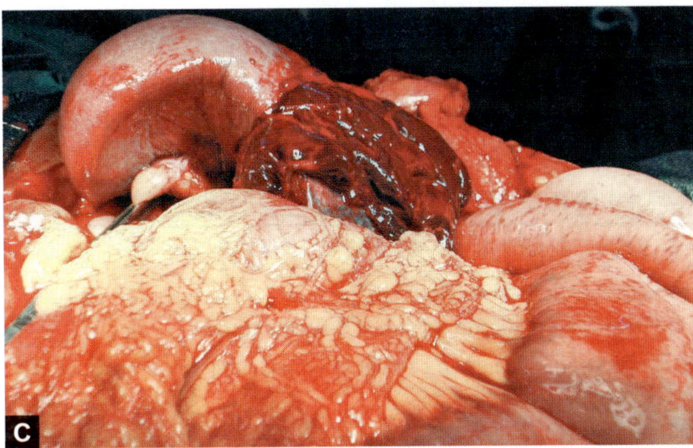

A to C: Splenic injury with splenic hematoma

93. Site of obstruction in portal system, in a patient with cirrhosis-liver:

a. Sinusoids
b. Extrahepatic portal vein
c. Post-sinusoidal
d. Hepatic vein

Increased resistance in portal hypertension

Presinusoidal	Sinusoidal	Postsinusoidal
Extrahepatic: portal/ splenic vein thrombosis Intrahepatic: schistosmiasis, sarcoidosis	Cirrhosis, hemochromatosis, Wilson's disease, congenital hepatic fibrosis	Budd-Chiari syndrome, congestive heart failure, veno-occlusive disease

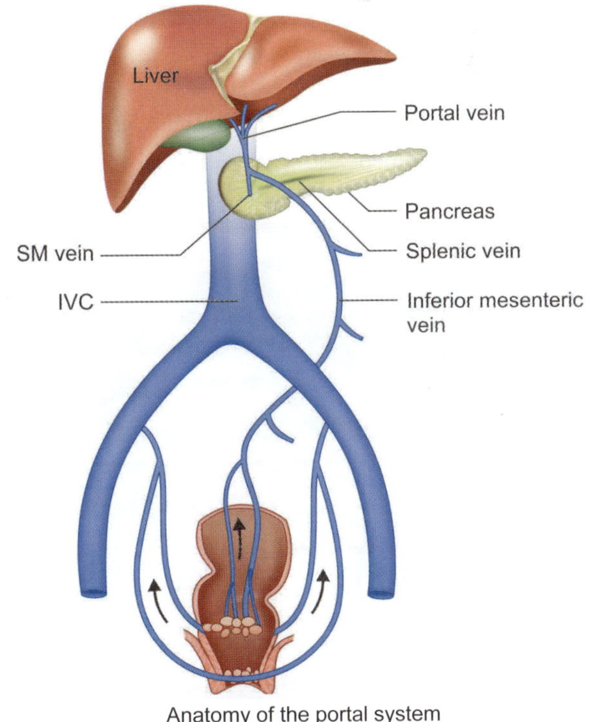

Anatomy of the portal system

Ans. 91. d. All of the above 92. c. CT scan 93. a. Sinusoids

94. NOT a cause of tender hepatomegaly:

a. Liver abscess b. Right heart failure
c. Typhoid fever d. Viral hepatitis

Typhoid presents initially with fever, chills, abdominal pain.

Typhoid
❑ *S typhi, S paratyphi* A, B and C
❑ Gram-negative flagellated bacilli
❑ Feco-oral route is commonest mode of spread
❑ Asymptomatic human carriers are most important reservoirs (*Typhoid Mary*)
❑ Peyer's patches, mesenteric lymph nodes, gallbladder, spleen, liver and bone marrow are commonly involved.

95. Splenectomy can lead to:

a. Leucopenia
b. DIC
c. Thrombocytopenia
d. Thrombocytopenia and leucopenia

Complications of splenectomy
❑ Hemorrhage and shock
❑ Hematemesis
❑ Pancreatitis
❑ Pancreatic fistula
❑ Gastric dilatation
❑ Left sided pleural effusion
❑ Left sided colonic injury
❑ Severe sepsis
❑ Changes in cellular component of blood
❑ DIC

96. Investigation of choice for acute pancreatitis:

a. X-ray abdomen b. CT scan
c. USG d. ERCP

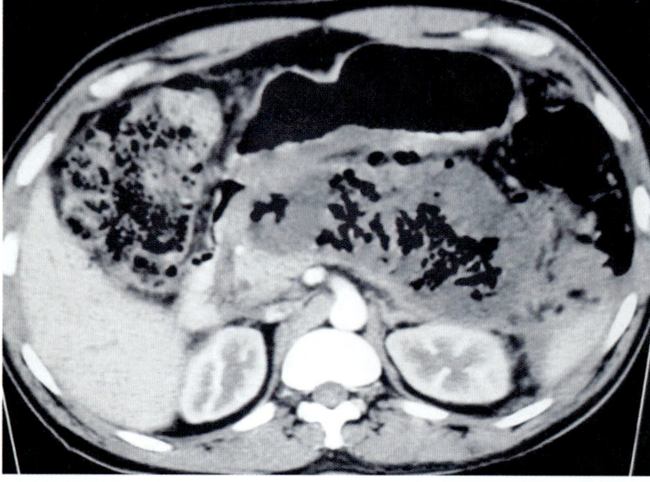

CT picture showing features of acute pancreatitis.

Spiral CT scan in acute pancreatitis—gold standard. It is done after 72 hours. To look for edema, altered fat and fascial planes, fluid collections, necrosis (non-enhancement area >30% or 3 cm), bowel distension, mesenteric edema and hemorrhage.

97. Charcoat triad is seen in:

a. Acute pancreatitis
b. Acute appendicitis
c. Acute hepatitis
d. Cholangitis

Effects of stones in CBD due to impaction

- Causes obstruction: Resulting in jaundice and pain
- Stasis: Resulting in infection, bacteremia and fever.

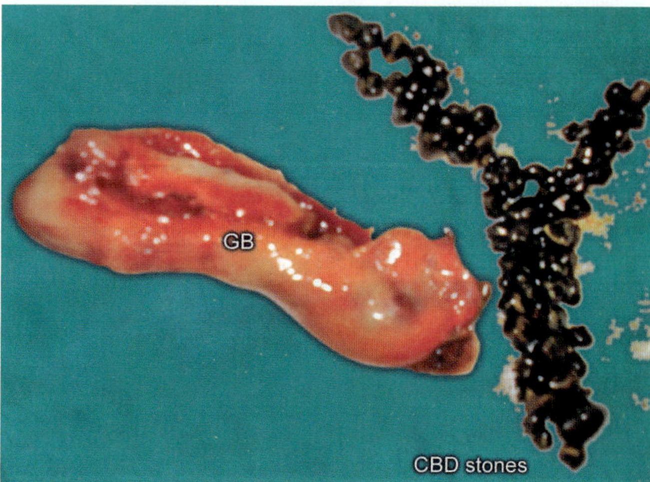

Multiple stones removed from common bile duct and hepatic ducts. They cause cholangitis. After stone removal patient needs choledochoduodenostomy/sphincteroplasty/choledochojejunostomy

98. Investigation for assessing injuries of biliary system:

a. USG
b. CT scan
c. HIDA scan
d. All of the above

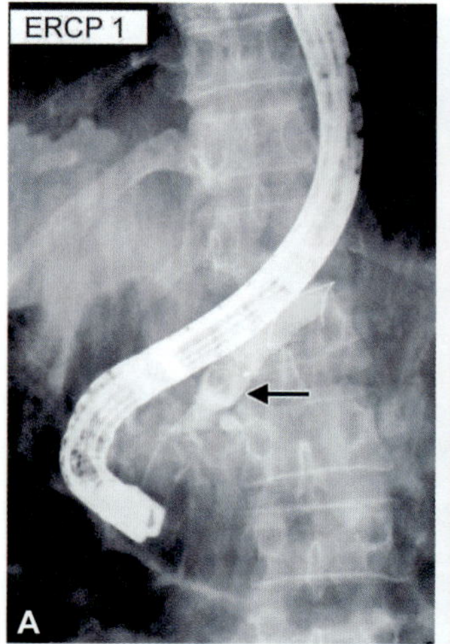

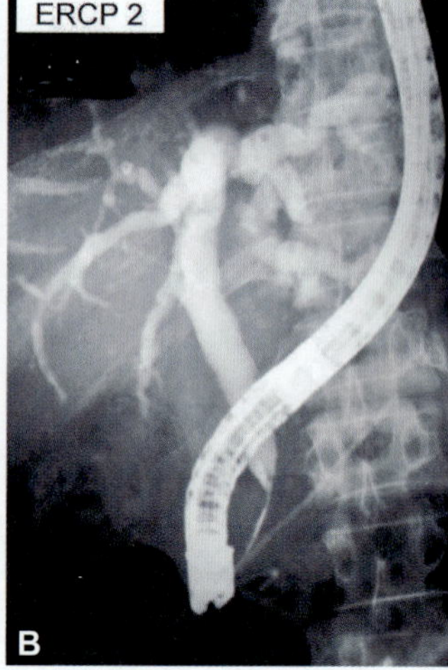

Ans. 94. c. Typhoid fever 95. b. DIC 96. b. CT scan 97. d. Cholangitis 98. d. All of the above

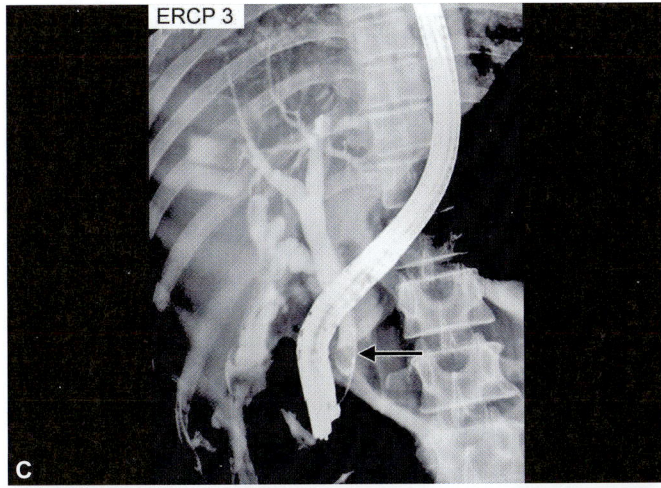

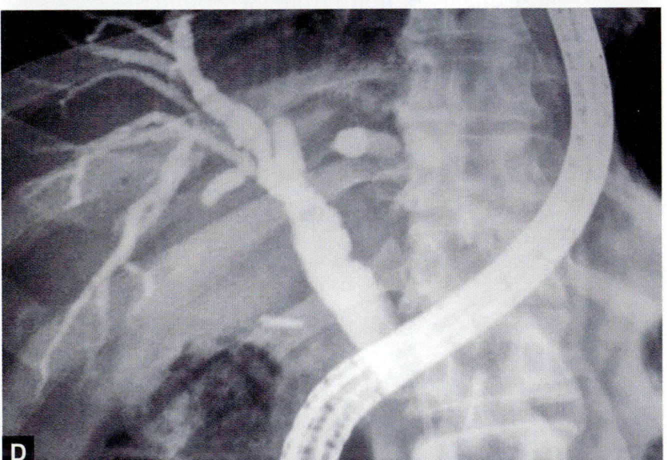

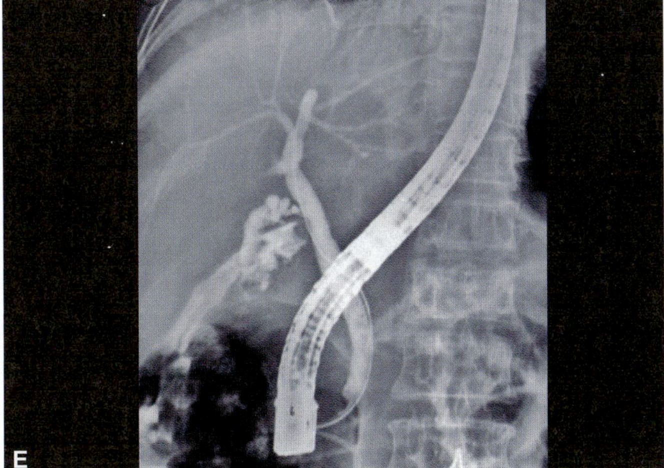

A to E: ERCP being done. Note the gastroduodenoscope with injection of dye. (A) Shows filling defect in the CBD. (B) Shows dilatation of biliary radicles. (C) Shows radiolucent stone (smooth filling defect) in distal CBD which can be removed through ERCP. Antibiotics should be given to prevent cholangitis.

Investigations in bile duct injuries

- LFT, coagulation profile
- USG abdomen
- Hepatobiliary scintigraphy
- CT arteriography is useful to identify associated hepatic artery or portal vein injury which is 20% in association with CBD injury
- PTC is the investigation of choice to identify site, nature, extent of stricture.
- ERCP is useful if injury is only partial where stenting cal also be done.

99. Best way to diagnose gallbladder stones:

a. USG b. Oral cholecystography
c. Percutaneous transhepatic cholangiography
d. Intravenous cholangiogram

On USG abdomen, gallstones are seen with posterior acoustic shadowing.

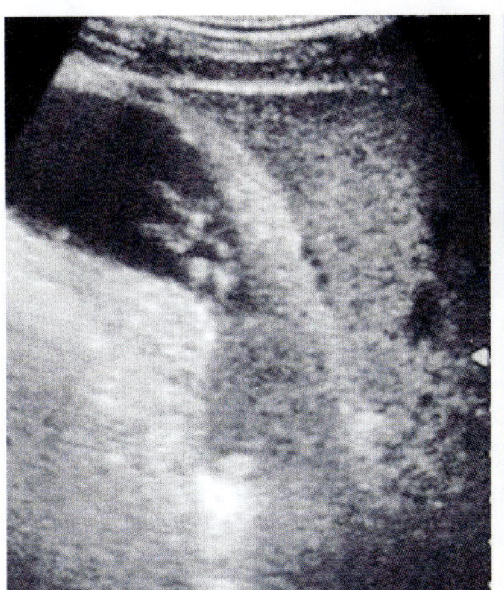

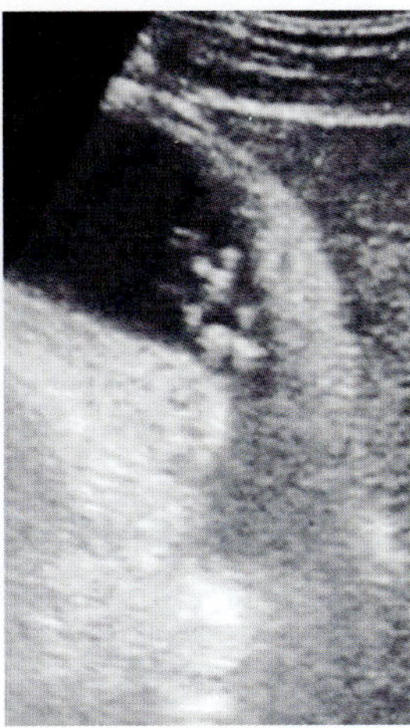

Ultrasound picture of visualisation of multiple gallstones.

100. Chronic and recurrent pancreatitis may be a feature of:

a. Tyrosinemia b. Methl-malonic acidemia
c. Maple syrup urine disease
d. Homocystinuria

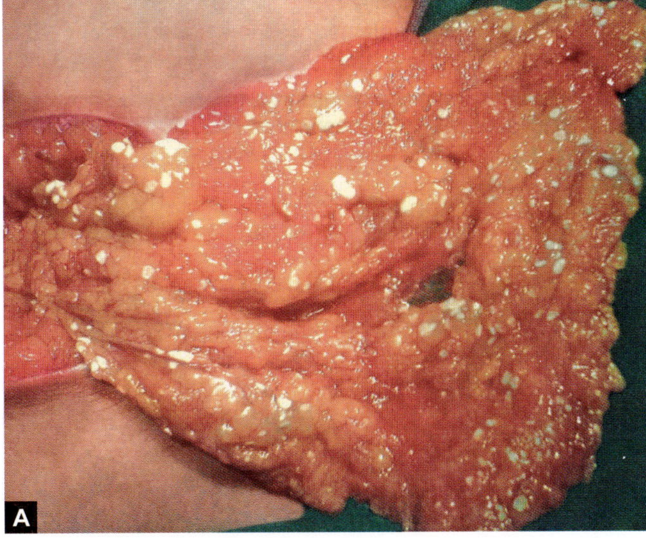

Ans. 99. **a.** USG 100. **d.** Homocystinuria

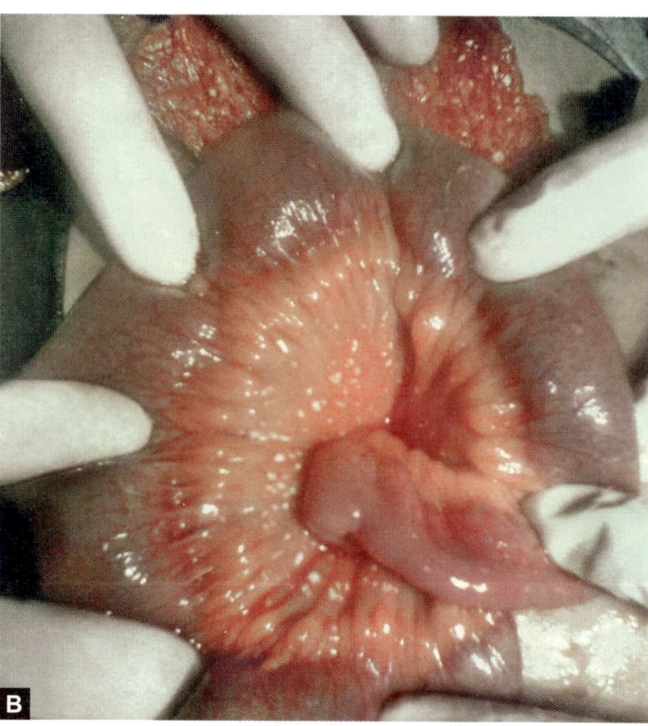

A and B: On table photos of acute pancreatitis. Note the typical saponification in the omentum and mesentery

Chronic relapsing pancreatitis in childhood is a rare entity. Etiologies usually considered include hereditary pancreatitis, hyperlipidemia, cystic fibrosis, hypercalcemia, congenital anomalies of the pancreatic duct as well as idiopathic chronic pancreatitis. An unusual and uncommon cause is homocystinuria.

101. MC site of cholangiocarcinoma:

a. Multifocal
b. Intrahepatic
c. Hilum
d. Distal biliary

Classification of cholangiocarcinoma: Intrahepatic -10%, perihilar – 65% and distal – 25%.

Classification of perihilar cholangiocarcinoma (Bismuth)
❑ Type I : Below the confluence of RHD and LHD
❑ Type II : Reaching the confluence of RHD and LHD
❑ Type III : Involving CHD and RHD/LHD
❑ Type IV : Involving confluence and both RHD and LHD or multicentric tumour

102. Charcot's triad is defined by all of the following EXCEPT:

a. Fever
b. Gallstones
c. Jaundice
d. Pain

Charcot's triad of ascending cholangitis
❑ Intermittent pain (may be colicky)
❑ Intermittent fever
❑ Intermittent jaundice

103. Most pathognomonic sign of impending burst abdomen:

a. Fever b. Shock
c. Pain d. Serosanguinous discharge

Clinical features of burst abdomen/abdominal dehiscence/ acute wound failure

- Sudden feeling of giving way from the wound—on 5th to 8th postoperative day often precipitated by bouts of severe cough
- Pinkish serosanguineous discharge (salmon colored large quality of fluid) from the wound.
- Often the coils of intestine are forced out of the wound.

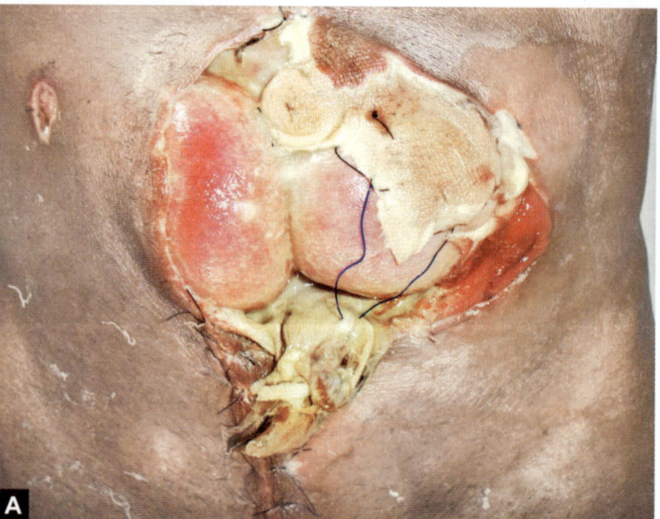

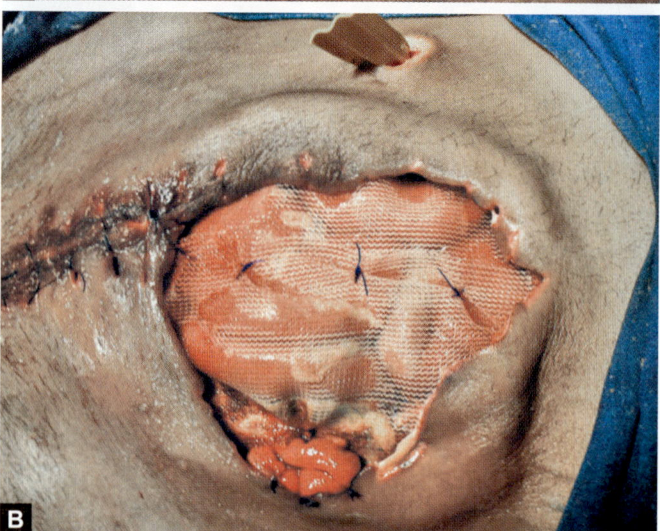

A and B: Burst abdomen wound exposing intestines outside. It is covered with a mesh later

Ans. **101. c.** Hilum **102. b.** Gallstones **103. d.** Serosanguinous...

104. Investigation, which can itself lead to acute pancreatitis:

a. USG b. CT scan
c. ERCP d. MRI scan

Complications of ERCP

- Pancreatitis
- Duodenal injury, perforation
- Cholangitis
- Bleeding from pancreaticoduodenal artery
- Sphincter stenosis

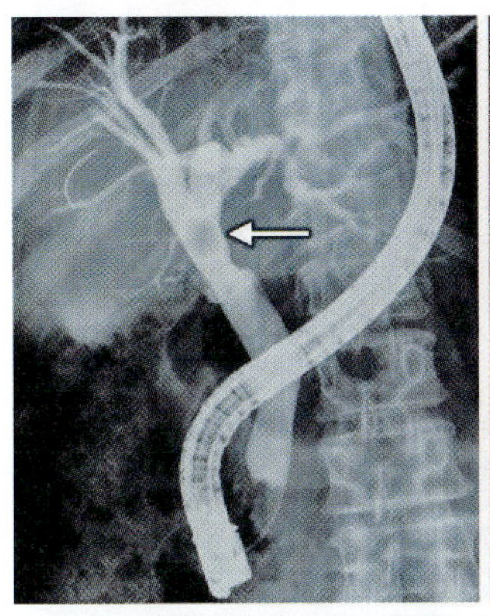
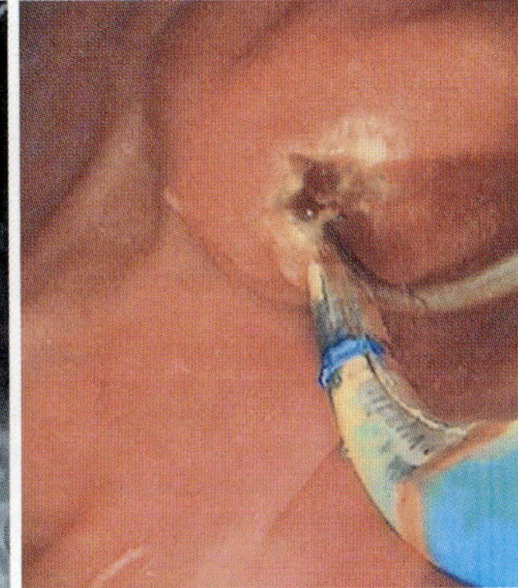

ERCP showing CBD stones. Endoscopic view of stenting is also seen

105. Indications of splenectomy are all EXCEPT:

a. Hereditary spherocytosis
b. Trauma
c. Polycythemia
d. Idiopathic thrombocytopenic purpura

Management of polycythemia

- Emergency treatment is by venesection
- Cytostatics (busulfan, hydroxyurea) are sometimes used if vensection is ineffective or contraindicated

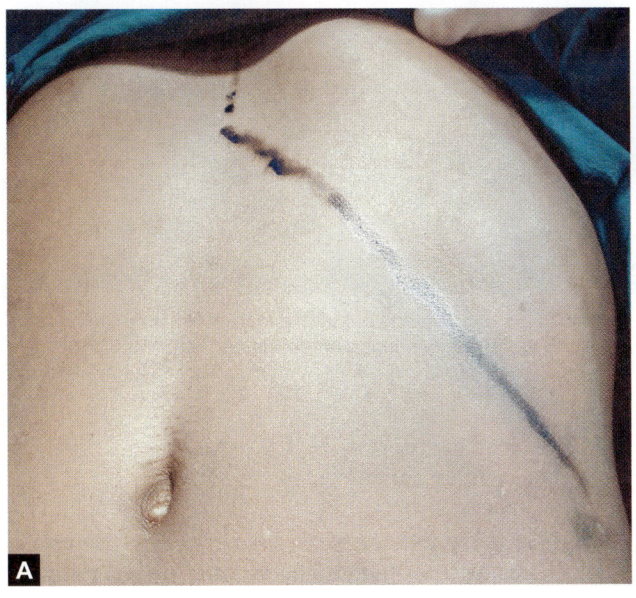

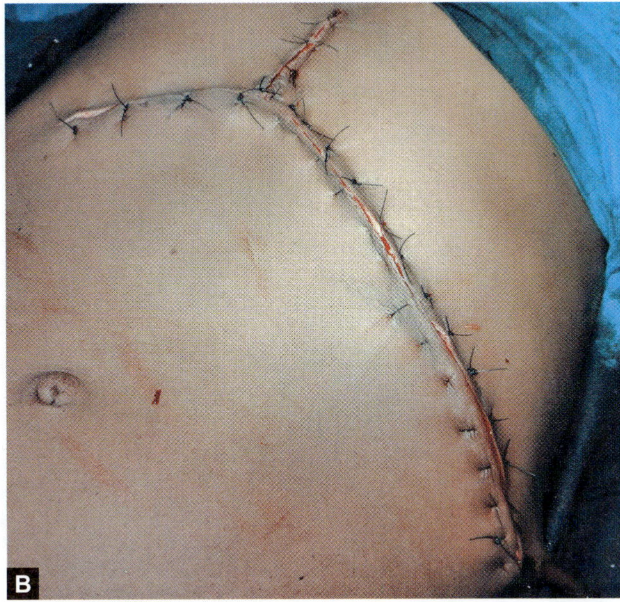

A and B: Incision for open splenectomy – left subcostal. Often in a massive spleen or adherent spleen incision need to be extended to opposite side and towards xiphisternum

106. Right hepatic duct does NOT drain:

a. Segment I b. Segment III
c. Segment V d. Segment VI

Segment III is a part of left lobe, drained by left hepatic duct.

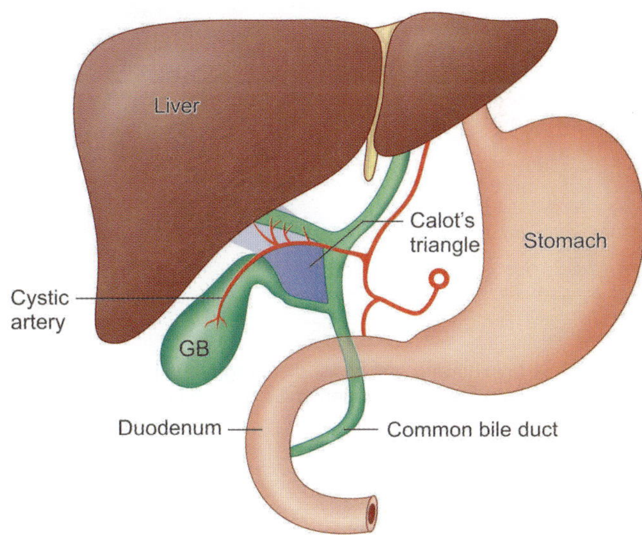

Anatomy of gallbladder

107. All of the following regarding diagnosis of acute peritonitis are correct EXCEPT:

a. Raised WBC count in peritoneal aspirate
b. Moderately raised amylase levels are diagnostic of peritonitis
c. CT scan may aid in diagnosis
d. Upright films shows free air under the diaphragm

Ans. **104. c.** ERCP **105. c.** Polycythemia **106. b.** Segment III **107. b.** Moderately raised...

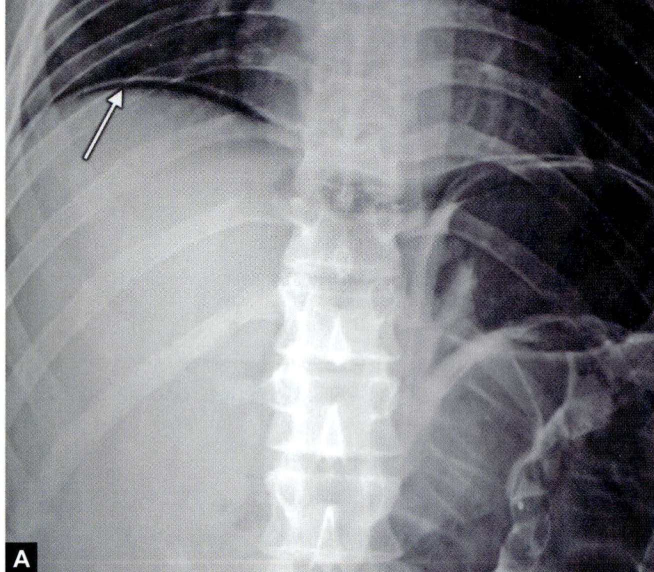

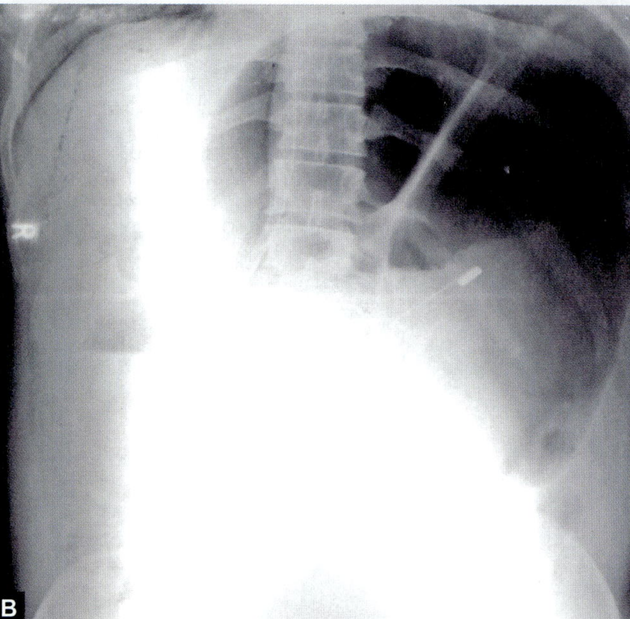

A and B: X-ray showing gas under diaphragm due to perforation. Ground glass appearance of peritonitis is seen in another X-ray

Serum amylase is raised in
- Salivary gland disease
- Acute pancreatitis
- Mesenteric ischemia
- Rupture of aortic aneurysm
- Intestinal obstruction
- Ectopic gestation
- Salpingitis
- Perforated duodenal ulcer (peritonitis)

108. Most sensitive and specific for acute pancreatitis amongst the following is:

a. S. amylase b. S. Alanine transaminase
c. S. lipase d. C-reactive protein

For diagnosing acute pancreatitis, serum lipase is more specific than amylase. Serum lipase level after rise, persists for longer period than amylase. Pancreas is the only source unlike amylase, hence more specific.

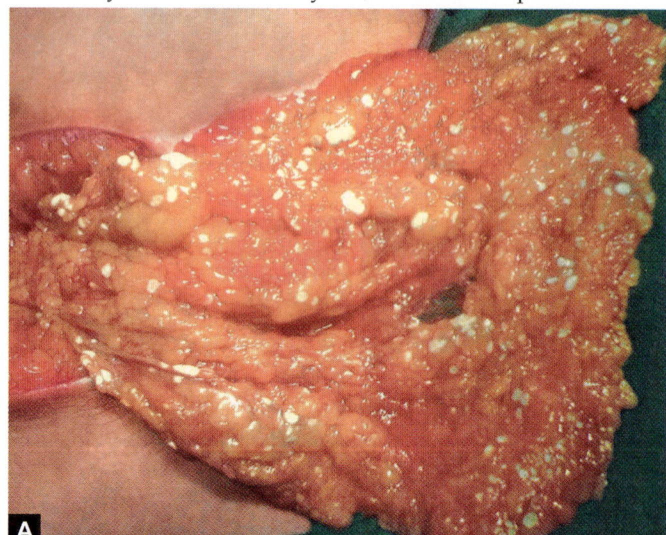

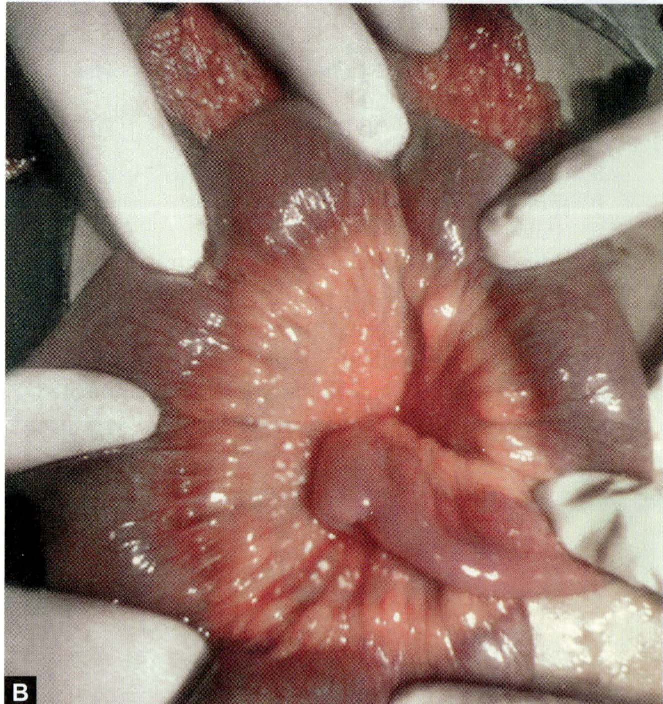

A and B: On table photos of acute pancreatitis. Note the typical saponification in the omentum and mesentery

109. Splenectomy is useful in:

a. Hemophilia
b. Polycythemia
c. Hereditary spherocytosis
d. Thalassemia

In hereditary spherocytosis, splenectomy prevents early RBC destruction thereby controlling anemia, jaundice

Ans. **108.** **c.** S. lipase **109.** **c.** Hereditary...

and also prevents further formation of leg ulcers. Splenectomy for HS is not done before the age of 6 years.

Indications for splenectomy		
Benefit is maximum/ very good	*Benefit is equivocal*	*Benefit may be there/low*
❑ Splenic injury ❑ Hereditary spherocytosis ❑ ITP ❑ Splenic cysts ❑ Splenic tumors ❑ Hypersplenism ❑ Segmental left sided portal hypertension	❑ AIHA (autoimmune hemolytic anemia) ❑ Tropical splenomegaly ❑ Felty's syndrome	❑ Thalassemia ❑ CML ❑ Gaucher's disease ❑ Hodgkin's lymphoma for staging laparotomy ❑ Sickle cell anemia

110. NOT a part of Charcot's triad:

a. Intermittent jaundice
b. Intermittent pain
c. Intermittent vomiting
d. Intermittent fever

Charcot's triad (ascending cholangitis)

- Intermittent fever
- Intermittent pain
- Intermittent jaundice

111. Reynold's pentad (fever, jaundice, right upper quadrant pain, septic shock and mental status changes) is observed in:

a. Pancreatitis
b. Cholecystitis
c. Hepatitis
d. Cholangitis

Reynold's pentad is seen in acute obstructive cholangitis (suppurative cholangitis). Here biliary tree contains pus.

Sometimes obstruction persists causing
❑ Persistent pain
❑ Persistent fever
❑ Persistent jaundice
❑ Shock (toxicity) and
❑ Altered mental status

112. MC retroperitoneal sarcoma:

a. Neural sheath sarcoma
b. Fibrosarcoma
c. Leiomyosarcoma
d. Liposarcoma

Malignant retroperitoneal tumor may be mesodermal (75%), neuroectodermal (24%) or embryonic remnant (1%) inorigin. Rarely it can be urologic or metastatic also. Sarcoma is the MC malignancy; in adult – liposarcoma is the MC retroperitoneal sarcoma (50%); leiomyosarcoma is 30%; malignanat nerve sheath tumor (5%); fibrosarcoma (5%); malignant fibrous histiocytoma (MFH – 10%) can also occur.

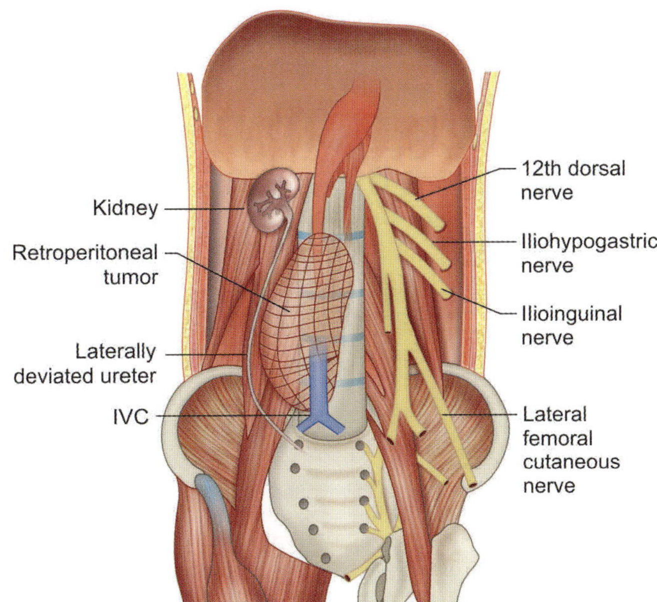

Retroperitoneal tumor can attain very large size often. It causes deviation of ureter laterally often may invade the ureter (In retroperitoneal fibrosis ureter is deviated medially). **It may invade or encase the IVC also causing IVC obstruction with features of bilateral edema feet, dilated lateral abdominal wall vein with upward direction flow of blood**

113. Casonis test is done for:

a. Meningitis
b. Syphilis
c. Hydatid disease
d. Gonorrhea

Casoni's test is done for hydatid cyst of liver. It is an intradermal test with 75% sensitivity.

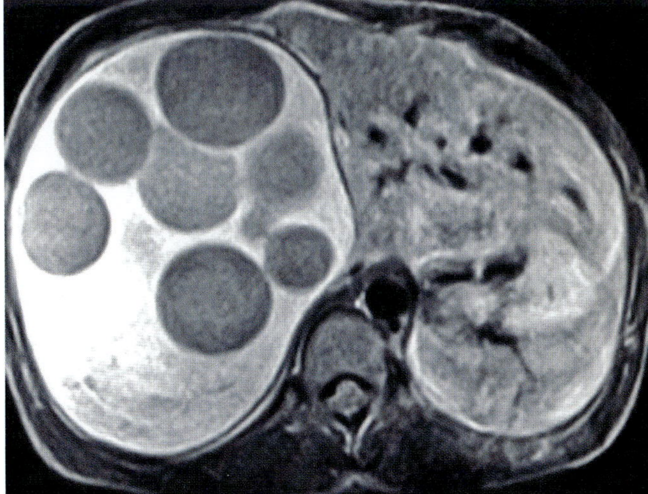

MRI picture of multiple hydatid cyst of liver—MRI is very useful investigation in hydatid cyst of liver

114. Pentad of pain, fever, jaundice, confusion and shock is seen in:

a. Pancreatitis
b. Hepatitis
c. Cholangitis
d. Appendicitis

Reynold's pentad is a feature of acute obstructive cholangitis/suppurative cholangitis.

Ans. 110. c. Intermittent... 111. d. Cholangitis 112. d. Liposarcoma 113. c. Hydatid disease 114. c. Cholangitis

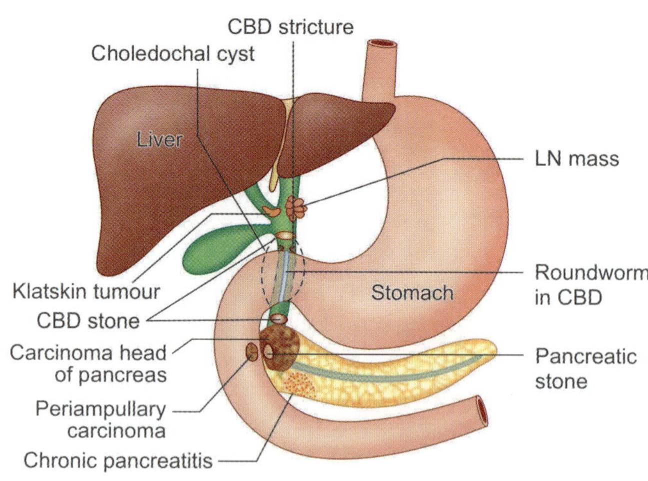

Different causes of obstructive jaundice (surgical jaundice)

115. Most common type of gallstone in India is:

a. Cholesterol b. Pigment
c. Mixed d. Both A and C

Black pigment stones are common in gallbladder. It is usually calcium bilirubinate, calcium phosphate and bicarbonate stone with a matrix. It is common in hemolytic disorders. They are common in Asia and Japan.

Altered GB function
- Stasis
- Poor emptying
- Poor absorption
- Infection

Supersaturated bile
- Female
- Fertile
- Fat
- Forty
- High calorie

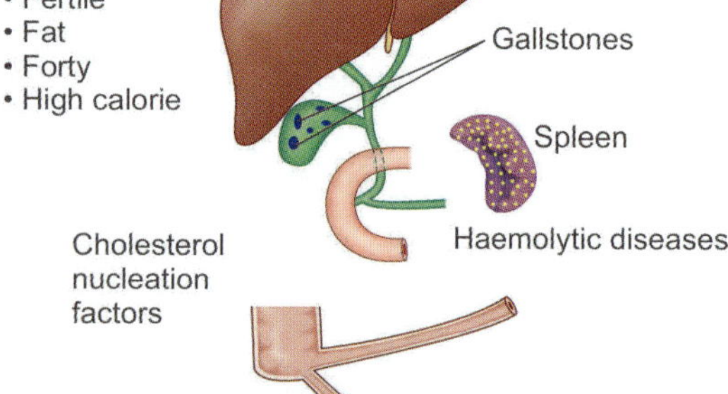

Cholesterol nucleation factors

Altered enterohepatic circulation
- Ileal resection
- Ileal diseases
- Altered bowel transit time
- Altered bowel flora
- Cholestyramine
- Deoxycholate

Diagram showing different causes of gallstone formation

116. Investigation of choice for hydatid disease is:

a. CT scan b. ELISA
c. Biopsy d. USG

CT scan abdomen is more accurate in identifying liver hydatid cyst characteristics, cart wheel like, multivesicular rosette like.

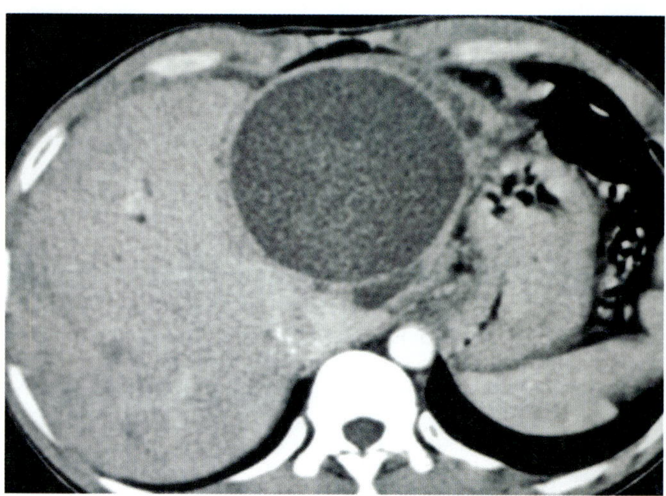

CT scan of hydatid disease of the liver

117. All of the following can cause postsplenectomy infection EXCEPT:

a. H. influenza b. N. meningitides
c. Klebsiella d. Streptococcus

As there is reduced IgM, tuftin, properdin and other antibodies after splenectomy, phagocytosis of encapsulated bacteria is defective. So the postsplenectomized patient is more prone for OPSI (overwhelming postsplenectomy infections) i.e. pneumococcal septicemia (commonest), N. meningitides, H. influenzae, Babesia microti infections.

Prevention of OPSI
❑ Life long prophylaxis using benzathine penicillin 12–24 lac units—controversial in adults
❑ Pneumococcal vaccine given 2–3 weeks prior to splenectomy—70% protection
❑ *H. influenzae* B type vaccine
❑ Meningococcal vaccine is given only to high-risk groups, as its effects are short-term. So it is not routinely given
❑ *Note: Protection by vaccine is not completely guaranteed*

118. Child's criteria is employed for:

a. AIDS b. Multiple myeloma
c. Cirrhosis d. Pancreatitis

Child's grading is used for selecting patients for surgery and predicting prognosis in varices. Surgery is contraindicated in Child C.

Child's grading of the severity of liver disease

Clinical and biochemical measurement	Points scored		
	1	2	3
Bilirubin (mg/dL)	< 2.0	2.0–3.0	> 3.0
Albumin (gm/dL)	> 3.5	3.0–3.5	< 3.0
Ascites	None	Controlled	Uncontrolled

Contd...

Ans. **115. b.** Pigment **116. a.** CT scan **117.** c. Klebsiella **118. c.** Cirrhosis

Contd...

Child's grading of the severity of liver disease			
Mental status	Normal	Disoriented	Coma
Nutrition	Very good	Good	Poor
Total Score	**< 6** *Child's 'A'* disease	**7–9** *Child's 'B'* disease	**10–15** *Child's 'C'* disease
(Pugh's modification)			
Prothrombin time seconds prolonged	Increase up to 3	Between 3–6	> 6

119. Management of infected pancreatic necrosis includes all of the following EXCEPT:

a. Percutaneous drainage
b. Pancreatic necrosectomy
c. Manage conservatively with antibiotics alone
d. Jejunostomy

Infection of the necrotic area (pancreatic abscess) usually occurs within 4 weeks. It is ideally conventionally treated with laparotomy, debridement is done by removing all necrotic tissue with adequate drainage for remaining viable exocrine function. Often repeated laparotomies are done once in 3 days until all necrotic materials are cleared and jejunostomy is done in final approach.

- Shock—Hypovolemic and septic
- Respiratory failure and ARDS—Common in 7 days
- Septicemia—Common after 7 days
- Hypocalcemia
- Disseminated intravascular coagulation (DIC)
- Acute renal failure
- Pancreatic pleural effusion (left sided 20%)
- Pancreatic pseudo aneurysm
- Pancreatic ascites
- Colonic stricture
- Pseudocyst of pancreas
- Chronic pancreatitis
- Splenic vein thrombosis
- Pancreatic abscess

120. Splenectomy is not done in:

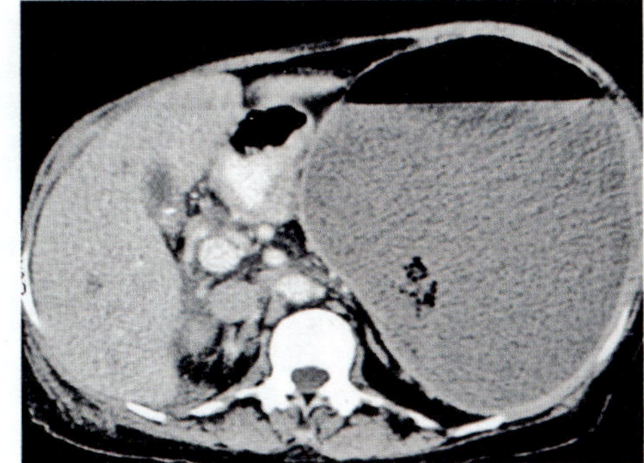

CT scan showing abscess in the spleen

a. Trauma
b. Tubercular abscess
c. Hereditary spherocytosis
d. Splenic abscess

ATT is used in case of TB causing splenic abscess

121. Which is NOT a cause for burst abdomen:

a. Abdominal operation lasting more than two hours
b. Incomplete suture
c. Infection
d. Poor general condition of patient

Factors related to burst abdomen

- Choice of suture materials used
- Method of closure; continuous closure is more likely to disrupt than interrupted sutures
- Upper midline and vertical wounds are more likely to disrupt than transverse
- Surgical wounds of peritonitis, acute abdomen, major surgeries like pancreatic, hepatic, gastric, surgeries for malignancies have a high incidence of disruption
- Severe cough, vomiting and distension in postoperative period
- Poor general condition of the patient—anemia, jaundice, hypoproteinemia, obesity, uremia and diabetes mellitus, old age, steroids, radiation, malignancy, chemotherapy.

122. Non-metabolic cause of abdominal pain:

a. DKA
b. Sickle cell anemia
c. Hyperparathyroidism
d. Porphyria

Sickle cell is a hereditary hemolytic anemia seen commonly in blacks wherein HbA is replaced by HbS (hence not a metabolic condition) leading to formation of crescent shaped red cells which is deformed and more prone for trapping in spleen and destruction. Patient present with anemia, pain abdomen and leg ulcers usually.

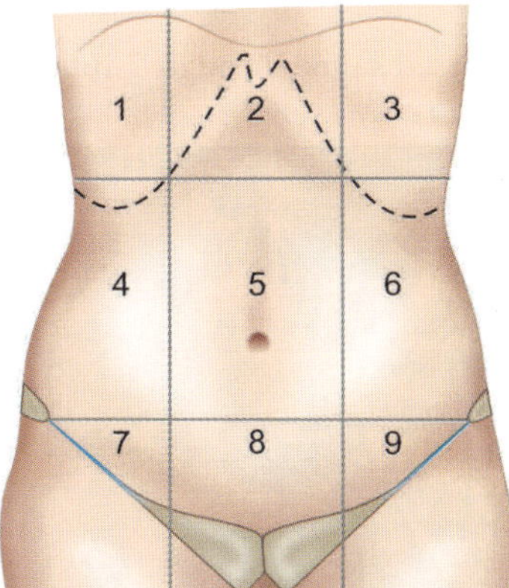

Regions in the abdomen

123. All of the following are features of Zollinger Ellison syndrome EXCEPT:

a. Intractable peptic ulcers
b. Severe diarrhea
c. Beta cell tumors of the pancreas
d. Very high acid output

Gastrinoma arise from non-beta cells (G cells) of the pancreas, which secrete high levels of gastrin.

Ans. **119. c.** Manage conser... **120. b.** Tubercular abscess **121. a.** Abdominal operation... **122. b.** Sickle cell anemia **123. c.** Beta cell tumors of the pancreas

Remember

- Gastrinomas are often associated with MEN syndrome and are multiple
- Sporadic gastrinomas are often solitary and then are malignant
- Gastrinoma often secretes ACTH
- Most common malignant endocrine pancreatic tumor is gastrinoma
- Gastrinoma causes ulcer of unusual nature (refractory/resistant); unusual recurrence (repeated and multiple); unusual number (multiple); unusual sites (2nd/3rd part duodenum/jejunum); unusual age (young and aged)

124. All of the following predict severity of acute pancreatitis EXCEPT:

a. Glasgow score ≥ 3
b. APACHE II score ≥ 9
c. CT severity index ≥ 6
d. C-reactive protein < 100

C-reactive protein (CRP) >210 mg/ L in first 4 days and >120 mg/ L in one week, in acute pancreatitis. This is one of the parameter used to assess the severity.

Ranson's prognostic criteria in gallstone pancreatitis	Ranson's prognostic criteria in non-gallstone pancreatitis	Glasgow-Imrie prognostic criteria	Acute physiology and chronic Health evaluation (APACHE II) score > 8 points predicts 11% to 18% mortality
On admission: ❑ Age > 70 years ❑ TC > 18,000/cu mm ❑ Blood sugar > 220 mg% ❑ LDH > 400 IU/L ❑ AST > 250 IU/100 mL	On admission: ❑ Age > 55 years ❑ TC > 16,000/cu mm ❑ Blood sugar > 200 mg% ❑ LDH > 700 IU/L ❑ AST > 250 IU/100 mL	On admission: ❑ Age > 55 years ❑ TC > 15,000/cu mm ❑ PaO_2 < 60 mm Hg ❑ Blood urea > 16 mmol/L (No response to IV fluids) ❑ Blood sugar > 200 mg% (no H/O diabetes)	❑ Equation includes the following factors: age, rectal temperature, mean arterial pressure, heart rate, PaO_2, arterial pH, serum potassium, serum sodium, serum creatinine, hematocrit, white blood cell count, Glasgow coma scale score.
Within 48 hours:	*Within 48 hours:*	*Within 48 hours:*	
❑ Hematocrit drop > 10% ❑ BUN rise > 2 mg% ❑ Serum calcium < 8 mg% ❑ Base deficit > 5 mEq/L ❑ Fluid sequestration > 4 L	❑ Hematocrit drop > 10% ❑ BUN rise > 5 mg% ❑ PaO_2 < 60 mm Hg ❑ Serum calcium < 8 mg% ❑ Base deficit > 4 mEq/L ❑ Fluid sequestration > 6 L	❑ Serum calcium < 2 mmol/L ❑ Serum albumin < 3.2 gm/dL ❑ LDH > 600 U/L ❑ AST / ALT > 600 U/L	❑ APACHE II modified (1996) ❑ LFT is added in biliary pancreatitis ❑ APACHE – O (Toh 1996) ❑ Obesity is added

125. After cholecystectomy, a small left over stone in the CBD is best treated by:

a. ERCP
b. ESWL
c. Heparinized saline through T-tube
d. Repeat surgery

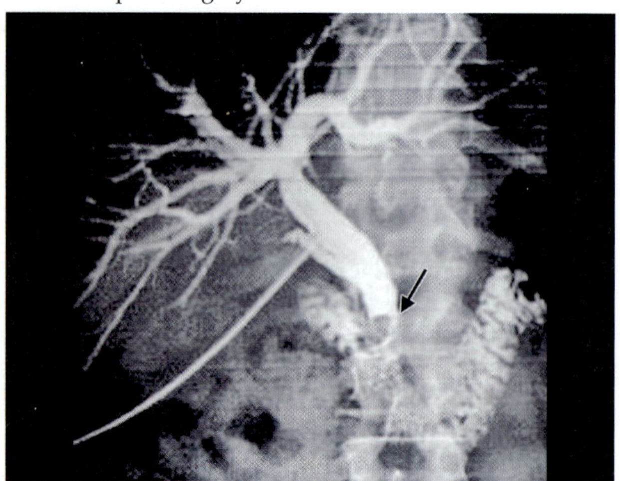

T-tube cholangiogram showing retained stone in the CBD (*Courtesy:* Dr Navin Chandra Shetty, HOD, Department of Radiodiagnosis, KMC, Mangalore)

ERCP is therapeutic for CBD stones, i.e. endocscopic papillotomy (sphincterotomy) and stone extraction through Dormia basket or balloon catheter; or fragmenting the stone and extraction; or removal through baby endoscope.

126. MC type of cancer gallbladder in a patient with gallstones:

a. Adenocarcinoma
b. Squamous carcinoma
c. Adenocarcinoma
d. None

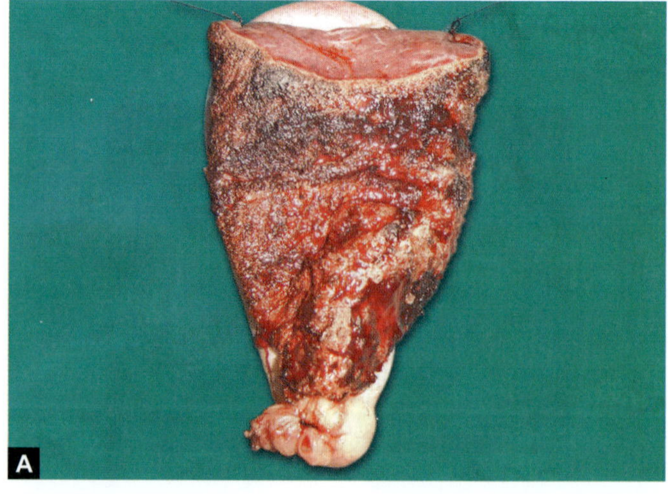

Ans. 124. **d.** C-reactive... 125. **a.** ERCP 126. **a.** Adenocarcinoma

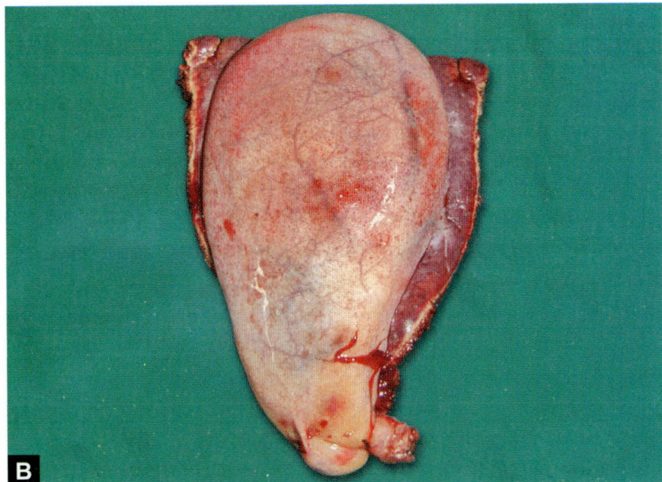

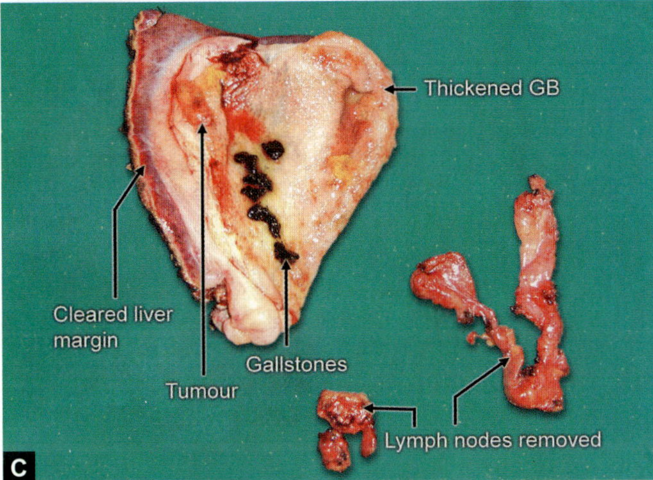

A to C: Specimen of gallbladder after extended cholecystectomy. Note the liver margin cleared of carcinoma, stone in the gallbladder and lymph nodes cleared.

90% of the carcinoma of gallbladder is associted with gallstones. Risk of developing carcinoma in gallstone disease is 7–10 times more than general population. Commonly it is adenocarcinoma (90%).

127. All of the following are true about OPSI (opportunistic postsplenectomy infections) EXCEPT:

a. Develop 1–5 year after splenectomy
b. Max risk is within 1 year of splenectomy
c. Begin with headache, myalgia and fever
d. May present with severe septic shock

OPSI is common in first 2 years after splenectomy. But it can occur any time. Risk persists for lifetime.

Treatment of OPSI
❑ Antibiotics like Cefoperazone, Ceftazidime, Amikacin
❑ Ventilatory support—ICU care
❑ Blood transfusion
❑ Immunoglobulin transfusion
❑ Nutrition (TPN) and maintaining of urine output

128. MC cysts of spleen are:

a. Hydatid cyst
b. Dermatoid cyst
c. Pseudocyst
d. Lymphangioma

Pseudocyst/secondary cysts account for 80% of splenic cysts. They are due to old trauma, malaria, tuberculosis, infectious mononucleosis, old parenchymal hematoma and syphilis.

Note:
❑ Commonest primary splenic neoplasm is hemangioma
❑ *Littoral cell angioma* is rare splenic tumor
❑ Lymphangioma, inflammatory pseudotumors are rare splenic tumors
❑ Hodgkin's lymphoma commonly involves spleen
❑ Secondaries in spleen are rare. Occasionally spread can occur from lungs, stomach, pancreas, breast, melanoma
❑ Primary malignant splenic tumors are exceedingly rare. Angiosarcoma is the most common primary tumor
❑ *Wandering spleen* is due to failure to form suspensory ligaments of spleen so that the spleen is *not* fixed in position. It is due to failure of dorsal mesogastrium to fuse with the posterior abdominal wall. It shows long splenic pedicle. It is prone for torsion and recurrent ischemia. It is common in females. CT scan is diagnostic. If there is no ischemia, *splenopexy* is done; if there is ischemia which is confirmed by absence of perfusion in CT scan, splenectomy is done.

GIT

129. Esophageal carcinoma is best diagnosed by:

a. CT scanning
b. USG chest
c. MRI
d. Endoscopic biopsy

Although an occlusive tumor may be suspected on a barium swallow or barium meal, the diagnosis is best made with an examination using an endoscope. This involves the passing of a flexible tube with a light and camera down the esophagus and examining the wall, and is called an esophagogastroduodenoscopy. Biopsies taken of suspicious lesions are then examined histologically for signs of malignancy.

130. ERCP can lead to:

a. Acute pancreatitis
b. Pseudo-pancreatic cyst
c. Chronic pancreatitis
d. Necrotizing pancreatitis

The major risk of an ERCP is the development of pancreatitis, which can occur in up to 5% of all procedures. This may be self limited and mild, but may require hospitalization, and rarely, may be life-threatening.

131. Achalasia cardia is characterized by all EXCEPT:

a. Bad smell from mouth
b. Regurgitation of food
c. Dysphagia more for liquids
d. Cork screw esophagus on barium meal

Ans. **127. b.** Max risk... **128. c.** Pseudocyst **129. d.** Endoscopic biopsy **130. a.** Acute pancreatitis
131. d. Cork screw esophagus on barium meal

Diffuse esophageal spasm is sometimes referred to as corkscrew esophagus, due to a characteristic appearance of the esophagus as a corkscrew on barium swallow X-rays.

132. Fistula-in-ano presents as:

a. Seropurulent discharge with occasional bleeding
b. Seropurulent discharge without bleeding
c. Painful bleeding with constipation
d. Painless bleeding with constipation

Anal fistulae symptoms

- Pain
- Discharge: Seropurulent; occasional bleeding
- Pruritus ani — itching
- Systemic symptoms if abscess becomes infected

133. Dysphagia, initially, more for liquids is a presenting feature of:

a. Barrett's esophagus
b. Diffuse esophageal spasm
c. Boerhaave syndrome
d. Achalasia cardia

Dysphagia is more for liquids in early stages of Achalasia cardia as solid foodstuff can dilate the Lower Esophageal Sphincter because of their weight.

134. True for anal canal are all EXCEPT:

a. One third above dentate line & two third below it
b. Extraperitoneal
c. Anoderm is painful
d. Keratinization throughout the length

Anal canal

- The anal canal is completely extraperitoneal.
- The length of the anal canal is about 4 cm (range, 3-5 cm).
- Epithelium in different segments:
  - *Upper third:* Columnar/ stratified columnar
  - *Middle third/ pecten:* Stratified squamous; without sebaceous & sweat glands
  - *Lower third:* Just like true skin (stratified squamous with keratinization; with sebaceous & sweat glands)

135. Arterial supply of fundus of stomach:

a. Right gastric artery
b. Short gastric artery
c. Left gastric artery
d. Left gastroduodenal artery

The lesser curvature of the stomach is supplied by the right gastric artery inferiorly, and the left gastric artery superiorly, which also supplies the cardiac region. The greater curvature is supplied by the right gastro-omental artery inferiorly and the left gastro-omental artery superiorly. The fundus of the stomach, and also the upper portion of the greater curvature, is supplied by the short gastric artery which arises from the splenic artery.

136. Anal carcinoma is best managed by:

a. Observation
b. Chemotherapy
c. 5-FU, irradiation followed by abdomino-perineal resection
d. Surgery alone

Current gold-standard therapy is chemotherapy and radiation treatment to reduce the necessity of debilitating surgery. This "combined modality" approach has led to the increased preservation of an intact anal sphincter, and therefore improved quality of life after definitive treatment. Current chemotherapy consists of continuous infusion 5-FU over four days with bolus mitomycin given concurrently with radiation. 5-FU and cisplatin are recommended for metastatic anal cancer.

137. Hour glass deformity of the stomach is seen in:

a. Lipoma
b. Gastric lymphoma
c. Gastric carcinoma
d. Gastric ulcer

One of the complications of gastric ulcer is hour glass contracture. It occurs exclusively in women, is due to cicatricial contracture of lesser curvature ulcer. Here the stomach is divided into two compartments.

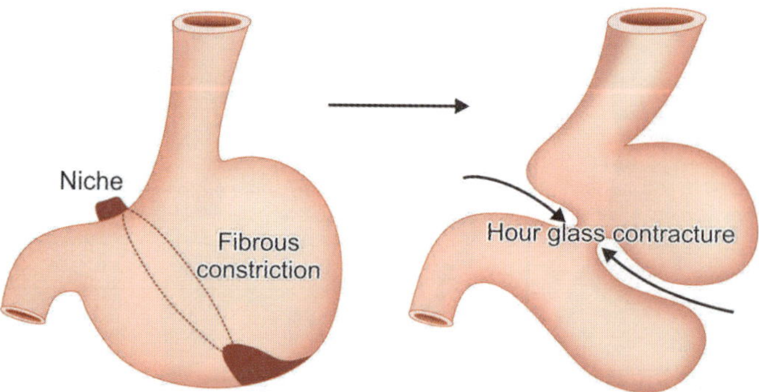

Hour glass contracture.

138. Diagnosis of Hirschsprung's disease:

a. Barium meal
b. Barium enema
c. Colonoscopy
d. Rectal biopsy

For diagnosing Hirschsprung's disease/congenital megacolon, biopsy from all the three zones is done to study the ganglions and hypetrophic nerve terminals in spasmodic segment. Starting from 2 cm above the dentate line, a full thickness rectal biopsy is ideal.

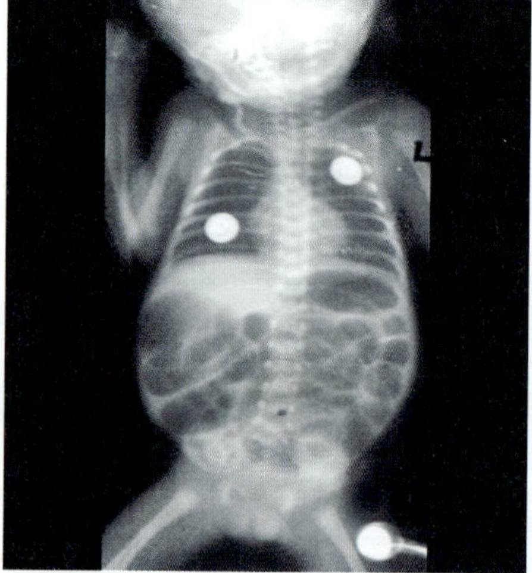

Newborn with Hirschsprung's disease with intestinal obstruction (*Courtesy:* Dr Vivek Prabhu, MCh, Mangalore)

Ans. 132. **a.** Seropurulent... 133. **d.** Achalasia cardia 134. **d.** Keratinization... 135. **b.** Short gastric artery 136. **c.** 5-FU, irradiation... 137. **d.** Gastric ulcer 138. **d.** Rectal biopsy

139. Condition which does NOT cause metabolic acidosis:

a. Renal failure
b. Ureterosigmoidostomy
c. Pancreatic/ biliary fistula
d. CHPS

Electrolyte imbalance seen in congenital hypertrophic pyloric stenosis is hypokalemic metabolic alkalosis.

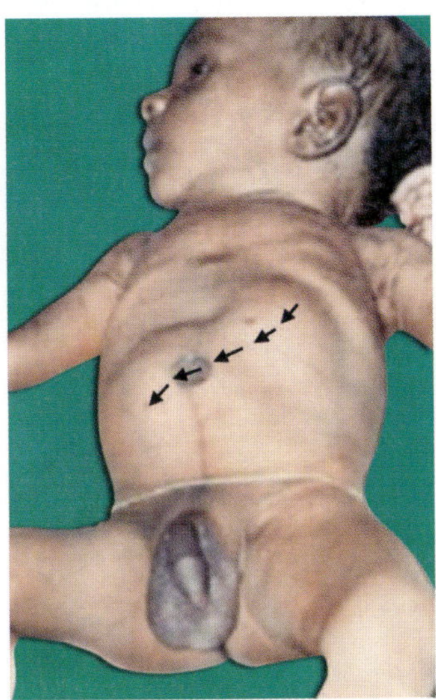

Visible gastric peristalsis.

140. Most common type of gastric sarcoma:

a. Lipoma
b. Glomus tumor
c. Leiomyosarcoma
d. Leioblastoma

Stomach is the MC site of gastrointestinal sarcoma. Leiomyosarcoma is the MC type of gastric sarcoma. Leiomyosarcoma is common in proximal stomach.

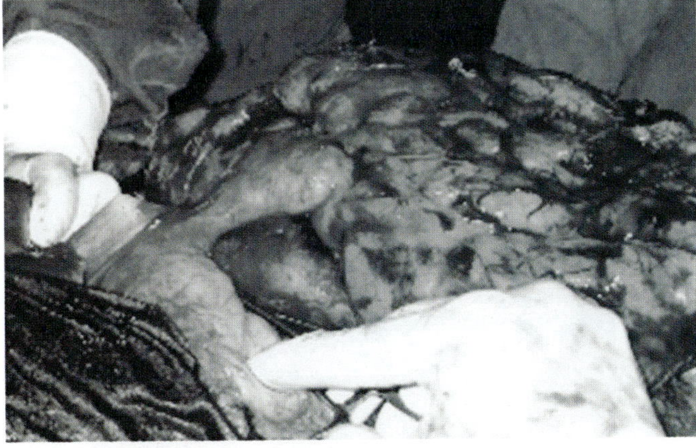

Gastric sarcomas

141. Surgery done for uncomplicated meconium ileus:

a. Ileostomy
b. Ladd's procedure
c. Bishop Koop operation
d. Instillation of peroxide

Meconium ileus
❑ Commonly associated with cystic disease of pancreas but not necessarily always
❑ Respiratory dysfunction
❑ Exocrine pancreatic insufficiency
❑ High salt in the sweat > 90 mmol/L
❑ Ileal obstruction
❑ Soap-bubble appearance in X-ray
❑ Gelatin in X-ray film will not get digested by patient's vomitus
❑ Bishop-Koop operation, ileostomy, dissolving ileal meconium pellets are required

142. Foreign body gets impacted in which part of esophagus:

a. Above the cricopharynx
b. Below the cricopharynx
c. In the middle of the esophagus
d. Cardiac part of the esophagus

Sites of impaction in esophagus

- Cervical constriction – C6
- Broncho-aortic constriction – T4
- Diaphragmatic constriction – T10
- Pre-existing malignancy or inflammatory stricture site

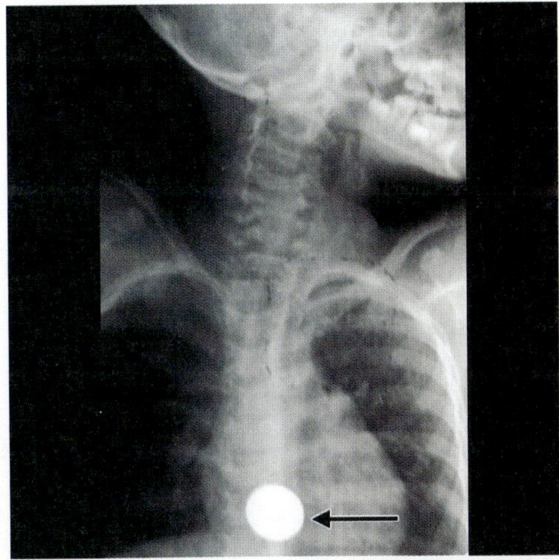

Foreign body (COIN) in the lower esophagus. Usually it can be removed by endoscope

143. Villous adenoma of rectum leads to loss of:

a. Potassium
b. Magnesium
c. Sodium
d. All of the above

Features of villous adenoma

- Bleeding per anum is usually chronic
- Anemia
- Diarrhea common in villous type; mucus discharge
- Electrolyte imbalance – hypokalemia
- Carcinomatous changes

Ans. 139. **d.** CHPS 140. **c.** Leiomyosarcoma 141. **c.** Bishop Koop... 142. **a.** Above the cricopharynx 143. **a.** Potassium

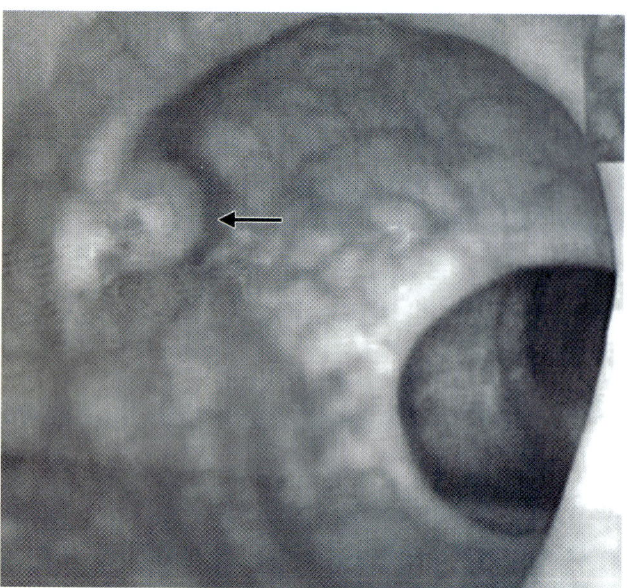

Colonoscopic view of colonic polyp

144. True for gastroschisis:

a. Herniation of abdominal contents through the body wall
b. Variant of gastric carcinoma
c. Anterior abdominal wall tumor
d. Omphalocele

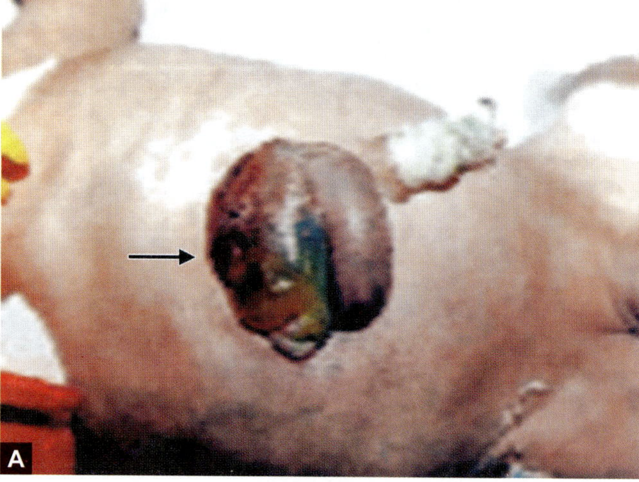

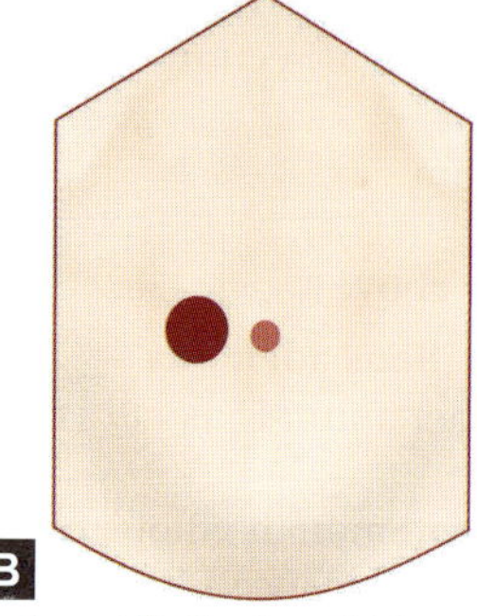

A and B: Gastroschisis

Gastroschisis/belly cleft is a defect of the anterior abdominal wall just lateral to the umbilicus. It is common in premature babies.

145. Bleeding tendency of esophageal varices depends on:

a. Gastroesophageal reflex b. Transhepatic pressure
c. Site and size of varices d. All of the above

Factors related to variceal bleed are—portal venous pressure; gastro-esophageal reflux causing ulceration; variceal size; variceal wall tension.

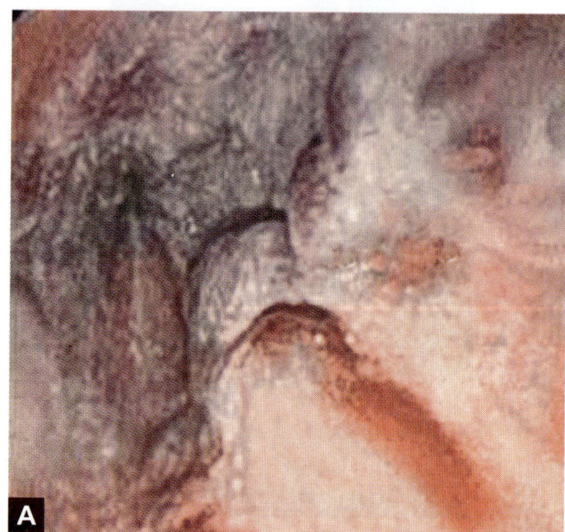

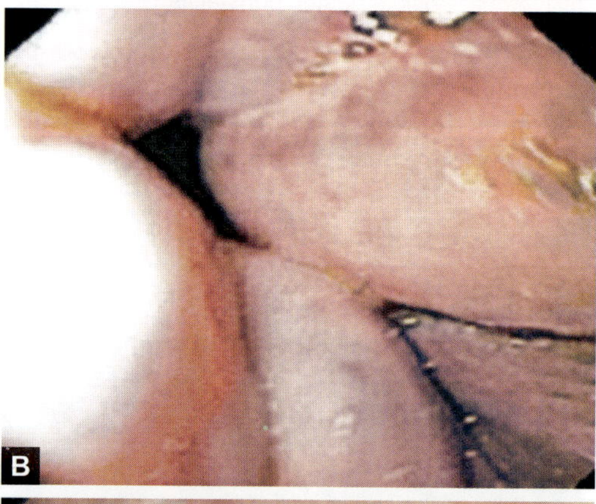

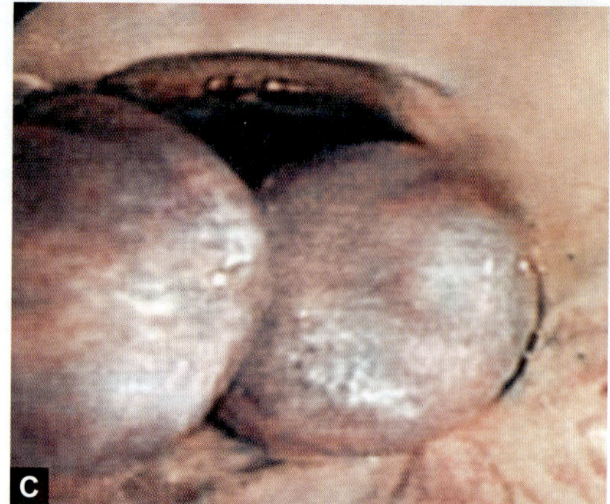

A to C: Different grades of esophageal varices—endoscopic views

Ans. **144.** **a.** Herniation of... **145.** **c.** Site and size of varices

146. **Routine management of paralytic ileus includes all of the following EXCEPT:**
   a. Electrolyte correction
   b. Nasogastric aspiration
   c. Parasympathomimetics
   d. Intravenous fluids

Do not stimulate the peristalsis ('Do not flog a tired horse') in paralytic ileus/adynamic intestinal obstruction.

Causes
❑ Postoperative
❑ Infective—pus, blood, bile, toxins, enteritis
❑ Uremia
❑ Hypokalemia
❑ Spinal injury
❑ Retroperitoneal hemorrhage
❑ Spinal surgery
❑ Plaster jacket

147. **Ideal management in an old and frail patient presenting with a mass situated 15 cm away from anal orifice:**
   a. Abdomino-perineal resection
   b. Colonoscopic removal
   c. Hartman's operation
   d. Anterior resection

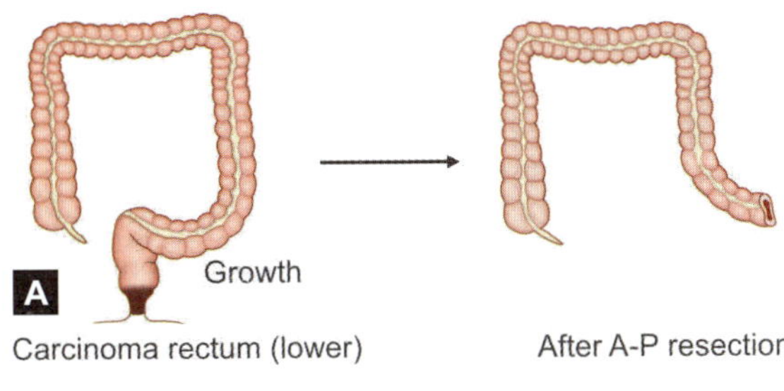

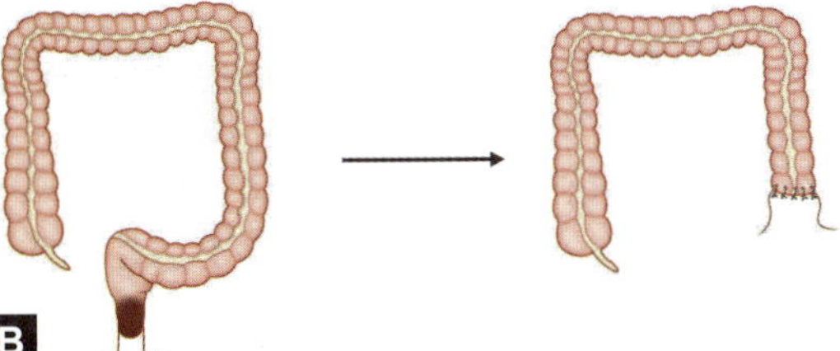

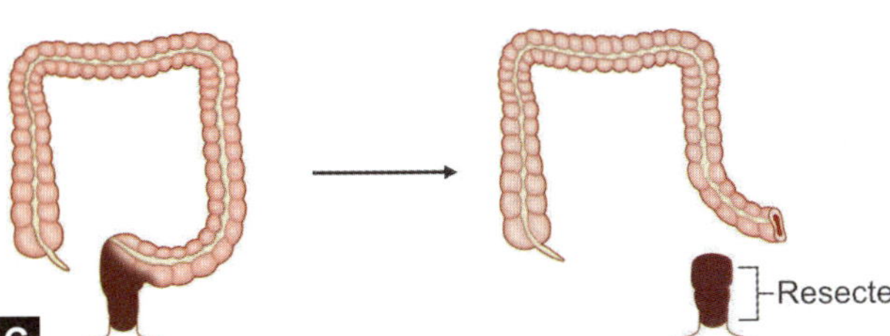

A to C: Surgeries for Ca rectum (A) A-P resection, (B) Anterior resection, (C) Hartmann's resection

Hartmann's operation is an excellent palliative procedure—done in elderly people who are not fit for major surgery like AP resection and also in locally advanced tumors. Here rectal growth is resected and upper end of the rectum is closed completely. Proximal colon is brought out as end colostomy.

148. **Late dumping syndrome is characterized by all of the following EXCEPT:**
   a. Colic
   b. Tremors and giddiness
   c. Hyperglycemia
   d. Epigastric fullness

Features of hypoglycemia (and NOT hyperglycemia) are seen in late dumping syndrome.

Types
1. ***EARLY DUMPING SYNDROME:***
❑ It is common and more severe type
❑ Incidence is 10%
❑ Vasomotor symptoms appear immediately after food, lasts for 30-40 minutes, aggravated by bulky food. It is relieved by lying down, aggravated by more food.
Clinical features:
❑ Sweating, tachycardia, colicky pain and diarrhea
❑ Hypotension and features of hypovolemia
Pathogenesis: It is a *primary disorder of carbohydrate metabolism* wherein initial transient hyperglycemia prevents further absorption of glucose, which in turn draws fluid from the bowel wall by high osmolarity resulting in increased intestinal activity, resulting in diarrhea and fall in blood volume.
Treatment: Small, dry, more frequent food, with avoidance of carbohydrates. Octreotide 100 μg given subcutaneously before meals is found to be beneficial
Surgical treatment:
❑ Conversion of Billroth II to Billroth I
❑ Interposition of reversed jejunal loop (*Henley's loop*)
❑ Early dumping syndrome can last for long time (many years)
2. ***LATE DUMPING SYNDROME***:
❑ It is of less severe type
❑ Incidence is 5%
❑ It usually occurs 2 hours after meal
❑ It is relieved by glucose and aggravated by exercise
Pathogenesis: Due to initial hyperglycemia insulin secretion is stimulated which in turn leads to hypoglycemia.
Clinical features:
❑ Tremor, fainting, nausea
❑ Features of hypoglycemia
Treatment: Symptoms are less severe and so treated conservatively, by giving glucose and food.

149. **NOT associated with Crohn's disease:**
   a. Fistula
   b. Stricture
   c. Sclerosing cholangitis
   d. Granuloma

Primary sclerosing cholangitis (PSC, 5%) is common in ulcerative colitis before 40 years of age; common in males; related to HLAB8 and DR3 (10 times).

MCQs with Short Explanations

Ans. 146. c. Parasympath... 147. c. Hartman's operation 148. c. Hyperglycemia 149. c. Sclerosing cholangitis

Differences between Crohn's disease and ulcerative colitis	
Crohn's disease	*Ulcerative colitis*
❑ It affects ileum and often colon but can involve any part of GIT—rectal sparing is common	❑ It affects rectum and colon from distal to proximal
❑ Full thickness—transmural disease	❑ It affects mucosa and sub-mucosa—not deeper
❑ Skip lesions are typical	❑ Skip lesions are not observed
❑ Granulomatous lesion on histology—deep ulcers; pseudopolyps are not found	❑ Not a granulomatous lesion—superficial ulcers, pseudopolyps are present
❑ Stricture and fistula are common	❑ Narrowing can occur but not very common
❑ Anal fissure and perianal abscess are more common	❑ Fissure and perianal disease can occur but not as common as in Crohn's disease
❑ May mimic appendicitis	❑ Will not mimic appendicitis
❑ Bleeding is not common	❑ Bleeding is common
❑ Fever is common	❑ Fever is uncommon
❑ Mass in RIF is common	❑ Mass is not a common feature
❑ Anal pathology very common	❑ Anal pathology is rare
❑ Discontinuous segmental asymmetrical colitis	❑ Continuous mucosal disease—colitis
❑ Toxic megacolon is rare	❑ Toxic megacolon is common
❑ Normal vascular pattern	❑ Distorted vascular pattern
❑ Fistula is very common	❑ Fistula is uncommon
❑ Recurrence is common after resection	❑ Total proctocolectomy cures the disease

150. Best treatment of Zollinger Ellison syndrome:

a. H_3 receptor antagonist
b. Excision of tumor alone
c. Partial gastrectomy
d. Total gastrectomy

Treatment options for gastrinomas

- 60% are curable
- Enucleation of tumors
- Distal pancreatectomy
- Pancreatico-duodenectomy
- Subtotal pancreatectomy
- Often total gastrectomy may be required

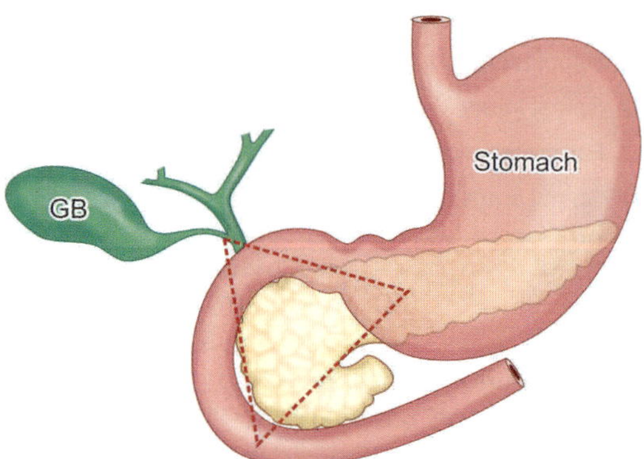

Passaros triangle.

151. Corkscrew esophagus is seen in:

a. Reflux esophagitis
b. Carcinoma esophagus
c. Diffuse esophageal spasm
d. Achalsia cardia

Diffuse esophageal spasm are incoordinated contractions of esophagus causing chest pain or dysphagia. Barium swallow X-ray shows corkscrew esophagus.

Causes of dysphagia		
Extraluminal causes	*Causes in the wall of oesophagus or other area*	*Causes in the lumen*
❑ Mediastinal nodes—secondaries/lymphoma/tuberculosis ❑ Aortic aneurysm ❑ Rolling hiatus hernia ❑ Thyroid enlargement—malignant ❑ Dysphagia lusoria ❑ Congenital anomalies ❑ Mediastinitis/mass	❑ Carcinoma esophagus ❑ Corrosive/tuberculous/inflammatory/congenital stricture esophagus ❑ GERD ❑ Achalasia cardia ❑ Plummer-Vinson syndrome ❑ Esophageal diverticulum ❑ Carcinoma posterior 1/3rd of tongue/pharynx ❑ Diffuse esophageal spasm ❑ Congenital anomalies ❑ Retropharyngeal abscess/peritonsillar abscess (Quinsy)/acute tonsillitis/pharyngitis	❑ Foreign body in the esophagus—coin/dentures/fish or meat bone *Other causes* Cranial causes (neurological): ❑ Bulbar palsy/infarction/hemiplegia ❑ Vertebro basilar insufficiency

152. Most common type of intussusception:

a. Coli-colic
b. Ileo-ileal
c. Ileo-colic
d. Ileal

Intussusception can be ileo-colic (MC type, 75%), colo-colic, ileo-ileocolic, colo-colic.

Ans. 150. b. Excision of... 151. c. Diffuse esophageal... 152. c. Ileo-colic

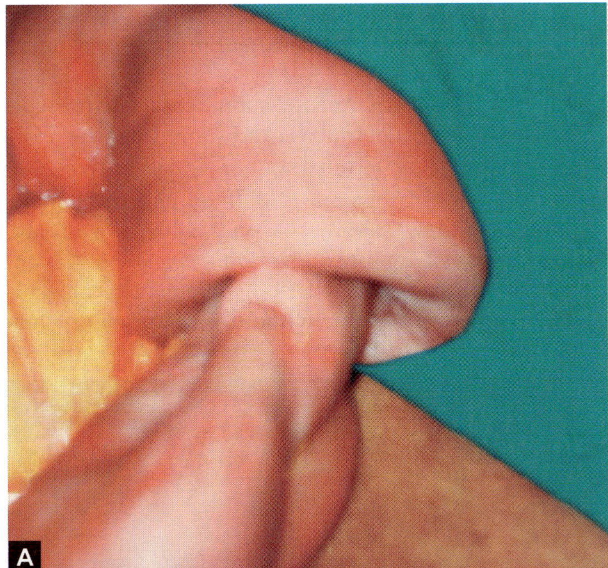

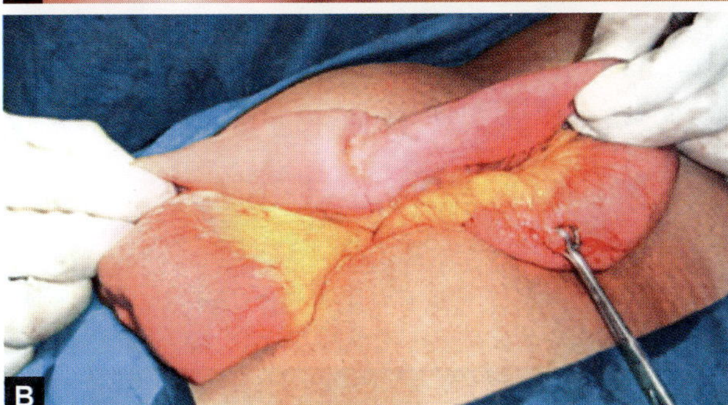

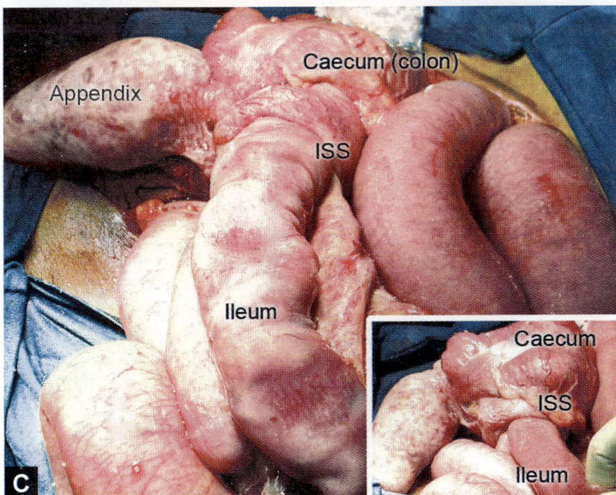

A to C: Intussusception in different patients. Different parts and apex point is also clearly seen

153. D-xylose test is diagnostic of:

a. Gastrinoma b. Bacterial overgrowth
c. Lactose intolerance d. Celiac disease

D-xylose absorption test is performed to diagnose conditions that present with malabsorption of the proximal small intestine due to defects in the integrity of the gastrointestinal mucosa. A decreased urinary excretion of D-xylose is seen in conditions involving the GI mucosa, such as small intestinal bacterial overgrowth and Whipple's disease.

Investigations for small bowel diseases
❑ Barium meal follow through
❑ Small bowel enema *(Enteroclysis)*
❑ Plain X-ray abdomen to see intestinal obstruction
❑ Selective splanchnic angiography to see vascular bleed or malformation (DSA)
❑ Isotope scintigraphy to see Meckel's diverticulum
❑ Estimation of fecal fat in 24 hours—normal is less than 7 gram
❑ *Schilling test* to find out the absorption of vitamin B_{12} from terminal ileum
❑ SeHCAT bile acid absorption test (selenium labelled) to find out the absorption of bile acids from the terminal ileum
❑ Many different breath tests are used to find out malabsorption, bacterial overgrowth and transit time
❑ Jejunal biopsy
❑ CT scans to see fistula, tumor, and spread
❑ Capsule endoscopy is very useful

154. Pseudopolyposis is seen in:

a. HIV b. Multiple myeloma
c. Ulcerative colitis d. Crohn's disease

To begin with (in ulcerative colitis), multiple minute ulcers (pin point ulcers) occur with proctitis and colitis → these ulcers extend into the deeper layer → spasm of the bowel → stricture of the colon → permanently contracted colon (pipe stem colon) → in between ulcers, epithelial thickening occurs which appears like polyps → pseudopolyposis.

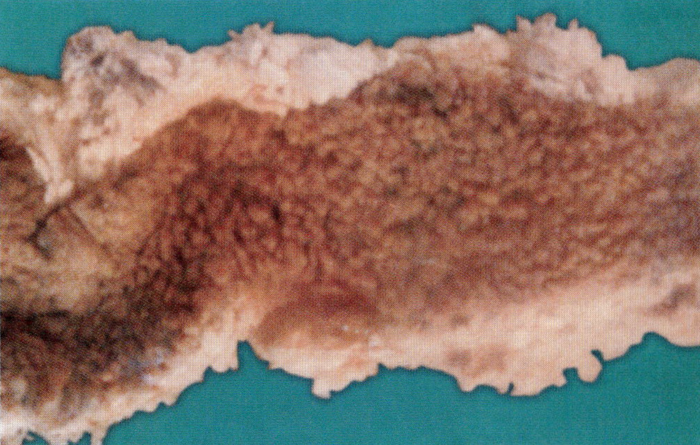

Multiple pseudopolyposis involving entire colon in ulcerative colitis. Disease involves only mucosa and submucosa

155. 'Double bubble' sign is seen in:

a. Hypertrophic pyloric stenosis
b. Duodenal atresia
c. Jejunal atresia
d. Ileal stenosis

Plain X-ray of duodenal atresia shows classic double-bubble sign with absence of air in the distal part.

Ans. **153. b.** Bacterial over... **154. c.** Ulcerative colitis **155. b.** Duodenal atresia

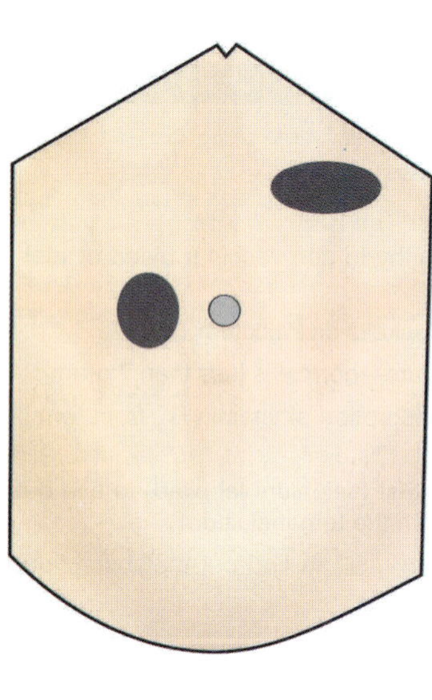

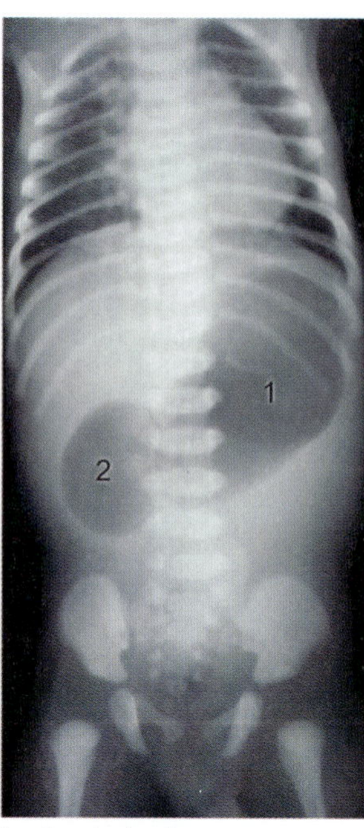

Double-bubble sign in duodenal atresia

156. All of the following are associated with carcinoid syndrome EXCEPT:

a. Asthma
b. Diarrhea
c. Flushing
d. Acute appendicitis

Presentation of carcinoid syndrome

Vasomotor	Flushing (80%) Cyanotic violaceous flush Red patchy flush
GIT	Diarrhea Hepatomegaly
Cardiac	Pulmonary stenosis Tricuspid incompetence Tricuspid stenosis Bronchospasm/asthma

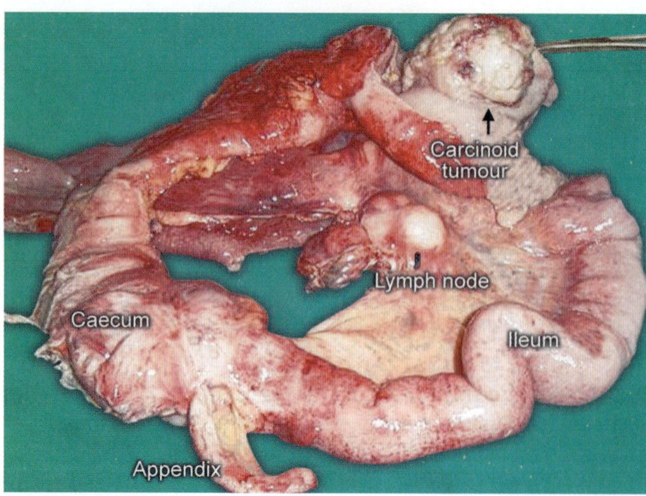

Carcinoid of ileum. It often presents when liver secondaries develop as carcinoid syndrome. Resection and anastomosis is the treatment

157. Does NOT indicate early gastric carcinoma:

a. Involvement of mucosa, submucosa and adjacent lymph nodes
b. Involvement of mucosa, submucosal and muscularis
c. Involvement of mucosa and submucosa
d. Involvement of mucosa

Early gastric carcinoma is defined as involvement of mucosa and/or submucosa only with or without involvement of lymph nodes – T1 + any N. Advanced gastric cancer is defined as involvement of muscularis and/ or serosa with or without involvement of lymph nodes.

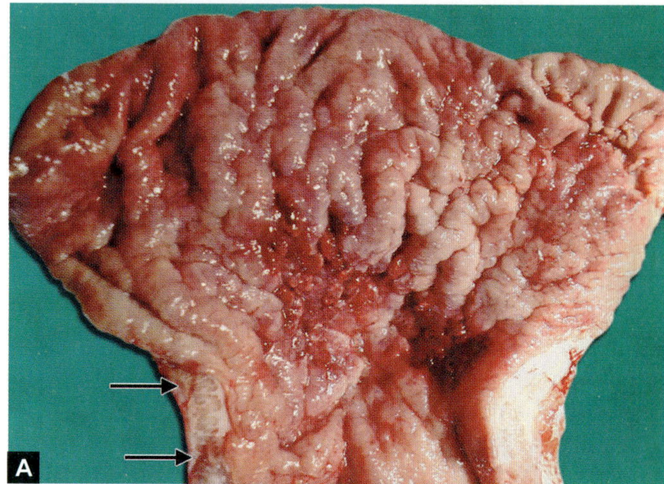

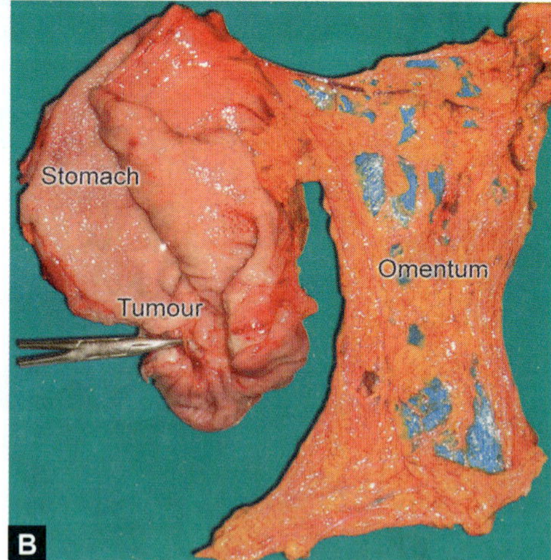

A and B: Specimen of stomach showing thickening of wall of part of the stomach with loss of rugosity. Omentum, proximal parts are also seen. Thickening is extending into serosa

158. Prepyloric/ channel ulcer in stomach is labeled as:

a. Type I
b. Type II
c. Type III
d. Type IV

Type III gastric ulcers are located in prepyloric region; incidence of 15% and shows high acid level.

Ans. 156. **d.** Acute appen... 157. **b.** Involvement of... 158. **c.** Type III

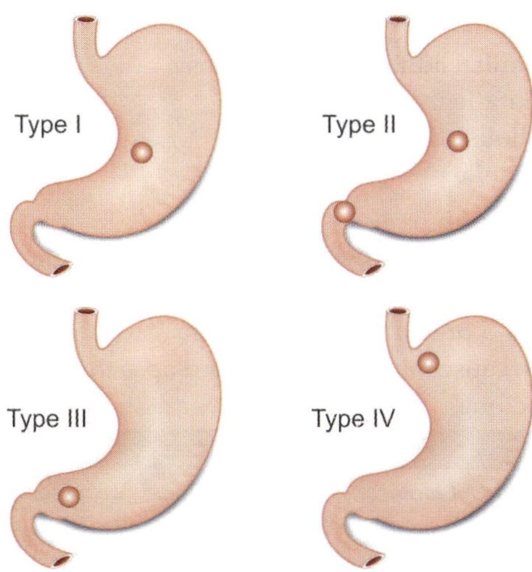

Types of gastric ulcer *(Daintree Johnson)*

159. NOT a permanent mucosal fold:

a. Plica semilunaris b. Spiral valve
c. Gastric rugae d. Transverse fold of rectum

The transverse folds of rectum (or Houston's valve) are semi-lunar transverse folds of the rectal wall that protrude into the rectum, not the anal canal as that lies below the rectum. Their use seems to be support the weight of fecal matter, and prevent its urging toward the anus, which would produce a strong urge to defecate.

160. A known case of colonic carcinoma presented with weakness, weight loss, anemia and a palpable abdominal mass. Most likely anatomic site is:

a. Ascending colon b. Left colon
c. Sigmoid colon d. Rectum

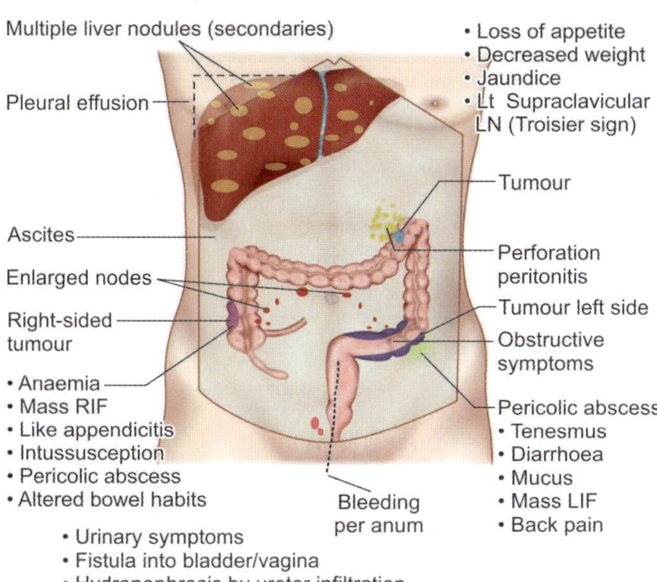

Clinical features of carcinoma of colon—diagrammatic representation

Right sided colon carcinomatous growth commonly presents with anemia, palpable mass in the right iliac fossa, which is not moving with respiration, mobile, non-tender, hard, well-localized with impaired resonant note.

161. MC cause of esophagitis:

a. Esophageal reflux
b. Spicy and hot food
c. Smoking
d. Alcohol

Types of reflux esophagitis

- Acute: Following burns, trauma, infection, peptic ulcer
- Chronic: Reflux of acid in sliding hernia, after gastric surgery, pregnancy

Grading
❑ Mucosal erythema
❑ Mucosal erythema + superficial ulceration
❑ Mucosal erythema + superficial ulceration + submucosal fibrosis
❑ Mucosal erythema + extensive ulceration + paramural fibrosis

162. Early complications seen in ileostomy:

a. Skin necrosis
b. Prolapse
c. Diarrhea
d. Obstruction

Skin excoriation is a major problem in stoma patients. It is basically due to leak adjacent to appliances.

Ileostomy
It is usually end ileostomy. But often loop ileostomy is also done
Indications:
❑ After total proctocolectomy for ulcerative colitis, total colonic Hirschsprung's diseases, Crohn's disease (occasionally), and total colectomy for carcinomas
❑ Loop ileostomy is done in critically ill patient with acute ileal conditions like multiple ileal perforations, ileal gangrene or distal fistulas or sepsis. It is temporary ileostomy
❑ Ileostomy is *placed in right iliac fossa* through the right rectus muscle.
❑ Ileostomy may be temporary (loop) or permanent (end)
❑ Brooke's classic end non continent ileostomy or Koch's continent ileostomy (with continent intra-abdominal pouch) are used
❑ Ileum should project as a spout at least 4 cm above the skin surface, which facilitates the effluent to pass directly into the bag
❑ Ileostomy usually acts in 48 hours
❑ Ileostomy bag, ileostomy care, nutrition and electrolyte management are important
❑ **Complications** like prolapse, stenosis, hemorrhage, retraction can occur

Ans. **159. d.** Transverse fold... **160. a.** Ascending colon **161. a.** Esophageal reflux **162. a.** Skin necrosis

163. MC site of curling's ulcer:

a. Esophagus
b. Stomach
c. Duodenum
d. Ileum

Curling ulcers occurs when burn injury is more than 35%. It is observed in the body and fundus, not in antrum and duodenum.

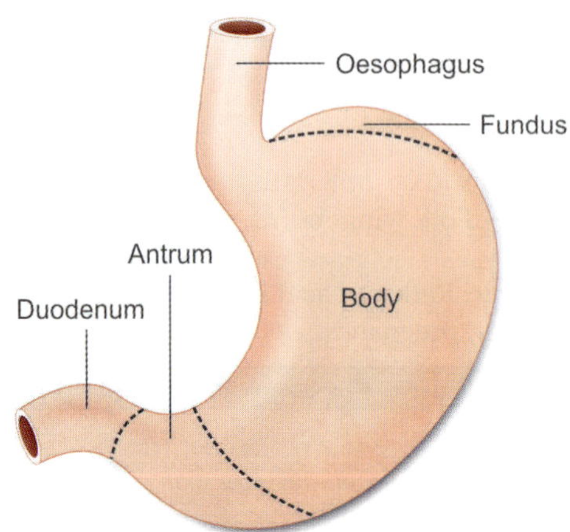

Parts of stomach

164. Cause of acute onset, large volume hematemesis in a patient with mild splenomegaly:

a. Gastric carcinoma
b. Barret's esophagus
c. Esophageal varices
d. Gastritis

Triad of portal hypertension

- Esophageal varices
- Splenomegaly
- Ascites

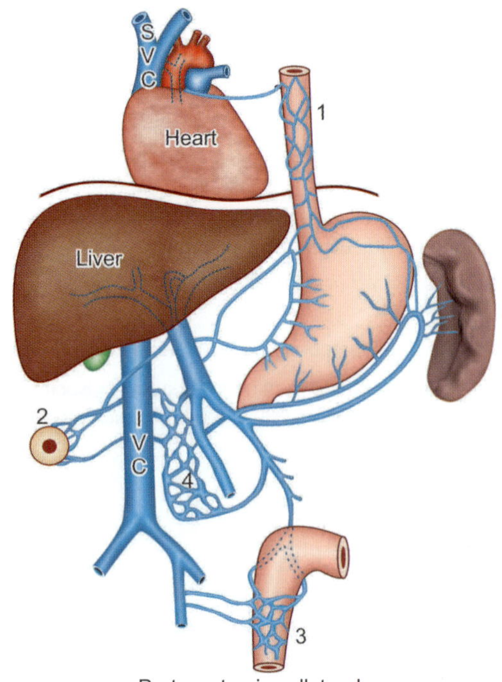

Portosystemic collaterals

165. NO risk of malignancy is with:

a. Familial adnomatous polyposis
b. Peutz-Jegher's syndrome
c. Villous adenoma
d. Juvenile polyp

Juvenile polyps

- Commonest polyps of colorectum in infants and children
- NOT a premalignant condition
- Can cause intussusception, prolapse through rectum, bleeding

Polyps			
Inflammatory	*Hyperplastic*	*Hamartomatous*	*Neoplastic*
Ulcerative colitis	(Metaplastic)	Peutz-Jegher syndrome	Adenomatous
Segmental colitis		Juvenile polyp	– Tubular
Dysenteric colitis		Cronkhite-Canada syndrome	– Tubulovillous
Crohn's disease			– Villous
Diverticulitis			Malignant (Carcinomatous)

166. Which of the following does NOT form boundary of gastrinoma triangle is between:

a. Pancreas and duodenum
b. CBD and pancreas
c. Gall bladder and CBD
d. CBD and duodenum

Gastrinoma is common in gastrinoma triangle/ Passaros triangle.

Three points forming Passaros triangle:
1. Junction between the head and neck of the pancreas
2. Junction of cystic duct with CBD
3. Junction between the 2nd and 3rd parts of the duodenum

167. Screening test, following genetic counseling, in a family with familial adenomatous polyposis/ FAP, is

a. APC gene
b. Occult blood in stool
c. Flexible sigmoidoscopy
d. Colonoscopy

About 80% of colorectal cancer arises from loss of heterozygosity (LOH) pathway. LOH pathway is due to APC gene defects (in FAP), K-ras mutation altering the cell cycle (K-ras binds to GTP/guanosine triphosphate, hydrolyze to GDP which inactivates G protein normally; K-ras mutation blocks GTP hydrolyze leading into permanently active forms of G protein causing carcinoma); loss of DCC tumor suppressor gene; mutation of tumor suppressor gene p53.

Ans. **163. b.** Stomach **164. c.** Esophageal varices **165. d.** Juvenile polyp **166. c.** Gallbladder and CBD **167. a.** APC gene

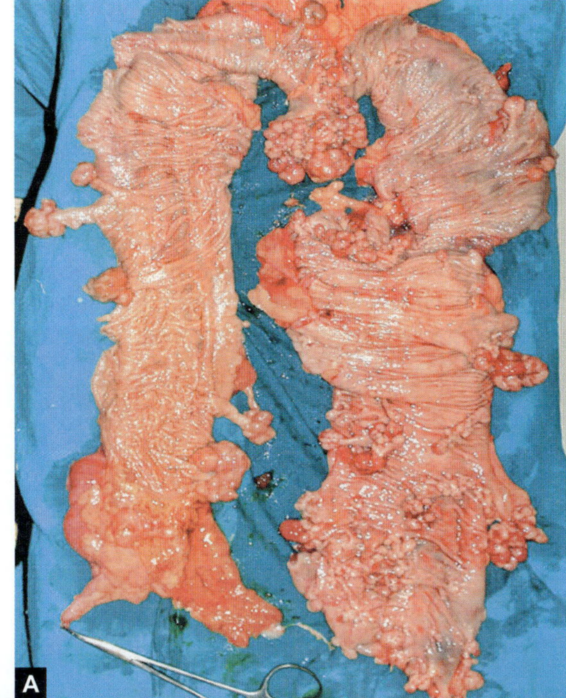

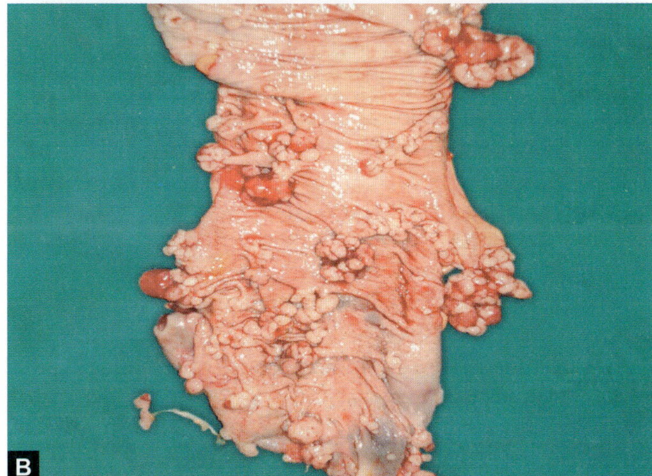

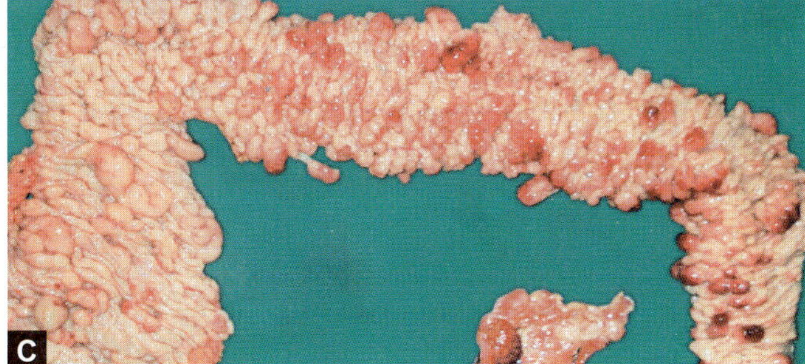

A to C: Multiple polyps extensively involving the colon

168. A patient presented with polyps in jejunum with a positive family history. He is also having pigmentation in mouth. Findings are suggestive of:

a. Hyperplastic polyp b. Turcot syndrome
c. Gardener's syndrome d. Peutz Jegher's syndrome

Peutz Jegher's polyp

- Common in small intestine (jejunum), but can also occur in large intestine
- Associated with melanomas of the oral mucosa, lips (lower lip) and occasionally in digits (not in tongue)
- It is autosomal dominant disease with germline defects in suppressor serine threonine kinase 11 (STK11)
- It can occasionally turn into malignancy.

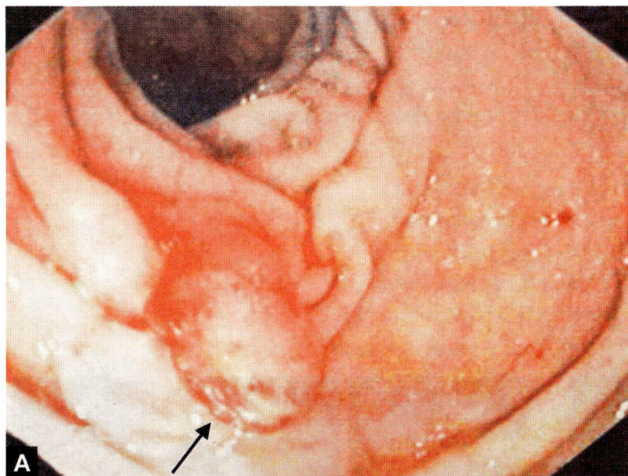

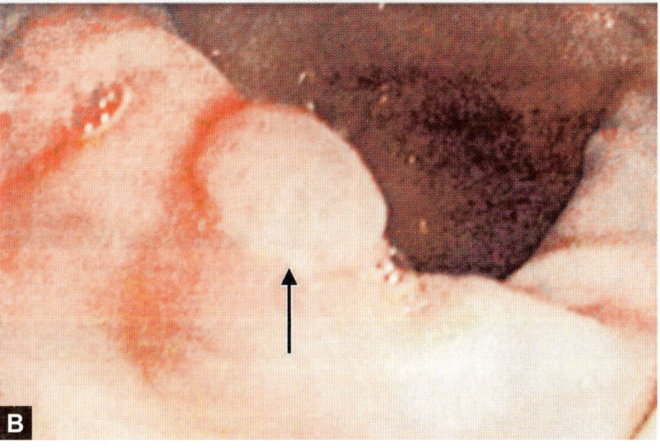

A and B: Colonoscopic view of polyp colon in two different patients.

169. Which of these is not a premalignant lesion of lesion:

a. Esophageal web b. Barrett's esophagus
c. Hiatus hernia d. Achalasia

Complications of rolling hernia

- Gangrene of the stomach
- Perforation into the mediastinum
- Perforation into the peritoneum
- Gastric volvulus
- Ischemic longitudinal ulcer in the herniated stomach in rolling hernia (Cameron ulcer)

Ans. 168. d. Peutz Jegher's... **169. c.** Hiatus hernia

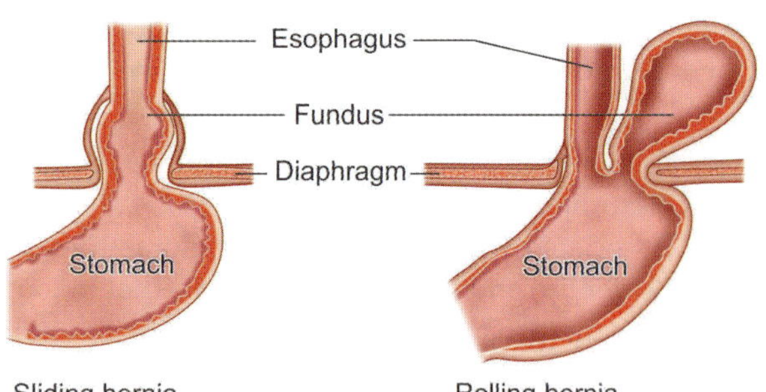

Sliding hernia Rolling hernia
Types of hiatus hernia.

170. In pyloric stenosis, the following changes are seen:
a. Hypokalemic, hyponatremic alkalosis
b. Hyperkalemia
c. Hyperkalemic, hyponatremic alkalosis
d. Hyperchloremic acidosis

Electrolytic changes in pyloric stenosis
- Hyponatremia
- Hypokalemia
- Hypomagnesemia
- Hypochloremia
- Metabolic alkalosis
- Paradoxical aciduria

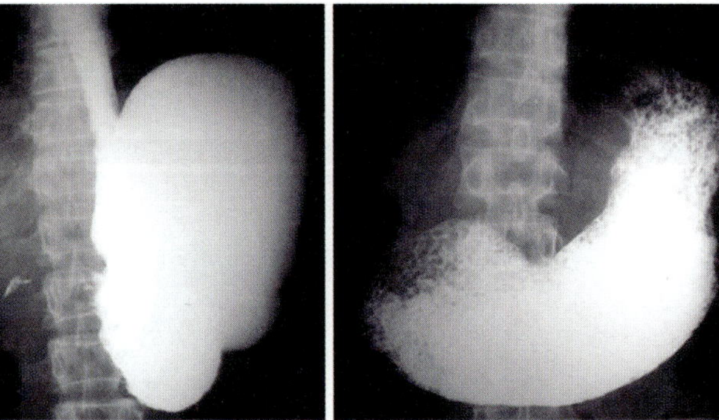

Barium meal pictures showing gastric outlet obstruction

171. Treatment of choice for small intestine carcinoma:
a. Radiotherpay
b. Chemotherapy
c. Surgery
d. None of the above

Surgical resection is the choice of therapy for small intestinal adenocarcinomas. Pancreatico-duodenectomy is done for duodenal tumors; for ileal/jejunal site tumors, radical resection with 10 cm margin with adjacent mesenteric clearance is done. Adenocarcinoma of terminal ileum is treated with right hemicolectomy.

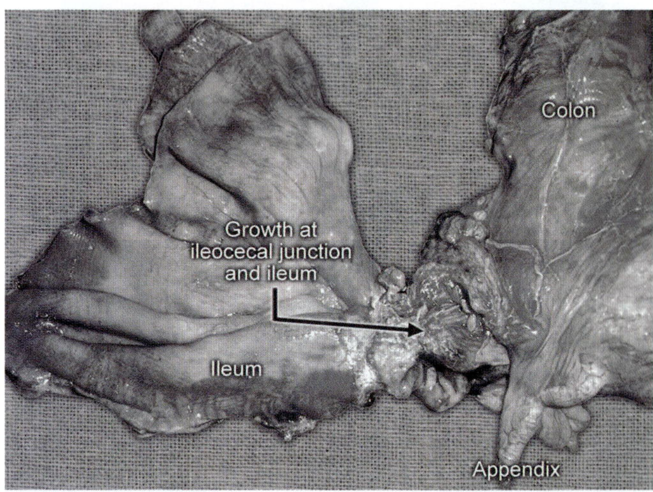

Carcinoma ileum near ileocecal junction. It (adenocarcinoma of ileum) carries poor prognosis. It is often on table diagnosis

172. Which of the following is a dynamic cause of intestinal obstruction:
a. Gallstone
b. Paralytic ileus
c. Mesenteric vascular obstruction
d. Ogilvie syndrome

Gallstone is an intra-luminal cause of dynamic type of intestinal obstruction.

	Dynamic		Adynamic
Outside the wall	*In the wall*	*In the lumen*	
❑ Hernia—25% ❑ Adhesions—40% ❑ Volvulus ❑ Intussusception	❑ Tuberculous stricture ❑ Crohn's disease ❑ Malignancy	❑ Gallstones ❑ Roundworm ❑ Inspissated feces ❑ Meconium ileus	❑ Cessation of peristalsis ❑ Postoperative period ❑ Electrolyte imbalance ❑ Spinal injuries ❑ Uremia ❑ Diabetes mellitus ❑ Retroperitoneal—hematomas and surgeries ❑ Renal surgeries ❑ Mesenteric ischemia ❑ Pseudo-obstruction

173. Entero-enteric fistula is seen in:
a. Ulcerative colitis
b. Crohn's disease
c. Both of the above
d. None of the above

Small bowel is the MC site of GI fistula. More than 75% are postoperative. Crohn's disease is the MC cause of spontaneous small bowel fistula in which 50% each are internal and external.

Ans. **170. a.** Hypokalemic... **171. c.** Surgery **172. a.** Gallstone **173. b.** Crohn's disease

Fistula may be due to:	*Physiological—based on quantity of daily output:*	*Fistula may be:*
❑ Complete disruption of anastomotic site ❑ Partial disruption ❑ Lateral fistula with distal obstruction ❑ Fistula in stricture bowel	❑ *High output*— > 500 mL/day—usually small bowel; 50% mortality; less chance of spontaneous closure. ❑ *Moderate output*—200–500 mL/day—colonic and small bowel mixed. ❑ *Low output*— < 200 mL/day—colonic; mortality is 15%; more chance of spontaneous closure.	*Favorable:* ❑ Site—oropharyngeal, esophsgeal, duodenal stump, pancreaticobiliary, jejunal, colonic. ❑ Cause—postoperative, appendicitis, diverticulitis. ❑ Low output, absence of sepsis, transferrin level more than 200 mg/dL. ❑ Healthy adjacent tissues with intestinal continuity, without distal obstruction. ❑ Fistula track more than 2 cm; bowel wall defect less than 1 cm^2. *Unfavorable:* ❑ Site—gastric, lateral duodenal, ileal. ❑ Cause—malignancy, inflammatory bowel disease. ❑ High output, poor nutrition, sepsis, transferrin < 200 mg/dL. ❑ Diseased adjacent bowel, presence of distal obstruction, large abscess, complete bowel disruption, radiation. ❑ Track < 1 cm; bowel wall defect > 1 cm^2. Track epithelialization, presence of foreign body.
Fistula may be: ❑ *End fistula* ❑ *Lateral fistula* **Fistula may be:** ❑ Single ❑ Multiple **Fistula may be:** ❑ *Simple* ❑ *Complicated*—if multiple tracks, track with an abscess, communication to more sites or more than one viscus. **Note:** Fistula of duration of more than 3 months is called as *chronic fistula*	**Fistula stoma categories:** *Category 1*: A single orifice fistula through an intact abdominal wall or healed scar with normal skin adjacent *Category 2*: Single or multiple fistulas passing through abdominal wall close to bony part or umbilicus or surgical scar *Category 3*: Fistula through a small dehiscence through the main wound *Category 4:* Fistula through a large dehiscence through main wound or dehiscence at the bottom of wound	

174. Sister Mary Joseph nodule is most commonly seen with:

a. Ovarian cancer
b. Stomach cancer
c. Colon cancer
d. Pancreatic cancer

Sister Mary Joseph's nodule is a secondary carcinoma. It is through lymphatics of the round ligament, primary being in the stomach, colon, ovary, uterus, breast (often blood spread).

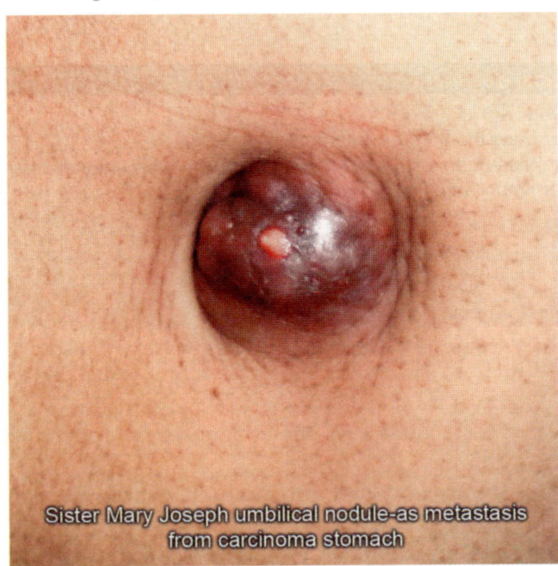

Sister Mary Joseph (Nee Julia Dempsey, Mayo Clinic USA) metastatic umbilical nodule from carcinoma stomach

175. True statement regarding Barrett's esophagus:

a. Patient present with severe symptoms
b. Normal pH profile
c. Increased risk of squamous cell carcinoma
d. Metaplastic change in the lining mucosa of the esophagus

Barrett's esophagus is the metaplastic changes in the mucosa of the esophagus as the result of GORD (gastroesophageal reflux disease). Squamous epithelium of lower end of the esophagus is replaced by diseased columnar epithelium (Columnar metaplasia).

Complications of Barrett's esophagus
❑ Ulcerations and stricture
❑ Dysphagia
❑ Bleeding
❑ Perforation
❑ Adenocarcinoma of O-G junction (25 times more common)

176. Which one of the following is a muscle splitting incision:

a. Gridiron
b. Rutherford-Morison's
c. Lower midline
d. Lanz

Approaches for appendicectomy

Approach	*Description*
Gridiron incision	Perpendicular incision at right spinoumbilical line at the McBurney's point
Rutherford-Morison's muscle cutting incision	Muscles are cut upwards and laterally

Contd...

Ans. 174. **b.** Stomach cancer 175. **d.** Metaplastic... 176. **b.** Rutherford...

Contd...

Approach	Description
Lanz crease incision	Centering at McBurney's point – cosmetically better
Right lower paramedian incision/ lower midline incision	When in doubt or when there is diffuse peritonitis

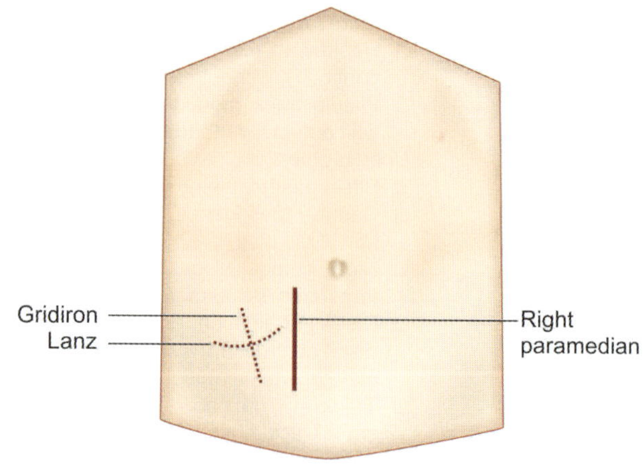

Approaches for appendicectomy

177. Regarding congenital hypertrophic pyloric stenosis, all are correct EXCEPT:

a. Weight loss
b. Diarrhea
c. Visible gastric peristalsis/ VGP
d. Ramstedt's operation done

Clinical features of congenital pyloric stenosis
❑ Vomiting
❑ VGP
❑ Palpable mass
❑ Constipation and dehydration

178. Ramstedt's operation is done for:

a. Congenital hypertrophic pyloric stenosis
b. Breast carcinoma
c. Thyroglossal cyst
d. Carcinoma stomach

Ramstedt's operation is done for CHPS, where after laparotomy, hypertrophied muscle is cut along the whole length adequately until the mucosa bulges out. Mucosa should not be opened (pyloromyotomy). If mucosa is injured, it should be sutured horizontally using interrupted vicryl or silk sutures.

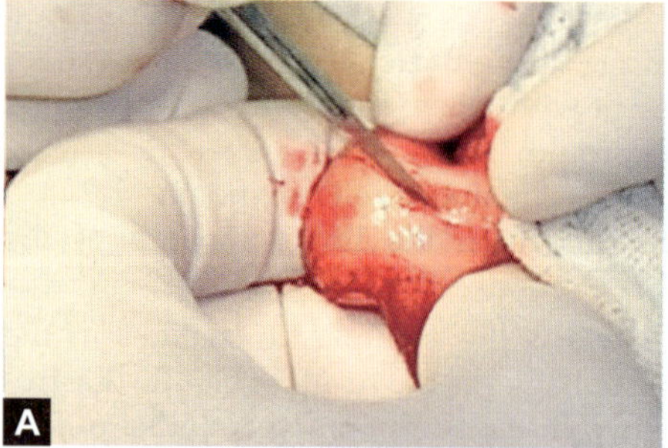

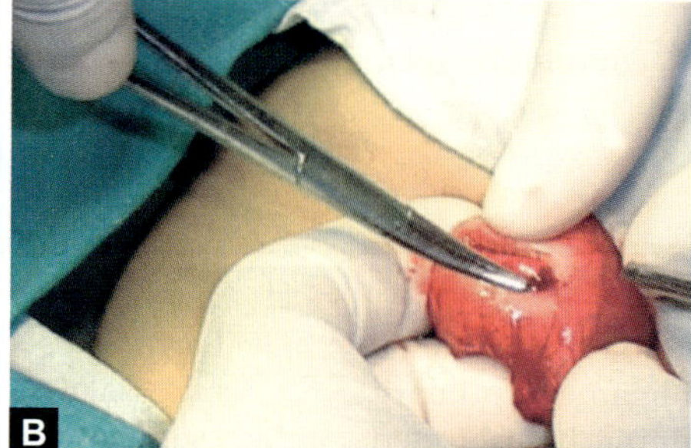

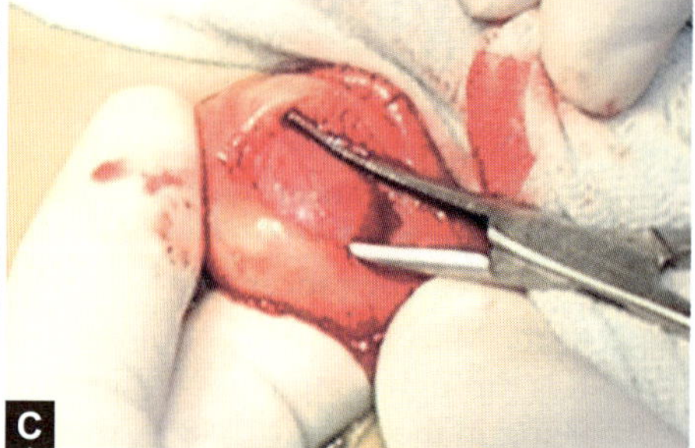

Ramstedt pyloromyotomy for congenital hypertrophic pyloric stenosis. Only muscular layer is cut to allow mucosa to bulge out

179. What should be done for an incidental carcinoid of 2.5 cms size detected in the appendix:

a. Right hemicolectomy
b. Appendicectomy
c. Appendicectomy followed by yearly HIAA estimation
d. Total colectomy

If carcinoid tumor is in the base of appendix or appendicular lesion >2 cm size or terminal ileum, right hemicolectomy is required.

Surgical treatment
❑ Appendix – Tip/lesion less than 2 cm but not involving base—appendicectomy – Lesion more than 2 cm/involving base—right hemicolectomy
❑ Gastroduodenum – Less than 1 cm—endoscopic resection – More than 1 cm—subtotal gastrectomy/pancreaticoduodenectomy

Contd...

Contd...

Surgical treatment
❑ *Small bowel lesion* – Less than 1 cm—segmental resection – More than 1 cm—radical resection with adjacent mesentery ❑ Terminal ileum—right hemicolectomy
❑ *Rectal lesion* – Less than 1 cm—endoscopic resection – 1 cm invasive—wide excision – More than 1 cm—anterior resection

180. Which of the following statement is NOT true for McBurney's incision:

a. Most suitable if the diagnosis of appendicitis is definite
b. If it is converted into a muscle cutting incision, it is called Rutherford Morison's incision
c. Inguinal hernia is a sequelae of the incision
d. The incision can be extended upwards or downwards

Ans. 177. **b.** Diarrhea 178. **a.** Congenital... 179. **a.** Right hemicolectomy 180. **d.** The incision can...

If McBurney's incision is extended superiorly, it would cut several segmental nerves, resulting in loss of sensation and paralysis of the muscles on the right side, which would in turn cause bulging of the abdominal wall.

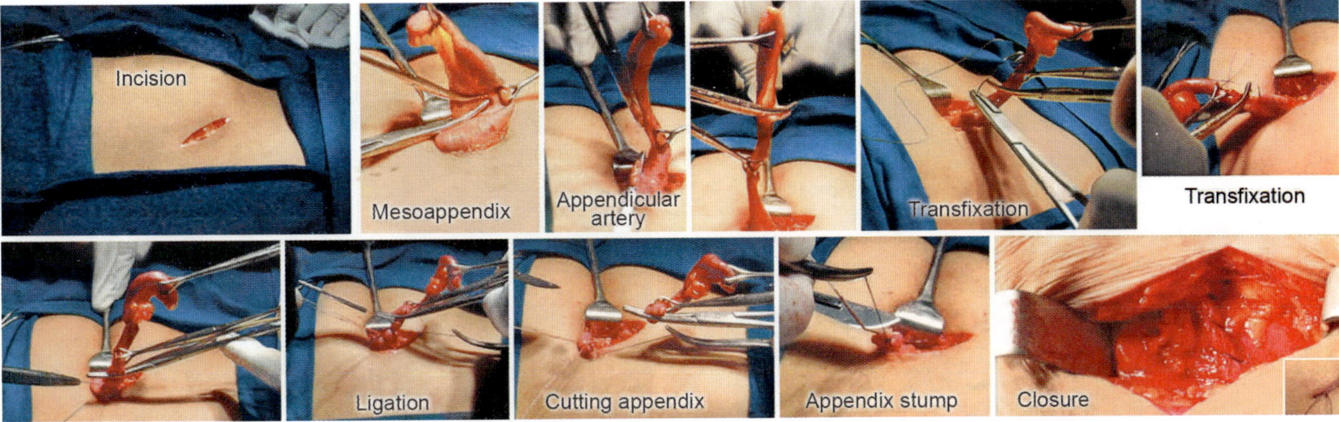

Steps in open appendicectomy. Note the base of appendix, mesoappendix; its ligation; transfixation of the base using 2 zero vicryl; cutting of appendix and closure of the wound. Burying is not essential; it is optional. Burying is done using silk/vicryl using purse string suture

181. True about carcinoid tumor are all EXCEPT:

a. Common in distal ¾ appendix
b. Carcinoid syndrome is due to malignant transformation
c. Distal 2/3 treatment of choice is appendicectomy
d. All of the above

It is the (first pass metabolism site) liver secondaries which causes carcinoid syndrome. Carcinoids of ovary, testis and retroperitoneum bypass the firstpass metabolism in liver and so causes syndrome without liver secondaries. Syndrome is due to release of 5-HT (serotonin), 5-HTP, histamine, dopamine, bradykinin, prostaglandin, kallikrein and substance P.

Medical treatment
❑ Mainly symptomatic
❑ Long acting somatostatin analogue—octreotide can be given—90% symptom palliation is achieved
❑ Slow release formulation of octreotide (*Sandostatin LAR*) is also used
❑ *Pasireotide* is 2nd generation octreotide which has got wide somatostatin receptor inhibition action (40 fold than octreotide) is said to be very effective
❑ Ketanserin (to control diarrhea), cyproheptadine, ondansetron are also effective
❑ Bevacizumab (antiangiogenesis factor), sunitinib (Tyrosine kinase inhibitor), everolimus (m TOR inhibitor) are other agents tried
❑ Others: Serotonin antagonists, antihistamines, alpha methyl dopa, 5-fluorouracil
❑ Bromocryptine, streptozocin, doxorubicin, dacarbazine, 5 FU, methylsergide, diphenoxylate hydrochloride, interferon
❑ Radiolabelled somatostatin analogue
❑ Indium 111 labelled pentetreotide is also effective

182. When 'spontaneous perforation' of the esophagus occurs as a result of severe barotrauma while a person vomits against a closed glottis, condition is known as:

a. Mallory-Weiss tear
b. Plummer Vinson syndrome
c. Kartagener syndrome
d. Boerhaave syndrome

Boerhaave's syndrome is a tear in the lower third of the esophagus which is occur when a person vomits against a closed glottis, causing leak into the mediastinum, pleural cavity and peritoneum.

Features of Boerhaave's syndrome

Presentations	*Differential diagnosis*	*Complications*
Sudden onset of symptoms	Myocardial infarction	Mediastinitis
Severe chest pain	Pancreatitis	Septicemia
Pain abdomen		Peritonitis
Subcutaneous emphysema Shock		Emphysema

'Crunching effect in the chest' is called as *Hamman's sign*.
Mackler's triad: (1) vomiting, (2) chest pain, (3) subcutaneous emphysema.

183. Commonest cause of esophageal perforation is:

a. Acid ingestion
b. Hyperemesis
c. Instrumentation
d. Carcinoma infiltrating

Esophageal perforation

- Instrumental injuries—commonest cause (75%), commonest site is just above the level of cricopharyngeus
- Foreign bodies
- Alkali injuries

Ans. 181. b. Carcinoid syndrome... 182. d. Boerhaave syndrome 183. c. Instrumentation

- Carcinoma esophagus (1%)
- Boerhaave's syndrome (15%)

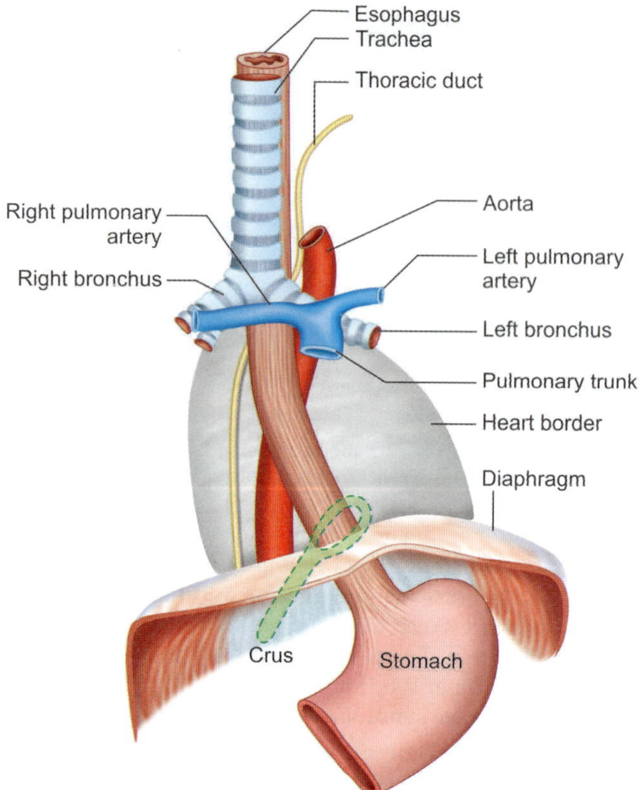

Anatomical relations of the esophagus

184. MC site of carcinoid tumor:

a. Appendix
b. Liver
c. Stomach
d. Rectum

Carcinoid tumor commonly occurs in appendix (45%), ileum (25%) and rectum (15%). Other (15%) sites are – other parts of GIT (including pancreas and biliary tract), bronchus and testis. In the ileum, it is almost always in the terminal 2 feet.

Foregut carcinoids—argyrophillic (cells can be stained with metallic silver only in the presence of reducing agent)
Midgut carcinoids—argentaffin (stained with metallic silver without a reducing agent) and argyrophillic both
Hindgut carcinoids—do not stain with silver

185. Commonest complication of Meckel's diverticulum is:

a. Bleeding
b. Perforation
c. Diverticulitis
d. Intussusception

Presentations in Meckel's diverticulum

- Asymptomatic – in majority cases
- Severe hemorrhage most common, seen in children aged 2 years or younger (Maroon colored blood)
- Intestinal obstruction due to bands/adhesions/ intussusceptions
- Perforation

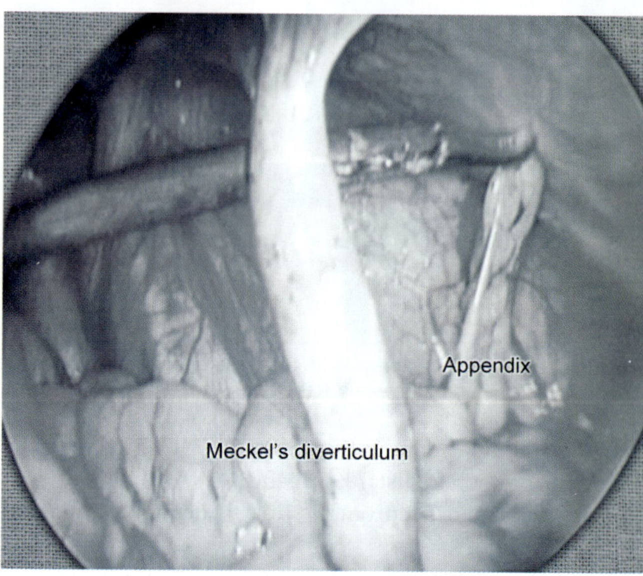

Laparoscopic view of Meckel's diverticulum. Patient presented with features of acute appendicitis. On laparoscopy, Meckel's diverticulum which was adherent to umbilicus by a cord was found. Appendix was identified separately. Appendicectomy and Mecklian diverticulectomy was done

186. Heller's operation is done in:

a. Achalasia cardia
b. Pyloric stenosis
c. Hirschprung's disease
d. Crohn's disease

Modified Heller's operation (Heller – German, 1913) is done for achalasia cardia (esophago-cardio-myotomy). Success rate is 85%.

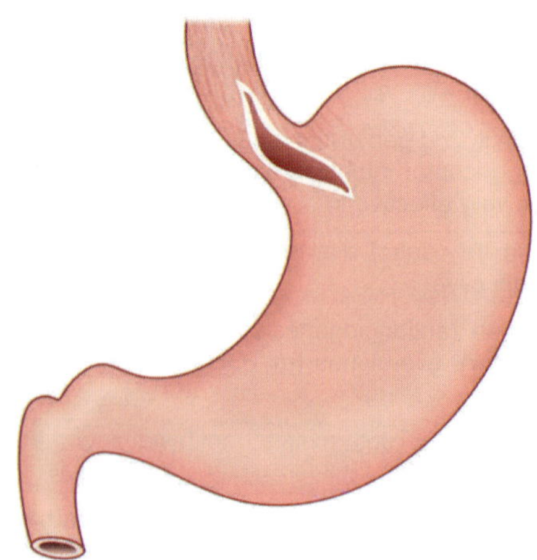

Heller's cardiomyotomy for achalasia cardia. Only circular muscle layer is cut longitudinally in OG junction until mucosa protrudes out without perforating the mucosa

Ans. **184. a.** Appendix **185. a.** Bleeding **186. a.** Achalasia cardia

187. True about left side colon carcinoma:
a. Anemia
b. Obstruction
c. Melena
d. Mass

Annular (stenosing) type of carcinoma colon is more common of left side. Here the growth spreads round the internal wall and so it often presents with intestinal obstruction.

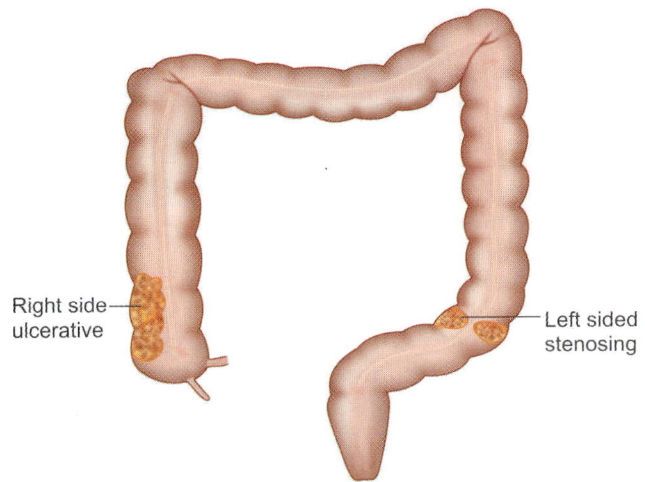

Carcinoma colon—types

188. Small intestine anastomosis is sutured by:
a. Non-absorbable in 2 layers
b. Absorbable in 2 layers
c. Inner absorbable and outer non-absorbable
d. Inner non-absorbable and outer absorbable

Vicryl is very good suture material for bowel anastomosis.

Uses of absorbable suture materials
❑ In bowel anastomosis like gastrojejunostomy, resection and anastomosis. Vicryl is used
❑ In cholecystojejunostomy (CCJ), choledocho-jejunostomy (CDJ), pancreaticojejunostomy. Vicryl is used
❑ In suturing muscle, fascia, peritoneum, subcutaneous tissue, mucosa
❑ In ligating pedicles. 1-zero chromic catgut or vicryl are used, e.g. ligation of pedicles during hysterectomy
❑ In circumcision, usually 3-zero plain or chromic catgut are used

189. Adenocarcinoma of esophagus is seen in:
a. Barrett's esophagus
b. Achalasia cardia
c. Scleroderma
d. Menetrier's disease

Lower 3 cm of esophagus is lined by columnar epithelium and so adenocarcinoma is common here. Barrett's esophagus metaplasia which occurs in lower third of esophagus is also more prone for adenocarcinoma.

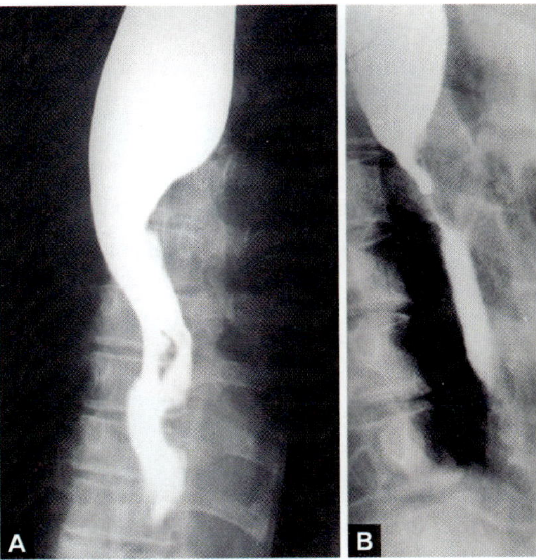

A and B: Barium swallow X-rays showing narrowing and irregularity in carcinoma esophagus

190. Commonest site of peptic ulcer perforation:
a. Anterior aspect of the first part of duodenum
b. Posterior aspect of the first part of duodenum
c. Greater curvature of the stomach
d. Lesser curvature

Anterior duodenal ulcer (DU) perforates commonly. In 80% of cases, there is a history of chronic DU. In 20% cases, it is silent perforation.

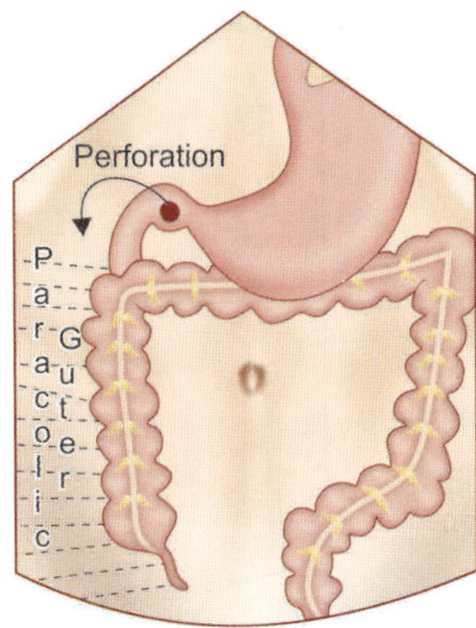

Spread in DU perforation

191. Which one of the following is NOT a premalignant condition for carcinoma of colon:
a. Familial adenomatous polyposis coli
b. Villous adenoma
c. Ulcerative colitis
d. Hamartomatous polyps

Juvenile polyp comes under hamartomatous polyps group and is not a premalignant condition.

Ans. 187. **b.** Obstruction 188. **b.** Absorbable... 189. **a.** Barrett's esophagus 190. **a.** Anterior aspect.. 191. **d.** Hamartomat...

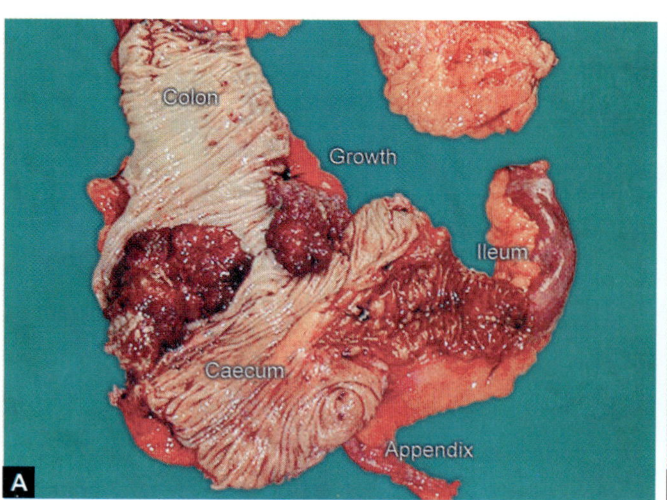

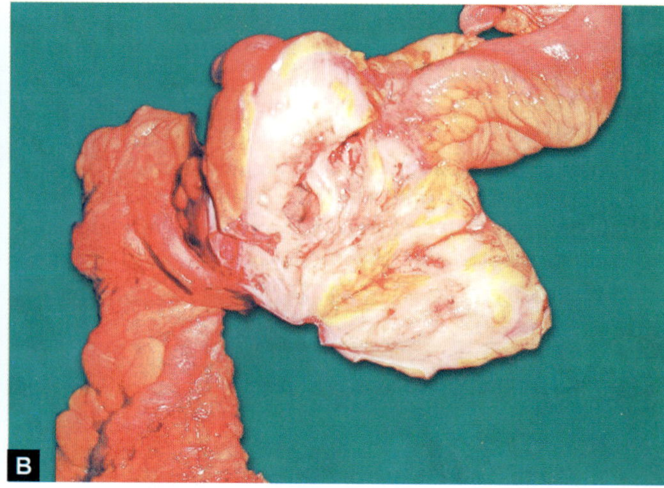

A and B: (A) Carcinoma cecum showing proliferative lesion. (B) Thickening of the wall is seen

192. Ochsner Sherren regimen is used in:

a. Appendicular abscess
b. Appendicular mass
c. Acute appendicitis
d. Pelvic abscess

Conservative (Ochsner Sherren Regimen) is used for appendicular lump/mass or periappendicular phlegmon. As nature has already localized the infection in appendicular mass, if now disturbed will causes fecal fistula. Appendicectomy is done after 6 weeks (interval appendicectomy).

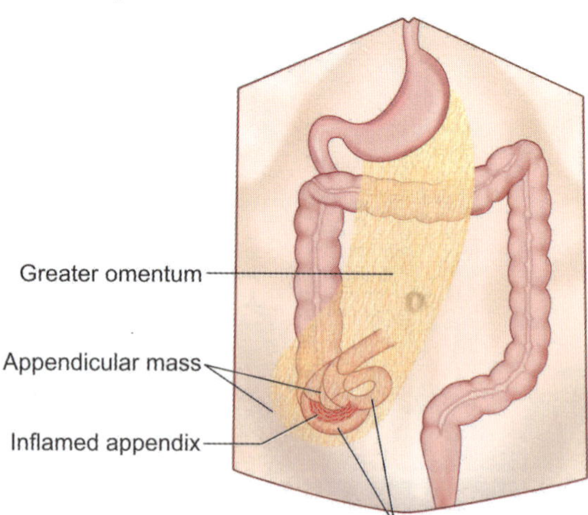

Appendicular mass is formed by dilated ileum; greater omentum; inflamed appendix and cecum. It is resonant, smooth, firm, and tender with well defined borders which does not move with respiration and does not have mobility

193. All of the following are true about achalasia cardia EXCEPT:

a. Bird beaks appearance
b. Absent air bubble in stomach
c. Decreased lower esophageal sphincter tone
d. Absent peristalsis in the body of esophagus

Esophageal manometry in achalasia cardia shows unrelaxed lower esophageal sphincter with high resting pressure/ tone – very useful and gold standard.

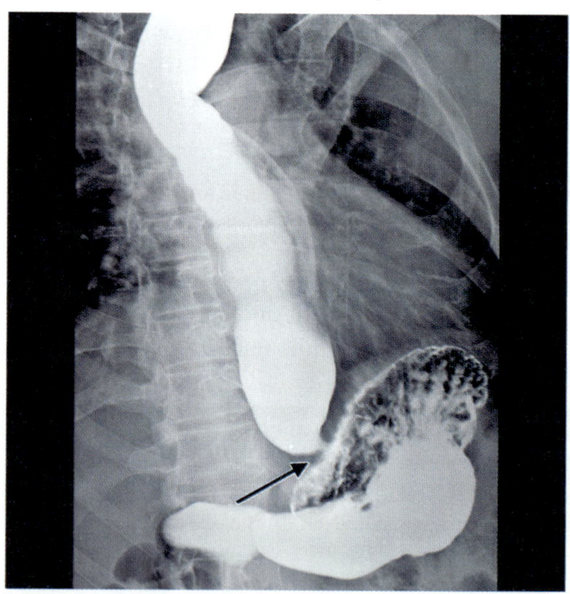

Barium swallow X-ray showing features of achalasia cardia

194. A patient after heavy drinking of alcohol presents with too much vomiting and hematemesis. Most likely diagnosis could be:

a. Mallory Weiss syndrome
b. Esophageal carcinoma
c. Achalasia cardia
d. Boerhaave syndrome

Mallory-Weiss syndrome is seen in adults with severe prolonged vomiting, causing longitudinal tear in the mucosa of stomach at and just below the cardia, leading to severe hematemesis. Violent vomiting often may be due to migraine or vertigo or following a bout of alcohol.

Ans. **192. b.** Appendicular... **193. c.** Decreased lower... **194. a.** Mallory Weiss...

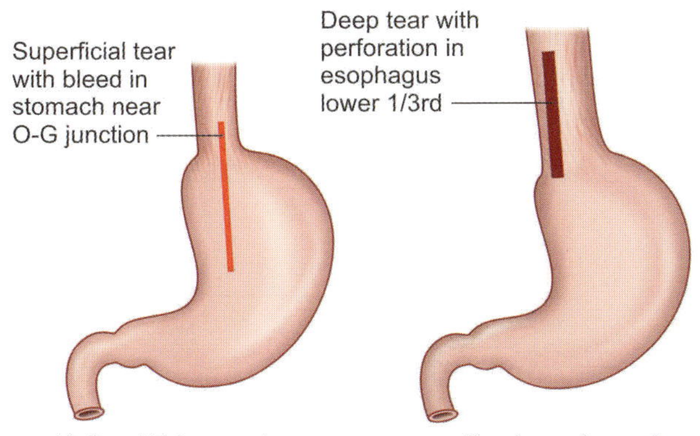

Diagrams showing Mallory-weiss syndrome and Boerhaave's syndrome

195. All of the following are common features of hemorrhoids EXCEPT:

a. Pain b. Anal irritation
c. Prolapse d. Bleeding

Clinical features of piles

- Bleeding—first symptom – 'splash in the pan' – 'bright red and fresh' – occurs during defecation
- Mass per anum/ prolapse
- Discharge – a mucoid discharge, causing irritation
- Pruritis
- Pain – may be due to prolapsed, infection or spasm

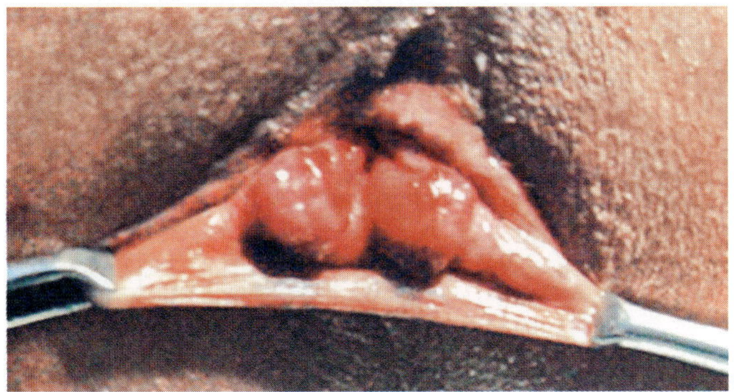

Parts of piles—plum coloured internal part and black cutaneous external component

HERNIA

196. True for femoral hernia are all EXCEPT:

a. Most common to strangulate
b. Absent cough impulse
c. More common in females
d. MC hernia in females

Femoral hernia is most common in females but most common hernia in females is indirect inguinal hernia (NOT femoral hernia)

197. Strangulation without obstruction is seen in:

a. Hernia-en-glissade b. Richter's hernia
c. Maydl's hernia d. Litter's hernia

Richter's hernia is a hernia in which the sac contains only a portion of the circumference of the intestine (small intestine). It mimics gastroenteritis with pain abdomen, diarrhea, toxicity and vomiting. There are no features of intestinal obstruction. Gangrene (strangulation) of part of bowel occurs, eventually leading to peritonitis.

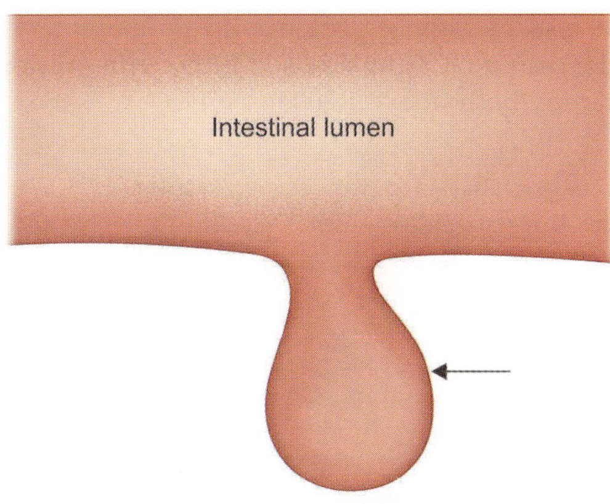

Richter's hernia.

198. NOT advisable in managing femoral hernia:

a. McEvedy's operation b. Truss
c. Lothenstein's operation d. Lockwood's operation

Rat tailed sprung truss is used in management of indirect inguinal hernia. Measurement is taken from the tip of greater trochanter to third piece of sacrum circumferentially. It may be used in elderly people who are not fit for anesthesia and surgery. Truss is absolutely contraindicated in femoral and sliding hernia.

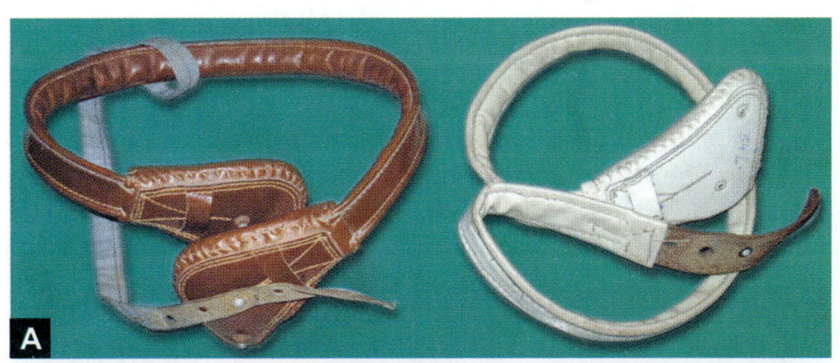

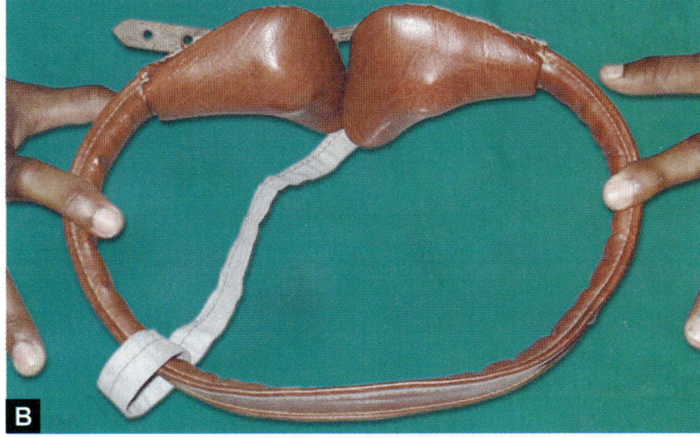

A and B: *Hernia truss*. It is used only when patient is not fit for surgery. It may precipitate strangulation. Before placing truss, contents of the hernia should be reduced completely

Ans. **195. a.** Pain **196. d.** MC hernia... **197. b.** Richter's hernia **198. b.** Truss

199. Viscera, forms posterior wall in which of the following hernia:

a. Lumbar hernia b. Sliding hernia
c. Epigastric hernia d. Femoral hernia

In sliding hernia/hernia-en-glissade, posterior wall of the sac is not only formed by the parietal peritoneum, but also by sigmoid colon with its mesentery on left side; cecum on right side and often with portion of the bladder (both sides) (1:2000).

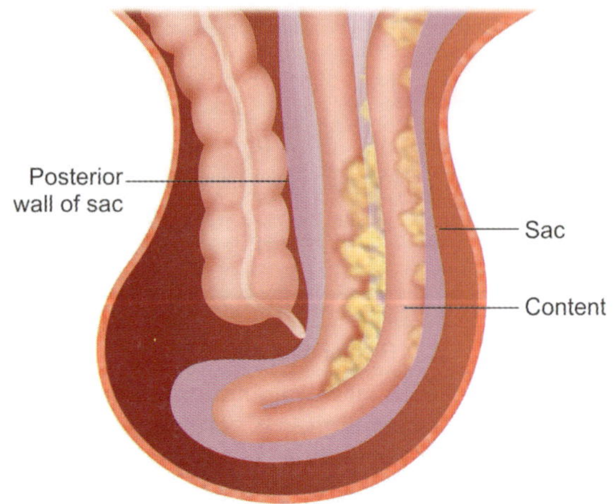

Sliding hernia (*Hernia-en-Glissade*)

200. The treatment of choice from inguinal hernia in infants is:

a. Herniotomy b. Herniorrhaphy
c. Truss d. Hernioplasty

In infants, whether it is hernia or hydrocele, only herniotomy is done through inguinal approach (Michaelis plank operation). In adults herniotomy (excision of sac) and herniorrhaphy or hernioplasty (ideal; strengthening of the posterior wall of inguinal canal either by repair or mesh.) is done.

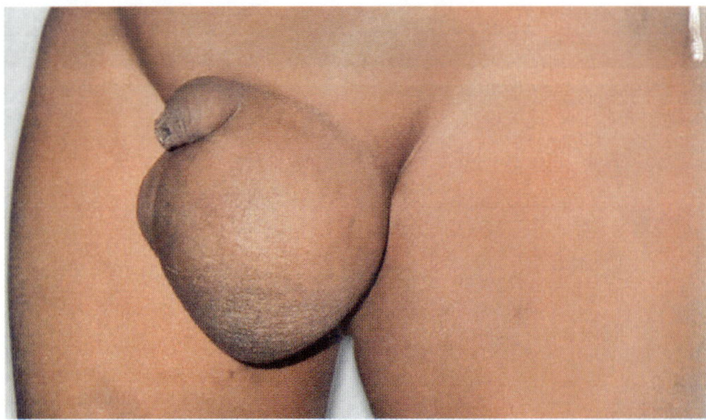

Inguinal hernia in 4-year-old child. Here just herniotomy is required. Repair is not done.

201. True for femoral hernia:

a. Occurs exclusively in females
b. Pregnancy is common cause
c. Does not strangulate
d. In males, associated with cryptorchidism

Etiology of femoral hernia includes wide femoral canal and multiple pregnancies.

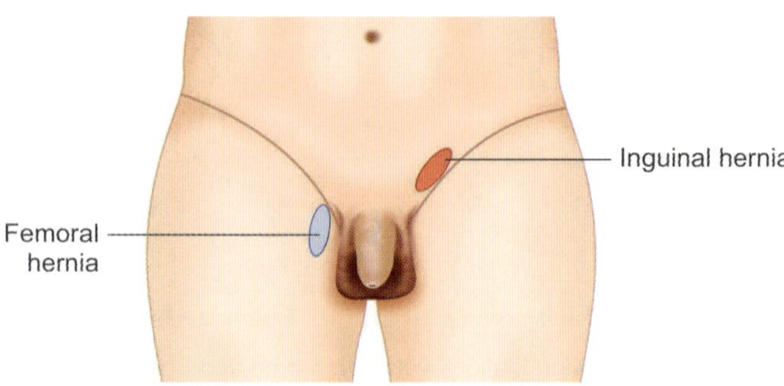

Hernia; inguinal hernia is above and medial to tubercle, and femoral hernia is below and lateral

202. Howship-Romberg sign is associated with:

a. Carcinoma rectum
b. Diaphragmatic hernia
c. Obturator hernia
d. Splenic rupture

Obturator hernia is hernia occurring through obturator canal between superior ramus of pubis and obturator membrane. Referred pain in knee joint through geniculate branch of obturator nerve signifies not only obturator hernia but also strangulation – Howship-Romberg sign (50%).

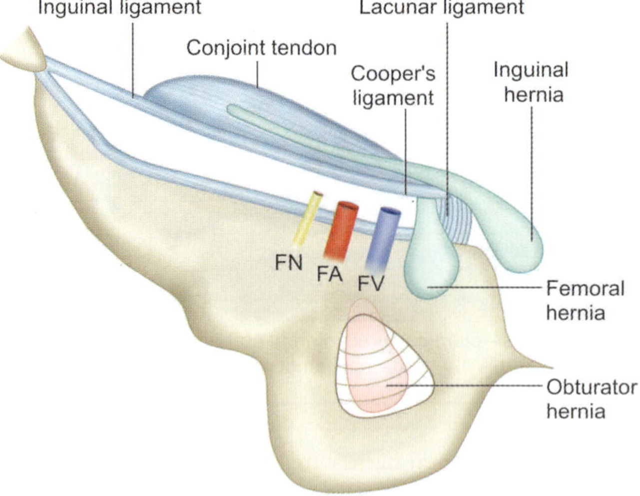

Obturator hernia through obturator canal in obturator foramen. Note also the locations of inguinal and femoral hernias

203. True statement regarding direct inguinal hernia:

a. Most common direct inguinal hernia in women
b. Direct hernia is medial to inferior epigastric artery
c. Repair of the transversalis fascia and the internal ring
d. Descends downwards and inwards towards the scrotum

Ans. 199. **b.** Sliding hernia 200. **a.** Herniotomy 201. **b.** Pregnancy is... 202. **c.** Obturator hernia 203. **b.** Direct hernia...

Direct hernia occurs through the posterior wall of the inguinal canal through 'Hesselbach's triangle' (bounded medially by the lateral border of rectus muscle, laterally by inferior epigastric artery, below by inguinal ligament). Sac is medial to the inferior epigastric artery.

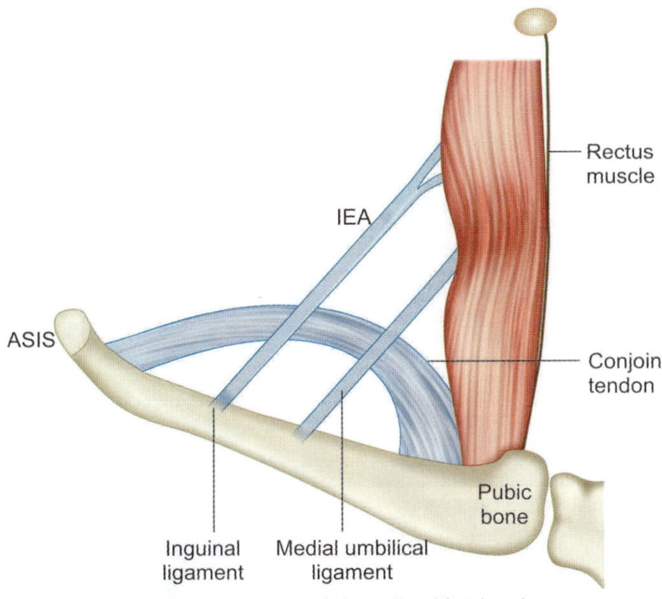

Surgical anatomy of Hesselbach's triangle

204. Mayo operation is done for:

a. Spigelian hernia
b. Femoral hernia
c. Richter's hernia
d. Umbilical hernia

Mayo's operation for umbilical hernia: Here horizontally opened rectus sheath is approximated as double breasting with upper flap overlapping lower flap in front. It is rarely done today.

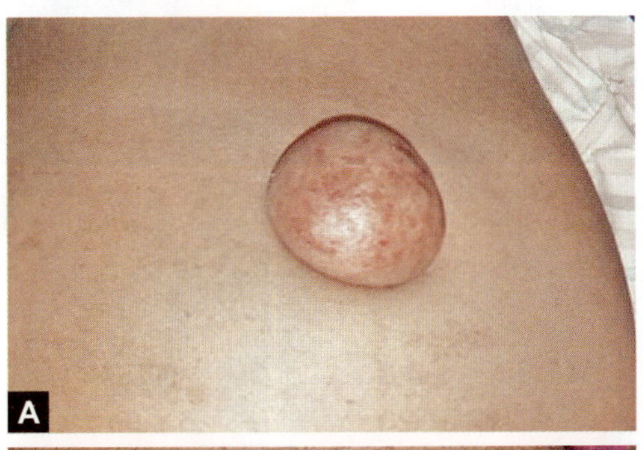

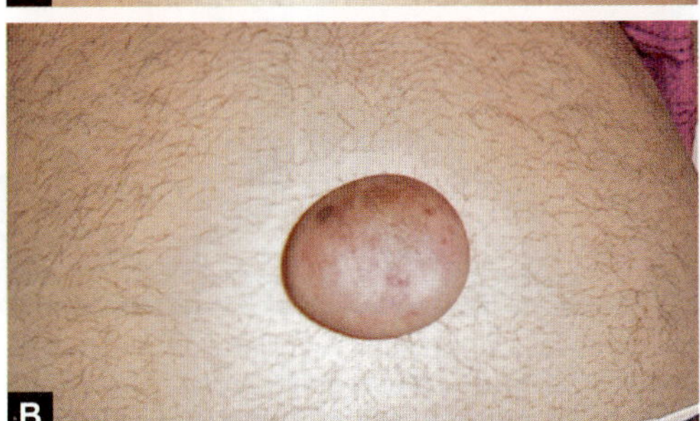

A and B: Umbilical hernia. Often it can attain large size

205. True about direct inguinal hernia are all EXCEPT:

a. It is more common in female
b. Less common than indirect
c. Direct hernia is less likely to undergo strangulation
d. Uncommon in children

Direct inguinal hernia is uncommon in females and children.

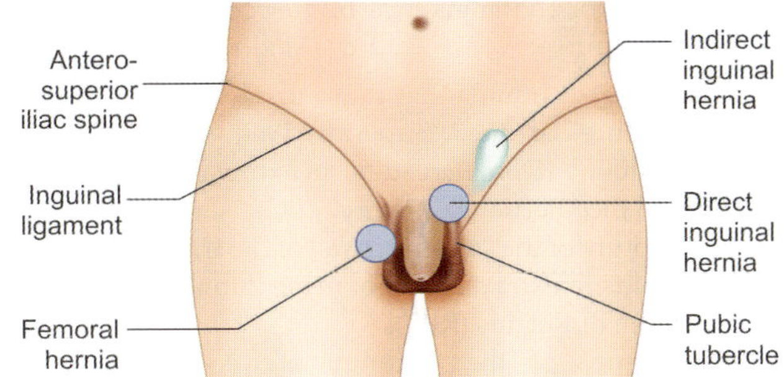

Location of direct and indirect inguinal hernia and femoral hernia

206. A 6 month old child presents with congenital inguinal hernia. Next step would be:

a. Observation
b. Wait for 3 years and operate
c. Operate immediately
d. Truss

Herniotomy is done in hernia in infants.

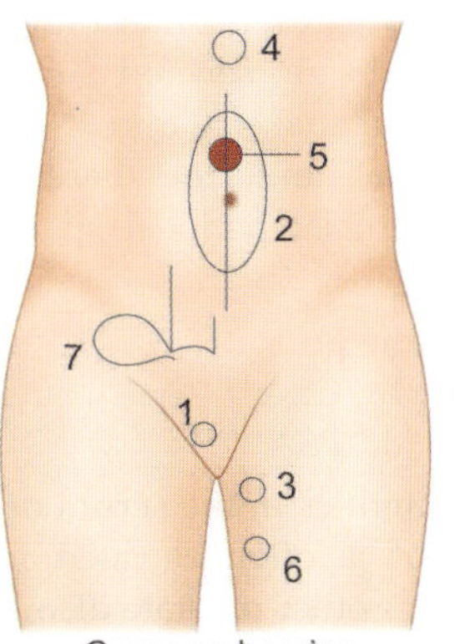

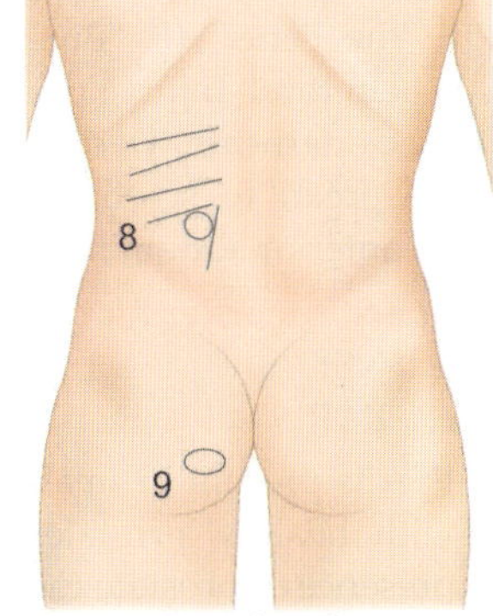

Common hernias
1. Inguinal
2. Incisional
3. Femoral
4. Epigastric
5. Umbilical

Rare hernias:
6. Obturator
7. Spigelian
8. Lumbar
9. Gluteal

Common and rare sites of hernias

GENITOURINARY SYSTEM

207. Feature of Struvite stones:

a. Because of high calcium diet
b. Painless hematuria is the initial presentation
c. Most common type of renal stones
d. Associated with alkaline urine

Struvite stones (also known as "infection stones", urease or triple-phosphate stones), form most often in the presence of infection by urea-splitting bacteria. Using

Ans. 204. **d.** Umbilical hernia 205. **a.** It is more common... 206. **c.** Operate immediately 207. **d.** Associated with...

the enzyme urease, these organisms metabolize urea into ammonia and carbon dioxide. This alkalinizes the urine, resulting in favorable conditions for the formation of struvite stones.

208. Rupture of urethra above the urogenital diaphragm, due to pelvic fracture will result in extravasation of urine in:

a. Anterior abdominal wall b. Retropubic space
c. Scrotum d. Medial aspect of thigh

Five areas of trauma that cause urine leakage

- Rupture of the "Superior Wall of the Urinary Bladder" (Dome) results in extravasation of urine into the "Peritoneal Cavity" (PC).
- Rupture of the "Anterior Wall of the Urinary Bladder" results in extravasation of urine into the "Retropubic Space of Retzius (RPS).
- Rupture of the "Urethra above the Urogenital Diaphragm"(UG) results in extravasation of urine into the "Retropubic space of Retzius".
- Rupture of the "Urethra below the Urogenital Diaphragm" results in extravasation of urine into the "Superficial Perineal space". (Extravasated urine within the superficial perineal space can extend into the scrotal, penile, and anterior abdominal wall areas)
- Rupture of the "Penile Urethra" with intact Buck Fascia results in extravasation of urine "Beneath the Deep Fascia of Buck" and will remain "Confined to the Penis" (If "Buck Fascia get severed" in Penile Urethral Injury, urine will make it into the space Underneath Dartos Fascia" and from here it can spread to scrotum, superficial perineal space and anterior abdominal wall)

209. Specific marker for carcinoma prostate:

a. NSE b. CEA
c. PAP d. PSA

PSA is present in small quantities in the serum of men with healthy prostates, but is often elevated in the presence of prostate cancer or other prostate disorders.

210. Tumour marker assessed to monitor the recurrence of carcinoma prostate in an elderly male treated by radiotherapy for carcinoma prostate:

a. AFP & CEA b. PSA only
c. PSA & CEA d. CEA only

PSA levels are monitored periodically (e.g., every 6–36 months) after treatment for prostate cancer — more frequently in patients with high-risk disease, less frequently in patients with lower-risk disease. If surgical therapy (i.e., radical prostatectomy) is successful at removing all prostate tissue (and prostate cancer), PSA becomes undetectable within a few weeks. A subsequent rise in PSA level above 0.2 ng/mL is generally regarded as evidence of recurrent prostate cancer after a radical prostatectomy.

211. First symptom of TB of kidney is:

a. Pain
b. Hesistancy
c. Increased frequency of micturition
d. Hematuria

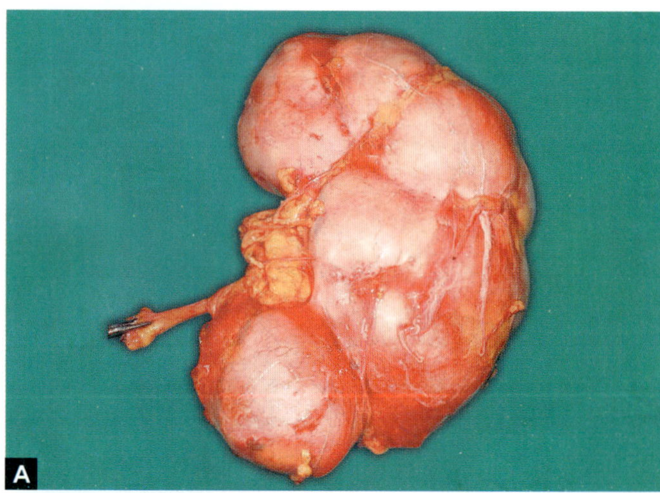

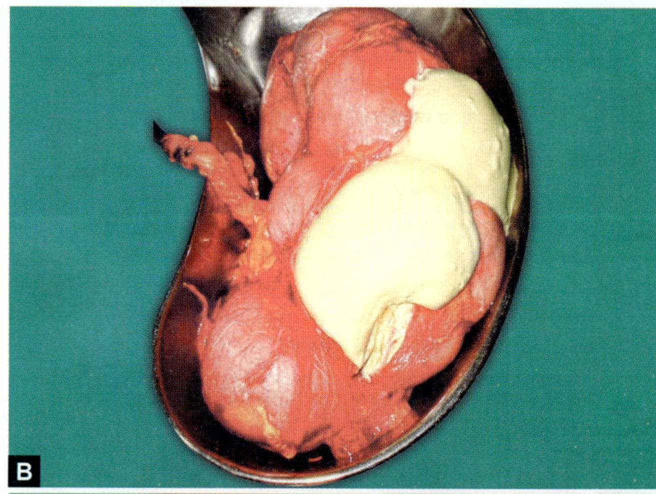

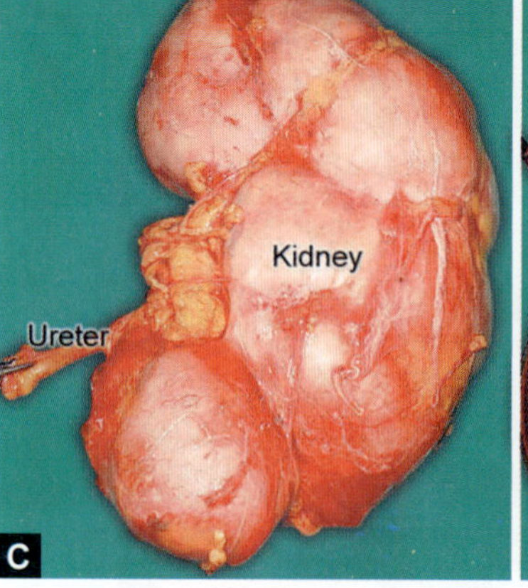

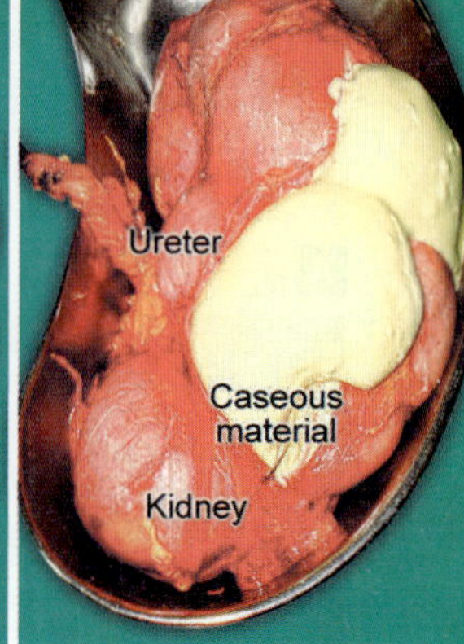

A to C: Specimen of kidney showing dilatation and caseous material as content. It is tuberculous pyonephrosis. Ureter is visualized in the specimen. Often there may be ureteric stricture due to tuberculosis

Ans. 208. b. Retropubic... 209. d. PSA 210. b. PSA only 211. c. Increased frequency...

Clinical features of renal TB

- Common in males
- Common on right side
- Frequency – both day and night
- Polyuria
- Sterile pyuria: Urine is palse and opalescent with presence of pus cells without organisms in an acid urine – a bacterial aciduria (other causes: Interstitial cystitis, chlamydia)

212. Cannon balls shadows in lungs are characteristic of:

a. Pheochromocytoma
b. Hypernephroma
c. Carcinoid
d. Seminoma testes

Renal cell carcinoma/Hypernephroma/Grawitz tumor/ Clear cell carcinoma/Internist tumor enters the renal vein as proliferative tumour thrombus, which extends into the IVC and later gets detached causing 'cannon ball secondaries' in the lung, which are often calcified. Once primary tumor is removed, secondaries may regress due to tumor immunity.

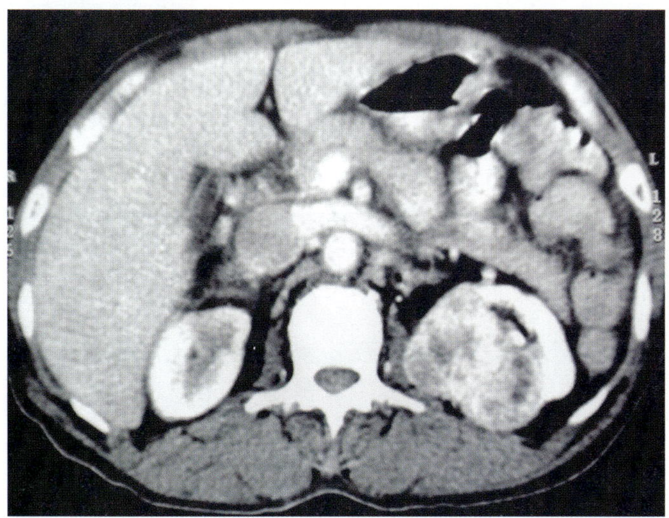

CT scan showing RCC—left sided

213. MC predisposing factor for pyelonephritis is:

a. Vesico-ureteric reflux
b. Posterior urethral valve
c. Calculi
d. Diabetes

Any structural abnormalities in the urinary tract, vesicoureteral reflux, kidney stones, urinary tract catheterization, ureteral stents or drainage procedures (e.g. nephrostomy), pregnancy, neurogenic bladder and BPH (in men) can cause inflammation of the kidney tissue, calcyes, and renal pelvis (pyelonephritis).

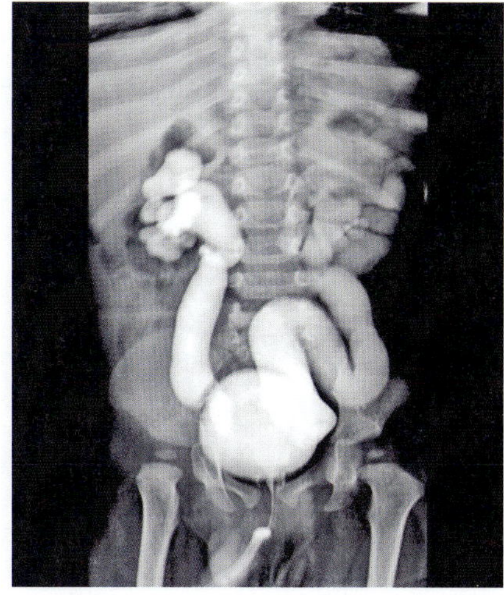

Micturating cystourethrogram (MCU) showing gross vesicoureteric reflux on both sides

214. Most malignant testicular tumor:

a. Seminoma
b. Choriocarcinoma
c. Teartocarcinoma
d. Teratoma

Pure choriocarcinoma of the testis represents the most aggressive pathologic variant of germ cell tumors in adults, characteristically with early hematogenous and lymphatic spread. Because of the early spread and inherent resistance to anticancer drugs, patients have poor prognosis.

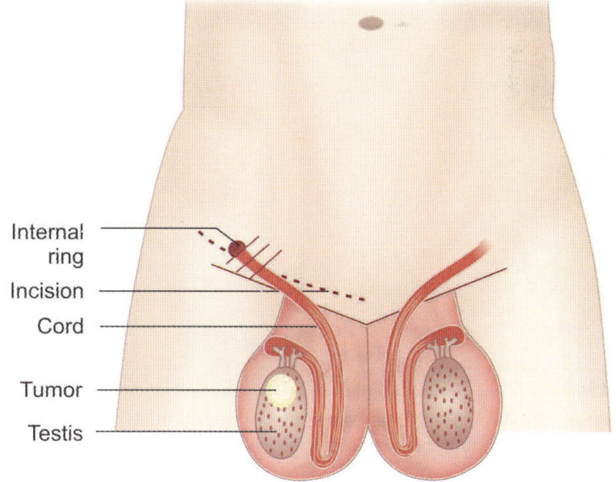

High orchidectomy is done for testicular tumor through inguinal approach. Not through scrotal incision. Cord is ligated at the level of the internal ring

215. NOT a feature of triad of Wilm's tumor:

a. Fever
b. Mass abdomen
c. Pain
d. Hematuria

Triad of Wilm's tumor/ nephroblastoma include mass, fever and hematuria. Mass abdomen is the commonest presentation.

Ans. **212. b.** Hypernephroma **213. a.** Vesico-ureteric reflux **214. b.** Choriocarcinoma **215. c.** Pain

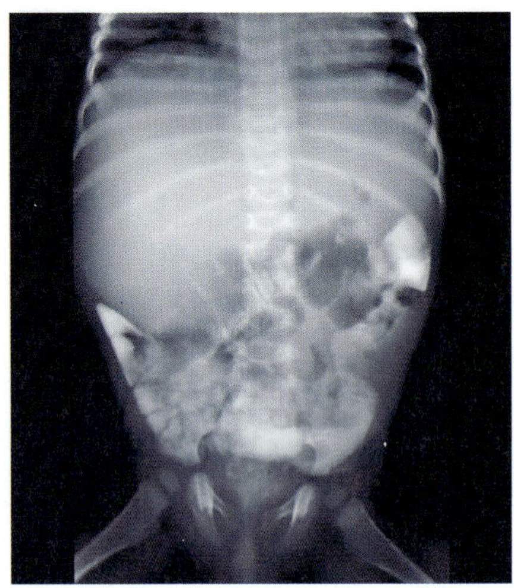
X-ray showing mass lesion in right abdomen. It could be Wilm's tumor

216. Serum acid phosphatase is raised in:
a. Osteosarcoma
b. Prostatic carcinoma
c. Paget's disease
d. Hyperparathyroidism

Prostatic fraction of acid phosphatase is increased in carcinoma prostate.

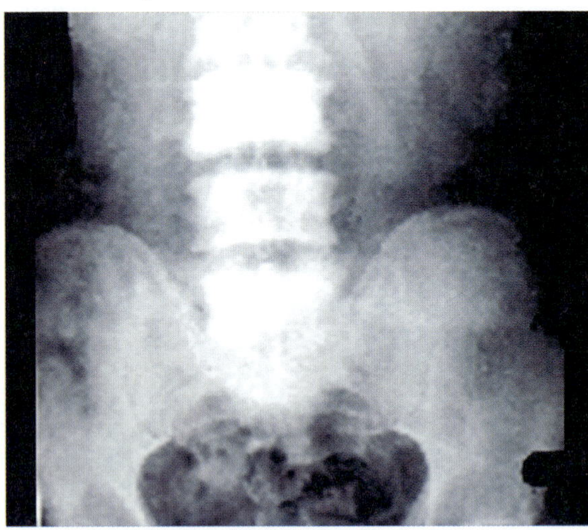
A plain X-ray AP view of lumbar spine in a patient with carcinoma prostate. Note the typical osteosclerotic secondaries

217. Most common tumor in undescended testes:
a. Teratoma
b. Seminoma
c. Both
d. None

Malignant transformation inundescended testis is 20 times more common than normally descended testis. It is higher in abdominal than in inguinally located testis. Seminoma is the most common malignancy in undescended testis.

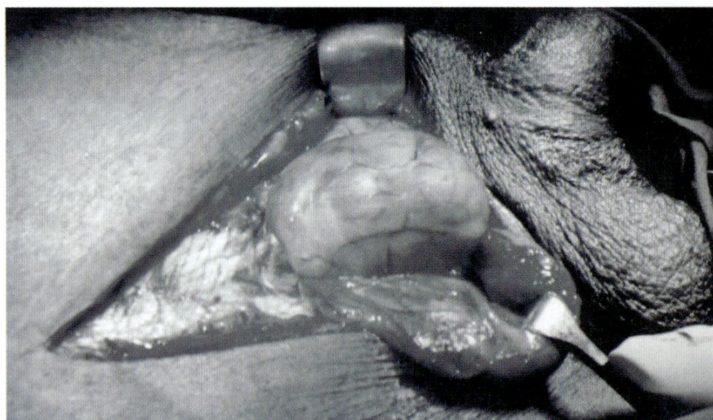
Undescended testis which has turned into seminoma testis

218. Mucus strings in urine suggests:
a. Pyelonephritis
b. Prostatitis
c. Cystitis
d. Urethritis

Clinical features of cystitis
- Painful urination, frequency, strangury, incomplete emptying, with often retention
- Occassionally hematuria may occur
- Burning urine, discolored foul smelling urine
- Fever, chills, rigors, suprapubic pain and tenderness and often joint pain.

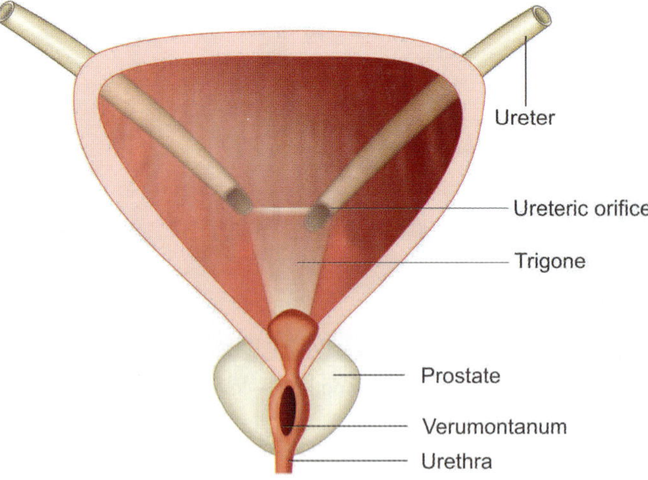

Urinary bladder—inner anatomy

219. Hydrocele is a type of:
a. Retention cyst
b. Distension cyst
c. Exudation cyst
d. Traumatic cyst

In the adult, a hydrocele is an accumulation of excessive secretion of the vaginal mucosa; exudates collect in the non-communicative vaginal cavities.

Ans. 216. **b.** Prostatic... 217. **b.** Seminoma 218. **c.** Cystitis 219. **c.** Exudation cyst

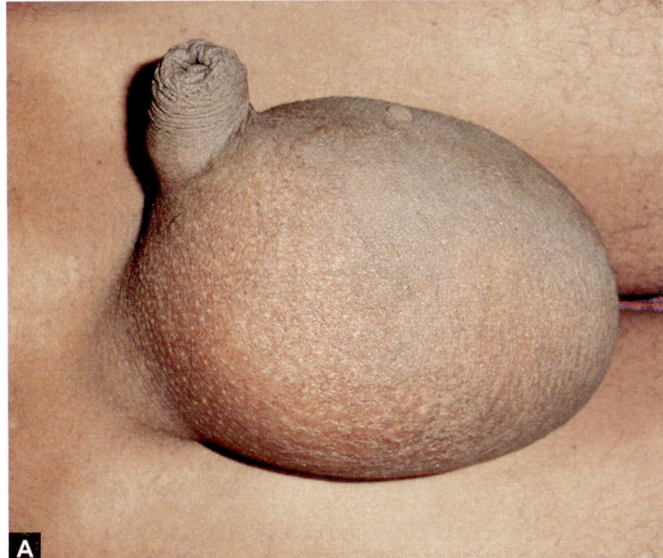

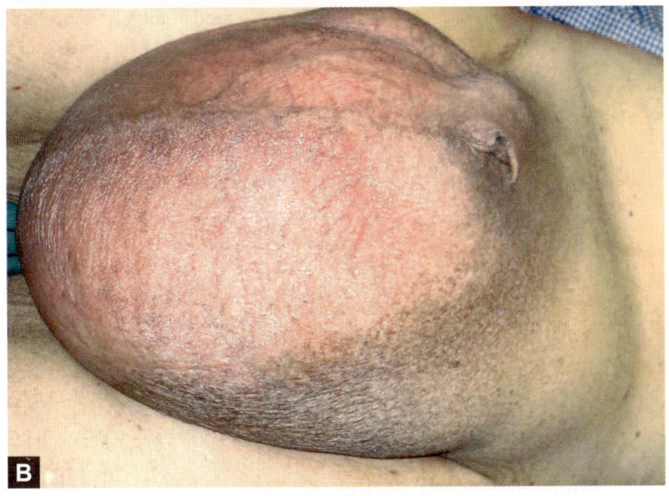

A and B: Hydrocele in two different patients. One is average sized; another is large and penis is buried into the hydrocele swelling

220. Drug NOT used for detrusor instability:

a. Tiaperetide
b. Flavoxate
c. Solifenacin
d. Duloxetine

Duloxetine is a serotonin-norepinephrine reuptake inhibitor (SNRI), which is mostly prescribed for major depressive disorder, generalized anxiety disorder, fibromyalgia and neuropathic pain.

221. Most important prognostic indicator of renal cell carcinoma:

a. Pathological staging
b. Size
c. Histological type
d. Nuclear grade

Prognosis of RCC

- Five year survival rate is 40%
- In early localized disease, it is 70–90%. In advanced and metastatic disease, it is 10-15%
- 5-year survival is 65% for stage I and II; 40% for stage III; 10% for stage IV.

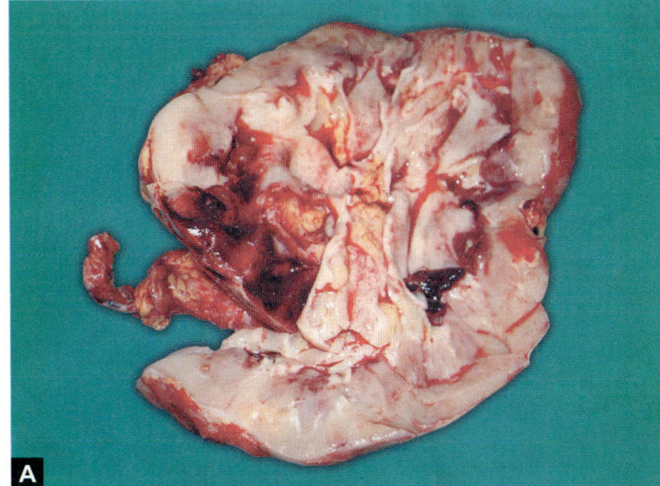

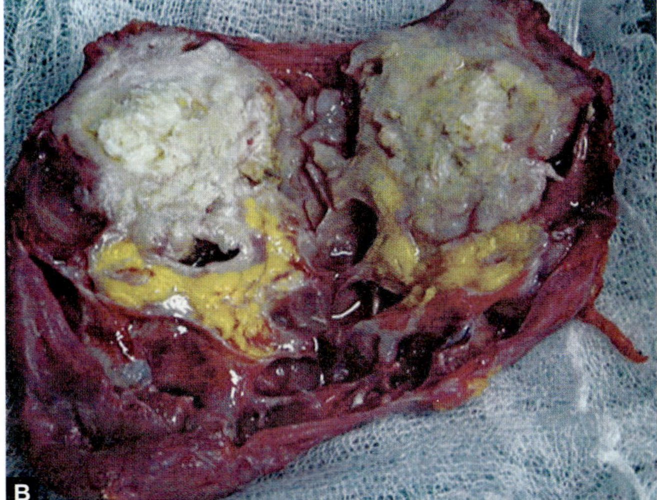

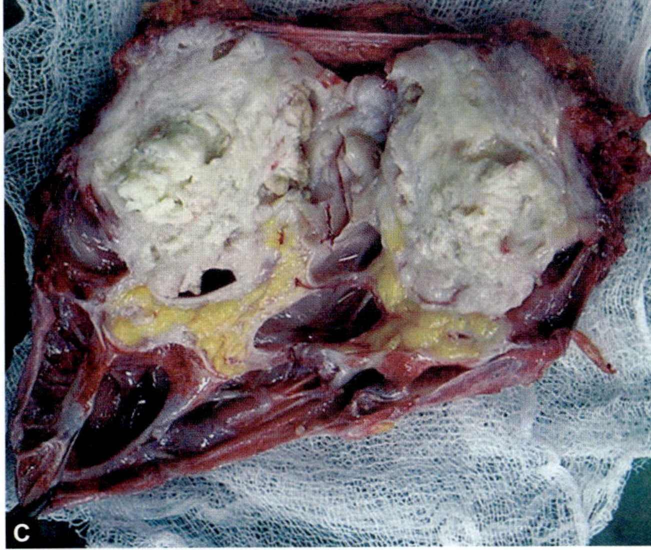

A to C: Renal cell carcinoma in upper pole of kidney—resected specimen. It is from two different patients

Ans. 220. **d.** Duloxetine 221. **a.** Pathological staging

222. Screening test for prostate carcinoma:

a. MRI enhanced imaging b. DRE and PSA
c. Prostatic specific antigen
d. Digital rectal examination

Screening of carcinoma prostate

- On per rectal examination, prostate feels hard, nodular, irregular often with loss of median groove
- Prostatic specific antigen/ PSA: More than 10 nmol/ mL is suggestive.

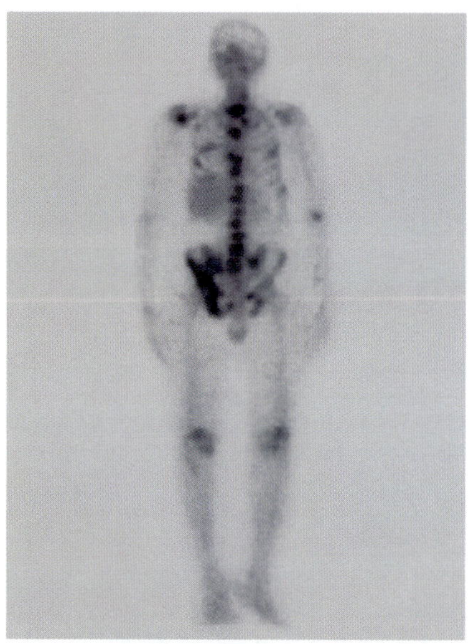

Carcinoma prostate showing skeletal secondaries in bone scan.

223. Ideal time for orchidopexy in case of undescended testes:

a. Neonatal period b. 1 year
c. 5–6 years d. Before puberty

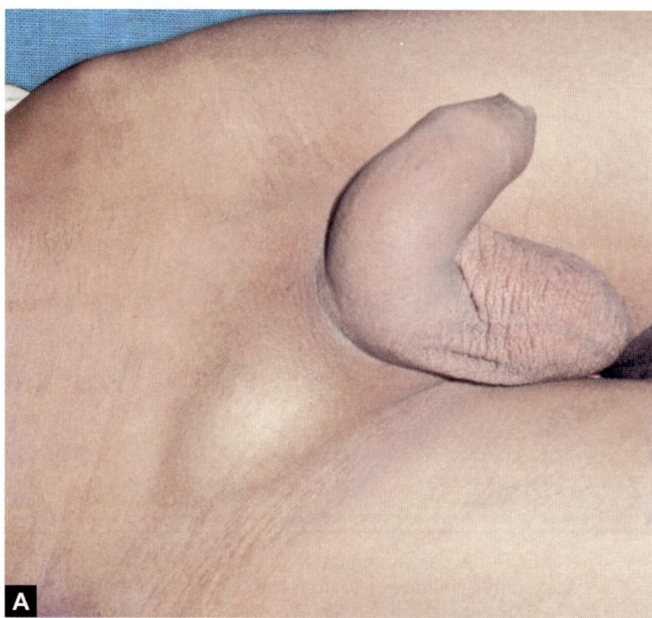

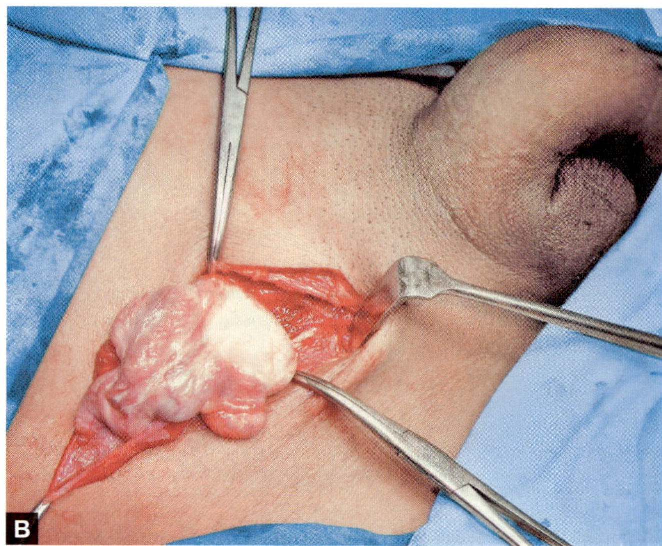

A and B: Undescended testis in the inguinal region. Right-sided scrotum is underdeveloped. On table finding seen in the same patient. Hernia is the common association.

For undescended testis (unilateral), surgery is done between two and four years of age. If bilateral cases, there should be a gap of 6 months. Orchidexopexy does not alter/reduce the risk of development of carcinoma of testis.

224. LDH is raised in:

a. Choriocarcinoma
b. Teratoma
c. Seminoma
d. All of the above

LDH level depends on growth rate/ cellular proliferation/ tumor burden. LDH is increased in 80% of advanced seminomas and 60% of non-seminomatous germ cell tumor (teratomas, endodermal sinus carcinoma/yolk sac tumor, choriocarcinoma, embryonal carcinoma)

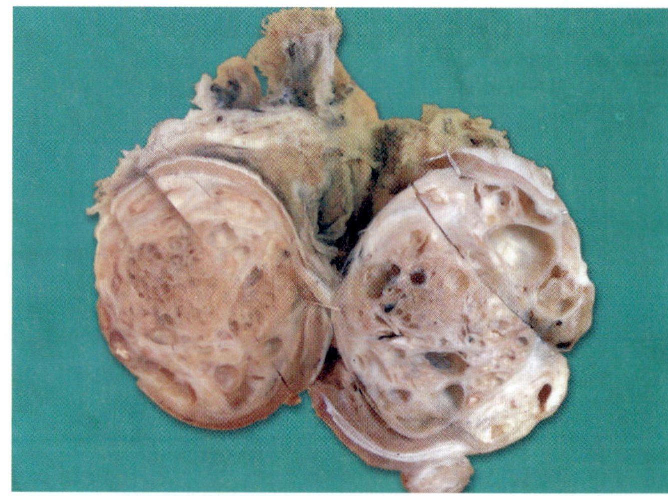

Specimen of testicular tumor. Note the cystic and solid areas of teratoma

Ans. 222. **b.** DRE and PSA 223. **b.** 1 year 224. **d.** All of the above

225. Lord's and Jabouley's operation is done for:

a. Rectal prolapse b. Fistula in Ano
c. Inguinal hernia d. Hydrocele

Treatment of hydrocele

- If the sac is small, thin and contains clear fluid, either Lord's pliaction, i.e. tunica is bunched into a 'ruff' by placing series of multiple interrupted chromic catgut sutures so as to make the sac to form fibrous tissues (It is relatively avascular and so hematoma will not occur).
- Or evacuation and eversion of the sac behind the testis (after eversion, everted sac is sutured with chromic catgut by continuous sutures) is done.
- Often the sac is excised partially and then eversion is done, which is called as Jabouley's operation.

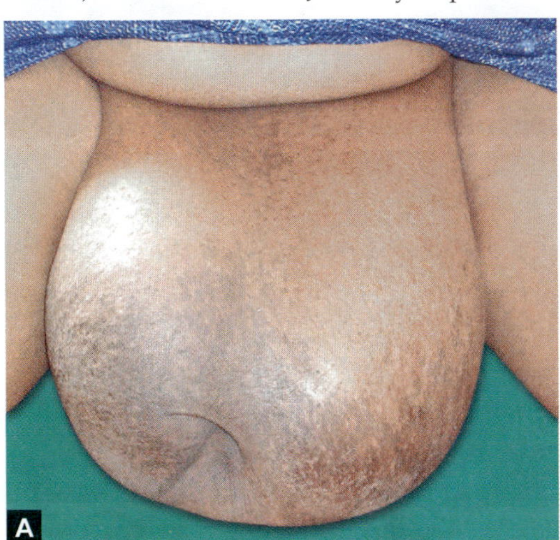

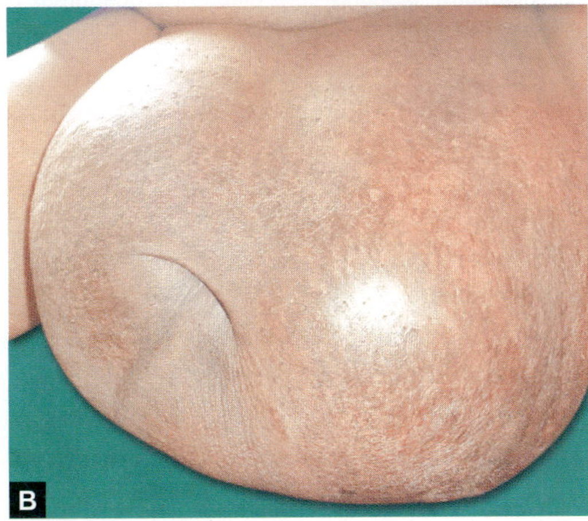

A and B: Massive hydrocele wherein penis is buried completely within the hydrocele area

226. 'Golf-hole' ureteric orifice is seen in:

a. Ureteric calculus b. Ureteral polyp
c. Tuberculosis of urinary bladder
d. Retroperitoneal fibrosis

Tuberculous cystitis eventually results in golf hole ureter and thimble bladder (cystoscopic findings). This is due to fibrosis causing rigid withdrawn dilated ureteric orifice looking like golf hole. Entire urinary bladder gets fibrosed, stiff and unable to dilate and accommodate urine causing thimble systolic bladder.

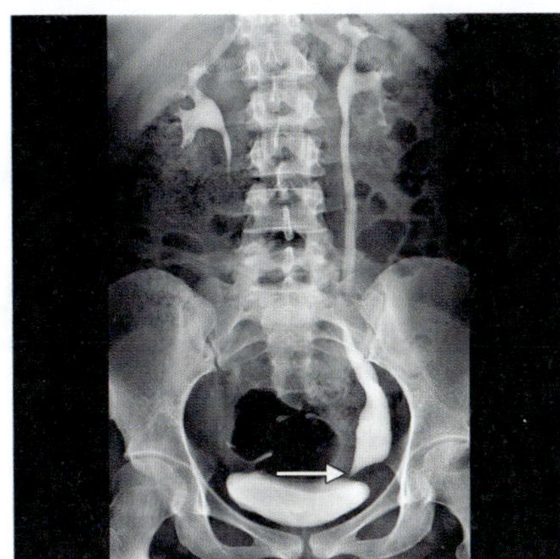

Stricture of left ureter lower part—IVU picture. Common cause is tuberculosis of ureter

227. Cause of bladder cancer are all EXCEPT:

a. Alcohol
b. Naphthylamine exposure
c. Cigarette smoking d. Cyclophosphamide

Etiology of transitional cell carcinoma include 3C's: **C**hemical carcinogens (2-Naphthylamine, aminobiphenyl, benzidine, chloro-O-toluidine, chloro-aniline), **C**igarette smoking and **C**yclophosphamide.

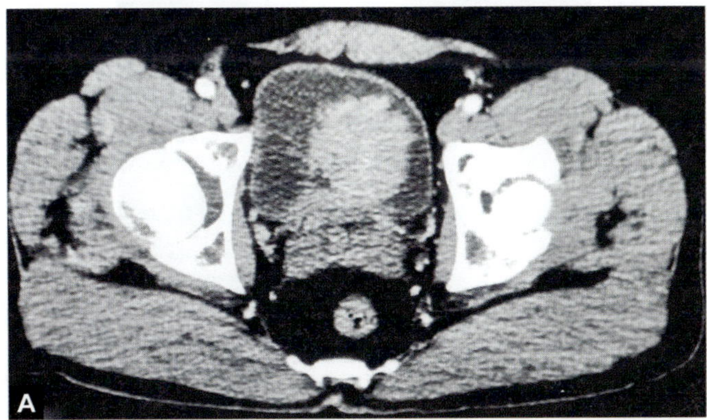

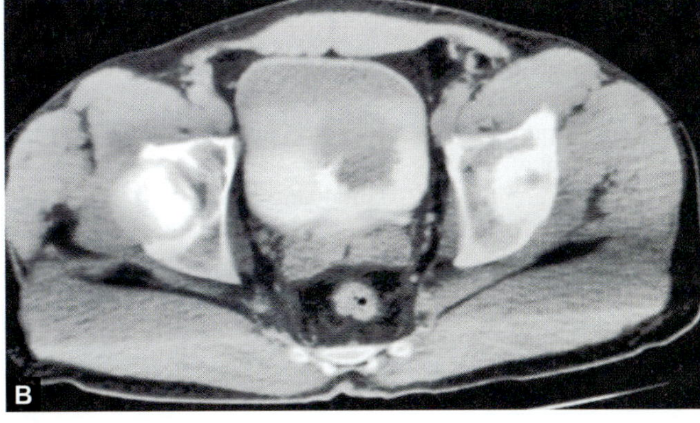

Ans. 225. **d.** Hydrocele 226. **c.** Tuberculosis... 227. **a.** Alcohol

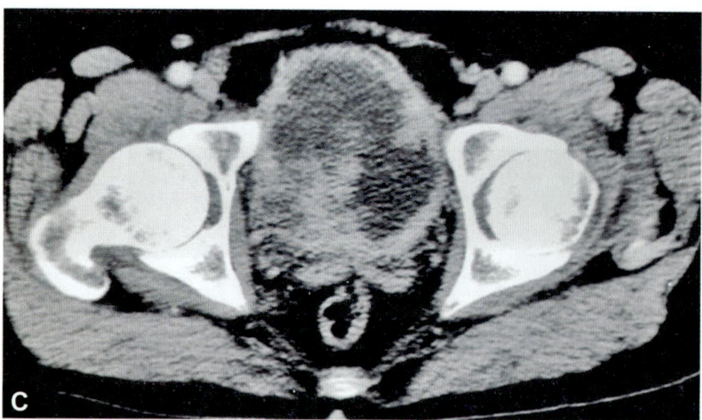

A to C: CT scan picture showing irregularity in bladder mucosa—carcinoma urinary bladder

228. In a patient suspected to be suffering from vesico-ureteric reflex, which one of the following radiological investigations may confirm the diagnosis:

a. Intravenous urography
b. Micturating cysto-urethrography
c. Pelvic ultrasound
d. Antegrade pyelography

MCU is indicated in vesico-ureteric reflux and posterior urethral valve.

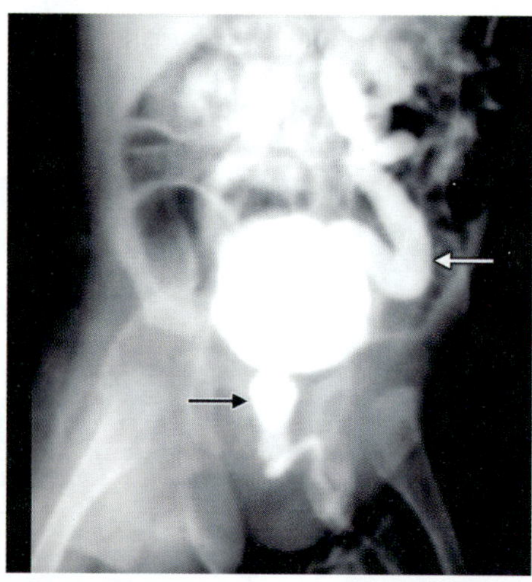

Micturating cystourethrogram showing concomitant existence of posterior urethral valve (causing dilatation of proximal urethra) and vesicoureteric reflux (left side)

229. 60-year-old undergoes TURP. After 3 days, patient develops altered sensitiveness and drowsiness. Most probable diagnosis is:

a. Hypernatremia   b. Hyponatremia
c. Stroke
d. Meningitis due to spinal anesthesia

Post-TURP complications

- Water intoxication with congestive cardiac failure – TURP syndrome
- Hyponatremia
- Hemorrhage
- Infection

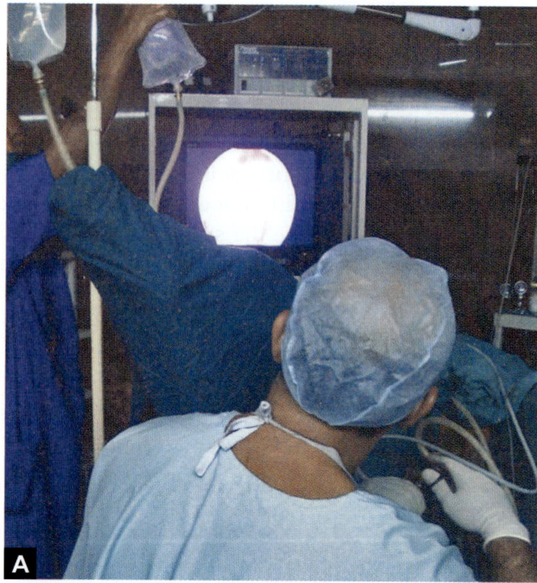

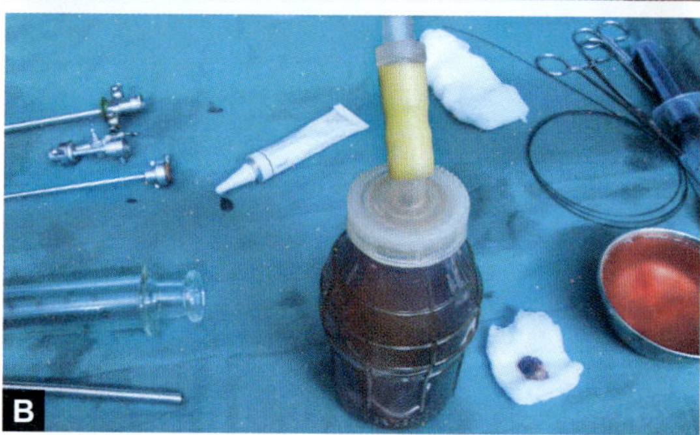

A and B: Endotherapy for BPH—TURP is the most common procedure; laser (holmium), stenting—are different procedures. TURP set is shown on the table with evacuator to remove fragmented prostate tissue

230. The common organism isolated in emphysematous pyelonephritis/ EPN is:

a. E. coli
b. Proteus
c. Pseudomonas
d. Klebsiella

Among the bacteria associated with EPN, Escherichia coli is isolated in 66% of patients and Klebsiella species are reported in 26%.

231. Renal calculi associated with proteus infection:

a. Uric acid
b. Triple phosphate
c. Calcium oxalate
d. Xanthine

Phosphate stone (10–15%) is either calcium phosphate or calcium, magnesium, ammonium phosphate stone usually occurring in an infected urine. Urea splitting organisms commonly cause stone formation, i.e. E. coli, Staphylococcus, Streptococcus, Proteus.

Ans. **228. b.** Micturating... **229. b.** Hyponatremia **230. a.** E. coli **231. b.** Triple phosphate

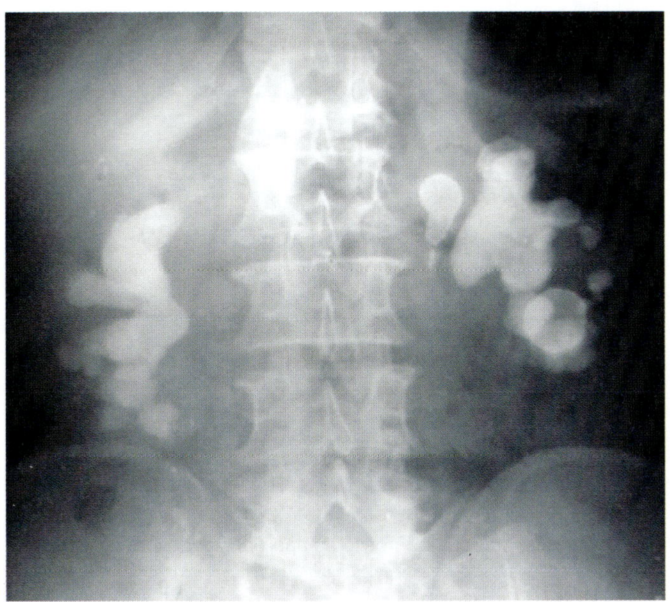

Bilateral staghorn calculi

232. In a patient with stage I (confined to mucosa and submucosa) transitional cell carcinoma of the urinary bladder, the recommended treatment is:

a. Transurethral resection of bladder tumour (TURBT)
b. Radical cystectomy
c. Radiation therapy
d. Systemic chemotherapy

Management of non-invasive tumor

- Endoscopic resection of tumour
- Intravesical chemotherapy using BCG, mitomycin-C, epirubicin, adriamycin, thiotepa, methotrexate
- Systemic chemotherapy: Using cisplatin, 5-FU, adriamycin, mitomycin
- Helmstein balloon degeneration for large papillary tumor.

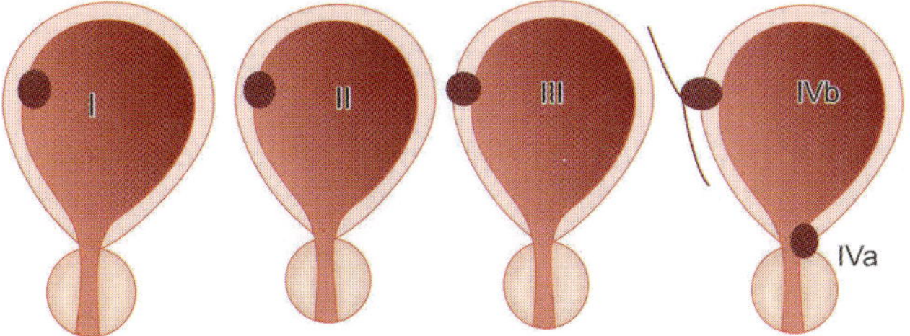

Staging of bladder tumor

233. A lady who presented with hematuria was found to have stage II transitional cell carcinoma of bladder. Which of the following statement about management of her condition is true:

a. Cystoscopic falguration is the standard treatment
b. 70% chance of requiring cystectomy in 5 years after TUR
c. History of smoking is NOT a risk factor
d. There is no role of chemotherapy

Surgery/partial cystectomy is done when the tumor is confined to fundus of the bladder and is single, with a margin of clearance of 2.5 cm. External beam radiotherapy and chemotherapy should be given.

Staging (Refer Fig. 26.104)	
Jewett-Strong-Marshall staging	
I	Tumor confined to subepithelial connective tissue
II	Muscle infiltration superficially
III	Full thickness muscle and perivesical tissue infiltrated, but mobile
IV	Fixed to adjacent organs
	IVa (prostate)
	IVb (pelvic wall)

234. FALSE regarding varicocele:

a. Varicosity of cremasteric veins
b. Left sided affected usually
c. Feels like a bag of worms
d. May lead to infertility

Varcicocele is dilatation and tortuosity of the pampiniform plexus of veins and so the testicular veins.

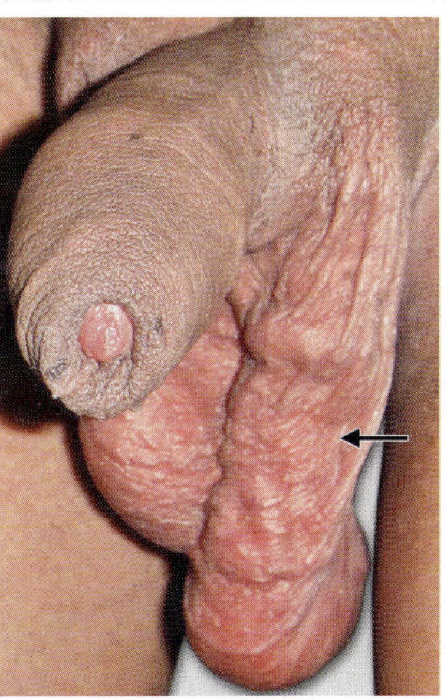

Clinical photo of left sided varicocele—'bag of worms' look

235. Commonest cause of ureteric injury during surgical operation is:

a. Abdomino-perineal resection
b. Hysterectomy
c. Prostatectomy
d. Colectomy

In females, uterine artery crosses the ureter from lateral to medial side, about 2 cm lateral to the cervix (this has to be remembered while ligating the uterine arteries in hysterectomy).

Ans. 232. a. Transurethral... **233. b.** 70% chance of req... **234. a.** Varicosity of... **235. b.** Hysterectomy

236. Prostatic carcinoma commonly arises from:

a. Central zone b. Peripheral zone
c. Transitional zone d. None of the above

Carcinoma prostate occurs in peripheral zone in prostatic gland proper, i.e. commonly in posterior lobe. So prostatectomy for BPH does not confer protection against development of carcinoma prostate.

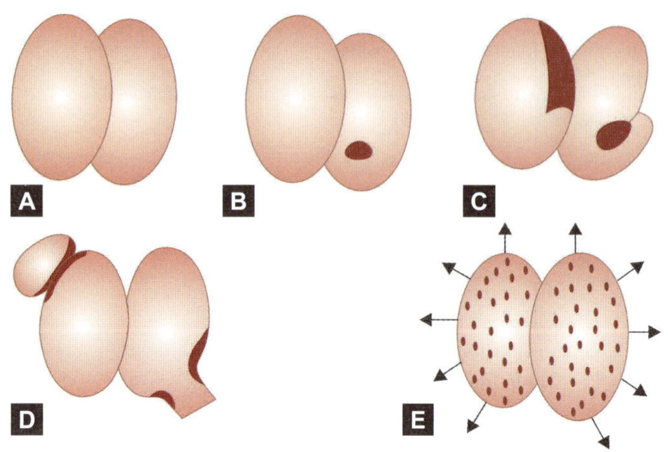

A to E: Staging of Ca prostate (A) Occult, (B) Stage I, (C) Stage II, (D) Stage III, (E) Stage IV

237. True regarding predisposing factors for penile carcinoma are all EXCEPT:

a. Paget's disease b. Genital warts
c. Circumcision d. Leucoplakia

Circumcision done during infancy confers total immunity against carcinoma penis.

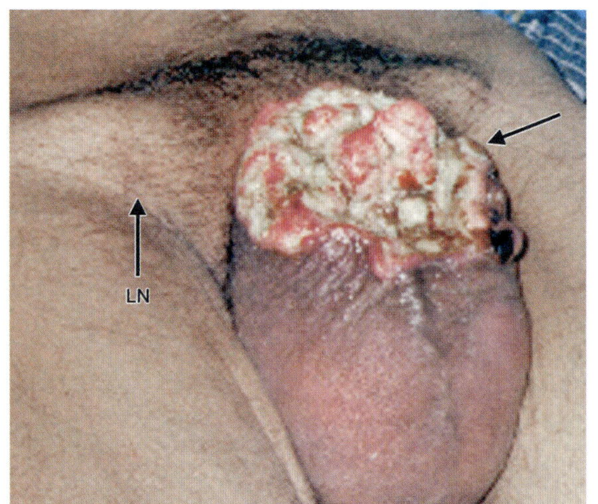

Carcinoma of penis causing destruction of entire penis

238. Undescended testis can lead to all of the following complications EXCEPT:

a. Torsion b. Sterility
c. Carcinoma d. Hypertrophy of testes

Testicular atrophy (NOT hypertrophy) is one of the complications of undescended testis.

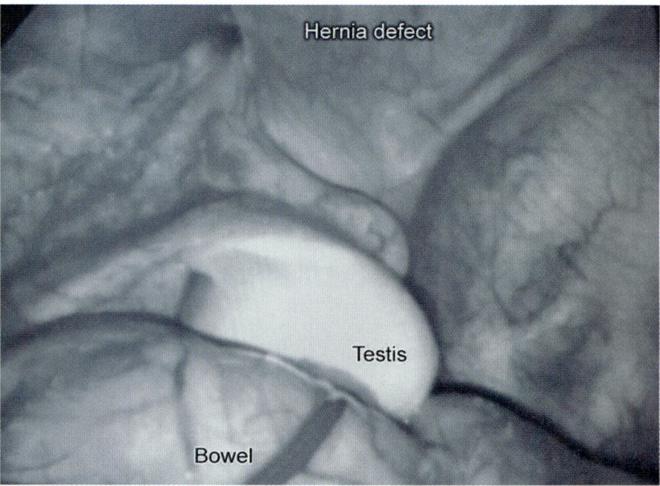

Laparoscopic view of undescended testis (abdominal testis). Note the inguinal hernial defect. Laparoscopic approach is becoming popular

THYROID

239. Which nerve can be injured (near superior thyroid artery) while operating for thyroid malignancy?

a. Right recurrent laryngeal nerve
b. Left recurrent laryngeal nerve
c. External branch of superior laryngeal nerve
d. Internal branch of superior laryngeal nerve

During thyroidectomy, Recurrent Laryngeal nerve injury may occur during the ligature of the inferior thyroid artery. To the medial side of superior thyroid artery are the Constrictor pharyngis inferior and the external branch of the superior laryngeal nerve (so liable to damage while doing thyroidectomy).

240. Occult thyroid malignancies are usually:

a. Anaplastic b. Papillary
c. Medullary d. Follicular

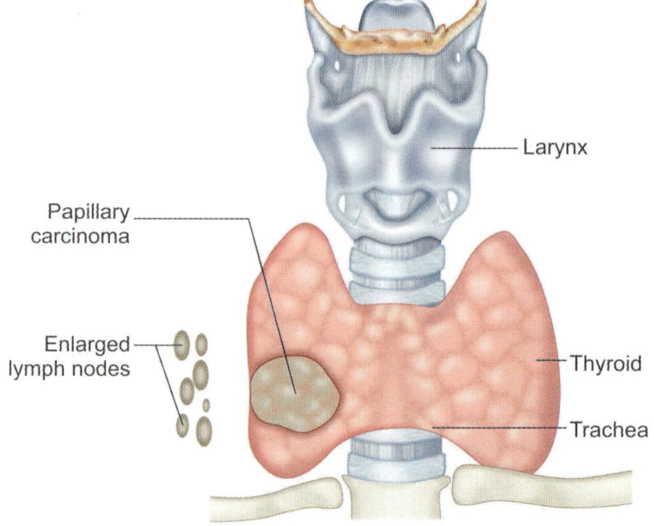

Papillary carcinoma of thyroid with nodal infiltration—diagrammatic representation

Ans. 236. **b.** Peripheral zone 237. **c.** Circumcision 238. **d.** Hypertrophy of... 239. **c.** External branch... 240. **b.** Papillary

Woolner classification of papillary carcinoma of thyroid

- Occult primary (<1.5 cm)
- Intrathyroidal
- Extrathyroidal

241. Medullary carcinoma of thyroid/MCT is most aggressive in:

a. Sporadic cases
b. MEN-IIb
c. MEN-IIa
d. MEN-I

MCT may be associated with MEN-II syndrome and pheochromocytoma and hypertension. MCT associated with MEN type IIB with pheochromocytoma (Sipple's disease) is most aggressive.

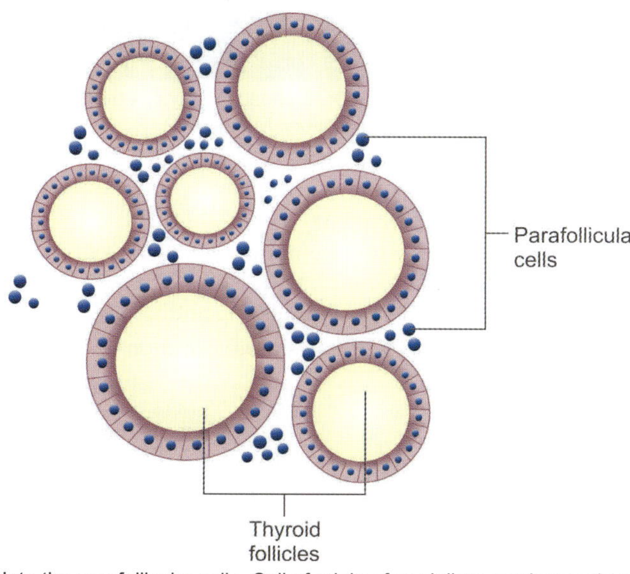

Note the parafollicular cells. Cell of origin of medullary carcinoma thyroid

242. Best management of a nodule of 2 cm in left thyroid, later found to be a papillary carcinoma:

a. Radiotherapy
b. Thyroidectomy with radical dissection
c. Total thyroidectomy
d. Hemi-thyroidectomy

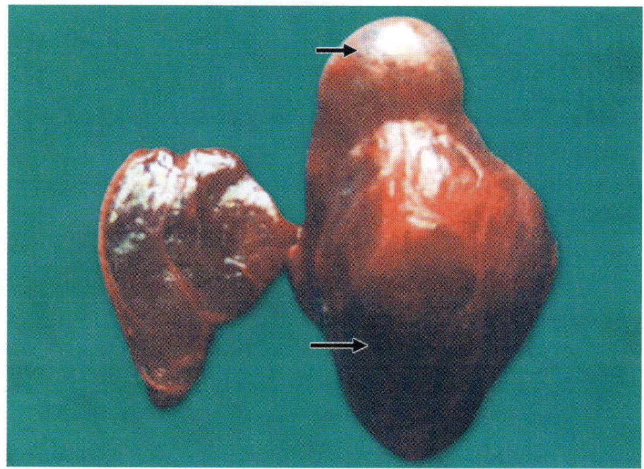

Papillary carcinoma thyroid, operated specimen

For papillary carcinoma of thyroid, total or near total thyroidectomy, with central node compartment dissection (level VI) is done.

243. Psammoma bodies are NOT seen in:

a. Follicular carcinoma of thyroid
b. Papillary carcinoma of thyroid
c. Serous cystadenoma of ovary
d. Meningioma

Psammoma bodies are seen in:
❑ Papillary carcinoma thyroid
❑ Meningioma
❑ Serous cystadenoma of ovary

244. Malignancy in a multinodular goiter is most often:

a. Follicular carcinoma
b. Papillary carcinoma
c. Anaplastic carcinoma
d. Medullary carcinoma

Complications of MNG

- Secondary thyrotoxicosis (30%)
- Follicular carcinoma of thyroid (10%)
- Hemorrhage in a nodule
- Tracheal obstruction, calcification
- Cosmetic problem

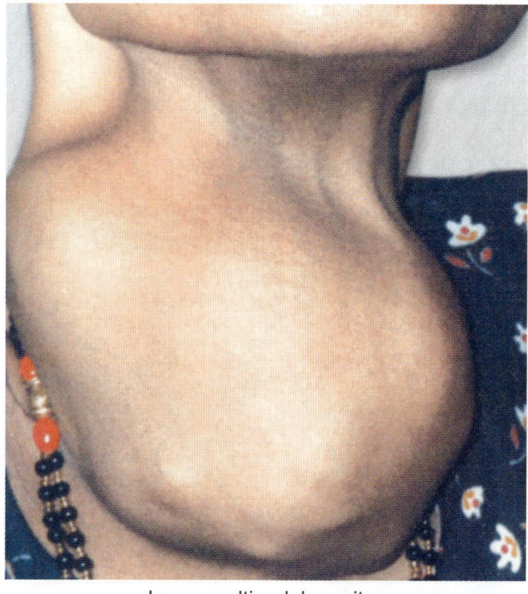

Large multinodular goiter

245. Treatment of choice in cold nodule of thyroid:

a. Subtotal thyroidectomy
b. Wait and watch
c. I-131
d. Hemithyroidectomy

Cold nodule is non-functioning nodule. It will not take up isotope (underactive). For non-toxic nodule due to any cause, hemithyroidectomy with complete removal of lateral lobe and whole of the isthmus is done.

Ans. 241. b. MEN-IIb 242. c. Total thyroidectomy 243. a. Follicular carc... 244. a. Follicular carcinoma
245. d. Hemithyroid...

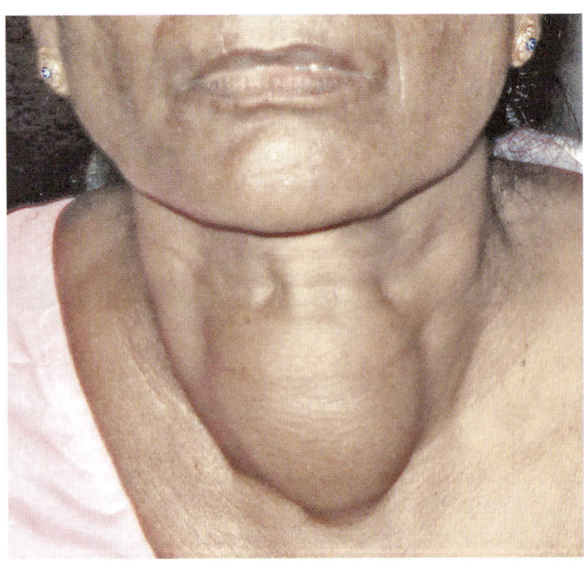

Solitary nodule thyroid involving isthmus

246. All of the following are symptoms of hyperthyroidism EXCEPT:

a. Voracious appetite b. Cold intolerance
c. Emotional disturbance d. Sleeplessness

Sympathetic overactivity in patient with thyrotoxicosis and hyperthyroidism causes dyspnea, palpitation, tiredness, heat intolerance, sweating, nervousness, increased appetite and decrease in weight.

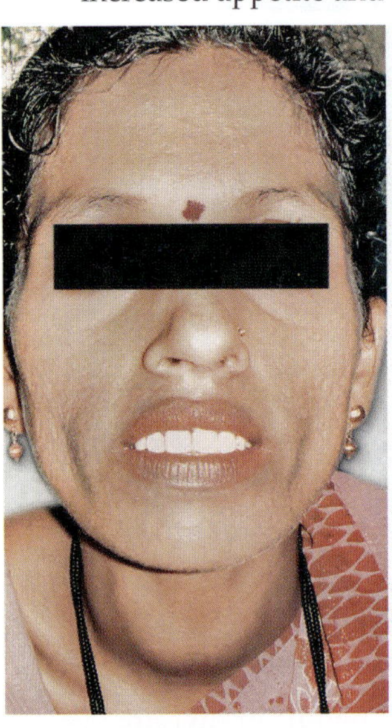

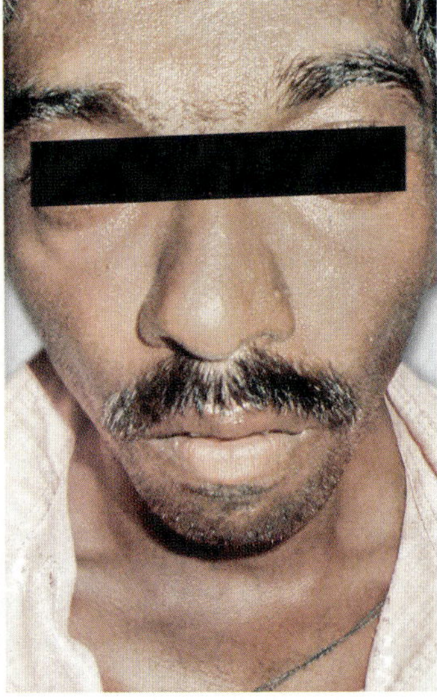

A and B: Graves disease in a female and male patient. Note the exophthalmos with clearly visible lower sclera

247. FNAC is NOT useful in which of the following thyroid carcinoma:

a. Medullary carcinoma
b. Follicular carcinoma
c. Papillary carcinoma
d. Lymphoma

Most often FNAC is inconclusive in follicular carcinoma, because capsular and angioinvasion, which are the main features in follicular carcinoma, cannot be detected by FNAC.

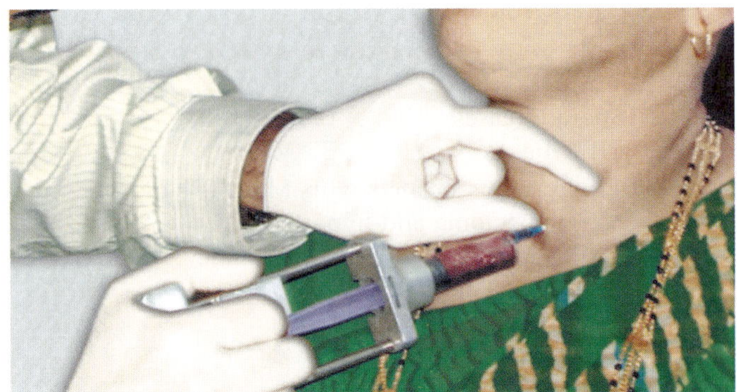

FNAC of thyroid (*Courtesy:* Dr Krishna Upadhya Pathologist, Nandikoor Laboratory, Mangalore)

248. All are true for Grave's disease EXCEPT:

a. Commoner in males
b. Eye signs are frequent
c. Family history of autoimmune endocrine disorders may be present
d. Presence of thyroid stimulating antibodies

Thyrotoxicosis is eight times more common in females.

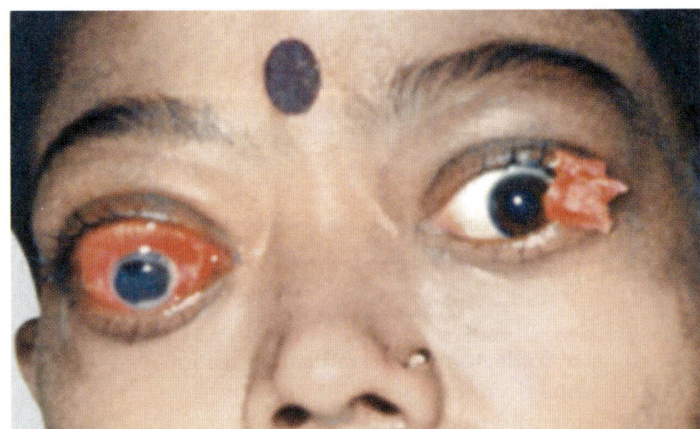

Malignant exophthalmos

BREAST

249. Stage 4 breast carcinoma, as per Manchester system involves:

a. Involvement of chest wall
b. Satellite lesions >4
c. Ulceration of skin surface
d. Spread to ipsilateral supraclavicular lymph nodes

Stage IV Manchester system

- Growth extends beyond the breast area;
- Fixation of the tumour to the chest wall;
- Fixation or matting of the axillary lymph nodes,
- Supraclavicular nodes involvement;
- Distant metastasis

Ans. **246. b.** Cold intolerance **247. b.** Follicular carcinoma **248. a.** Commoner in males **249. d.** Spread to ipsilateral...

250. As per TNM staging, 3 cm breast carcinoma and involving 4 ipsilateral axillary lymph nodes would be:

a. Stage IIA	b. Stage IIB
c. Stage IIIA	d. Stage IIIB

Stage IIIA describes invasive breast cancer in which either

- No tumor is found in the breast or the tumor may be any size; cancer is found in 4 to 9 axillary lymph nodes or in the lymph nodes near the breastbone (found during imaging tests or a physical exam) OR
- The tumor is larger than 5 centimeters; small groups of breast cancer cells (larger than 0.2 millimeter but not larger than 2 millimeters) are found in the lymph nodes OR
- The tumor is larger than 5 centimeters; cancer has spread to 1 to 3 axillary lymph nodes or to the lymph nodes near the breastbone (found during a sentinel lymph node biopsy)

251. Prognostic factor of most significance in breast carcinoma:

a. HER2/ Neu	b. Histological grading
c. Tumour staging	d. Elston score

Whereas microscopic typing & grading are important to understand the prognosis of a breast cancer, clinical staging is a guide to treatment.

252. Lymphatic from left upper quadrant of breast does NOT drain into:

a. Internal mammary	b. Apical
c. Central	d. Anterior axillary

25% of lymphatics, mainly from the medial half of the breast, into 2nd, 3rd and 4th intercostals space internal mammary lymph nodes. Internal mammary nodes are located in retrosternal intercostals spaces 1–2 cm lateral to the sterna margin.

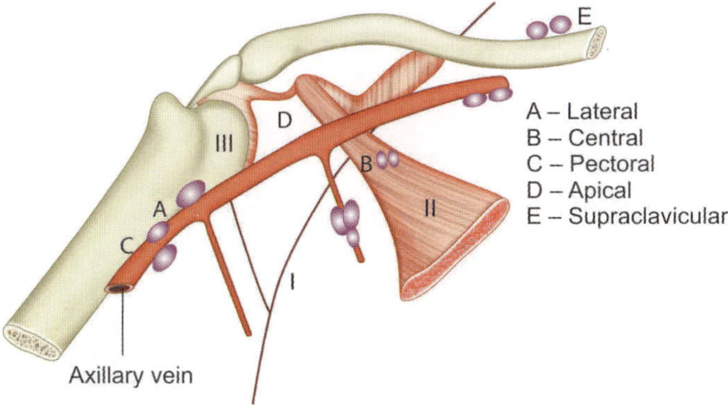

Surgical levels of lymph nodes in the axilla draining the breast

253. Which investigation is important in breast conservation surgery:

a. Tumor markers
b. Sentinel lymph node biopsy
c. Total body scan
d. Serum calcium

The first axillary node draining the breast (by direct drainage) is designated as the sentinel lymph node/ SLN. SLN is the first node involved by tumor cells and presence or absence of its histological involvement, when assessed will give a predictive idea about the further spread of tumor to other nodes. The incidence of involvement of other nodes with SLN is less than 3% and so if SLNB (SLN biopsy) is negative, nodal dissection can be avoided but regular follow-up is needed.

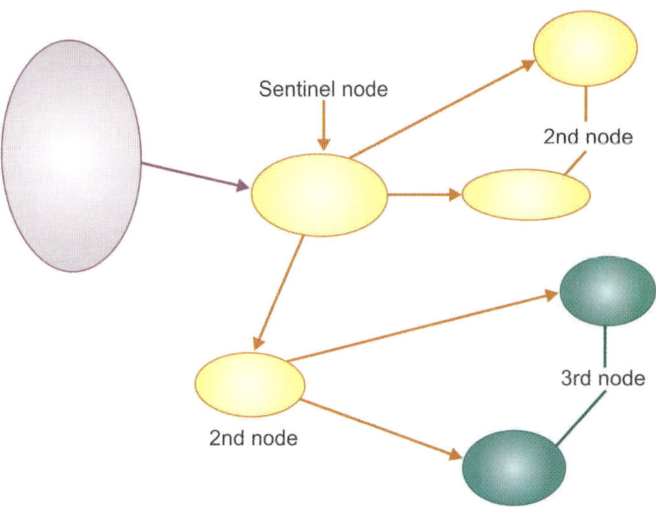

Sentinel lymph node biopsy (SLNB) of breast. Note: Spread by skipping the sentinel node is less than 3%

254. Carcinoma breast with best prognosis:

a. Medullary carcinoma
b. Intraductal carcinoma
c. Colloid carcinoma
d. Schirrous carcinoma

Colloid carcinoma produces abundant mucin, both intra and extracellularly carrying better prognosis.

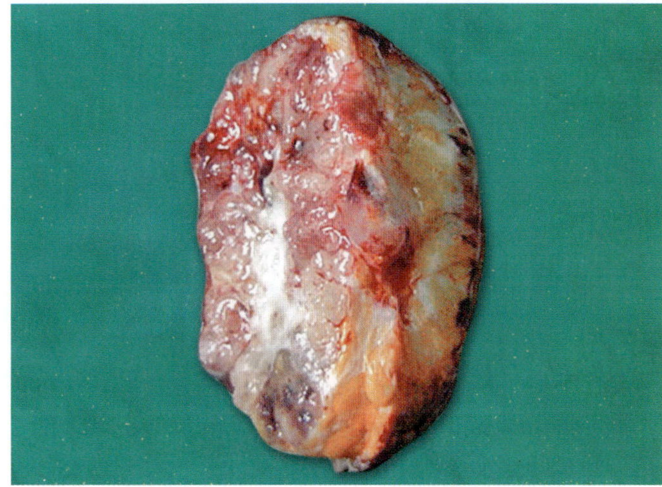

Specimen of carcinoma breast. Cut section showing tumor tissue of scirrhous type (most common type)

Ans. 250. c. Stage IIIA	251. b. Histological grading	252. a. Internal mammary	253. b. Sentinel lymph node...
254. c. Colloid carcinoma

255. Agent NOT used for treating breast carcinoma:

a. Tamoxifen
b. Cisplatin
c. DES
d. Letrozole

Cisplatin is used to treat various types of cancers, including sarcomas, some carcinomas (e.g. small cell lung carcinoma, squamous cell carcinoma of the head and neck and ovarian cancer), lymphomas, bladder cancer, cervical cancer, and germ cell tumors.

Drugs used in hormone therapy

Drug	*Mechanism of action*	*Dose*	*Adverse effects*
Tamoxifen	Antiestrogen	20 mg	Nausea, weight gain, hot flushes, vaginal bleeding, bone pain, amenorrhea
Medroxyprogesterone	Progestogen	400 mg	Nausea, flushing, vaginal bleeding
Aminoglutethimide	Aromatase inhibitor	250 mg QID	Rash, dizziness, lethargy, Cushing facies
Arimidex	Aromatase inhibitors	1 mg	Lethargy, GI upset
Letrozole	Aromatase inhibitor	2.5 mg OD	Vaginal dryness, hot flushes,vaginal bleeding, cardiovascular problem
Zoladex (Goserelin)	LHRH agonist	3.6 mg monthly	Amenorrhea, nausea. It is expensive
Diethylstilbestrol	Estrogen	15 mg daily	Fluid retention, vomiting, thrombosis, hypercalcemia
Fluoxymestrone	Androgen	30 mg daily	Masculinization, nausea

It is more beneficial in ER +ve patient; perimenopausal patient with node +ve; postmenopausal patient.
Presently ***Tamoxifen and Oophorectomy*** are the commonly used methods.

256. The tumor which may occur, following wide local excision and radiotherapy for mammary Ca is:

a. Leiomyosarcoma
b. Squamous cell Ca
c. Basal cell Ca
d. Lymphangiosarcoma

Lymphangiosarcoma (Stewart-Treve's syndrome) of upper limb can develop in patient's who have developed lymphoedema after mastectomy with axillary clearance. Usually it occurs 3–5 years after development of lymphoedema.

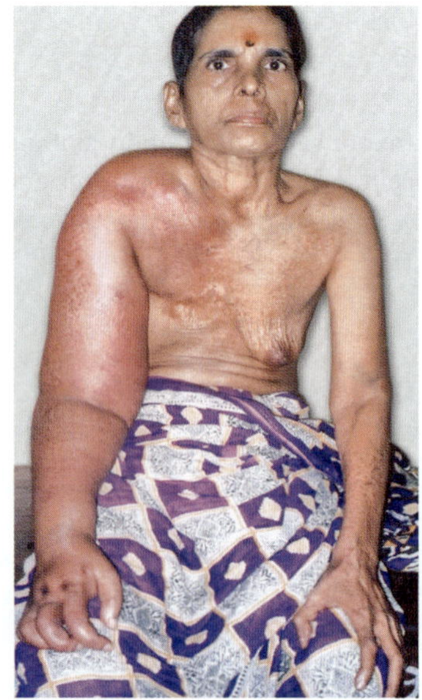

Postmastectomy lymphoedema. Note the mastectomy scar

257. Paget's disease of the nipple is:

a. Infection
b. Dermatitis
c. Neoplasia
d. Hypopigmentation

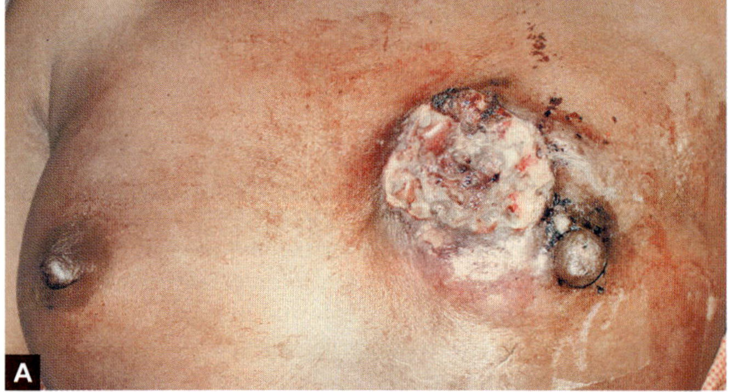

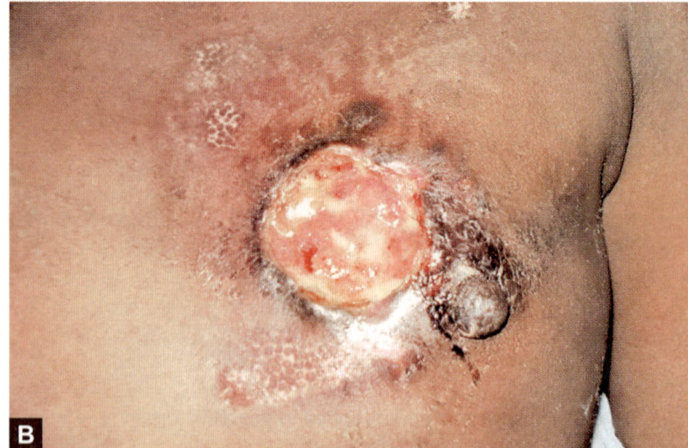

A and B: Paget's disease of the breast

Paget's disease of the nipple is superficial manifestation of an intraductal carcinoma. The malignancy spreads within the duct up to the skin of the nipple and down into the substance of the breast. It mimics eczema of nipple and areola.

Ans. 255. **b.** Cisplatin 256. **d.** Lymphangiosarcoma 257. **c.** Neoplasia

258. Triple assessment for carcinoma breast includes:
a. History, clinical examination and mammogram
b. History, clinical examination and FNAC
c. USG, Mammogram and FNAC
d. Clinical examination, Mammogram and FNAC

Triple assessment includes
- Clinical assessment
- Radiological imaging USG/MRI/mammography (after 40 years)
- Cytological or histological analysis FNAC/core biopsy.

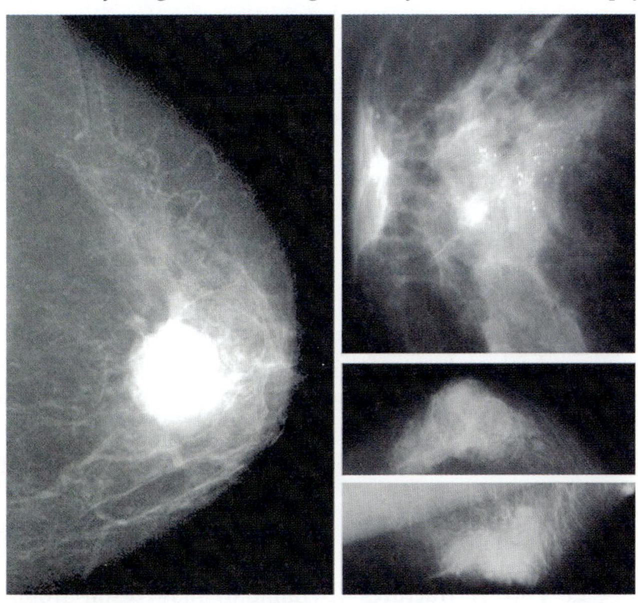

Different mammography pictures, craniocaudal and mediolateral films showing mass lesion, microcalcification (*Courtesy:* Dr Ganesh, MDRD, Mangalore)

259. Treatment of cystosarcoma phyllodes is:
a. Radical mastectomy
b. Incissional biopsy
c. Simple mastectomy
d. Modified radical mastectomy

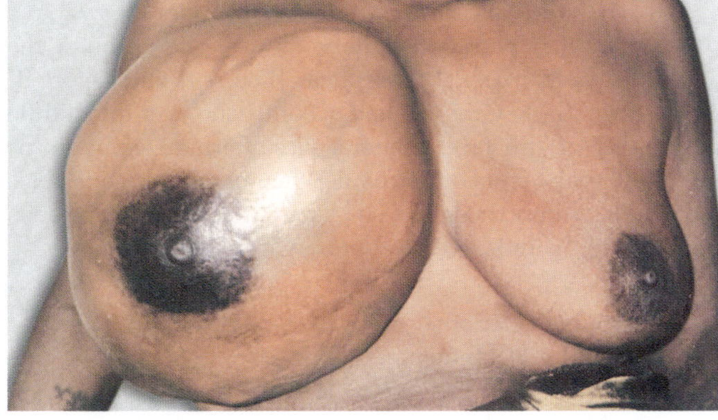

Cystosarcoma phyllodes of right breast. Note the dilated veins. Tumor occupies the entire breast

Treatment of phyllodes tumor
- Excision or subcutaneous mastectomy is done
- If malignant (sarcoma), total mastectomy is indicated.

260. Paget's disease of breast, following are true EXCEPT:
a. Treated by simple mastectomy
b. Represents underlying malignancy
c. Presents as eczema
d. Cytology is not diagnostic

Histologically, Paget's disease contains large, ovoid, clear Paget's cells with malignant features. Paget's hyperchromatic cells are located in rete pegs of epidermis containing intracellular mucopolysaccharides as clear halo in cytosol.

Differences between Paget's disease and eczema of nipple

	Paget's disease		*Eczema*
1.	Unilateral	1.	Bilateral
2.	Edges are distinct	2.	Edges are indistinct
3.	Itching absent	3.	Itching present
4.	Seen in menopausal women	4.	Occurs during the time of lactation
5.	Vesicles absent	5.	Vesicles present
6.	Nipple is usually destroyed	6.	Nipple is usually intact
7.	Underlying lump is usually present	7.	No underlying lump

261. True about sentinel lymph node biopsy/ SLNB are all EXCEPT:
a. Contraindicated if axillary LN is involved
b. Blue dye injected
c. It is done to avoid inadvertent axillary LN biopsy
d. Radioactive dye is used

SLNB is contraindicated in patients who are allergic to vital blue dye or radio-colloid, in pregnancy and in inflammatory carcinoma of the breast.

SLNB is done in:
❑ Carcinoma breast
❑ Carcinoma penis
❑ Malignant melanoma

262. The most frequently used procedure for diagnosing palpable breast masses is:
a. Core-cutting needle biopsy
b. Fine needle aspiration
c. Excisional biopsy
d. Incisional biopsy

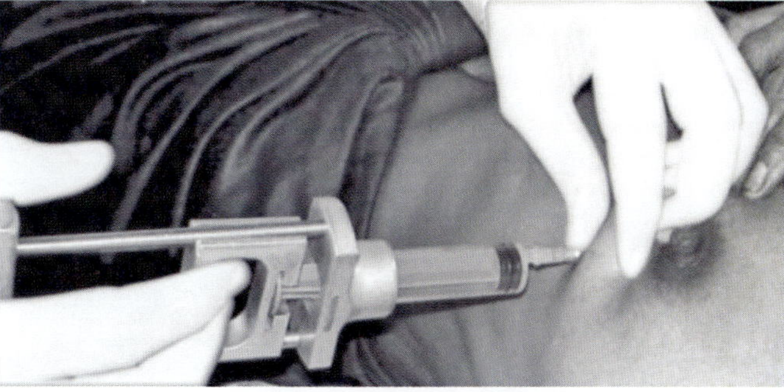

FNAC of breast lump

Ans. 258. **d.** Clinical... 259. **c.** Simple mastectomy 260. **d.** Cytology is not... 261. **a.** Contraindicated if... 262. **b.** Fine needle aspiration

FNAC is least painful, can be done on OPD basis, reliable and cheaper. Malignant deposits will not occur along FNAC track (only contraindication for FNAC is testicular tumor).

263. Commonest site of carcinoma of the breast:
a. Lower inner quadrant b. Nipple
c. Upper inner quadrant d. Upper outer quadrant

Most common site of carcinoma breast is upper outer quadrant (60%) because breast tissue is more in this quadrant.

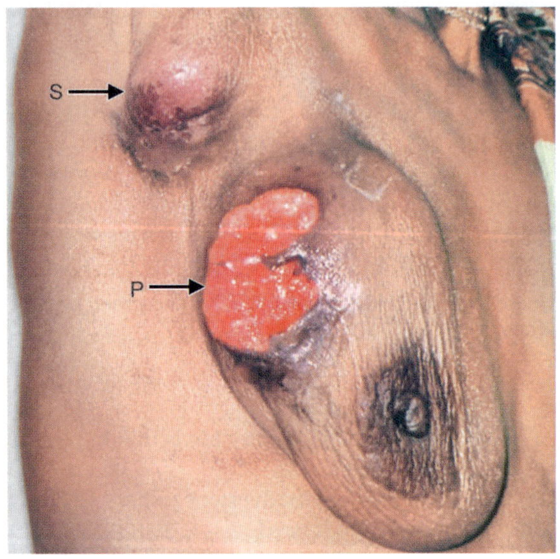

Carcinoma right breast with ulceration in the primary (P) with axillary lymph node secondaries (S)

264. A lady presented with breast carcinoma. On investigation, it is noticed that other breast is also involved. Likely histological subtype is:
a. Inflammatory carcinoma b. Colloid carcinoma
c. Lobular carcinoma d. In situ carcinoma

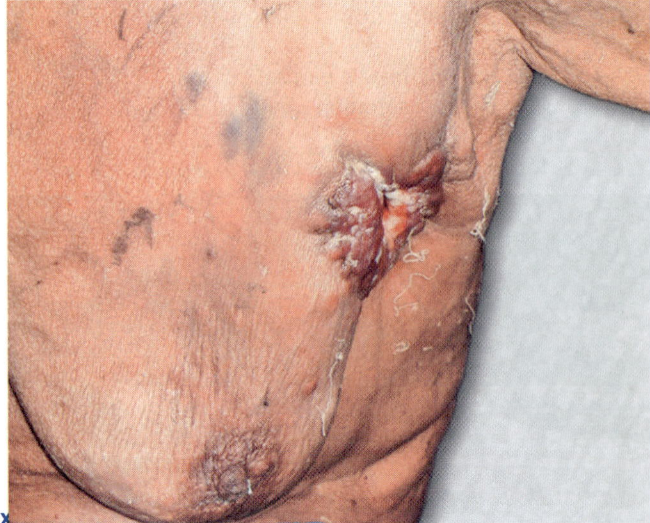
Carcinoma breast involving axillary tail of Spence

Lobular carcinoma in situ/LCIS, multifocal breast cancer, family history are risk for development of bilateral breast cancer. There is 5 fold increases in 2nd breast cancer on opposite side in a female, who has had breast cancer on ipsilateral side.

HEAD-NECK

265. Raised intracranial pressure is characterised by:
a. Hypertension & bradycardia
b. Hypotension & tachycardia
c. Hypertension & tachycardia
d. Hypotension & bradycardia

An increase in intracranial pressure/ICP, most commonly due to head injury leading to intracranial hematoma or cerebral edema, can crush brain tissue, shift brain structures, contribute to hydrocephalus, cause brain herniation, and restrict blood supply to the brain. It is a cause of reflex bradycardia. One of the main dangers of increased ICP is that it can cause ischemia by decreasing cerebral perfusion pressure/ CPP. Once the ICP approaches the level of the mean systemic pressure, cerebral perfusion falls. The body's response to a fall in CPP is to raise systemic blood pressure and dilate cerebral blood vessels.

266. Fracture of face involving middle area manifest as all EXCEPT:
a. Proptosis b. Lengthening of face
c. Epistaxis d. Ecchymosis

Le Fort II fractures (pyramidal) may result from a blow to the lower or mid maxilla and usually involve the inferior orbital rim. Such a fracture has a pyramidal shape and extends from the nasal bridge at or below the nasofrontal suture through the frontal processes of the maxilla, inferolaterally through the lacrimal bones and inferior orbital floor and rim through or near the inferior orbital foramen, and inferiorly through the anterior wall of the maxillary sinus; it then travels under the zygoma, across the pterygomaxillary fissure, and through the pterygoid plates. Manifests as [Lefort II and Lefort III (common)] - Gross edema of soft tissue over the middle third of the face, bilateral circumorbital ecchymosis, bilateral subconjunctival hemorrhage, epistaxis, CSF rhinorrhoea, dish face deformity, diplopia, enophthalmos (NOT proptosis), cracked pot sound.

267. Commonest cause for hyperparathyroidism is:
a. Single adenoma
b. Multiple adenoma
c. Single gland adenoma
d. Multiple gland adenoma

Primary hyperparathyroidism
- Adenoma (75–90%)
- Hyperplasia (20–24%)
- Carcinoma, rare (1%)

Ans. 263. **d.** Upper outer... 264. **c.** Lobular carcinoma 265. **a.** Hypertension... 266. **a.** Proptosis 267. **a.** Single adenoma

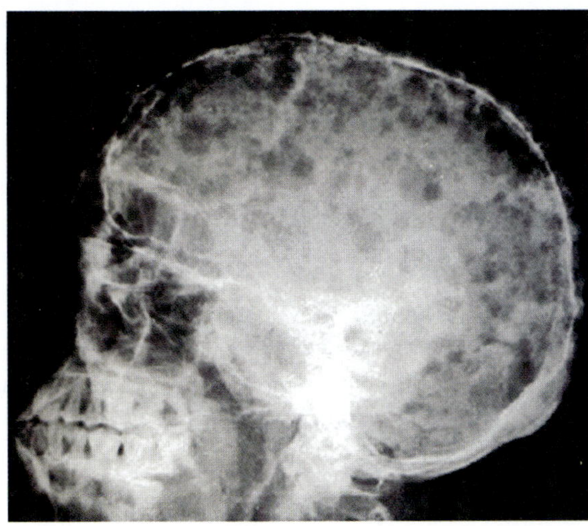

Plain X-ray skull. Note the characteristic salt-pepper appearance of the skull bone

268. Commonest site of thyro-glossal cyst:

a. At the level of cricoids cartilage
b. Subhyoid
c. Suprahyoid
d. At the level of hyoid

Possible sites of thyroglossal cyst

- Beneath the foramen cecum
- In the floor of mouth
- Suprahyoid
- Subhyoid – comonest site
- On the thyroid cartilage – 2nd common site

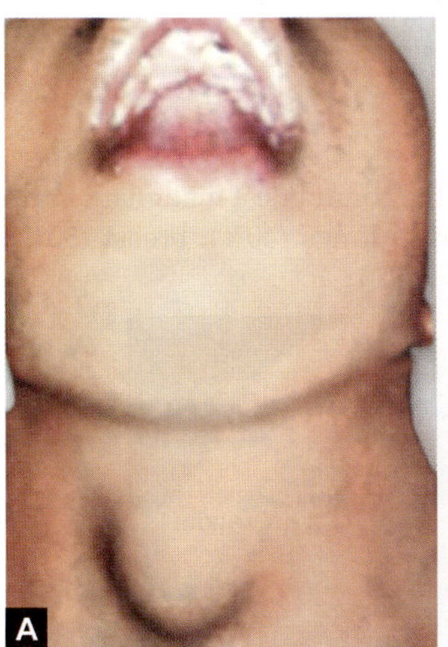

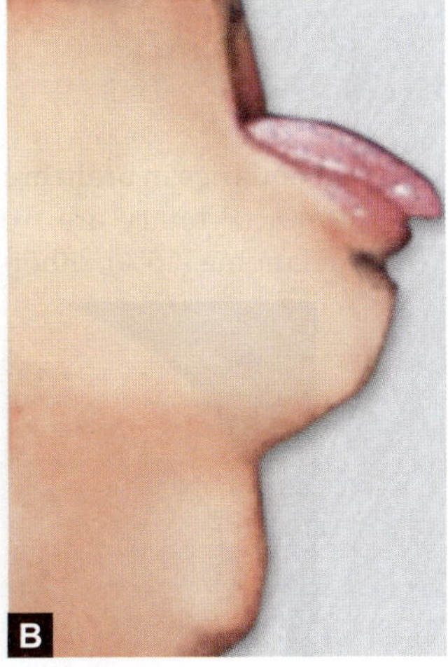

A and B: Thyroglossal cyst

269. Mild head injury is having a Glasgow Coma Scale/ GCS of:

a. 3–5
b. 5–8
c. 8–10
d. 13–15

Mild head injury has a GCS of 13–15

Glasgow coma scale

Eye opening		*Verbal response*		*Motor response*	
Spontaneous	–4	Oriented	–5	Obeys commands	–6
To speech	–3	Confused	–4	Localises pain	–5
To pain	–2	Inappropriate words	–3	Flexion to pain	–4
None	–1	Incomprehensible words	–2	Abnormal flexion	–3
		None	–1	Extension to pain	–2
				None	–1

Total score-15
Mild head injury: score 13–15
Moderate head injury: 9–12
Severe head injury: less than 8 (3–8)

270. According to GCS, a verbal score of 1 indicates:

a. No response
b. Inappropriate words
c. Incomprehensible sounds
d. Disoriented response

Verbal response in GCS is 1, there is no response.

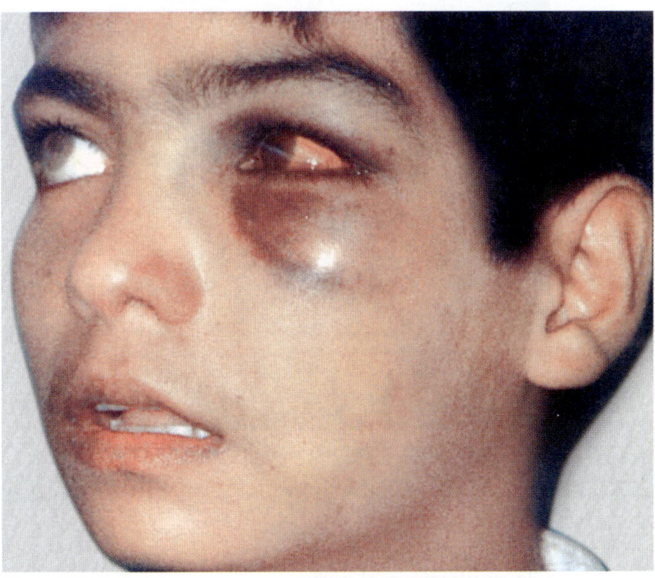

Patient with head injury having black eye

271. What develops in an unerupted tooth:

a. Dentigerous cyst
b. Dental cyst
c. Caries
d. Adamintinoma

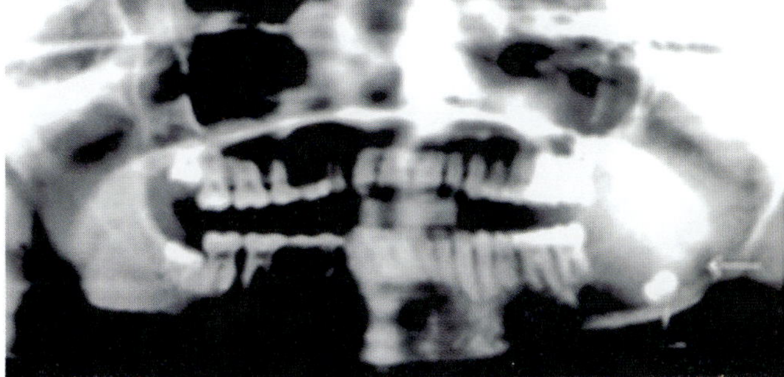

Orthopantomogram showing dentigerous cyst

Ans. **268. b.** Subhyoid **269. d.** 13-15 **270. a.** No response **271. a.** Dentigerous cyst

Dentigerous cyst/follicular odontome is a unilocular cystic swelling arsing in relation to the dental epithelium from an unerupted tooth.

272. Swelling of deep parotid gland presents as a swelling in:

a. Temporal region b. Floor of mouth
c. Neck d. Parietal region

When deep lobe of parotid is involved, swelling is commonly located in the lateral wall of pharynx, posterior pillar and over the soft palate – 10%. Deep lobe tumor passes through Patey's stylomandibular tunnel pushing tonsils, pharynx, soft palate often without any visible swelling or only small swelling when only deep lobe tumor is present.

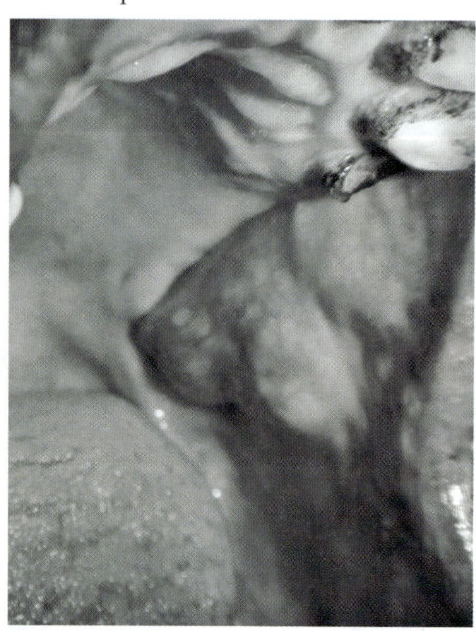

Deep lobe tumor of parotid is examined per orally

273. Nerve NOT damaged in Submandibular gland surgery for removal of stones:

a. Hypoglossal nerve
b. Glossopharyngeal nerve
c. Mandibular branch of facial nerve
d. Lingual nerve

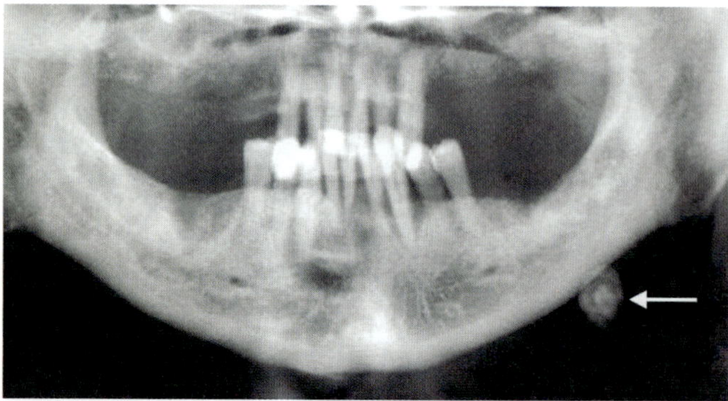

X-ray (OPG) showing left sided submandibular salivary stone

Complications of submandibular gland excision surgery (sialadenectomy) include injury to marginal mandibular nerve, lingual nerve and hypoglossal nerve. There may be injury to nerve to mylohyoid causing anesthesia over submental skin.

274. Probable cause of sudden death in a case of superficial injury to neck:

a. Injury to trachea
b. Bleeding from subclavian artery
c. Air embolism through external jugular vein
d. Injury to phrenic nerve

Traumatic opening of major veins sucking air inside, causing embolism, may lead to sudden death.

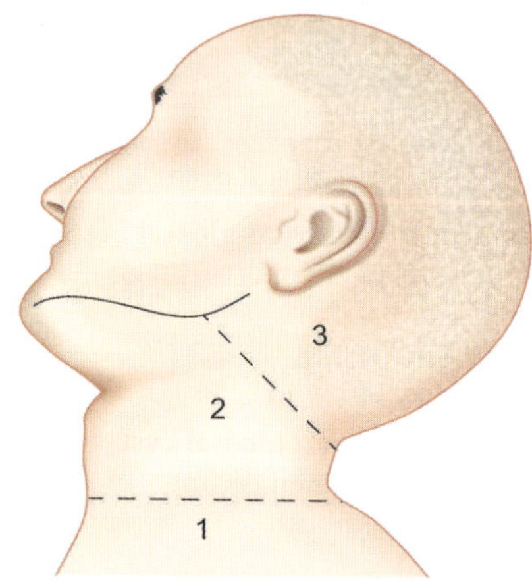

Neck trauma zones

275. Most common primary source of metastasis to brain is:

a. Thyroid
b. Lung
c. Liver
d. Breast

Secondaries in brain are the commonest malignant brain tumor. Primary are from – lungs (40%), breast (30%), melanoma (15%), others (15%).

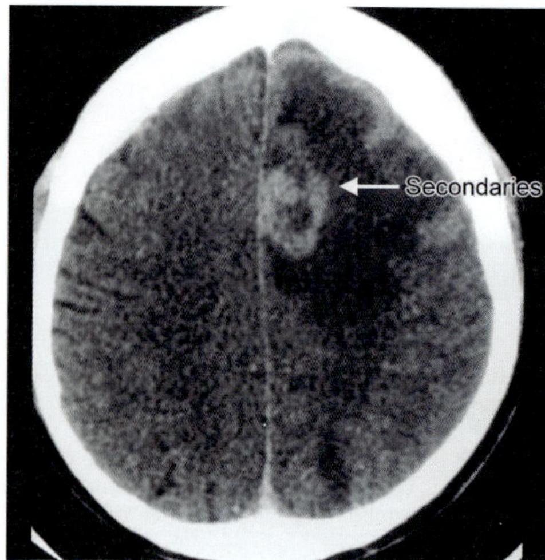

CT scan head showing brain secondaries

Ans. 272. c. Neck 273. b. Glossopharyngeal... 274. c. Air embolism... 275. b. Lung

276. Commonest site of sialectasis is:

a. Internal jugular chain   b. Submandibular
c. Sublingual   d. Parotid

Sialectasis is an aseptic dilatation of salivary ductules causing grape-like (cluster-like) dilatations. It is common in parotids; often bilateral. Sialogram is diagnostic (grape or cluster-like dilatations).

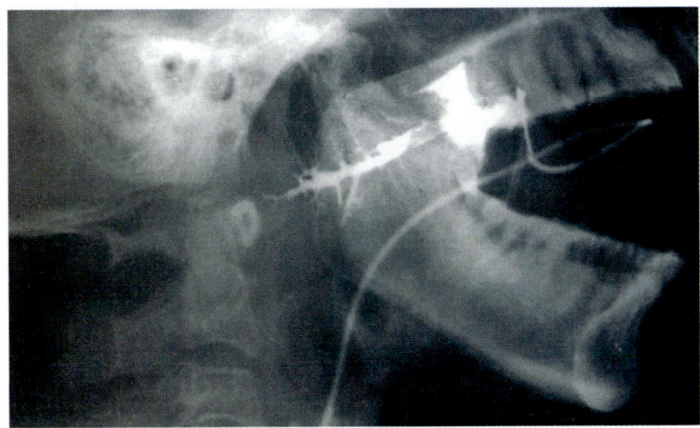

Sialogram X-ray done to visualize the ductal pattern in parotid

277. In radical neck dissection surgery, structure preserved is:

a. Submandibular gland
b. Sternocleidomastoid muscle
c. External jugular vein
d. Phrenic nerve

Classical radical neck dissection is resection of lymph nodes (level I to V), fat, fascia, sternomastoid muscle, omohyoid muscle, internal jugular vein, external jugular vein, accessory nerve, submandibular gland, lower part of parotid, prevertebral fascia – 'en-block' (Criles' operation).

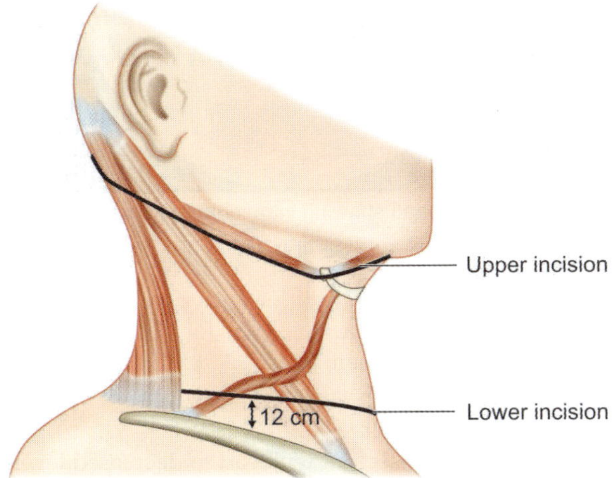

MacFee incision for radical neck dissection. Upper incision is from mastoid process along the line of digastric to hyoid bone point, then upwards to chin. Lower incision is parallel to clavicle 2 cm above from anterior margin of trapezius to midline

278. Sebaceous cyst is a:

a. Mucous cyst   b. Epidermoid cyst
c. Extravasation cyst   d. Distension cyst

Sebaceous cyst/epidermoid cyst is a retention cyst. It is due to blockge of the duct of sebaceous gland, causing a cystic swelling.

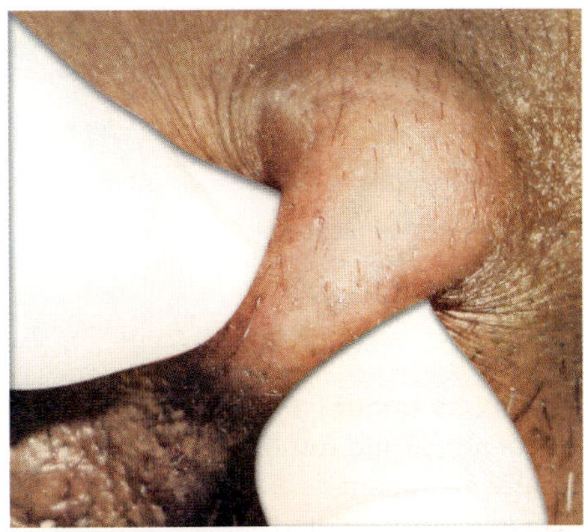

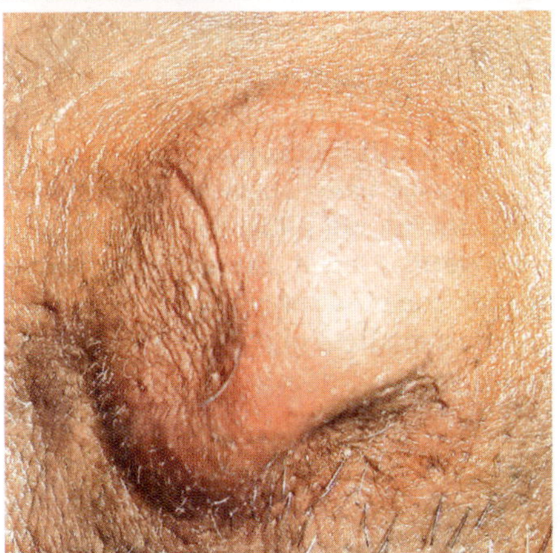

Sebaceous cyst showing moulding sign

279. MC cyst of jaw is:

a. Follicular cyst   b. Radicular cyst
c. Dentigerous cyst   d. Odontogenic keratocyst

Dental cyst/radicular cyst/periapical cyst occurs under the root of the chronically infected dead erupted tooth.

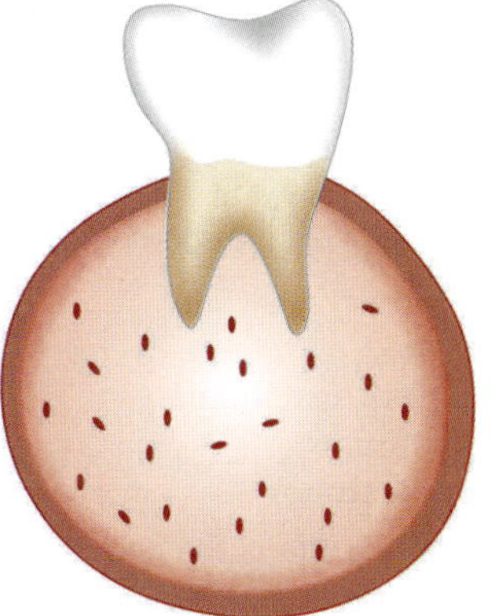

Dental cyst.

Ans. 276. **d.** Parotid   277. **d.** Phrenic nerve   278. **b.** Epidermoid cyst   279. **b.** Radicular cyst

280. Sardonic grin is associated with:

a. Rabies b. Tetanus
c. Bell's palsy d. Hemiplegia

Risus sardonicus (smiling facies) is tetanus is due to spasm of the facial muscle – zygomaticus major. Look as if patient is smiling.

Symptoms
❑ *Trismus* is the most common symptom
❑ Jaw stiffness, pain and stiffness in the neck and back muscles
❑ Anxiousness, sweating
❑ Headache, delirium, sleeplessness
❑ Dysphagia
❑ Dyspnea

281. Mixed salivary tumor is:

a. 50% of all parotid tumors
b. Locally malignant
c. Firm and encapsulated
d. Slowly growing and lobular

Pleomorphic adenoma/mixed salivary tumor is a single painless, smooth, firm, lobulated, mobile swelling in front of the parotid with positive curtain sign (As the deep fascia is attached above to the zygomatic bone, it acts as a curtain, not allowing the parotid swelling to move above that level). Even though it is capsulated, tumor may come out as pseudopods and may extend beyond the main limit of the tumor tissue.

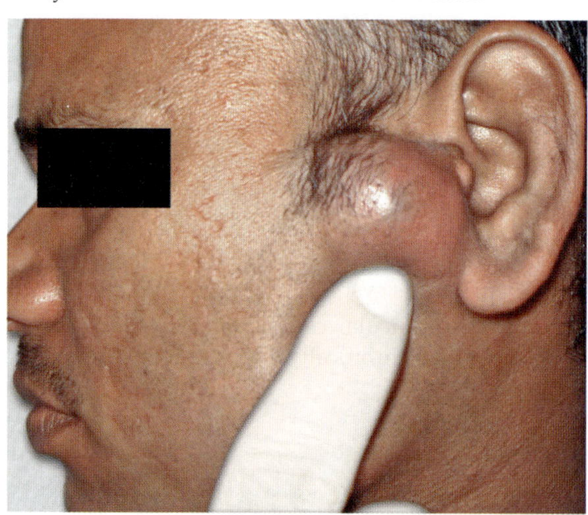

Pleomorphic adenoma showing *curtain sign*

282. MC parotid tumor:

a. Metastasis
b. Adenoidcystic carcinoma
c. Warthin's tumor
d. Pleomorphic tumor

Pleomorphic adenoma is the commonest of the salivary gland tumor in adult. It is 80% common. More common in parotids (80%).

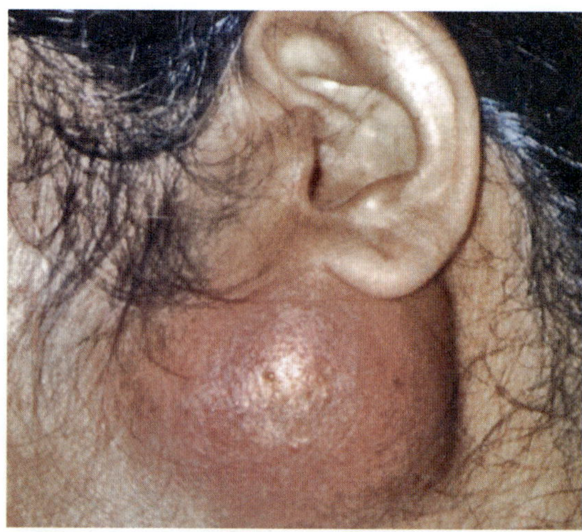

Typical parotid tumor—a pleomorphic adenoma

283. MC neurologic abnormality occurring with head injury:

a. Convulsions b. Altered consciousness
c. Ocular nerve palsy d. Hemiplegia

In head injury, any impact creates shearing forces in the brain causing damage to the neurons, supporting tissues and blood vessels. This leads to loss of consciousness, focal neurological deficits etc.

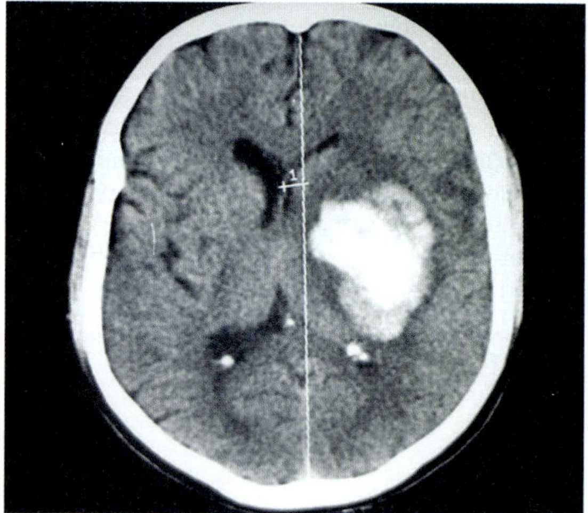

CT scan head showing intracerebral hematoma

284. NOT seen in a case of accidental transection of pituitary stalk as a result of injury:

a. Hypothyroidism
b. Hyperprolactinemia
c. Diabetes insipidus
d. Diabetes mellitus

Accidental transection will lead to decreased levels and decreased effects of all pituitary hormones. Since insulin comes from beta cell of pancreas, so it will remain unaffected and hence no chances of development of diabetes mellitus.

Ans. 280. **b.** Tetanus 281. **c.** Firm and encapsulated 282. **d.** Pleomorphic tumor 283. **b.** Altered consciousness 284. **d.** Diabetes mellitus

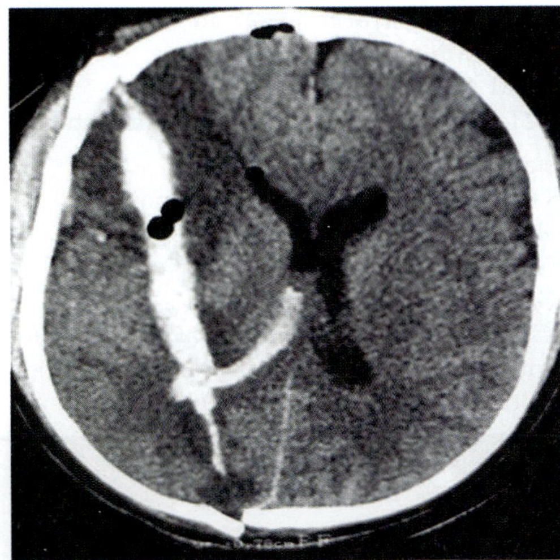

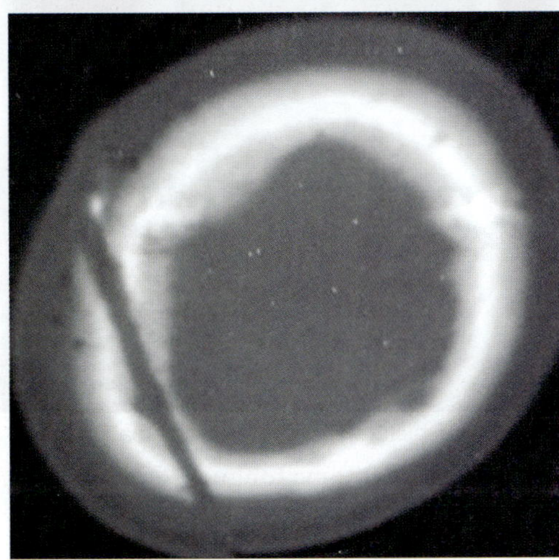

CT scan head showing sharp head injury causing through and through cut across skull and brain. Patient survived and went home

285. Which is used to define penetrating neck injury/ PNI:

a. Through and through wound
b. Breach of platysma
c. Injury to vital structures
d. 2 cm depth of wound

PNI refer to neck injuries resulting from gunshot wounds, stab wounds, or penetrating debris, such as glass or shrapnel, that penetrate the platysma muscle. PNI can injury to the aerodigestive and neurovascular systems.

Triage algorithm
Step One (Assess physiological impact)
Measure vital signs and level of consciousness
❑ By Glasgow coma scale
❑ Systolic blood pressure
❑ Respiratory rate
❑ Revised trauma score. It is based on airway, laryngeal injury, spine injury, maxillofacial injury
Step Two (Assess anatomical impact)
❑ All penetrating injuries to head, neck, thorax, major burns, fracture bones, pelvic fractures, paralysis
Step Three (Assess mechanism)
❑ Automobile accidents, crash or blast injuries, high energy injuries, fall from more than 20 feet. Bullet injury
Step Four (Assess history)
❑ Patient's age below 5 years or age more than 55 years
❑ Cardiac diseases, respiratory and metabolic diseases
❑ Pregnancy
❑ Patients with bleeding disorders
❑ Immunosuppressed individuals
Based On These Steps Consider To Shift The Patient To Trauma Center And Trauma Team Should Be Kept Alert.
It is important in multiple and mass casualities (fire, blasts, automobile accidents, train accidents).

286. A patient with head injury opens eyes on painful stimulus, uses inappropriate words and localizes pain. What is his GCS score:

a. 8
b. 10
c. 12
d. 14

Eye opening of painful stimuli is 2, inappropriate words in verbal response is 3 and localizing pain in motor response is 5.

Primary lesions	*Secondary lesions*
❑ Diffuse neuronal damage ❑ Shearing lesions ❑ Contusions ❑ Lacerations	Brain swelling ❑ Edema, venous con-gestion, hypoxia Intracranial hemorrhage ❑ Extradural ❑ Subdural ❑ Intracerebral Infections ❑ Open head injury – Generalized meningitis – Subdural empyema ❑ Closed head injury – Pott's puffy tumor
Cerebral concussion	*Cause of death in head injury*
❑ Temporary physiological paralysis of nervous system ❑ Loss of consciousness ❑ Post-traumatic amnesia ❑ Full recovery is expected ❑ Residual complications may develop	❑ Brain hypoxia ❑ Coning ❑ Diffuse severe irreversible ne-uronal injury ❑ Death may be due to other in-juries like abdo-minal/thoracic ❑ Metabolic changes ❑ Aspiration in unconscious patient

287. Commonest site of branchial cyst:

a. Lower 1/3rd of sternomastoid on anterior border
b. Lower 1/3rd of sternomastoid on posterior border
c. Upper 1/3rd of sternomastoid on anterior border
d. Upper 1/3rd of sternomastoid on posterior border

Ans. 285. b. Breach of... 286. b. 10 287. c. Upper 1/3rd of...

Branchial cyst presents as a swelling in the neck beneath the anterior border of upper third of sternocleidomastoid muscle. It is smooth, soft, fluctuant, often transilluminant with a sensation of 'Half-filled double hot water bottle'.

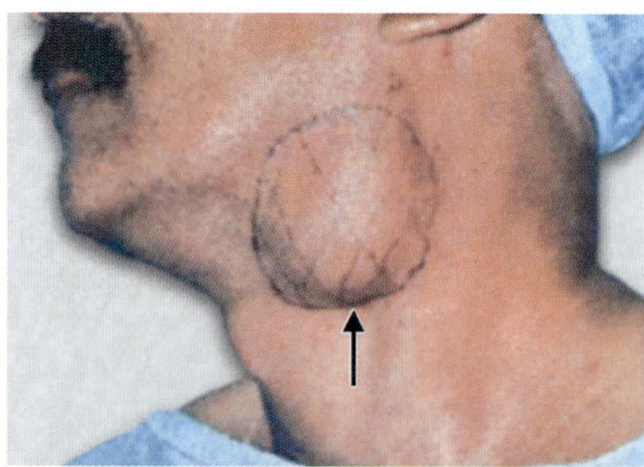

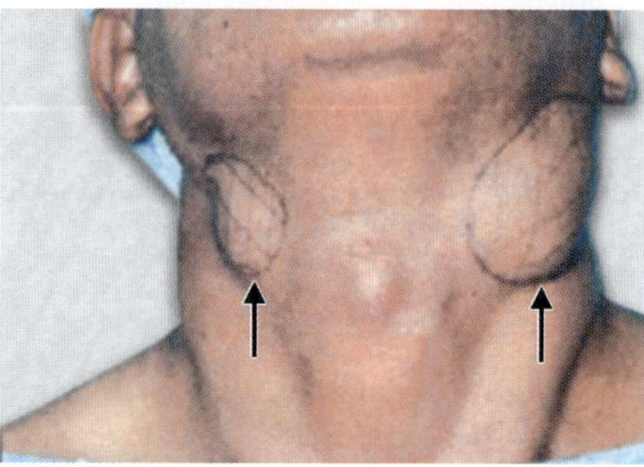

Branchial cyst—both sides

288. Hyoid bone is closely associated to:

a. Bronchogenic cyst
b. Cystic hygroma
c. Thyroglossal cyst
d. Ranula

Thyroglossal cyst is a swelling in the neck in any part along the line of thyroglossal tract. Subhyoid location is the commonest site.

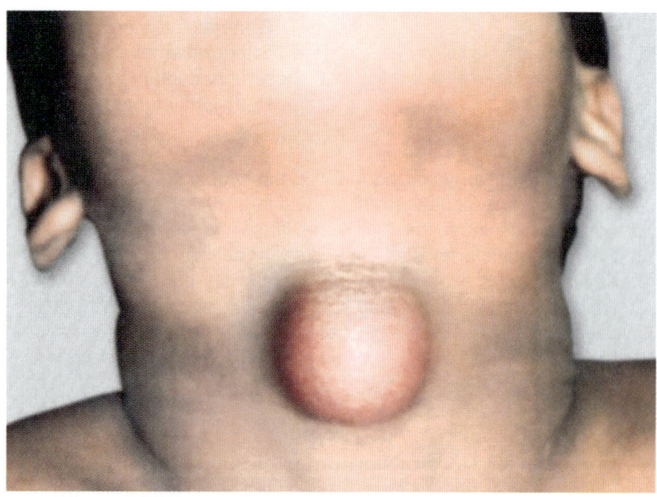

Thyroglossal cyst in a boy. It is a midline swelling with a 'TUG' feeling while protruding the tongue out

289. Presence of calcification on an intracranial lesion is best made out by:

a. MRI
b. USG
c. CT scan
d. Contrast study

Advantages of CT scan

- One to 2 mm sized sections are possible
- Amount of exposure to radiation is less
- More accurate, sensitive, and specific
- Small lesions are also detected
- CT guided biopsies are done at present, safely
- Intracranial calcifications can be studied as in calcified neurocysticercosis.

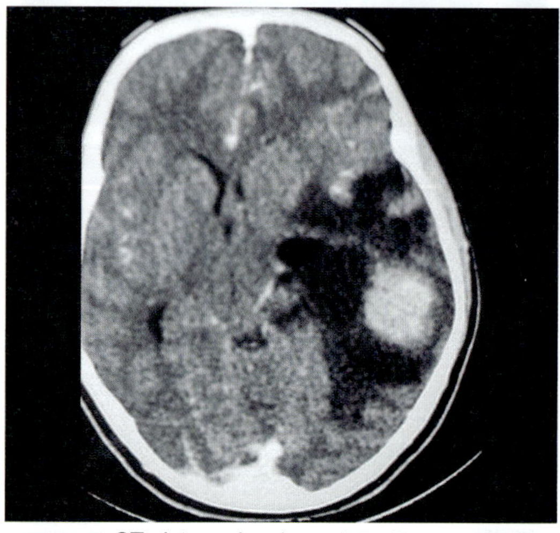

CT picture showing astrocytoma.

290. NOT true for carcinoma tongue:

a. Lateral border is involved
b. Cervical lymph node involvement
c. Commonly adenocarcinoma
d. Tobacco chewing is a risk factor

MC histological type of carcinoma tongue is squamous cell carcinoma.

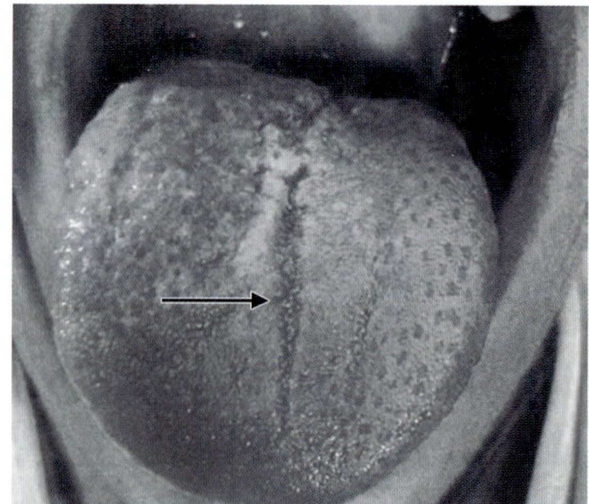

Tongue showing fissuring. Fissuring is one of the presentations of carcinoma tongue

Ans. **288. c.** Thyroglossal... **289. c.** CT scan **290. c.** Commonly...

291. A 60-year-old patient with a history of fall presents with headache and progressive neurological deterioration. The diagnosis is:

a. Acute subdural hemorrhage
b. Extradural hemorrhage
c. Chronic subdural hemorrhage
d. Fracture skull

Chronic subdural haematoma

- Common in old age, with history of minor trauma.
- Patient presents with confusion, disorientation, gradually with altered level of consciousness and drowsiness.
- Later convulsions, features of intracranial hypertension and features of coning develop.

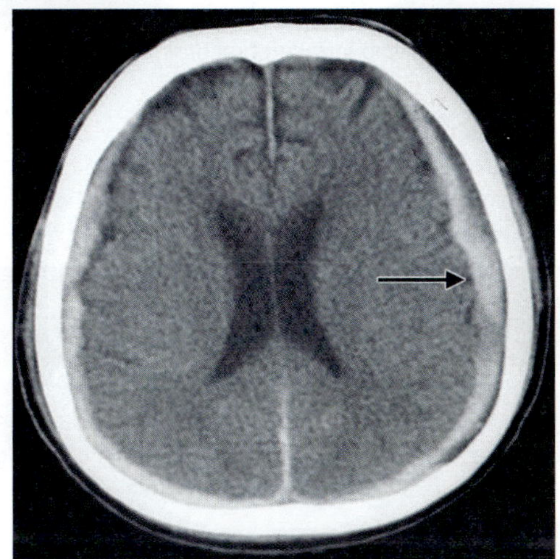

CT scan head showing subdural hematoma with concavo-convex lesion

292. MC cause of acute subdural hematoma:

a. Middle meningeal artery tear
b. Rupture of cortex vein
c. Internal carotid artery tear
d. Rupture of internal jugular vein

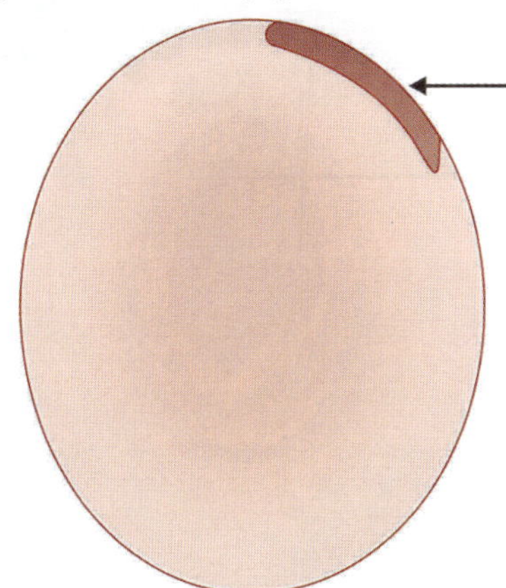

Subdural hematoma. Note the concavo-convex configuration of the lesion

Acute subdural hematoma is a collection of blood between the brain and dura. It is due to injury of the cortical veins and often due to laceration of cortex of brain which bleeds and blood gets collected in the subdural space forming a hematoma.

293. Commonest tumor of parotid gland:

a. Adenoma
b. Pleomorphic adenoma
c. Squamous cell carcinoma
d. Warthin's tumor

Eighty percent salivary neoplasms are in the parotids of which 80% are benign; 80% of these are pleomorphic adenomas.

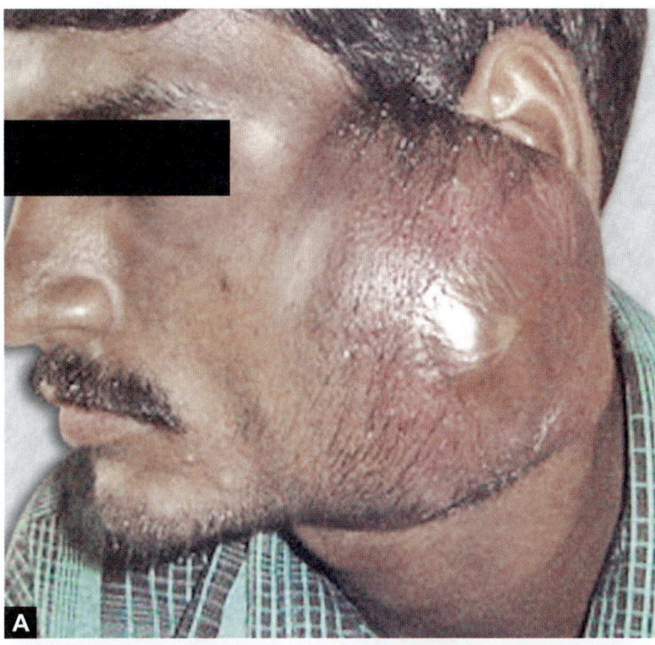

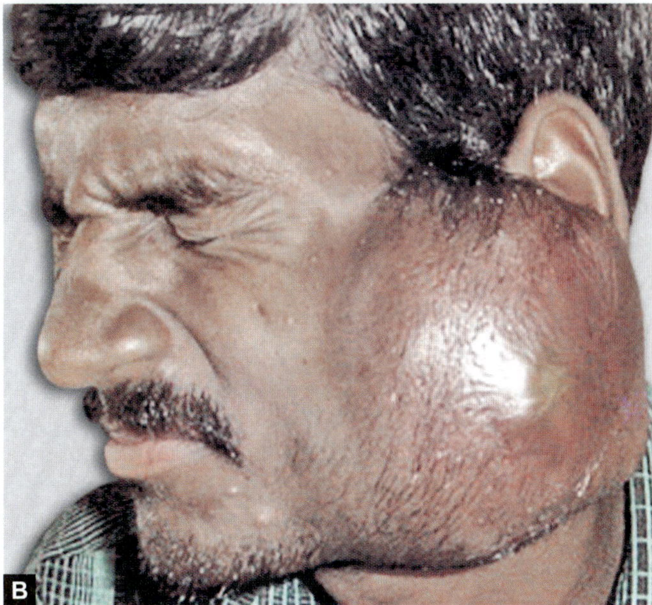

Ans. 291. c. Chronic... **292. b.** Rupture of cortex vein **293. b.** Pleomorphic...

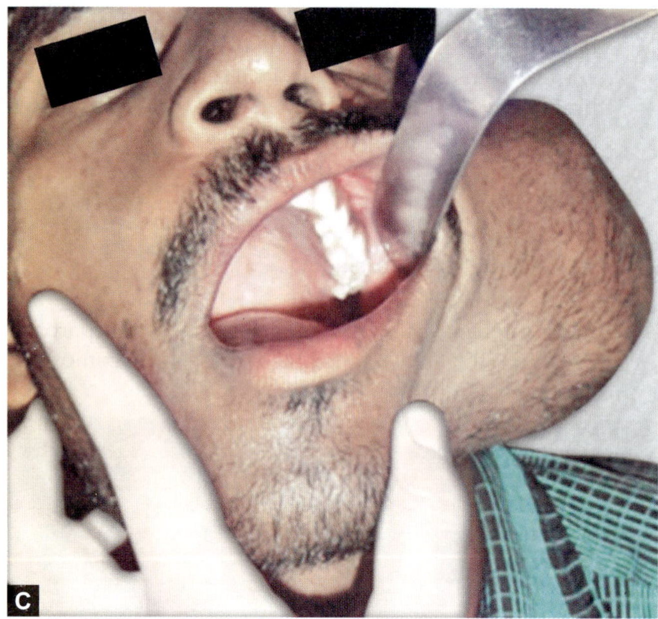

A to C: Recurrent parotid tumor which has attained large size. Note facial nerve is intact. Duct orifice should be inspected using retractor

294. Dentigerous cyst arises from:
- a. An unerupted tooth
- b. Apex of an infected tooth
- c. Nasopalatine cysts
- d. Solitary bone cyst

Dentigerous cyst/follicular odontome occur over the crown of unerupted tooth. It is commonly seen in relation to premolars or molars.

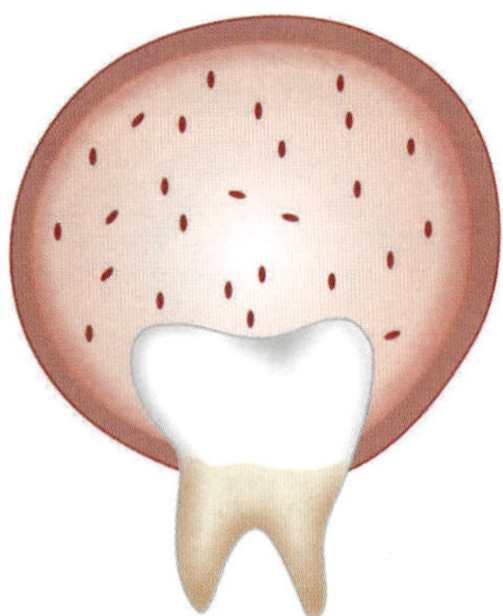

Dentigerous cyst

295. NOT a feature of raised intracranial tension:
- a. Altered sensorium
- b. Papilloedema
- c. Convulsions
- d. Tachycardia

Raised intracranial pressure causes bradycardia, hypertension and vomiting. Raised intracranial pressure may precipitate coning and thus aggravates brain ischemia.

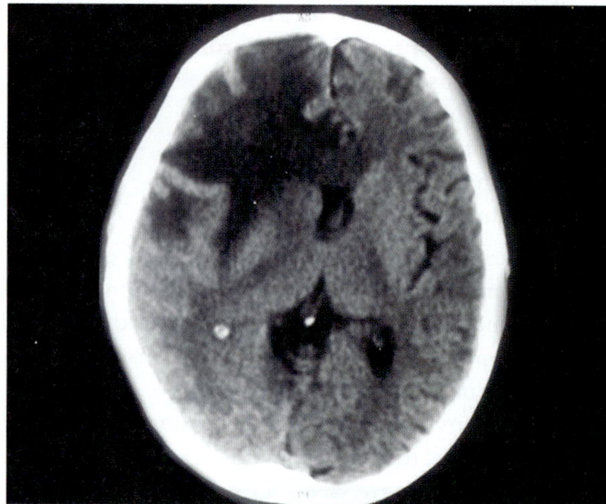

CT scan showing intracerebral brain hemorrhage

296. Lucid interval is classically seen in:
- a. Intracerebral hematoma
- b. Acute subdural hemorrhage
- c. Chronic subdural hemorrhage
- d. Extradural hemorrhage

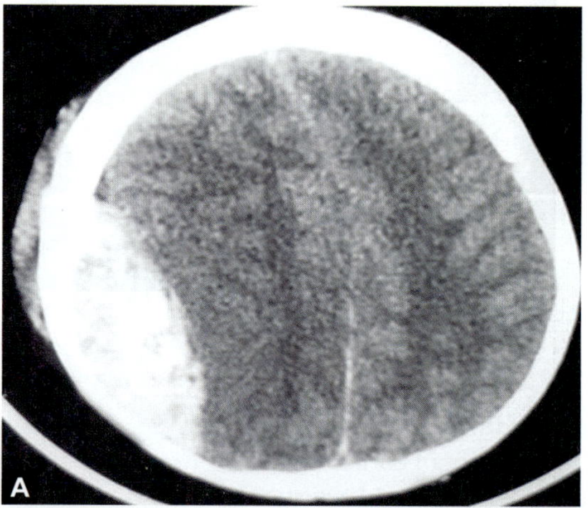

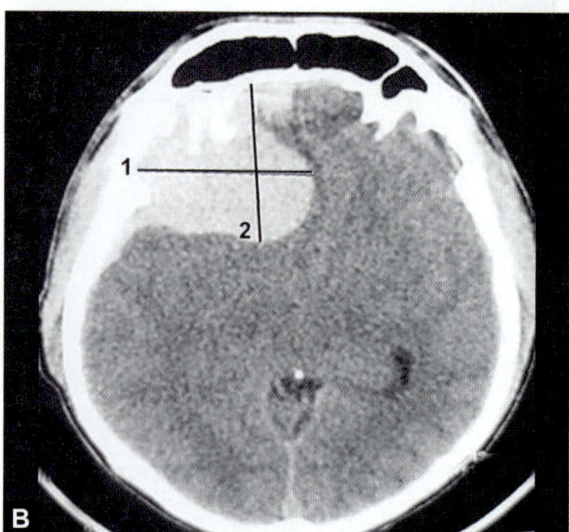

A and B: CT scan head showing extradural hematoma with biconvex lesion

Ans. **294. a.** An unerupted... **295. d.** Tachycardia **296. d.** Extradural...

Clinical features of extradural hematoma

- History of transient loss of consciousness following a history of blow or fall
- Patient soon regains consciousness and again after 6–12 hours, start deteriorating (lucid interval).

297. Cystic, compressible, translucent swelling in the posterior triangle of neck:

a. Cystic hygroma b. Branchial cyst
c. Thyroglossal cyst d. Dermoid cyst

Clinical features of cystic hygroma

- Swelling is present at birth in the posterior triangle of neck causing obstructed labor
- Swelling is smooth, soft, fluctuant (cystic), partially compressible, brilliantly transilluminant. It is not reducible completely.

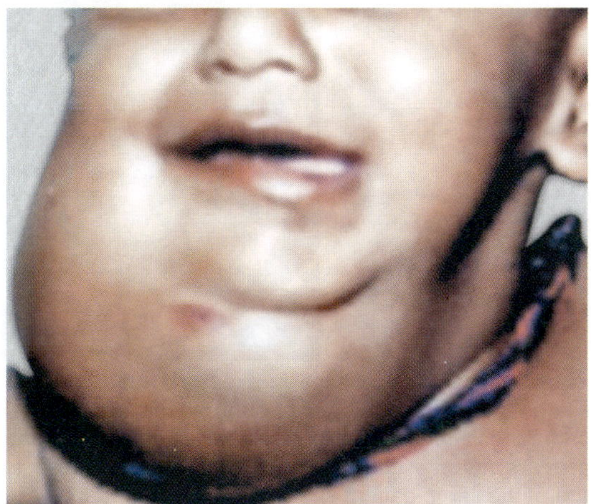

Cystic hygroma

298. All of the swelling moves with deglutition EXCEPT:

a. Thyroglossal cyst b. Thyroid swelling
c. Branchial cyst
d. Tuberculous lymph nodes

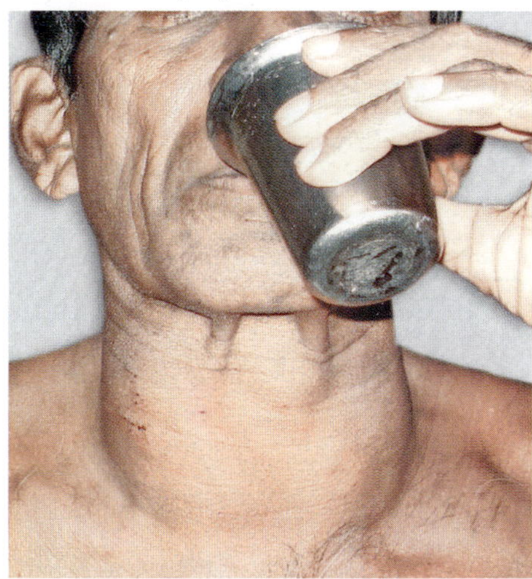

Thyroid swelling moves on deglutition because of attachment of pretracheal fascia through Berry's ligament to cricoid cartilage and to constrictor muscles

Branchial cyst is present in neck beneath the anterior border of upper third of sternomastoid muscle and hence does not move with swallowing/deglutition movement.

LUNGS

299. Probable cause of hypoventilation in a patient who sustained multiple injuries as a result of RTA:

a. Damage to lungs b. Damage to ribs
c. Damage to respiratory centre
d. Damage to vasomotor centre

The **respiratory center** (RC) is located in the medulla oblongata, which is the lowermost part of the brain stem. The RC receives controlling signals of neural, chemical and hormonal nature and controls the rate and depth of respiratory movements of the diaphragm and other respiratory muscles. Injury to this center may lead to center respiratory failure, which necessitates mechanical ventilation

300. FALSE for flail chest:

a. Overlapping should be treated with open reduction
b. Intubation should be done if PO_2 is less than 40% with 60% O_2
c. Paradoxical breathing is not observed in conscious patient
d. Fracture of at least three ribs bilaterally

Flail segment moves independent of the adjacent thoracic cage. During inspiration, flail segment moves inwards (unlike normal thoracic cage which moves outward), and during expiration the segment moves outwards (unlike normal cage which moves inward). This is paradoxical respiration.

Flail chest

Derangements	Types	Problems
❑ Paradoxical respiration ❑ Mediastinal flutter ❑ Pendular movement of air ❑ Pulmonary contusion	❑ Anterior—near costochondral junction ❑ Lateral—in rib shafts ❑ Posterior—safer, due to support of scapula	❑ Cardiac arrest ❑ Respiratory failure ❑ Hemothorax ❑ Infection ❑ ARDS

SURGICAL ONCOLOGY

301. Most radiosensitive tumour:

a. Wilm's tumour
b. Osteosarcoma
c. Non-Hodgkins lymphoma
d. Seminoma

Management of seminoma

- Modern radiotherapy techniques as well as one or two cycles single-agent carboplatin have been shown to reduce the risk of relapse in stage I seminoma (Regardless of treatment strategy, stage 1 seminoma has nearly a 100% cure rate).

Ans. **297. a.** Cystic hygroma **298. c.** Branchial cyst **299. c.** Damage to... **300. c.** Paradoxical breathing... **301. d.** Seminoma

- Stage 2 seminoma is indicated by the presence of retroperitoneal metastasis. Such cases require radiotherapy or, in advanced cases, combination chemotherapy.

302. Commonest premalignant lesion:

a. Nevus spilus b. Junctional nevus
c. Dysplastic nevus d. Blue nevus

Junctional moles are immature and unstable and can turn malignant. In fact majority of the malignant melanoma begin in junctional naevus.

303. Other than galactorrhoea, which of the following is commonly seen in Prolactinoma?

a. Hypothyroidism b. Headache
c. Amenorrhoea d. Menorrhagia

Symptoms of prolactinoma

- Amenorrhea
- Galactorrhea (infrequent in men)
- Loss of axillary and pubic hair
- Hypogonadism, gynecomastia, erectile dysfunction (in males)

304. Sentinel node biopsy is NOT done in:

a. Malignant melanoma b. Ocular cancer
c. Colon carcinoma d. Breast cancer

The **sentinel lymph node** is the hypothetical first lymph node or group of nodes draining a cancer. In case of established cancerous dissemination it is postulated that the sentinel lymph node/s is/are the target organs primarily reached by metastasizing cancer cells from the tumor. The main uses are in breast cancer and malignant melanoma surgery, although it has been used in other tumor types (colon cancer) with a degree of success.

305. N-myc gene is seen in:

a. Nephroblastoma b. Wilm's tumor
c. Retinoblastoma d. Neuroblastoma

Prognosis in neuroblastoma

- It depends on staging of the neuroblastoma – 1, 2A, 2B, 3, 4, 4S
- Low-risk has got 3 years survival – 90%; intermediate risk – 70% and high-risk group has got 30%
- Factors are—age of the child; stage of the disease; Shimada's histology; N-myc amplification status (more means high-risk); DNA ploidy; neurotrophin receptor Trk A (increased is favorable); neutrophin receptor Trk B (increased is unfavorable).

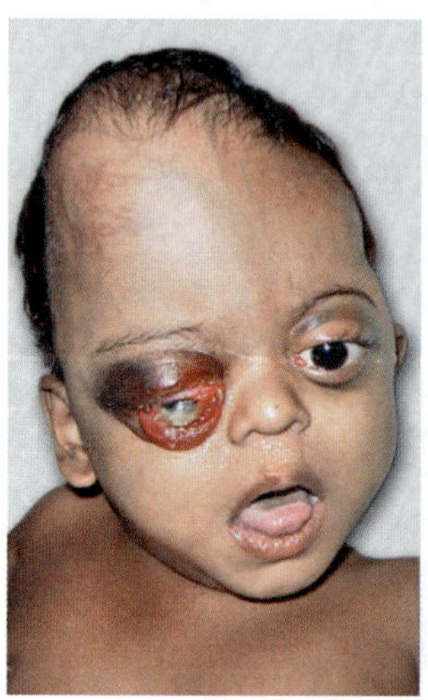

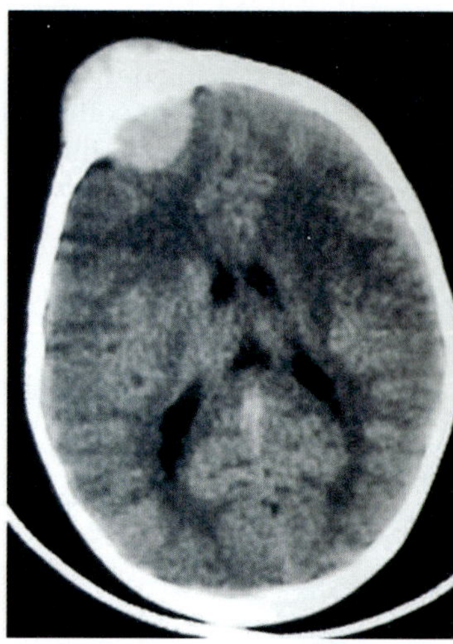

Figure shows typical secondaries in skull and orbit with primary in adrenal gland. Such patients carry poor prognosis. *Racoon's eye sign* is infraorbital ecchymosis due to secondaries in retro-orbital region. Dancing eye syndrome and opsomyoclonus are other eye features. CT picture of the same patient shows obvious secondaries

306. The term universal tumor refers to:

a. Adenoma b. Papilloma
c. Fibroma d. Lipoma

Lipoma is called as universal tumor (ubiquitous tumor) as it can occur anywhere in the body (except in brain).

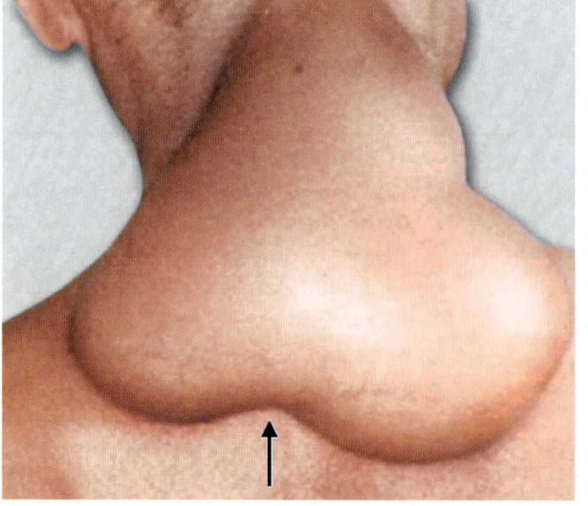

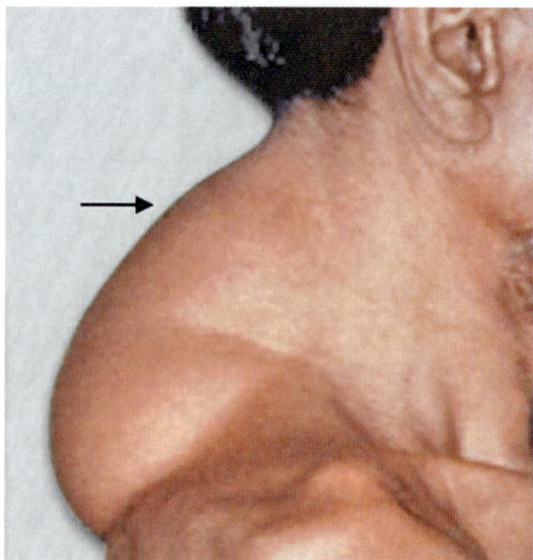

Large lipoma in the nape of neck

Ans. 302. **b.** Junctional... 303. **c.** Amenorrhoea 304. **b.** Ocular cancer 305. **d.** Neuroblastoma 306. **d.** Lipoma

307. Marjolin ulcer is:

a. Squamous cell Ca from scar
b. Adenoma of scar
c. TB ulcer
d. Amoebic ulcer

Marjolin's ulcer is a slow growing locally malignant lesion—a very well differentiated squamous cell carcinoma occurring in an unstable scar of long duration. It is commonly seen in chronic venous ulcer scar. Often it is observed in burns scar and scar of previous snake bite.

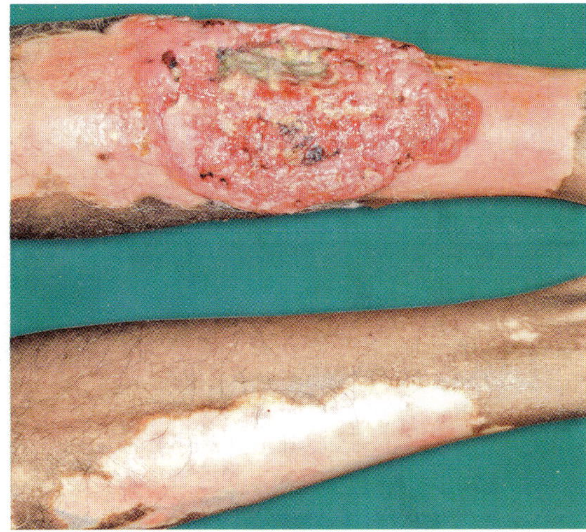

Marjolin's ulcer in a chronic unstable scar (of long duration) in the leg. It does not spread through lymphatics

308. Glomus tumor is seen in:

a. Finger b. Liver
c. Adrenal d. Pituitary

Glomus tumour/ glomangioma is often seen in limbs and common in nail-beds near the finger tips, as purple red swelling. It does not turn into malignancy.

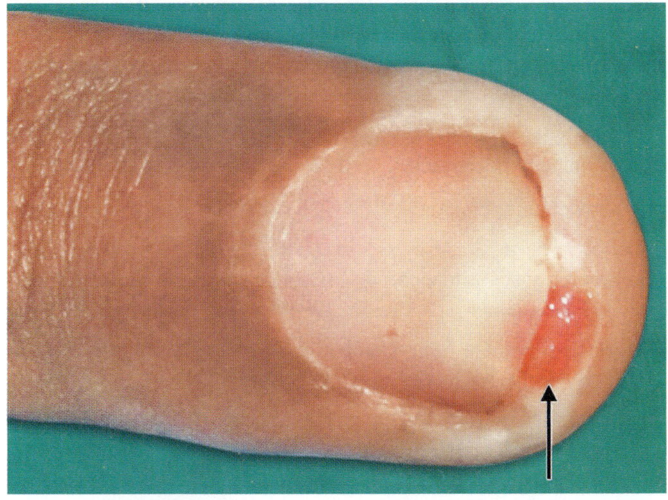

Glomus tumor in finger tip—subungual region

309. Treatment of choice for desmoids tumor:

a. Local excision b. Radiotherapy
c. Wide excision and radiotherapy
d. Wide excision

Desmoid tumor is encapsulated, hard, fibroma, presently classified under aggressive fibromatosis. Wide excision of the tumor with a margin of 2.5 cm is done along with placement of a mesh to the abdominal defect.

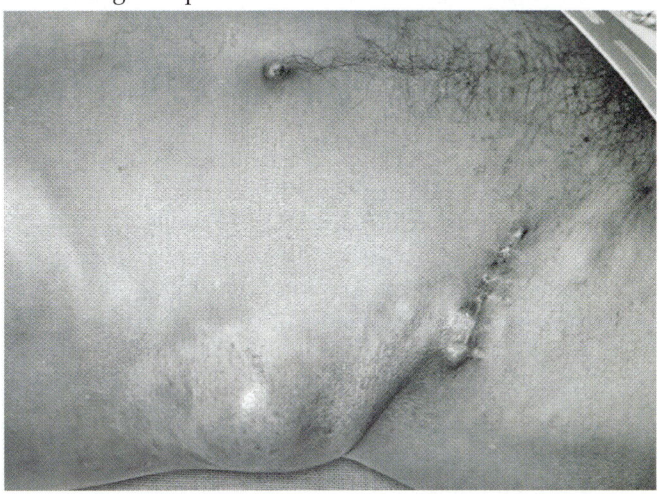

Recurrent abdominal wall tumor. It may be fibromatosis or recurrent dermatofibroma

310. Smoking is NOT associated with:

a. Urinary bladder carcinoma
b. Nasopharynx carcinoma
c. Larynx carcinoma
d. Esophagus carcinoma

Nasopharynx carcinoma is caused by Ebstein Barr virus.

Trotter's triad
❑ Unilateral deafness
❑ Immobile elevated soft palate
❑ Pain in the distribution of trigeminal nerve

311. MC tumor of anterior mediastinum:

a. Thymoma b. Lymphoma
c. Germ cell tumor d. Thyroid tumors

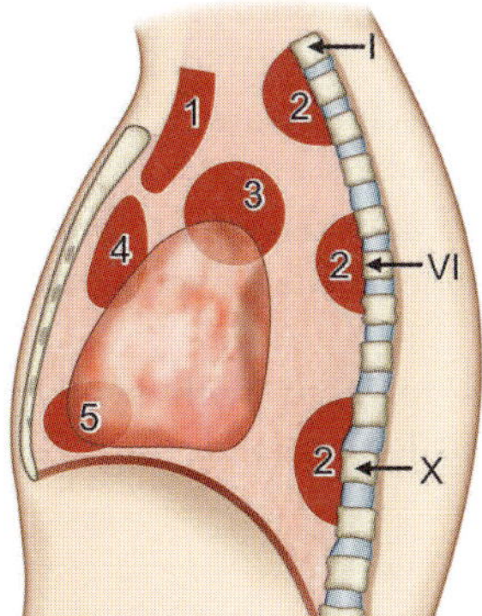

1. Retrosternal goitre
2. Neural tumours (neurofibroma) meningocele, meningomyelocele
3. Lymphoma, foregut, duplication
4. Teratoma/ thymoma/ lymphoma
5. Pleuropericardial cyst

Sites of mediastinal tumors

Ans. **307. a.** Squamous cell **308. a.** Finger **309. d.** Wide excision **310. b.** Nasopharynx carcinoma **311. a.** Thymoma

Thymomas are the most common tumours of the anterosuperior mediastinum in the adult.

MISCELLANEOUS

312. Tinel sign is done in:

a. Axonotemesis
b. Complete transection of nerve
c. Degeneration of nerve
d. Regeneration of nerve

Tinel's sign

- It is referred to as "distal tingling on percussion" or DTP.
  - This distal sign of regeneration can be expected during different stage of somatosensory recovery.
- It is also a way to detect irritated nerves.
  - It is performed by lightly tapping (percussing) over the nerve to elicit a sensation of tingling or "pins and needles" in the distribution of the nerve.

313. True statements regarding Keloid are all EXCEPT:

a. Hyperkeratotic
b. Most common on sternum
c. Familial
d. Self limiting

Removing the keloid is one treatment option; however, it may result in more severe consequences: the probability that the resulting surgery scar will also become a keloid is high, usually greater than 50% (Keloid is a recurrent entity; NOT self limiting).

314. Xenograft is:

a. Organ from self
b. Organ from mother or father
c. Organ from twins
d. Organ from any other species

Graft taxonomy

- Autologous: The donor skin is taken from a different site on the same individual's body (also known as an autograft).
- Isogeneic: The donor and recipient individuals are genetically identical (e.g., monozygotic twins, animals of a single inbred strain; isograft or syngraft).
- Allogeneic: The donor and recipient are of the same species (human→human, dog→dog; allograft).
- Xenogeneic: The donor and recipient are of different species (e.g., bovine cartilage; xenograft or heterograft).
- Prosthetic: Lost tissue is replaced with synthetic materials such as metal, plastic, or ceramic (prosthetic implants)

315. Hoffman's sign is seen in:

a. Upper motor neuron lesion
b. Deep venous thrombosis
c. Nerve degeneration
d. Nerve regeneration

A Hoffmann (or **Tinel's sign**) is a tingling sensation triggered by a mechanical stimulus in the distal part of an injured nerve. This sensation radiates peripherally, from the point where it is triggered to the cutaneous distribution of the nerve. The tingling response can be compared with that produced by a weak electric current, as in **transcutaneous electrical nerve stimulation (TENS)**.

316. Intravenous antibiotics for prophylaxis should be given:

a. Anytime
b. With pre-medication
c. Night before surgery
d. Post-operatively

Preoperative treatment

- Control of respiratory and cardiac diseases
- Improvement of hemoglobin status, if anemia is present
- Preoperative antibiotics are given
- Blood should be kept ready for major surgeries
- Starvation for 4 hours for liquids and six hours for solids
- Bladder and bowel should be emptied to prevent soiling on the operation table. Urinary catheter may be passed and enema may be given
- Dentures, contact lenses, jewellery must be removed
- Surgical area should be cleaned and properly prepared.

317. In treatment of hand injuries, the greatest priority is:

a. Repair of tendons
b. Repair of skin cover
c. Repair of nerves
d. All

Primary repair of tendons and nerves are of lesser priority in untidy injuries. Priority is wound debridement/ wound excision and early skin cover.

In hand

Do's	*Don'ts*
Do examine hand carefully	Do not incise every infected digit
Do think of other diagnosis	Do not make puncture incisions or over pads
Do wait for abscess to localise	Do not injure the digital nerves or vessels
Do place adequate length and depth of incisions	Do not place incisions crossing the crease line
Do immobilise, elevate the hand	Do not close human bites or lacerated wounds
Do give antibiotics and proper dressings	Do not forget to send pus for culture and sensitivity

Ans. 312. **d.** Regeneration... 313. **d.** Self limiting 314. **d.** Organ from any... 315. **d.** Nerve regeneration
316. **b.** With pre... 317. **b.** Repair of skin cover

318. In case of acute abdominal trauma, best guideline for quick replacement of fluid is:

a. Pulse
b. Hemoglobin
c. Urine output
d. CVP

In case of abdominal trauma, evaluation of the extent of the injury must be done; number of organs injured and severity of injury; hematocrit assessment (hemoglobin drop up to 6 gm% is tolerated well with adequate tissue oxygenation. Rapid drop of hemoglobin needs adequate number of blood to be kept ready for transfusion, like 5/10/bottles or more); central line for volume replacement; urinary catheterization; administration of systemic antibiotics.

Categorise the patient	
I: Deceased II: Walking wounded III: Immobile wounded IV: Trapped wounded	
Tag the patient accordingly	
Red color	Immediate treatment is required
Yellow color	Urgent treatment is required
Green color	Delayed treatment is required
Blue color	Expectant treatment is required
Black color	Deceased
Airway	*Breathing*
Chin lift	100% oxygen
Jaw thrust	Assess bilateral chest raise
Nasal airway	Assess breath sounds
Oral airway	Use pulse oximetry
Endotracheal intubation	Treat flail chest, pneumothorax
Tracheostomy	Intercostal tube drainage
(assess airway patency)	
Circulation	*Disability evaluation*
Monitor vitals	Neurological examination
Heart sounds	Glasgow coma scale
ECG	Pupillary reaction
IV fluids blood transfusion	
Treatment of shock	
Control of external bleed	
Use two IV lines—14G/16G	
Expose the Patient	Fingers and Tubes
Fully	Examine all orifices like P/R,
Undress the patient	P/V, etc.

Contd...

Contd...

Categorise the patient	
Hypothermia assessment	Use required tubes like catheter,
Assess injuries	Ryle's tube
Examine joints, bones, abdomen, other systems	
Look for identification marks	

319. NOT a site for keloid formation:

a. Back
b. Sternum
c. Face
d. Ear

Common site of keloid are over the sternum, upper arm, chest wall, lower neck in front.

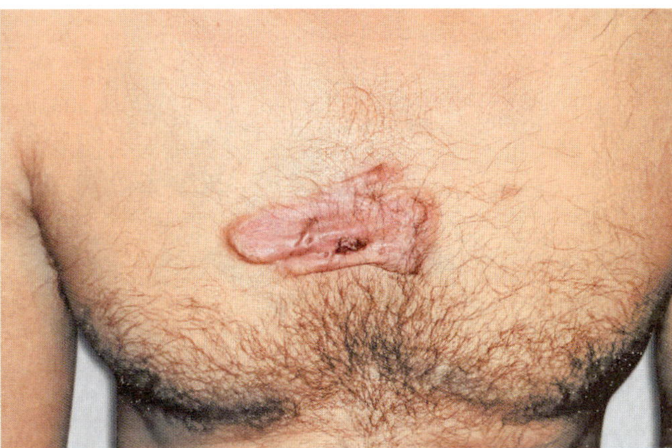

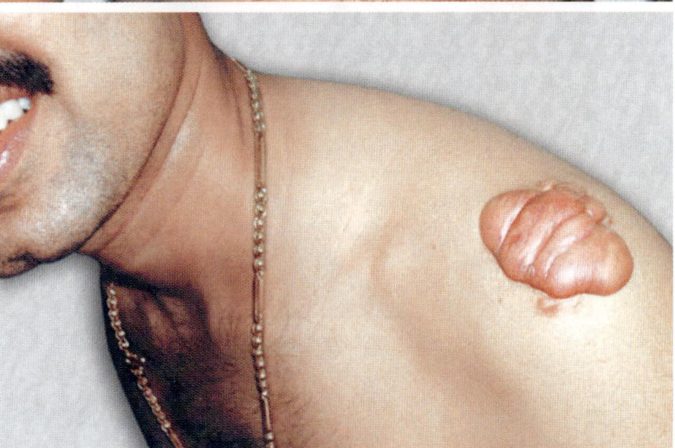

Keloid in chest below the sternum and upper part of arm near shoulder—common sites of occurrence

320. Chronic thick walled pyogenic abscess may be due to all EXCEPT:

a. Presence of foreign body
b. Prolonged antibiotic therapy
c. Virulent strains of organism
d. Inadequate drainage

Virulent strains of organism will cause acute infection.

Ans. **318. c.** Urine output **319. c.** Face **320. c.** Virulent strains...

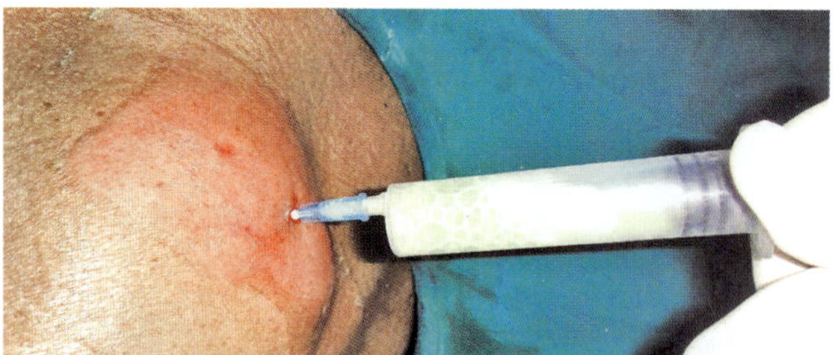

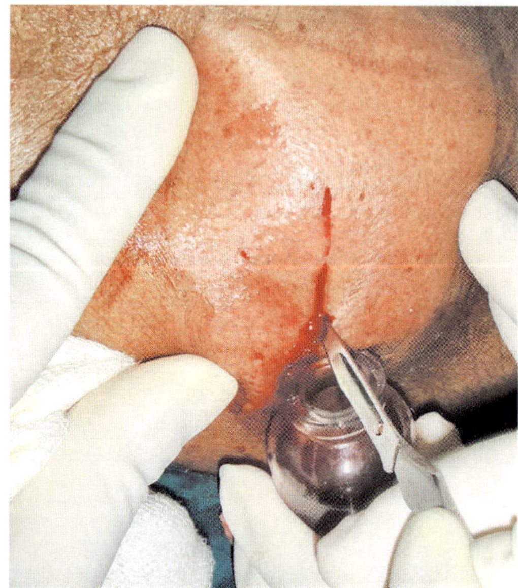

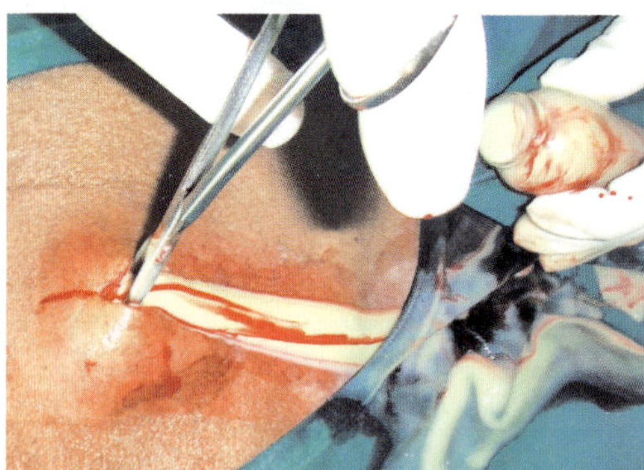

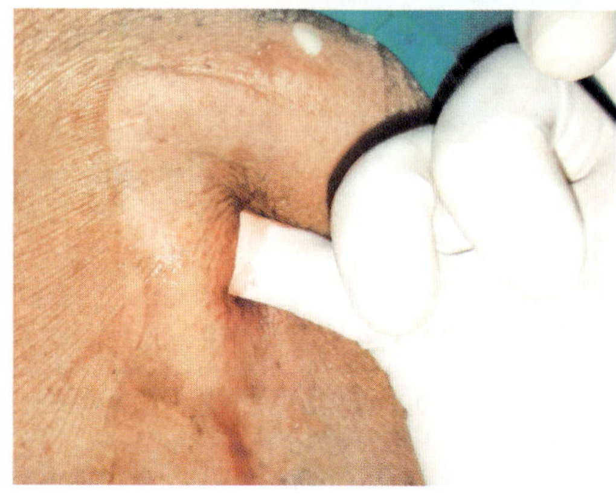

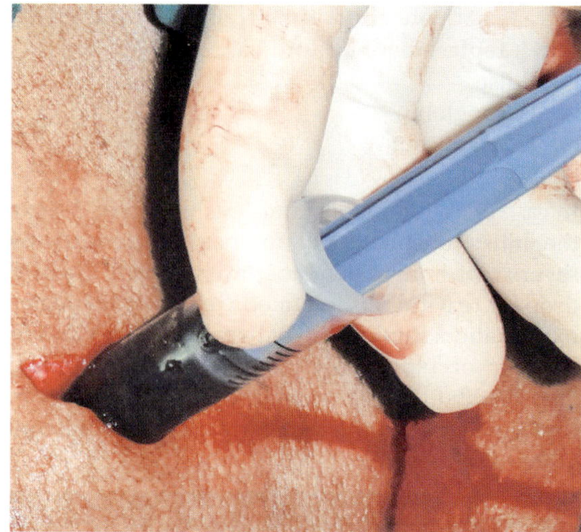

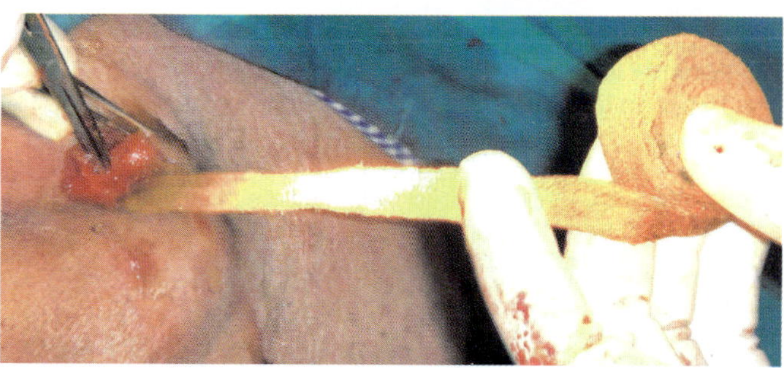

Technique of incision and drainage of a pyogenic abscess. Abscess should be aspirated first to get pus; No. 11 blade is used to incise; using sinus forceps pyogenic membrane is opened; pus is collected for culture; loculi are broken using sinus forceps and little finger; cavity is irrigated with *normal saline (ideal)* and povidone iodine; cavity is packed with roller gauze; wound is not sutured

321. Painless effusion in joints in congenital syphilis is called:

a. Clutton's joint
b. Banton's joint
c. Charcoat's joint
d. Synovitis

Manifestations of tertiary/ late stage syphilis

- Gummatous ulcer
- Perforation of nasal septum/ palate
- Clutton's joint
- Sabre tibia
- Neurosyphilis (tabes dorsalis)
- Aneurysm of arch of aorta

322. A boil is due to staphylococcal infection of:

a. Hair follicle
b. Sweat gland
c. Subcutaneous tissue
d. Epidermis

Boil/furuncle is an acute staphylococcal infection of a hair follicle with perifolliculitis which usually proceeds to suppuration and central necrosis.

Ans. 321. a. Clutton's joint **322. a.** Hair follicle

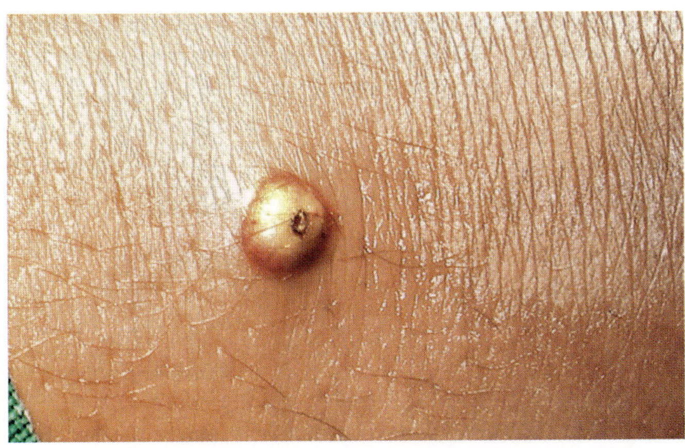

Furuncle/boil are infection of hair follicle with perifolliculitis due to *Staphylococcus aureus*

323. Commonest site of meningomyelocele:

a. Cervical b. Thoracic
c. Lumbar-sacral d. None of the above

In myelomeningocele, part of the cord or cauda equina or both present as median cystic swelling at back. It is common in lumbosacral region.

Meningocele	*Meningomyelocele*
❑ Membranes content	❑ Membranes with nerve roots
❑ Soft, cystic	❑ Soft to firm
❑ Brilliantly transilluminant	❑ Nontransilluminant
❑ Longitudinal furrow absent	❑ Longitudinal furrow is seen due to adherence of nerve roots
❑ No neurological defect	❑ Trophic ulcer, bowel/urine incontinence, motor problems
❑ Good prognosis after repair	❑ Neurological deficit present
	❑ Not good results

324. Catgut is derived from intestine of:

a. Sheep b. Cat
c. Human d. All of the above

Plain catgut is derived from submucosa of jejunum of sheep. It is yellowish white in color.

325. When do we start antibiotics to prevent post-operative infection:

a. 2 days before surgery
b. After surgery
c. 1 week before surgery
d. 1 hour before surgery and continue after surgery

Antibiotics are given pre-operatively and continued for 1-2 weeks after surgery.

326. Congenital sensorineural deafness with abnormal iodine metabolism and goiter in children is:

a. Nome's syndrome
b. Gradenigo's syndrome
c. Pendred's syndrome
d. Cogan's syndrome

Pendred syndrome is characterized by defective organification of iodine, goiter and sensorineural deafness (typically associated with malformation of the inner ear bony labyrinth).

327. Pendred's syndrome is due to a defect in:

a. Chromosome 7p b. Chromosme 7q
c. Chromosome 8p d. Chromosome 8q

Mutation of the pendrin gene (chromosome 7q) causes Pendred syndrome, an autosomal recessive disorder.

328. MC complication of immunosuppression is:

a. Malignancy b. Graft rejection
c. Infection d. Thrombocytopenia

Complications
❑ Infection—commonest
❑ Malignancy—squamous cell carcinoma, lymphoma, Kaposi's sarcoma
❑ Nephrotoxicity
❑ Bone marrow toxicity
❑ GIT toxicity
❑ Neurotoxicity

329. Highest chances of success in renal transplant is seen when the donor is:

a. Identical twin b. Father
c. Mother d. Sister

Highest chances of success in any transplantation (renal) is seen when the donor is the identical twin.

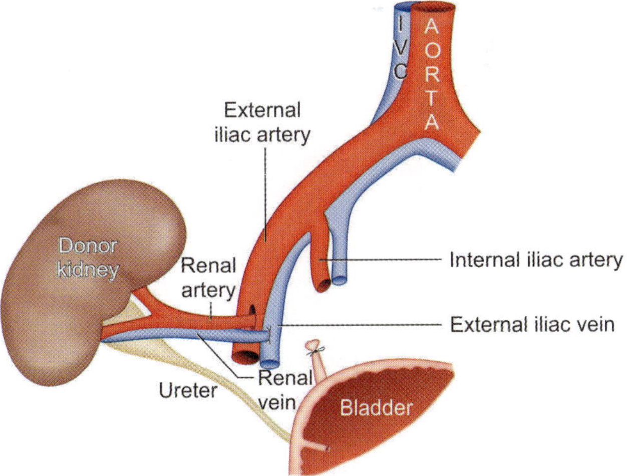

Renal transplantation

330. Transplant of kidney from mother to son is an example of:

a. Autograft b. Allograft
c. Isograft d. Xenograft

A graft is said to be allograft if there is tissue transfer between two genetically different members, e.g. kidney transplantation (human to human) (Homograft).

Ans. 323. c. Lumbar-sacral 324. a. Sheep 325. d. 1 hour before... 326. c. Pendred's syndrome
327. b. Chromosme 7q 328. c. Infection 329. a. Identical twin 330. b. Allograft

Major histocompatibility complex (MHC)
❑ MHC is located in chromosome number 6
❑ Individual will have two HLA (*Human Leucocyte Antigens*) genes inherited from each parents, which together called as HLA types
❑ Class I— HLA is HLA-A, HLA-B and HLA-C. Intracellular antigens
❑ Class II—HLA is HLA-DP, HLA-DQ and HLA- DR. Extracellular antigens
❑ HLA-DR is most important in kidney transplantation

331. Amputated digits are preserved in:

a. Cold saline b. Cold Ringer Lactate
c. Ice in plastic bag d. Deep freezer

The best way to preserve the amputated part is to wrap it in gauze moistened with saline (salt water), place the wrapped part in a plastic sealable bag, and put the bag on ice.

332. Foramen of Bochdalek is related to:

a. Duramater b. Diaphragm
c. Urogenital diaphragm d. Mediastinum

Foramen of Bochdalek is a developmental defective condition, due to the failure of fusion of pleuroperitoneal canal leaving a direct communication between pleura and peritoneum on left side.

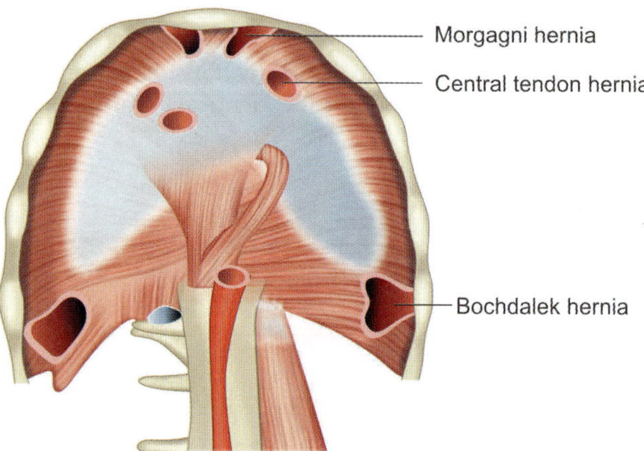

Anatomy of diaphragm showing different sites where hernia can occur

333. Hyperacute graft rejection is due to:

a. Preformed antibodies b. T lymphocytes
c. Macrophages d. B lymphocytes

Hyperacute graft rejection occurs within minutes or hours. It is observed typically with xenogeneic grafts and, in rare instances (for example ABO incompatibility) with allogeneic grafts. It is caused by pre-existing antibodies directed to components of the graft, typically endothelial cells.

334. Infection in renal transplant patient is usually due to:

a. CMV b. HIV
c. Herpes d. Salmonella

Opportunistic infections are common with immunosuppression. Cytomegalovirus (CMV) infection is common causing pneumonia, hepatitis, pancreatitis, GI problems.

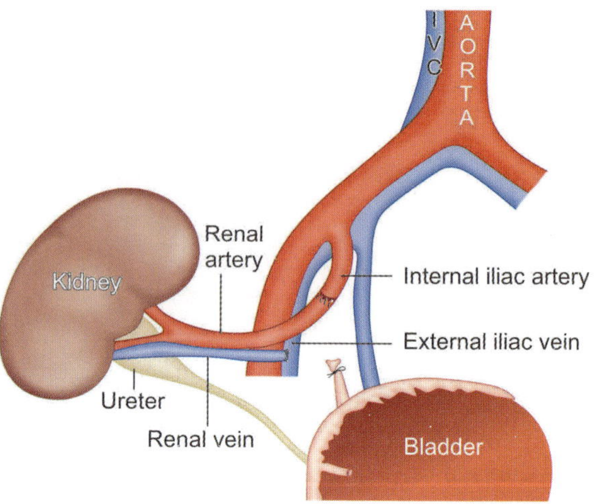

Another method of getting arterial perfusion of the transplanted kidney by suturing (*Carrel stitch*) external iliac artery to renal artery side-to-end

335. Transplantation of which of the following is most often associated with hyperacute rejection:

a. Heart b. Kidney
c. Lungs d. Liver

Hyperacute rejection of the renal allograft occurs within hours of the transplant; nephrectomy is indicated.

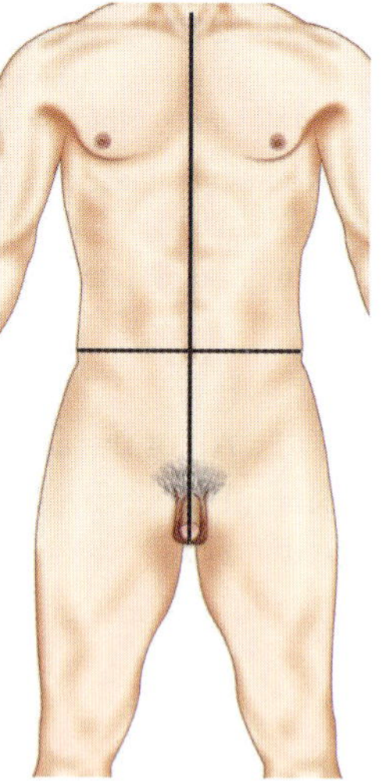

Incision from manubrium as sternotomy to pubic symphysis with a horizontal part above umbilicus

Incision for organ procurement.

336. Cocks peculiar tumor is:

a. Papilloma b. Infected sebaceous cyst
c. Cylindroma d. Squamous cell Ca

Surface of sebaceous cyst may get ulcerated leading to formation of a painful, fungating mass with discharge called as – Cock's peculiar tumor—often resembles epithelioma. It is a misnomer as it is not a true tumor. It is a chronic granuloma on an ulcerated surface of a sebaceous cyst.

Ans. 331. **c.** Ice in plastic bag 332. **b.** Diaphragm 333. **a.** Preformed... 334. **a.** CMV
335. **b.** Kidney 336. **b.** Infected sebaceous...

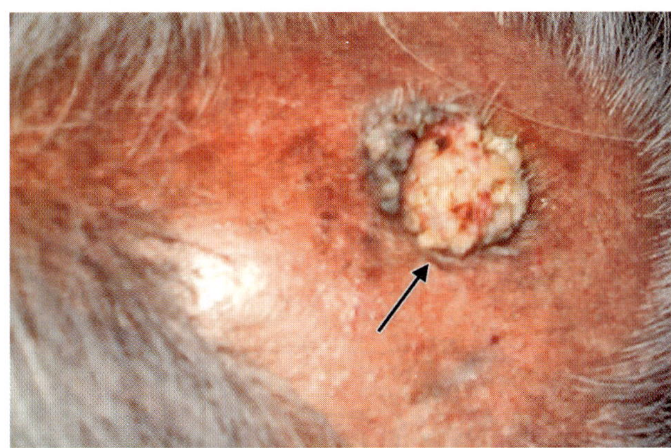

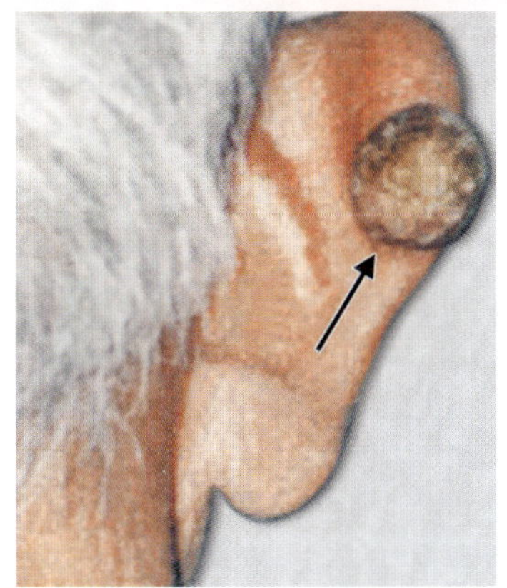

Cock's peculiar tumor over scalp and ear

337. A young patient presented with dyspnea, bleeding and petechial hemorrhage in the chest after 2 days following fracture shaft femur of right side. Most likely cause is:

a. Air embolism
b. Fat embolism
c. Pulmonary thromboembolism
d. Amniotic fluid embolism

Fat embolism is commonly seen after fracture femur, tibia, or multiple fractures and occasionally following electroconvulsive therapy, usually occurs in 72 hours. Clinical features include tachypnea, petechial hemorrhages in the skin etc.

338. Pseudo-claudication is due to compression of:

a. Popliteal artery   b. Cauda equina
c. Tibial artery   d. Femoral artery

Neurogenic claudication (NC), also known as pseudo-claudication, is a common symptom of lumbar canal stenosis, or inflammation of the nerves emanating from the spinal cord. In some patients with severe compression of the nerve roots, the NC is not intermittent but painfully present.

339. Which of the following is a regressing tumor:

a. Portwine stain   b. Strawberry angioma
c. Venous angioma   d. Plexiform angioma

Strawberry hemangioma may start at birth or child is normal at birth; between one to three weeks it appears as red mark which rapidly increases in size in 3 months to form strawberry/raspberry hemangioma. After one year of age, it slowly begins to disappear, and completely in 7–8 years (70% in 7 years).

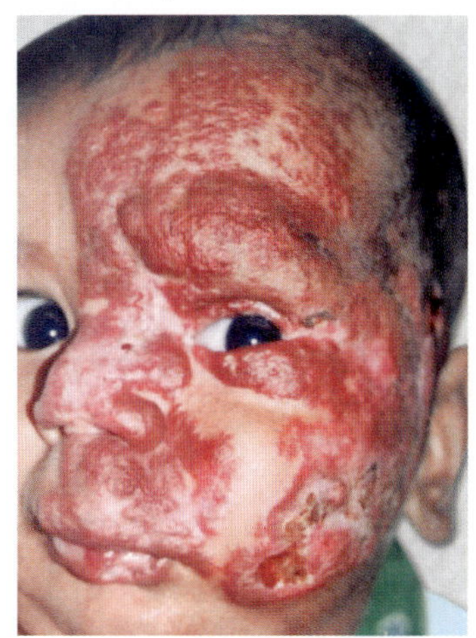

Strawberry hemangioma

340. Split thickness skin graft is NOT taken up by:

a. Fat   b. Muscle
c. Deep fascia   d. Skull bone

SSG cannot be done over bone, tendon, cartilage, joint.

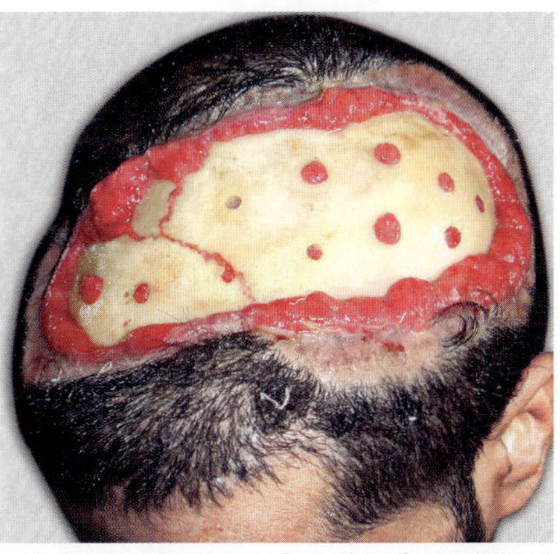

Multiple burr holes done to promote formation of granulation tissue from vascular diploe of the skull. Once granulation tissue covers the entire defect, skin grafting can be placed

341. Split skin grafts in young children should be harvested from:

a. Buttocks   b. Thigh
c. Trunk   d. Upper limb

Donor area for SSG is commonly thigh, occasionally arm, leg and forearm.

342. Basal cell carcinoma spreads by:

a. Lymphatics   b. Hematogenous
c. Direct spread   d. None of the above

Ans. **337. b.** Fat embolism **338. b.** Cauda equina **339. b.** Strawberry angioma **340. d.** Skull bone
341. b. Thigh **342. c.** Direct spread

In BCC, no lymph node or blood spread occurs. Due to large sized tumor cells/tumour cluster, it does not spread through lymphatics. But it erodes deeply into local tissues including cartilages, bones causing extensive local destruction. Hence the name "rodent ulcer" is given.

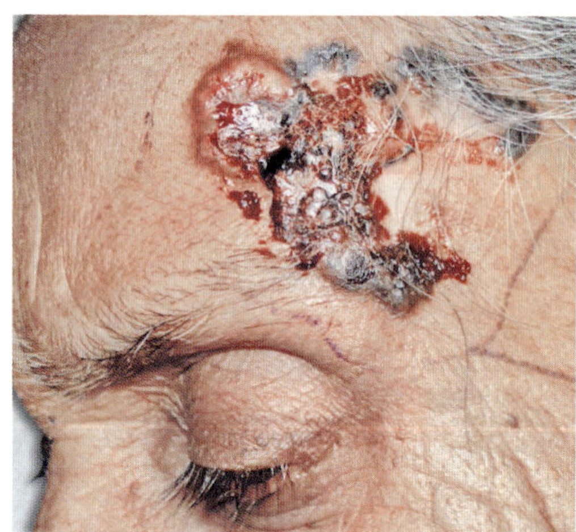

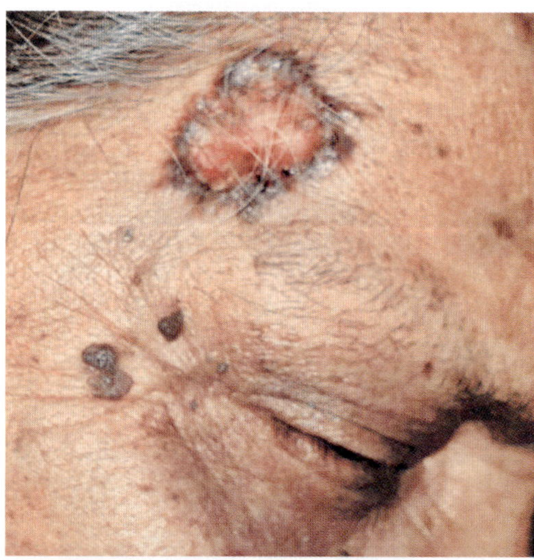

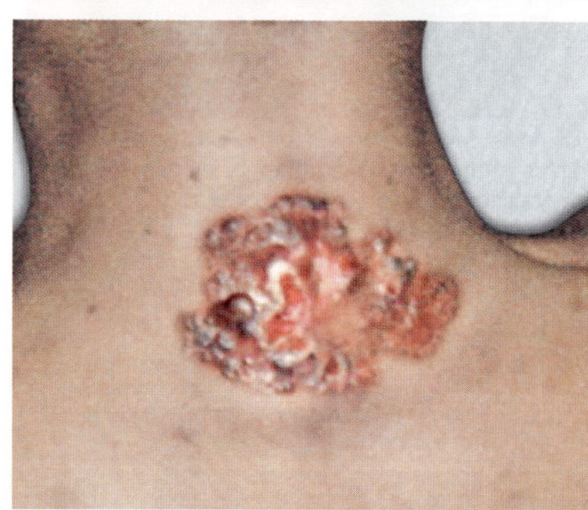

Basal cell carcinoma in different locations. Note the nodularity and ulceration. Note the beaded edge

343. Full thickness graft can NOT be obtained from:

a. Supraclavicular
b. Groin
c. Post-auricular
d. Axilla

Common sites of donor area for full thickness graft

- Post-auricular area
- Supraclavicular area
- Groin crease area

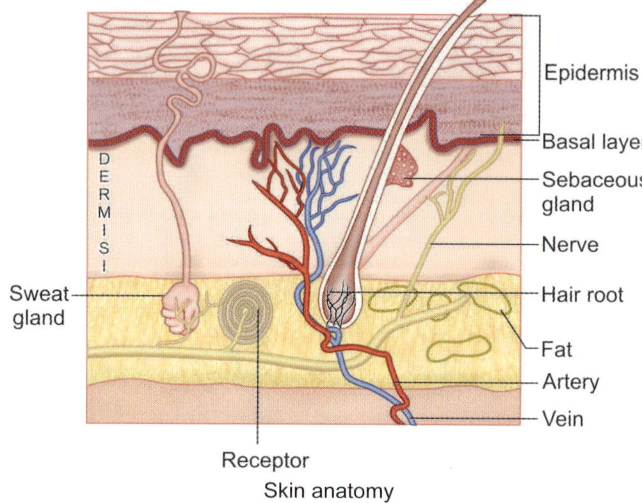

Skin anatomy

344. Felon is:

a. Midpalmar space infection
b. Terminal pulp space infection
c. Infection of the ulnar bursa
d. Infection of the radial bursa

Terminal pulp space infection/felon is the second MC hand infection (25%). It is usually caused by a minor injury like finger prick.

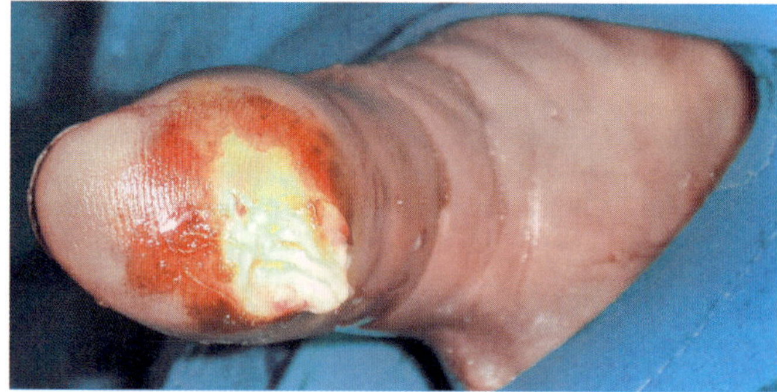

Pulp space infection

345. Prolapsed intervertebral disc (PID) is most common at:

a. C2-C3
b. T10-T11
c. L2-L3
d. L4-L5

In lumbosacral region, discs between L5 and S1; L4 and L5 are commonly affected impinging first sacral nerve and 5th lumbar nerve respectively.

Ans. **343. d.** Axilla **344. b.** Terminal pulp space... **345. d.** L4-L5

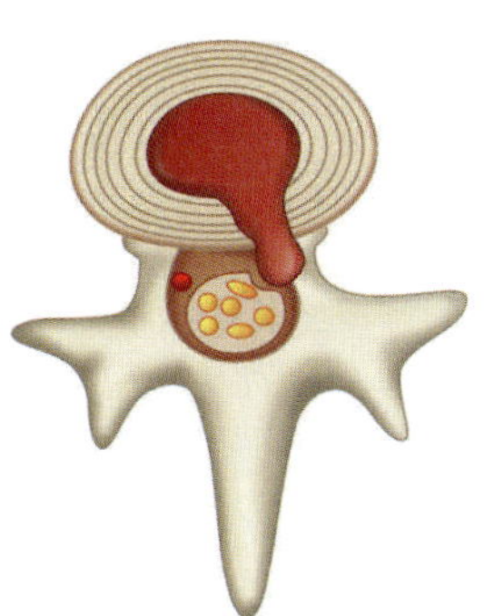
Intervertebral disc prolapse

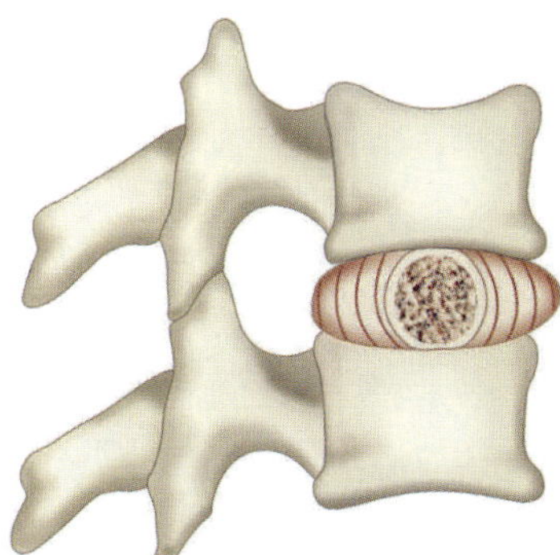
Vertebra with nucleus pulposus and annulus fibrosis

Intervertebral disc prolapse

346. The most important sign in Volkman's ischemic contracture:

a. Pain
b. Pallor
c. Numbness
d. Obliteration of radial pulse

Clinical features of acute phase of VIC

- Pain (persistent pain in the forearm, hand and fingers – ominous symptom)
- Pallor
- Puffiness (due to edema)
- Pulseless (absence of radial pulse; but its presence does not rule out the onset of impending contractures)
- Paresis

347. Characteristics of SIRS include all of the following EXCEPT:

a. Leukocytosis
b. Thrombocytopenia
c. Infectious or non-infectious cause
d. Oral temperature more than 38°C

Systemic inflammatory response syndrome

- It is a part of severely decompensated reversible shock which eventually leads to MODS (multiorgan dysfunction syndrome), a state of irreversible shock wherein patient is anuric, drowsy, cold and terminally ill.
- It is final common pathway in shock due to any cause (trauma, sepsis, endotoxemia, burns) where there is failure of inflammatory localization with vasodilatation, increased endothelial permeability with damage, thrombosis, leucocyte migration and activation.

348. A Wolfe graft is:

a. Partial thickness skin graft
b. Pinch skin graft
c. Small full thickness skin graft
d. Pedicle graft

Full thickness graft (Wolfe graft) includes both epidermis + full dermis. It is used over the face, eyelid, hands, fingers and over the joints.

349. MC type of renal transplantation in India is:

a. Allograft
b. Autograft
c. Isograft
d. Xenograft

Three types of donors

- Living related donors
- Living nonrelated donors
- Cadaver donors (Individuals with severe brain injury resulting in brain death).

350. Best treatment of strawberry angioma is:

a. Sclerosants
b. Corticosteroids
c. Masterly inactivity
d. Excision

Since strawberry hemangioma disappear completely in 7–8 years, so wait and watch is the best policy.

351. Most effective step in treatment of gas gangrene is:

a. Hyperbaric oxygen
b. Debridement
c. Debridement and wound closure
d. Antibiotics

Therapy of gas gangrene should be concentrated in managing dehydration, hypotension, infection, toxemia by hydration, fresh whole blood transfusion, passive immunization, antibiotics, and hyperbaric oxygen, doing radical wound excision with removal of all dead tissues (debridement) with foreign body or amputation with critical care.

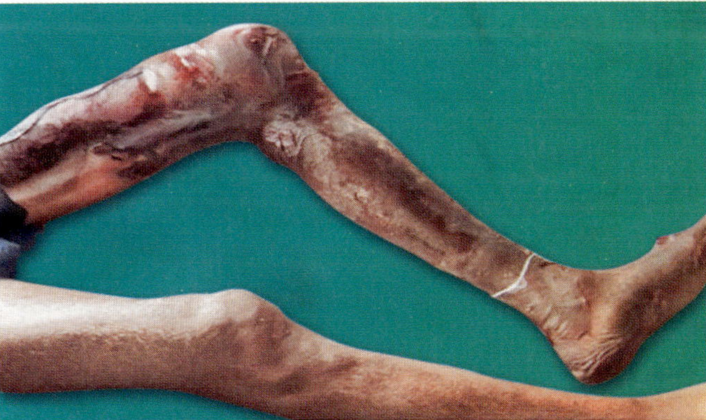

Gas gangrene involving entire leg extensively. Note the black/khaki colored area. Patient died of toxemia

352. Epidermal cyst is lined by:

a. Transitional epithelium
b. Stratified squamous epithelium
c. Columnar epithelium
d. Cuboidal epithelium

Epidermoid cyst/sebaceous cyst contains yellowish white cheesy material with fat and epithelium. It has putty like consistency, with a parasite in the wall of the sebaceous cyst – Demodex folliculorum. It is lined by only epidermal layer of squamous epithelium.

Ans. **346. a.** Pain **347. b.** Thrombocytopenia **348. c.** Small full... **349. a.** Allograft **350. c.** Masterly... **351. b.** Debridement **352. b.** Stratified...

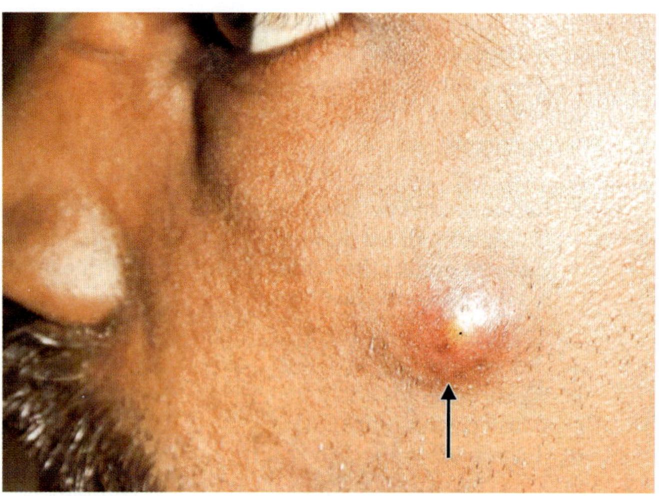

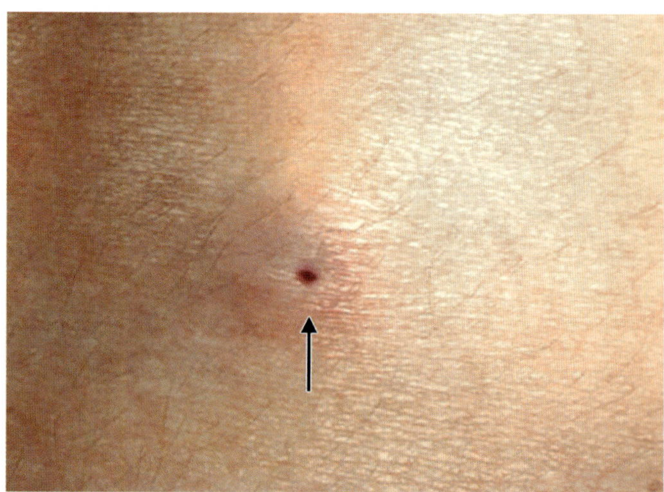

Small sebaceous cysts in face and back with typical punctum over the summit

ANSWERS WITH REFERENCES

BURNS

1. **Ans. (d) Hyperthermia**
Ref: S Das's Surgery, 4/e p53

2. **Ans. (a) Consider intravenous resuscitation in children with burns greater than 15% TBSA**
Ref: SRB's Surgery 4/e p131

3. **Ans. (a) 1%**
Ref: SRB's Surgery 4/e p130

4. **Ans. (d) Extremely painful**
Ref: SRB's Surgery, 4/e p131

5. **Ans. (c) 3 weeks**
Ref: SRB's Surgery 4/e p131

6. **Ans. (b) Painless**
Ref: SRB's Surgery 4/e p134

7. **Ans. (d) Hyperthermia**
Ref: SRB's Surgery 4/e p131

8. **Ans. (b) Painful**
Ref: SRB's Surgery 4/e p132

9. **Ans. (a) Fluid resuscitation**
Ref: SRB's Surgery 4/e p132

10. **Ans. (b) Hypovolumic shock**
Ref: SRB's Surgery 4/e p134

11. **Ans. (c) Ringer lactate**
Ref: SRB's Surgery 4/e p132

12. **Ans. (b) Physical burn injury to the airways above the larynx**
Ref: SRB's Surgery 4/e p133

13. **Ans. (c) Handwashing**
Ref: SRB's Surgery 4/e p135

14. **Ans. (c) Blister formation**
Ref: SRB's Surgery 4/e p131

15. **Ans. (d) Peripheral pulse and circulation**
Ref: SRB's Surgery 4/e p133

16. **Ans. (a) 1%**
Ref: SRB's Surgery 4/e p134

17. **Ans. (d) (% body surface area) × (weight in Kgs) × 4 = Volume in ml**
Ref: SRB's Surgery 4/e p131

18. **Ans. (c) Circumferential full thickness burns**
Ref: SRB's Surgery 4/e p139

VASCULAR SYSTEM

19. **Ans. (d) Varicose veins**
Ref: S Das's Surgery, 4/e p205

20. **Ans. (d) Small acral vessels of limb are involved which result in hypohydrosis**
Ref: S Das's Surgery, 4/e p176

21. **Ans. (c) Normal saline**
Ref: S Das's Surgery, 4/e p30

22. **Ans. (c) Filariasis**
Ref: SRB's Surgery 4/e p259

23. **Ans. (a) Direct pressure over the wound**
Ref: SRB's Surgery 4/e p122

24. **Ans. (b) Swabs/ suction bottles**
Ref: SRB's Surgery 4/e p122

25. **Ans. (c) Hypercalcemia**
Ref: SRB's Surgery 4/e p126

26. **Ans. (c) Buerger's disease**
Ref: SRB's Surgery 4/e p186

27. **Ans. (d) All of the above**
Ref: SRB's Surgery 4/e p232

28. **Ans. (c) Hypovolemic shock**
Ref: SRB's Surgery 4/e p122

29. **Ans. (d) All of the above**
Ref: SRB's Surgery 4/e p111

30. **Ans. (d) Anterior and posterior tibial artery**
Ref: SRB's Surgery 4/e p187

31. **Ans. (b) Rise in temperature**
Ref: SRB's Surgery 4/e p233

32. **Ans. (c) Sickle cell anemia**
Ref: SRB's Surgery 4/e p234

33. **Ans. (a) Duplex scanning**
Ref: SRB's Surgery 4/e p234

34. **Ans. (c) Aneurysm**
Ref: SRB's Surgery 4/e p202

35. **Ans. (c) Ethanol**
Ref: SRB's Surgery 4/e p242

36. **Ans. (c) Osteoarthritis**
Ref: SRB's Surgery 4/e p188

37. **Ans. (a) Injury to intra abdominal solid organ**
Ref: SRB's Surgery 4/e p150

38. **Ans. (b) May lead to lung infarction**
Ref: SRB's Surgery 4/e p232

39. **Ans. (b) White, blue, red**
Ref: SRB's Surgery 4/e p189

40. **Ans. (b) Hematocrit**
Ref: SRB's Surgery 4/e p126

41. **Ans. (b) Factor VIII**
Ref: SRB's Surgery 4/e p125

42. **Ans. (a) 20–24 deg C for 5 days**
Ref: SRB's Surgery 4/e p124

43. **Ans. (b) Dilutional thrombocytopenia**
Ref: SRB's Surgery 4/e p127

44. **Ans. (a) 24 hours**
Ref: SRB's Surgery 4/e p124

45. **Ans. (c) Pancreatic carcinoma**
Ref: SRB's Surgery 4/e p252

46. **Ans. (d) Fibromuscular hyperplasia**
Ref: Internet resources

47. **Ans. (c) Large arteries**
Ref: SRB's Surgery 4/e p187

48. **Ans. (b) Bradycardia**
Ref: SRB's Surgery 4/e p116

49. **Ans. (d) Cervical rib**
Ref: SRB's Surgery 4/e p458

50. **Ans. (d) Congenital**
Ref: SRB's Surgery 4/e p226

51. **Ans. (c) Related to venous refilling after emptying a length of vein**
Ref: Internet resources

52. **Ans. (b) Pain in the leg only on exercise**
Ref: SRB's Surgery 4/e p176

53. **Ans. (a) 1st part**
Ref: SRB's Surgery 4/e p217

54. **Ans. (b) Popliteal artery**
Ref: SRB's Surgery 4/e p208

55. **Ans. (b) Superficial temporal**
Ref: SRB's Surgery 4/e p225

56. **Ans. (b) Atherosclerosis**
Ref: SRB's Surgery 4/e p202

57. **Ans. (a) L1**
Ref: SRB's Surgery 4/e p195

58. **Ans. (c) Cardiac arrhythmias**
Ref: SRB's Surgery 4/e p227

59. **Ans. (c) Christmas disease**
Ref: SRB's Surgery 4/e p129

60. **Ans. (d) Adson's test**
Ref: SRB's Surgery 4/e p239

61. **Ans. (d) Radial artery**
Ref: SRB's Surgery 4/e p458

62. **Ans. (d) Deep vein thrombosis**
Ref: SRB's Surgery 4/e p235

63. **Ans. (b) Intermittent claudication**
Ref: SRB's Surgery 4/e p193

64. **Ans. (b) Atherosclerosis**
Ref: SRB's Surgery 4/e p177

65. **Ans. (c) Is familial**
Ref: SRB's Surgery 4/e p257

66. **Ans. (a) Antibiotic and rest**
Ref: SRB's Surgery 4/e p40

67. **Ans. (d) 0.3**
Ref: SRB's Surgery 4/e p177

68. **Ans. (a) Duplex ultrasound imaging**
Ref: SRB's Surgery 4/e p241

69. **Ans. (b) Acidosis, hypothermia, hyperkalemia**
Ref: SRB's Surgery 4/e p127

70. **Ans. (b) Pain in limbs on taking very first step**
Ref: SRB's Surgery 4/e p176

ABDOMEN

71. **Ans. (c) Amoebic liver abscess**
Ref: S Das's Surgery, 4/e p885

72. **Ans. (d) Ranson criteria**
Ref: S Das's Surgery, 4/e p962

73. **Ans. (c) Serum bilirubin**
Ref: Internet resources

74. **Ans. (d) All of the above**
Ref: S Das's Surgery, 4/e p1031

75. **Ans. (a) Spleen**
Ref: SRB's Surgery 4/e p148

76. **Ans. (d) 7.5 cm**
Ref: SRB's Surgery 4/e p670

77. **Ans. (b) Nucleotide scan**
Ref: SRB's Surgery 4/e p542

78. **Ans. (d) Fatty liver**
Ref: SRB's Surgery 4/e p628

79. **Ans. (c) Bile duct obstruction**
Ref: SRB's Surgery 4/e p853

80. **Ans. (a) Observation**
Ref: SRB's Surgery 4/e p736

81. **Ans. (b) Insulinoma**
Ref: SRB's Surgery 4/e p756

82. **Ans. (d) Pain in upper abdomen**
Ref: SRB's Surgery 4/e p728

83. **Ans. (b) Hemangioma**
Ref: SRB's Surgery 4/e p642

84. **Ans. (d) 8**
Ref: SRB's Surgery 4/e p628

85. **Ans. (a) Malignancy**
Ref: SRB's Surgery 4/e p737

86. **Ans. (c) Acute appendicitis**
Ref: SRB's Surgery 4/e p679

87. **Ans. (b) USG**
Ref: SRB's Surgery 4/e p681

88. **Ans. (d) Trauma**
Ref: SRB's Surgery 4/e p704

89. **Ans. (b) Acute pancreatitis**
Ref: SRB's Surgery 4/e p728

90. **Ans. (a) Hypercalcemia**
Ref: SRB's Surgery 4/e p727

91. **Ans. (d) All of the above**
Ref: SRB's Surgery 4/e p727

92. **Ans. (c) CT scan**
Ref: SRB's Surgery 4/e p714

93. **Ans. (a) Sinusoids**
Ref: SRB's Surgery 4/e p651

94. **Ans. (c) Typhoid fever**
Ref: SRB's Surgery 4/e p928

95. **Ans. (b) DIC**
Ref: SRB's Surgery 4/e p715

96. **Ans. (b) CT scan**
Ref: SRB's Surgery 4/e p730

97. **Ans. (d) Cholangitis**
Ref: SRB's Surgery 4/e p691

98. **Ans. (d) All of the above**
Ref: SRB's Surgery 4/e p672

99. **Ans. (a) USG**
Ref: SRB's Surgery 4/e p685

100. **Ans. (d) Homocystinuria**
Ref: SRB's Surgery 4/e p733

101. **Ans. (c) Hilum**
Ref: SRB's Surgery 4/e p702

102. **Ans. (b) Gallstones**
Ref: SRB's Surgery 4/e p691

103. **Ans. (d) Serosanguinous discharge**
Ref: SRB's Surgery 4/e p789

104. **Ans. (c) ERCP**
Ref: SRB's Surgery 4/e p692

105. **Ans. (c) Polycythemia**
Ref: SRB's Surgery 4/e p721

106. **Ans. (b) Segment III**
Ref: SRB's Surgery 4/e p670

107. **Ans. (b) Moderately raised amylase levels are diagnostic of peritonitis**
Ref: SRB's Surgery 4/e p604

108. **Ans. (c) S. lipase**
Ref: SRB's Surgery 4/e p733

109. **Ans. (c) Hereditary Spherocytosis**
Ref: SRB's Surgery 4/e p720

110. **Ans. (c) Intermittent vomiting**
Ref: SRB's Surgery 4/e p

111. **Ans. (d) Cholangitis**
Ref: SRB's Surgery 4/e p691

112. **Ans. (d) Liposarcoma**
Ref: SRB's Surgery 4/e p765

113. **Ans. (c) Hydatid disease**
Ref: SRB's Surgery 4/e p639

114. **Ans. (c) Cholangitis**
Ref: SRB's Surgery 4/e p695

115. **Ans. (b) Pigment**
Ref: SRB's Surgery 4/e p680

116. **Ans. (a) CT scan**
Ref: SRB's Surgery 4/e p639

117. **Ans. (c) Klebsiella**
Ref: SRB's Surgery 4/e p722

118. **Ans. (c) Cirrhosis**
Ref: SRB's Surgery 4/e p659

119. **Ans. (c) Manage conservatively with antibiotics alone**
Ref: SRB's Surgery 4/e p732

120. **Ans. (b) Tubercular abscess**
Ref: SRB's Surgery 4/e p723

121. **Ans. (a) Abdominal operation lasting more than two hours**
Ref: SRB's Surgery 4/e p789

122. **Ans. (b) Sickle cell anemia**
Ref: SRB's Surgery 4/e p773

123. **Ans. (c) Beta cell tumors of the pancreas**
Ref: SRB's Surgery 4/e p757

124. **Ans. (d) C-reactive protein < 100**
Ref: SRB's Surgery 4/e p734

125. **Ans. (a) ERCP**
Ref: SRB's Surgery 4/e p593

126. **Ans. (a) Adenocarcinoma**
Ref: SRB's Surgery 4/e p700

127. **Ans. (b) Max risk is within 1 year of splenectomy**
Ref: SRB's Surgery 4/e p722

128. **Ans. (c) Pseudocyst**
Ref: SRB's Surgery 4/e p734

GIT

129. **Ans. (d) Endoscopic biopsy**
Ref: S Das's Surgery, 4/e p818

130. **Ans. (a) Acute pancreatitis**
Ref: S Das's Surgery, 4/e p958

131. **Ans. (d) Cork screw esophagus on barium meal**
Ref: S Das's Surgery, 4/e p811

132. **Ans. (a) Seropurulent discharge with occasional bleeding**
Ref: Shenoy's Surgery, 2nd ed., p-530

133. **Ans. (d) Achalasia cardia**
Ref: S Das's Surgery, 4/e p809

134. **Ans. (d) Keratinization throughout the length**
Ref: S Das's Surgery, 4/e p1069

135. **Ans. (b) Short gastric artery**
Ref: S Das's Surgery, 4/e p827

136. **Ans. (c) 5-FU, irradiation followed by abdomino-perineal resection**
Ref: S Das's Surgery, 4/e p1103

137. **Ans. (d) Gastric ulcer**
Ref: SRB's Surgery 4/e p882

138. **Ans. (d) Rectal biopsy**
Ref: SRB's Surgery 4/e p949

139. **Ans. (d) CHPS**
Ref: SRB's Surgery 4/e p876

140. **Ans. (c) Leiomyosarcoma**
Ref: SRB's Surgery 4/e p917

141. **Ans. (c) Bishop Koop operation**
Ref: SRB's Surgery 4/e p993

142. **Ans. (a) Above the cricopharynx**
Ref: SRB's Surgery 4/e p868

143. **Ans. (a) Potassium**
Ref: SRB's Surgery 4/e p962

144. **Ans. (a) Herniation of abdominal contents through the body wall**
Ref: SRB's Surgery 4/e p794

145. **Ans. (c) Site and size of varices**
Ref: SRB's Surgery 4/e p655

146. **Ans. (c) Parasympathomimetics**
Ref: SRB's Surgery 4/e p1000

147. **Ans. (c) Hartman's operation**
Ref: SRB's Surgery 4/e p1028

148. **Ans. (c) Hyperglycemia**
Ref: SRB's Surgery 4/e p897

149. **Ans. (c) Sclerosing cholangitis**
Ref: SRB's Surgery 4/e p957

150. **Ans. (b) Excision of tumor alone**
Ref: SRB's Surgery 4/e p757

151. **Ans. (c) Diffuse esophageal spasm**
Ref: SRB's Surgery 4/e p840

152. **Ans. (c) Ileo-colic**
Ref: SRB's Surgery 4/e p995

153. **Ans. (b) Bacterial overgrowth**
Ref: SRB's Surgery 4/e p923

154. **Ans. (c) Ulcerative colitis**
Ref: SRB's Surgery 4/e p955

155. **Ans. (b) Duodenal atresia**
Ref: SRB's Surgery 4/e p990

156. **Ans. (d) Acute appendicitis**
Ref: SRB's Surgery 4/e p939

157. **Ans. (b) Involvement of mucosa, submucosal and muscularis**
Ref: SRB's Surgery 4/e p905

158. **Ans. (c) Type III**
Ref: SRB's Surgery 4/e p879

159. **Ans. (d) Transverse fold of rectum**
Ref: Internet resources

160. **Ans. (a) Ascending colon**
Ref: SRB's Surgery 4/e p969

161. **Ans. (a) Esophageal reflux**
Ref: SRB's Surgery 4/e p848

162. **Ans. (a) Skin necrosis**
Ref: SRB's Surgery 4/e p959

163. **Ans. (b) Stomach**
Ref: SRB's Surgery 4/e p870

164. **Ans. (c) Esophageal varices**
Ref: SRB's Surgery 4/e p652

165. **Ans. (d) Juvenile polyp**
Ref: SRB's Surgery 4/e p961

166. **Ans. (c) Gallbladder and CBD**
Ref: SRB's Surgery 4/e p757

167. **Ans. (a) APC gene**
Ref: SRB's Surgery 4/e p963

168. **Ans. (d) Peutz Jegher's syndrome**
Ref: SRB's Surgery 4/e p963

169. **Ans. (c) Hiatus hernia**
Ref: SRB's Surgery 4/e p848

170. **Ans. (a) Hypokalemic, hyponatremic alkalosis**
Ref: SRB's Surgery 4/e p877

171. **Ans. (c) Surgery**
Ref: SRB's Surgery 4/e p937

172. **Ans. (a) Gallstone**
Ref: SRB's Surgery 4/e p983

173. **Ans. (b) Crohn's disease**
Ref: SRB's Surgery 4/e p944

174. **Ans. (b) Stomach cancer**
Ref: SRB's Surgery 4/e p791

175. **Ans. (d) Metaplastic change in the lining mucosa of the esophagus**
Ref: SRB's Surgery 4/e p849

176. **Ans. (b) Rutherford-Morison's**
Ref: SRB's Surgery 4/e p1011

177. **Ans. (b) Diarrhea**
Ref: SRB's Surgery 4/e p877

178. **Ans. (a) Congenital hypertrophic pyloric stenosis**
Ref: SRB's Surgery 4/e p877

179. **Ans. (a) Right hemicolectomy**
Ref: SRB's Surgery 4/e p940

180. **Ans. (d) The incision can be extended upwards or downwards**
Ref: SRB's Surgery 4/e p1012

181. **Ans. (b) Carcinoid syndrome is due to malignant transformation**
Ref: SRB's Surgery 4/e p940

182. **Ans. (d) Boerhaave syndrome**
Ref: SRB's Surgery 4/e p857

183. **Ans. (c) Instrumentation**
Ref: SRB's Surgery 4/e p839

184. **Ans. (a) Appendix**
Ref: SRB's Surgery 4/e p939

185. **Ans. (a) Bleeding**
Ref: SRB's Surgery 4/e p924

186. **Ans. (a) Achalasia cardia**
Ref: SRB's Surgery 4/e p852

187. **Ans. (b) Obstruction**
Ref: SRB's Surgery 4/e p967

188. **Ans. (b)** Absorbable in 2 layers
Ref: SRB's Surgery 4/e p1256

189. **Ans. (a)** Barrett's esophagus
Ref: SRB's Surgery 4/e p841

190. **Ans. (a)** Anterior aspect of the first part of duodenum
Ref: SRB's Surgery 4/e p888

191. **Ans. (d)** Hamartomatous polyps
Ref: SRB's Surgery 4/e p99

192. **Ans. (b)** Appendicular mass
Ref: SRB's Surgery 4/e p1015

193. **Ans. (c)** Decreased lower esophageal sphincter tone
Ref: SRB's Surgery 4/e p851

194. **Ans. (a)** Mallory Weiss syndrome
Ref: SRB's Surgery 4/e p856

195. **Ans. (a)** Pain
Ref: SRB's Surgery 4/e p1039

HERNIA

196. **Ans. (d)** MC hernia in females
Ref: S Das's Surgery, 4/e p1119, 1134

197. **Ans. (b)** Richter's hernia
Ref: SRB's Surgery 4/e p835

198. **Ans. (b)** Truss
Ref: SRB's Surgery 4/e p812

199. **Ans. (b)** Sliding hernia
Ref: SRB's Surgery 4/e p821

200. **Ans. (a)** Herniotomy
Ref: SRB's Surgery 4/e p807

201. **Ans. (b)** Pregnancy is common cause
Ref: SRB's Surgery 4/e p822

202. **Ans. (c)** Obturator hernia
Ref: SRB's Surgery 4/e p834

203. **Ans. (b)** Direct hernia is medial to inferior epigastric artery
Ref: SRB's Surgery 4/e p812

204. **Ans. (d)** Umbilical hernia
Ref: SRB's Surgery 4/e p830

205. **Ans. (a)** It is more common in female
Ref: SRB's Surgery 4/e p802

206. **Ans. (c)** Operate immediately
Ref: SRB's Surgery 4/e p797

GENITOURINARY SYSTEM

207. **Ans. (d)** Associated with alkaline urine
Ref: S Das's Surgery, 4/e p1192

208. **Ans. (b)** Retropubic space
Ref: S Das's Surgery, 4/e p1283

209. **Ans. (d)** PSA
Ref: S Das's Surgery, 4/e p1261

210. **Ans. (b)** PSA only
Ref: S Das's Surgery, 4/e p1274

211. **Ans. (c)** Increased frequency of micturition
Ref: SRB's Surgery 4/e p1082

212. **Ans. (b)** Hypernephroma
Ref: SRB's Surgery 4/e p1101

213. **Ans. (a)** Vesico-ureteric reflux
Ref: SRB's Surgery 4/e p1117

214. **Ans. (b)** Choriocarcinoma
Ref: SRB's Surgery 4/e p1169

215. **Ans. (c)** Pain
Ref: SRB's Surgery 4/e p1099

216. **Ans. (b)** Prostatic carcinoma
Ref: SRB's Surgery 4/e p1126

217. **Ans. (b)** Seminoma
Ref: SRB's Surgery 4/e p1162

218. **Ans. (c)** Cystitis
Ref: SRB's Surgery 4/e p1105

219. **Ans. (c)** Exudation cyst
Ref: SRB's Surgery 4/e p1151

220. **Ans. (d)** Duloxetine
Ref: Internet resources

221. **Ans. (a)** Pathological staging
Ref: SRB's Surgery 4/e p1101

222. **Ans. (b)** DRE and PSA
Ref: SRB's Surgery 4/e p1127

223. **Ans. (b)** 1 year
Ref: SRB's Surgery 4/e p1162

224. **Ans. (d)** All of the above
Ref: SRB's Surgery 4/e p1167

225. **Ans. (d)** Hydrocele
Ref: SRB's Surgery 4/e p1149

226. Ans. (c) Tuberculosis of urinary bladder
Ref: SRB's Surgery 4/e p1083

227. Ans. (a) Alcohol
Ref: SRB's Surgery 4/e p1114

228. Ans. (b) Micturating cysto-urethrography
Ref: SRB's Surgery 4/e p1069

229. Ans. (b) Hyponatremia
Ref: SRB's Surgery 4/e p1124

230. Ans. (a) E. coli
Ref: Internet resources

231. Ans. (b) Triple phosphate
Ref: SRB's Surgery 4/e p1098

232. Ans. (a) Transurethral resection of bladder tumor (TURBT)
Ref: SRB's Surgery 4/e p1113

233. Ans. (b) 70% chance of requiring cystectomy in 5 years after TUR
Ref: SRB's Surgery 4/e p1113

234. Ans. (a) Varicosity of cremasteric veins
Ref: SRB's Surgery 4/e p1157

235. Ans. (b) Hysterectomy
Ref: SRB's Surgery 4/e p1066

236. Ans. (b) Peripheral zone
Ref: SRB's Surgery 4/e p1126

237. Ans. (c) Circumcision
Ref: SRB's Surgery 4/e p1143

238. Ans. (d) Hypertrophy of testes
Ref: SRB's Surgery 4/e p1163

THYROID

239. Ans. (c) External branch of superior laryngeal nerve
Ref: S Das's Surgery, 4/e p659

240. Ans. (b) Papillary
Ref: SRB's Surgery 4/e p511

241. Ans. (b) MEN-IIb
Ref: SRB's Surgery 4/e p518

242. Ans. (c) Total thyroidectomy
Ref: SRB's Surgery 4/e p511

243. Ans. (a) Follicular carcinoma of thyroid
Ref: SRB's Surgery 4/e p512

244. Ans. (a) Follicular carcinoma
Ref: SRB's Surgery 4/e p493

245. Ans. (d) Hemithyroidectomy
Ref: SRB's Surgery 4/e p494

246. Ans. (b) Cold intolerance
Ref: SRB's Surgery 4/e p

247. Ans. (b) Follicular carcinoma
Ref: SRB's Surgery 4/e p512

248. Ans. (a) Commoner in males
Ref: SRB's Surgery 4/e p503

BREAST

249. Ans. (d) Spread to ipsilateral supraclavicular lymph nodes
Ref: S Das's Surgery, 4/e p720

250. Ans. (c) Stage IIIA
Ref: S Das's Surgery, 4/e p721; CSDT, 12/e p311t

251. Ans. (b) Histological grading
Ref: S Das's Surgery, 4/e p720

252. Ans. (a) Internal mammary
Ref: SRB's Surgery 4/e p547

253. Ans. (b) Sentinel lymph node biopsy
Ref: SRB's Surgery 4/e p579

254. Ans. (c) Colloid carcinoma
Ref: SRB's Surgery 4/e p566

255. Ans. (b) Cisplatin
Ref: SRB's Surgery 4/e p585

256. Ans. (d) Lymphangiosarcoma
Ref: SRB's Surgery 4/e p584

257. Ans. (c) Neoplasia
Ref: SRB's Surgery 4/e p567

258. Ans. (d) Clinical examination, Mammogram and FNAC
Ref: SRB's Surgery 4/e p547

259. Ans. (c) Simple mastectomy
Ref: SRB's Surgery 4/e p552

260. Ans. (d) Cytology is not diagnostic
Ref: SRB's Surgery 4/e p567

261. Ans. (a) Contraindicated if axillary LN is involved
Ref: SRB's Surgery 4/e p579

262. **Ans. (b) Fine needle aspiration**
Ref: SRB's Surgery 4/e p

263. **Ans. (d) Upper outer quadrant**
Ref: SRB's Surgery 4/e p568

264. **Ans. (c) Lobular carcinoma**
Ref: SRB's Surgery 4/e p567

HEAD-NECK

265. **Ans. (a) Hypertension & bradycardia**
Ref: CSDT, 12/e p865

266. **Ans. (a) Proptosis**
Ref: CSDT, 12/e p1236

267. **Ans. (a) Single adenoma**
Ref: SRB's Surgery 4/e p532

268. **Ans. (b) Subhyoid**
Ref: SRB's Surgery 4/e p487

269. **Ans. (d) 13-15**
Ref: SRB's Surgery 4/e p1175

270. **Ans. (a) No response**
Ref: SRB's Surgery 4/e p1174

271. **Ans. (a) Dentigerous cyst**
Ref: SRB's Surgery 4/e p384

272. **Ans. (c) Neck**
Ref: SRB's Surgery 4/e p442

273. **Ans. (b) Glossopharyngeal nerve**
Ref: SRB's Surgery 4/e p436

274. **Ans. (c) Air embolism through external jugular vein**
Ref: SRB's Surgery 4/e p146

275. **Ans. (b) Lung**
Ref: SRB's Surgery 4/e p1183

276. **Ans. (d) Parotid**
Ref: SRB's Surgery 4/e p434

277. **Ans. (d) Phrenic nerve**
Ref: SRB's Surgery 4/e p480

278. **Ans. (b) Epidermoid cyst**
Ref: SRB's Surgery 4/e p80

279. **Ans. (b) Radicular cyst**
Ref: SRB's Surgery 4/e p385

280. **Ans. (b) Tetanus**
Ref: SRB's Surgery 4/e p50

281. **Ans. (c) Firm and encapsulated**
Ref: SRB's Surgery 4/e p442

282. **Ans. (d) Pleomorphic tumor**
Ref: SRB's Surgery 4/e p443

283. **Ans. (b) Altered consciousness**
Ref: SRB's Surgery 4/e p1175

284. **Ans. (d) Diabetes mellitus**
Ref: SRB's Surgery 4/e p1176

285. **Ans. (b) Breach of platysma**
Ref: SRB's Surgery 4/e p143

286. **Ans. (b) 10**
Ref: SRB's Surgery 4/e p1174

287. **Ans. (c) Upper 1/3rd of sternomastoid on anterior border**
Ref: SRB's Surgery 4/e p460

288. **Ans. (c) Thyroglossal cyst**
Ref: SRB's Surgery 4/e p487

289. **Ans. (c) CT scan**
Ref: SRB's Surgery 4/e p1241

290. **Ans. (c) Commonly adenocarcinoma**
Ref: SRB's Surgery 4/e p418

291. **Ans. (c) Chronic subdural hemorrhage**
Ref: SRB's Surgery 4/e p1179

292. **Ans. (b) Rupture of cortex vein**
Ref: SRB's Surgery 4/e p1179

293. **Ans. (b) Pleomorphic adenoma**
Ref: SRB's Surgery 4/e p444

294. **Ans. (a) An unerupted tooth**
Ref: SRB's Surgery 4/e p384

295. **Ans. (d) Tachycardia**
Ref: SRB's Surgery 4/e p1180

296. **Ans. (d) Extradural hemorrhage**
Ref: SRB's Surgery 4/e p1178

297. **Ans. (a) Cystic hygroma**
Ref: SRB's Surgery 4/e p465

298. **Ans. (c) Branchial cyst**
Ref: SRB's Surgery 4/e p490

LUNGS

299. **Ans. (c) Damage to respiratory centre**
Ref: BDC, Vol-III, 3rd ed., p-253

300. **Ans. (c) Paradoxical breathing is not observed in conscious patient**
Ref: SRB's Surgery 4/e p1196

SURGICAL ONCOLOGY

301. **Ans. (d) Seminoma**
Ref: S Das's Surgery, 4/e p1316

302. **Ans. (b) Junctional nevus**
Ref: S Das's Surgery, 4/e p110

303. **Ans. (c) Amenorrhoea**
Ref: CSDT, 12/e p908

304. **Ans. (b) Ocular cancer**
Ref: S Das's Surgery, 4/e p730; CSDT, 12/e p1345

305. **Ans. (d) Neuroblastoma**
Ref: SRB's Surgery 4/e p541

306. **Ans. (d) Lipoma**
Ref: SRB's Surgery 4/e p71

307. **Ans. (a) Squamous cell Ca from scar**
Ref: SRB's Surgery 4/e p24

308. **Ans. (a) Finger**
Ref: SRB's Surgery 4/e p82

309. **Ans. (d) Wide excision**
Ref: SRB's Surgery 4/e p791

310. **Ans. (b) Nasopharynx carcinoma**
Ref: SRB's Surgery 4/e p423

311. **Ans. (a) Thymoma**
Ref: SRB's Surgery 4/e p1206

MISCELLANEOUS

312. **Ans. (d) Regeneration of nerves**
Ref: S Das's Surgery, 4/e p245

313. **Ans. (d) Self limiting**
Ref: S Das's Surgery, 4/e p123

314. **Ans. (d) Organ from any species**
Ref: CSDT, 12/e p1351

315. **Ans. (d) Nerve regeneration**
Ref: S Das's Surgery, 4/e p245

316. **Ans. (b) With pre-medication**
Ref: SRB's Surgery 4/e p1232

317. **Ans. (b) Repair of skin cover**
Ref: SRB's Surgery 4/e p166

318. **Ans. (c) Urine output**
Ref: SRB's Surgery 4/e p144

319. **Ans. (c) Face**
Ref: SRB's Surgery 4/e p11

320. **Ans. (c) Virulent strains of organism**
Ref: SRB's Surgery 4/e p44

321. **Ans. (a) Clutton's joint**
Ref: SRB's Surgery 4/e p28

322. **Ans. (a) Hair follicle**
Ref: SRB's Surgery 4/e p46

323. **Ans. (c) Lumbar-sacral**
Ref: SRB's Surgery 4/e p1188

324. **Ans. (a) Sheep**
Ref: SRB's Surgery 4/e p

325. **Ans. (d) 1 hour before surgery and continue after surgery**
Ref: SRB's Surgery 4/e p1232

326. **Ans. (c) Pendred's syndrome**
Ref: Internet resources

327. **Ans. (b) Chromosme 7q**
Ref: Internet resources

328. **Ans. (c) Infection**
Ref: SRB's Surgery 4/e p1229

329. **Ans. (a) Identical twin**
Ref: SRB's Surgery 4/e p355

330. **Ans. (b) Allograft**
Ref: SRB's Surgery 4/e p353

331. **Ans. (c) Ice in plastic bag**
Ref: Internet resources

332. **Ans. (b) Diaphragm**
Ref: SRB's Surgery 4/e p1212

333. **Ans. (a) Preformed antibodies**
Ref: Internet resources

334. **Ans. (a) CMV**
Ref: SRB's Surgery 4/e p355

335. **Ans. (b) Kidney**
Ref: SRB's Surgery 4/e p354

336. **Ans. (b) Infected sebaceous cyst**
Ref: SRB's Surgery 4/e p82

337. **Ans. (b) Fat embolism**
Ref: SRB's Surgery 4/e p201

338. **Ans. (b) Cauda equina**
Ref: Internet resources

339. **Ans. (b) Strawberry angioma**
Ref: SRB's Surgery 4/e p222

340. **Ans. (d) Skull bone**
Ref: SRB's Surgery 4/e p1176

341. **Ans. (b) Thigh**
Ref: SRB's Surgery 4/e p

342. **Ans. (c) Direct spread**
Ref: SRB's Surgery 4/e p305

343. **Ans. (d) Axilla**
Ref: SRB's Surgery 4/e p293

344. **Ans. (b) Terminal pulp space infection**
Ref: SRB's Surgery 4/e p161

345. **Ans. (d) L4-L5**
Ref: SRB's Surgery 4/e p1190

346. **Ans. (a) Pain**
Ref: SRB's Surgery 4/e p169

347. **Ans. (b) Thrombocytopenia**
Ref: SRB's Surgery 4/e p117

348. **Ans. (c) Small full thickness skin graft**
Ref: SRB's Surgery 4/e p344

349. **Ans. (a) Allograft**
Ref: SRB's Surgery 4/e p355

350. **Ans. (c) Masterly inactivity**
Ref: SRB's Surgery 4/e p

351. **Ans. (b) Debridement**
Ref: SRB's Surgery 4/e p53

352. **Ans. (b) Stratified squamous epithelium**
Ref: SRB's Surgery 4/e p79

PRACTICE QUESTIONS

BURNS

1. **Large area of burns over head and neck can be effectively managed by:**
   a. Dressings only
   b. Immediate surgery
   c. Intravenous fluids only
   d. Topical agent application only
2. **After a burn injury, patient developed blisters. This is which degree of burns:**
   a. First
   b. Second
   c. Third
   d. Fourth
3. **Which of the following is NOT true for partial thickness burn:**
   a. Either first/ second degree burn
   b. Blisters
   c. Insensitive
   d. Red
4. **Rule of Nine was given by:**
   a. Rutherford
   b. Wallace
   c. Theirsch
   d. Lund and Browder
5. **What could be the most probable cause of death in a patient with severe burns:**
   a. Sepsis
   b. Hypoxia
   c. Malnutrition
   d. Hypovolemia
6. **An old patient, who suffered 70% burns was not enterally feeded. What could be the most likely cause of death in such a patient:**
   a. Dehydration
   b. Malnutrition
   c. Electrolyte imbalance
   d. Bacterial infection
7. **Which of the following is FALSE regarding burn patient:**
   a. Hemetemesis may be seen in extensive burns
   b. Exposure method of treatment for head and neck burn
   c. Stridor may be present
   d. Infection is most commonly caused by pseudomonas
8. **Which of the following is NOT commonly used for managing burn patients:**
   a. Hypotonic solutions
   b. Albumin
   c. 25% Dextrose
   d. Hartmann solution
9. **Perineum burns is what % of total area:**
   a. 1%
   b. 9%
   c. 11%
   d. 19%

VASCULAR SYSTEM

10. **Characteristic sign and symptoms of hypovolumic shock appears when the amount of blood loss is more than:**
    a. 40%
    b. 30%
    c. 20%
    d. 10%
11. **Which of the following condition present as warm, pulsatile compressible swelling:**
    a. Arterio-venous fistula
    b. Varicose veins
    c. Thromboangitis obliterans
    d. Septic shock
12. **Investigation of choice in a victim of penetrating injury abdomen and unstable hemodynamic parameters:**
    a. FAST/ Focussed abdominal sonar trauma
    b. Diagnostic peritoneal lavage/ DPL
    c. Exploratory laparotomy
    d. CT scan
13. **Crush syndrome results into:**
    a. Fat embolism
    b. Air embolsim
    c. Renal failure
    d. Heart failure
14. **Most likely complication, while cannulating internal juglar vein for CVP measurement:**
    a. Pnuemothorax
    b. Ventricular arrhythmias
    c. Pulmonary thromboembolism
    d. Arterial puncture

Ans.
1. **d.** Topical agent app... 2. **b.** Second 3. **c.** Insensitive 4. **b.** Wallace
5. **d.** Hypovolemia 6. **c.** Electrolyte imbalance 7. **d.** Infection is most... 8. **a.** Hypotonic solutions
9. **a.** 1% 10. **a.** 40% 11. **a.** Arterio-venous fistula 12. **b.** Diagnostic peritoneal...
13. **c.** Renal failure 14. **a.** Pnuemothorax

15. Which of the following is ideally given to a RTA patient with Systolic BP of 80 mm Hg and pulse of 108/ minute:
a. Plasma
b. Normal saline
c. Blood transfusion
d. 5% Dextrose

16. Site of pain in thromboangitis obliterans are all EXCEPT:
a. Calf region
b. Foot region
c. Toes region
d. Hip region

17. Thromboangitis disease involves all of the following EXCEPT:
a. Nerve b. Lymphatics
c. Small arteries d. Vein

18. Which of the type of shock may present with normal cardiac output:
a. Septic b. Anaphylactic
c. Neurogenic d. Hemorrhagic

19. Parameter used to assess renal perfusion during shock:
a. Central venous pressure
b. Urinary output
c. Pulmonary capillary wedge pressure
d. Hemoglobin

20. Which of the vein is NOT used for putting central line:
a. External jugular vein
b. Internal juguar vein
c. Basilic vein
d. Subclavian vein

21. Which of the following is NOT a feature of varicose veins:
a. Ulceration b. Dragging pain
c. Heaviness d. Ischemia

ABDOMEN

22. Most specific marker for pancreatitis:
a. Serum amylase
b. Liver function test
c. Serum lipase
d. Serum creatinine

23. A patient came with severe abdominal pain in right lower quadrant. Which scan should be done first:
a. USG b. CT
c. MRI d. X-ray

24. Which of the following s NOT a component of APACHE II scoring system:
a. Glagom coma scale
b. Arterial pH
c. Mean BP
d. Serum amylase

25. A young patient, who recently travelled, presented with fever with chills. On examination, pain in right upper abdominal quadrant can be elicited. Hepatomegaly was also noticed. Percussion revealed right sided pleural effusion. Most likely diagnosis:
a. Pyogenic liver abscess
b. Amoebic liver abscess
c. Infected hydatid cyst
d. Malignancy

26. A young lady presented with pain in right hypochondrium. On examination she was having high grade fever. On per abdominal examination, she caught her breath while exhaling. Most likely diagnosis :
a. Acute pancreatitis
b. Chronic cholecystitis
c. Acute appendicitis
d. Chronic pancreatitis

27. Which of the following is indicated in a patient with severe, deep liver injury:
a. Total hepatectomy
b. Hemi-hepatectomy
c. Hepatic artery ligation
d. Packing with mops

28. A patient presented to the emergency surgery department with history of abdominal trauma. He is having abdominal distension, respiratory distress and features of shock. Management of such a case:
a. Laparoscopy
b. Shift for CT scan abdomen
c. Emergency laparotomy
d. Wait and watch

29. Location of Klatskin tumour:
a. Gall bladder
b. Common hepatic duct
c. Common bile duct
d. Junction of CBD with CHD

30. Common cause of acute cholecystitis:
a. Fatty diet
b. Gallstones
c. Renal stones
d. Acute pancreatitis

Ans. **15. b.** Normal saline **16. d.** Hip region **17. b.** Lymphatics **18. a.** Septic
19. b. Urinary output **20. a.** External jugular vein **21. d.** Ischemia **22. c.** Serum lipase
23. a. USG **24. d.** Serum amylase **25. b.** Amoebic liver abscess **26. b.** Chronic cholecystitis
27. d. Packing with mops **28. c.** Emergency laparotomy **29. b.** Common hepatic duct **30. b.** Gallstones

31. Which of the following presents as a swelling in left iliac fossa and may show cross fluctuation:
a. Carcinoma sigmoid colon
b. Splenic trauma
c. Ectopic kidney
d. Psoas abscess

32. A patient presented with mass in right hypochondrium. On palpation, the liver is soft, smooth but tender. Right sided pleural effusion was also noticed. Most likleyy diagnosis:
a. Amoebic liver abscess
b. Hepatocellular carcinoma
c. Acute cholecystitis
d. Liver secondaries

33. A young male presented with features of jaundice and discomfort in right hypochondrium. On examination, thrill was elicited on three-finger test. Most likely diagnosis:
a. Amoebic liver abscess
b. Pyogenic liver abscess
c. Hydatid cyst
d. Hepatocellular carcinoma

34. An old male presented with jaundice. On examination the gall bladder was distended size 10X8 cm. Which of the following is LEAST possible diagnosis:
a. Common bile duct stones
b. Carcinoma head of pancreas
c. Periampullary carcinoma
d. None

35. A patient had history of acute pancreatitis one month back. Now he is presenting with abdominal pain and a lump in epigastrium, which is soft, smooth and non-mobile. Most likely diagnosis:
a. Enlarged left lobe of liver
b. Hydatid cyst of liver
c. Carcinoma stomach
d. Pancreatic pseudocyst

36. A chronic alcoholic patient presented with sudden onset of abdominal pain which is referred to back. There is associated vomiting and high grade fever. On inspection, hemorrhagic spots and ecchymosis was noticed in the flanks. Per abdominally, there is rebound tenderness, guarding and rigidity. Which of the following is likely diagnosis:
a. Acute appendicitis b. Acute cholecystitis
c. Acute pancreatitis d. Acute hepatitis

37. Which of the following incisions of acute appendicectomy is given perpendicular to McBurney's point:
a. Rutherford Morison's
b. Lanz crease
c. Gridiron
d. Right lower paramedian

38. Patient involved in road traffic accident and sustained trauma to left side of abdomen. X-ray abdomen showed elevation of left side of diaphragm. Most likely injured structure:
a. Stomach b. Spleen
c. Pancreas d. Adrenal

39. Chain of lakes appearance is seen in which condition:
a. Acute pancreatitis
b. Chronic pancreatitis
c. Pancreatic pseudocyst
d. Pancreatic carcinoma

GIT

40. A young patient was involved in an assault and sustained abdominal injury. Erect X-ray abdomen showed presence of free air under diaphragm. Which of the following organ might have been injured:
a. Spleen b. Intestine
c. Liver d. Lung

41. All of the following are features of congenital hypertrophic pyloric stenosis EXCEPT:
a. Projectile vomiting b. Paradoxical aciduria
c. Billous vomiting d. Metabolic alkalosis

42. A 70 year old patient shows symptoms similar to hypertrophic pyloric stenosis. Which of the following condition is responsible for this:
a. Jejunal obstruction b. Duodenal ulcer
c. CBD stone d. Pancreatic pseudocyst

43. All of the following are common complications of Barrett's esophagus EXCEPT:
a. Ulceration b. Stricture
c. Bleeding d. Squamous malignancy

44. Prevention of colorectal carcinoma can be possible by intake of:
a. Red meat
b. Saturated fat
c. NSAID
d. Less fibre diet

Ans. 31. **d.** Psoas abscess 32. **a.** Amoebic liver abscess 33. **c.** Hydatid cyst 34. **a.** Common bile duct stones
35. **d.** Pancreatic pseud... 36. **c.** Acute pancreatitis 37. **c.** Gridiron 38. **b.** Spleen
39. **b.** Chronic panc... 40. **b.** Intestine 41. **c.** Billous vomiting 42. **b.** Duodenal ulcer
43. **d.** Squamous mal... 44. **c.** NSAID

45. All of the following are examples of mesenteric cysts EXCEPT:
a. Mesothelial cyst
b. Enterogenous cyst
c. Chylolymphatic cyst
d. Epidermoid cyst

46. Which of the following is the best investigation to evaluate dysphagia:
a. Barium meal
b. Barium swallow
c. Barium enema
d. Barium meal follow through

47. Which type of metaplasia is commonly observed in lower end of esophagus in a heavy smoker:
a. Gastric type
b. Goblet cells intestinal type
c. Colonic type
d. Anal type

48. Oesophageal carcinoma invades trachea. This is which stage:
a. T1 b. T2
c. T3 d. T4

49. Earliest diagnosis of development of intestinal malignancy in a case of Peutz Jeghers syndrome is possible by:
a. X-ray abdomen
b. Routine colonoscopy
c. CT scan
d. CT angiography

50. MC histological type of anal cancer:
a. Adenocarcinoma
b. Squamous
c. Transitional
d. Mixed

51. A 2 year old female child presented with bleeding with maroon coloured blood. Most likely diagnosis:
a. Intussusception
b. Meckel's diverticulum
c. Duodenal atresia
d. Hirschsprung's disease

52. Saint's triad al triad EXCEPT:
a. Gallstone
b. Hiatal hernia
c. Diverticulosis
d. Carcinoma gall bladder

HERNIA

53. A patent processus vaginalis results in which type of hernia:
a. Bubonocele type indirect inguinal
b. Funicular type indirect inguinal
c. Scrotal type indirect inguinal
d. Direct inguinal

54. A young female presented with sudden severe lower abdominal pain with abdominal distension. On examination, a tender and non-reducible swelling was noticed in inguinal region. Cough impulse test was negative. Most probable diagnosis:
a. Strangulated hernia b. Testicular torsion
c. Scrotal abscess d. Epididymo-orchitis

55. Hernia in which the lumen of that portion of colon occupying hernia sac is blocked by faeces:
a. Littre's hernia
b. Reducible hernia
c. Maydl's hernia
d. Incarcerated hernia

56. An old patient presented with direct inguinal hernia. Intra-operatively an indirect hernia was also seen. Diagnosis:
a. Maydl's hernia b. Velpau hernia
c. Petit hernia d. Saddle hernia

57. Which of the following is known as double sac hernia:
a. Richters hernia
b. Coopers hernia
c. Littres hernia
d. Spigelian hernia

GENITOURINARY

58. Ureteric stones in lower part are best removed by:
a. ESWL/ Extracorporeal shock wave lithotripsy
b. PCNL/ Percutaneous nephrolithotomy
c. Flushing
d. Dormia basket

59. A patient presented with undescended testis and indirect inguinal hernia. On examination the testis were found to be totally atrophied. Best surgical management of such a case would be:
a. Orchidectomy plus inguinal ligament repair
b. Orchidopexy alone
c. Orchidopexy with inguinal hernia repair
d. Orchidectomy alone

Ans. **45. d.** Epidermoid cyst **46. b.** Barium swallow **47. b.** Goblet cells intestinal type
48. d. T4 **49. b.** Routine colonoscopy **50. b.** Squamous **51. b.** Meckel's diverticulum
52. d. Carcinoma gall... **53. c.** Scrotal type indirect... **54. a.** Strangulated hernia **55. d.** Incarcerated hernia
56. d. Saddle hernia **57. b.** Coopers hernia **58. d.** Dormia basket **59. c.** Orchidopexy with...

60. MC histology of Urinary bladder carcinoma:
a. Squamous b. Columnar
c. Transitional d. Cuboidal

61. Stone formed in the urinary bladder in presence of infection with proteus:
a. Uric acid stones b. Cystine stones
c. Phosphate stones d. Oxalate stones

62. Value of serum PSA > 10 ng/ ml suggest the diagnosis of:
a. Benign prostatic hypertrophy
b. Prostatic carcinoma
c. Prostatitis
d. All of the above

63. A young adult male presented with red and swollen testes. Marked swelling of epididymis gave an impression as if testes is separated from epididymis. Elevation of scrotal sac also relieves pain. Most probable diagnosis:
a. Torsion of testes
b. Fourniers gangrene
c. Epididymo-orchitis
d. Malignancy of testes

64. Stage III penile carcinoma involves:
a. Shaft of penis
b. Movable inguinal lymph nodes metastasis
c. Unmovable inguinal lymph node metastasis
d. Prepuce

65. A young male child presented with scrotal swelling which increase in size to maximum by evening and resolves by next morning. Most likely diagnosis:
a. Scrotal abscess
b. Congenital hydrocoele
c. Scrotal cyst
d. Epididymo-orchitis with effusion

66. A 6 year old child tends to pull penile skin while passing urine. The stream is poor. On examination, erythema and edema over the prepuce was also noticed. Findings suggest the diagnosis of:
a. Hypospadias b. Urethral calculi
c. Posterior uretheral valved. Phimosis

67. In a patient with testicular carcinoma, which of the following is the investigationof choice to check lymph node metastasis:
a. CT abdomen b. USG
c. Tumour markers d. Open surgery

68. Which of the following is the specific tumour marker for prostate cancer:
a. AFP
b. beta-HCG
c. PSA
d. CEA

THYROID

69. Investigation of choice for solitary thyroid nodule:
a. CT scan b. MRI
c. FNAC d. X-ray

70. Which of the following is a feature of Grave's dieases:
a. Cold intolerance
b. Proptosis
c. Bradycardia
d. Hung up reflexes

71. MEN-II syndrome is related to which thyroid tumour:
a. Papillary b. Anaplastic
c. Medullary d. Follicular

72. Radiosensitive thyroid carcinoma:
a. Papillary carcinoma
b. Medullary carcinoma
c. Anaplastic carcinoma
d. Follicular carcinoma

BREAST

73. Which of the following condition presents as greenish discharge from breast:
a. Duct papilloma b. Carcinoma breast
c. Duct ectasia d. Fibroadenoma

74. A 20 years old lady presented with a smooth, non-tender and freely movable lump in right breast. Diagnosis:
a. Cystosarcoma phylloides
b. Duct ectasia
c. Fibroadenoma
d. Peau'd orange

75. Obstruction of dermal lymphatics in carcinoma breast will lead to:
a. Breast abscess b. Breast cyst
c. Fibroadenoma d. Peau'd orange

76. Best management of a young lady with infiltrating breast carcinoma of 1 cm and $T_1N_0M_0$ stage:
a. Radical mastectomy
b. Simple mastectomy
c. Extended radical mastectomy
d. Wait and watch

Ans. 60. c. Transitional 61. c. Phosphate stones 62. d. All of the above 63. c. Epididymo-orchitis
64. b. Movable inguinal... 65. b. Congenital hydrocoele 66. b. Urethral calculi 67. a. CT abdomen
68. c. PSA 69. c. FNAC 70. b. Proptosis 71. c. Medullary
72. c. Anaplastic carc... 73. c. Duct ectasia 74. c. Fibroadenoma 75. d. Peau'd orange
76. b. Simple mastectomy

77. Breast cancer with best prognosis:
a. Medullary b. Tubular
c. Inflammatory d. Scirrhous

HEAD-NECK

78. Delayed primary suturing is done in how many days:
a. 2-7 days b. 10-14 days
c. 3 weeks d. 1 month

79. A child with past history of recurrent dental infections, now presents with pain, thickening and discharging sinus from angle of mouth. He was put on antibiotics, but not resolved even after antibiotics. Further management:
a. Wait and watch
b. ATT
c. Mandibulectomy
d. Biopsy

80. Maxillary process does not join with median nasal process. This will result in:
a. Cleft palate
b. Cleft lip on side
c. Cleft lip in centre
d. Both cleft lip and cleft palate

81. Motor response is graded as 4 in Glasgow Coma Scale if the response is:
a. Withdrawl by flexion
b. Decorticate posturing
c. Decerebrate posturing
d. Extension

82. In GCS, score of 3 indicates:
a. Death
b. Severe head injury
c. Coma
d. Healthy

83. Most likely condition which presents as a sinus in neck, often producing mucous discharge and which moves with deglutition:
a. Branchial sinus
b. Pilonidal cyst
c. Thyroglossal fistula
d. Sublingual dermoid cyst

84. Which of the following condition is brilliantly transilluminant:
a. Branchial cyst
b. Thymic cyst
c. Ranula
d. Enlarged lymph node

85. Maximum score in GCS:
a. 5 b. 10
c. 15 d. 20

86. A patient with head injury has eye opening to pain stimuli, inappropriate words and abnormal flexion. This indicates:
a. Normal
b. Mild head injury
c. Moderate head injury
d. Severe head injury

LUNGS

87. What is the common cause of acute lung injury because of blood transfusion:
a. Noscomial infection
b. HLA mediated
c. Auto-immune
d. Genetic predisposition

SURGICAL ONCOLOGY

88. All of the following cancers commonly metastasize to liver EXCEPT:
a. Lung b. Prostate
c. Basal cell carcinoma d. Colon

89. Which of the following does NOT come under APUDomas:
a. Parathyroid tumours
b. Insulinoma
c. Bronchial carcinoid
d. Glucagonoma

90. MC tumour in posterior mediastinum:
a. Neurofibroma
b. Thymoma
c. Pericardial cyst
d. Lymphoma

91. MC carcinoma in white skinned people exposed to sunlight:
a. Squamous cell carcinoma
b. Keloid
c. Basal cell carcinoma
d. Melanoma

92. Desmoid tumour arises from:
a. Lymphatics
b. Collagen
c. Blood vessels
d. Musculo-aponeurotic tissue

Ans. **77. b.** Tubular **78. a.** 2-7 days **79. c.** Mandibulectomy **80. b.** Cleft lip on side
81. a. Withdrawl by... **82. b.** Severe head injury **83. c.** Thyroglossal fistula **84. c.** Ranula
85. c. 15 **86. d.** Severe head injury **87. c.** Auto-immune **88. c.** Basal cell carcinoma
89. c. Bronchial car... **90. a.** Neurofibroma **91. c.** Basal cell carcinoma **92. d.** Musculo-aponeurotic...

MISCELLANEOUS

93. **A patient sustained penetrating chest injury on left side at the level of 5th intercostals space in midaxillary line. Which of the following structure will be LEAST damaged:**
    a. Diaphragm
    b. Liver
    c. Stomach
    d. Lungs

94. **A patient is on total par-enteral nutrition. What % of energy is supplied by glucose in intravenous fluid fluids:**
    a. 20
    b. 30
    c. 40
    d. 50

95. **True for pericardium:**
    a. Pericardium has 2 layers
    b. Phrenic nerve innervates it
    c. Prevent excessive dilatation of heart
    d. All of the above

96. **A youg adult with RTA presented to the emergency department with swelling over face and no passage of urine since last 4 hours. On clinical examination, swelling and crepitus was felt on face, neck and chest. Most likely diagnosis:**
    a. Renal shut down
    b. Lung laceration
    c. Gas gangrene
    d. Fracture base of skull

97. **Pseudocyst differs from true cyst in terms of:**
    a. Size
    b. Lining
    c. Complications
    d. Presentation

98. **First step in management of blood group mismatch while transfusing blood:**
    a. Immediately stop blood transfusion
    b. I/V Steroids
    c. I/V fluids
    d. Alkalization of urine

99. **Location of nucleus ambiguus:**
    a. Medulla
    b. Pons
    c. Midbrain
    d. Paracentral lobule

100. **A patient presented with a single painful ulcer in the axilla with undermined edges. Which of the following is likely diagnosis:**
    a. Basal cell carcinoma
    b. Squamous cell carcinoma
    c. Aphthous ulcer
    d. Tuberculous ulcer

Ans. 93. **b.** Liver 94. **d.** 50 95. **d.** All of the above 96. **b.** Lung laceration
97. **b.** Lining 98. **a.** Immediately stop... 99. **a.** Medulla 100. **d.** Tuberculous ulcer

IMAGE-BASED QUESTIONS

1. **Management of this condition:**

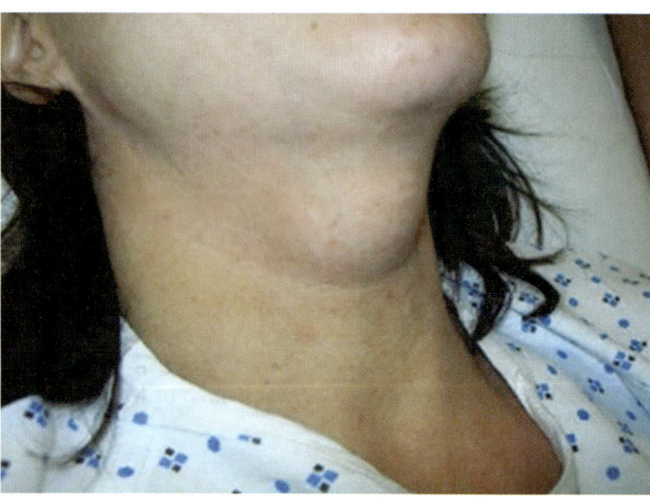

a. Hemithroidectomy b. Total thyroidectomy
c. Radioiodine ablation d. Sitrunk operation

Thyroglossal cyst should be managed by Sistrunk operation, where excision of cyst and also full tract up to the foramen cecum is done along with removal of central part of the hyoid bone, as the tract passes through it.

2. **Which of the following is FALSE for this condition:**

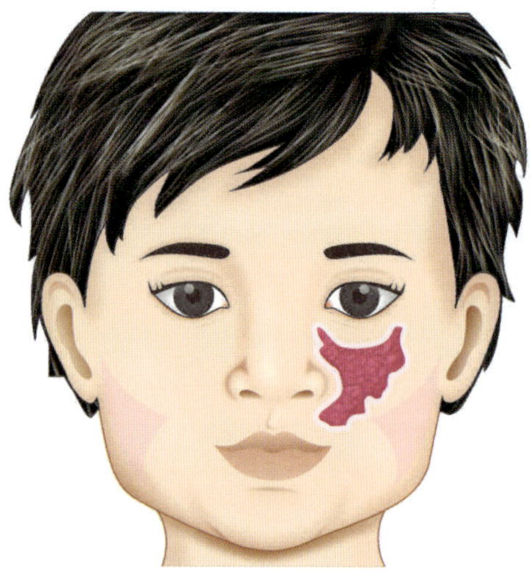

a. Presents at birth
b. Resolve spontaneously
c. May be associated with Sturge-Weber syndrome
d. Capillary malformation

Port-wine stain (naevus flammeus) presents at birth and persists throughout life without any change. Spontaneous regression will not occur.

3. **MC complication of this condition:**

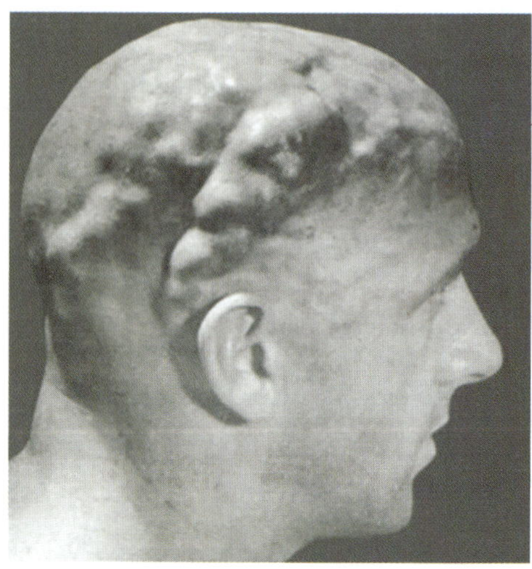

a. Embolism b. Thrombosis
c. Hemorrhage d. Malignancy

Ulceration is the eventual problem in cirsoid aneurysm, which will lead to uncontrollable hemorrhage.

4. **Investigation of choice for this condition:**

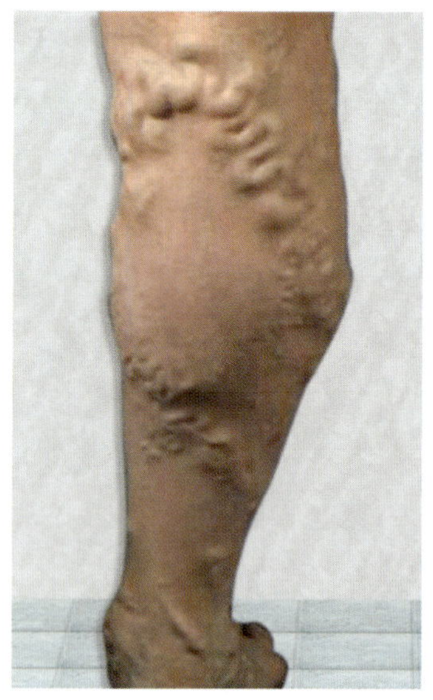

a. Venous doppler b. Duplex scan
c. Venography d. Plethysmography

Duplex scan is a highly reliable ultrasound Doppler imaging technique (here high resolution B mode ultrasound imaging and Doppler ultrasound is used) for varicose veins, which along with direct visualization of veins, gives the functional and anatomical information, and also color map.

5. Name the clinical test shown:

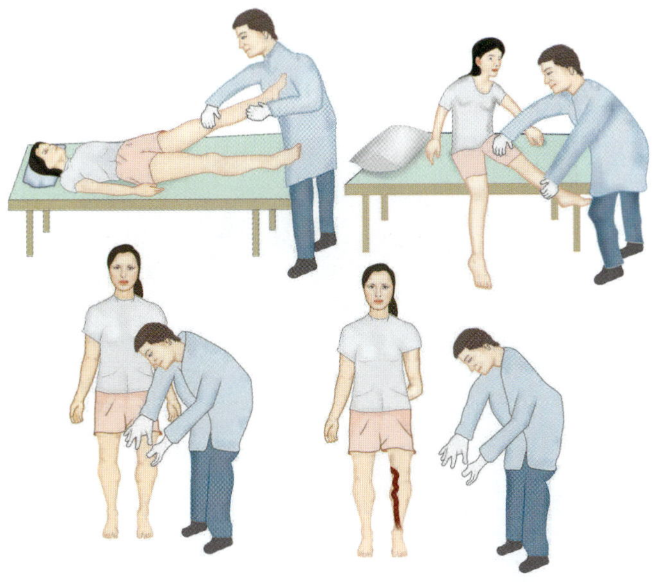

a. Perthe's test
b. Fegan's test
c. Brodie-Trendelenburg test
d. Tourniquet test

In Brodie-Trendelenburg test-I, vein is emptied by elevating the limb and a tourniquet is tied just below the sapheno-femoral junction (or using thumb, saphenofemoral junction is occluded). Patient is asked to stand quickly. When tourniquet or thumb is released, rapid filling from above signifies saphenofemoral incompetence.

6. Which of the following is FALSE for the condition shown:

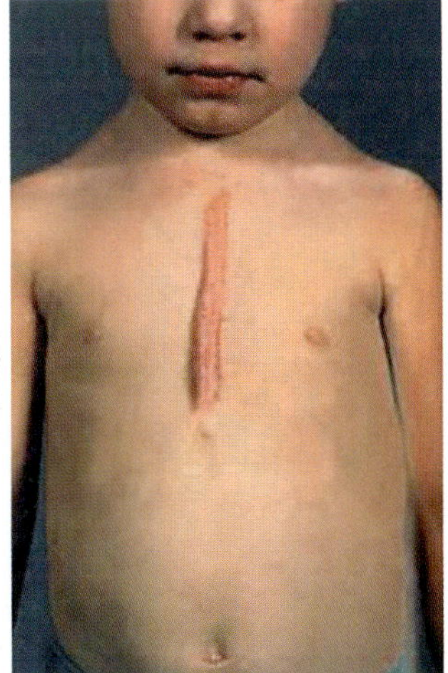

a. Common in blacks
b. Common over sternum
c. Can be completely cured
d. Extends into adjacent normal skin

Recurrence rate for keloid is very high – more than 50%.

7. Management of choice for the condition shown:

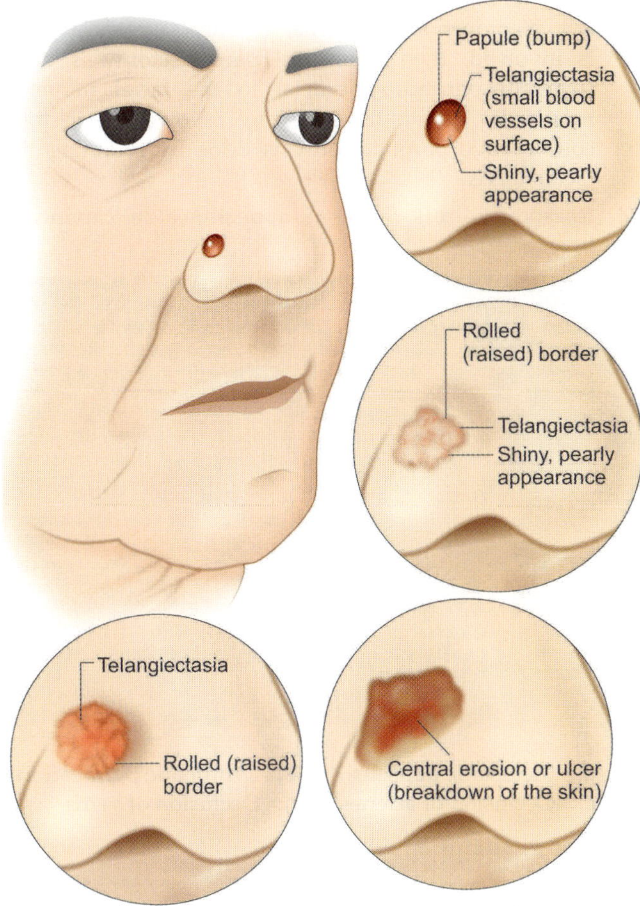

a. Radiotherapy
b. Chemotherapy
c. Laser surgery
d. Wide excision

Wide excision (1 cm clearance) with skin grafting, primary suturing or flap (Z plasty, rhomboid flap, rotation flap) is the procedure of choice for basal cell carcinoma.

8. Management of choice for this condition:

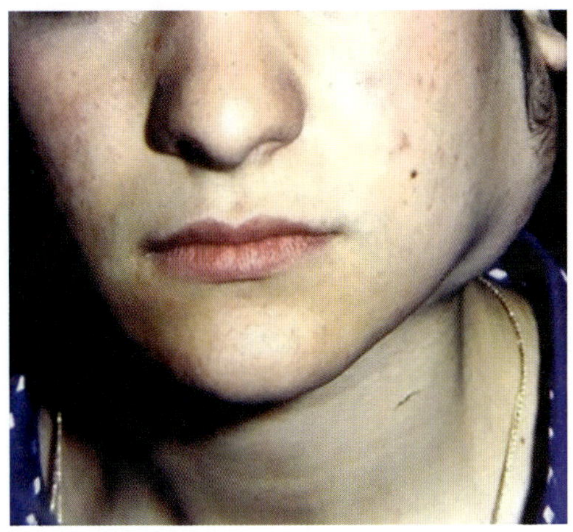

a. Radiotherapy b. Chemotherapy
c. Surgery d. Wait and watch

For pleomorphic adenoma, if only superficial lobe is involved, then superficial parotidectomy is done (wherein parotid superficial to the facial nerve is removed). If both the lobes are involved, then total conservative parotidectomy is done by retaining the facial nerve.

9. Reason for this cause of appearance in carcinoma breast:

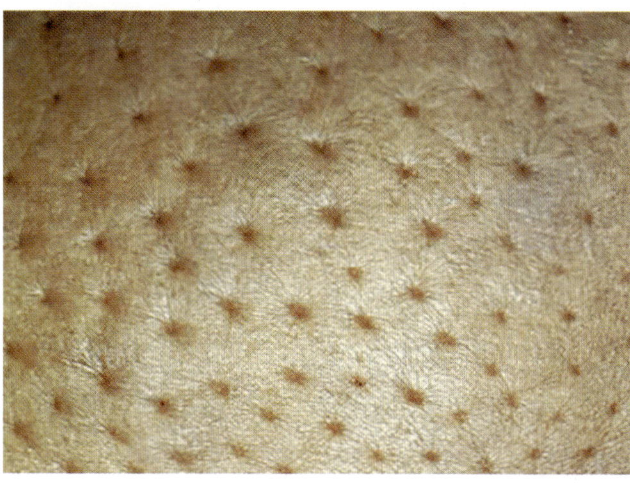

a. Metastatic deposits b. Lymphatic permeation
c. Occlusion of arteries d. Occlusion of veins

Due to obstruction of dermal lymphatics, openings of the sebaceous glands and hair follicles get buried in the edema giving rise to orange peel appearance (Peau d'orange).

10. Tissue of origin of this condition:

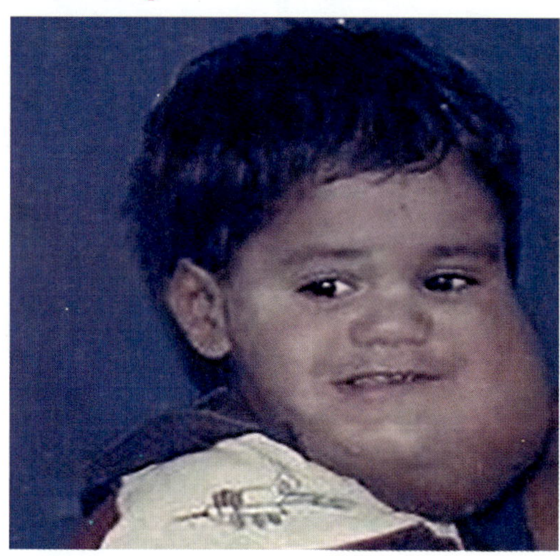

a. Neural b. Arterial
c. Vascular d. Lymphatic

Cystic hygroma/cavernous lymphangioma is a cystic swelling due to sequestration of a portion of jugular lymphatic system, during the development period in utero.

MCQ POINTS

S. No.	Question statements	Answer
1.	Initial investigation for breast lump	***FNAC***
2.	Thyroid tumor, associated with MEN II syndrome	***Medullary***
3.	Bilateral breast carcinoma	***Lobular***
4.	Vascular malformation which regresses	***Strawberry angioma***
5.	MC cause of false aneurysm	***Trauma***
6.	Sign indicative of deep venous thrombosis	***Homan sign***
7.	Gold standard method of diagnosing varicose veins	***Doppler USG***
8.	Sign associated with arteriovenous fistula	***Nicoladoni Branham sign***
9.	Mode of healing in dirty incised and unsutured wound	***Primary***
10.	MC site of keloid	***Sternum***
11.	MC site of basal cell carcinoma	***Face/ inner canthus of eye***
12.	MC soft tissue tumor in a child	***Rhabdomyosarcoma***
13.	MC benign parotid gland tumor	***Pleomorphic adenoma***
14.	Treatment of pleomorphic adenoma	***Superficial parotid ectomy***
15.	Cause of peau'd orange	***Lymphatic permeation***
16.	Treatment of choice for cystic hygroma	***Excision***
17.	Retention cyst of sublingual gland is known as	***Ranula***
18.	Thyroid carcinoma which may secrete calcitonin	***Medullary***
19.	Cork screw appearance of esophagus on barium swallow is seen in	***Diffuse esophageal spasm***
20.	X-ray appearance of achalasia cardia	***Bird beak appearance***
21.	Tumor associated with Barrett's esophagus	***Adenocarcinoma***
22.	MC type of esophageal carcinoma	***Squamous***
23.	MC cause of peptic ulcer disease	***H. pylori***
24.	GIT ulcers, seen in severe burns	***Curling's***
25.	MC malignant tumor of appendix	***Argentaffinoma***
26.	Source of bleeding in duodenal ulcer	***Gastroduodenal artery***
27.	Meckel's diverticulum is a remnant of … duct	***Vitello-intestinal***
28.	MC site of colorectal carcinoma	***Rectum***
29.	MC cause of acute pancreatitis	***Gallstones***
30.	MC site of pancreatic carcinoma	***Head***
31.	MC site of gastrinoma	***Duodenum***
32.	Whipple's triad is seen in	***Insulinoma***
33.	MC cause of overwhelming post splenectomy infections	***Streptococcus pneumoniae***
34.	Union of superior mesenteric and splenic vein forms …vein	***Portal vein***
35.	Anchovy sauce pus is seen in	***Amoebic liver abscess***
36.	PAIR technique is used in the management of	***Hydatid cyst***
37.	MC marker for hepatocellular carcinoma	***Alphafetoprotein***
38.	Subtype of hepatocellular carcinoma carrying best prognosis	***Fibrolamellar***
39.	MC cause of obstructive jaundice	***CBD stone***

S. No.	Question statements	Answer
40.	Stone which grows in alkaline urine	***Struvite***
41.	MC type of renal cell carcinoma	***Clear cell Ca***
42.	Schistosomiasis may predispose to …type of urinary bladder carcinoma	***Squamous***
43.	Thimble bladder is suggestive of….infection	***TB***
44.	MC cause of urinary obstruction in male infant	***Posterior uretheral valve***
45.	MC carcinoma of the testes in young age group	***Teratoma***
46.	Prostatic carcinoma arises from …zone	***Peripheral***
47.	Metastasis of prostatic carcinoma to vertebra is through ….. vertebral venous plexus	***Batesons***
48.	Triad of pain, jaundice and melena is seen in	***Hemobilia***
49.	MC endocrine tumor of pancreas	***Insulinoma***
50.	Management of annular pancreas	***Duodeno-jejunostomy/duodeno-duodenostomy***
51.	Source of bleeding in duodenal ulcer	***Gastroduodenal artery***
52.	Meckel's diverticulum is a remnant of … duct	***Vitello-intestinal***
53.	MC site of colorectal carcinoma	***Rectum***
54.	MC cause of acute pancreatitis	***Gallstones***
55.	MC site of pancreatic carcinoma	***Head***
56.	MC site of gastrinoma	***Duodenum***
57.	Whipple's triad is seen in	***Insulinoma***
58.	MC cause of overwhelming post splenectomy infections	***Streptococcus pneumoniae***
59.	Union of superior mesenteric and splenic vein forms …vein	***Portal vein***
60.	Anchovy sauce pus is seen in	***Amoebic liver abscess***
61.	PAIR technique is used in the management of	***Hydatid cyst***
62.	MC marker for hepatocellular carcinoma	***Alphafetoprotein***
63.	Subtype of hepatocellular carcinoma carrying best prognosis	***Fibrolamellar***
64.	MC cause of obstructive jaundice	***CBD stone***
65.	Stone which grows in alkaline urine	***Struvite***
66.	MC type of renal cell carcinoma	***Clear cell Ca***
67.	Schistosomiasis may predispose to …type of urinary bladder carcinoma	***Squamous***
68.	Thimble bladder is suggestive of….infection	***TB***
69.	MC cause of urinary obstruction in male infant	***Posterior uretheral valve***
70.	MC carcinoma of the testes in young age group	***Teratoma***
71.	Prostatic carcinoma arises from …zone	***Peripheral***
72.	Metastasis of prostatic carcinoma to vertebra is through ….. vertebral venous plexus	***Batesons***
73.	Triad of pain, jaundice and melena is seen in	***Hemobilia***
74.	MC endocrine tumor of pancreas	***Insulinoma***
75.	Management of annular pancreas	***Duodeno-jejunostomy/duodeno-duodenostomy***
76.	Fluid of choice for burns patients	***Ringer lactate***
77.	Palmar surface of hand represents what … %	***1%***
78.	MC vessels to be affected in Buergers disease	***Small and medium sized arteries***
79.	Nicoladoni Branham sign is seen in	***Arterio-Venous fistula***

S. No.	Question statements	Answer
80.	Best guideline to check adequacy of fluid replacement	***Urinary output***
81.	MC complication of pseudopancreatic cyst	***Infection***
82.	MC ruptured organ in blunt injury to abdomen	***Spleen***
83.	Charcoat triad is seen in	***Acute cholangitis***
84.	Best way to diagnose gallbladder stones	***USG***
85.	Reverse 3 sign on barium studies is seen in	***Ca head of pancreas***
86.	Hirschprungs disease is diagnosed by	***Rectal biopsy***
87.	MC cause of peptic ulcer disease	***H. pylori***
88.	Metabolic disturbance seen with pyloric stenosis	***Hypochloremic hypokalemic metabolic alkalosis***
89.	Ochsner Sherren regimen is used for	***Appendicular lump***
90.	MC site of volvulus is	***Sigmoid colon***
91.	Sister Mary Joseph nodule is most commonly seen with	***Gastric Ca***
92.	Spigelian hernia is seen at the level of	***Arcuate line***
93.	IOC for Vesicoureteral reflux/ VUR	***MCUg/ VCUG***
94.	Example of radiolucent stone is	***Uric acid***
95.	Adder head appearance on excretory urography is seen in	***Ureterocoele***
96.	Lords and Jaboulay procedure is done for	***Hydrocoele***
97.	Golf hole ureteric orifice is seen in	***TB***
98.	MC type of hypospadias	***Glandular***
99.	Amyloid deposition is seen in ..type of thyroid carcinoma	***Medullary***
100.	MC type of breast carcinoma	***Ductal***
101.	MC route of infection to liver	***Ascending (from biliary tract)***
102.	Components of Saints triad	***Gallstones, hiatus hernia and diverticulosis***
103.	MC site of gallstone ileus	***Ileum***
104.	Meniscus sign on cholangiography is seen in	***CBD stone***
105.	Type IV collagen is found in:	***Basement membrane***
106.	Hypokalemia with hypertension is a feature of:	***Primary hyperaldosteronism/ Conn's syndrome***
107.	Neuromuscular irritability is a feature of:	***Hypocalcemia***
108.	Flask shaped ulcers in GIT:	***Amoebic liver abscess***
109.	Investigation of choice for lump:	***Biopsy***
110.	Investigation of choice for acute cholecystitis:	***HIDA scan (2. USG)***
111.	MC predisposing factor for carcinoma of gallbladder:	***Gallstones***
112.	Lords plication is done for:	***Hydrocoele***
113.	Least malignant thyroid tumor:	***Papillary***
114.	Hunterian ligature operation is done for:	***Aneurysm***
115.	MC site of curling ulcer (point 48):	***Stomach***
116.	Skip lesions are a feature of:	***Crohn's disease***
117.	Smoking may predispose to …type of urinary bladder carcinoma	***Squamous***
118.	Which vaccine is indicated in carcinoma urinary bladder	***BCG***
119.	Dukes classification is employed for:	***Rectal Ca***
120.	MC carcinoma of the testes in young age group	***Teratoma***

S. No.	Question statements	Answer
121.	Benign Prostatic Hypertrophy arises from …zone	***Periurethral***
122.	Best way to prevent DVT in post operative period:	***Heparin***
123.	Triad of pain, jaundice and fever is seen in	***Acute cholangitis***
124.	Gas used for creating pneumoperitoneum:	***Carbon-di-oxide***
125.	MC organism associated with emphysematous pyelonephritis:	***E. coli***
126.	Invertogram is done for:	***Anorectal malformations/ imperforate anus***
127.	Diagnosis of vesicouretric reflex:	***MCUG/ VCUG***
128.	Chronic burrowing ulcer is caused by:	***Microaerophilic streptococci***
129.	Communicating track between two epithelial surfaces is known as:	***Fistula***
130.	Undermined edge is seen in ………………………. ulcer	***TB***
131.	Epidural hematoma is because of rupture of:	***Middle meningeal artery***
132.	Lisfranc's amputation is through which level of foot	***Tarsometatarsal***
133.	Vitamin K dependent factors are	***Factor 2, 7, 9, 10***
134.	Union of superior mesenteric and splenic vein forms portal vein behind………..	***Neck of pancreas***
135.	Cleft lip operation is done at:	***3-6 months***

CHAPTER

5

ORTHOPEDICS

KEY POINTS

Malignancy Features

- Codman's triangle: Triangular area of subperiosteal new bone at the tumour host junction seen in osteosarcoma.
- Sunray appearance: New bone laid along the blood vessels within the tumour growing centrifugally seen in osteosarcoma.
- Onion peel appearance: New bone formation in layers, seen in Ewing's sarcoma.

Fracture Eponyms (Fracture and bone involved)

- Barton's fracture: Distal radius, intra—articular
- Colles': Distal radius, extra articular with dorsal tilt
- Smith's: Distal radius, extra articular with volar tilt
- Galleazzi's: Distal ½ radius, with dislocation of distal radioulnar joint.
- Monteggia: Proximal ½ of ulna with dislocation of radial head
- Chauffeur's: Radial styloid
- Night stick: Shaft ulna
- Bennett's: Base of 1st metacarpal, intra articular
- Rolando: Base of 1st metacarpal, extra articular (T/Y configuration)
- Boxer's fracture: Neck 5th metacarpal
- Mallet: Avulsion tendon from distal phalanx
- Hangman's: Second cervical vertebra
- Malgaigne's: Pelvic disruption, injury on one side
- Bumper: Lateral condyle of tibia
- Cotton: Trimalleolar ankle fracture
- Pott's: Bimalleolar ankle fracture
- Aviators: Neck of talus fracture
- March: Fracture shaft of 2nd metatarsal
- Jone's: Fracture bases of 5th metatarsal
- Side sweep fracture/Baby car facture: Elbow injury sustained when one puts one's elbow projecting out of a car
- Massonaise's fracture: Fracture of neck of fibula
- Pilon fracture: Comminuted intra articular fracture of the neck of fibula
- Clay shoveller fracture: Avulsion fracture of the spinous process of vertebra
- Straddle fracture: Bilateral ischiopubic rami fracture

Stages of Fracture Healing

- Stage of hematoma: Less than 1 week
- Stage of granulation tissue formation: 2–3 weeks
- Stage of callus: 4–12 weeks
- Stage of remodeling: 1–2 years
- Stage of modeling: Many years

Bone Grafts

- Autogenous graft: Graft is taken from the patient himself, from sites like iliac crest, upper end of tibia, fibula.
- Allogenous graft: Can be obtained form cadavers (Cadaveric graft)—Allogenous grafts from the mother are used when a child's bone reserves are not enough to fill a big gap. Also the bone preserved by deep freezing, by decalcifying or formalin preservation can be used for allogenous bone grafting.
- Xenografting: Bone grafts from some other species are used.
- Artificial bones: Hydroxyapatite derived from corals.

Splints Used in Nerve Injuries

- Axillary nerve: Shoulder abduction splint
- Radial nerve palsy: Cock-up splint
- Sciatic nerve palsy: Foot drop splint

Nerve Injuries

- Neurapraxia: Physiological disruption of nerve conduction in the absence of structural changes, complete spontaneous recovery occurs.
- Axonotmesis: Axons are damaged but the internal structure is preserved. Spontaneous recovery possible.
- Neurotmesis: Structure of the nerve is damaged by actual cutting Nerve repair is required, no spontaneous recovery.

Nerve Degeneration

- Proximal part undergoes primary or retrograde degeneration.
- Part of the neuron distal to point of injury undergoes secondary or Wallerian degeneration
- The rate of recovery of axon is 1 mm/day
- Motor march—the nearest to the site of injury recovers first followed by others form proximal to distal.

Nerve Palsies

- Wrist drop: Radial nerve palsy
- Foot drop: Common peroneal nerve palsy
- Winging of scapula: Paralysis of serratus anterior in long thoracic never palsy
- Main- en- griffe/Claw hand: Paralysis of lumbricals in ulnar nerve palsy
- Ape thumb: Paralysis of opponens pollicis in median nerve palsy
- Pointing index: Paralysis of flexor digitorum superficialis in median nerve palsy
- Crutch palsy/Saturday night: Radial nerve
- Honeymoon palsy: Median nerve palsy

Muscle Wasting in Nerve Injuries

- Flat shoulder: Axillary nerve
- Flat thenar eminence: Median nerve
- Flat hypothenar eminence: Ulnar nerve
- Hollowing between metacarpals: Ulnar nerve
- Thigh washing: Femoral nerve
- Calf wasting: Sciatic nerve

Common Sites of Avascular Necrosis

- Fracture neck femur: Necrosis femoral head
- Fracture Scaphoid waist: Necrosis of proximal pole of Scaphoid
- Fracture neck talus: Necrosis of body of talus

Carrying Angle of Elbow

- Normal in males: 11 degree
- In females: 14 degree

Three Bony Relationship

- Three points relationship in elbow is formed by: Medial epicondyle, Lateral epicondyle and Tip of olecranon
- Tip of radius is considered as fourth point
- When elbow is flexed to 90 degree, these points forms a near isosceles triangle, whereas on extension, they lie in a straight line
- They are important in diagnosing injuries around elbow joint
- Maintained in supracondylar fractures and disturbed in posterior dislocation of elbow

Shoulder Dislocation

- Shoulder dislocation: Commonest joint to dislocate
- Bankart's lesion: Stripping of the glenoidal labrum and periosteum from the anterior surface of glenoid and scapular neck
- Hill-Sachs lesion: Depression on the humeral head in its posterolateral quadrant due to impingement by anterior edge of the glenoid on the head.

Management of Clubfoot by Age

- 0–1 months: Manipulation by mother
- 1–6 months: Manipulation with plaster cast (Ponseti casting)
- ½–3 years: Posterolateral soft tissue release
- 4–8 years: Evan's surgary (posteromedial soft tissue release with calcaneocuboid fusion
- 8–11 years: Wedge tarsectomy
- > 12 years: Triple arthrodesis
- Already operated: Ilizarov technique

Older Method of Manipulation in CTEV (Kites Method; NOT used nowadays)

- A - Adduction
- I - Inversion
- E - Equinus
- If not corrected in this order then it can lead to Rocker bottom feet

Premalignant Bone Lesions

- Paget's disease
- Dipahysial aclasia
- Enchondromatosis
- Postradiation

Remember

- Most common bone tumour: Secondaries (metastasis) from other regions
- Most common benign bone tumour: Osteochondroma
- Most common true benign bone tumour: Osteoid osteoma
- Most common primary bone malignancy: Multiple myeloma, followed by osteosarcoma

Acute Osteomyelitis

- Treatment within 48 hours off onset of symptoms: Conservative (antibiotics)

- Beyond 48 hours: Surgical exploration
- Sequestrum: Dead bone, surrounded by infected granulation tissue
- Involucrum: Dense sclerotic bone overlying sequestrum

Tubercular Arthritis of Hip Joint

- Stage 1/Stage of synovitis or stage of apparent lengthening: Flexion, abduction, external rotation
- Stage 2/Stage of arthritis or stage of apparent shortening: Flexion, adduction, internal rotation.
- Stage 3/Stage of erosion or stage of true shortening: Flexion, adduction, internal rotation

Clinical Features of Rickets

- Craniotabes (earliest manifestation of rickets)
- Bossing of frontal and parietal bones
- Delayed closure of fontanelle
- Rachitic rosary—prominent costochondral junction
- Harrison's groove horizontal depression along the lower border of chest corresponding to diaphragm
- Pigeon breast—forward projection of sternum
- Pot belly—hypotonia of abdominal muscles.
- Ewing's sarcoma is the most radiosensitive tumour, but not most radiocurable tumour

Remember

- Epiphyseal enlargement: JRA
- Epiphyseal widening: Rickets
- Epiphyseal dysgenesis: Hypothyroidism

Some Conditions

- Osteogenesis imperfect: Tendency for frequent fracture, due to brittleness of bones. Autosomal dominant inheritance. Associated with blue sclera, joint laxity and otosclerosis.
- Diaphysial aclasia: Multiple exostoses, Multiple cartilage capped bony outgrowths from the metaphysic of long bones. Inherited as autosomal dominant. X-ray shows trumpet shaped metaphysic and bony projections.
- Osteopetrosis/Marble-bone disease/Albers—Schonberg disease: Dense but brittle bones
- Paget's disease/Ostetis deformans: Progressive tendency for one or more bones to bend, get thickened and spongy, followed by increased density and hardening. Pathological fractures and malignant change can occur.
- Histiocytosis X: Proliferation of histiocytes in the bones, includes Eosinophilic granuloma, Hand-Schuller Christian disease, Litterer Siwe disease
- Achondroplasia: Trident hand, Globular skull, Dwarfism and Prognathism.

Radiological Signs of Scurvy (Usually Studied In Knee Joints)

- Wimberger's sign/Signet ring/halo sign: Sclerotic rim around epiphysis
- White line of Frankel: Zones of provisional calcification
- Trummerfeld's zone: Radiolucent cortex proximal to white line
- Pelkan spur/Corner sign: Marginal metaphyseal infarction with healing
- Pencil thin cortex: Cortical thinning
- Ground glass shaft: Rarification of cortical bone
- Scorbutic rosary: Sharp elevation at costochonadral junction
- Raised periosteum: Subperiosteal haematoma.

Diagnostic Criteria of Rheumatoid Arthritis (RA)

If 4 or more criteria are present, it is RA

- Morning stiffness
- Swelling of 3 or more specified joints
- Swelling of joints in the hand and wrist
- Symmetric swellings
- Rheumatoid nodule
- Rheumatoid factor [positive]
- Erosion or unequivocal periarticular osteropenia on X-ray

RA Associated Syndromes

- Felty's syndrome: Rheumatoid arthritis, Splenomegaly, Neutropenia and High titres of rheumatoid arthritis
- Caplan's syndrome: Rheumatoid arthritis and Pneumoconiousis
- Still's disease: Rheumatoid arthritis, Splenomegaly, Leucocytosis, Rash and Rheumatoid factor absent

Joints Commonly Affected in RA

- Metacarpophalangeal joint
- Proximal interphalangeal joint
- Wrist
- Knees
- Elbows
- Ankles

Neural Tube Defects

- Spina bifida occulta: Mildest and the commonest. Failure of the fusion of vertebral arches results in bifid spinous process.

- Spina bifida aperta: Failure of fusion of not only vertebral arches but also soft tissue, skin and meninges
- Meningocele: Protrusion of meninges through a defect in the neural arch. Contains only CSF
- Meningomyelocele: Protrusion of meninges with some neural element
- Syringomyelocele: Spinal cord with dilated central canal (Syringomyelia) lies within the meningial sac
- Myelocele: Central canal opens to the exterior.

Miscellaneous Conditions

- Tennis elbow: Lateral epicondylitis, pain and tenderness at the lateral epicondyle of the humerus due to inflammation at the origin of extensor muscles of forearm.
- Golfer's elbow: Medial epicondylitis, pain and tenderness at the medial epicondyle of the humerus due to Inflammation at the origin of flexor tendons of foremen.
- De Quervain's tenovaginitis: Pain and swelling over the radial styloid process. Inflammation of the common sheath of abductor pollicis longus and extensor pollicis longus tensons. Tenderness is elicited by adducting the thumb.
- Meralgia paresthetica: Paresthesia in the area of skin supplied by lateral cutaneous nerve of thigh as it gets trapped beneath the fascia.
- Gamekeeper's thumb: Tear of ulnar collateral ligament of thumb digital nerve.
- Jumper's knee: Tendonitis of quadriceps apparatus
- Madelung deformity: Development ulnar and volar tilt of distal end of radius with dorsal dislocation of ulna (manus valgus)
- Dupyuytren's Contracture: Contracture of palmar aponeurosis Flexion deformity of one or more fingers due to thickening and shortening of the palmar aponeurosis.
- Frog hand: Infection of midpalmar space, resulting in deep palmar abscess. Edema of dorsum of hand Inderphalangeal joint movements are not painful, while metacarphalangeal joints movements are painful.

Degree of Sprain

- First: Tear of only few fibers
- Second: From third to almost the fibres of ligaments are disrupted, movements are disrupted, movements are normal
- Third: Complete tear of ligament

Charcot's Joint

- Diabetic arthropathy: Foot joint
- Tabes dorsalis: Knee and hip
- Diabetes mellitus: Foot
- Syringomyelia: Upper limb

Some Tests

- Oschner's clasping test: Interlock the digits of both the hands and flex the metacarpophalangeal and interphalangeal joints. In median nerve palsy, lateral part of flexor digitorum profundus, will get paralysed leading to pointing index.
- Hook sign: Suppurative tenosynovitis Metacarpophalangeal joint movement in not painful while interphalangeal movement are painful.
- Book test/Froment's sign: In ulnar nerve paralysis, adductor pollicis will be paralyzed and the patient will not be able to grasp the book between the thumb and index finger.
- Simon's test: Diagnostic of ruptured tendo Achilles
- Kanavel's sign: Seen in ulnar bursa infection point of maximum tenderness is over the part lying between transverse palmar creases.

MCQs WITH SHORT EXPLANATIONS

ORTHOPEDIC TRAUMA

1. **A patient came to orthopedics emergency room with a history of road traffic accident. You are working as an intern. Which of the following findings of the patient would you inform to your orthopedic PG resident with priority?**
   a. Intra-articular fracture
   b. Multiple abrasions of 20 cm
   c. Compound fracture
   d. Blackening of patient's toes

   If the blood supply is grossly insufficient, gangrene occurs.

Vascular injuries and skeletal trauma.

Vessel injured	*Trauma*
Femoral	Fracture lower third of femur
Popliteal	Supracondylar fracture of the femur
Posterior tibial	Dislocation of the knee, Fracture tibia
Subclavian	Fracture-dislocation of the shoulder
Brachial	Supracondylar fracture of the humerus

2. **Which of the following correlates well to perilunate dislocation?**
   a. Both lunate and capitate are out of plane
   b. Lower end of radius, scaphoid and capitate are in alignment but lunate is out of plane
   c. Lower end of radius, lunate are in alignment but rest of carpals is out of plane
   d. Both scaphoid and capitate are in plane

   In perilunate dislocation, the lunate remains in position and the rest of the carpal bones dislocates dorsally.

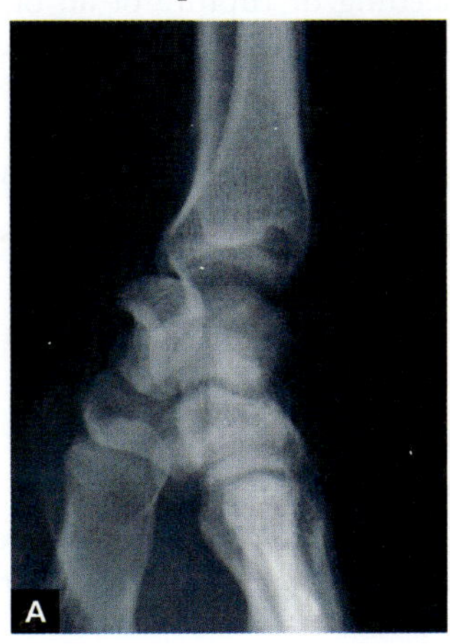

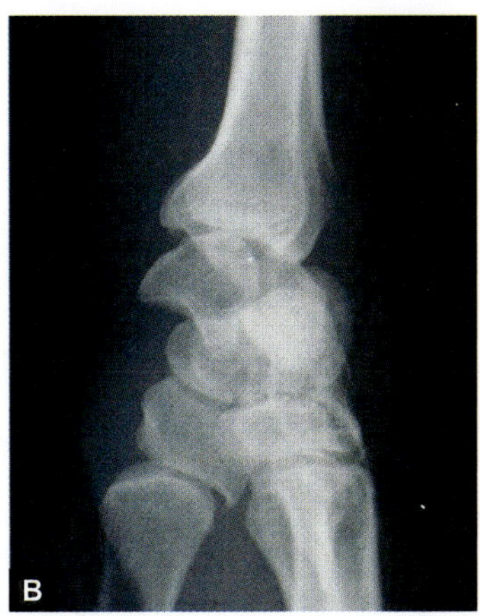

Lateral views of the wrist X-rays showing (A) Lunate dislocation; and (B) Perilunate dislocation.

3. **A child presented to the orthopedics OPD with complains of deformity, pain and swelling at ankle joint. There was past history of road traffic accident 2 years back involving the ankle joint. Imaging studies were done. Clinical and imaging findings are suggestive of:**

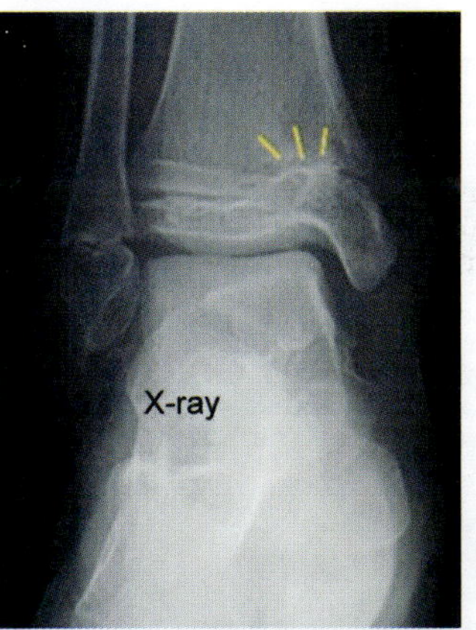

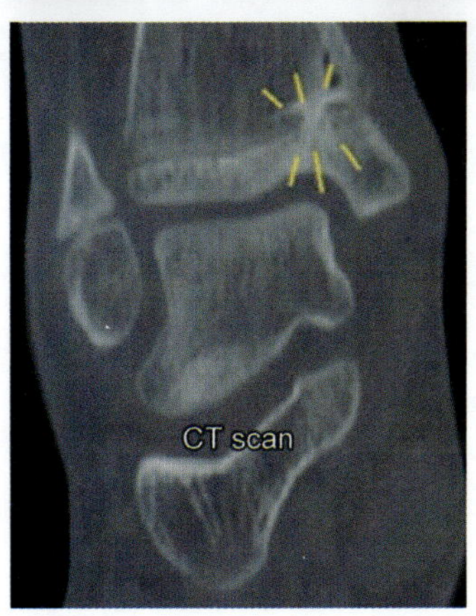

Ans. 1. **d.** Blackening... 2. **c.** Lower end of radius... 3. **a.** Missed epiphyseal...

a. Missed epiphyseal injury
b. Chronic osteomyelitis
c. Ewing's sarcoma
d. Osteogenic sarcoma

Growth disturbances in epiphyseal injuries (leading to deformity) are a common complication.

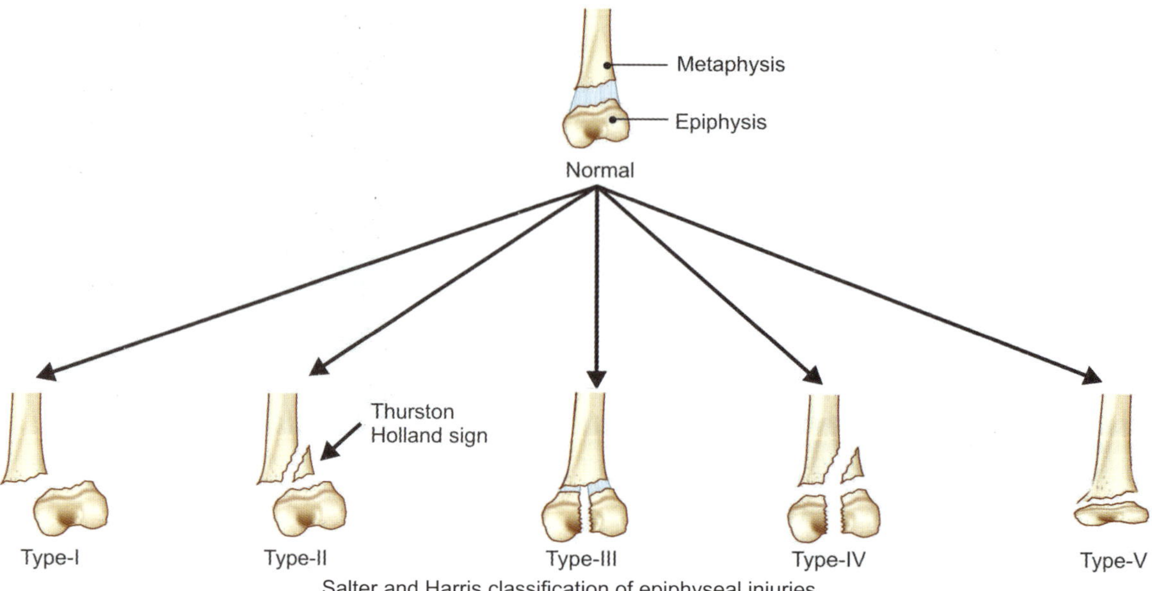

Salter and Harris classification of epiphyseal injuries

4. Which of the following bone will be commonly fractured if a elderly patient has FOSH (fall on outstretched hand) injury?

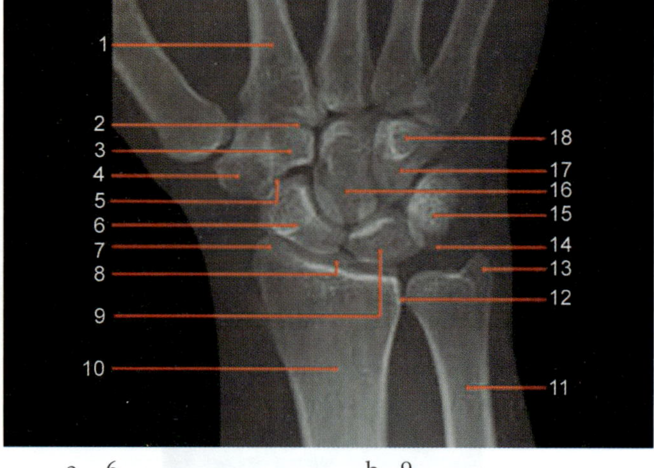

a. 6
b. 9
c. 10
d. 11

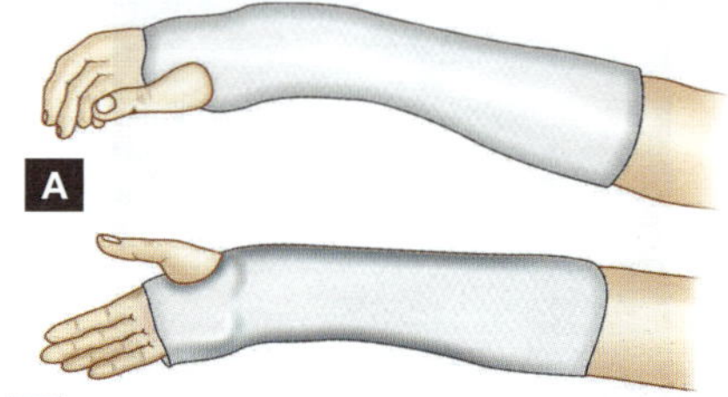

Colles' cast. (A) In palmar flexion. (B) In ulnar deviation

Colles' fracture is the commonest fracture in people over forty years of age, and is particularly common in women because of post-menopausal osteoporosis. It nearly always results from a fall on out-stretched hand.

5. A 1-year-old child presents with multiple fractures seen in various stages of healing. The most probable diagnosis in this case is:

a. Scurvy
b. Rickets
c. Battered baby syndrome
d. Sickle cell disease

Physical examination of a child with battered child syndrome/BCS with detect injuries such as bruises, burns, swelling, retinal hemorrhages, internal damage such as bleeding or rupture of an organ, fractures of long bones or spiral fractures that result from twisting, and fractured ribs or skull. The presence of injuries at different stages of healing (i.e., having occurred at different times) is nearly indicative of BCS.

6. Medial meniscus is more vulnerable to injury than lateral meniscus because of:

a. Its fixity to tibial collateral ligament
b. Its semicircular shape
c. Action of adductor magnus
d. Its attachment to fibrous capsule

The medial meniscus gets torn more often because it is less mobile (being fixed to the medial collateral ligament).

Ans. **4. c.** 10 **5. c.** Battered baby... **6. a.** Its fixity to tibial...

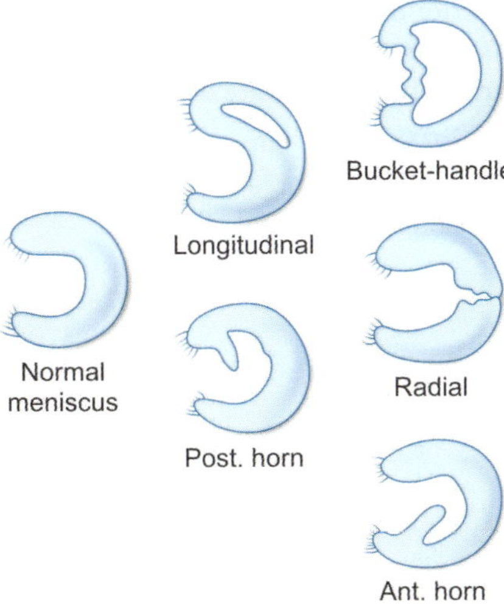

Types of meniscus tear.

7. **MC complication of extracapsular fracture of neck of femur is:**
   a. Non-union
   b. Ischemic necrosis
   c. Malunion
   d. Pulmonary complications

Extracapsular fracture neck of femur is also known as intertrochanteric fractures. Inter-trochanteric fractures always unite, but because of possible failure in keeping the fragments aligned, these often malunite. Malunion give rise to coxa vara (decreased femoral neck-shaft angle), shortening and the leg in external rotation.

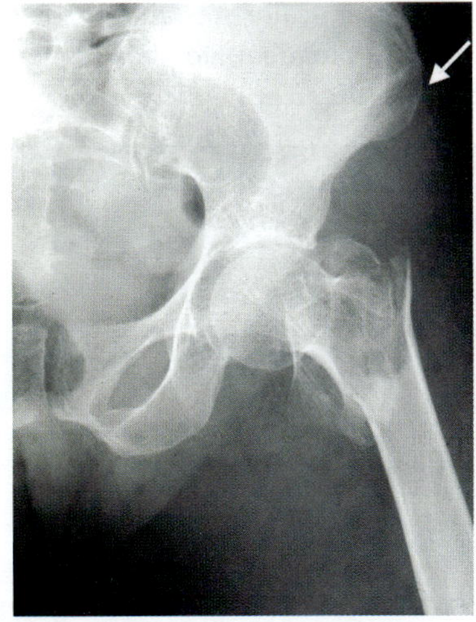

X-ray of the hip, AP view, showing inter-trochanteric fracture.

8. **An army recruit, smoker and 6 months into training started complaining of pain at posterior medial aspect of both legs. There was acute point tenderness and the pain was aggravated on physical activity. The most likely diagnosis is:**
   a. Burger's disease
   b. Gout
   c. Lumbar canal stenosis
   d. Stress fracture

Stress fracture is a special type of fracture sustained due to the chronic repetitive injury (stress) causing a break in bony trabeculae. These often present as only pain and may not be visible on X-rays.

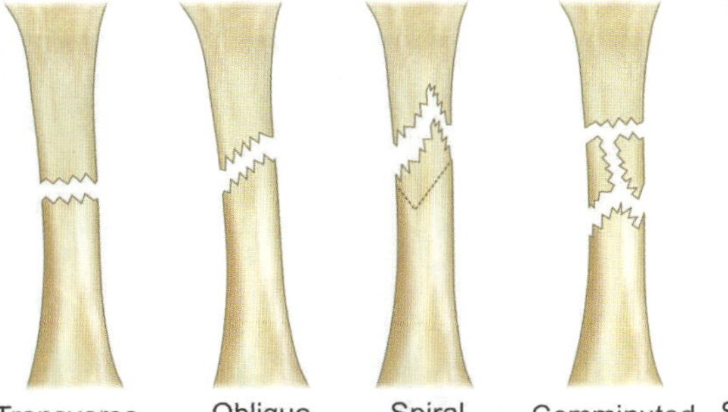

Patterns of fractures.

9. **A 3-year-old child falls from 2 metres height. On X-ray, no abnormality was detected. After 2 years, the child presents with calcaneal valgus. Probable cause is:**
   a. Undiagnosed
   b. Tibial epiphyseal plate injury
   c. Avascular necrosis of talus
   d. Rocker bottom foot

Epiphyseal injury is a group of injuries seen in a growing skeleton. An injury involving the growth plate result in deformities due to irregular growth. Shortening may occur because of premature epiphyseal closure.

Essential features of epiphyseal injuries (Salter and Harris classification).

Type	*Example*	*Treatment*	*Prognosis*
I	Radial neck epiphysis separation	Closed reduction	Good
II	Lower end radius epiphysis	Closed reduction	Good
III	Medial malleolus epiphysis	Open reduction	Growth disturbance can occur
IV	Lateral condyle of humerus	Open reduction	Growth disturbance common
V	Lower tibial epiphysis injury	Conservative	Growth disturbance always

10. **Jefferson fracture occurs at which vertebra:**
    a. C1 b. C2
    c. C1, C2 d. C2, C3

Jefferson's fracture is fracture of the first cervical vertebra.

11. **Least common complication of Colles' fracture:**
    a. Malunion

Ans. 7. **c.** Malunion 8. **d.** Stress fracture 9. **b.** Tibial epiphyseal... 10. **a.** C1

b. Non-union
c. Stiffness of fingers
d. Sudecks dystrophy

A Colles' fracture always unites, but malunion occurs in a large proportion of cases. The cause of malunion is redisplacement of the fracture within the plaster so that a 'dinner fork' deformity results.

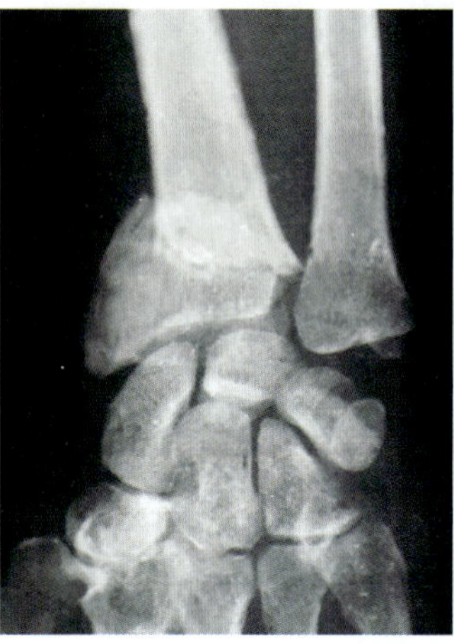
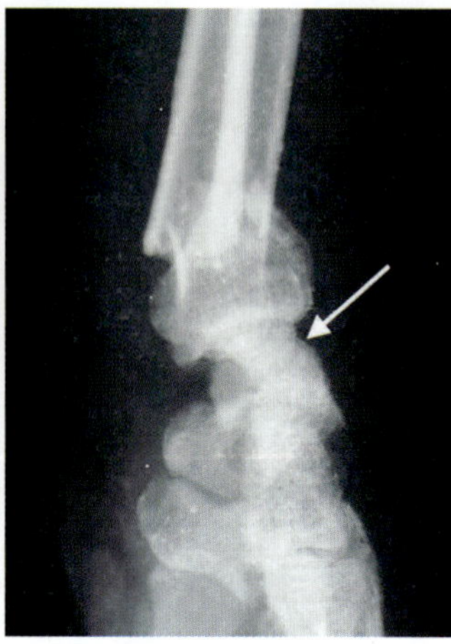

X-ray of the wrist, AP and Lateral views, showing a Colles' fracture. Note that the distal articular surface of the radius faces dorsally (tilted dorsally).

12. Treatment of acute myositis ossificans:
a. Active mobilization
b. Passive immobilization
c. Infrared therapy
d. Immobilization

In the early active stage of myositis the limb should be rested, and NSAID is given. In late stages, it is possible to regain movement by physiotherapy. In some cases, once the myositic mass matures, surgical excision of the bone mass may help regain movement.

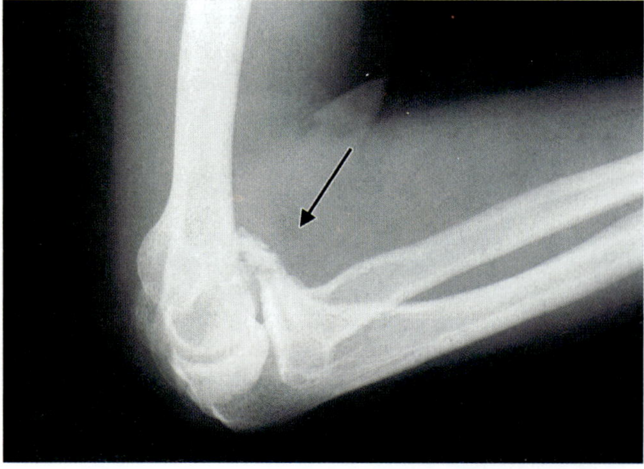

X-ray of the elbow showing myositis ossificans.

13. Triangular relation of elbow is maintained in:
a. Fracture ulna
b. Anterior dislocation of elbow
c. Posterior dislocation of elbow
d. Supracondylar fracture of humerus

Since the fracture in supracondylar humerus is above the condyles, the three bony points relationship is maintained as in a normal elbow.

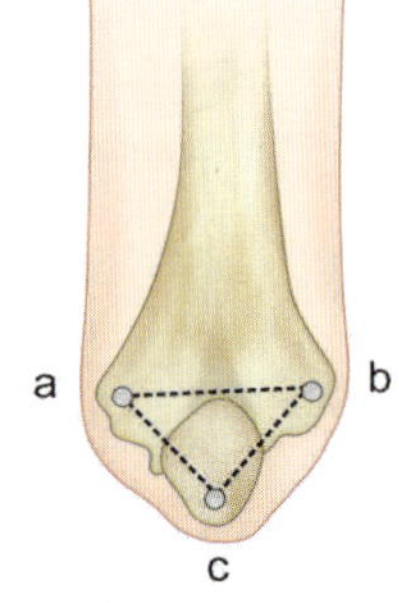

Flexed elbow (looking form behind)

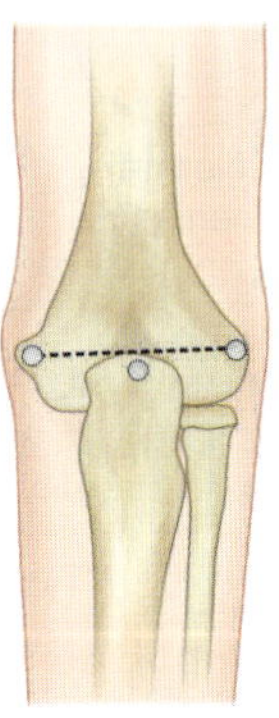

Extended elbow

Three bony points relationship. (a) Medial epicondyle, (b) Lateral epicondyle, (c) Tip of olecranon.

14. Most commonly, recurrent dislocation is seen with:
a. Shoulder
b. Patella
c. Elbow
d. Hip

The shoulder joint is the commonest joint to undergo recurrent dislocation. This results from the following causes: (i) anatomically unstable joint, e.g. in Marfan syndrome; (ii) inadequate healing after the first dislocation, or (iii) an epileptic patient.

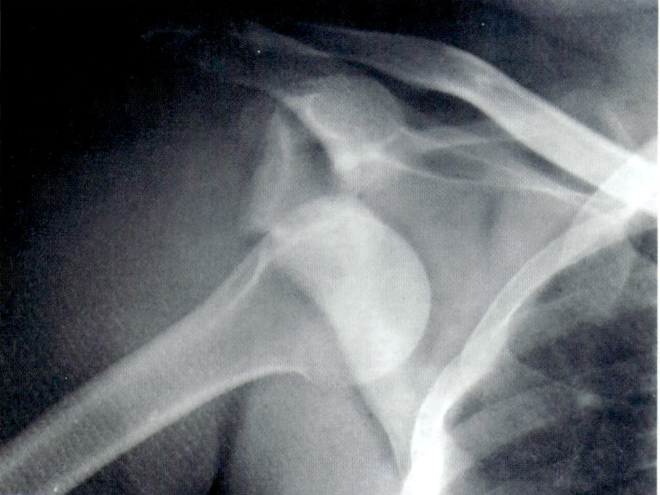

X-ray of the shoulder, AP view, showing anterior dislocation of the shoulder.

15. A patient with recurrent dislocation of the shoulder presents to the hospital. The doctor tries to abduct his

Ans. 11. b. Non-union 12. d. Immobilization 13. d. Supracondylar... 14. a. Shoulder

arm and to extend the elbow and external rotation, but the patient doesn't allow to do so. This test is called:

a. Dugas test
b. Hamilton test
c. Callaway's test
d. Apprehension test

Apprehension test is a test to detect an unstable shoulder. The shoulder is abducted and externally rotated. As the examiner loads the shoulder along the long axis of the arm, the patient becomes apprehensive, and tries to resist any further movement by using his hand or by making the shoulder stiff by muscle spasm.

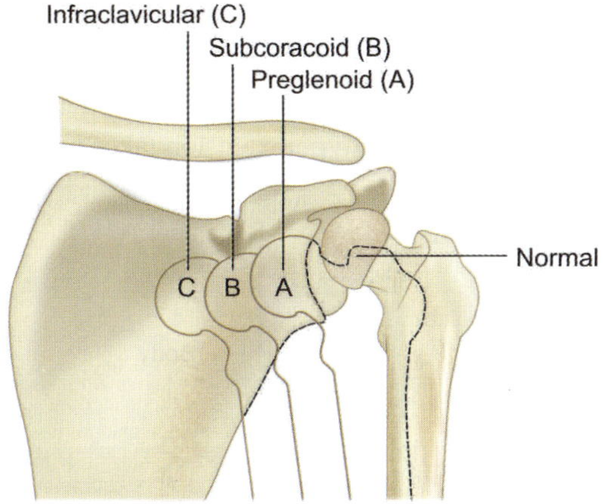

Types of anterior dislocation of shoulder.

16. A 24-year-old male, known epileptic, presented following a seizure with pain in the right shoulder region. Examination revealed that the right upper limb was aducted and internally rotated and the movements could NOT be performed. Likely diagnosis is:

a. Posterior dislocation of shoulder
b. Luxatio erecta
c. Intrathoracic dislocation of shoulder
d. Subglenoid dislocation of shoulder

A posterior dislocation of the shoulder may result from a direct blow on the front of the shoulder, driving the head backwards. More often, however, posterior dislocation is the consequence of an electric shock or an epileptiform convulsion.

17. All of the following are complications of a malunited Colles' fracture EXCEPT:

a. Rupture of flexor pollicis longus tendon
b. Reflex sympathetic dystrophy (RSD)
c. Carpal tunnel syndrome
d. Carpal instability

Rupture of the extensor pollicis longus tendon is an extremely rare complication and occurs a long time after the Colles' fracture has united. It is either due to loss of blood supply to the tendon at the time of fracture, or due to friction the tendn is subjected to every time it moves over a malunited fracture.

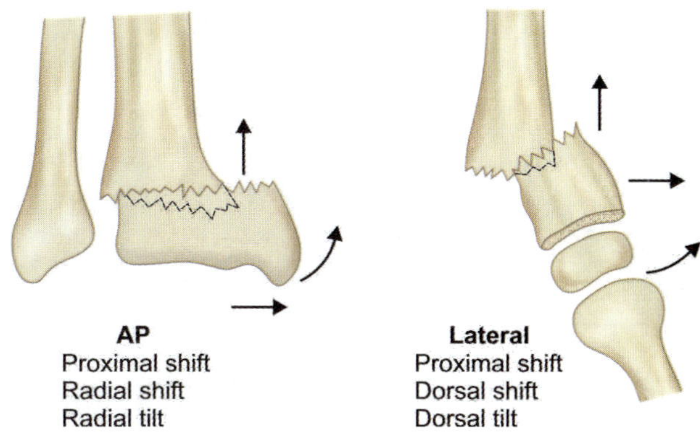

Displacements in Colles' fracture.

18. Flexion, adduction and internal rotation are characteristic posture in:

a. Anterior dislocation of hip joint
b. Posterior dislocation of hip joint
c. Fracture femoral head
d. Fracture shaft femur

An isolated posterior dislocation of the hip is easy to diagnose. The patient presents with a history of severe trauma followed by pain, swelling and deformity (flexion, adduction and internal rotation).

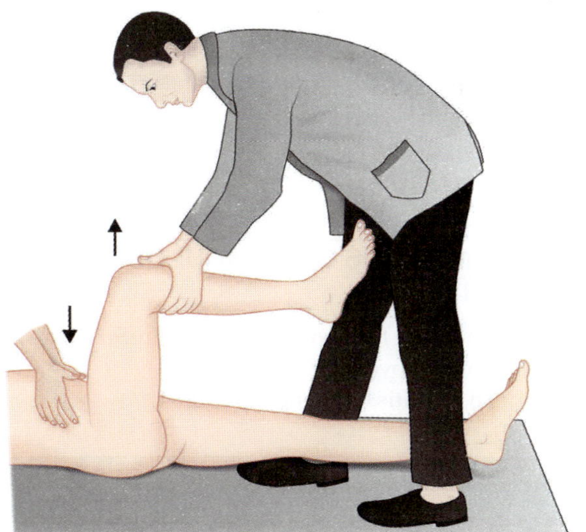

Technique of reduction of hip dislocation.

19. Cotton's fracture involves:

a. Ankle
b. Foot
c. Knee
d. Spine

Cotton's fracture is trimalleolar fracture at ankle joint (medial, lateral and posterior malleoli).

Ans. 15. **d.** Apprehension... 16. **a.** Posterior dislocation... 17. **a.** Rupture of flexor... 18. **b.** Posterior dislocation... 19. **a.** Ankle

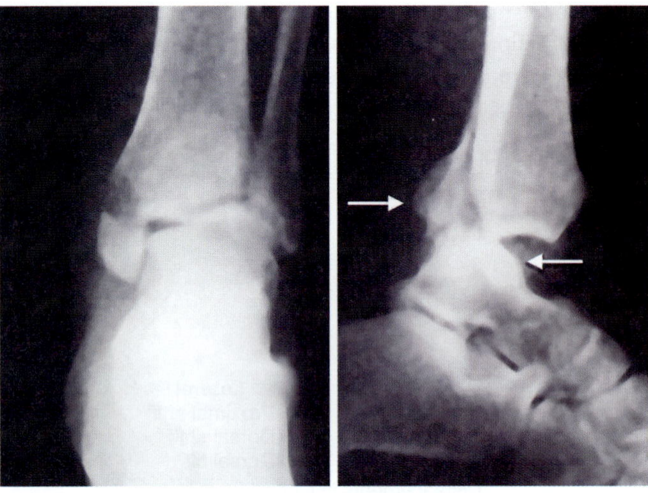

X-rays of the ankle, AP and lateral views, showing an ankle injury (Note, the talus is subluxated, and there is a fracture of the posterior malleolus).

20. Boxer's fracture involves:

a. Metacarpal
b. Carpal
c. Tarsal
d. Metatarsal

Fracture through the neck of the metacarpal commonly affects the neck of the fifth metacarpal. The distal fragment is titled forwards. It is usually sustained when a closed fist hits against a hard object (Boxer's fracture).

21. Whiplash injury is related to:

a. Lumbar spine
b. Thoracic spine
c. Sacral spine
d. Cervical spine

Whiplash injury is cervical spine injury where sudden flexion followed by hyperextension takes place.

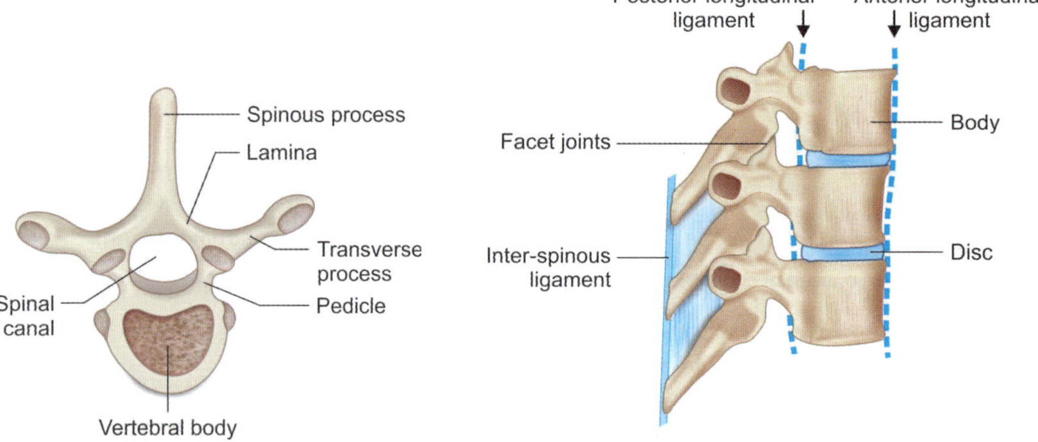

Anatomy of the spine.

INFLAMMATIONS OF MUSCULOSKELETAL SYSTEM

22. Which of the following defines Tom-Smith arthritis?

a. Chronic pyogenic arthritis
b. TB arthritis of infancy
c. Septic arthritis of infancy
d. Rheumatoid arthritis of infancy

Septic arthritis in infancy (Tom-Smith arthritis) is a septic arthritis of the hip seen in infants. At this age, the head of the femur is cartilaginous and is rapidly and completely destroyed by the pyogenic process.

Synovial fluid examination.

Points	*Normal*	*Non-inflammatory*	*Inflammatory*	*Septic*
Gross examination				
Volume (mL)	Often < 3.5 mL	Often > 3.5 mL	Often > 3.5 mL	> 3.5 mL
❑ Viscosity	High	High	Low	Variable
❑ Colour	Colourless	Straw yellow	Yellow	Variable
❑ Clarity	Transparent	Transparent	Translucent	Opaque
Examination in lab				
WBC count	< 200	200–2000	2000–7500	> 10000
PMN leucocytes	< 25%	<25%	>50%	>75%

Contd...

Ans. **20. a.** Metacarpal **21. d.** Cervical spine **22. c.** Septic arthritis...

Contd...

Points	Normal	Non-inflammatory	Inflammatory	Septic
Culture	–	–	–	+
Mucin clot	Firm	Firm	Friable	Friable
Glucose level	Equal to blood glucose	Nearly equal to blood glucose	< 25 mg% of blood glucose	> 25 mg% of blood glucose
Crystal examination	Positive in Gout — Sodium biurate.		Positive in Pseudogout–Ca pyrophosphate	

23. Which of the following is NOT a feature of seronegative rheumatoid arthritis?

a. Joint pain and swelling
b. Distal interphalangeal joints is most commonly affected
c. Symmetrical
d. Affection of multiple joints

The joints most commonly affected in RA are the metacarpophalangeal joints, particularly that of the index finger.

Joints affected in Rheumatoid arthritis.	
Common	❑ MP joints of hand ❑ PIP joints of fingers ❑ Wrists, knees, elbows, ankles
Less common	❑ Hip joint ❑ Temporomandibular joint
Uncommon	❑ Atlanto-axial joint ❑ Facet joints of cervical spine

24. The most common sequelae of TB spondylitis in an adolescent is:

a. Fibrous ankylosis
b. Bony ankylosis
c. Pathological dislocation
d. Chronic osteomyelitis

Fibrous ankylosis is a common outcome of healed tuberculosis of the joints, except in the spine where bony ankylosis follows more often.

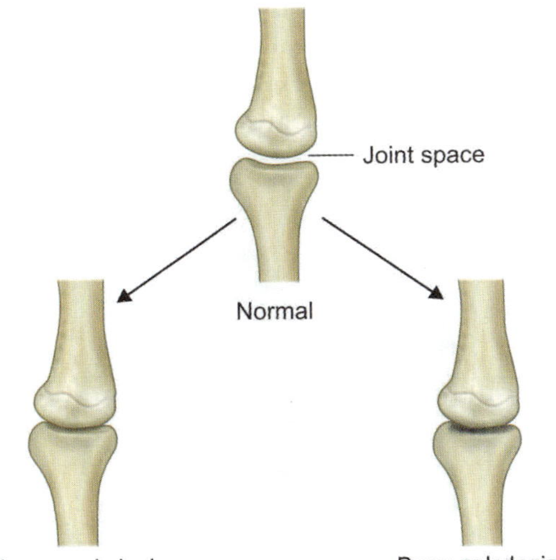

Types of ankylosis.

25. All are seen in chronic osteomyelitis EXCEPT:

a. Sequestrum
b. Amyloidosis
c. Myositis ossificans
d. Sinus tract malignancy

Myositis ossificans/post-traumatic ossification is ossification of the haematoma around a joint, resulting in the formation of a mass of bone restricting joint movements, often completely.

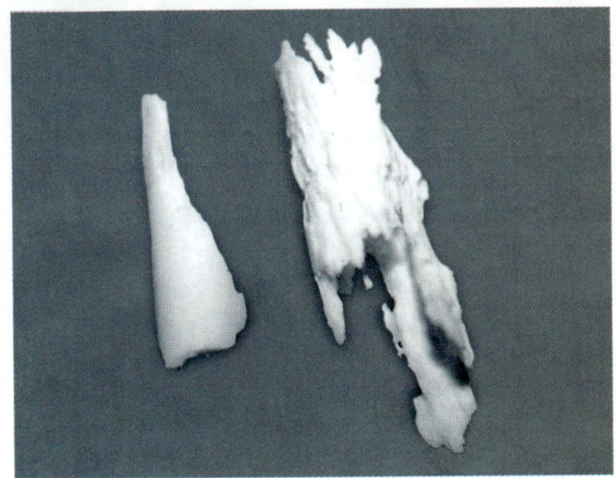

Bone sequestra (Note the rough outer surface).

26. Which of the following statements about tubercular osteomyelitis is NOT true:

a. It is a type of secondary osteomyelitis
b. Sequestrum is uncommon
c. Periosteal reaction is characteristic
d. Inflammation is minimal

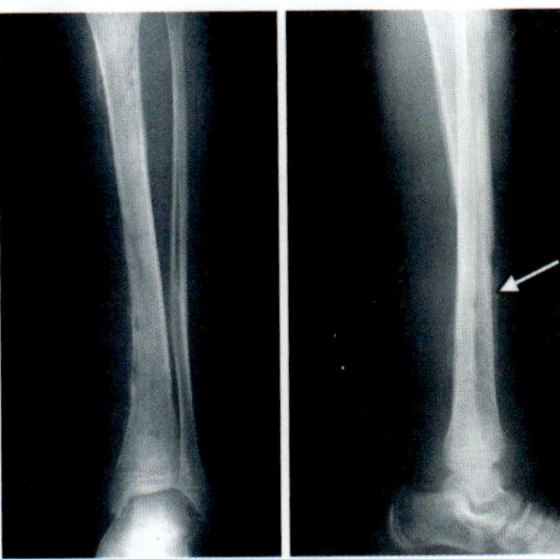

X-ray of leg, AP and Lateral views, showing acute osteomyelitis of tibia (Note early periosteal reaction–arrow).

A tubercular osteomyelitis presents as a well-defined area of bone destruction, typically with minimal reactive new bone formation. This is unlike a pyogenic infection, where reactive periosteal new bone formation is an important feature.

Ans. 23. **b.** Distal inter... 24. **b.** Bony ankylosis 26. **c.** Myositis ossificans 26. **c.** Periosteal reaction...

27. In RA, pathology starts in:

a. Articular cartilage
b. Synovium
c. Capsule
d. Muscles

In RA, initially the synovium becomes oedematous, filled with fibrin exudates and cellular infiltrates. There is an increase in synovial fluid.

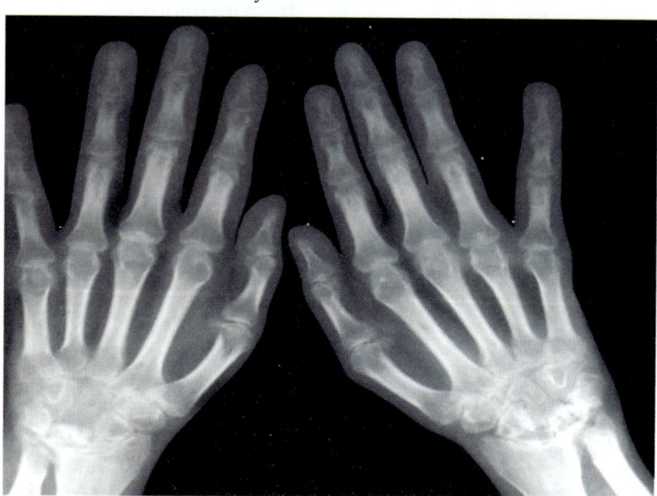

X-rays of both hands, AP view, showing juxta-articular rarefaction.

28. HLA B27 is associated with:

a. RA
b. Anklyosing spondylitis
c. Osteoarthritis
d. Gouty arthritis

The exact aetiology of AS is not known. A strong association has been found between a genetic marker—HLA-B27 and this disease. Whereas, the incidence of HLA-B27 is less than 1% in general population, it is present in more than 85% of patients with AS.

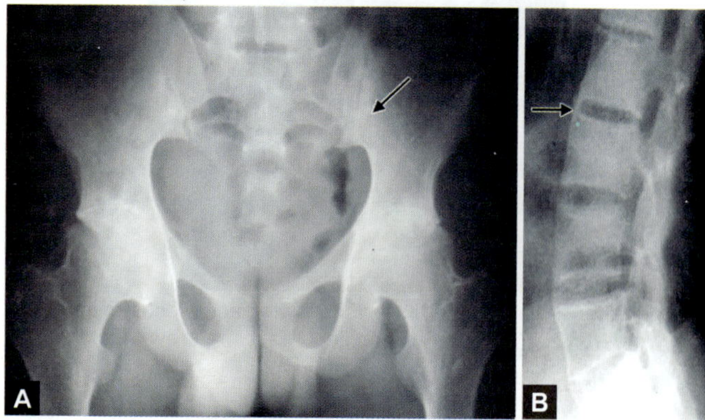

X-rays showing changes in ankylosing spondylitis. (A) X-ray of the pelvis, AP view, showing bilateral SI joint and hip involvement (B) X-ray of the lumbar spine, Lateral view, showing calcification of the ligaments.

29. Spina ventosa is:

a. Tubercular dactylitis
b. TB sacrococcygeal joint
c. TB lumbosacral joint
d. TB spinal cord

Spina ventosa is the name given to tuberculosis of the phalanges of hand. The affected phalanx swells up like a balloon. An X-ray typically shows a lytic lesion distending the phalanx, and a lot of new bone formation.

Musculo-skeletal tuberculosis.

Tissue	*Disease*	*Remarks*
Bone		
Long bone	TB osteomyelitis	Tibia commonly affected
Short bone (phalanges)	Tubercular dactylitis	Also called *spina ventosa*
Spine	TB spondylitis	Also called Pott's disease
Joint		
Arthritis	TB arthritis	Hip joint commonly affected
Synovium	Synovial TB	Knee-commonest site
Others		
Tendon (synovium)	TB tenosynovitis of flexor tendons at wrist	Compound palmar ganglion
Bursae	TB bursitis of trochanteric bursa	Trochanteric bursitis

30. Triple deformity of the knee is a complication of:

a. Tuberculosis
b. Osteoarthritis
c. Septic arthritis
d. All of the above

In TB knee, long standing distension of the joint and destruction of the ligaments produces subluxation of the tibia. The tibia flexes, slips backwards and rotates externally on the femoral condyles (triple subluxation).

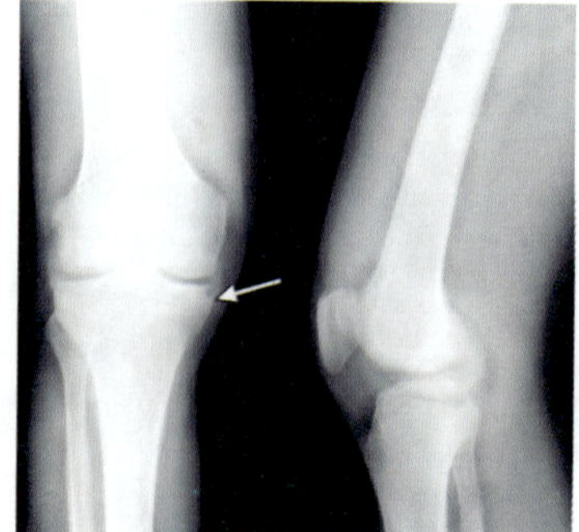

X-ray of the knee, AP and Lateral views, showing changes in tuberculosis of the knee (Note, reduction in joint space and marginal erosions—arrow).

Ans. 27. **b.** Synovium 28. **b.** Anklyosing spondylitis 29. **a.** Tubercular dactylitis 30. **a.** Tuberculosis

31. **MC site of osteomyelitis in children:**
a. Diaphysis b. Metaphysis
c. Epiphysis d. Growth plate

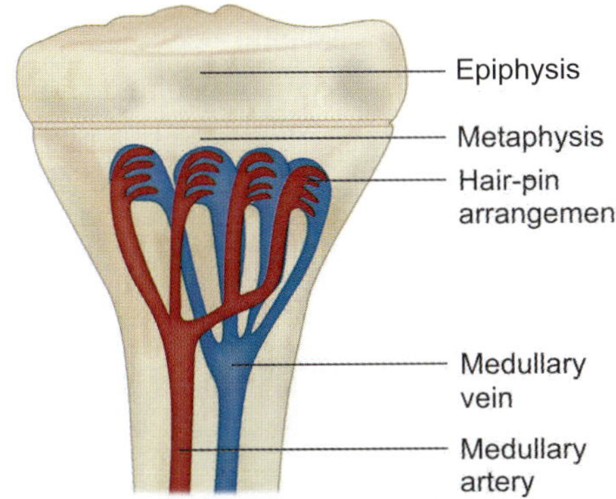

Vascular arrangement at metaphysis of a long bone.

Vessels in metaphysis of the long bone are arranged in the form of loop (hair-pin arrangement). The blood stasis resulting from such an arrangement is probably responsible for the metaphysis being a favourite site for bacteria to settle, and thus a common site for osteomyelitis.

OTHER NON-TRAUMATIC CONDITIONS

32. **A male child presented to the orthopedics OPD with non-suppurative osteomyelitis. He is a known case of sickle cell anemia. Which of the following organism would be responsible for causing osteomyelitis in such a case?**
a. Staphylococcus
b. Streptococcus
c. Pseudomonas
d. Salmonella

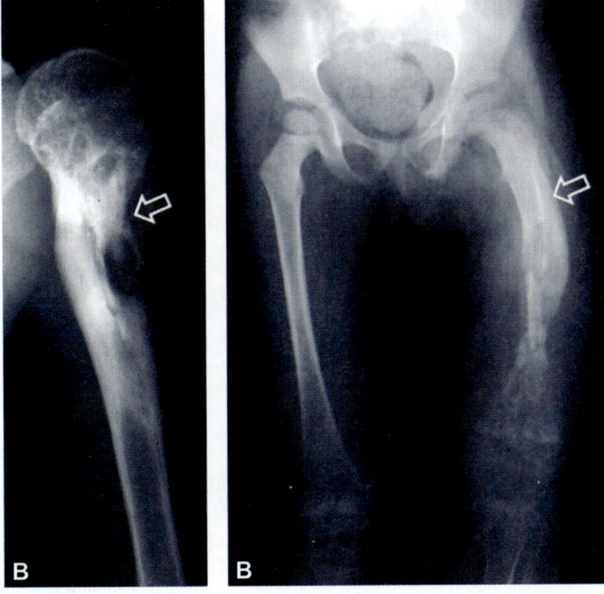

X-rays showing different sizes of sequestra in osteomyelitis.

Salmonella osteomyelitis occurs during the convalescent phase after an attack of typhoid fever. It is a subacute type of osteomyelitis, usually occurring in the ulna, tibia, or vertebra. Often, multiple bones are affected, sometimes bilaterally symmetrical. The disease occurs more commonly in children with sickle cell anemia.

33. **Which of the following set of muscles are commonly affected in De-Quervain's tenosynovitis?**
a. Adductor pollicis longus and flexor pollicis brevis
b. Adductor pollicis longus and extensor pollicis brevis
c. Abductor pollicis longus and flexor pollicis brevis
d. Abductor pollicis longus and extensor pollicis brevis

De-Quervain's tenosynovitis is a condition characterized by pain and swelling over the radial styloid process. It results from inflammation of the common sheath of abductor pollicis longus and extensor pollicis brevis tendons.

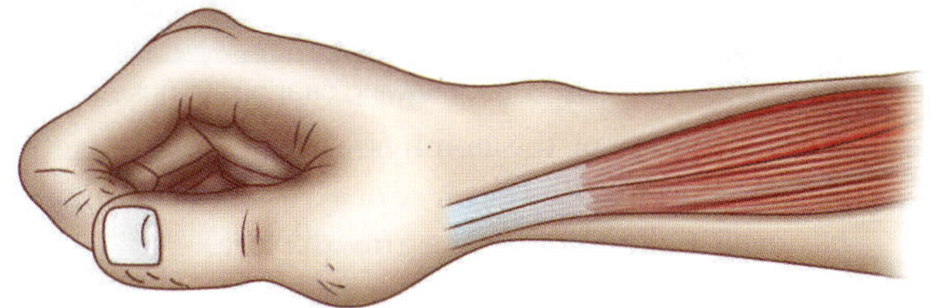

De-Quervain's tenosynovitis (affected tendon sheaths).

34. **Which of the following is NOT fused in triple arthrodesis in CTEV?**
a. Tibiotalar
b. Calcaneocuboid
c. Talonavicuar
d. Talocalcaneal

Triple arthrodesis (for CTEV) consists of the fusion of three joints of the foot (subtalar, calcaneocuboid and talonavicular), after taking suitable wedges to correct the deformity.

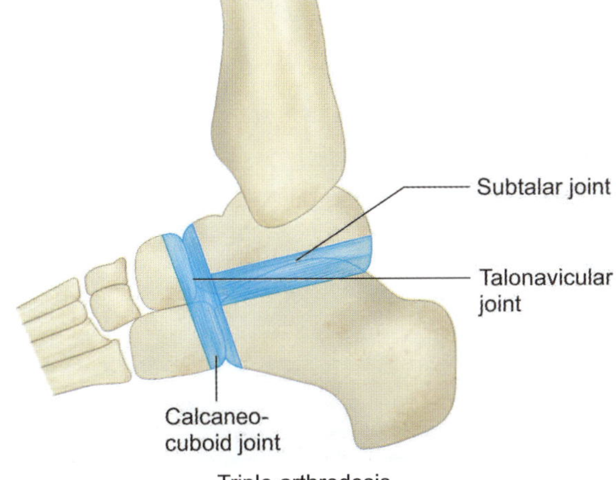

Triple arthrodesis.

Ans. 31. **b.** Metaphysis 32. **d.** Samonella 33. **d.** Abductor pollicis... 34. **a.** Tibiotalar
35. **a.** Rickets

35. Epiphyseal enlargement is a feature of:

a. Rickets
b. Ankylosing spondylitis
c. Spondyloepiphyseal dysgenesis
d. Scurvy

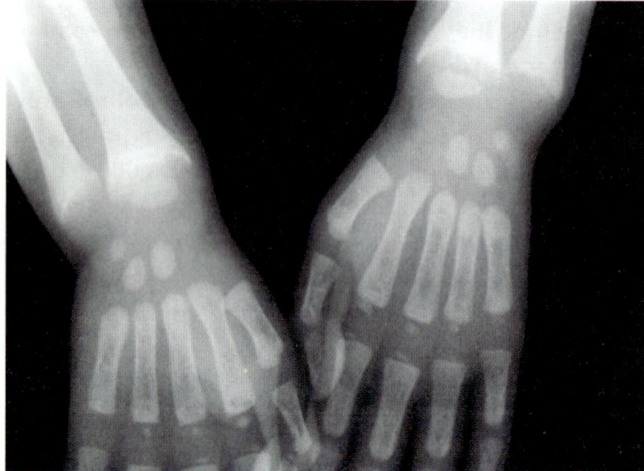

X-ray of the wrists, AP view, showing changes in rickets.

Normal width of the epiphyseal plate is 2–4 mm. In rickets, it is increased because of excessive accumulation of uncalcified osteoid at the growth plate.

36. Osteomalacia is:

a. Normal osteoid and defective mineralization
b. Abnormal osteoid and normal mineralization
c. Abnormal osteoid with abnormal mineralization
d. Abnormal bone deposition

Osteomalacia, which means softening of the bones, is the adult counterpart of rickets. It is primarily due to deficiency of vitamin D. This results in failure to replace the turnover of calcium and phosphorous in the organic matrix of bone. Hence, the bone content is demineralised and the bony substance is replaced by soft osteoid tissue.

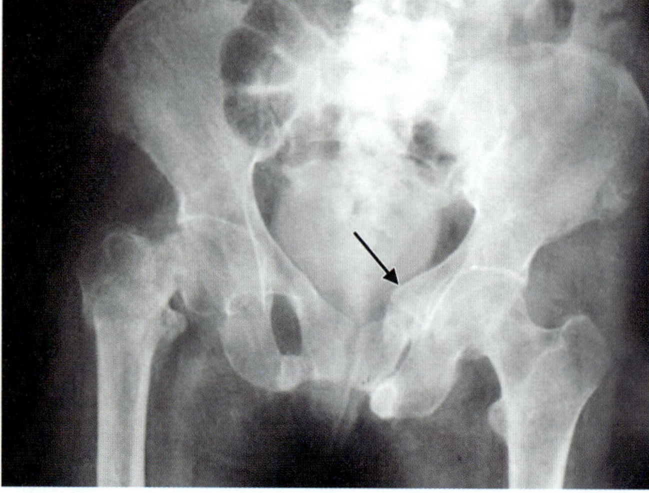

X-ray of pelvis showing 'loosers zones' on the pubic rami.

37. Primary osteoarthritis affects all EXCEPT:

a. Hip joint
b. Knee joint
c. Distal interphalangeal joint
d. Metacarpophalangeal joint

Primary osteoarthritis occurs in a joint de novo. It occurs in old age, mainly in the weight bearing joints (knee and hip). In a generalized variety, the trapeziometacarpal joint of the thumb and the distal inter-phalangeal joints of the fingers are also affected. Primary OA is commoner than secondary OA.

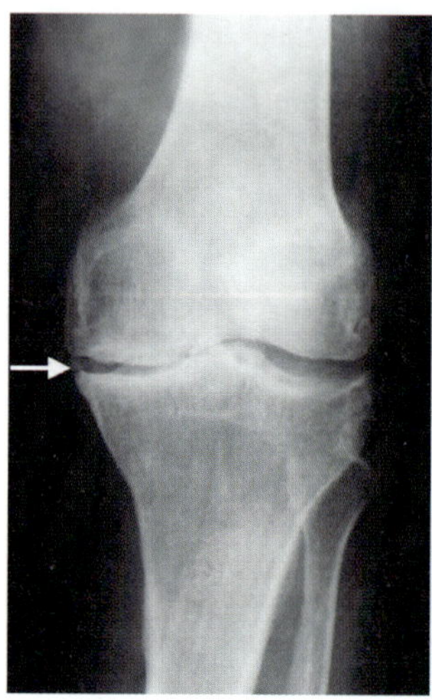

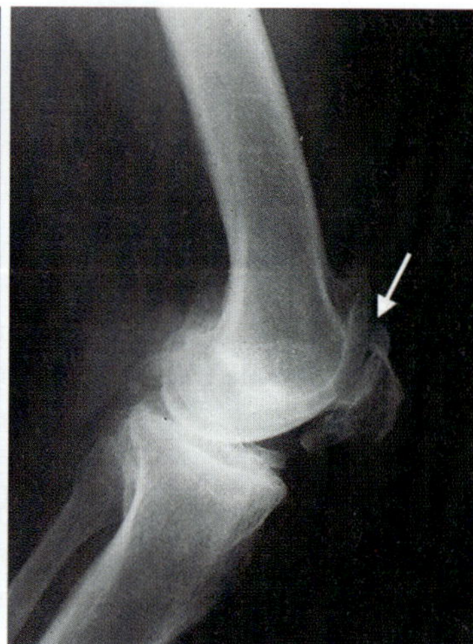

X-rays of the knee, AP and Lateral views, showing osteoarthritis of the knee (Note reduction in joint space on the medial side, osteophyte formation—arrow).

38. Pain and tenderness over the lateral condyle of humerus with painful dorsiflexion of the wrist is indicative of:

a. Golfer's elbow
b. Tennis elbow
c. Pitcher's elbow
d. Cricket elbow

Tennis elbow (lateral epicondylitis) is a condition characetrized by pain and tenderness at the lateral epicondyle of the humerus due to non-specific inflammation at the origin of the extensor muscles of the forearm.

39. True for Duchennes muscular dystrophy/DMD:

a. Autosomal recessive
b. Autosomal dominant
c. Muscle wasting disorder
d. Milder form

Muscular dystrophy comprises of a group of heterogenous disorders that share in common: (i) bilateral, usually symmerical, topographically patterned loss of strength and muscle wasting; (ii) progression over several years; and (iii) largely non-specific laboratory and histologic evidence of myofibril necrosis.

Ans. **36. a.** Normal osteoid... **37. d.** Metacarpoph... **38. b.** Tennis elbow **39. c.** Muscle wasting...

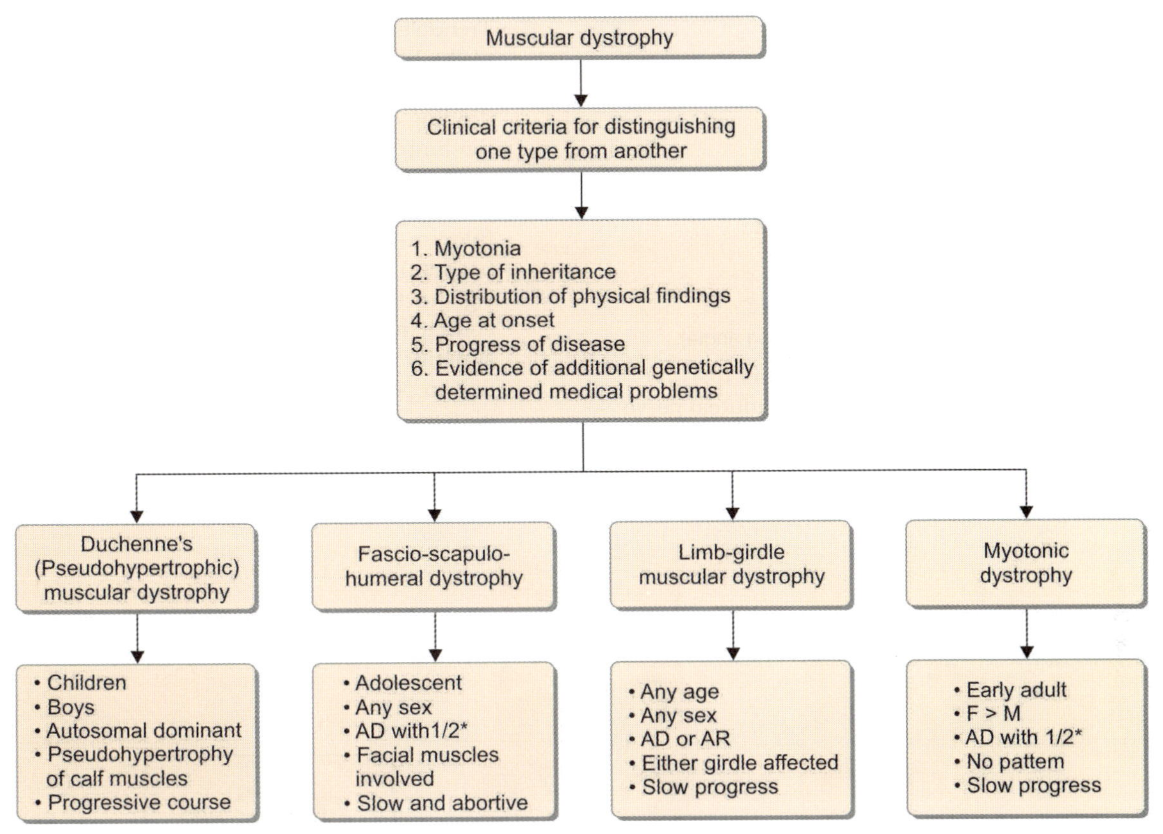

* Incomplete penetrance, AD – autosomal dominant AR – autosomal recessive

Muscular dystrophy—How to distinguish various types?

40. Tophi are seen in:

a. Gout
b. Pseudogout
c. Ankylosing spondylitis
d. Rheumatoid arthritis

Tophus is a deposit of crystalline uric acid and other substances at the surface of joints or in skin or cartilage, typically as a feature of gout.

Other rheumatological diseases.	
Gout	Disturbed purine metabolism leading to excessive accumulation of uric acid in the blood—an inherited disorder; or impaired excretion of uric acid by the kidneys. The result is accumulation of *sodium biurate* crystals in some soft tissues. Tissues of predilection are cartilage, tendon, bursa Patient, usually beyond 40 years of age, presents as (i) arthritis—MP joint of the big toe being a *favourite site*, onset is acute, pain is severe; (ii) bursitis—commonly of the olecranon bursa; or (iii) tophi formation deposit of uric acid salt in the soft tissue Confirmation of diagnosis—urate crystals

Contd...

Contd...

Other rheumatological diseases.	
	in the aspirate from a joint or bursa, high serum uric acid levels Treatment—NSAIDs, uricosuric drugs, uric acid inhibitors.
Pseudo-gout	*Sodium pyrophosphate* crystal deposition Symptoms like those of gout *Meniscus calcification* may be seen on X-rays of the knee Treatment—NSAIDs.

PERIPHERAL NERVE INJURIES

41. Tardy ulnar nerve palsy is seen with malunited:

a. Lateral humeral condyle fracture
b. Supracondylar fracture
c. Medial humeral condyle fracture
d. Fracture capitullum

Diminished growth at the lateral side of distal humerus epiphysis (because of fracture lateral humeral condyle) results in a cubitus valgus deformity. This may result in late ulnar nerve palsy (tardy ulnar nerve palsy) because of friction neuritis of the ulnar nerve as it moves over the medial epicondyle, everytime the elbow is flexed and extended.

Ans. 40. **a.** Gout 41. **a.** Lateral humeral

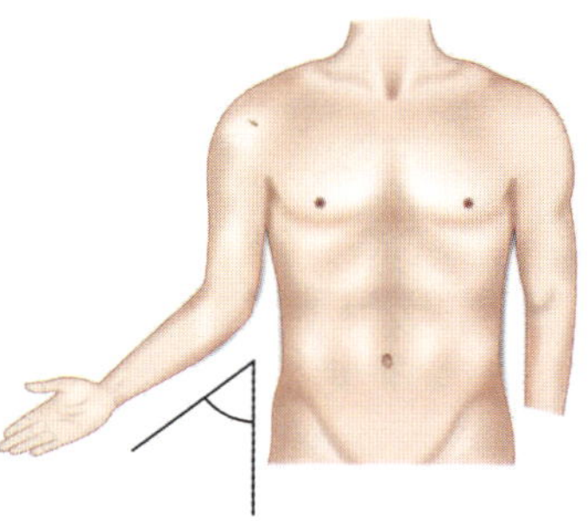

Cubitus valgus deformity (Increased carrying angle).

42. Trendelenburg's test is positive in injury to:

a. Superior gluteal nerve b. Inferior gluteal nerve
c. Pudendal nerve d. Obturator nerve

Trendelenburg's test is a test to establish the stability of the hip. A hip is stable if the abduction mechanism of the hip is effective in preventing the pelvis from dipping on the opposite side, when weight is borne on the limb. Any failure in the effectivity of the abductor mechanism causes dipping of the ASIS on the opposite (normal) side. This could occur if: (a) there is no fulcrum—e.g. dislocation of the hip, destruction of the head; (b) ineffective lever-arm (the neck of the femur)—e.g. fracture of the neck of the femur; (c) ineffective contraction of the abductor muscles (supplied by superior gluteal nerve)—e.g. weakness of the muscles due to polio or abductor muscles (gluteus medius and gluteus minimus) acting ineffectively through a short lever-arm (as in coxa vara).

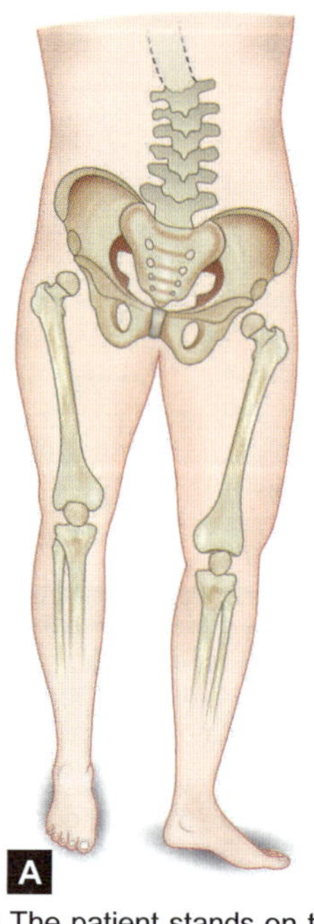

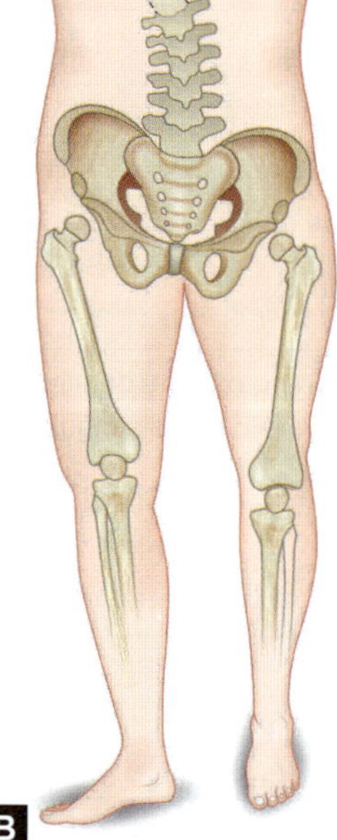

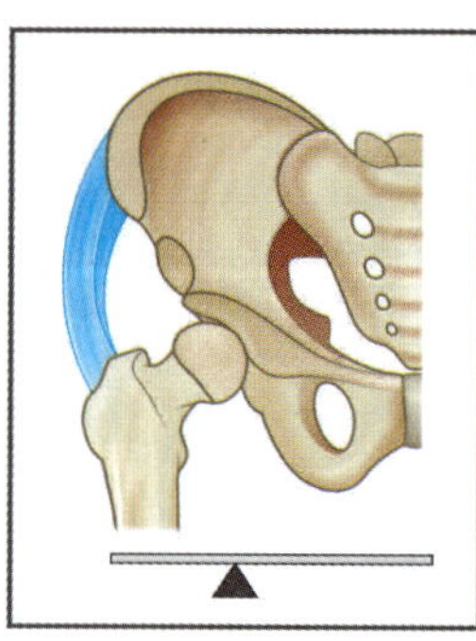

Trendelenburg's test. (A) The patient stands on the normal limb, the opposite ASIS goes up. (B) The patient stands on the affected limb, the opposite ASIS dips down. Box shows the abductor mechanism.

43. Ulnar nerve injury results in:

a. Ape thumb deformity
b. Wrist drop
c. Clawing of fingers
d. Pointing index

Claw hand (Main- en- griffe) means hyperextension at the metacarpophalangeal joints and flexion at the proximal and distal inter-phalangeal joints. This occurs due to the paralysis of the lumbricals, which flex the metacarpophalangeal joints and extend the inter-phalangeal joints.

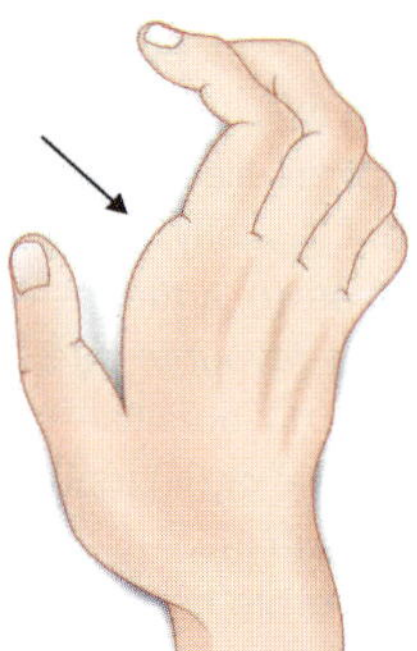

Claw hand (hyperextension at the MP joint).

Ans. **42. a.** Superior gluteal... **43. c.** Clawing of fingers

44. Fractures of fibular neck may involve:

a. Tibial nerve
b. Sciatic nerve
c. Common peroneal nerve
d. Sural nerve

The foot remains in plantar flexion due to weakness of the dorsiflexors. It occurs in common peroneal nerve palsy. Common peroneal nerve is commonly involved in fractures of fibular neck.

Nerve injuries and skeletal trauma.

Nerve	Trauma	Effect
Axillary nerve	Dislocation of the shoulder	Deltoid paralysis
Radial nerve	Fracture shaft of the humerus	Wrist drop
Median nerve	Supracondylar fracture of humerus	Pointing index
Ulnar nerve	Fracture medial epicondyle humerus	Claw hand
Sciatic nerve	Posterior dislocation of the hip	Foot drop due to weakness of dorsiflexors of the foot
Common peroneal nerve	Knee dislocation Fracture of neck of the fibula	Foot drop

45. Cock-up splint is used in injuries of:

a. Ulnar nerve
b. Radial nerve
c. Axillary nerve
d. Common peroneal nerve

The first procedure to be adopted in every case of nerve injury is to splint the limb in the position which will most effectively relax the affected muscles.

Common splints/braces and their uses.

Name	Use
Cramer-wire splint	Emergency immobilisation
Thomas splint	Fracture femur-anywhere
Bohler-Braun splint	Fracture femur-anywhere
Aluminium splint	Immobilisation of fingers
Dennis Brown splint	CTEV
Cock-up splint	Radial nerve palsy
Knuckle–bender splint	Ulnar nerve palsy
Toe-raising splint	Foot drop
Volkmann's splint	Volkmann's ischaemic contracture (VIC)
Four-post collar	Neck immobilisation
Aeroplane splint	Brachial plexus injury
SOMI brace	Cervical spine injury
ASHE (Anterior spinal hyper extension) brace	Dorso-lumbar spinal injury
Taylor's brace	Dorso-lumbar immobilisation
Milwaukee brace	Scoliosis
Boston brace	Scoliosis
Lumbar corset	Backache

ORTHOPEDIC ONCOLOGY

46. Fallen fragment sign is a radiological feature of:

a. Ewing's sarcoma
b. Simple bone cyst
c. Giant cell tumour
d. Aneurysmal bone cyst

The *fallen fragment sign* refers to the presence of a bone fracture fragment resting dependently in a cystic bone lesion. This finding is said to be pathognomonic for a simple (unicameral) bone cyst following a pathological fracture.

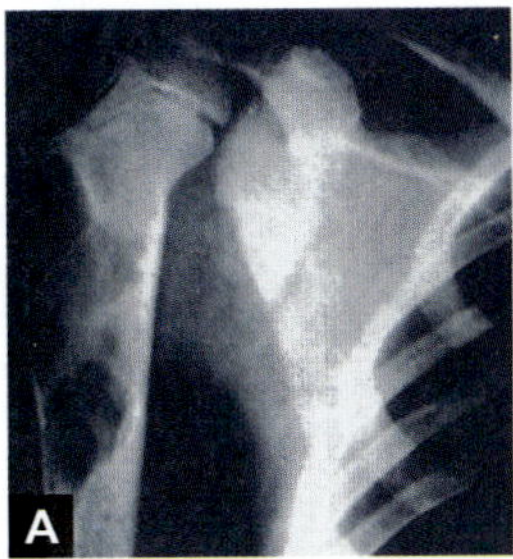

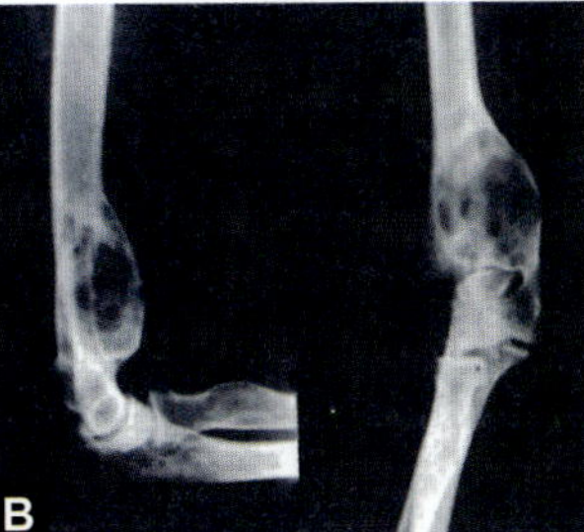

Simple bone cyst　Aneurysmal bone cyst
X-rays showing bone cysts

47. A 15-year-old boy presented with mass in the distal femur. X-ray from the lesion showed features of codman's triangle and sunray appearance. The diagnosis is:

a. Osteosarcoma
b. Ewing's sarcoma
c. Osteoclastoma
d. Chondroblastoma

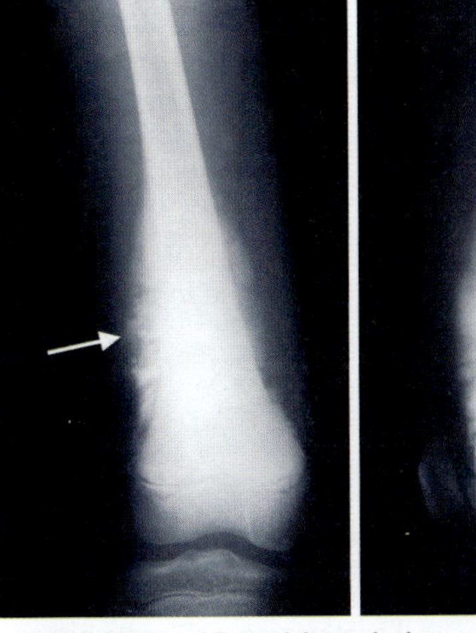

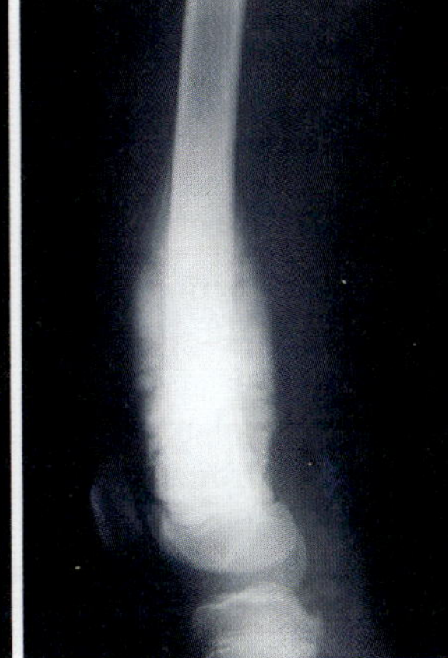

X-ray of the femur, AP and lateral views showing osteosarcoma of lower end of the femur (Note the metaphyseal origin and lot of new bone formation).

Ans. 44. c. Common... 45. b. Radial nerve 46. b. Simple bone cyst 47. a. Osteosarcoma

Radiological examination in osteosarcoma

- An area of irregular destruction in the metaphysis, sometimes overshadowed by the new bone formation
- Periosteal reaction
- Codman's triangle
- Sun-ray appearance

48. Radioresistant tumour:

a. Ewing's sarcoma b. Retinoblastoma
c. Osteosarcoma d. Neuroblastoma

Treatment of osteosarcoma include local control of the tumour (by surgical ablation/amputation) or control of distant macro or micro-metastasis (done by adjuvant chemotherapy, immunotherapy etc.).

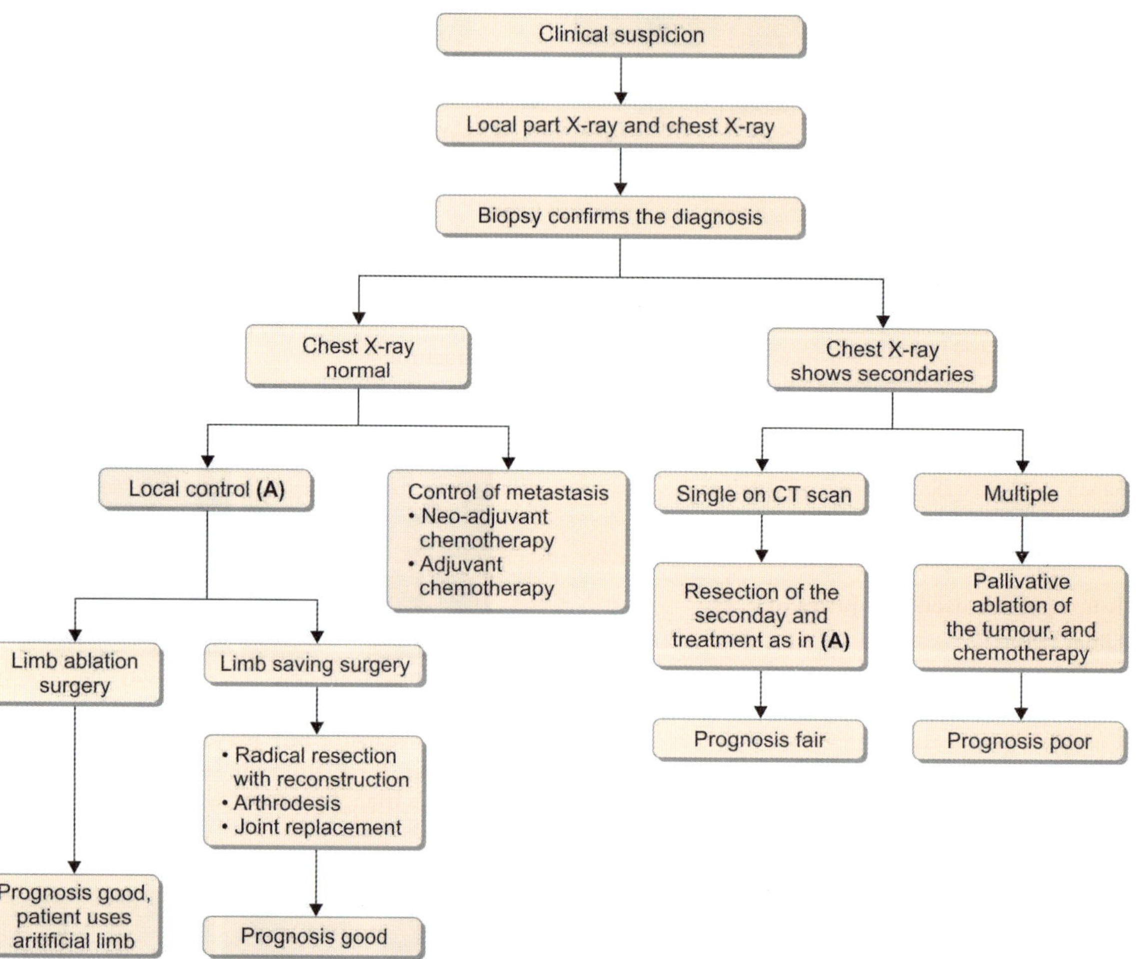

Treatment plan for osteosarcoma.

49. All are the predisposing factors of osteogenic sarcoma EXCEPT:

a. Paget's disease of bone b. Radiation
c. Viral infection d. Bone infarction

Premalignant bone lesions

- Paget's disease
- Diaphysial achalasia
- Enchondromatosis
- Post-radiation

Types of lesions radiographically.

Type of lesion	*Aggression*	*Examples*
Geographic lesion: well-defined lesion	Least aggressive	Simple bone cyst
Moth eaten: Less well-defined with a moth eaten appearance	More aggressive	Low grade osteosarcoma, Giant cell tumour
Permeative lesion: least defined	Most aggressive	Telengiectatic osteosarcoma

50. All of the following are true about exostosis EXCEPT:

a. It occurs at the growing end of bone
b. Growth continues after skeletal maturity
c. It is covered by cartilaginous cap
d. Malignant transformation may occur

Ans. 48. c. Osteosarcoma 49. c. Viral infection 50. b. Growth continues...

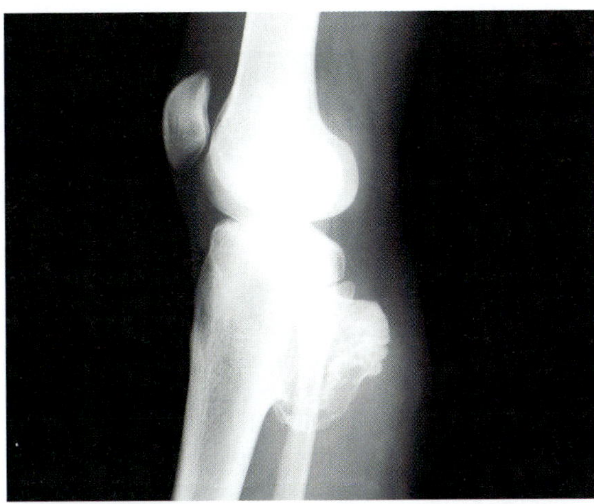
X-ray of knee, lateral view, showing osteochondroma from upper end of tibia.

Osteochondroma (exostosis) is the commonest benign "tumour" of the bone. It is not a true neoplasm since its growth stops with cessation of growth at the epiphyseal plate. A rapid increase in the size of the tumour, if it continues to grow beyond the period of epiphyseal plate fusion or appearance of pain in a hitherto painless swelling may be suggestive of malignant transformation.

51. MC bony tumour:

a. Metastasis
b. Osteosarcoma
c. Ewing's sarcoma
d. Osteoclastoma

Metastatic tumours in the bone are commoner than the primary bone tumours. The tumours most commonly metastasizing to bone are carcinoma of the lung in the male and carcinoma of the breast in the female.

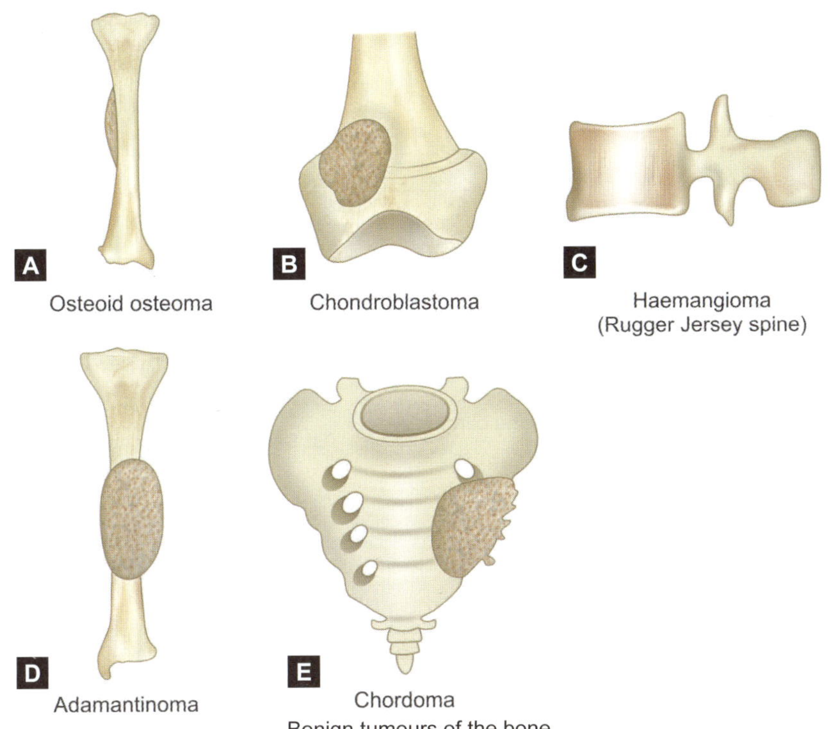

Benign tumours of the bone.

52. Soap bubble appearance is seen in:

a. Multiple myeloma
b. Giant cell tumour
c. Fibrous dysplasia
d. Osteoid osteoma

Soap bubble appearance is a radiological feature of giant cell tumour, where the tumour is homogenously lytic with trabeculae of the remnants of bone traversing it, giving rise to a loculated appearance.

Differential diagnosis of a solitary bone lesion.

Features	*Giant cell tumour*	*Simple bone cyst*	*Aneurysmal bone cyst*	*Fibrous dysplasia*
Age	20–40 yrs.	< 20 yrs.	10–40 yrs.	20–30 yrs.
Common bones	Lower femur, Upper tibia Lower radius	Upper humerus Upper femur	Tibia Humerus	Neck of the femur Tibia
Location	Epiphysis	Metaphysis	Metaphysis	Metaphysis

Contd...

Ans. **51. a.** Metastasis **52. b.** Giant cell tumour

Contd...

Features	Giant cell tumour	Simple bone cyst	Aneurysmal bone cyst	Fibrous dysplasia
X-ray	Soap-bubble appearance, eccentrically placed	Maximum width less than width of the growth plate	Distending lesion, 'ballooning' the bone	Multi-loculated Ground-glass appearance Trabeculations++
Treatment preferred	Excision	Curettage and bone graft	Curettage and bone graft	Curettage and bone graft

MISCELLANEOUS

53. Investigation of choice in traumatic paraplegia:

a. MRI
b. CT scan
c. Myelography
d. Spine X-ray

CT and MRI scan may be indicated in cases of traumatic paraplegia with incomplete paralysis, particularly if it is increasing. It is also indicated in cases where no bony lesions are visible on plain X-rays. MRI has become the imaging modality of choice for these cases.

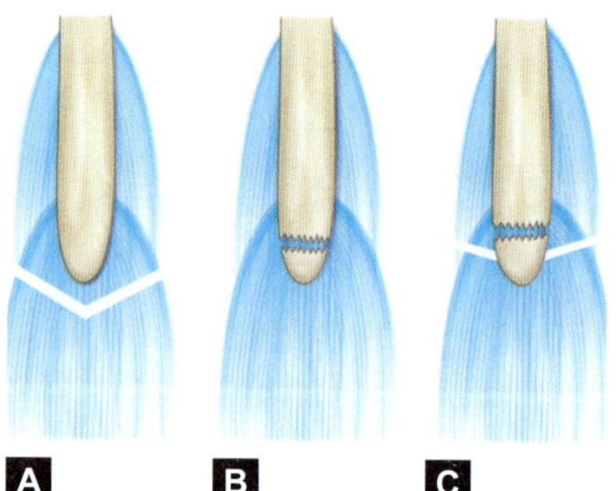

Pathology of neural injury. (A) Only roots affected, (B) Only the cord affected, (C) Roots + cord affected.

54. Deposition of homogentisic acid in joints is seen in:

a. Psoriasis
b. Haemophilia
c. Charcot's joint
d. Ochronosis

Ochronosis is the syndrome caused by the accumulation of homogentisic acid in connective tissues. The condition was named after the yellowish (ocher-like) discoloration of the tissue seen on microscopic examination.

Types of arthritis.
Monoarthritis
❑ Pyogenic arthritis
❑ Tubercular arthritis
❑ Haemophilic arthritis
❑ Secondary osteoarthritis
❑ Gout—sometimes
Polyarthritis
❑ Rheumatoid arthritis
❑ Rheumatic fever
❑ Juvenile chronic polyarthritis
❑ Primary osteoarthritis
❑ Seronegative spondarthritis

Ans. **53. a.** MRI **54. d.** Ochronosis

ANSWERS WITH REFERENCES

ORTHOPEDIC TRAUMA

1. **Ans. (d)** Blackening of patient's toes
   Ref: Maheshwari's Orthopedics, 5/e p44

2. **Ans. (c)** Lower end of radius, lunate are in alignment but rest of carpals is out of plane
   Ref: Maheshwari's Orthopedics, 5/e p116

3. **Ans. (a)** Missed epiphyseal injury
   Ref: Maheshwari's Orthopedics, 5/e p58

4. **Ans. (c)** 10
   Ref: Maheshwari's Orthopedics, 5/e p113

5. **Ans. (c)** Battered baby syndrome
   Ref: Internet resources

6. **Ans. (a)** Its fixity to tibial collateral ligament
   Ref: Maheshwari's Orthopedics 5/e p151

7. **Ans. (c)** Malunion
   Ref: Maheshwari's Orthopedics 5/e p138

8. **Ans. (d)** Stress fracture
   Ref: Maheshwari's Orthopedics 5/e p2

9. **Ans. (b)** Tibial epiphyseal plate injury
   Ref: Maheshwari's Orthopedics 5/e p58

10. **Ans. (a)** C1
    Ref: Maheshwari's Orthopedics 5/e p3

11. **Ans. (b)** Non-union
    Ref: Maheshwari's Orthopedics 5/e p112

12. **Ans. (d)** Immobilization
    Ref: Maheshwari's Orthopedics 5/e p52

13. **Ans. (d)** Supracondylar fracture of humerus
    Ref: Maheshwari's Orthopedics 5/e p96

14. **Ans. (a)** Shoulder
    Ref: Maheshwari's Orthopedics 5/e p91

15. **Ans. (d)** Apprehension test
    Ref: Maheshwari's Orthopedics 5/e p90

16. **Ans. (a)** Posterior dislocation of shoulder
    Ref: Maheshwari's Orthopedics 5/e p89

17. **Ans. (a)** Rupture of flexor pollicis longus tendon
    Ref: Maheshwari's Orthopedics 5/e p112

18. **Ans. (b)** Posterior dislocation of hip joint
    Ref: Maheshwari's Orthopedics 5/e p131

19. **Ans. (a)** Ankle
    Ref: Maheshwari's Orthopedics 5/e p162

20. **Ans. (a)** Metacarpal
    Ref: Maheshwari's Orthopedics 5/e p118

21. **Ans. (d)** Cervical spine
    Ref: Maheshwari's Orthopedics 5/e p265

INFLAMMATIONS OF MUSCULOSKELETAL SYSTEM

22. **Ans. (c)** Septic arthritis of infancy
    Ref: Maheshwari's Orthopedics, 5/e p177

23. **Ans. (b)** Distal interphalangeal joints is most commonly affected
    Ref: Maheshwari's Orthopedics, 5/e p287

24. **Ans. (b)** Bony ankylosis
    Ref: Maheshwari's Orthopedics 5/e p183

25. **Ans. (c)** Myositis ossificans
    Ref: Maheshwari's Orthopedics 5/e p172

26. **Ans. (c)** Periosteal reaction is characteristic
    Ref: Maheshwari's Orthopedics 5/e p170

27. **Ans. (b)** Synovium
    Ref: Maheshwari's Orthopedics 5/e p288

28. **Ans. (b)** Anklyosing spondylitis
    Ref: Maheshwari's Orthopedics 5/e p292

29. **Ans. (a)** Tubercular dactylitis
    Ref: Maheshwari's Orthopedics 5/e p182

30. **Ans. (a)** Tuberculosis
    Ref: Maheshwari's Orthopedics 5/e p201

31. **Ans. (b)** Metaphysis
    Ref: Maheshwari's Orthopedics 5/e p168

OTHER NON-TRAUMATIC CONDITIONS

32. **Ans. (d)** Samonella
    Ref: Maheshwari's Orthopedics, 5/e p169

33. **Ans. (d)** Abductor pollicis longus and extensor pollicis brevis
    Ref: Maheshwari's Orthopedics, 5/e p303

34. **Ans. (a) Tibiotalar**
Ref: Maheshwari's Orthopedics 5/e p216

35. **Ans. (a) Rickets**
Ref: Maheshwari's Orthopedics 5/e p311

36. **Ans. (a) Normal osteoid and defective mineralization**
Ref: Maheshwari's Orthopedics 5/e p312

37. **Ans. (d) Metacarpophalangeal joint**
Ref: Maheshwari's Orthopedics 5/e p296

38. **Ans. (b) Tennis elbow**
Ref: Maheshwari's Orthopedics 5/e p302

39. **Ans. (c) Muscle wasting disorder**
Ref: Maheshwari's Orthopedics 5/e p233

40. **Ans. (a) Gout**
Ref: Maheshwari's Orthopedics 5/e p293

PERIPHERAL NERVE INJURIES

41. **Ans. (a) Lateral humeral condyle fracture**
Ref: Maheshwari's Orthopedics 5/e p104

42. **Ans. (a) Superior gluteal nerve**
Ref: Maheshwari's Orthopedics 5/e p348

43. **Ans. (c) Clawing of fingers**
Ref: Maheshwari's Orthopedics 5/e p64

44. **Ans. (c) Common peroneal nerve**
Ref: Maheshwari's Orthopedics 5/e p46

45. **Ans. (b) Radial nerve**
Ref: Maheshwari's Orthopedics 5/e p25

ORTHOPEDIC ONCOLOGY

46. **Ans. (b) Simple bone cyst**
Ref: Maheshwari's Orthopedics, 5/e p249

47. **Ans. (a) Osteosarcoma**
Ref: Maheshwari's Orthopedics 5/e p240

48. **Ans. (c) Osteosarcoma**
Ref: Maheshwari's Orthopedics 5/e p242

49. **Ans. (c) Viral infection**
Ref: Maheshwari's Orthopedics 5/e p235

50. **Ans. (b) Growth continues after skeletal maturity**
Ref: Maheshwari's Orthopedics, 5/e p248

51. **Ans. (a) Metastasis**
Ref: Maheshwari's Orthopedics 5/e p236

52. **Ans. (b) Giant cell tumour**
Ref: Maheshwari's Orthopedics 5/e p237

MISCELLANEOUS

53. **Ans. (a) MRI**
Ref: Maheshwari's Orthopedics 5/e p276

54. **Ans. (d) Ochronosis**
Ref: Maheshwari's Orthopedics 5/e p286

PRACTICE QUESTIONS

TRAUMA

1. Thurstons Holland sign is a feature of Salter Harris type:

a. I b. II
c. III d. IV

2. Hill-Sachs lesion is observed in:

a. Glenoidal labrum tears
b. Posterior dislocation of shoulder joint
c. Recurrent anterior dislocation of shoulder joint
d. Posterolateral surface of humeral shaft

3. Comminuted fracture is caused by which type of injuries?

a. Bending force
b. Tapping force
c. Compressing force
d. Twisting force

INFLAMMATIONS

4. Inflammatory arthritis is characterized by:

a. Fever
b. Morning stiffness
c. Swelling
d. Inability to move

5. Triple deformity of the knee includes:

a. Extension, anterior subluxation and internal rotation of tibia
b. Flexion, posterior subluxation and internal rotation of tibia
c. Flexion, posterior subluxation and external rotation of tibia
d. Extension, posterior subluxation and external rotation of tibia

OTHER NON-TRAUMATIC CONDITIONS

6. Brittle bone disease is another name for:

a. Osteoporosis
b. Osteopetrosis
c. Osteogenesis imperfecta
d. Paget's disease

7. MC site of gout:

a. Great toe
b. Small toe
c. Thumb
d. Little finger

PERIPHERAL NERVE INJURIES

8. A highly drunk adult male slept on the chair with arm hanging by the side of arm rest. Next morning he realized that he is NOT able to dorsiflex the wrist. Physician diagnosed him as a case of Saturday night palsy. What kind of nerve injury is this:

a. Neuropraxia b. Axonotmesis
c. Neurotmesis d. None of the above

ONCOLOGY

9. Age group affected in Ewing's sarcoma:

a. 0–5 years b. 5–20 years
c. 20–30 years d. >30 years

MISCELLANEOUS

10. Splaying of metaphysis is seen in:

a. Scurvy b. Rickets
c. Cretinism d. Down syndrome

Practice Questions

Ans. 1. **b.** II 2. **c.** Recurrent anterior... 3. **c.** Compressing force 4. **b.** Morning stiffness
5. **c.** Flexion, posterior... 6. **b.** Osteopetrosis and **c.** Osteogenesis imperfecta 7. **a.** Great toe
8. **a.** Neuropraxia 9. **b.** 5–20 years 10. **b.** Rickets

IMAGE-BASED QUESTIONS

1. **Age group commonly affected in the condition shown below:**

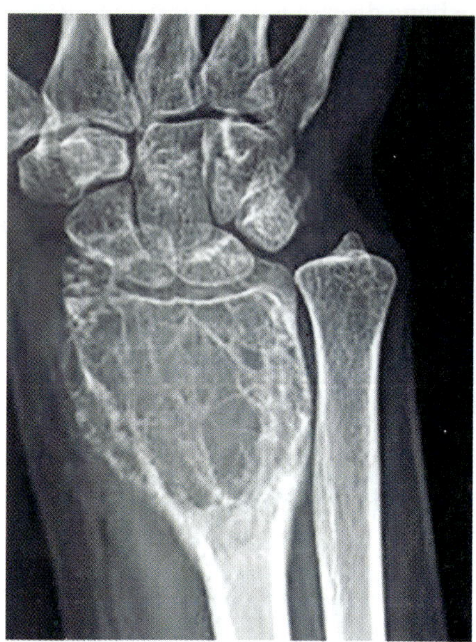

Giant cell tumour is commonly seen in 20-40 years of age.

a. 10–20 years b. 20–40 years
c. 40–60 years d. 60–80 years

2. **Radiological feature shown in the image below:**

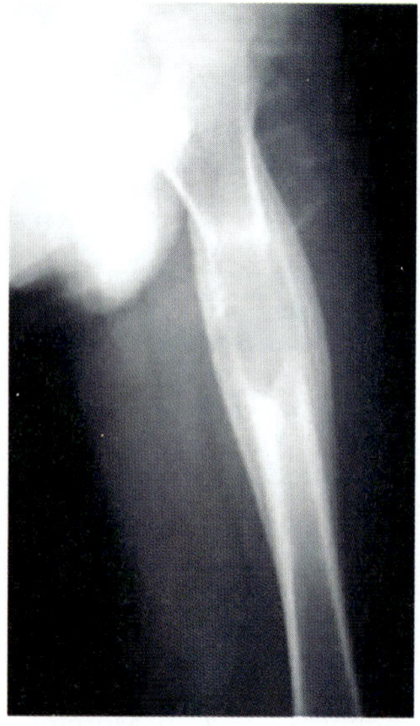

a. Soap bubble appearance
b. Codman's triangle
c. Onion peel appearance
d. Sun-ray appearance

In a typical case of Ewing's sarcoma, there is a lytic lesion in the medullary zone of the midshaft of a long bone, with cortical destruction and new bone formation in layers—onion peel appearance.

3. **Management of the fracture shown below:**

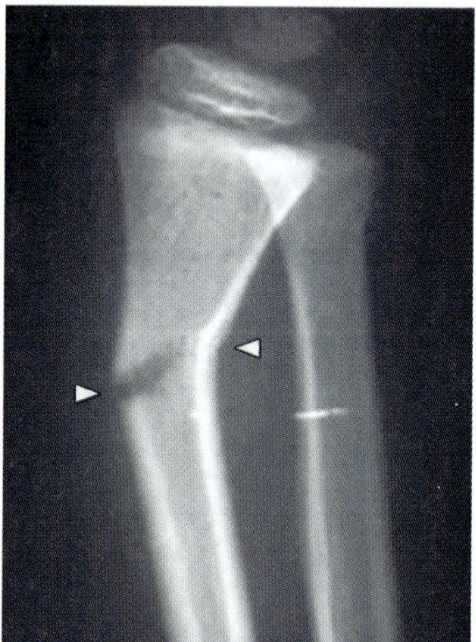

a. Closed reduction b. Open reduction
c. Internal fixation d. Observation

Greenstick fractures are managed by closed reduction by manipulation under general anaesthesia, and immobilisation in an above-elbow plaster cast.

4. **Management of the fracture shown below:**

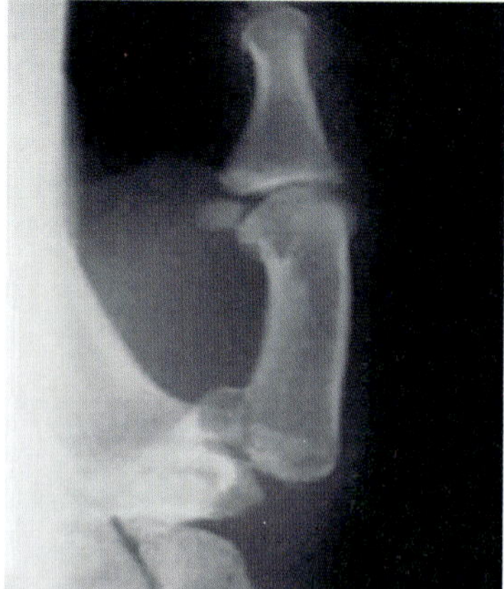

a. Closed reduction and cast
b. Closed reduction and fixation
c. Observation
d. Excision of trapezium

Bennet's fracture-dislocation needs accurate reduction and restoration of the smooth joint surface. This is because, being an intra-articular fracture, if not reduced accurately, it will lead to incongruity of the articular surfaces.This would increase the chances of developing osteoarthritis. This can be done by closed reduction/ open reduction with K-wire fixation.

5. Such splint is used in which nerve injury?

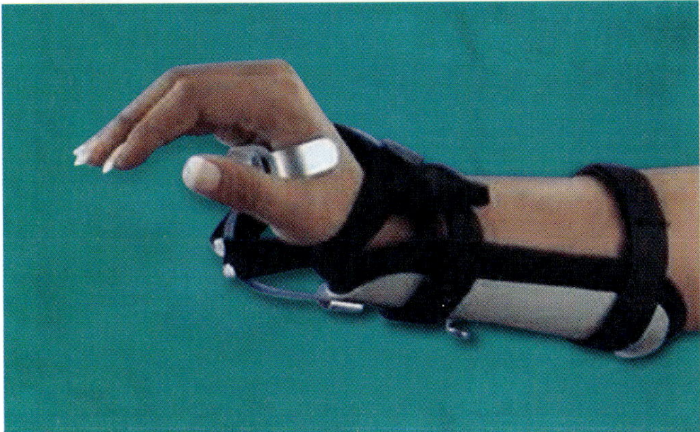

a. Ulnar nerve
b. Median nerve
c. Radial nerve
d. Axillary nerve

Cock-up splint is used for radial nerve palsy.

6. Splint shown is used for which condition?

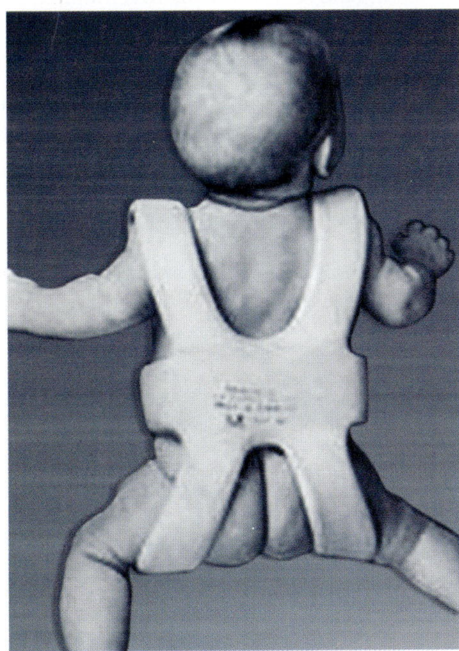

a. Fracture neck of femur
b. Developmental dysplasia of hip
c. Perthes disease
d. Coxa vara

While managing DDH, once the hip has been reduced by closed or open methods, Von Rosen's splint is used for maintaining the head of femur inside the acetabulum. It can be removed once the acetabulum develops to a round shape.

7. Which nerve palsy can result in this kind of appearance?

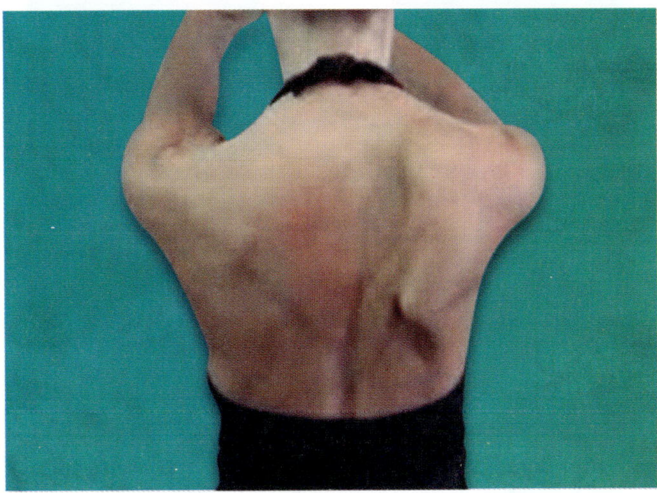

a. Long thoracic nerve
b. Thoracodorsal nerve
c. Suprascapular nerve
d. Subscapular nerve

The serratus anterior muscle can be examined by asking the patient to push against a wall with both hands. The medial border of the scapula on the affected side will become prominent (winging of scapula). Serratus anterior muscle is supplied by long thoracic nerve.

8. Which nerve is injured?

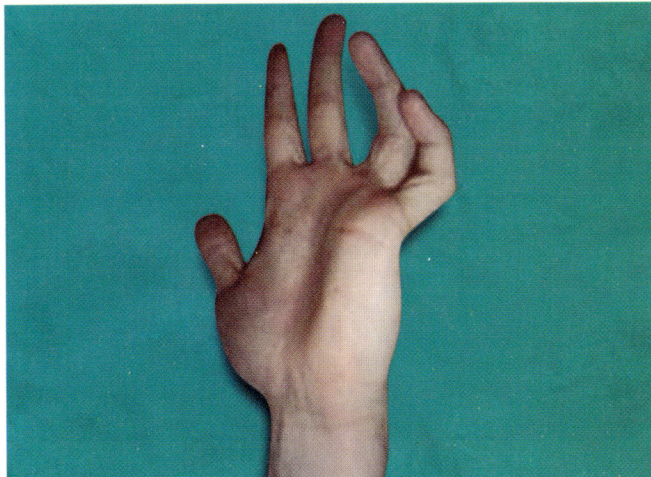

a. Radial nerve
b. Median nerve
c. Ulnar nerve
d. Ulnar + median nerve

In ulnar nerve palsy, only the medial two fingers develop clawing while all the four finger develop clawing in combined median and ulnar nerve palsies. Clawing may not become apparent in the early post-injury period.

9. Which nerve is injured?

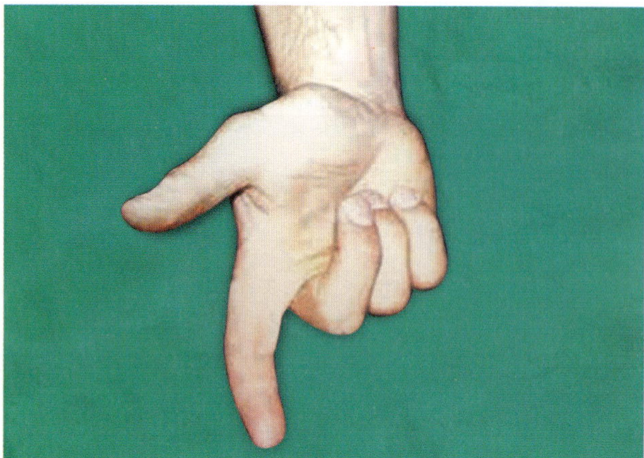

a. Median nerve
b. Ulnar nerve
c. Radial nerve
d. Axillary nerve

On asking the patient to make a fist, it is noticed that the index finger remains straight (pointing index). This is due to paralysis of both the flexors (digitorum superficialis and lateral half of the digitorum profundus) of the index finger, which occurs in median nerve palsy at the level proximal to the elbow. The other fingers can be flexed by functioning medial side of the flexor digitorum profundus, supplied by the ulnar nerve.

10. X-ray is suggestive of:

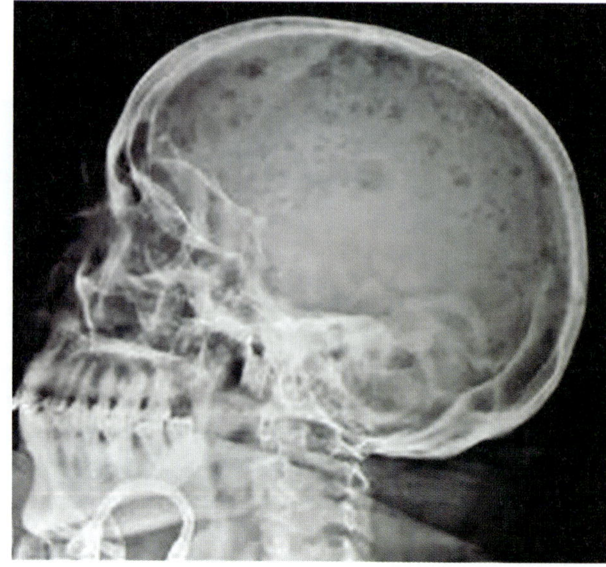

a. Thalassemia
b. Sickle cell anemia
c. Multiple myeloma
d. Secondaries

Multiple punched out lesions in the skull and other flat bones is suggestive of multiple myeloma.

MCQ POINTS

S. No.	Question statements	Answers
1.	IOC for traumatic paraplegia	MRI
2.	Tardy ulnar nerve palsy is seen with	Fracture lateral humeral condyle
3.	Gun stock deformity is seen with	Malunited supracondylar fracture humerus
4.	Bamboo spine is radiological sign of	Ankylosing spondylitis
5.	Splaying and widening of metaphysis is radiological sign of	Rickets
6.	Galeazzi fracture involves...bone	Distal radius
7.	MC complication of fracture neck of femur	Non-union
8.	Carpal tunnel syndrome is due to compression of…nerve	Median nerve
9.	Nerve injured in shoulder dislocation	Axillary nerve
10.	Wrist drop is seen in lesion of...nerve	Radial nerve
11.	Foot drop may be a manifestation of fracture...	Neck of fibula
12.	Ewing's sarcoma involves...part of bone	Diaphysis
13.	MC cause of acute osteomyelitis	Staph aureus
14.	MC symptom of TB spine	Backache
15.	Radiological features of osteosarcoma	Sunray appearance and Codman triangle
16.	Cock up splint is used for…nerve injury	Radial nerve
17.	Hanging cast is used for fractures of…	Shaft of humerus
18.	Winging of scapula is due to involvement of …nerve	Long thoracic nerve
19.	Punched out lytic lesion is radiological feature of	Multiple myeloma
20.	Barlow test is done for	Developmental dysplasia of hip
21.	Fracture radial styloid process is known as	Chauffeur's fracture
22.	Milwaukee brace is used for	Scoliosis
23.	Looser's zone is a radiological feature of	Osteomalacia
24.	Dead piece of bone lying in infected granulation tissue is known as	Sequestrum
25.	Prepatellar bursitis is known as	Housemaid's knee
26.	MC bone to be involved in Pott's disease:	Vertebrae
27.	House maid's knee is due to inflammation of ... bursa:	Prepatellar bursa
28.	Nerve likely to be injured in fracture shaft of humerus	Radial nerve
29.	Swan neck and Z-deformity of fingers is seen in which ... arthritis	Rheumatoid
30.	MC extra-articular manifestation of Ankylosing spondylitis:	Anterior uveitis
31.	Forward slipping of one vertebrae over other is known as:	Spondylolisthesis
32.	Heterotopic bone formation in a muscle belly is known as:	Myositis ossificans
33.	Nerve injured in anterior dislocation of shoulder:	Axillary nerve
34.	Tenderness in anatomical snuff box suggests fracture of:	Scaphoid
35.	Recurrent dislocation of patella occurs commonly on which side:	Lateral
36.	Example of atavistic epiphyses	Coracoid process
37.	Cubital tunnel syndrome is due to compression of which nerve:	Ulnar nerve
38.	Tumour that usually stops growing in size with physeal closure:	Exostosis/osteochondroma
39.	MC bone sarcoma in children:	Ewing's sarcoma
40.	Nerve MC injured in maxillary fractures:	Infraorbital nerve
41.	HLA antigen linked to anterior uveitis:	HLA B27

S. No.	Question statements	Answers
42.	Tension band wiring is best done for fractures of:	Olecranon and patella
43.	MC fractured bone of face:	Nasal
44.	Tarsal tunnel syndrome is due to compression of which nerve:	Posterior tibial nerve
45.	Which type of infection usually results in bony ankylosis:	TB of spine and pyogenic infection
46.	LeFort classification is used for fractures of which bone:	Maxilla
47.	Potts puffy tumour is also known as:	Chronic frontal osteomyelitis
48.	Tinel sign suggests ... of nerve:	Regeneration
49.	Around elbow, which epiphyses ossifies first:	Capitellum
50.	Hill-Sach lesion is seen in recurrent dislocation of which joint:	Shoulder
51.	A young male presented with joint pain and backache. X-ray of the spine shows evidence of sacroiliatis. Diagnosis:	Ankylosing spondylitis
52.	Most characteristically involved joint in Rheumatoid arthritis:	Metacarpophalngeal joint
53.	MC cause of multiple fractures in childhood:	Osteogenesis imperfecta
54.	Pointing index is due to injury to which nerve:	Median nerve
55.	Fracture upper third ulna with dislocation of superior radioulnar joint is known as ... fracture dislocation:	Monteggia fracture dislocation
56.	Flexion, adduction and internal rotation of lower limb suggests the diagnosis of:	Posterior dislocation of hip
57.	Boxers muscle is:	Serratus anterior
58.	Sun-ray appearance is suggestive of which bony tumour:	Osteosarcoma
59.	Subperiosteal resorptions are seen in which metabolic disorder:	Hyperparathyroidism
60.	MC organism responsible for acute osteomyelitis in sickle cell anemia:	Salmonella
61.	Bautonniere's deformity is seen in:	Rheumatoid arthritis
62.	'Pseudo-fractures' are suggestive of:	Osteomalacia
63.	TB spine is also known as:	Pott's disease
64.	Spindle shaped expansion of the bone in TB dactylitis is known as:	Spina ventosa
65.	Kienbock's disease is avascular necrosis of:	Lunate
66.	Nerve damaged in fracture supracondylar humerus:	Median nerve (anterior interosseous branch)
67.	Claw hand is a manifestation of:	Ulnar nerve (+ median nerve in complete clawing)
68.	Blow-out injuries with ptosis are characteristic of:	Orbit
69.	Sausage digits are seen in:	Psoriasis
70.	Ape thumb deformity is seen in:	Median nerve
71.	Fracture neck of femur in an elderly is managed by:	Hemireplacement arthroplasty
72.	MC joint to dislocate in human body:	Shoulder
73.	Part of a long bone commonly affected in acute osteomyelitis:	Metaphysis
74.	Example of pressure epiphyses:	Femoral head
75.	MC type of TB spine	Paradiscal

CHAPTER 6

PEDIATRICS

KEY POINTS

Weight

- Average birth weight: 3 kg
- Newborn gains weight at the rate of 25 grams per day for the first 3 months
- Doubling of weight occurs at 5 months
- Tripling by 1 year
- Quadruples by 2 years.

Height

- Average newborn length: 50 cm
- Increases by 25 cm in first year
- Then by 12.5 cm in second year
- Then 6 cm in third year
- Child is 100 cm tall at end of fourth year.

Head Circumference

- Head circumference at birth is 35 cm
- Circumference of chest is 3 cm less than head circumference at birth
- Equals head circumference by 1 year of age.

Other Parameters

- At birth the upper segment is to lower segment ratio is 1.7
- Normal temperature of neonate is 36.5–37.5 degrees
- Normal heart rate: 100–160/min
- Normal respiratory rate is: 40–60/ min
- Anterior fontanelle: 0.5 cm in diameter.

Gross Motor (Age in Months)

- 3: Neck
- 6: Sitting with support
- 8: Sitting without support
- 9: Standing with support
- 11: Crawling
- 12: Standing without support
- 13: Walking with support
- 18: Running
- 24: Walking upstairs
- 36: Riding a tricycle

Fine Motor (Age in Months)

- 3: Grasping
- 3: Intentional reaching with bidextrous grasp
- 7: Palmar
- 9: Pincer

Language (Age in Months)

- 1: Turns head to sound
- 3: Cooing
- 6: Monosyllables
- 9: Bisyllables
- 12: 2 words with meaning
- 24: Simple sentences
- 36: Story telling

Social (Age in Months)

- 2: Social smile
- 3: Recognizes
- 6: Smiles at mirror image
- 9: Waves bye-bye
- 12: Plays a simple ball game
- 15: Identifies body parts
- 36: Knows gender

Low Birth Weight

- Low birth weight: < 2500 g
- At risk low birth weight: < 2000 g
- Very low birth weight: < 1500 g
- Very very low birth weight/ extremely low birth weight: < 1000 g

WHO Growth Charts

- Upper curve: Median for boys–50th percentile of Boston/ Harvard standards
- Lower curve: Median for girls–3rd percentile of Boston/ Harvard standards

Government of India Growth Chart

- First curve: 50th percentile, *i.e.* 80 percent
- Second curve: 70 percent
- Third curve: 60 percent
- Fourth curve: 50 percent

Formula for Weight

- 3 months to 1 year: (age + 9)/2
- 1–6 years: (2 x age)+8
- 6–12 years: {(7x age) -5}/2

Order of Puberty in Girls

- Thelarche
- Adrenarche
- Height
- Menarche

Gestational Age

- Small for gestational age: < 10th percentile for that gestational age
- Appropriate for gestational age: 10th–90th percentile for respective gestational age
- Large for gestational age: > 90th percentile

Term

- Preterm: < 37 weeks/ < 258 days
- Term: 37–42 weeks/ 259–294days
- Post-term: > 42 weeks/ > 294 days

Wellcome Classification, Using Harvard Standards

- Children between 60–80 percent of expected weight without edema: Underweight
- Children between 60–80 percent of expected weight with edema: Kwashiorkor
- Children below 60 percent of expected weight without edema: Marasmus
- Children below 60 percent of expected weight with edema: Marasmic kwashiorkor

IAP Grading of PEM

- Grade 1: 70–80: percent of 50th percentile
- Grade 2: 60–70: percent of 50th percentile
- Grade 3: 50–60: percent of 50th percentile
- Grade 4: <50: percent of 50th percentile

Shakeer's Tape (Color Zone: Mid-arm Circumference: Interpretation (for Children between 1 and 5 Years)

- Green: > 13.5 cm: Well nourished
- Yellow: 12.5–13.5cm: Borderline
- Red zone: <12.5 cm: Malnourished

Kwashiorkor

- Flag sign—Alternate bands of hypopigmented and normally pigmented hair
- Flaky paint dermatosis—hypopigmented patches of skin desquamate to expose raw hypopigmented skin

Breast Milk

- 70 cal /100 mL
- Proteins 1.1g / 100 mL, 7 gram lactate/ 100 mL
- Expressed breast milk can be stored at
- Room temperature of 8 hours
- In refrigerator for 24 hours
- In cold room for 3 months

WHO Classification of Xerophthalmia

- X1A: Conjunctival xerosis
- X1B: Bitot's spots
- X2: Corneal xerosis
- X3B: Keratomalacia
- XN: Night blindness
- XF: Fundal changes
- XS: Corneal scarring

Treatment of Vitamin A Deficiency

- **In endemic areas**
- 2 lac units immediately
- 2 lac units on second day
- 2 lac units after 14 days
- **Infants (less than 1 year)**
  - Should be given 1 lac IU along with measles vaccine
  - Water miscible retinol palmitate injection can be given in those with continuous vomiting.

Signs of Latent Tetany

- *Trousseau's sign*: Carpal spam is elicited by occluding brachial artery, by inflating pressure cuff for 3 minutes. Carpal spasm is seen as flexion at the wrist and metacarpophalangeal joints, extension of proximal and distal interphalangeal joints, adduction of thumb and fingers.
- *Chvostek sign*: When facial nerve is tapped at the angle of mandible
- *Weiss' sign*: Facial muscles go into spasm (twitching of nose or lips)

- *Peroneal sign*: The peroneal sign consists of dorsiflexion and abduction of the foot on tapping the peroneal nerve on the lateral surface of the fibula just before the knee.
- *Erb sign*: Increased electric irritability of motor nerves in tenany.

Immunization Schedule as per IAP

- Birth – 15 days: BCG, OPV zero dose, hepatitis B 1st dose
- 6–8 weeks: OPV1, DPT1, hepatitis B 2nd dose, HB 1st dose
- 10–12 weeks: OPV2, DPT 2, HIB 2nd dose
- 14–16 weeks: OPV3 DPT 3, hepatitis B 3rd dose, HIB 3rd dose
- 9 months completed: Measles
- 15–18 months: DPT and OPV booster dose, 1, MMR vaccine
- 4–6 year: 2nd booster dose of OPV and DPT
- 10 years: Tetanus toxoid
- 16 years: Tetanus toxoid

Ophthalmia Neonatorum

- Gonococcal, Chemical: < 48 hours
- Other bacteria: 2–3 days
- H. Simplex: 5–7 days

Late Manifestations of Syphilis

Stigmata of initial lesions	Late hypersensitivity reactions
Hutchinson's teeth	Interstitial keratitis
Frontal bossing	Nerve deafness
Short maxilla	Clutton's joint
Saddle nose	
High arched palate	
Enlargement of sternoclavicular portion of clavicle	
Protuberant mandible	
Radiating perioral scars/rhagades	
Saber tibia	
Mulberry molars	

Hutchinson's Triad–Congenital Syphilis

- Hutchinson's teeth
- Interstitial keratitis
- 8th nerve deafness

Unconjugated Hyperbilirubinemia

- Crigler–Najjar syndrome UDP glucuronyl transferase deficiency
- Gilbert's syndrome – Decreased activity of UDPGT
- Decreased hepatic uptake of bilirubin

Conjugated Hyperbilirubinemia

- Rotors syndrome and Dubin-Johnson syndrome—deficiency in excretion
- A cardinal feature of Dubin–Johnson syndrome is accumulation in Lysosome of centrilobular hepatocytes of dark, coarsely granular pigment. As a result, liver may be grossly black in color; the pigment is derived from epinephrine metabolites that are not excreted normally
- Clinical jaundice in neonate, when bilirubin level is more than 5 mg/dL

Pathological Jaundice

- Clinical jaundice appearing in first 24 hours
- Increase in level of total bilirubin by more than 0.5 mg/dL/ hr
- Total bilirubin > 15 mg /dL
- Direct bilirubin >2 mg/dL

Tachypnea

- 0–2 months: more than 60 /min
- 2 months to 12 months: more than 50 /min
- 1–5 years: more than 40/min

Nadas' Criteria for Diagnosis of Heart Disease (Presence of 1 Major or 2 Minor Criteria are Essential for Diagnosis)

Major criteria	Minor criteria
Systolic murmur of grade III or more	Systolic murmur less than grade II
Diastolic murmur	Abnormal S2
Cyanosis	Abnormal X-ray
Congestive cardiac failure	Abnormal blood pressure

Condition in which there can be CCF without Cardiac Enlargement

- Congenital mitral stenosis
- Cor triatriatum
- Obstructive variety of total anomalous pulmonary venous connection

Holt-Oram Syndrome

- Thumb hypoplasia
- Hypoplasia of clavicle
- ASD
- First degree heart block

Pentalogy of Fallot

- TOF + ASD

Systemic Pulmonary Shunts

- Blalock-Taussig: Subclavian artery—Pulmonary artery anastomosis
- Pott's shunt: Descending aorta—Pulmonary artery
- Waterson's shunt: Ascending aorta—Right pulmonary artery

- Modified B—T Shunt: Same as above but uses Gore-tex conduit
- Glenn: SVC with right pulmonary artery

Sickle Cell Anemia

- Vaso-occlusive crisis/Painful crisis: Due to blockade of end organ capillaries resulting in ischemia, pain and organ damage.
- Aplastic crisis: Acute worsening of anemia producing pallor, tachycardia and fatigue; precipitated by *Parvovirus B* 19 infection. Erythropoiesis is stopped for 2–3 days.
- Splenic sequestration crisis: Acute painful enlargement of spleen

HbH Disease

- Deletion of 3 alpha gene

Loss of alpha gene	Manifestation
1	Silent carrier state
2	Alpha thalassemia trait
3	Hemoglobin disease
4 (all)	Hydrops fetalis
Acute ITP	**Chronic ITP**
4-6 weeks of duration	>6 months/year
Acute onset	Insidious onset
Antecedent infection is common	Not so
Spontaneous remission in majority	Unlikely

Most Common Malignancies in Children in Descending Order

- Leukemia
- Lymphoma
- Brain tumors
- Neuroblastoma
- Retinoblastoma
- Wilm's tumor

Brain Tumors in Children

- Most common. Subtentorial–cerebellar astrocytoma: also has best prognosis
- Medulloblastoma – Second most common; most radiosensitive
- Most common supratentorial–craniopharyngioma
- Worst prognosis is seen with—Glioblastoma multiforme

Classification of Mental Retardation by IQ

- Mild: 50–70
- Moderate: 35–50
- Severe: 20–35
- Profound: <20

Causative Agents of Meningitis

- Neonate: Group *B Streptococci*
- < 2 months: *E.coli*
- 2 months to 2.5 years: *H. influenza*
- 2.5 years – 20 years: Meningococci
- >20 years: Pneumococcus

Duchenne Muscular Dystrophy

- Pseudohypertrophic muscular dystrophy
- Cause by mutation in the gene, located at p21 that encodes dystrophin
- X-linked recessive disorder
- Valley sign-groove between supraspinatus and teres minor increases on abduction on shoulder

Gowers' Sign

- The sign descries a patient that has to use his or her hands and arms to "walk" up his or her own body from a squatting position due to lack of hip and thigh muscle strength

  There are three Gowers' Signs.
- Pain along the compressed sciatic nerve on passive dorsiflexion of the foot.
- The irregular contraction of the pupil in early tabes (Argyll Robertson).
- The climbing up the legs signs in Duchenne dystrophy.

Level of Intelligence and IQ Range

- Idiot: 0–24
- Imbecile: 25–49
- Moron: 50–69
- Borderline: 70–79
- Low normal: 80–89
- Normal: 90–109
- Superior: 110–119
- Very superior: 120–139
- Near genius: 140 and over

Acute Low Respiratory Tract Infection

- 'No pneumonia' is when patient is having cough and cold but NO fast breathing, NO chest indrawing or NO indicators of severe illness
- 'Pneumonia' is said to be present if respiratory rate is 60 or more in less than 2 months of age; 50 or more in 2–12 months and 40 or more in 12–60 months of age (treated by cotrimoxazole at home)
- 'Severe pneumonia' if there is chest indrawing (treated by I/V or I/M penicillin at hospital)
- 'Very severe pneumonia' is indicated by presence of severe chest indrawing and inability to feed (treated by I/V chloramphenicol at hospital).

MCQs WITH SHORT EXPLANATIONS

GROWTH

1. **Likely age of a child who sits in tripod fashion, has bidextrous approach, recognizes strangers and can spell out monosyllables:**
   a. 7
   b. 12
   c. 9
   d. 10

   A child sits with own support (tripod) and holds objects with bidextrous grasp at 5 months. Child speaks monosyllables at 6 months. He shows anxiety on meeting strangers as he becomes 7-8 months old.

2. **Height of a newborn doubles at:**
   a. 1 year
   b. 2 years
   c. 3 years
   d. 4 years

   On an average, the ideal length of a full-term infant at birth is 50 cm. It rises to 60 cm at 3 months, 70 cm at 9 months, 75 cm at one year, 90 cm at 2 years, 95 cm at 3 years and 100 cm at 4 years. Thereafter, the child gains little over 5 cm every year until 10 years. With the onset of puberty, remarkable acceleration in height gain occurs.

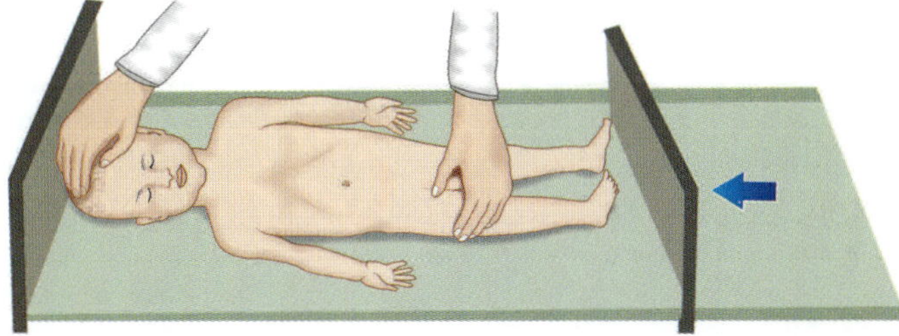

Infantometer. In case this kind of an infantometer is not available, the purpose is served with a fabricated infantometer employing a book at the head-end and another at the foot-end of the infant (in lying down posture)

3. **Weight of a child triples at:**
   a. 6 months
   b. 1 year
   c. 18 months
   d. 2 years

   On an average, ideal birth weight is said to be around 3.25 kg. The newborn loses up to 10% of his weight during the first week. It is, however regained by the age of 10 days. After this, weight gain occurs at a rate of 25 to 30 gram a day for the first 3 months and 40 gram a month during the rest of the first year of life. The infant double his birthweight by the age of 5 months and trebles it by one year.

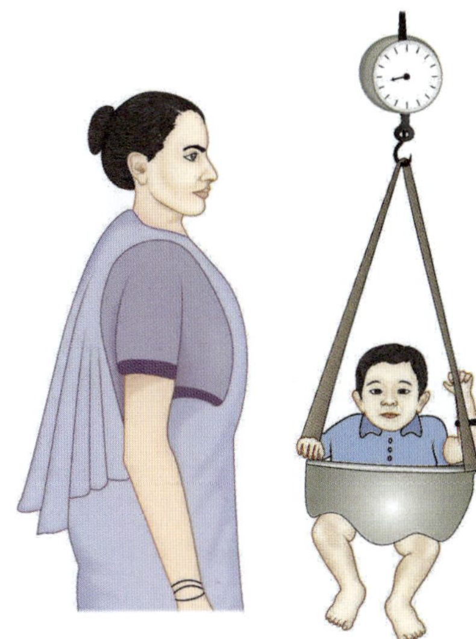

Hanging scale for weight recording in field practice

4. **An 8-month-old baby will be able to do which of the following:**
   a. Stable sitting
   b. Pincer grasp
   c. Stands without support
   d. Says mama

   By 7-8 months, a child can sit without support.

Important normal milestones	
Gross motor	
Head/neck holding	3 months
Sitting (with support)	5 months
Sitting (without support)	7-8 months
Standing (with support)	9 months
Walking with support	10 months
Crawling/creeping	11 months
Standing (without support)	12 months
Walking (without support)	13 months
Running	18 months
Climbing upstairs	24 months
Riding cycle	36 months
Fine motor	
Grasping a rattle (when placed in hand)	4 months
Reaching out for a bright object (intentional reaching) and grasps it with both hands (bidextrous grasp)	5 months

Contd...

Ans. 1. **a.** 7 2. **d.** 4 years 3. **b.** 1 year 4. **a.** Stable sitting

Contd...

Important normal milestones	
Holding an object with crude grasp from palm (palmar grasp)	7 months
Holding a small object between index finger and thumb (pincer grasp)	9 months
Personal/social	
Social smile	4-8 weeks
Recognition of mother	3 months
Smiling at mirror image	6 months
Waving "bye-bye"	9 months
Playing a simple ball game	1 year
Knowing gender	3 years
Language	
Turning head to sound (rattle, ball)	1 month
Cooing	3 months
Monosyllables (ma, pa, ba)	6 months
Bisyllables (mama, papa, baba)	9 months
Two words with meaning	1 year
Simple sentence	2 years
Telling a story	3 years
Account of recent events	4 years

5. Normal weight of infant at 1 year from birth is:

a. Doubled b. Tripled

c. Quadrupled d. Variable increase

$$\text{Weight (kg) at 3 to 12 months} = \frac{\text{age (months)} + 9}{2}$$

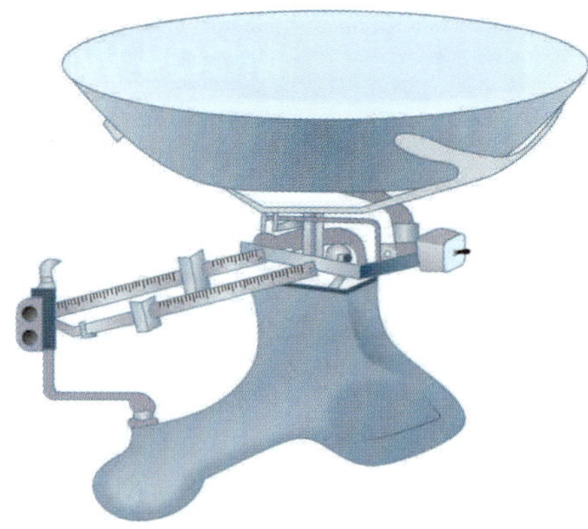

A conventional beam balance scale for weight recording in hospital and clinic practice

6. Earliest indication of sexual maturation in females:

a. Maturation of breasts b. Thelarche

c. Pubarche d. Menarche

Order of morphological changes in girls

- Accelerated gain in weight and height
- Breast changes like pigmentation of areola and enlargement of breast tissue and nipple (thelarche)
  - Increase in pelvic girth
- Appearance of pubic hair
- Activity of axillary sweat glands
- Appearance of axillary hair
- Onset of menstruation (menarche). The first bleed occurs usually 2 years after the first manifestation of puberty
- Abrupt slowing of gain in height

Developmental characteristics of three phases of adolescence			
Characteristics	*Early adolescence*	*Middle adolescence*	*Late adolescence*
Age (years)	10 to 13	14 to 16	17 to 20
SMR	1 to 2	3 to 5	5
Somatic development	Secondary sex characters, onset of rapid growth, awkward	Height growth peaks, body shape and configuration change, acne appears, menarche, spermarche	Slower growth
Sexual development	Sexual interest much more than sexual activity	Sexual drive surges, experimentation, questions of sexual orientation	Consolidation of sexual identity
Cognitive and motor absolutism development	Concrete operations, conventional morality	Appearance of abstract thoughts, self-centered, questioning more	Idealism,
Self-concept	Preoccupation with changing body, self-conscious	Concern with attractiveness, increasing introspection	Relatively stable body image
Family independence, secure base	Struggles for greater independence	Struggles for acceptance of greater autonomy	Practical family remains
Peers possicommitment	Same sex groups, conformity, cliques	Dating, peer group less important	Intimacy
Relationship to society	Middle-school adjustment	Gauging skills and opportunities	Career decisions (dropout college, work)

Ans. **5. b.** Tripled **6. b.** Thelarche

7. **Height of children in 2–10 years of age is increased by:**
a. 2 cm/year b. 4 cm/year
c. 6 cm/year d. 10 cm/year

Child attains a height of 100 cm at 4 years. Thereafter, the child gains little over 5 cm every year until 10 years. With the onset of puberty, remarkable acceleration in height gain occurs.

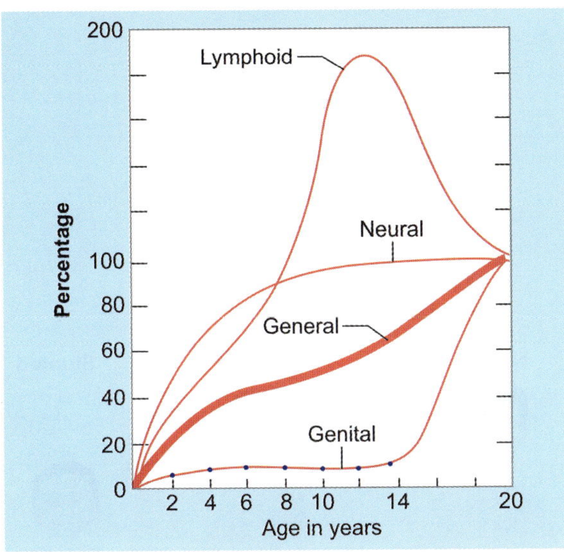

Major types of postnatal growth curves

8. **A normal healthy child has a height of 100 cm and weight of 16 kg. What is his most likely age:**
a. 3 years b. 4 years
c. 5 years d. 6 years

Height (cm) at 2 to 12 years = age (years) × 6 + 77
Weight (kg) at 1 to 6 years = age (years) × 2 + 8

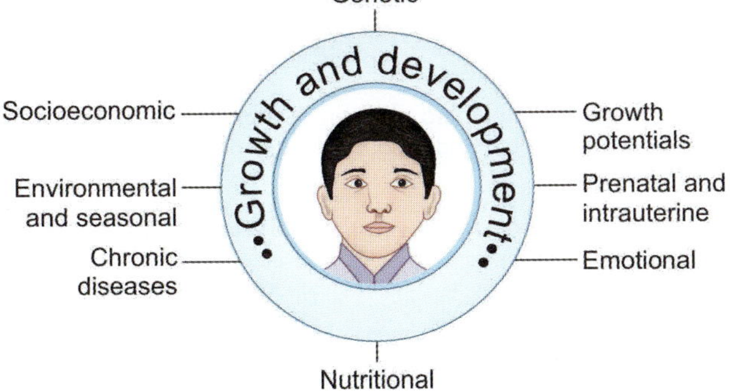

Factors influencing growth and development

9. **Head control is possible in an infant by:**
a. 1 month
b. 2 months
c. 3 months
d. 6 months

Head/ neck holding is possible by 3 months.

10. **Order of development of secondary sexual characteristic in male:**
a. Testicular development → pubic hair → axillary hair → beard
b. Pubic hair à testicular development → axillary hair → beard
c. Testicular development → beard → pubic hair → axillary hair
d. Axillary hair → pubic hair → beard → testicular development

Order of morphological changes in boys
- Accelerated gain in weight and height
- Enlargement of external genitalia
- Appearance of pubic hair followed by hair in axilla, upper lip, groin, thigh, and between pubis and umbilicus. Facial hair appear about 2 years after the pubic hair
- Changes in voice
- Nocturnal discharge of seminal fluid
- Abrupt slowing in gain in height

Three phases of puberty growth spurt	
Phase 1	Moderate gain in height velocity in the prepubescent phase
Phase 2	Both height and weight show rapid gain in the pubescent phase
Phase 3	Growth velocity shows deceleration though weight gain continues in the postpubescent phase

11. **A female child has recently learned to eat with spoon without spilling; to dress and undress herself with supervision and to understand that she is a girl. These skills are FIRST mastered between the ages:**
a. 2 and 3 years b. 3 and 4 years
c. 4 and 5 years d. 5 and 6 years

A child knows his/ her gender by 3 years.

12. **Child speaks sentences at:**
a. 1 year b. 2 years
c. 3 years d. 4 years

A child speaks simple sentence by 2 years.

13. **Height of 100 cm is attained by a child at:**
a. 1 year b. 2 years
c. 3 years d. 4 years

A child attains a height of 100 cm at 4 years.

14. **A baby knows his gender at the age of:**
a. 1 year b. 2 years
c. 3 years d. 4 years

A child knows gender by the age of 3 years.

15. **A child of 3 years will be able to:**
a. Copy circle b. Copy rectangle
c. Copy cross d. Copy triangle

A child can copy a circle at the age of 3 years.

Ans. 7. **c.** 6 cm/ year 8. **b.** 4 years 9. **c.** 3 months 10. **a.** Testicular development... 11. **a.** 2 and 3 years 12. **b.** 2 years 13. **d.** 4 years 14. **c.** 3 years 15. **a.** Copy circle

16. **A child of 4 years can do all of the following EXCEPT:**
    a. Skip
    b. Goes down stairs one foot per step
    c. Tell a story
    d. Copies triangle

    A child can copy a triangle by 5 years of age.

NUTRITION

17. **Mid-upper arm circumference (MUAC) measurement indicating severe malnutrition:**
    a. 12.5 cm b. 10.5 cm
    c. 14.5 cm d. 9.5 cm

    MUAC interpretation
    - >13.5 cm: Satisfactory nutritional status
    - 12.5 to 13.5 cm: Mild to moderate nutrition
    - <12.5 cm: Severe malnutrition

18. **Albumin levels in mild degree of malnutrition:**
    a. 2 g/dL b. 2.5 g/dL
    c. 3 g/dL d. 3.5 g/dL

    Mild malnutrition
    - Two of the following criteria must be met
      - Serum albumin > 2.9 to 3.4 g/dL*
      - Weight is 80 to 89% of IBW
      - Weight is 85 to 95% of usual weight

19. **Vitamin D deficiency is manifested as:**
    a. Scurvy b. Night blindness
    c. Beri-Beri d. Rickets

    Vitamin D deficiency produces rickets. Disturbed metabolism and poor synthesis of vitamin D from the skin, malabsorption state, diarrheal disease and excessive phylate with low calcium and low phosphate content of the diet may well be other causes of rickets in malnourished children.

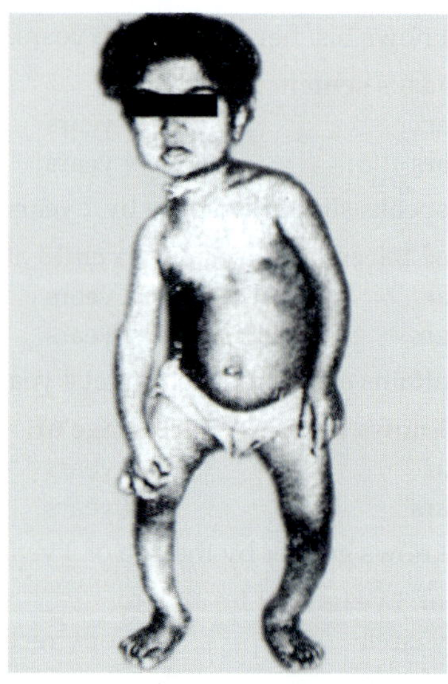

Gross bowleg deformity of rickets. Note widening of ankles and "double malleoli"

20. **Malnutrition is assessed clinically by:**
    a. Mid arm circumference b. Weight for age
    c. Body mass index d. All of the above

    Anthropometric indices for assessment of nutritional status
    - Age-dependent
      - Weight for age
      - Height for age
    - Age-independent
      - Weight for height
      - Mid-arm circumference
      - Chest/head circumference ratio
      - Triceps skin fold thickness
      - Mid-upper-arm/ height ratio
      - QUAC-stick method
      - Shakir tape method
      - Quetelet index
      - Dugdale index

Normal Wasted Stunted

	Normal	Wasted	Stunted
Weight/age%	100	70	70
Weight/height%	100	70	100
Height/age%	100	100	84

Normal, wasted and stunted children. Weight-forage is low in both wasted child and the stunted child. But weight per height is not affected in the stunted child

21. **Vitamin associated with hemolytic anemia in preterm babies:**
    a. Vitamin K b. Vitamin E
    c. Vitamin C d. Vitamin A

    The commonest manifestation of vitamin K deficiency is what is known as the hemorrhagic disease of the newborn. Its causes include a low level of vitamin K in breast milk, hepatic immaturity and inadequate synthesis of vitamin K in the GIT by the bacterial flora.

22. **FALSE for Kwashiorkor:**
    a. Edema
    b. Patchy depigmentation of hair
    c. Fatty liver
    d. Fatty infiltration of pancreas

Ans. 16. **d.** Copies triangle 17. **a.** 12.5 cm 18. **d.** 3.5 g/ dL 19. **d.** Rickets
20. **d.** All of the above 21. **a.** Vitamin K 22. **d.** Fatty infiltration of pancreas

A classical case of Kwashiorkor is dull, apathetic and miserable, evincing hardly any interest in the surroundings. His growth is stunted and there is marked muscle wasting with some retention of subcutaneous fat. He has pitting edema over the legs and feet and perhaps over certain other parts of the body. There may be diarrhea, skin and hair changes, anemia and vitamin deficiency signs. Liver is, as a rule, enlarged due to fatty change.

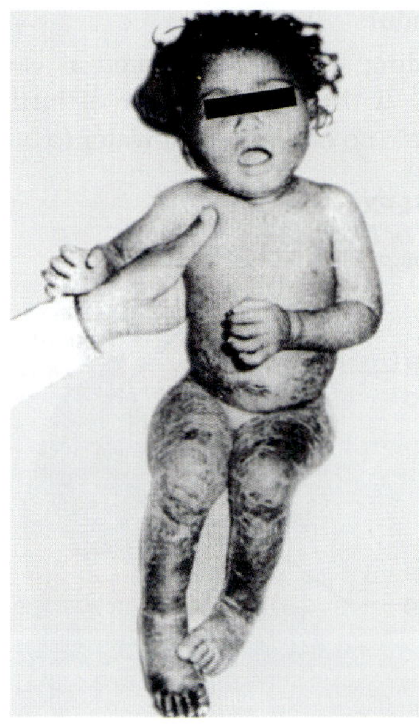

Kwashiorkor in a toddler. Note the classical flaky-pain dermatosis and massive edema. Absence of hair changes reflects acute nature of the ailment

23. Specific sign of Kwashiorkor is:

a. Pitting edema b. Weight loss
c. Flag sign d. Muscle wasting

One of the essential feature of kwashiorkor is hypoalbuminemic pitting edema, at least over the pretibial region.

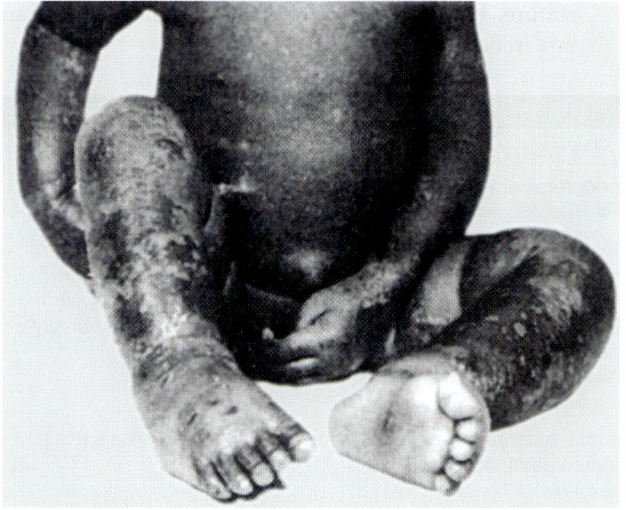

Typical flaky-paint dermatosis and gross edema of kwashiorkor

24. Prelacteal feed given just after birth is:

a. Cow's milk b. Honey
c. Water d. None

The basic food for infant feeding is milk. Breast feeding is the most natural method and, in fact, the supreme gift. Artificial feeding should not be the first choice, except for a compulsive situation.

Situations where breastfeeding may be avoided
In Mother
❑ Chronic diseases such as active tuberculosis, leprosy, malignancy, beriberi, AIDS, etc. Many authorities advocate continuing breastfeeding in the first two provided chemotherapeutic coverage is being given.
❑ Mothers stubbornly addicted to alcohol or heavy doses of some drugs. Those on heavy metals, phenobarbital, hydantoin, steroids, etc. should also not be allowed to breastfeed their babies.
❑ Psychosis.
❑ Local conditions, e.g. breast abscess, cracked nipples, etc. Breastfeeding must be resumed as soon as possible.
In Infant
❑ Gross prematurity of the baby or other conditions in which the newborn cannot suckle.
❑ Inborn errors such as phenylketonuria, galactosemia or lactose intolerance.
❑ *Breast-milk jaundice*, provided that serum bilirubin approaches critical level.
❑ Biological mother may avoid breastfeeding an infant who is to be passed on to another couple.

25. All of the following are the features of scurvy EXCEPT:

a. Hyperkeratosis
b. Ecchymosis of lower limbs
c. Hypoglycemia
d. Bleeding gums

Clinical features of scurvy

- Infantile scurvy
  - Gross irritability
  - Excessive crying
  - Pseudoparalysis
  - Palpable subperiosteal hemorrhage
  - Hemorrhage may occur into the skin and mucous membranes
  - Hemorrhages into the gums may result in spongy, swollen, bluish purple gums, especially about the erupted teeth
- Childhood scurvy
  - Follicular hyperkeratosis with development of minute hemorrhages at the root of the hair follicles
  - Bleeding into the skin, leading to petechiae or even large purpuric swellings, and guns may occur but subperiosteal hemorrhages are infrequent

Ans. **23. a.** Pitting edema **24. d.** None **25. c.** Hypoglycemia

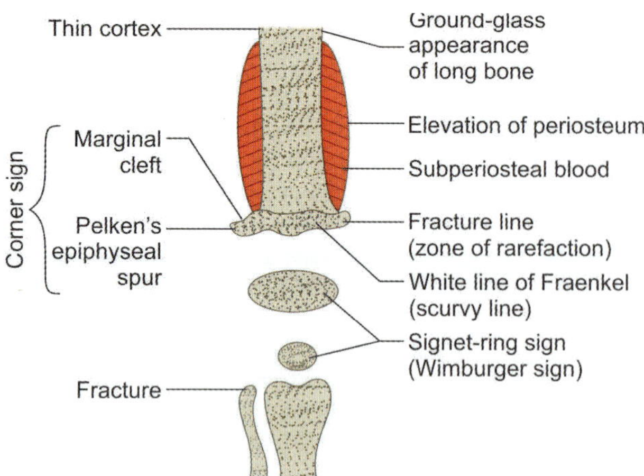

Diagrammatic representation of radiological picture of scurvy

26. A child of age 9 needed prophylaxis of vitamin A. The dose and route of administration is:

a. 1,000,000 IU intramuscularly
b. 1,000,000 IU orally
c. 2,000,000 IU intramuscularly
d. 2,000,000 IU orally

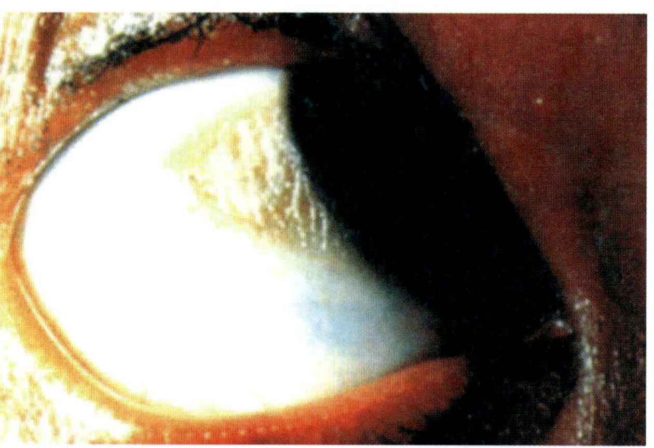

Bitot's spot. Note the position of the lesion and its shape. The foamy deposit lies on top of a patch of pigmented conjunctiva

According to the National Vitamin A Prophylaxis Program, all children in the age group 6 months to 6 years in the target areas should receive 2,000,000 IU of vitamin A (in an oily base) orally every six months.

27. Breastfeeding should be initiated within:

a. Half an hour
b. One hour
c. One and a half hours
d. Two hours

Breastfeeding should be initiated as early as possible, preferably within half an hour of birth. It should be "exclusive" (no other food or water to be given).

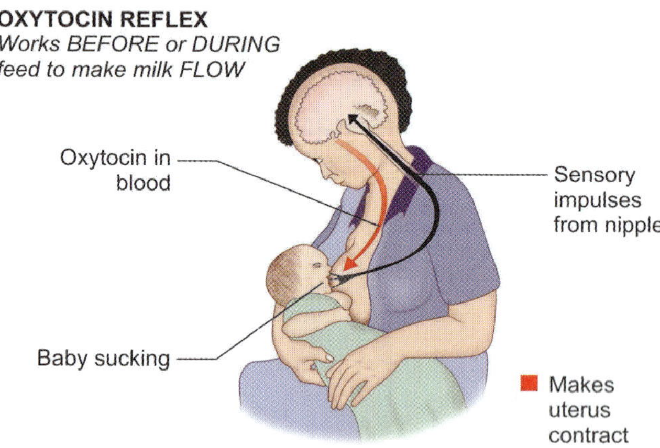

Oxytocin milk ejection reflex

28. A child with alopecia, hyperpigmentation, dermatitis in genitals and mouth with hypogonadism is most likely to have deficiency of:

a. Copper
b. Zinc
c. Iron
d. Magnesium

Zinc deficiency may play an important role in the etiology of the syndrome of growth retardation with short stature, hypogonadism, hepatosplenomegaly and anemia in boys.

Salient features of important minerals/trace elements/micronutrients

Mineral/ trace element	*Source*	*Deficiency*	*Excess*
Iron	Green vegetables, meat, yolk, whole grains, nuts, legumes. Milk, especially breastmilk, is a poor source.	Microcytic-hypochromic anemia	Hemosiderosis; poisoning
Zinc	Cheese, nuts, grains, meat, fish	Dwarfism with iron-deficiency anemia, hyperpigmentation, hepatosplenomegaly, hypogonadism; acrodermatitis enteropathica: poor wound healing; depressed immunocompetence, ITS, LBW,	Gastrointestinal upset, copper deficiency, reduced high density lipoprotein
Copper	Legumes, nuts, whole grains, meat, liver, oyster (shell-fish)	Refractory anemia, osteoporosis, neutropenia, depigmentation, ataxia, raised serum cholesterol	Indian childhood cirrhosis (ICC)

Contd...

Ans. **26. d.** 2,000,000 IU... **27. a.** Half an hour **28. b.** Zinc

Contd...

Mineral/ trace element	*Source*	*Deficiency*	*Excess*
Magnesium	Cereals, legumes, nuts, meat, milk	Tetany	None
Calcium	Milk and its products, fish, green leafy vegetables	Tetany rickets	Renal stones, heart block
Phosphorus	Milk and its products, fish, green leafy vegetables	Rickets	Tetany
Iodine	Sea-foods, vegetables from iodine-rich soil, iodized salt	Goiter, cretinism	Goiter
Fluoride	Sea-food, tea	Dental caries	Fluorosis
Chromium	Drinking water, animal foods, yeast	Impaired glucose tolerance; diabetes mellitus in animals	None

29. Firstly given to a severely malnourished child:

a. Vitamin A b. 10% albumin
c. Dextrose d. ReSoMal

Intravenous fluid therapy is usually needed in severe dehydration in malnourished child. Initially, Ringer lactate or N/2 saline in 5% dextrose, 30 mL/kg in 2 hours.

Serious complications of advanced PEM	
Complications	*Remarks*
Superadded	Both overt and hidden: Septicemia, pneumonia, diarrhea, pyoderma, scabies, UTI, tuberculosis infections.
Dehydration and dyselectrolytemia	Usually complicating accompanying diarrhea, often with lactose intolerance.
Hypothermia	An unattended rectal temperature of < 35 degree Celsius may prove fatal, causing sudden infant death syndrome (SIDS)
Hypoglycemia	It contributes to poor response to nutritional therapy and carries a poor prognosis.
CCF	It is usually precipitated by excessive intake of sodium and fluid or severe anemia. Since cardiac size is invariably small in PEM, even a normal sized heart in X-ray should arouse suspicion of CCF.
Anemia	Moderate to severe anemia may result from malnutrition as such or such factors as superadded infection(s), contributing to development of CCF.
Bleeding	DIC may complicate the clinical picture.
Sudden infant death syndrome (SIDS)	Sudden death 4-7 days after admission. Usually, the cause remains unclear.

30. Fluid given to a 10-month-old child with severe dehydration is:

a. 45 mL/ kg/ hour b. 30 mL/ kg/ hour
c. 15 mL/ kg/ hour d. 5 mL/ kg/ hour

Quick correction of severe dehydration is done with IV fluids (preferably Ringer's lactate) in a hospital. For <1 year child, 30 mL/ kg is given within first hour followed by 70 mL/ kg over net 5 hours.

Composition of ReSoMal compared to standard ORS and hypoosmolar ORS (mmol/L)			
	ReSoMal	*Standard ORS*	*Hypoosmolar ORS*
Sodium	45	90	
Potassium	40	20	
Chloride	70	80	
Citrate	7	10	
Magnesium	3	–	
Zinc	0.3	–	
Copper	0.045		
Total osmolarity	300	311	
Recommended regimen for ReSoMal is 75–100 mL/kg in 12 hours. It may be given orally or through nasogastric tube.			

31. Large doses of vitamin K administered to a newborn result in:

a. Shortened bilirubinemia b. Bulgingofthefontanelles
c. Hypoprothrombinemia d. Hemolytic anemia

Excessive administration of vitamin K may cause hemolytic anemia, hyperbilirubinemia and kernicterus, especially in preterm and G-6-PD deficient infants.

32. About scurvy, all are true EXCEPT:

a. Subperiosteal hematomas with tenderness
b. Separation of epiphysis
c. Raised serum alkaline phosphatase
d. Gingival bleeding

Ans. **29. c.** Dextrose **30. b.** 30 mL/ kg/ h **31. d.** Hemolytic anemia **32. c.** Raised serum alkaline...

Biochemical findings of rickets include raised alkaline phosphatase (except in malnourished children), usually a normal serum calcium and a reduced phosphorous.

Daily requirement for vitamins	
Vitamins	*Requirement*
A	1,500 to 5,000 IU
B_1 (thiamine)	0.5 to1.5 mg
B_2 (riboflavin)	0.5 to 2.5 mg
Niacin (niacinamide, nicotinamide, nicotinic acid)	0 to 20 mg
B_6 (pyridoxine)	0.4 to 1.4 mg
B_{12} (cyanocobalamin)	1 to 1.5 mcg
Folic acid	25 to 1000 mcg
C	30 to 50 mg
D	400 IU
E	4 to 5 IU

33. The most common cause of short stature:

a. Constitutional
b. Systemic diseases
c. Hypothyroidism
d. Growth hormone deficiency

Primary short stature is usually due to an intrinsic defect in the skeletal system as a result of some genetic or prenatal damage (say, IUGR). Here, potential for normal bone growth is impaired though skeletal age is unaffected. Main effect is on diaphyseal growth.

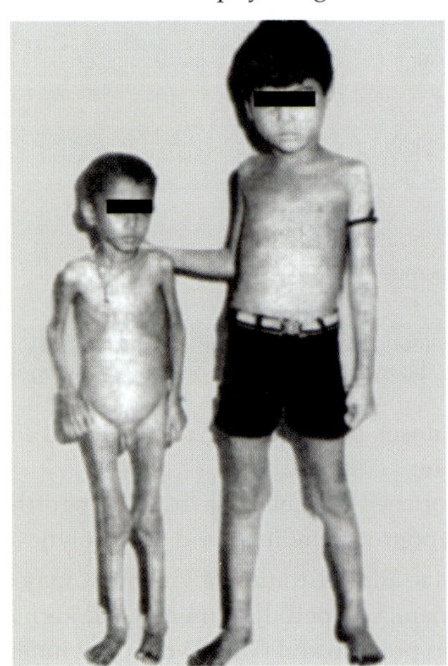

Short stature in a child with acute on chronic PEM (nutritional dwarfing) against a control (both 5.5-year-old)

34. Low osmolarity ORS has (as compared to WHO-ORS):

a. Low glucose and high sodium
b. Low glucose and low sodium
c. Low glucose and low potassium
d. Low glucose and high potassium

Recently, WHO has done well to introduce a low osmolarity ORS cut down risk of hypernatremia which earlier restricted its wide usage in neonates and infants. This formulation provides a total osmolarity of 245 mOSM/ L compared to the standard WHO formulation with 311 mOsm/ L. It is supposed to lower stool output, shorten diarrheal duration and reduce vomiting.

Low osmolarity ORS vis-a-vis standard ORS		
Component	*Standard ORS*	*Low osmolarity ORS*
Contents		
Sodium chloride	3.5 g	2.6 g
Sodium bicarbonate (citrate)	2.5 g (2.9 g)	2.9 g
Potassium chloride	1.5 g	1.5 g
Glucose	20.0 g	13.5 g111
Osmolarity		
Sodium	90 mmol	75 mmol
Chloride	80 mml	65 mmol
Citrate	10 mmol	10 mmol
Potassium	80 mmol	20 mmol
Glucose	111 mmol	75 mmol
Total osmolarity	311	245
Replacement of sodium bicarbonate by trisodium citrate dihydrite (2.9 g) undoubtedly enhances the shelf-life of the ORS but also makes it more expensive. The ORS thus prepared provides 10 mmol/L of citrate in place of 30 mmol/L of bicarbonate (one mmol citrate = 3 mmol base)		

35. Recommended dietary allowances for infant of 6 months to 12 months (per kg):

a. 100 kilocalories/day energy and 1.5 gram/day protein
b. 100 kilocalories/day energy and 3.5 gram/day protein
c. 200 kilocalories/day energy and 1.5 gram/day protein
d. 200 kilocalories/day energy and 3.5 gram/day protein

Daily requirement of calories under 1 year of age is 110 kilocalories per kg whereas daily requirement of the proteins is 1.5 to 2.6 g/ kg.

Daily requirement for calories	
Age range (years)	*Requirement k calorie per kg*
Under 1 (average)	110
1 to 3	100
4 to 6	90
7 to 9	80
10 to 12	70
13 to 15	60
16 to 19	50
Adult	40

Ans. **33. a.** Constitutional **34. b.** Low glucose... **35. a.** 100 kilocalories/day energy...

36. Calorie provided while managing a severe malnutrition case:

a. 50 kcal/ kg/ day
b. 100 kcal/ kg/ day
c. 150 kcal/ kg/ day
d. 200 kcal/ kg/ day

The nutritional correction, the cornerstone of treatment of severe acute malnutrition (SAMN) is carried by providing high protein and high energy diet. A daily intake of 100 kcal/ kg/ day of expected weight (150–200 kcal/ kg/ day of actual weight) and 3 g/kg of proteins calculated with reference to the actual weight should be achieved in very first week. This target is reached slowly, beginning with just 100 kcal/ kg/ day at the start.

WHO classification of PEM		
Criteria	*Moderate PEM*	*Severe PEM*
Symmetrical edema	No	Yes
Weight for height Index of wasting)	70-79% of expected Wasting)	< 70% of expected (Severe wasting)
Height for age (Index of stunting)	85-89% of expected (Stunting)	< 85% of expected (Severe stunting)

37. True regarding child with PEM:

a. Low total body sodium, reduced ECF volume
b. Low total body sodium, increased ECF volume
c. High total body sodium, reduced ECF volume
d. High total body sodium, increased ECF volume

Total body water is increased in PEM, irrespective whether it is of kwashiorkor or marasmic type. Unlike potassium depletion, sodium is retained by the body. Sodium retention is primarily extracellular though muscle, skin, brain and viscera, too, are affected.

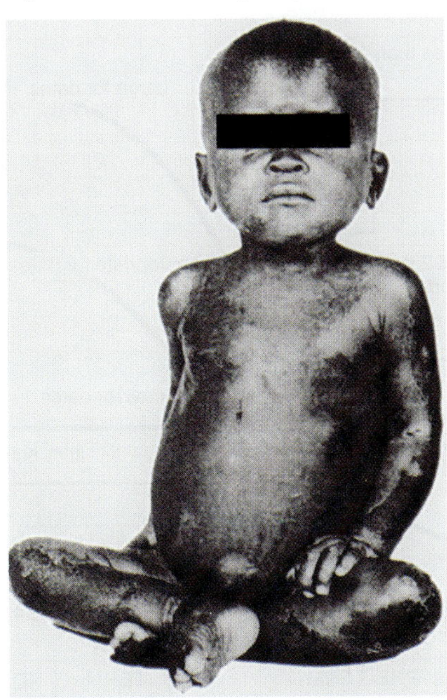

Kwashiorkor, showing characteristic features

38. Dose of vitamin A, on 1st day, for a 9-month-old child with malnutrition:

a. 50,000 IU
b. 1 lakh IU
c. 1.5 lakh IU
d. 2 lakh IU

For children under 1 year and under 8 kg weight at any age, half the dose of vitamin A as indicated for children 1 to 6 years and above is given.

WHO/UNICEF treatment schedule of xerophthalmia	
Children 1 to 6 years and above	
Immediately on diagnosis	200,000 IU vitamin A (O)
The following day	200,000 IU vitamin A(O)
Four weeks later	200,000 IU vitamin A(O)
Children under 1 year and under 8 kg weight at any age Half the doses as indicated for children 1 to 6 years and above For night blindness or Bitot Spot	
Treat with a daily dose of	10,000 IU of vitamin A(O) for 2 weeks
Note: If there is a persistent vomiting or profuse diarrhea, an intramuscular injection of 100,000 IU of water-miscible vitamin A (but not an oil-based preparation) may be substituted for the first dose.	

39. True for vitamin D resistant rickets:

a. No end organ resistance to calcitriol
b. X linked recessive
c. Defect in proximal tubular reabsorption
d. Hyperphosphatemia and high calcitriol

Causes of type II refractory rickets

- Poor intake or absorption of phosphates
- Defective reabsorption of phosphates by the renal tubules
  - Fanconi syndrome
  - Familial hypophosphatemic vitamin D refractory rickets
  - Isolated phosphaturia
  - Renal tubular acidosis
  - Oncogenous tumors (oncogenous rickets) as in von Recklinghausen disease
  - Epidermal nevus syndrome

Clues to diagnosis of refractory rickets	
Clue	*Diagnosis*
Clinical	
Familial	Familial hypophosphatemic vitamin D refracting rickets, 1-OH deficiency vitamin D-dependent rickets, renal tubular acidosis (distal)
Manifesting before 6 months of age	Familial conditions like Fanconi syndrome, cystinosis, 1-hydroxylase deficiency
Manifesting after 6 months of age but before 12 months	X-linked dominant vitamin D refractory rickets
Manifesting in early childhood	Renal tubular acidosis

Contd...

Ans. **36. b.** 100 kcal/ kg/day **37. d.** High total body... **38. b.** 1 lakh IU **39. c.** Defect in proximal...

Contd...

Clue	Diagnosis
Manifesting in late childhood	Renal osteodystrophy, glycine phosphaturia
Gross muscle weakness	Renal tubular acidosis, glycine phosphaturia
Renal/ureteric colic	Renal stone, renal tubular acidosis
Nausea, vomiting, lethargy	Renal osteodystrophy, renal tubular acidosis, hypophosphatasia
Mental deficiency, buphthalmos	Lowe syndrome
Highly pigmented skin, cystine crystals in cornea on slit lamp exam	Cystinosis
Sutural diastasis, short ribs, cutaneous dimples, hypotonia, failure to thrive	Hypophosphatasia
Lab investigations	
Low phosphate with amino aciduria	Vitamin D deficiency secondary to malabsorption, liver disease, chronic anticonvulsant therapy
Low phosphate without amino aciduria, isolated	Familial hypophosphatemic vitamin D refractory rickets, oncogenic phosphaturia, normal pH tumors
Low pH	Renal tubular acidosis
High phosphate	Renal osteodystrophy.

NEWBORN

40. All are included in APGAR score EXCEPT:

a. Respiratory rate b. Color
c. Motor activity d. Heart rate

Respiratory effort (NOT respiratory rate) is included in APGAR score

41. All are useful for prenatal diagnosis of Down syndrome EXCEPT:

a. Reduced femur length
b. Nuchal fold translucency of more than 3 mm
c. Associated ASD
d. Prolonged and increased umbilical blood flow

USG findings and risk of Down syndrome

- Nuchal fold thickness >6 mm: Likelihood ratio: 17
- Hypoplastic nasal bone/absence of a nasal bone has a likelihood ratio of 83
- Echogenic intracardiac focus: Likelihood ratio: 1.5
- Echogenic bowel: Likelihood ratio: 6.1
- Shortened humerus: Likelihood ratio: 7.5
- Shortened femur: Likelihood ratio: 2.7
- Single umbilical artery: Only considered a soft marker if other abnormalities are present. In an otherwise normal 2nd trimester ultrasound it is NOT a marker of aneuploidy.
- Mild pyelectasis : Weak association with aneuploidy.

42. A 2-year-old child presented with severe dehydration. Amount of fluid to be given is:

a. 30 mL in 60 min b. 30 mL in 30 min
c. 70 mL in 360 min d. 70 mL in 180 min

Intravenous fluid therapy in severe dehydration

Age	First give	Then give
<12 months	30 mL/kg in 1 hour	70 mL/kg in 5 hours
12 months – 5 years	30 mL/kg in 30 minutes	70 mL/kg in 2 hours 30 minutes

43. All are features of Down syndrome EXCEPT:

a. Hypotonia
b. Brushfield spots
c. Mental retardation
d. Dolicocephaly

Head findings in Down syndrome

- Brachycephaly (NOT dolicocephaly)
- Oblique palpebral fissures.
- Epicanthic folds.
- Ring of iris speckles-Brushfield's spots.
- Ears set low, folded or stenotic meatus.
- Flat nasal bridge.

44. Very low birth weight is less than:

a. 500–1000 g b. 1000–1500 g
c. 1500–2000 g d. 2000–2500 g

The term, very low birth weight, refers to a birth weight between 1,000 g and 1,500 g, and extremely low birth weight to a birth weight less than 1,000 g.

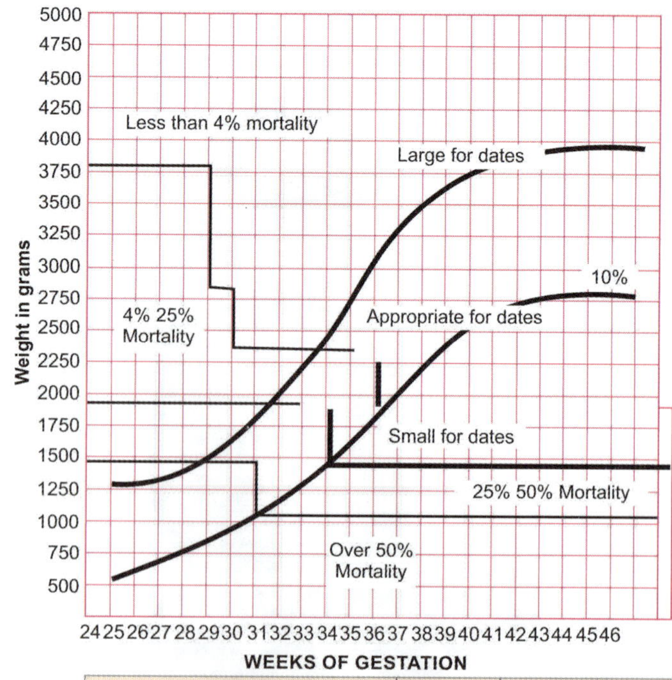

Practical classification of newborns by weight and gestational age

Ans. **40. a.** Respiratory rate **41. d.** Prolonged and... **42. b.** 30 ml in 30 min **43. d.** Dolicocephaly **44. b.** 1000–1500 g

45. Jaundice at birth or within 24 hours of birth is due to:
a. Erythroblastosis
b. Congenital hyperbilirubinemia
c. Biliary atresia
d. Physiological

When hemolysis in utero is less intense, deep jaundice appears during the first 12 to 24 hours (icterus gravis).

Important causes of neonatal jaundice based on age of onset
First Day
❑ Rh and ABO incompatibilities (hemolytic disease of the newborn)
❑ Intrauterine infections like toxoplasmosis and cytomegalic inclusion disease
❑ G-6-PD deficiency
❑ Hereditary spherocytosis
❑ Drug administration to mother (vitamin K, sulfisoxazole, salicylates)
❑ Homozygous alpha-thalassemia
Second and Third Days
❑ Physiologic
❑ Hyperbilirubinemia of newborn
❑ Birth asphyxia
❑ Cephalhematoma
❑ Acidosis
❑ Hypothermia
❑ Hypoglycemia
❑ Drugs
❑ Familial nonhemolytic icterus as in Crigler-Najjar disease
❑ Gilbert disease, Dubin-Johnson syndrome
Fourth to Seventh Days
Septicemia
❑ Syphilis
❑ Toxoplasmosis
❑ Cytomegalic inclusion disease
❑ Extrahepatic atresia of bile duct
❑ Breast-milk jaundice
After First Week
❑ Septicemia
❑ Extrahepatic atresia of bile duct
❑ Hereditary spherocytosis
❑ Neonatal hepatitis
❑ Drug-induced hemolytic anemia
❑ Galactosemia
Persistent Jaundice during First Month
❑ Inspissated bile syndrome
❑ Cretinism
❑ Congenital hypertrophic pyloric stenosis

46. A neonate after 12 hours of birth passes black colored meconium. Most likely condition:
a. Hirschsprung's disease
b. Fibrocystic disease of pancreas
c. Intestinal hemorrhage
d. Normal

Within 12 to 24 hours, the infant passes dark meconium. In 2 to 3 days, stools change color to yellow-green and are loose and frequent. These are called "transitional stools" and are perfectly normal in infants fed on mother's milk.

47. Most appropriate approach to a neonate presenting with vaginal bleeding on day 4 of life:
a. Administration of vitamin K
b. Investigation for bleeding disorder
c. No specific therapy
d. Administration of 10 mL/kg of fresh frozen plasma over 4 hours

Withdraw of maternal bleeding supply may cause slight vaginal bleeding on the third day. It disappears by seventh day and is harmless.

48. A neonate born to infected hepatitis B mother, should be treated with:
a. Isolation
b. Immunoglobulin
c. Hepatitis B vaccine
d. Immunoglobulin and hepatitis B vaccine

Passive immunization against hepatitis B can be achieved by administering specific anti-HBs gamma globulins for short term immediate protection in such situations as accidental needleprick, neonate of a HBsAg-positive mother. Newborns of mothers who are chronic HBsAg carriers should also receive hepatitis B vaccine (Engerix-B, Shanvac-B, HBvac, Envac, Hepavax).

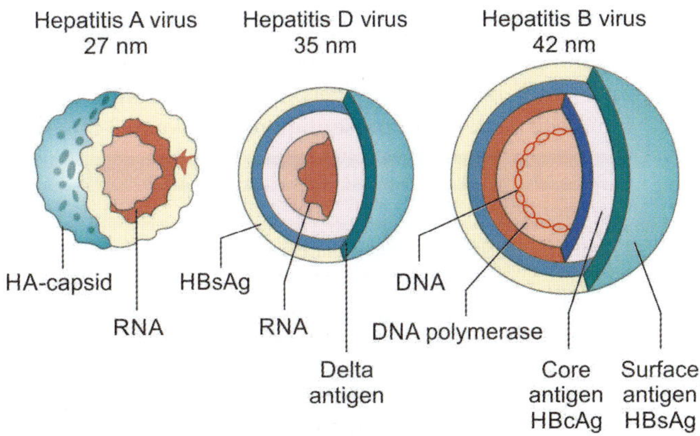

Diagrammatic representation of structures of hepatitis A, B and D viruses

Ans. 45. a. Erythroblastosis 46. d. Normal 47. c. No specific therapy 48. d. Immunoglobulin...

49. Condition that does NOT present with cyanosis at birth:

a. TOF
b. Transposition of great vessels
c. PDA
d. Tricuspid atresia

Cyanotic congenital heart disease (Right-to-left shunt)

- Decreased pulmonary blood flow
  - Tetralogy of Fallot
  - Tricuspid atresia
  - Transposition of great arteries with
    - VSD and PS
    - DORV with PS
    - Ebstein anomaly
- Increased pulmonary blood flow
  - Transposition of great arteries
  - Persistent truncus arteriosus

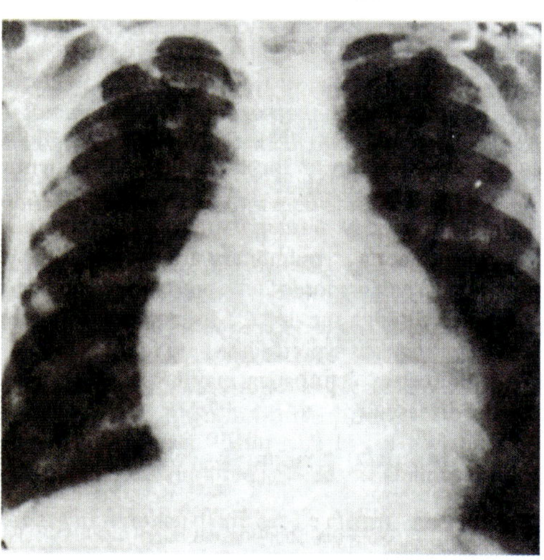

X-ray chest showing cardiomegaly, prominent aortic arch and pulmonary artery in patent ductus arteriosus (PDA)

50. NOT a cause of vomiting on 1st day of baby's life:

a. Pyloric stenosis
b. Esophageal atresia
c. Aerophagy
d. Amniotic gastritis

The typical presentation is with onset of non-bilious vomiting starting anytime between 1–8 weeks of age and which progressively becomes forceful and "projectile". The peak age of presentation is between 3-5 weeks.

Causes of vomiting in various age groups	
Newborn	
Benign	Swallowed air due to erratic feeding, possetting, swallowed amniotic fluid or blood.
Organic	Septicemia or other infections, such as meningitis, intrauterine infections causing encephalitis, otitis, gastroenteritis; congenital obstructive defects of the GIT, birth trauma, birth defects of the CNS, hypoglycemia, galactosemia.
Early Infancy	
Benign	Faulty feeding, too much crying, loneliness.
Organic	Infections such as meningitis, encephalitis, URI, whooping cough, gastroenteritis, congenital hypertrophic pyloric stenosis, hiatal hernia, pylorospasm, cow milk allergy, space-occupying lesions, diabetes, uremia, galactosemia.
Late Infancy and Childhood	
Benign	Forcing the feed, as an attention-seeking device in upset parent-child relationship, motion sickness, cyclic vomiting.

51. All of the following are components of APGAR score EXCEPT:

a. Heart rate
b. Respiratory efforts
c. BP
d. Muscle tone

First put forward by Professor Virginia Apgar, a renowned New York-based anesthesiologist, in 1953, Apgar score is a quantitative assessment of neonate's condition at birth, especially with reference to the respiratory, circulatory and neurologic status.

Apgar scoring system

Clinical features	*Score 0*	*Score 1*	*Score 2*
Appearance (Color)	Blue or pale	Body pink, limbs blue	Pink all over
Pulse (Heart rate)	Nil	Less than 100 per minute	Over 100 per minute
Grimace (Response to catheter put into nostril or stimulation of sole of foot)	Nil	Grimace or feeble cry	Cry or sneezing
Activity and tone	Limp	Some flexion of limbs	Active movements
Respiration	Nil	Slow, irregular	Good, strong cry

52. MC cause of cholestatic jaundice in newborn is:

a. Hypoplasia of biliary tract
b. Neonatal hepatitis
c. Choledochal cyst
d. Physiological

The term, neonatal cholestasis syndrome, should be restricted to conjugated hyperbilirubinemia persisting beyond a fortnight. The two most important causes are neonatal hepatitis syndrome and extrahepatic biliary atresia. Neonatal hepatitis, or the so-called giant-cell arteritis, may manifest any time during the first six weeks of life.

Ans. **49. c.** PDA **50. a.** Pyloric stenosis **51. c.** BP **52. b.** Neonatal hepatitis

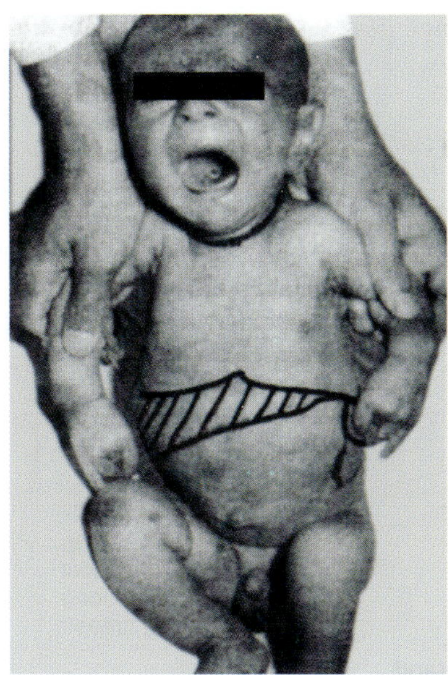

Neonatal hepatitis

53. Which of the following is NOT the correct sign of good attachment of a baby to the breast:

a. Baby's mouth wide open
b. Lower areola more visible
c. Baby's lower lip everted
d. Baby's chin touching the breast

Good attachment on infant's mouth on mother's areola and nipple is indicated by

- Infant's mouth wide open
- Infant's lower lip turned outward
- Infant's chin touches mother's breast
- Most of the areola inside infant's mouth

PROLACTIN
Secreted AFTER feed to produce NEXT feed

Sensory impulses from nipple
Prolactin in blood
Baby sucking
More prolactin secreted at night
Suppresses ovulation

Prolactin milk-secreting reflex

CONGENITAL DISORDER

54. Earliest congenital anomaly to be detected on USG:

a. Anencephaly b. Spina bifida
c. Duodenal atresia d. Hydrocephalus

Anencephaly may be sonographically detectable as early as 10 weeks. Ultrasound can be a noninvasive, cost effective and fast method to detect anencephaly and has an accuracy of approximating 100% at 14 weeks.

55. A 25-year-old lady delivered a small for age child at 38 weeks of pregnancy. On examination, the newborn was having bloody rhinorrhea, abdominal distension, wrinkled skin and maculopapular rash. There is past history of abortions and stillbirths. Most probable diagnosis:

a. Congenital rubella
b. Congenital toxoplasmosis
c. Congenital syphilis
d. Neonatal pemphigus

Features of congenital syphilis

- Snuffles, aka "syphilitic rhinitis", which appears similar to the rhinitis of the common cold, except it is more severe, lasts longer, often involves bloody rhinorrhea, and is often associated with laryngitis
- Petechiae
- Other skin rash
- Enlarged liver (abdominal distension)
- Enlarged spleen (abdominal distension).

56. NOT a common manifestation of congenital rubella:

a. Deafness b. PDA
c. Aortic stenosis d. Mental retardation

Congenital defects in CR include cardiovascular malformations (patent ductus arteriosus), microcephaly, cataracts and microphthalmia. Late sequelae include deafness, mental retardation, thyroid disorders, diabetes mellitus, degenerative brain disease, infantile autism etc.

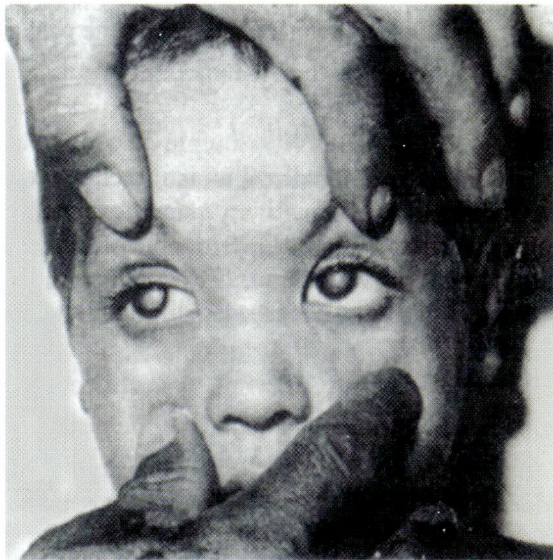

Congenital cataract (bilateral). The child had several other features of congenital rubella syndrome, including mental retardation, deafness, patent ductus arteriosus, syndactyly and hepatosplenomegaly

Ans. 53. **b.** Lower areola... 54. **a.** Anencephaly 55. **c.** Congenital syphilis 56. **c.** Aortic stenosis

57. Triple test for diagnosis of Down syndrome includes all EXCEPT:

a. Beta HCG b. Alpha fetoprotein
c. Serum HPL d. Serum estriol

AFP levels are low in Down syndrome whereas beta-HCG and serum estriol levels are raised.

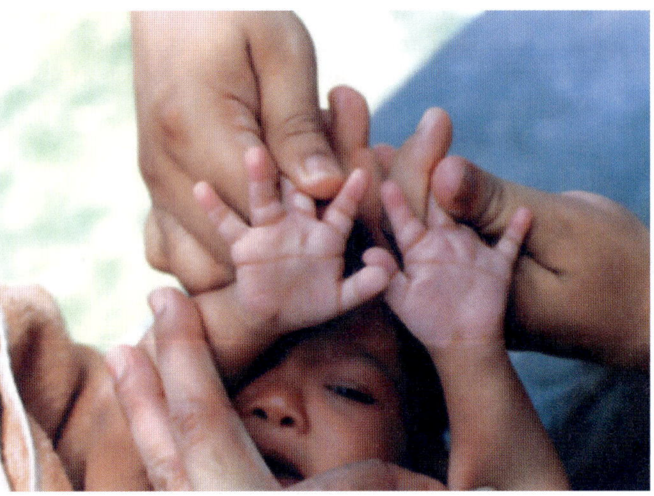

Simian (single palmar) crease in Down syndrome

58. Recurrent respiratory infection does NOT occur in:

a. Tetralogy of Fallot
b. Atrial septal defect
c. Ventricular septal defect
d. Bronchiectasis

Manifestations of Fallot tetralogy usually become evident after the closure of the ductus arteriosus begins. Cyanosis of lips and nailbeds (blue baby) and dyspnea are the earliest presenting features. As the child grows, he feels comfortable while lying down or in squatting position only. Anoxic, hypoxic or blue (hypercyanotic) spells may occur due to cerebral anoxia.

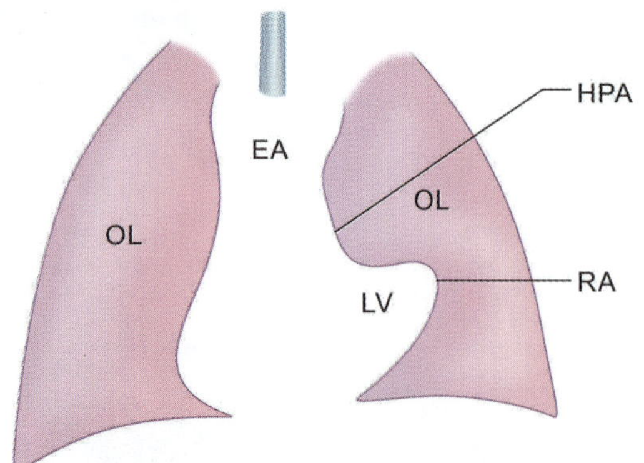

Classical X-ray appearance of Fallot's tetralogy. Note the boot-shaped heart

EA-Enlarged aorta
RV-Right ventricle
HPA-Hypoplastic pulmonary artery
RA-Raised apex
OL-Oligemic lung
LV-Left ventricle

59. MC congenital defect in Down syndrome:

a. PDA
b. ASD
c. Atrioventricular septal defect
d. VSD

Congenital heart disease (usually atrioventricular canal, VSD or ASD: rarely TOF) is usually seen in Down's syndrome.

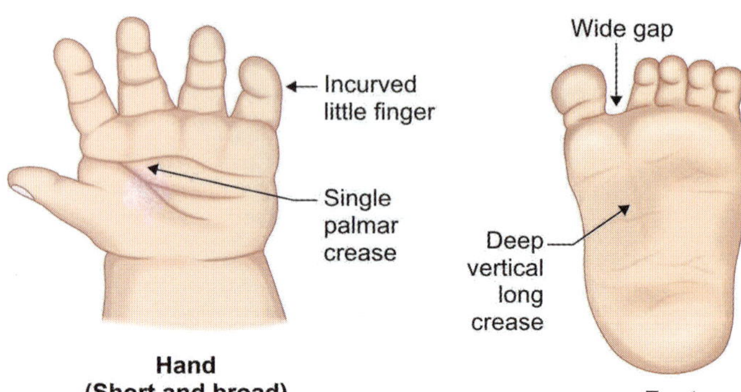

Hand and sole of foot in Down syndrome

60. All of the following are associated with Down syndrome EXCEPT:

a. Sensory hearing loss b. VSD
c. Hypothyroidism d. Duodenal atresia

Sensori-neural hearing loss is a feature of congenital rubella syndrome.

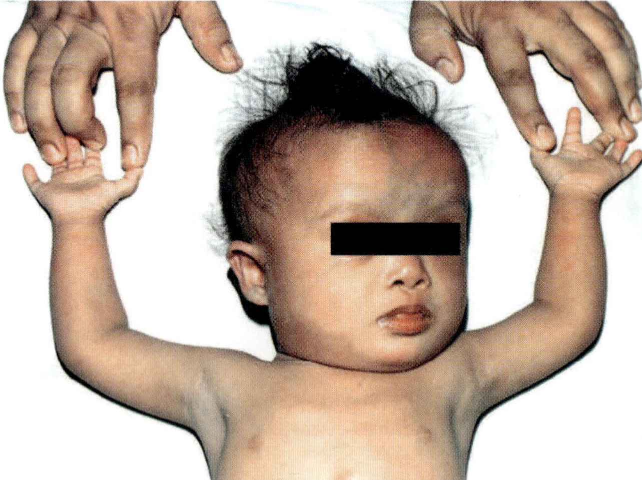

Down syndrome. Note the characteristic facial features

61. MC cause of heart failure in infancy:

a. Congenital heart disease
b. Pericarditis
c. Rheumatic fever
d. Myocarditis

By definition, congestive cardiac failure (CCF), means failure on the part of the heart to maintain an output necessary for the needs of the body at rest or during

Ans. **57. c.** Serum HPL **58. a.** Tetralogy of Fallot **59. c.** Atrioventricular... **60. a.** Sensory hearing loss **61. a.** Congenital heart disease

stress following myocardial failure. In constrictive pericarditis, the cause of peripheral circulatory congestion lies in the definite mechanical obstruction and not in myocardium.

Causes of CCF according to age	
Fetus	Severe anemia from fetomaternal transfusion or hemolysis, tachycardia (supraventricular or ventricular), complete heart block
Newborn	Transposition of great vessels, aortic atresia, coarctation of aorta, patent ductus arteriosus, pulmonary stenosis/atresia, hypoplastic left heart syndrome.
1 to 2 months	Transposition of great vessels, endocardial cushion defects, ventricular septal defect, patent ductus arteriosus, aortic stenosis, coarctation of aorta, anomalous pulmonary venous connection.
3 to 6 months	Endocardial fibroelastosis, transposition of great vessels, ventricular septal defect, coarctation of aorta.
6 to 12 months	Endocardial fibroelastosis, ventricular septal defect.
1 to 4 years	Carditis, anemia, nephrotic syndrome, acute nephritis, endocardial fibroelastosis, atrial or ventricular septal defect.
4 to 12 years and later	All foregoing causes plus rheumatic heart disease.

62. Congenital rubella causes all EXCEPT:

a. Hydrocephalus
b. Cardiac defects
c. Cataract
d. Deafness

Neonatal manifestations include low birth weight, hepatosplenomegaly, icterus, hemolytic anemia, thrombocytopenic purpura, petechiae or maculopapular rash, and osteitis.

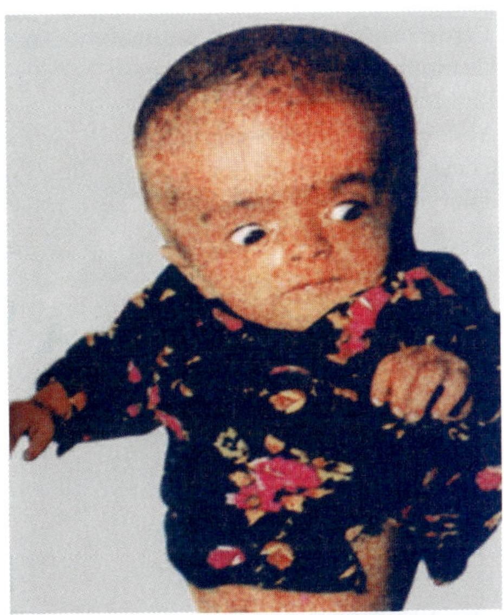

Congenital hydrocephalus. Note the "sunset" sign in the eyes in addition to enlarged head (43 cm) in this neonate

CVS DISORDER

63. MC cause of systemic hypertension in children:

a. Lactic acidosis
b. Nephrotic syndrome
c. Acute glomerulonephritis
d. Coarctation of aorta

In children, the hypertension is due to secondary causes in over 90% of case. Among them renal causes account for about 75% of cases. The essential hypertension, hypertension without any known underlying disease, accounts for only 5-10% of cases in children.

Causes of transient hypertension in children	
Common causes	*Others*
❑ Acute post streptococcal glomerulonephritis Hemolytic uremic syndrome Anaphylactoid purpura	Increased intracranial pressure Guillain–Barré syndrome Poliomyelitis
❑ Post renal transplant/urological surgery Hypervolemia Renal trauma	Hypernatremia Corticosteroids/contraceptive administration Familial dysautonomia Postcoarctation repair

64. Single heart sound (S2) is heard in:

a. Transposition of great vessels
b. Ebstein's anomaly
c. Tetralogy of Fallot
d. Eisenmenger's syndrome

Auscultatory findings in TOF

- Typical murmur is loud short systolic, at left sterna border in third space (usually not accompanied by a thrill)
- The murmur is soft rather than harsh in very severe degree of the disease.
- P_2 is usually single

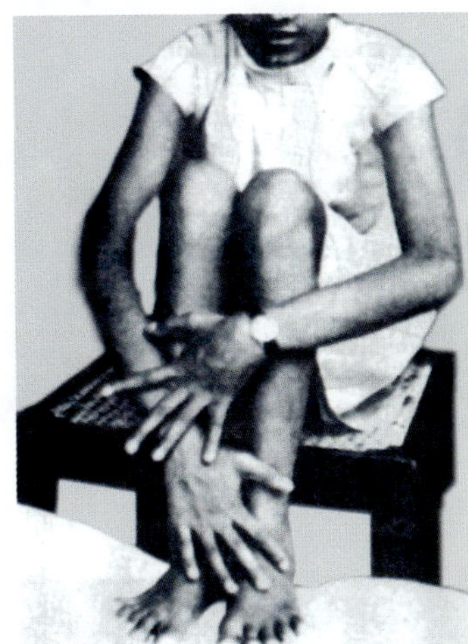

Gross clubbing in a girl with Fallot's tetralogy

Ans. **62. a.** Hydrocephalus **63. c.** Acute glomerulone... **64. c.** Tetralogy of Fallot

65. Rib notching of 4-9th rib with double bulging is seen in:

a. Aortic aneurysm
b. Aortic dissection
c. Co-arctation of aorta
d. Diaphragmatic hernia

X-ray chest findings of COA include some left ventricular enlargement, notching of the ribs caused by intercostals collaterals and "E" sign on barium swallow. The first arch of the "E" is due to dilatation of aorta before the coarctation, the second due to postnecrotic dilatation and the middle due to the coarctation per se.

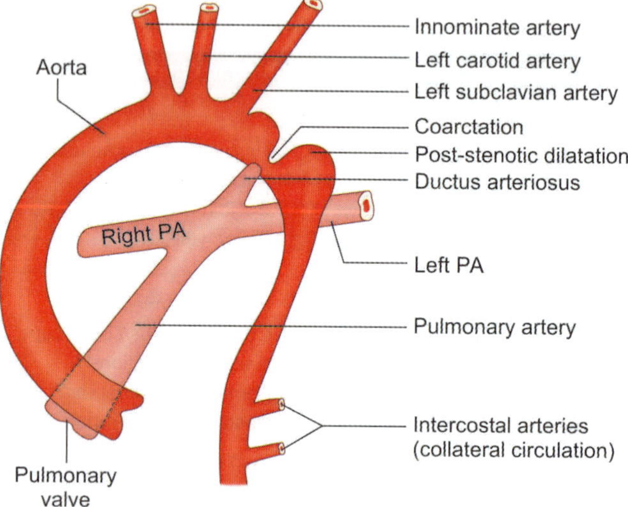

Adult (postductal) type of coarctation of aorta. Note the collaterals which spare the infant from left ventricular failure

66. All of the following are features of chest radiography in Tetralogy of fallot EXCEPT:

a. Boot shaped heart shadow
b. In 80% right sided arch of aorta
c. Oligemic lung fields
d. Right atrial enlargement

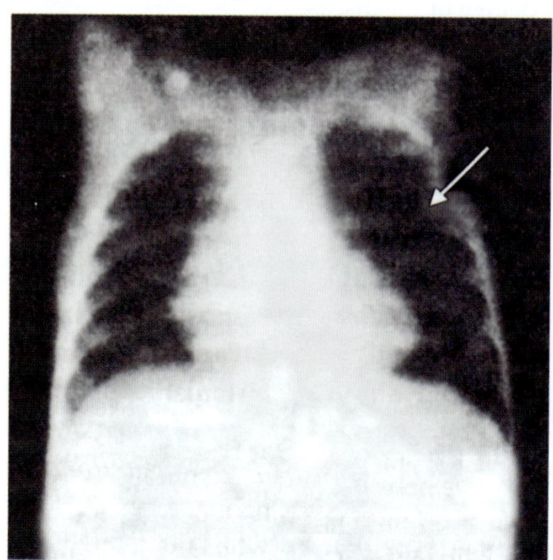

Chest X-ray in Fallot's tetralogy. Note the bootshaped heart and oligemic lung fields

X-ray chest of TOF reveals oligemic lung fields (poorly vascularized lungs), a small boot-shaped heart (Coeur en sabot) with the tip of the boot turned up above the diaphragm (because of right ventricular hypertrophy), and concavity of the pulmonary artery segment (small pulmonary conus). One in every 4 or 5 cases of Fallot tetralogy has right aortic arch.

67. LEAST useful in the management of TOF:

a. Anastomosis of a systemic artery with pulmonary artery
b. Modified Blalock-Taussig shunt
c. Administer 100% oxygen
d. None of the above

General measures in the management of TOF include correction of iron deficiency anemia, and dehydration and an appropriate antibiotic for bacterial infection. Nevertheless, the best approach is to refer the child for surgical treatment as soon as he starts having anoxic spells.

Selective treatment of hypercyanotic spells
1. Comfort the child and place in knee-chest position.
2. Administer humidified O_2 by face mask
3. Give morphine, 0.1–0.2 mg/kg. (IV)
4. Begin IV fluid replacement and volume expansion (if child is anemic, administer blood)
5. Treat acidosis with sodium bicarbonates
6. Administer propranolol, 0.1 to 0.2 mg/kg (IV)
7. Increase systemic vascular resistance by IV administration of vaso-pressors like methoxamine or phenylephrine. Titrate dose to increase systemic systolic blood pressure by 20%. In no case this step should be allowed to postpone surgical intervention
8. Operate to repair defect or to establish systemic-to-pulmonary artery anastomosis

68. NOT true regarding Ebstein anomaly:

a. Cyanotic congenital heart disease
b. Right ventricular hypertrophy
c. Abnormality of tricuspid valve
d. Chest X-ray shows right atrial and ventricular enlargement

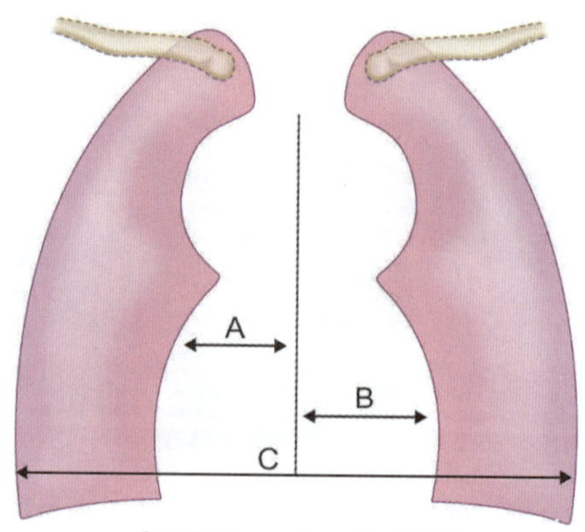

Cardiothoracic ratio OSC

Ans. 65. **c.** Coarctation o... 66. **b.** In 80% right sided... 67. **c.** Administer 100%... 68. **b.** Right ventricular...

The abnormal tricuspid valve (all cusps except anterior) divides the right ventricle into two parts, an atrialized part that is continuous with the right atrium and a normal portion consisting of myocardial tissue. As a result, right atrium becomes huge.

INFECTIOUS DISEASES

69. A HIV positive symptomatic newborn child would receive all vaccines EXCEPT:

a. Mumps vaccine
b. Measles
c. Tetanus
d. BCG

Children with symptomatic HIV infection should not be given oral polio vaccine or BCG. Children with asymptomatic HIV infection should receive BCG in addition to the vaccines mentioned above.

70. A 2-year-old male child was brought to the emergency department with a history of cough and fever for 5 days. He was unable to drink water for last 24 hours. On examination, the child was having weight of 5 kg and respiratory rate of 45/minute with fever. As per IMNCI, the child will be classified as:

a. No pneumonia
b. Pneumonia
c. Severe pneumonia
d. Very severe pneumonia

'Very severe pneumonia' is indicated by presence of cyanosis, severe chest indrawing and inability to feed (treated by I/V chloramphenicol at hospital)

71. To diagnose HIV infection in a 2 months old child, which one is NOT used:

a. p24 antigen
b. DNA PCR
c. Viral culture
d. ELISA

The definitive diagnosis of HIV infection in children born to HIV infected mothers is cumbersome due to the following reasons. An HIV infected mother transmits her IgG antibodies to the newborn transplacentally. Children born to infected mothers are usually antibody positive at birth, but only 15-30 percent are actually infected. Maternally transmitted antibodies usually dip to undetectable levels in 9 months but occasionally remain at significant levels until 18 months; hence IgG antibody tests are not reliable indicators of infection status in a child before 18 months of age. Therefore, presence of antibody beyond this period is necessary to consider the child infected, specially in an asymptomatic child. Now tests are available that can diagnose definite HIV infection even in newborn. Viral diagnostic assays, such as HIV DNA or RNA PCR, HIV culture, or HIV p24 antigen immune dissociated p24 (ICD-p24) are useful in the young infant. Detection of p24 antigen is less sensitive.

PEDIATRIC ONCOLOGY

72. MC hematological malignancy in children:

a. ALL
b. AML
c. CLL
d. CML

About 98% of children suffering from leukemia have acute type of the disease. Mostly it is lymphocytic leukemia (ALL) which accounts for 76% of the cases. Acute nonlymphocytic leukemia (ANLL) is responsible for 20% and chronic myelocytic leukemia (CML) and others together form a meager 4%.

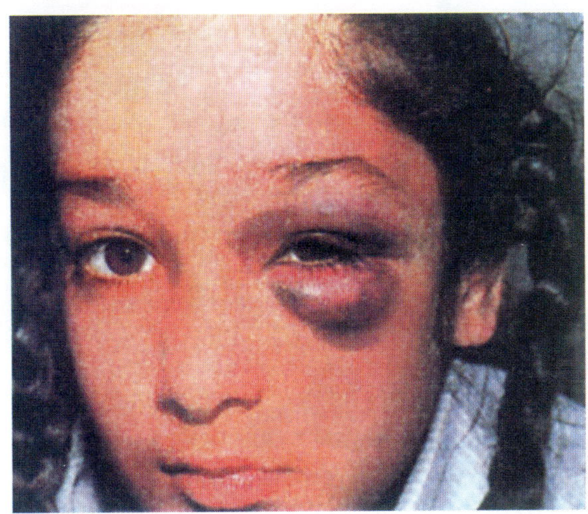

ALL. Note the black eye. The patient had severe anemia, sternal tenderness, generalized adenopathy and hepatosplenomegaly. Bone marrow was full of "blast" cells

73. MC malignant neoplasm of infancy is:

a. Malignant teratoma
b. Neuroblastoma
c. Wilm's tumor
d. Hepatoblastoma

Neuroblastoma is a malignant tumor arising from sympathetic ganglia or adrenal medulla. The common locations of neuroblastoma are the abdomen and the chest.

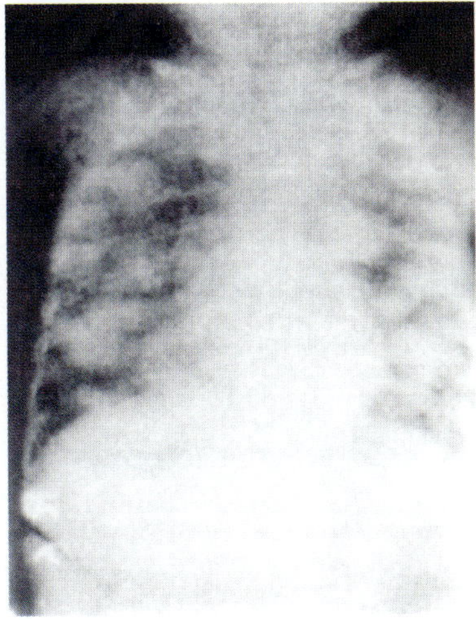

Secondaries in lungs from neuroblastoma

74. MC malignancy in children is:

a. Retinoblastoma
b. Lymphoma and leukemia
c. Wilm's tumor
d. Neuroblastoma

Ans. 69. **d.** BCG 70. **d.** Very severe pneum... 71. **d.** ELISA 72. **a.** ALL
73. **b.** Neuroblastoma 74. **b.** Lymphoma and leukemia

MCQs with Short Explanations

According to a conservative estimate, nearly 50,000 children suffer from cancer every year. In terms of frequency, leukemias (33%) top the list followed by brain tumors (20%) and lymphoma (12%).

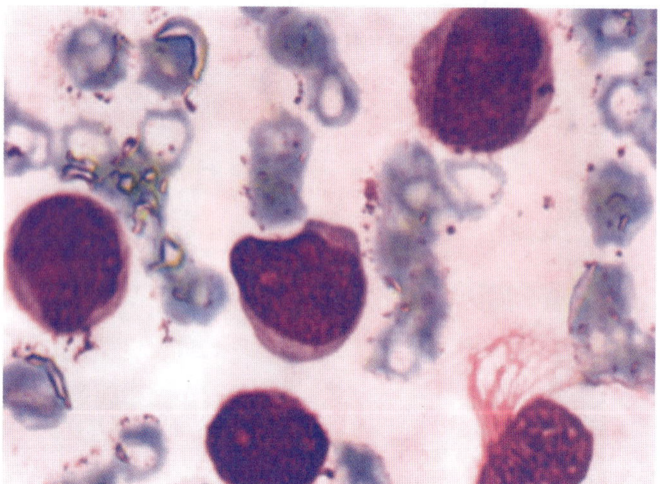

Bone marrow in ALL. Note the large number of blast cells

75. Most common malignancy of the childhood:

a. CLL b. ALL
c. CML d. AML

ALL accounts for 76% of the cases of all the leukemia in childhood.

Categories of childhood leukemia
Acute lymphocytic leukemia (ALL)
1. Standard-risk ALL (Null cell)
2. High-risk ALL – T-Cell ALL – B-Cell ALL
Acute nonlymphocytic leukemia (ANLL) M1 (myeloblastic, no maturation) M2 (myeloblastic, some maturation) M3 (hypergranular promyelocytic) M4 (myelomonocytic) M5 (monocytic) M6 (erythroleukemia)
Chronic myelocytic leukemia (CML) 1. Adult form – Chronic phase – Blast crisis 2. Juvenile form—Congenital leukemia

76. MC inherited childhood tumor:

a. Wilm's tumor b. Retinoblastoma
c. Neuroblastoma d. Leukemia

This rare ocular tumor, though the commonest ocular neoplasm of childhood, usually develops in the posterior portion of the retina. All children with bilateral disease and 10–20% with unilateral disease have a genetic predisposition. The retinoblastoma gene is located on chromosome 13.

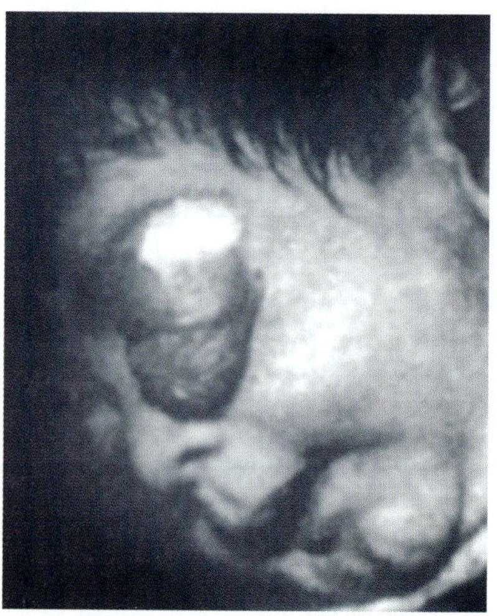

Unilateral retinoblastoma

77. NOT true for Wilm's tumor:

a. Most commonly metastasizes to lung
b. Presents as abdominal mass
c. Hematuria is the presenting symptoms
d. Present after 5 years of age

Wilm's tumor (nephroblastoma) is by and large next only to neuroblastoma in frequency of occurrence among the solid tumors of infancy and childhood. Almost half of the sufferers older than 2 years show metastases. About one-fourth under 2 years too have some metastases.

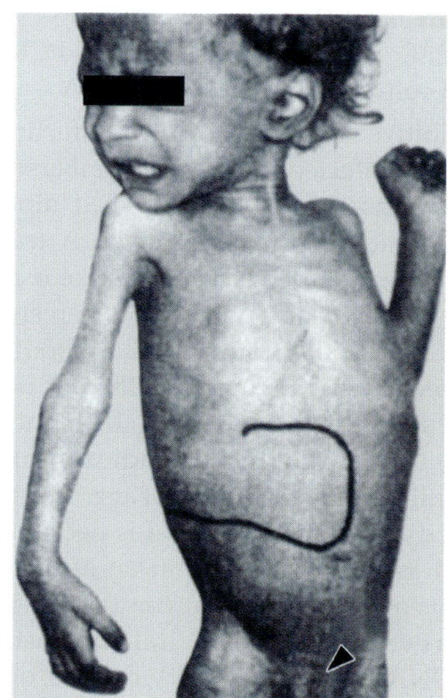

Wilms' tumor

78. MC thyroid neoplasm in children is:

a. Thyroid lymphoma b. Medullary carcinoma
c. Follicular carcinoma d. Papillary carcinoma

Age of presentation of

- Thyroid lymphoma: Older patients
- Medullary carcinoma: Middle age

Ans. 75. **b.** ALL 76. **b.** Retinoblastoma 77. **d.** Present after 5 years... 78. **d.** Papillary carcinoma

- Follicular carcinoma: 30–50 years
- Papillary carcinoma: 20–40 years

79. A malignant tumor of childhood that frequently metastasizes to bone marrow most often is:

a. Wilm's tumor
b. Neuroblastoma
c. Adrenal gland tumors
d. Granulosa cell tumor of ovary

Early metastases constitute the hallmark of the neuroblastoma. Bone marrow examination may show secondary deposits, i.e. neuroblasts, which may simulate leukemia.

Evans clinical staging system for neuroblastoma	
Stage I	Tumor confined to organ or structure of origin
Stage II	Tumor extending in continuity beyond organ or structure of origin but not crossing the midline; regional nodes on homolateral side may be involved
Stage III	Tumor extending in continuity beyond the midline; original nodes may be involved bilaterally; bilateral extension of midline disease
Stage IV	Remote disease involving selection, organs, soft tissue, distant nodes, and so on
Stage V	Patients who would otherwise be stage I or II, i.e. with small and/or resectable primary tumor, but who have remote disease confined only to one or more of the following sites: liver, skin or bone marrow (not bone)

80. Wilm's tumor is NOT associated with:

a. Bilateral polycystic kidney
b. Undescended testes
c. Hemihypertrophy
d. Aniridia

Wilm's tumor is embryonal in origin and develops within the kidney parenchyma, distorting it and invading the surrounding tissues. Existence of certain congenital anomalies predisposes to its development.

Accompaniments of Wilms' tumor
❑ Ambiguous genitalia
❑ Undescended testes
❑ Hypospadias
❑ Duplication of ureter or kidney
❑ Horse-shoe kidney
❑ Aniridia
❑ Hemihypertrophy
❑ Beckwith syndrome

81. True regarding Wilm's tumor are all EXCEPT:

a. MC malignant tumor of the kidneys
b. Frequency similar in boys and girls
c. Presents commonly between 5–10 years of age
d. Bilateral affection may be seen

Wilm's tumor is commonly seen between 2–5 years.

Clinical staging for Wilms' tumor (NWTS Group)	
Stage I	Limited to the kidneys; can be fully excised with capsular surface intact
Stage II	Extends beyond the kidney but can be fully excised
Stage III	Residual nonhematogenous extension of the tumor, confined to the abdomen following surgery
Stage IV	Hematogenous metastases, most frequently involving the lung
Stage V	Bilateral kidney involvement in 5 to 10% cases

MISCELLANEOUS

82. Best way to diagnosing Post streptococcal glomerulonephritis:

a. Mild proteinuria, high cholesterol and normal ASO titer
b. Mild proteinuria, high cholesterol and high ASO titer
c. Mild proteinuria, hematuria and normal ASO titer
d. Mild proteinuria, hematuria and high ASO titer

Acute glomerulonephritis is characterized by the sudden appearance of hematuria, proteinuria, red blood cell casts in the urine, edema, and hypertension with or without oliguria. ASO titers are frequently used to document streptococcal infection, but a more sensitive test is the streptozyme test, which tests antibodies to ASO, anti–DNAse B, AHase, and anti-NAD.

83. All are problems of pre-school age children EXCEPT:

a. Pica
b. Stuttering
c. Truancy
d. Sleep disturbances

Truancy is any intentional unauthorized or illegal absence from compulsory education. It is absences caused by students of their own free will, and usually does not refer to legitimate "excused" absences, such as ones related to medical conditions.

84. The most common presentation of neonatal meningitis is:

a. Bulging fontanelles
b. Nuchal rigidity
c. Poor feeding
d. Convulsion

In newborns and small infants, pyogenic meningitis may have insidious onset with meagre symptoms like refusal to take feed, fever and irritability. Some may have convulsions. These, especially in the presence of bulging anterior fontanel, should arouse suspicion of meningitis.

Age wise etiology of pyogenic meningitis
Under 2 months
❑ Gram-negative organisms, especially *E. coli*
❑ Group B beta-Streptococcus hemolyticus
❑ Listeria monocytogenes
2 months to 6 years
❑ *H. influenzae*
❑ *Pneumococcus*

Contd...

Ans. 79. **b.** Neuroblastoma
80. **a.** Bilateral polycystic kidney
81. **c.** Presents commonly between 5-10 years of age
82. **d.** Mild proteinuria, hematuria and high ASO titre
83. **c.** Truancy
84. **c.** Poor feeding

Contd...

Age wise etiology of pyogenic meningitis
❑ *N. meningitidis*
Beyond 6 years
❑ Pneumococcus
❑ *N. meningitidis*

85. MC cause of diarrhea in children:

a. Vibrio cholera b. *E. coli*
c. Rotavirus d. Pneumococcus

Recent evidence has indicated that viruses, such as rotavirus and Norwalk and Norwalk-like agents, are responsible for majority of the acute diarrhea in infants and young children.

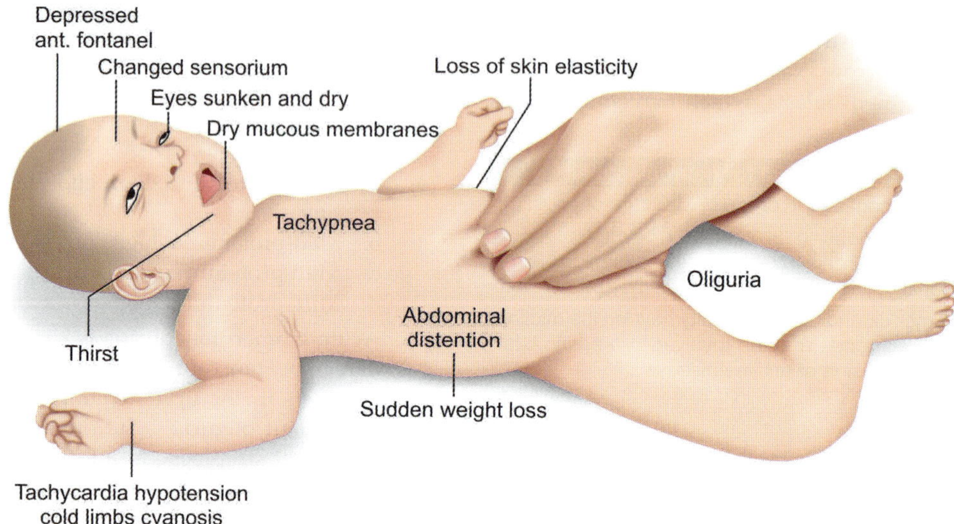

Severe diarrheal dehydration. Note the classical features

86. MC cause of bacterial pneumonia in children is:

a. *Streptococcus pyogenes*
b. *Hemophilus influenzae*
c. *Streptococcus pneumoniae*
d. *Staphylococcus aureus*

Pneumococcaol pneumonia accounts for 90% of bacterial pneumonias in childhood. After first year of life, it is responsible for virtually all bacterial pneumonias.

Predisposing factors for chronic pneumonia
Immunodeficiency
❑ PEM
❑ HIV
Congenital respiratory malformations
❑ Tracheoesophageal fistula
❑ Gastroesophageal reflux
Congenital heart disease
❑ Ventricular septal defect
Defective clearance of airway secretions
❑ Cystic fibrosis
Chronic pulmonary diseases
❑ Tuberculosis
❑ Bronchiectasis
❑ Asthma

87. A child with diarrhea has deep and rapid respiration. Most likely diagnosis is:

a. Respiratory acidosis b. Respiratory alkalosis
c. Metabolic acidosis d. Metabolic alkalosis

In significant metabolic acidosis (pH <7.2), respiration becomes deep and rapid (Kussmaul breathing) and the child becomes drowsy, confused and stuporous. In severe acidosis, peripheral vasodilation, vascular collapse and shock may follow.

Normal levels of blood pH, pCO$_2$ and HCO$_3$		
	Blood levels	
Criteria	*Venous*	*Arterial*
pH	7.35-7.40	7.38-7.45
PCO$_2$	45-50 torr	35-45 torr
HCO3	24-25 mEq/L	23-27 mEq/L

88. Nocturnal enuresis may be considered normal up to:

a. 3 years
b. 4 years
c. 5 years
d. 6 years

The term, enuresis, denotes normal urinary bladder emptying at a wrong place and time at least twice a month after the age of 5 years. Nocturnal enuresis refers to bedwetting.

Ans. **85. c.** Rotavirus **86. c.** Streptococcus... **87. c.** Metabolic acidosis **88. c.** 5 years

89. The coagulation profile in a 13-year-old girl with menorrhagia having von Willebrand disease is:

a. Isolated prolonged PTT with a normal PT
b. Isolated prolonged PT with a normal PTT
c. Prolongation of both PT and PTT
d. Prolongation of thrombin time

vWD is an autosomal disorder is characterized by disproportionate bleeding following minor trauma as observed in hemophilia. A noteworthy point is that whereas ristocetin-induced aggregation is normal in classic hemophilia, it is reduced in vWD.

Situations in which clotting time and bleeding time are prolonged	
Prolonged CT	
With high PT	Factor VII deficiency
With high APTT	Factor VIII, IX, XI and XII deficiency, von Willebrand's disease
With high PT and APTT	Vitamin K deficiency, advanced liver disease, DIC, factors V, X, fibrinogen deficiency.
Prolonged BT	
With low platelet count	ITP, drug-induced purpura, leukemia or bone marrow.
With normal platelet count	Henoch-Schonlein purpura

90. A child aged 2 years presents with nonspecific symptoms suggestive of anemia. Peripheral smear shows target cells. He has microcytic hypochromia picture and Hb of 6 g%. There is positive family history. Next investigation is:

a. NESTROFT test
b. HbA1c estimation
c. Hb electrophoresis
d. Osmotic fragility test

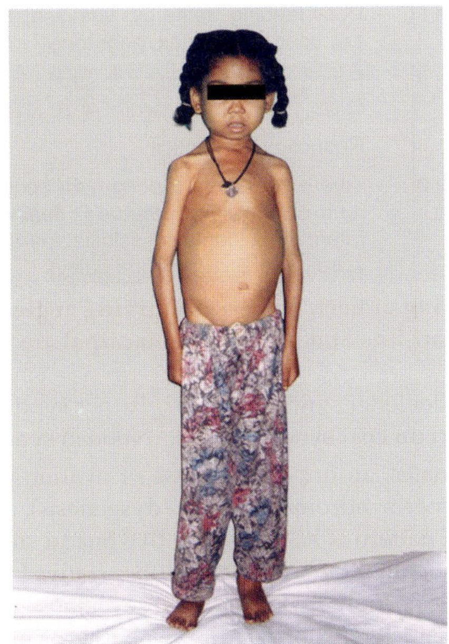

Thalassemia major. Note hemolytic facies and growth retardation. She had considerable splenohepatomegaly

Diagnosis of thalassemia

- Blood picture
  - Microcytic hypochromic anemia
  - Anisocytosis, poikilocytosis, moderate basophilic stippling, nucleated and fragmented erythrocytes, target cells, large number of normoblasts and increased number of reticulocytes
- Bone marrow
  - Erythroid hyperplasia
- Osmotic fragility
  - Reduced fragility (there is resistance to hemolysis in very dilute, i.e. hypotonic solution)
- Hb electrophoresis
  - Fetal hemoglobin exceeds 40% of the total.

91. MC cause of death in diphtheric child:

a. Septicemia
b. Tonsillitis
c. Myocarditis
d. Third nerve palsy

Prognosis of diphtheria is guarded. Almost 50% of the cases die if left untreated. With recommended treatment, mortality is around 4 to 5% and is usually the result of myocarditis.

Various complications occurring in diphtheria
❑ Bronchopneumonia
❑ Nephritis (mere albuminuria in early stages)
❑ Myocarditis: It may occur any time during the course of the disease. The early development is a bad prognostic sign.
❑ Paralysis about 12 to 21% of the cases suffer from the postdiphtheretic paralysis somewhere between first and sixth week of illness. The following are the various types seen:
a. Pharyngeal and palatal paralysis are manifested by nasal voice, dysphagia, nasal regurgitation, and failure to lift the palate.
b. Ocular paralysis occurs late and is second in frequency. It is manifested in the form of diplopia, squint, ptosis, ophthalmoplegias, etc.
c General paralysis occurs quite late. There may be quadriplegia, paralysis of the neck muscles and respiratory embarrassment, as a result of involvement of the diaphragm from phrenic nerve paralysis. Even CSF protein may be elevated. This complication closely simulates Guillain-Barré syndrome.
❑ Vasomotor disturbances in the form of hypotension and cardiac failure 2 to 3 weeks after onset of the disease occur rarely.
❑ Gastritis
❑ Hepatitis

92. Subacute sclerosing panencephalitis is a complication of:

a. Pertussis
b. Diphtheria
c. Measles
d. Pneumonia

Ans. **89. a.** Isolated prolonged PTT with a normal PT **90. c.** Hb electrophoresis
91. c. Myocarditis **92. c.** Measles

Very rarely, subacute sclerosing panencephalitis (SSPE), a universally fatal disease, may result as long-term sequelae on an average of 6 years (range 3-6 years) after the attack of measles. It is characterized by myoclonic jerks and mental deterioration. It behaves like a degenerative disorder.

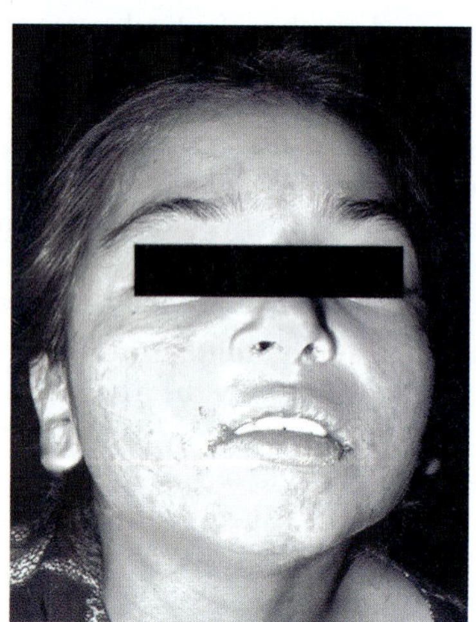

Measles: Note the classical pink, blotchy, irregular macular rash first involving the face and retroauricular area

93. DOC for mycoplasma pneumonia is:

a. Erythromycin b. Ampicillin
c. Gentamicin d. Ciprofloxacin

Primary atypical pneumonia resulting from mycoplasma pneumoniae is treated with erythromycin or tetracyclines in case of grown-up children.

Indication of microbiologic examination of body secretions in diagnosis of respiratory disease	
Secretions	*Indications*
Sputum, tracheal, bronchial, gastric microscopy/culture	Lung abscess, bronchiectasis, cystic fibrosis, tuberculosis, *Pneumocystis carinii* pneumonia
Nasal cytology for eosinophils	Allergic rhinitis, nasobronchial allergy
Special iron stains of bronchial secretions	Hemosiderosis

94. Treatment of choice in bronchiolitis in children is:

a. Ribavirin b. Amantadine
c. Vidarabine d. Zidovudine

The only recognized antiviral drug for RSV infection is ribavirin aerosol which should be administered early in the course of the disease in very sick or high-risk infants.

95. Steroids are useful in:

a. Minimal change disease
b. Rapidly progressive glomerulonephritis
c. Membranous glomerulonephritis
d. Post-streptococcal glomerulonephritis

Corticosteroids constitute the cornerstone of management of nephrotic syndrome. About 80 to 85% of children with nephrotic syndrome are of "minimal lesion", or "corticosteroid-responsive" type. The term, "minimal change nephrotic syndrome" (MCNS) is currently considered most appropriate for this condition.

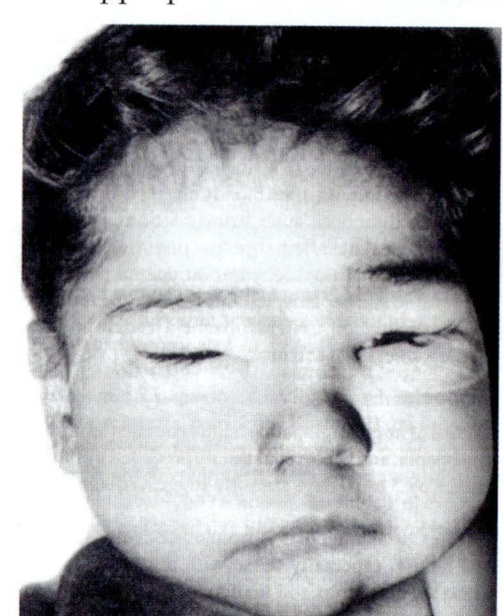

Nephrotic syndrome, showing gross periorbital edema

96. NOT a cause of craniotabes:

a. Kernicterus b. Syphilis
c. Hydrocephalus d. Rickets

Kernicterus: Unconjugated (indirect) bilirubin is neurotoxic, especially to basal ganglia in full-term neonates and to cranial nerve nuclei and thalamus in preterm neonates with birth weight <1500 g.

Staging of kernicterus (bilirubin encephalopath)	
Stage I	Poor feeding, lethargy, vomiting, high-pitched cry, poor Moro reflex, poor tone
Stage II	Fever, seizures, rigidity, opisthotonos,oculogyric crisis, paralysis of upward gaze, even death
Stage III	Reduction in spasticity
Stage IV	This is the stage of long-term sequelae in the form of spasticity, athetosis, deafness, mental retardation, dental dysplasia, paralysis of upward gaze, etc. (cerebral palsy)

97. Webbing of neck, increased carrying angle, low posterior hair line and short 4th metacarpal are characteristic of:

a. Klinefelter syndrome b. Turner syndrome
c. Cri du chat syndrome d. Noonan syndrome

In females, an important cause of ovarian dysfunction is Turner syndrome (gonadal dysgenesis). Its chromosomal pattern is XO with negative buccal smear though occasionally XO/ XX pattern with negative buccal smear may be encountered. Delayed or even absent secondary sex characters, short stature, webbing of neck, cubitus valgus and mental retardation are its important clinical features.

Ans. 93. **a.** Erythromycin 94. **a.** Ribavirin 95. **a.** Minimal change... 96. **a.** Kernicterus 97. **b.** Turner syndrome

Salient features of leading chromosomal disorders			
Syndromes	*Chromosomal aberration*	*Incidence*	*Manifestations*
Down syndrome	Trisomy 21 translocation mosaicism	1 in 600–800 births	Mongolian facies, simian crease, slanted palpebral apertures, hypotonia etc.
Patau syndrome	Trisomy 13	1 in 20,000 births	Cleft lip, polydactyly and flexed fingers, hemangiomas, broad, flat nose, low-set malformed ears, microcephaly, microphthalmia, hypoplastic or absent ribs, genital and visceral anomalies, including cardiac and cerebral
Edward syndrome	Trisomy 18	1 in 8,000 births	LBW, closed fists, narrow hips with poor abduction, rocker-bottom feet, microcephaly, microphthalmia, cardiac and renal anomalies, mental retardation; 95% mortality in infancy
Mosaicism	Trisomy 8	Not known	Long face with high forehead, broad upturned nose, thick everted lower lip, low-set ears, high-arched/ cleft palate, microretrognathia, osteoarticular anomalies, moderate mental retardation
Turner syndrome cardiovascular	Loss (total or a part) of sex chromosome Pattern: 45, XO	1 in 8,000 livebirths	Short stature, peripheral edema, lymphadema, extra skin fold/webbing of neck, renal and anomalies, gonadal dysplasia, some learning disability, absence of sex characters, infertility, treatment with estrogens
Klinefelter syndrome	An extra X chromosome Pattern: 47, XXY Variants with more than X chromosomes may occur	1.3 in 1,000 livebirths; 80 in 1,000 in mentally retarded; 100-200 in 1,000 in infertile males	Relatively tall stature, gynecomastia, slow development of secondary sex characters, azoospermia, small testes, infertility, psychosocial, behavior maladjustment, mental retardation; treatment replacement therapy with testosterone
XYY males minor	Additional Y chromosome(s)	1 in 1,000 livebirths	Relatively tall stature, behavioral problems, infrequently genital anomalies, radioulnar dysostosis and prolonged PR interval
Fragile X syndrome	Fragile site at Xq 27,3 of distal long arm of chromosome X; due to change in size of DNA sequence (alleic expansion)	Commonest cause of mental retardation in males	Mental retardation, long face with prominent jaw and large ears, macroorchidism

98. Duchenne muscular dystrophy is a disease of:

a. Neuromuscular junction
b. Sarcolemmal protein
c. Muscle contractile protein
d. Disuse atrophy due to muscle weakness

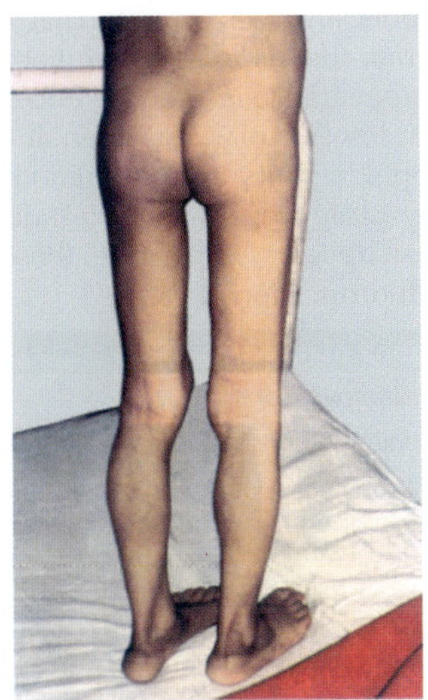

Pseudohypertrophic muscular dystrophy. Note the remarkably bulky calf muscles

Pathologic changes in DMD include various stages of necrosis of muscle fibers, phagocytosis of degenerating fibers, abnormally small fibers and increase in fat and endomysial connective tissue. There are signs of regeneration which eventually disappear.

99. MC cause of meningitis in post-neonatal period:

a. *Klebsiella*
b. *Streptococcus pneumoniae*
c. *Staphylococcus aureus*
d. *Mycobacterium tuberculosis*

In our country, *H. influenzae* and Pneumococcus are the leading causative agents. Meningococcus, Staphylococcus and Streptococcus are less common.

100. FALSE regarding attention deficit hyperactivity disorder/ADHD:

a. Lack of concentration
b. Impulsivity
c. Mental retardation
d. Hyperactivity

Diagnosis of ADHD is mainly clinical. At least 6 symptoms of hyperactivity-impulsiveness or inattentiveness are required.

Ans. 98. **b.** Sarcolemmal... 99. **b.** Streptococcus... 100. **c.** Mental retardation

Diagnostic criteria in ADHD
Inattention
At least six of the following criteria for a minimal of six months:
1. Often fails to give close attention to details or makes careless mistakes in school work or other activities.
2. Often has difficulty in sustaining attention in tasks or play activity.
3. Often doesn't seem to listen where spoken to directly.
4. Often doesn't follow through instructions and fails to finish schoolwork, chores, duties in workplace (not due to oppositional behavior or failure to understand instructions).
5. Often has difficulty in organizing tasks and activities.
6. Often avoids, dislike, or is reluctant to engage in tasks that require sustained mental effort (such as schoolwork or homework).
7. Often loses things necessary for talks or activities, e.g. toys, school assignments, pencils, books, tools, etc.
8. Often easily distracted by extranuous stimuli.
9. Often forgetful in daily activities.
Hyperactivity/Impulsivity
At least six of the following criteria for a minimal of six months:
1. Often fidgets with hands or squirms in seat.
2. Often leaves seat in the classroom or other situations in which remaining seated is expected.
3. Often runs about or climbs excessively in situations in which it is inappropriate.
4. Often has difficulty in playing or in engaging in leisure activities.
5. Often "on the go" or acts as if "driven by a motor".
6. Often talks excessively.
7. Impulsivity
8. Often blurts out answers before questions have been completed.
9. Often has difficulty awaiting turn.
10. Often interrupts or intrudes on others, e.g. bursts into conversation or games.

101. A 5-year-old child suffering from nephrotic syndrome is responding well to steroid therapy. What will be the findings on light microscopy:

a. No findings
b. Basement membrane thickening
c. Hypercelular glomeruli
d. Fusion of foot processes

Minimal change disease shows no changes on light microscopy whereas on electron microscopy shows loss of foot processes.

Side effects of chronic steroid therapy
Electrolytes: Fluid retention (edema), hypokalemia
Disfiguring: Round facial contour, cervicodorsal hump (buffalo), anterocervical hump (Turkey), and pigmentation, hirsutism, baldness, kyphosis
Disquieting: Muscle wasting, hypertension, glycosuria, menstrual disturbances
Enjoyable: Euphoria, increased appetite
Disturbing: Insomnia, polyuria, headache, thinning of skin with development of striae and bruising, myopathy, poor wound healing
Alarming: Epigastric discomfort, intercurrent infections, osteoporosis, psychosis

102. NOT a cause of delayed eruption of teeths:

a. Progeria
b. Hyperthyroidism
c. Hypopituitarism
d. Rickets

Delayed eruption of first tooth (up to as late as 15 months) in a normal child is also seen. Likewise, late appearance of other teeth may also be there. Among the possible factors responsible for delayed dentition, familial and/ or racial tendency, poor nutritional status, rickets and osteogenesis imperfect are important. Very infrequently, a child may have an absolute non-eruption of teeth (anodontoid) which is a classical feature of ectodermal dysplasia.

Temporary (primary) teething	
Birth	*Nil*
6 to 7 months	Central incisors
By 10 months	Laterals incisors
1 to 1½ years	First molars
l¼ to 1¾ years	Cuspids (Canines)
2 to 3 years	Second molars

103. Koplik spot is a feature of:

a. Measles
b. Tetanus
c. Diphtheria
d. Mumps

Koplik's spots are seen in catarrhal stage. These are fine, tiny grain-like papules on faint erythematous base. Their first appearance is over the buccal mucosa, opposite the first lower molar, and then at other sites in the mouth. Koplik's spots are pathognomonic of measles and usually disappear by about 5th day, usually a day after the rash appears. In practice, these are observed in only a small proportion of cases.

Complications of measles
Immediate Complications
❑ Otitis media tops the list of respiratory complications.
❑ Tracheobronchitis, laryngotracheobronchitis, bronchiolitis, bronchopneumonia subcutaneous emphysema* etc. Rarely, measles virus may spread to the lung parenchyma, causing the so-called "giant-cell pneumonia" which may prove fatal. Measles pneumonia in AIDS may occur without any rash. It often proves fatal.
❑ Stomatitis, enteritis and even cancrum oris (noma), especially in malnourished children.

Contd...

Ans. 101. a. No findings **102. b.** Hyperthyroidism **103. a.** Measles

Contd...

Complications of measles
❑ Activation of existing tuberculosis with transient loss of hypersensitivity to tuberculin.
❑ Keratitis and corneal ulceration secondary to vitamin A deficiency that commonly follows measles.
❑ Bleeding diathesis, the so-called hemorrhagic measles. It has a stormy onset with high fever, convulsions, delirium, coma and bleeding. Also termed "black measles", it has a fatal outcome.
❑ Appendicitis
❑ Malnutrition
❑ Encephalitis is rare (just 0.1 percent) but the most dreadful of all. The survivors are invariably left with residual sequelae, including mental retardation.
❑ Remaining CNS complications such as Guillain-Barré syndrome, cerebral thrombophlebitis, hemiplegia, and retrobulbar neuritis are still rarer. – Acute glomerulonephritis – Steven-Johnson syndrome – Decreased cell-mediated immunity and anergy (during few weeks after attack)
❑ Transient ECG changes and myocarditis (uncommon)
Late Complication
❑ Very rarely, subacute sclerosing panencephalitis (SSPE), a universally fatal disease, may result as a long-term sequelae on an average of 6 years (range 3-6 years) after the attack of measles. It is characterized by myoclonic jerks and mental deterioration. It behaves like a degenerativee disorder
* Other cause of subcutaneous emphysema include trauma, asthma, pertussis, foreign body, violent cough, etc.

104. MC cause of nephrotic syndrome in children:

a. Congenital
b. Hemolytic uremic syndrome
c. Chronic glomerulonephritis
d. Minimal change disease

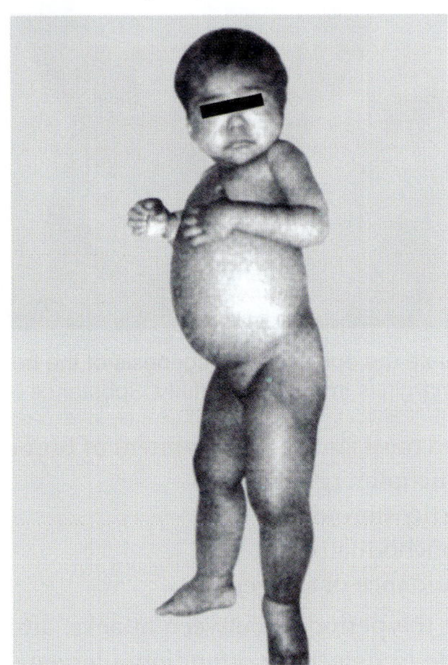

Nephrotic syndrome, showing generalized edema

About 80 to 85% of children with nephrotic syndrome are of "minimal lesion", or "corticosteroid-responsive" type.

105. Best method to diagnose childhood HIV:

a. Western blot
b. ELISA
c. PCR
d. All

Seropositivity alone, unless it is persists beyond 15 months, cannot be counted for establishing diagnosis of perinatal HIV infection. On the other hand, actually infected infants may turn out to be seronegative at 15 months. The ELISA and Western blot tests, therefore, have limited diagnostic value in perinatal AIDS. Culture and polymerase chain reaction (PCR) are recommended for early and dependable diagnosis of perinatal HIV infection.

World Health Organization (WHO) criteria for diagnosis of pediatric AIDS in developing countries such as India
Major Criteria
❑ Weight loss or abnormally slow growth
❑ Chronic diarrhea for over 1 month
❑ Prolonged or intermittent pyrexia for over 1 month
Minor Criteria
❑ Generalized lymphadenopathy
❑ Oropharyngeal candidiasis
❑ Recurrent common bacterial infections
❑ Persistent cough for over 1 month
❑ Generalized dermatitis
❑ Confirmed HIV infection in the mother
Note: The existence of 2 major and 2 minor criteria in the absence of other known causes of immunodeficiency is diagnostic of AIDS

106. FALSE regarding phenylketonuria:

a. Provocative protein meal test helps in the diagnosis
b. Tyrosine becomes essential amino acid in the diet
c. Serum phenylalanine is increased and urinary phenylpyruvate level is increased
d. Phenylalanine should be completed stopped in the diet

A low phenylalanine diet must begin before the baby is 2 weeks old, maintaining the serum phenylalanine at about 8 mg/dL, if mental retardation is to be prevented.

Classification of inborn errors of metabolism
Amino Acid Metabolism Phenylketonuria (PKU), tyrosinosis, albinism, alkaptonuria, cystinosis (including deToni-Fanconi syndrome), cystinuria, homocystinuria, Hartnup disease, maple syrup disease, lysine intolerance.
Carbohydrate Metabolism Congenital lactose intolerance, galactosemia, glycogen storage disease (glycogenosis), diabetes mellitus, scurvy, gargylism. Morquio disease.

Contd...

Ans. 104. **d.** Minimal change... 105. **c.** PCR 106. **d.** Phenylalanine should be completed stopped...

Classification of inborn errors of metabolism
Lipid Metabolism Abetalipoproteinemia, progressive lipodystrophy, lipidosis (Gaucher disease, Neimann-Pick disease. Tay-Sachs disease, hyperlipo-proteinemia).
Protein Metabolism Immunoglobulin deficiencies, absent clotting factors (hemophilia, Christmas disease, afibrogenemia, hypoprothrombinemia), metal-binding protein deficiency (Wilson hepatolenticular degeneration), alpha-1-antitrypsin deficiency (neonatal hepatitis).
Pigment Metabolism Porphyrias, methemoglobinemia, albinism, Waardenburg syndrome, Crigler-Najjar disease, Dubin-Johnson disease, Gilbert disease, Rotor syndrome, primary hemochromatosis.
Unknown Biochemical Defect Osteogenesis imperfecta, Marfan syndrome, achondroplasia, Ehlers-Danlos syndrome.

107. Negri bodies are seen in:

a. Rubella b. Mumps
c. Rabies d. Measles

The pathologic hallmark of rabies is the Negri body that is found in neurons.

Two groups of slow virus infections
Conventional
❑ Subacute sclerosing panencephalitis (SSPE)
❑ Progressive rubella panencephalitis (PRP)
❑ AIDS encephalopathy
❑ Rabies
❑ Cytomegalovirus (CMV) encephalitis
❑ Kozhevnikov's epilepsy
❑ Tropical spastic paraparesis (TSP)/HTLV-I-associated myeopathy (HAM)
❑ Progressive multifocal leukoencephalitis (PML)
❑ (?) Rasmusson chronic encephalitis
Unconventional
❑ Kuru
❑ Creutzfeldt-Jakob disease (CJD)
❑ Gerstmann-Straussler syndrome (GSS)

108. Management of thalassemia major:

a. Iron, blood transfusion and desferrioxamine
b. Blood transfusion and desferrioxamine
c. Folic acid and desferrioxamine
d. Blood transfusion and iron therapy

Allogenic bone marrow transplantation using a matched sibling donor is currently the curative treatment of thalassemia. This form of treatment is expensive and not easily available. In the absence of transplant, transfusion-chelation (desferrioxamine) therapy is the only effective treatment.

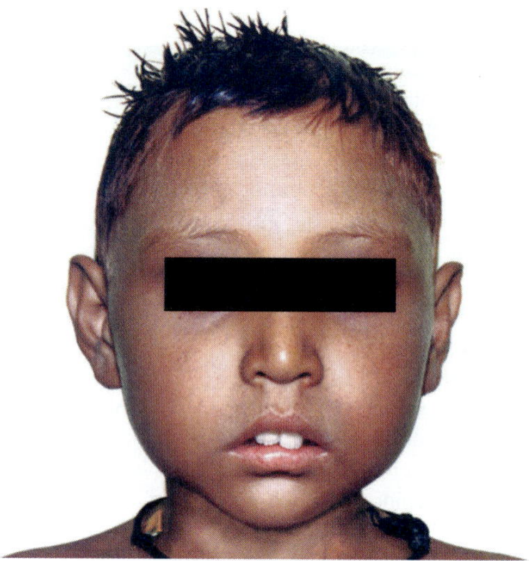

Thalassemia major, showing hemolytic facies

109. Epiphyseal dysgenesis is a pathognomonic feature of:

a. Hyperthyroidism
b. Hypothyroidism
c. Hyperparathyroidism
d. Hypoparathyroidism

In hypothyroidism, X-ray studies are done for bone age and presence of epiphyseal dysgenesis. The latter is seen as numerous foci of ossification, mostly in the head of femur and at times, in the head of humerus.

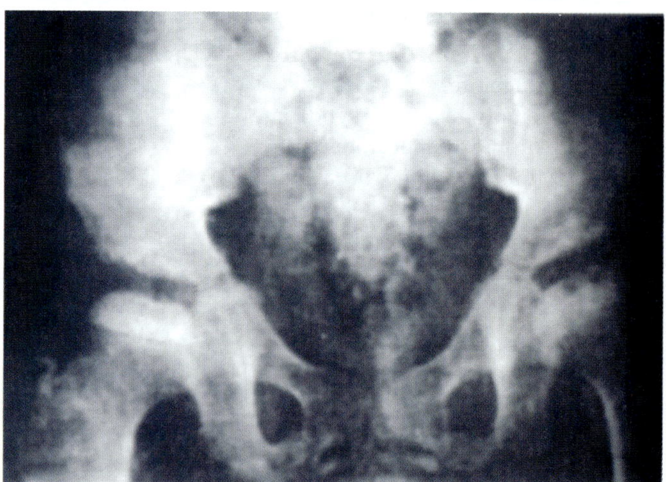

Cretinism. Note the epiphyseal dysgenesis of the head of femur. Epiphyseal margin is irregular and fluffy. Substance is fragmented

110. Best and most successful treatment of bronchial asthma:

a. Anticholinergics
b. Corticosteroids
c. Bronchodilators
d. Avoidance of antigen

During the period in between attacks, attempts should be made to detect the offending allergen, to avoid this and, if possible, to hyposensitize the patient.

Ans. 107. **c.** Rabies 108. **b.** Blood transfusion... 109. **b.** Hypothyroidism 110. **d.** Avoidance of antigen

Pharmacological management (long-term) of different grades of asthma
Mild intermittent (episodic) asthma: Oral or inhaled salbutamol or terbutaline as and when required Mild persistent asthma: Inhaled short-acing beta2 agonists plus inhaled steroids
Moderate persistent asthma *Severe persistent asthma:* Inhalation steroids plus long-acting beta- agonist and/or slow release theophylline. Add on therapy with montelukast yields better control. Poor control is an indication for oral steroids (low dose alternate day prednisolone).

111. Acute stage of poliomyelitis lasts for:

a. 1–1 days b. 10–15 days
c. 2–4 weeks d. 1–2 years

The incubation period is 7 to 14 days (range 5-35 days).

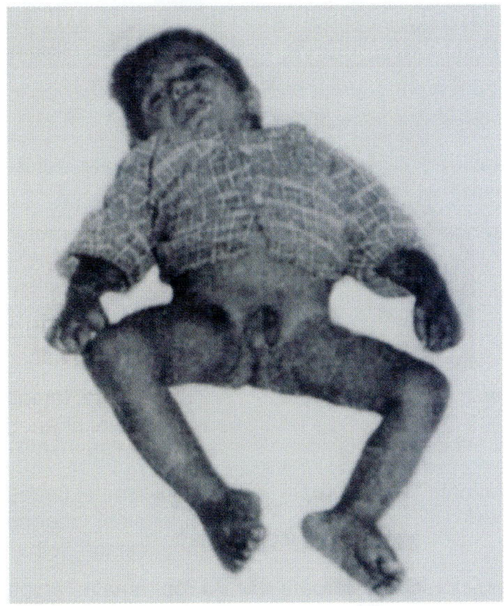

Paralytic polio of both legs. Note the characteristic "frog" position

112. True about administration of corticosteroids for fetal lung maturity all of the following EXCEPT:

a. Repeat dose if the women remain undelivered after the first course
b. Decreased risk of enterocolitis and intracranial hemorrhage
c. Contra-indicated in eclampsia
d. Indicated in women with preterm labor between 24-34 weeks of gestation

Prevention of Hyaline Membrane Disease

- Administration of steroids (dexamethasone or betamethasone) 48 to 72 hours before delivery in case of fetuses of 32 week or less gestation, especially if lecithin in amniotic fluid indicates immaturity of the fetal lungs.
- Administration of one dose of surfactant into trachea of premature neonates during 24 hours after birth. It reduces mortality from HMD.

Causes of neonatal respiratory distress	
Maternal	Toxemia, severe anemia, cardiovascular disease, abnormal uterine contractions, anesthesia or drugs
Obstructive	Aspirated material, macroglossia, glossoptosis, choanal atresia, vascular rings pressing on trachea, goiter, diaphragmatic hernia, tracheoesophageal fistula
Pulmonary	Idiopathic respiratory distress syndrome, pneumonia, pneumothorax, pneumomediastinum, pulmonary edema or hemorrhage, pleural effusion, atelectasis, Wilson-Mikity syndrome*, bronchopulmonary dysplasia*, wetlung syndrome**
Neurologic	Central depression due to birth trauma, anesthesia, drugs, intracranial hemorrhage, phrenic nerve paralysis, intercostal muscle paralysis as in congenital poliomyelitis, Werdnig-Hoffmann disease, myasthenia gravis
Cardiac	Congestive cardiac failure
Metabolic	Acidosis, alkalosis, organic acidemia

* These two conditions occurring in SFD, appear to result from oxygen toxicity. The prognosis is poor. Many of the affected infants die from a progressive respiratory illness like cor pulmonale or CCF.

** This almost benign condition is characterized by perihilar congestion and clears on its own in 2 to 4 days. Poor lymphatic clearing of alveoli appears to be the cause. The other name given to this condition is transient tachypnea of the newborn.

113. FALSE for Hemophilia A:

a. Decreased VIII factor b. Raised PTT
c. Raised PT d. Normal BT

Blood tests in hemophilia

- Clotting time is prolonged
- Bleeding time and prothrombin times are normal
- Clot retraction is also normal
- Prothrombin consumption is low
- Thromboplastin generation is high
- Confirmation of the diagnosis is by specific factor assay

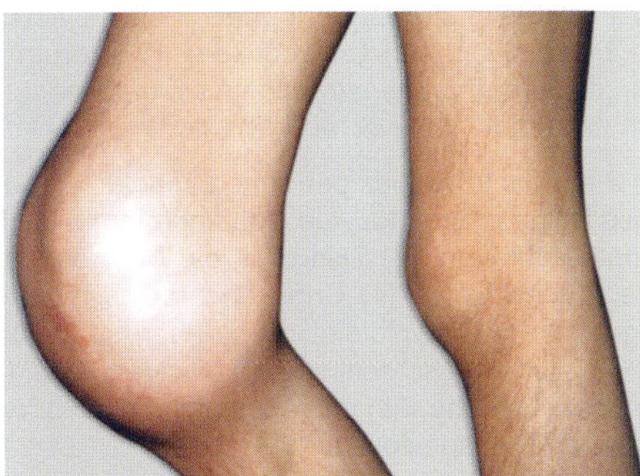

Hemophilia. Note the muscle atrophy and nearly fixed unstable joints from degenerative changes following repeated hemorrhages (hemarthrosis) in a child suffering from classical hemophilia

Ans. 111. b. 10-15 days **112. a.** Repeat dose if the women remain undelivered... **113. c.** Raised PT

114. 100% oxygen will NOT improve cyanosis in which of the following:

a. Bronchial asthma
b. Tetralogy of fallot
c. Eosinophilic pneumonia
d. Interstitial lung disease

Humidified oxygen is given in hypercyanotic spells of TOF (and not 100% oxygen).

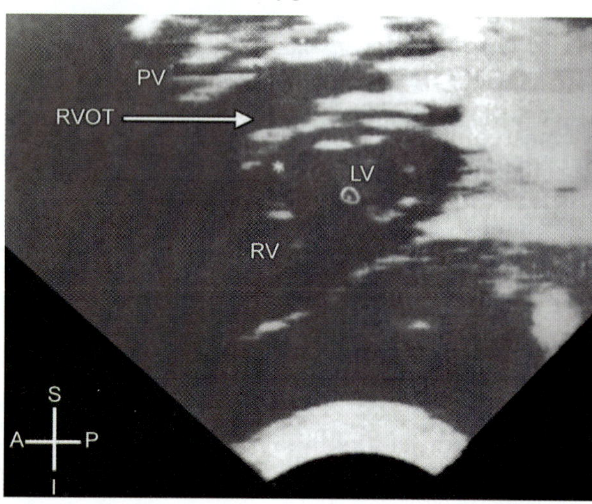

Echocardiography (two-dimensional) in tetralogy of Fallot (TOF)

115. A case of nephritis presents with hematuria and hemoptysis. Antinuclear membrane antibodies are present. Likely diagnosis is:

a. Goodpasture syndrome
b. Nephritic syndrome
c. Nephrotic syndrome
d. Guillain-Barre syndrome

Goodpasture syndrome, only occasionally seen in pediatric practice, is characterized by pulmonary alveolar hemorrhage (clinically presenting as hemoptysis and secondary anemia) and nephritis. Accompanying manifestations may include dyspnea, cough and pyrexia. Progressive renal failure is common.

Stepwise investigations of gross hematuria
Step 1 relates to studies performed in all subjects: (1) Complete blood count, (2) Urine culture, (3) Serum creatinine level, (4) 24-hour urine collection for creatinine, protein, calcium, (5) Serum C3 level, and (6) Ultrasound or IVP.
Step 2 relates to studies performed in selected subjects: (1) DNase B titer or streptozyme test if hematuria is of less than 6 months duration, (2) Skin or throat cultures when appropriate, (3) ANA titer, (4) Urine erythrocyte morphology, (5) Coagulation studies/platelet count when suggested by history, (6) Sickle cell screening in all black patients, (7) Voiding cystourethrography with presence of infection or when lower tract lesion is suspected.
Step 3 relates to invasive procedures such as renal biopsy and cystoscopy.

Contd...

Contd...

Stepwise investigations of gross hematuria
Renal biopsy is indicated for: (1) Persistent high grade microscopic hematuria, (2) Microscopic hematuria plus any of the following: diminished renal function, proteinuria exceeding 150 mg/day (0.15 g/day), hypertension, and second episode of gross hematuria.
Cytoscopy is indicated for pink to red hematuria, dysuria, and sterile urine culture.

116. DOC for simple partial seizures:

a. Phenytoin
b. Valproate
c. Carbamazepine
d. Phenobarbitone

Carbamazepine, though expensive, is of special value in grand mal epilepsy, and temporal lobe seizures to counter the usual problem of psycho-somatic deterioration.

Anticonvulsant choice based on seizure type in intractable/refractory epilepsy

Seizure type Generalized	*First choice*	*Other options*
Infantile spasm	Corticotropin	Topiramate, zonisamide, vigabatrin
Absence	Ethosuccimide	Valproate, lamotrigine, zonisamide
Atonic	Valproate	Topiramate, lamotrigine, phenytoin, phenobarbitone, zonisamide, felbamate
Tonic	Valproate	Topiramate, lamotrigine, phenytoin, phenobarbitone, zonisamide, felbamate
Myoclonic	Valproate	Topiramate, lamotrigine, phenytoin, phenobarbitone, zonisamide, felbamate
Tonic-clonic	Valproate	Topiramate, lamotrigine, phenytoin, phenobarbitone, zonisamide, felbamate
Partial Generalized or not	Carbamazepine	Oxcarbazepine, or not lamotrigine, topiramate, phenytion, levetiracetam, zonisamide tiagabine, gabapentin, valproate, phenobarbitone felbamate

117. LEAST observed laboratory findings in neonatal sepsis:

a. Raised C-reactive proteins
b. Neutrophilia
c. Increased ESR
d. Increased immature cells

Diagnosis of neonatal septicemia

- TLC <5,000/ mm^3
- Band/ total neutrophil count ratio >0.16
- m-ESR >15 mm
- Positive CRP
- Presence of two or more above mentioned parameters means positive sepsis screen

Ans. **114. b.** Tetralogy of... **115. a.** Goodpasture synd... **116. c.** Carbamazepine **117. b.** Neutrophilia

- A repeat screen in indicated in case of a negative result after 12 hours; every 48 hours in ventilated neonates.

Clinical clues to etiologic diagnosis	
Clues	*Organisms*
Such superficial infections as pyoderma, abscess, conjunctivitis, umbilical sepsis, osteomyelitis; onset of manifestations after 72 hours of birth	*Staphylococcus*
Grayish-black gangrenous lesions over skin	*Pseudomonas*
Peripartum flu-like maternal illness, gastroenteritis, meconium-stained liquor amnii, baby is unwell right at birth with limpness and develops respiratory difficulty, apneic spells, rash and hepatosplenomegaly on the first day	*Listeria*
Maternal fever during labor, prolonged rupture of membranes (PRM); respiratory distress within 3 hours of birth, apneic spells, shock	*Streptococcus group B*

118. Precocious puberty is seen in:

a. Neuroblastoma
b. McCunne Albright syndrome
c. Addison's disease
d. Hyperthyroidism

Development of secondary sex characters, much before the anticipated age, is referred to as precocious puberty. In tropical areas, the age landmark for boys is 9 and for girls 8 years.

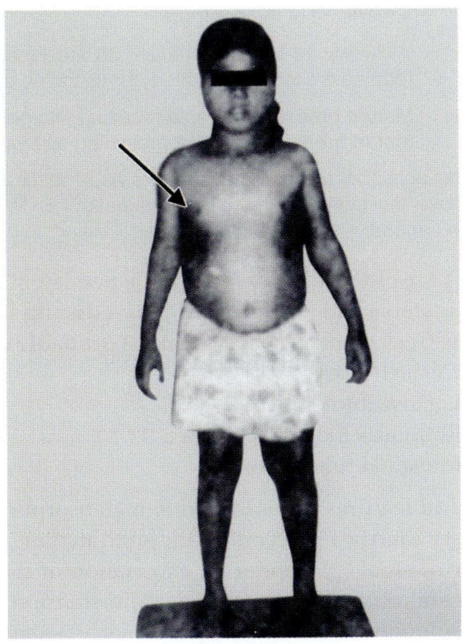

Precocious puberty, showing, noteworthy breast enlargement, in a 7-year-old girl

119. A 3.5 kg baby born to a diabetic mother develops seizures at 16 hours. Likely cause is:

a. Hypocalcemia
b. Hypomagnesemia
c. Hypoxia
d. Hypoglycemia

Neonatal seizures are usually secondary to HIE (hypoxic ischemic encephalopathy), hypocalcemia, hypoglycemia or septicemia with meningitis.

Etiology of neonatal seizures
Developmental neurologic problems Congenital hydrocephalus, microcephaly, cerebral dysgenesis, porencephaly, polymicrogyria, pachygyria, hydrencephaly, lissencephaly, agenesis of corpus collosum.
Perinatal complications HIE, birth asphyxia, birth injuries (especially with CNS involvement), intracranial bleed (IVH, SAH)
Perinatal infections Meningitis, septicemia, intrauterine infections (STORCH)
Metabolic problems Hypocalcemia, hypoglycemia, hypomagnesemia, hypo- or hypernatremia, pyridoxine dependency, severe hyperbilirubinemia with kernicterus (bilirubin encephalopathy), inborn errors of metabolism (amino acid metabolism, organic acidemias)
Drugs Neonates born to mothers with narcotic addiction (narcotic withdrawal syndrome), theophylline, propylene glycol, advertent injection of local anesthesia
Idiopathic

120. Commonest virus causing diarrhea in infants is:

a. Poliovirus
b. Adenovirus
c. Rotavirus
d. Rhabdovirus

Viral causes of diarrhea are rotavirus, Norwalk and allied viruses, enterovirus, Influenza virus, measles virus etc.

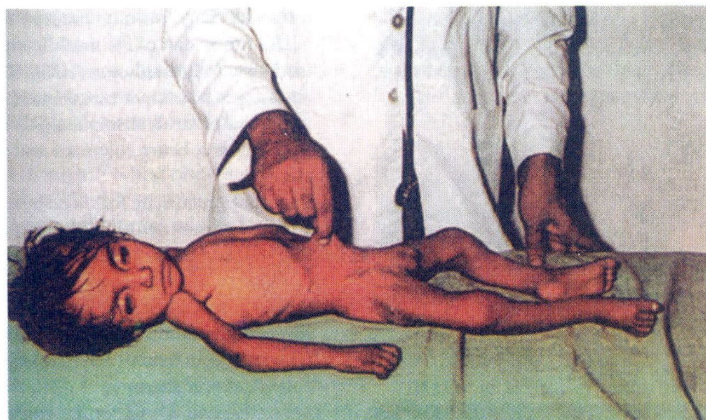

Severe diarrheal dehydration. Note the characteristic features, including moribund state with shock, acidosis and anuria. ORS, hailed as the most important medical advance of the 20th century, has the potential of saving 10,000 children each day—the child population that could otherwise die from diarrheal dehydration

121. Koplik's spots are seen in:

a. Typhoid
b. Measles
c. Mumps
d. Polio

Koplik spots are pathognomonic of measles.

Ans. 118. b. McCunne Alb... 119. d. Hypoglycemia 120. c. Rotavirus 121. b. Measles

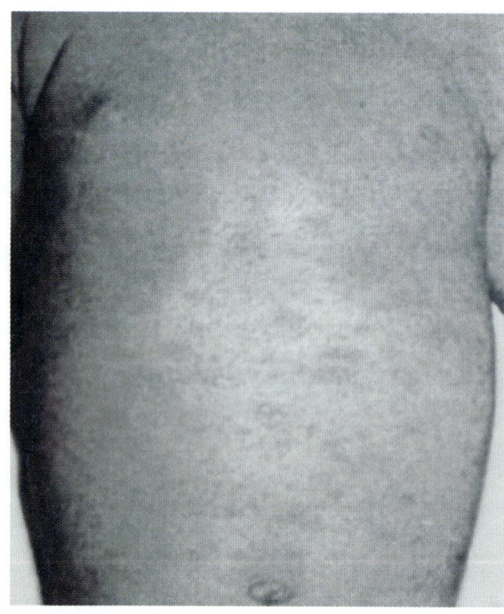

Measles. Note the light-brown staining (pigmentation) left behind as the rash is gone away

122. MC cause of acute infantile gastroenteritis:

a. Rotavirus b. Norwalk virus
c. *E. coli* d. Adenovirus

Rotavirus, also termed GEV (gastroenteritis virus) and Due virus, is the most frequently encountered virus in diarrheal stools of children. Four established serotypes of rotavirus account for 20-40% of acute diarrhea.

Etiology of pediatric acute diarrhea	
A. Enteric Infections	
Bacteria	*E. coli, Shigella, Salmonella, Staphylococcus, Cholera vibrio, Yersinia enterocolitica, Campylobacter jejuni, Clostridium difficile, Aeromonas hydrophilia. Vibrio parahemolyticus, Plesiomonas shigelloides.*
Viruses	*Rotavirus, Norwalk and allied viruses, enterovirus. Influenza virus, measles virus.*
Parasites	*Ent. histolytica, Giardia lamblia, Cryptosporidium, H. nana, malaria*
Fungi	*Candida albicans.*
Parental	URI, otitis media, tonsillitis, pneumonia, urinary tract infection.
B. Dietetic/Nutritional: Overfeeding, starvation, food allergy, food poisoning.	
C. Drugs: Antibiotics	
D. Nonspecific.	

123. In females, growth spurt is maximum in:

a. Tanner's breast stage IV, Pubic hair stage IV
b. Tanner's breast stage III, Pubic hair stage III
c. Tanner's breast stage II, Pubic hair stage II
d. Tanner's breast stage I, Pubic hair stage I

Tanner's sexual maturity rating (SMR) quantifies sexual growth from 1 to 5. In case of boys, genitalia and pubic hair and in case of girls, genitalia and breasts are prime considerations. No sexual growth (prepubescent stage) means SMR 1 whereas full sexual growth means SMR 5.

Tanner's sexual maturity rating (SMR)	
Pubic hair stages for boys and girls	
PH-1	Preadolescent, no pubic hair
PH-2	Sparse growth of long, pigmented hair at base of penis (boys) and bilaterally along medial border of labia (girls)
PH-3	Hair, which begin to curl and develop increased pigmentation, spread laterally in boys and over mons pubis in girl.
PH-4	Hair become coarse and involve more area
PH-5	Hair spread medial side of thigh.
Genitalia stages for boys	
G-I	Testes, scrotum and penis of small size
G-2	Testes and penis slightly enlarged, scrotum develops red hue
G-3	Testes, scrotum and penis further enlarge
G-4	Penis enlarged in breadth and develop glans; scrotal skin become dark
G-5	Mature adult sized penis, testes* and penis
Breast development stages in girls	
B-I	Preadolescent, elevated papilla
B-2	Breast bud forms, elevated beast and papilla, increased areolar diameter
B-3	Further enlargement of breast and areola without separation of the contours
B-4	Well-defined breast contour with areola and papilla forming a seconday mound above the concur
B-5	Mature breast with areola receding into general contour of breast and papilla projecting as nipple.
* The objective tool for measuring size of testis (over and above the convesitional clinical palpation) is Prader's orchidometer	

124. A-2-year-old child presents with persistent diarrhea, acidic stools and presence of 1% of reducing substances in the fresh stools. What is the most probable diagnosis:

a. Cystic fibrosis
b. Lactose intolerance
c. Rotavirus induced diarrhea
d. Intestinal tuberculosis

Clinical features of disaccharide malabsorption include watery diarrhea with only little solid matter, acid character of stool (pH under 6), excoriation of the perianal area and buttocks, and abdominal distension and pain. The abdominal cramps are particularly a feature of lactose intolerance in older children and result from excessive gas production.

Ans. 122. **a.** Rotavirus 123. **b.** Tanner's breast stage... 124. **b.** Lactose intolerance

Four phases of evaluation of the child with chronic diarrhea/malabsorption	
Phase I	History and physical examination with special reference to onset of diarrhea and its relationship with various factors (excessive carbonated drinks/ fruit juices, supplementary milk feeds, cereals), specific amount of fluids ingested/day, nutritional status, etc. Meticulous stool examination (ova and cysts, pH, reducing substances, fat globules) Stool culture Stool for *Cl. difficile toxia* Blood studies (CBC, ESR, electrolytes, BUN, creatinine
Phase II	Fat balance studies for daily stool fat or steatocrit D-xylose test Sweat chloride test Stool osmolality and electrolytes, phenophthalein, magnesium sulfate, phosphate Breath H_2 tests
Phase III	Barium meal/enema to exclude anatomic defects small intestinal biopsy/colonic biopsy by endoscopic studies Sigmoidoscopy/colonoscopy
Phase IV	Hormonal studies Neurotransmittal studies (vasoactive intestinal polypeptide, gastrin, secretin, 5-hydroxyindole-acetic assays)

125. DOC of myoclonic epilepsy in children:

a. Valproic acid
b. Carbamazepine
c. Ethosuximide
d. Lamotrigine

First choice for myoclonic seizures is valproate and second line drugs are topiramate, lamotrigine, phenytoin, phenobarbitone, zonisamide and felbamate.

New international classification of convulsions
Partial Seizures
I. *Simple* – With motor signs (Jacksonian or focal motor) – With somatosensory or special sensory i.e. visual, auditory, olfactory, vertiginous, gustatory, symptoms (sensory seizures) – With autonomic manifestations (abdominal epilepsy, epileptic equivalent)
II. *Complex*
Generalized Seizures
I. Absence seizures – Typical (Petit mal) – Atypical (Petit mal variant or complex Petit mal)
II. Myoclonic seizures
III. Atonic seizures (akinetic seizures or drop attacks)
IV. *Tonic-clonic seizures (grand mal, major motor seizures, generalized convulsive seizures)*

126. Apnea in infants is defined as cessation of respiration for at least:

a. 10 seconds
b. 20 seconds
c. 30 seconds
d. 40 seconds

Recurrent neonatal apnea (apneic spells) is characterized by intermittent respiratory pause of more than 20 seconds or apnea (sudden cessation of respiration) followed by cyanosis, bradycardia and limpness with unresponsiveness to tactile stimuli.

127. A child with history of diarrhea, is having convulsions. Most likely cause:

a. Hypokalemia
b. Hyperkalemia
c. Hyponatremia
d. Hypernatremia

Manifestations of diarrhea secondary to CNS disturbances are prominent in all types of severe dehydration. Hypertonic dehydration has more of these. Early irritability, alternating with apathy, may progress to restlessness, clouding of consciousness, delirium or stupor, lethargy and coma. Convulsions can occur at any stage. The high viscosity of blood may cause as serious a complication as cerebral thrombosis. In addition to cerebral thrombosis, conditions that may cause seizures in acute diarrhea or AGE include marked hyponatremia, rapid correction of hypernatremia, hypocalcemia, hypomagnesemia, encephalitis and shigellosis.

Clinical picture in certain special situations

Conditions	*Physical signs*
Acidosis	Breathing increased in depth and rate
Alkalosis	Breathing decreased in depth and rate; latent or manifest tetany.
Hypokalemia	Abdominal distention, paralytic ileus hypotonia, hyporeflexia; mental apathy; ECG changes.
Hyperkalemia	Fibrillation or paralysis of skeletal muscles; ECG changes
Hypocalcemia	Tetany; paralytic ileus
Hypercalcemia	Hypotonia; fecal masses
Hypomagnesemia	Tetany; muscular twitching
Hypermagnesemia	CNS depression; hyporeflexia

128. True for cephalhematoma:

a. Common
b. Located in subcutaneous plane
c. Limited by suture line
d. Resolves within 3 days

Ans. 125. **a.** Valproic acid 126. **b.** 20 seconds 127. **c.** Hyponatremia 128. **c.** Limited by suture line

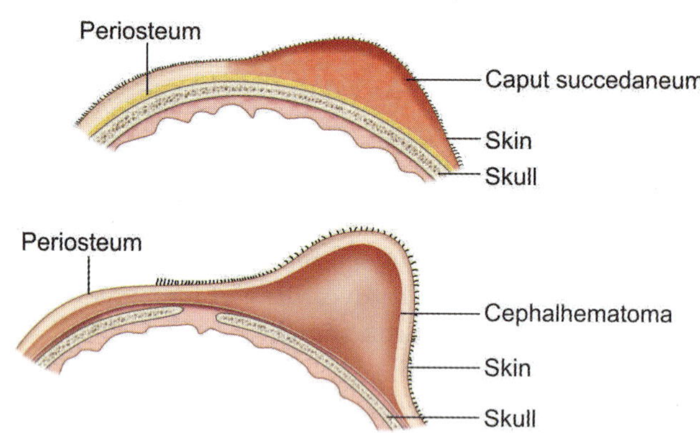

Development of caput succedaneum and cephalhematoma. Caput succedaneum: serosanginous fluid collection in the soft tissue, not limited by suture lines, disappears speedily. Cephalhematoma: Collection is blood, between skull bone and overlying pericranium, limited by suture line; disappears slowly in a few weeks

Whereas intracranial hemorrhage is a serious condition, cephalhematoma is rather benign, self-limiting and resolves in a few weeks time. The swelling is nonpulsatile, does not increase in size on crying, and does not cross a suture line. The most common site is the parietal or occipital bone. It needs no treatment.

129. Hypsarrhythmia occurs in:

a. Neonatal seizures
b. Partial seizures
c. Congenital juvenile convulsions
d. Infantile spasms

In infantile myoclonic epilepsy, also called salaam seizures or west syndrome, the baby (usually under 6 months of age) has massive attacks of flexion of the head, once or as many as 100 times a day. In the primary type child is microcephalic and mentally retarded. EEG shows typical hypsarrhythmia.

Drugs commonly employed in recurrent convulsions	
Phenobarbital	3 to 5 mg/kg/day in I or 2 divided doses
Diphenylhydantoin	5 to 8 mg/kg/day in 2 divided doses
Carbamazepine	10 to 20 mg/kg/day in 2 or 3 divided doses
Sodium valporate	15 to 20 mg/kg/day in 3 or 4 divided doses
Ethosuximide	10 to 20 mg/kg/ day in 2 divided doses
Clonazepam	0.01 to 0.3 mg/kg/day in 3 divided doses

130. MC cause of otitis media in children:

a. *Staphylococcus*
b. *Streptococcus pneumoniae*
c. *Moraxella*
d. *Streptococcus pyogenes*

The common etiologic organisms in order of frequency are S. pneumoniae, H. influenzae and Moraxella catarrhalis (these are responsible for 75% of the cases), S. aureus, group A Streptococcus, Alpha Streptococcus, P. aeruginosa and group B Streptococcus.

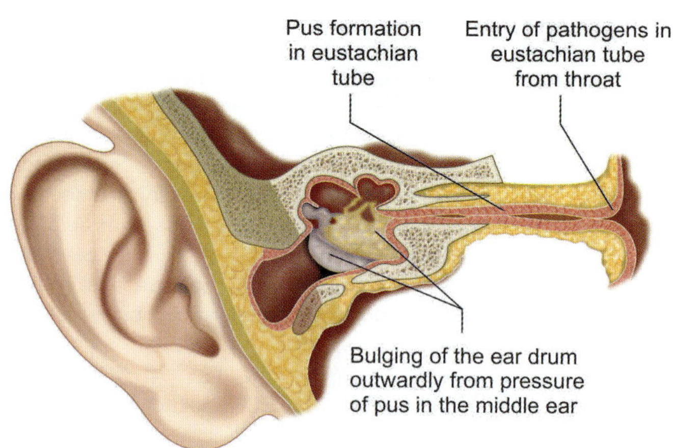

Acute otitis media (an artist's representation)

131. Which of the following is an indicator of pneumonia:

a. Chest indrawing
b. Respiratory rate of 60 or more in less than 2 months of age
c. Respiratory rate of 50 or more in less than 2 months of age
d. Respiratory rate of 40 or more in less than 2 months of age

The cut-off point for high respiratory rate is over 60 per minute up to 2 months of age, over 50 per minute between 2 months to 12 months, and 40 per minute between 12 months to 5 years.

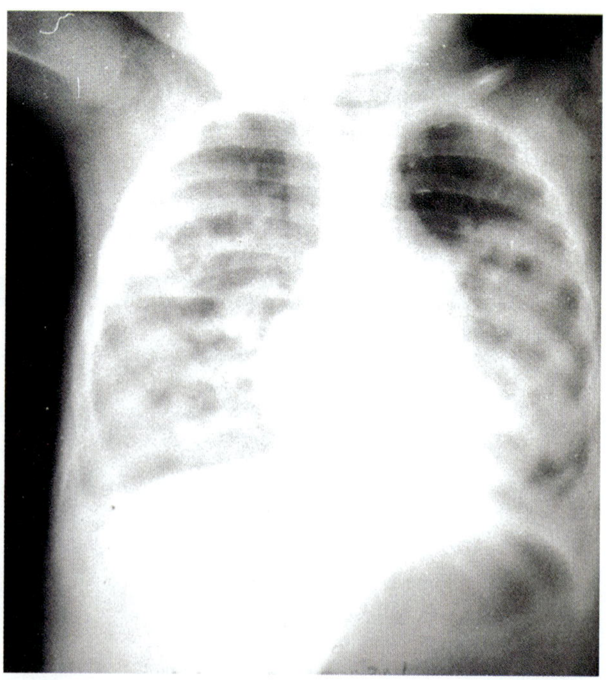

Staphylococcal pneumonia: Demonstration of pneumatoceles is regarded pathognomonic of staphylococcal pneumonia. It usually occurs during infancy secondary to staphylococcal infection elsewhere in the body. Unless, treated energetically, serious complications are a rule

Ans. **129. d.** Infantile spasms **130. b.** *Streptococcus...* **131. b.** Respiratory rate of 60 or more in less...

132. Earliest to reduce in iron deficiency anemia:
a. TIBC
b. Total body iron stores
c. Free erythroprotoporphyrin
d. Reticulocyte count

On the basis of biochemical and hematological changes iron deficiency anemia is graded into 3 stages: Stage I – Depletion of iron stores (ferritin is decreased, transferring saturation, serum iron and hemoglobin are normal), Stage II – Depletion of transport iron (transferring saturation and serum iron also reduced, Hb is normal) and Stage III- State of IDA (frank features of IDA).

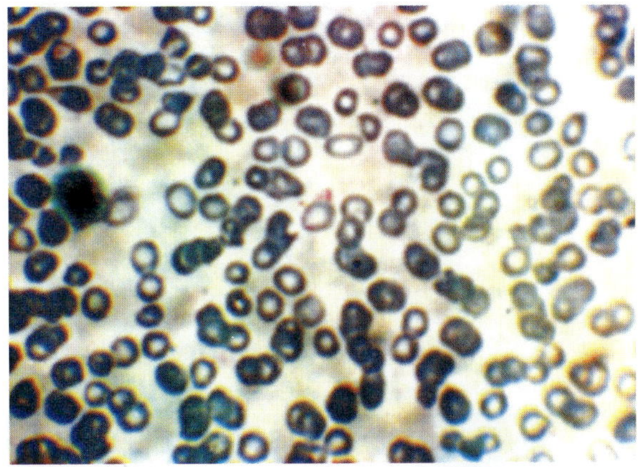

Peripheral blood film showing microcytic-hypochromic picture with, anisocytosis and poikilocytosis in IDA

133. NOT a cause of meningitis in neonates:
a. E. coli
b. Listeria
c. Pneumococcus
d. Meningococci

Pyogenic meningitis is neonates of <2 months age is caused by Gram-negative organisms, esp E. coli, Group B beta-streptococci hemolyticus and Listeria monocytogenes.

134. Temperature of a child in severe hypothermia:
a. 37°C
b. 36.0–36.4°C
c. 32.0–35.9 °C
d. Less than 32°C

Severe hypothermia is when the body temperature is below 32°C. Mild – moderate hypothermia is temperature between 32°C and 36°C.

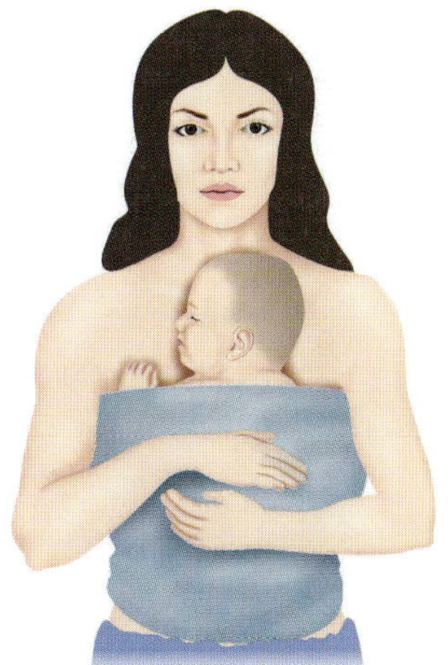

Kangaroo mother care (KMC): Note that the baby is held upright against the mother's skin and between the breasts and covered with mother's clothes plus an additional shawl/blanket. A belt around mother's waist may assist in keeping the baby in position

135. Most common cause of nephrotic syndrome in children:
a. Mesangial proliferative glomerulonephritis
b. Minimal change disease
c. Focal segmental glomerulosclerosis
d. Membranous nephropathy

In children, minimal change disease (nil deposit disease) is the MC cause of nephrotic syndrome.

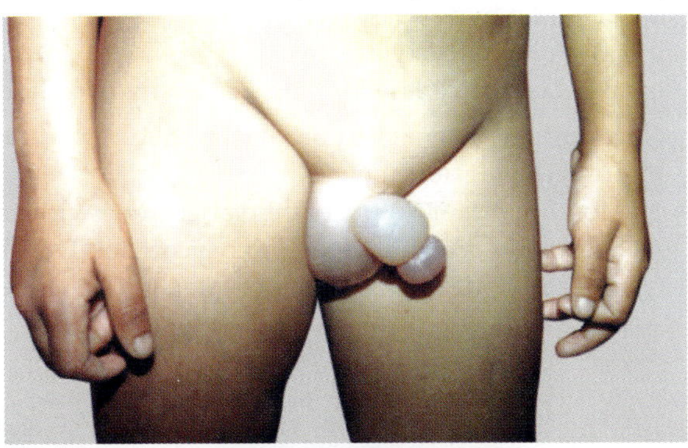

Nephrotic syndrome: Note generalized edema, including hydrocele and involvement of the penis

136. Drug NOT useful in the management of acute asthma in children:
a. Theophylline
b. Morphine
c. Steroids
d. Salbutamol

Morphine is not used in managing asthma.

Drugs employed in asthma

Drugs	Oral dose	Parenteral dose	Aerosol dose
Beta-2 adrenergic agonists			
Salbutamol (Albuterol)	0.1 mg/kg/dose 3 to 4 times/day	7.5 µg/kg in 5 to 10 min, then 0.1 µg/min, increase	100 to 200 mcg (1 to 2 puffs) every 1 to 5 hrs every 15 min by 0.1 mcg/kg up to 0.4 µg/kg/min (IV) 650 µg (1 or 2 puffs)

Contd...

Ans. **132. b.** Total body iron... **133. d.** Meningococci **134. d.** Less than 32°C **135. b.** Minimal change disease **136. b.** Morphine

Contd...

Drugs	*Oral dose*	*Parenteral dose*	*Aerosol dose*
Metapreterenol (Orceprenaline)	0.3 to 9.5 mg/kg/dose 3 to 4 times/day		
Terbutaline	0.075 mg/kg/dose	0.005 mg/kg dose (IV) 3 to 4 times/day	250 mcg (1 or 2 puffs)
Theophyllines			
Aminophylline	4 to 6 mg/kg/dose	6 mg/kg followed	
		3 to 4 times/day	by 0.9 mg/kg/hr
Theophylline	4 to 5 mg/kg/dose		
	3 to 4 times/day		
Steroids			
Prednisolone	1 to 2 mg/kg/day		
Hydrocortisone		8 to 10 mg/kg followed by	
		1 mg/kg/hr	
		or 3 mg/kg every 6 hr	
Beclomethasone			1 to 2 puffs 3 to 4 times/day
			maximum 10 puffs/day
Ketotifen	0.25 to 0.5 mg BD		1 to 2 puffs 6 hrly; 1 to 2 puffs
Cromoglycate			20 minutes before exercise in EIA

137. A male child presents with hypertension, hyperpigmentation and virilization. He is most likely to have:

a. 17 alpha hydoxylase deficiency
b. 21 alpha hydroxylase
c. 3 beta hydroxylase
d. 11 beta hydroxylase

Congenital adrenal hyperplasia due to 11-beta-hydroxylase deficiency

- Most important feature of this variety too is virilization
- Because of accumulation of deoxycortisol (DOC), hypertension develops sooner or later.

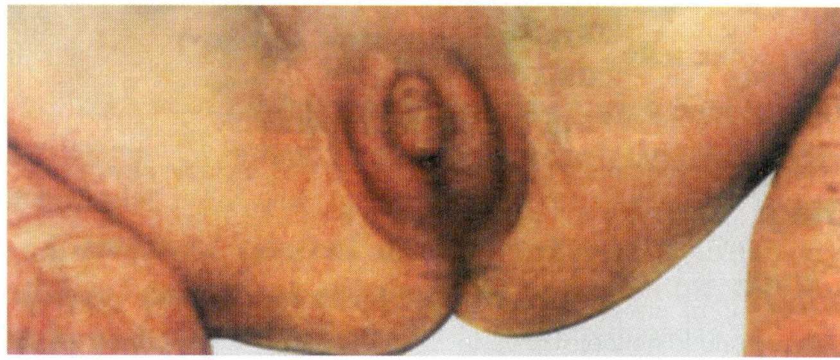

Congenital adrenal hyperplasia. Note the ambiguous genitalia

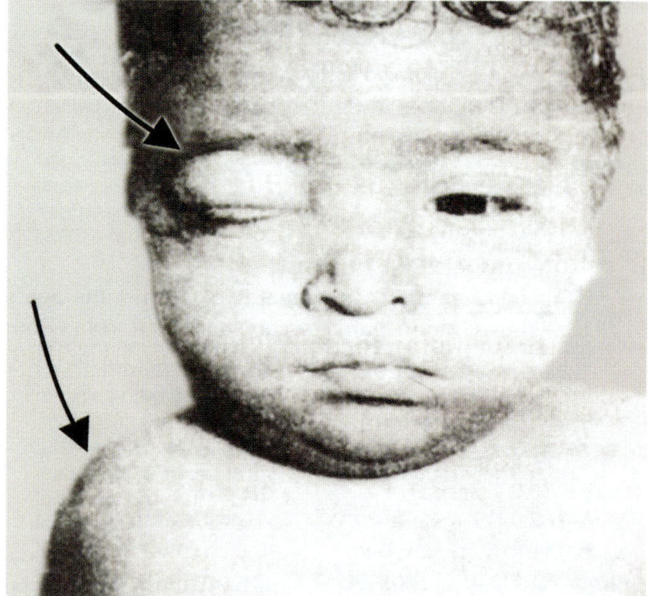

Subcutaneous emphysema in an infant with bronchopneumonia

138. A 6 month child with cough is having respiratory rate of 50/ min. This indicates:

a. No pneumonia
b. Pneumonia
c. Severe pneumonia
d. Very severe pneumonia

The cut-off point for high respiratory rate is over 60 per minute up to 2 months of age, over 50 per minute between 2 months to 12 months, and 40 per minute between 12 months to 5 years.

139. All of the following are true for Turner's syndrome EXCEPT:

a. Height of more than 145 cm
b. Webbing of neck
c. Increased carrying angle
d. Coarctation of aorta may be seen

Person with Turner's syndrome has a short stature (less than 145 cm).

Ans. 137. **d.** 11 beta hydro... 138. **b.** Pneumonia 139. **a.** Height of more than 145 cm

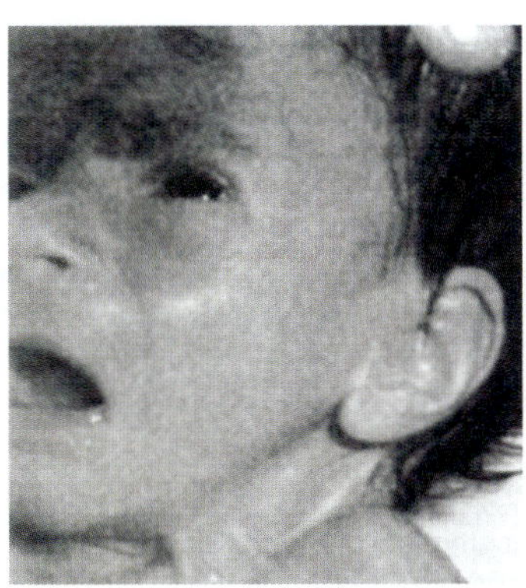

Turner syndrome. Note the classical webbing of the neck

140. Fluid intake by a 8 kg boy should be:

a. 700 mL b. 800 mL
c. 900 mL d. 1 L

The daily fluid requirements in children are calculated as follows:

Up to 10 kg = 100 mL/kg
10–20 kg = 50 mL/kg
>20 kg = 20 mL/kg

141. Children born to SLE affected mothers may develop:

a. Complete heart block
b. Transposition of great vessels
c. TOF d. ASD

Third-degree heart block/complete heart block may be congenital and has been linked to the presence of lupus in the mother. It is thought that maternal antibodies may cross the placenta and attack the heart tissue during gestation.

Cardiovascular anomalies in various syndromes/ extracardiac lesions	
Apert syndrome	VSD
Carpenter syndrome	PDA
CHARGE association (coloboma, heart disease, retardation, genital and ear anomalies)	VSD, ASD, PADA, TOF, ECD
CHILD (congenital hemi-dysplasia, ichthyosiform erythroderma, limb defects)	Miscellaneous
Congenital hypertrophic subaortic stenosis	VSD, PDA
Congenital rubella	PDA, peripheral pulmonic stenosis
Crouzon syndrome	PDA, COA
Cutis laxa	Pulmonary hypertension PA Stenosis
deLange syndrome	VSD
DiGeorge sequence	Aortic arch anomalies, conotruncal anomalies
Down syndrome	VSD, ECD, ASD
Ellis-Van Crevald syndrome	Single atrium, ADS
Familial dwarfism and nevi	Cardiomyopathy
Familial elfin facies, mental retardation, infantile hypercalcemia	Supravalvular AS
FAVS (facio-auriculo-vertebral spectrum)	TOF, VSD
Fetal alcohol syndrome	ASD, VSD
Fetal hydantoin syndrome	VSD, ASD, COA, PDA
Fetal valproate syndrome	COA, hypoplastic left side of the heart, AS, PA, VSD
Holt-Oram syndrome	Familial ASD
Infants of diabetic mother	Hypertrophic cardiomyopathy, VSD, conotruncal anomalies
Jarvell-Lange-Nielsen syndrome	Prolonged QT
Kartagener syndrome	Dextrocardia
Laurence-Moon-Biedl syndrome	Variable, including TOF
Marfan syndrome	Aortic or pulmonary artery dilatation, MI
Noonan syndrome	PS, ASD, cardiomyopathy
Progeria	Accelerated atherosclerosis
Rubinstein-Taybi syndrome	PDA
Rubella syndrome	PDA, PS
Thrombocytopenia and absent radius) (TAR)	ASD, TOF
Treacher Collins	VSD, PDA, ASD
Tuberous sclerosis	Myocardial rhabdomyoma
Ehler-Danlos syndrome	Arterial dilatation
Gargolism	Multivalvular and coronary artery disease
Morquio-Ulrich	Aortic incompetence
Ostegenesis imperfecta	Aortic incompetence
Trisomy 13-15	VSD, PDA, ASD
Trisomy 16-18	VSD, PDA, PS
Turner syndrome	COA, PS, AS
VATER association (vertebral, anal, tracheo-esophageal, radial and renal anomalies)	VSD, TOF, ECD

142. Capillary refill time in a child with shock will be:

a. Shortened b. Remains same
c. Prolonged d. None of the above

Clinical features of neonatal shock include marked pallor despite adequate hematocrit, lethargy, irritability, hypotonia, circumoral grayish discoloration, cold-clamy skin of limbs, difference of >2.5°C between core and surface temperatures, capillary refill time >2 seconds, tachycardia, tachypnea and sclerema.

Ans. 140. b. 800 mL **141. a.** Complete heart block **142. c.** Prolonged

Etiology of neonatal shock
Hypovolemic Shock *Blood loss:* Antepartum (twin to twin transfusion, fetomaternal transfusion, placenta previa), Intrapartum (ICH, birth trauma, excessive bleeding, umbilical vessels), Postpartum (DIC, IVH)
Fluid and electrolyte loss: Vomiting, diarrhea, phototherapy, hyperthermia, poor fluid intake, iatrogenic renal disease, abdominal surgery
Distributive Shock *Infections:* Septicemia *CNS:* Trauma (neurogenic shock), HIE *Drugs:* Phenobarbital, muscle relaxants, anethetics
Cardiogenic Shock *Myocardial Dysfunction:* CCF, viral myocarditis, cardiomyopathy, arrhythmias, myocardial depressants (hypoglycemia, acidosis, sepsis) *Outflow (Mechanical) Obstruction:* Pneumo- or hemopericardium, tension pneumothorax, diaphragmatic hernia, severe interstitial emphysema, pulmonary embolism *Congenital Heart Disease:* TOF (severe), TOGA, HLHS, TA, PDA, AS, COA, PA with intact ventricular septum.

143. Brachycephaly is due to the fusion of:

a. Parietal suture b. Sagittal suture
c. Lamboid suture d. Coronal suture

Brachycephaly, the cephalic disorder is known as **flat head syndrome**, and results from premature fusion of the coronal sutures (craniosynostosis) or from external deformation (plagiocephaly). The coronal suture is the fibrous joint that unites the frontal bone with the two parietal bones of the skull. The parietal bones form the top and sides of the skull. This feature can be seen in Down syndrome.

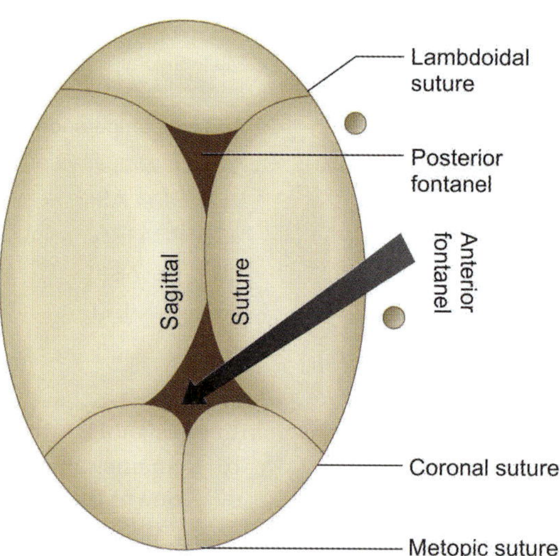

Skull top, showing fontanels and sutures

144. NOT a cause of unconjugated hyperbilirubinemia:

a. Rotor's syndrome b. Spherocytosis
c. Galactosemia d. Breast milk jaundice

Rotor syndrome, also called **Rotor type hyperbilirubinemia**, is a rare, relatively benign autosomal recessive bilirubin disorder. It is a distinct, yet similar disorder to Dubin–Johnson syndrome — both diseases cause an increase in conjugated bilirubin.

Causes of unconjugated hyperbilirubinemia
Physiologic
Pathologic
Increased Production of Bilirubin
❑ *Hemolytic disease of the newborn:* Rh isoimmunization, ABO incompatibility, minor blood group incompatibility
❑ Hereditary spherocytosis
❑ *Nonspherocytic hemolytic anemia:* G-6-PD deficiency, pyruvate kinate deficiency, alpha-thalassemia
❑ *Acquired hemolysis disorders:* Vitamin K3-induced hemolysis, microangiopathies
❑ Septicemia
❑ *Increased enterhepatic circulation:* Intestinal obstruction, congenital hypertrophic pyloric stenosis, meconium ileus paralytic ileus, Hirschsprung disease
Decreased Clearance of Bilirubin
❑ *Inborn errors of metabolism:* Familial nonhemolytic jaundice (Crigler-Najjar syndrome) type I and II, Gilbert disease
❑ *Medications:* Vitamin K3
❑ *Hormones:* Breastmilk jaundice, hypothyroidism, hypopituitarism

145. Most important cause of under-5 mortality:

a. Trauma b. Respiratory infections
c. Malnutrition d. Diarrhea

Acute **respiratory illnesses**, such as pneumonia, are the largest single cause of **death** in children **under five**.

146. NOT a cause of unconjugated hyperbilirubinemia:

a. Physiological jaundice
b. Dubin Johnson syndrome
c. Hypothyroidism
d. Hemolytic anemia

Dubin–Johnson syndrome (DJS) is a rare, autosomal recessive, benign disorder that causes an isolated increase of conjugated bilirubin in the serum. Classically, the condition causes a black liver due to the deposition of a pigment similar to melanin.

147. Berger nephropathy is due to mesangial deposition of:

a. IgA and C3 b. IgE and C3
c. IgD and C3 d. Fibrin and C3

Histologically, IgA nephropathy may show mesangial widening and focal and segmental inflammation. Diffuse mesangial proliferation or crescentic glomerulonephritis may also be present. Immunoflourescence shows mesangial deposition of IgA often with C3 and properdin and smaller amounts of other immunoglobulins (IgG or IgM). Early components of the classical complement pathway (C1q or C4) are usually not seen.

Ans. **143. d.** Coronal suture **144. a.** Rotor's syndrome **145. b.** Respiratory infections **146.b.** Dubin Johnson syndrome **147. a.** IgA and C3

148. Fast breathing in a child of 3 year is (respiratory rate/minute):

a. More than 30
b. More than 40
c. More than 50
d. More than 60

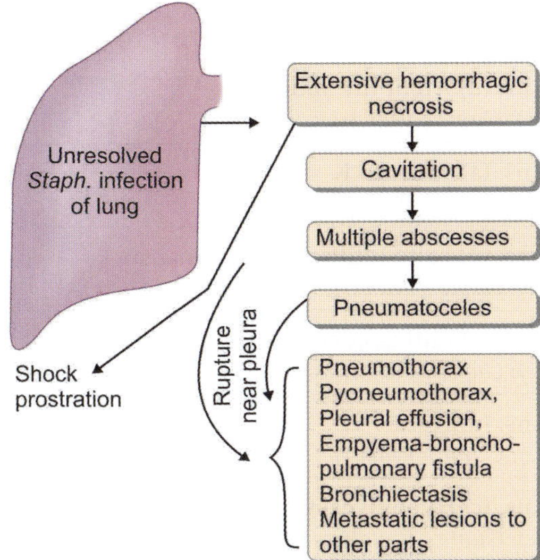

Natural history of development of complications in staphylococcal pneumonia

The cut-off point for high respiratory rate is over 60 per minute up to 2 months of age, over 50 per minute between 2 months to 12 months, and 40 per minute between 12 months to 5 years.

149. Most common cause of death in Klinefelter syndrome:

a. Suicide
b. Respiratory problems
c. Cardiovascular problems
d. Infections

Testicular hypofunction or deficiency (hypogonadism) is an important finding in the Klinefelter syndrome. Such a patient has XXY chromosomal pattern with positive buccal smear, looks more of a male, is tall and may have gynecomastia. Testes are just rudimentary. Infections is the MC cause of death.

150. MC form of intracranial hemorrhage in preterm neonates is:

a. Subarachnoid hemorrhage
b. Intraparenchymal hemorrhage
c. Subdural hemorrhage
d. Subependymal hemorrhage

The pathogenesis of intraventricular hemorrhage in the newborn includes that of subependymal hemorrhage (SEH), the single most common pathologic alteration seen in the infants.

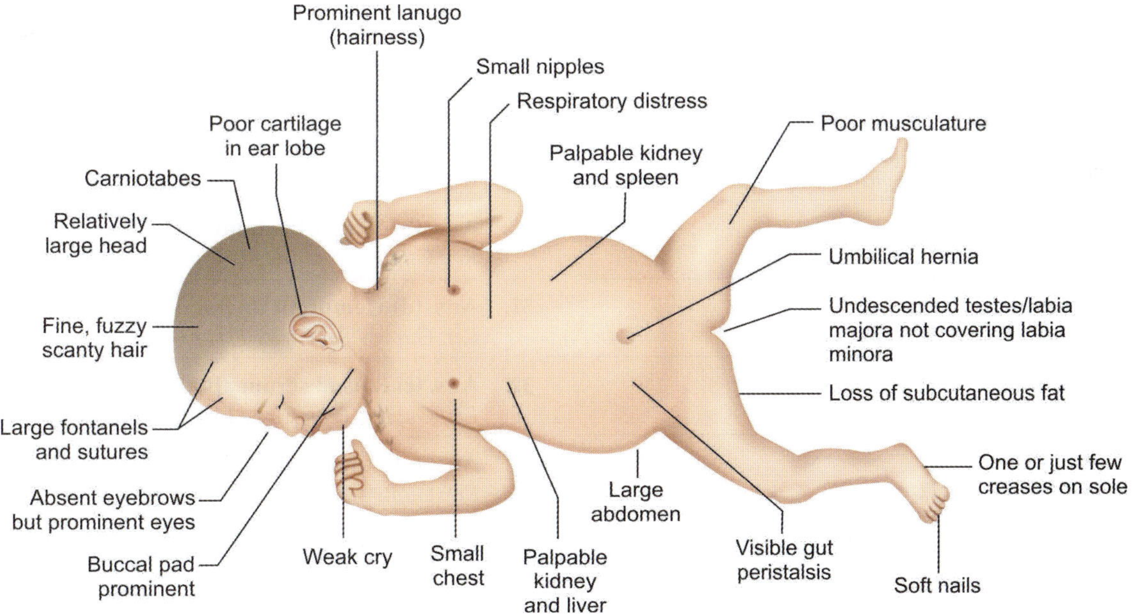

Special features of a preterm baby

MCQs with Short Explanations

Ans. 148. b. More than 40 **149. d.** Infections **150. d.** Subependymal hemorrhage

ANSWERS WITH REFERENCES

GROWTH

1. **Ans. (a) 7**
   Ref: Ghai's Paediatrics, 6/e p46, 47
2. **Ans. (d) 4 year**
   Ref: Gupte's Pediatrics 11/e p30
3. **Ans. (b) 1 year**
   Ref: Gupte's Pediatrics 11/e p29
4. **Ans. (a) Stable sitting**
   Ref: Gupte's Pediatrics 11/e p37
5. **Ans. (b) Tripled**
   Ref: Gupte's Pediatrics 11/e p29
6. **Ans. (b) Thelarche**
   Ref: Gupte's Pediatrics 11/e p61
7. **Ans. (c) 6 cm/ year**
   Ref: Gupte's Pediatrics 11/e p28
8. **Ans. (b) 4 years**
   Ref: Gupte's Pediatrics 11/e p25
9. **Ans. (c) 3 months**
   Ref: Gupte's Pediatrics 11/e p37
10. **Ans. (a) Testicular development → pubic hair → axillary hair → beard**
    Ref: Gupte's Pediatrics 11/e p62
11. **Ans. (a) 2 and 3 years**
    Ref: Gupte's Pediatrics 11/e p (Figure)
12. **Ans. (b) 2 years**
    Ref: Gupte's Pediatrics 11/e p37
13. **Ans. (d) 4 years**
    Ref: Gupte's Pediatrics 11/e p30
14. **Ans. (c) 3 years**
    Ref: Gupte's Pediatrics 11/e p37
15. **Ans. (a) Copy circle**
    Ref: Internet resources
16. **Ans. (d) Copies triangle**
    Ref: Internet resources

NUTRITION

17. **Ans. (a) 12.5 cm**
    Ref: Park's PSM, 21/e p592
18. **Ans. (d) 3.5 g/dL**
    Ref: Internet resources
19. **Ans. (d) Rickets**
    Ref: Gupte's Pediatrics 11/e p164
20. **Ans. (d) All of the above**
    Ref: Gupte's Pediatrics 11/e p140
21. **Ans. (a) Vitamin K**
    Ref: Gupte's Pediatrics 11/e p168
22. **Ans. (d) Fatty infiltration of pancreas**
    Ref: Gupte's Pediatrics 11/e p142
23. **Ans. (a) Pitting edema**
    Ref: Gupte's Pediatrics 11/e p143
24. **Ans. (d) None**
    Ref: Gupte's Pediatrics 11/e p116
25. **Ans. (c) Hypoglycemia**
    Ref: Gupte's Pediatrics 11/e p162
26. **Ans. (d) 2,000,000 IU orally**
    Ref: Gupte's Pediatrics 11/e p156
27. **Ans. (a) Half an hour**
    Ref: Gupte's Pediatrics 11/e p116
28. **Ans. (b) Zinc**
    Ref: Gupte's Pediatrics 11/e p112
29. **Ans. (c) Dextrose**
    Ref: Gupte's Pediatrics 11/e p146
30. **Ans. (b) 30 mL/ kg/ hour**
    Ref: Gupte's Pediatrics 11/e p182
31. **Ans. (d) Hemolytic anemia**
    Ref: Gupte's Pediatrics 11/e p168
32. **Ans. (c) Raised serum alkaline phosphatase**
    Ref: Gupte's Pediatrics 11/e p111
33. **Ans. (a) Constitutional**
    Ref: Gupte's Pediatrics 11/e p43
34. **Ans. (b) Low glucose and low sodium**
    Ref: Gupte's Pediatrics 11/e p457
35. **Ans. (a) 100 kilocalories/ day energy and 1.5 gram/ day protein**
    Ref: Gupte's Pediatrics 11/e p110
36. **Ans. (b) 100 kcal/ kg/ day**
    Ref: Gupte's Pediatrics 11/e p140
37. **Ans. (d) High total body sodium, increased ECF volume**
    Ref: Gupte's Pediatrics 11/e p141

38. **Ans. (b)** **1 lakh IU**
Ref: Gupte's Pediatrics 11/e p158

39. **Ans. (c)** **Defect in proximal tubular reabsorption**
Ref: Gupte's Pediatrics 11/e p167

NEWBORN

40. **Ans. (a)** **Respiratory rate**
Ref: Ghai's Paediatrics, 6/e p144

41. **Ans. (d)** **Prolonged & increased umbilical blood flow**
Ref: Sumer Sethi's Radiology, 5/e p49

42. **Ans. (b)** **30 mL in 30 min**
Ref: Ghai's Paediatrics, 6/e p274t

43. **Ans. (d)** **Dolicocephaly**
Ref: Ghai's Paediatrics, 6/e p592

44. **Ans. (b)** **1000–1500 g**
Ref: Gupte's Pediatrics 11/e p206

45. **Ans. (a)** **Erythroblastosis**
Ref: Gupte's Pediatrics 11/e p228

46. **Ans. (d)** **Normal**
Ref: Gupte's Pediatrics 11/e p202

47. **Ans. (c)** **No specific therapy**
Ref: Gupte's Pediatrics 11/e p203

48. **Ans. (d)** **Immunoglobulin and Hepatitis B vaccine**
Ref: Gupte's Pediatrics 11/e p487

49. **Ans. (c)** **PDA**
Ref: Gupte's Pediatrics 11/e p365

50. **Ans. (a)** **Pyloric stenosis**
Ref: Gupte's Pediatrics 11/e p473

51. **Ans. (c)** **BP**
Ref: Gupte's Pediatrics 11/e p196

52. **Ans. (b)** **Neonatal hepatitis**
Ref: Gupte's Pediatrics 11/e p235

53. **Ans. (b)** **Lower areola more visible**
Ref: Gupte's Pediatrics 11/e p115

CONGENITAL DISORDER

54. **Ans. (a)** **Anencephaly**
Ref: Dutta's Obstetrics, 7/e p408

55. **Ans. (c)** **Congenital syphilis**
Ref: Dutta's Obstetrics, 7/e p295

56. **Ans. (c)** **Aortic stenosis**
Ref: Gupte's Pediatrics 11/e p254

57. **Ans. (c)** **Serum HPL**
Ref: Gupte's Pediatrics 11/e p412

58. **Ans. (a)** **Tetralogy of Fallot**
Ref: Gupte's Pediatrics 11/e p367

59. **Ans. (c)** **Atrioventricular septal defect**
Ref: Gupte's Pediatrics 11/e p411

60. **Ans. (a)** **Sensory hearing loss**
Ref: Gupte's Pediatrics 11/e p411

61. **Ans. (a)** **Congenital heart disease**
Ref: Gupte's Pediatrics 11/e p357

62. **Ans. (a)** **Hydrocephalus**
Ref: Gupte's Pediatrics 11/e p424

CVS DISORDER

63. **Ans. (c)** **Acute glomerulonephritis**
Ref: Gupte's Pediatrics 11/e p395

64. **Ans. (c)** **Tetralogy of Fallot**
Ref: Gupte's Pediatrics 11/e p366

65. **Ans. (c)** **Coarctation of aorta**
Ref: Gupte's Pediatrics 11/e p375

66. **Ans. (b)** **In 80% right sided arch of aorta**
Ref: Gupte's Pediatrics 11/e p367

67. **Ans. (c)** **Administer 100% oxygen**
Ref: Gupte's Pediatrics 11/e p368

68. **Ans. (b)** **Right ventricular hypertrophy**
Ref: Gupte's Pediatrics 11/e p354

INFECTIOUS DISEASES

69. **Ans. (d)** **BCG**
Ref: Ghai's Paediatrics, 6/e p224

70. **Ans. (d)** **Very severe pneumonia**
Ref: Ghai's Paediatrics, 6/e p352

71. **Ans. (d)** **ELISA**
Ref: Ghai's Paediatrics, 6/e p222

PEDIATRIC ONCOLOGY

72. **Ans. (a)** **ALL**
Ref: Gupte's Pediatrics 11/e p556

73. **Ans. (b)** **Neuroblastoma**
Ref: Gupte's Pediatrics 11/e p564

74. **Ans. (b)** **Lymphoma and leukemia**
Ref: Gupte's Pediatrics 11/e p558

75. **Ans. (b)** **ALL**
Ref: Gupte's Pediatrics 11/e p555

76. **Ans. (b)** **Retinoblastoma**
Ref: Gupte's Pediatrics 11/e p568

77. **Ans. (d) Present after 5 years of age**
Ref: Gupte's Pediatrics 11/e p562

78. **Ans. (d) Papillary carcinoma**
Ref: Shenoy's Surgery, 2/e p266

79. **Ans. (b) Neuroblastoma**
Ref: Gupte's Pediatrics 11/e p564

80. **Ans. (a) Bilateral polycystic kidney**
Ref: Gupte's Pediatrics 11/e p562

81. **Ans. (c) Presents commonly between 5-10 years of age**
Ref: Gupte's Pediatrics 11/e p563

MISCELLANEOUS

82. **Ans. (d) Mild proteinuria, hematuria & high ASO titre**
Ref: Ghai's Paediatrics, 6/e p447

83. **Ans. (c) Truancy**
Ref: Ghai's Paediatrics, 6/e p58

84. **Ans. (c) Poor feeding**
Ref: Gupte's Pediatrics 11/e p416

85. **Ans. (c) Rotavirus**
Ref: Gupte's Pediatrics 11/e p449

86. **Ans. (c) Streptococcus pneumoniae**
Ref: Gupte's Pediatrics 11/e p327

87. **Ans. (c) Metabolic acidosis**
Ref: Gupte's Pediatrics 11/e p177

88. **Ans. (c) 5 years**
Ref: Gupte's Pediatrics 11/e p49

89. **Ans. (a) Isolated prolonged PTT with a normal PT**
Ref: Gupte's Pediatrics 11/e p540

90. **Ans. (c) Hb electrophoresis**
Ref: Gupte's Pediatrics 11/e p533

91. **Ans. (c) Myocarditis**
Ref: Gupte's Pediatrics 11/e p274

92. **Ans. (c) Measles**
Ref: Gupte's Pediatrics 11/e p250

93. **Ans. (a) Erythromycin**
Ref: Gupte's Pediatrics 11/e p322

94. **Ans. (a) Ribavirin**
Ref: Gupte's Pediatrics 11/e p269

95. **Ans. (a) Minimal change disease**
Ref: Gupte's Pediatrics 11/e p518

96. **Ans. (a) Kernicterus**
Ref: Gupte's Pediatrics 11/e p238

97. **Ans. (b) Turner syndrome**
Ref: Gupte's Pediatrics 11/e p646

98. **Ans. (b) Sarcolemmal protein**
Ref: Gupte's Pediatrics 11/e p661

99. **Ans. (b) Streptococcus pneumoniae**
Ref: Gupte's Pediatrics 11/e p416

100. **Ans. (c) Mental retardation**
Ref: Gupte's Pediatrics 11/e p48

101. **Ans. (a) No findings**
Ref: Gupte's Pediatrics 11/e p519

102. **Ans. (b) Hyperthyroidism**
Ref: Gupte's Pediatrics 11/e p35

103. **Ans. (a) Measles**
Ref: Gupte's Pediatrics 11/e p252

104. **Ans. (d) Minimal change disease**
Ref: Gupte's Pediatrics 11/e p518

105. **Ans. (c) PCR**
Ref: Gupte's Pediatrics 11/e p267

106. **Ans. (d) Phenylalanine should be completed stopped in the diet**
Ref: Gupte's Pediatrics 11/e p647

107. **Ans. (c) Rabies**
Ref: Gupte's Pediatrics 11/e p264

108. **Ans. (b) Blood transfusion and desferrioxamine**
Ref: Gupte's Pediatrics 11/e p533

109. **Ans. (b) Hypothyroidism**
Ref: Gupte's Pediatrics 11/e p628

110. **Ans. (d) Avoidance of antigen**
Ref: Gupte's Pediatrics 11/e p339 (Box 21.2)

111. **Ans. (b) 10-15 days**
Ref: Gupte's Pediatrics 11/e p257

112. **Ans. (a) Repeat dose if the women remain undelivered after the first course**
Ref: Gupte's Pediatrics 11/e p216

113. **Ans. (c) Raised PT**
Ref: Gupte's Pediatrics 11/e p544

114. **Ans. (b) Tetralogy of fallot**
Ref: Gupte's Pediatrics 11/e p367

115. **Ans. (a) Goodpasture syndrome**
Ref: Gupte's Pediatrics 11/e p509 (Box 26.1)

116. **Ans. (c) Carbamazepine**
Ref: Gupte's Pediatrics 11/e p434

117. **Ans. (b) Neutrophilia**
Ref: Gupte's Pediatrics 11/e p224

118. **Ans. (b) McCunne Albright syndrome**
Ref: Gupte's Pediatrics 11/e p631

119. **Ans. (d) Hypoglycemia**
Ref: Gupte's Pediatrics 11/e p238

120. **Ans. (c) Rotavirus**
Ref: Gupte's Pediatrics 11/e p447

121. **Ans. (b) Measles**
Ref: Gupte's Pediatrics 11/e p251

122. **Ans. (a) Rotavirus**
Ref: Gupte's Pediatrics 11/e p445

123. **Ans. (b) Tanner's breast stage III, Pubic hair stage III**
Ref: Gupte's Pediatrics 11/e p62

124. **Ans. (b) Lactose intolerance**
Ref: Gupte's Pediatrics 11/e p462 (Box 24.1)

125. **Ans. (a) Valproic acid**
Ref: Gupte's Pediatrics 11/e p432

126. **Ans. (b) 20 seconds**
Ref: Gupte's Pediatrics 11/e p219

127. **Ans. (c) Hyponatremia**
Ref: Gupte's Pediatrics 11/e p448

128. **Ans. (c) Limited by suture line**
Ref: Gupte's Pediatrics 11/e p190

129. **Ans. (d) Infantile spasms**
Ref: Gupte's Pediatrics 11/e p433

130. **Ans. (b) Streptococcus pneumoniae**
Ref: Gupte's Pediatrics 11/e p681

131. **Ans. (b) Respiratory rate of 60 or more in less than 2 months of age**
Ref: Gupte's Pediatrics 11/e p329

132. **Ans. (b) Total body iron stores**
Ref: Gupte's Pediatrics 11/e p526

133. **Ans. (d) Meningococci**
Ref: Gupte's Pediatrics 11/e p416

134. **Ans. (d) Less than 32°C**
Ref: Gupte's Pediatrics 11/e p211

135. **Ans. (b) Minimal change disease**
Ref: Gupte's Pediatrics 11/e p518

136. **Ans. (b) Morphine**
Ref: Gupte's Pediatrics 11/e p336

137. **Ans. (d) 11 beta hydroxylase**
Ref: Gupte's Pediatrics 11/e p634

138. **Ans. (b) Pneumonia**
Ref: Gupte's Pediatrics 11/e p328

139. **Ans. (a) Height of more than 145 cm**
Ref: Gupte's Pediatrics 11/e p646

140. **Ans. (b) 800 mL**
Ref: Ghai's Pediatrics, 8th ed., p-294

141. **Ans. (a) Complete heart block**
Ref: Gupte's Pediatrics 11/e p360

142. **Ans. (c) Prolonged**
Ref: Gupte's Pediatrics 11/e p218

143. **Ans. (d) Coronal suture**
Ref: Gupte's Pediatrics 11/e p32

144. **Ans. (a) Rotor's syndrome**
Ref: Gupte's Pediatrics 11/e p229

145. **Ans. (b) Respiratory infections**
Ref: Internet resources

146. **Ans. (b) Dubin Johnson syndrome**
Ref: Gupte's Pediatrics 11/e p229

147. **Ans. (a) IgA and C3**
Ref: Internet resources

148. **Ans. (b) More than 40**
Ref: Gupte's Pediatrics 11/e p329

149. **Ans. (d) Infections**
Ref: Gupte's Pediatrics 11/e p631

150. **Ans. (d) Subependymal hemorrhage**
Ref: Gupte's Pediatrics 11/e p205

PRACTICE QUESTIONS

GROWTH

1. **Anterior fontanel fuses by:**
   a. 6 months b. 18 months
   c. 36 months d. 72 months

NUTRITION

2. **A 1-year-old female patient presented with excessive crying, pain in extremities and bleeding from gums. She is apprehensive to move her limbs. Most probable diagnosis:**
   a. Rickets
   b. Scurvy
   c. Osteogenesis imperfecta
   d. Osteomyelitis
3. **All of the following are features of marasmus EXCEPT:**
   a. Old men look b. Wasting
   c. Loose folds of skin d. Apathy

NEWBORN

4. **Which of the following step is indicated in neonatal resuscitation:**
   a. Put extremely cold water on back
   b. Gentle stroking on back
   c. Tickling the sole
   d. Hanging in head down position
5. **Which of the following is an indication for chest compression in neonate while doing cardiopulmoary resuscitation:**
   a. Irregular breathing with heart rate of 80/min after 30 seconds
   b. Regular breathing with heart rate of 80/min after 30 seconds
   c. Heart rate of less than 60/ min with AMBU bag respiration for 30 seconds
   d. Regular breathing with heart rate more than 100/ min but cyanotic
6. **Physiological jaundice in preterm babies last for:**
   a. 7 days b. 10 days
   c. 14 days d. 21 days

CONGENITAL DISORDERS

7. **Congenital rubella syndrome/ CRS is associated with:**
   a. Coarctation of aorta
   b. Ventricular septal defect
   c. Patent ductus arteriosus
   d. Atrial septal defect
8. **Congenital rubella syndrome does NOT include:**
   a. Cataract
   b. Sensori-neural hearing loss
   c. Cardiac defects
   d. Macro-ophthalmia

CVS DISORDERS

9. **Which of the following condition presents with mid-diastolic murmur with presystolic accentuation:**
   a. Mitral regurgitation
   b. Mitral stenosis
   c. Aortic regurgitation
   d. Aortic stenosis

INFECTIOUS DISEASES

10. **Retrobulbar neuritis is a complication of:**
    a. INH b. Rifampin
    c. Ethambutol d. Streptomycin
11. **FALSE statement for mumps:**
    a. Orchitis is a common complication
    b. Incubation period of 16 days
    c. High chances of recurrence
    d. Generalized infection may occur

PAEDIATRIC ONCOLOGY

12. **Probable diagnosis of a case presenting with enlargement of cervical lymph nodes which have a rubbery feel:**
    a. Non-Hodgkin's lymphoma
    b. Hodgkin's lymphoma
    c. Neuroblastoma
    d. Wilm's tumor

Ans.
1. b. 18 months **2.** b. Scurvy **3.** d. Apathy **4.** c. Tickling the sole
5. c. Heart rate of less than 60... **6.** c. 14 days **7.** c. Patent ductus arteri... **8.** d. Macro-ophthalmia
9. b. Mitral stenosis **10.** c. Ethambutol **11.** c. High chances of... **12.** b. Hodgkin's lymphoma

MISCELLANEOUS

13. Most definite method of estimating GFR
- a. Serum creatinine
- b. Serum insulin
- c. Serum creatine
- d. Serum inulin

14. Which of the following is NOT a content of breast milk:
- a. Lactaglobulin
- b. Lactoalbumin
- c. Whey protein
- d. Lymphocytes

15. Treatment of choice for Kawasaki disease:
- a. Steroids
- b. Intravenous immunoglobulins
- c. Immunosuppressants
- d. NSAIDs

16. Best management of a 3-year-old child with diurnal enuresis and soiling of clothes:
- a. Urethroplasty
- b. Catheterization for a week
- c. Emergency circumcision
- d. Behavioural modification

Ans. **13.** c. Serum creatine **14.** a. Lactaglobulin **15.** b. Intravenous immun... **16.** d. Behavioural modification

IMAGE-BASED QUESTIONS

1. Spot diagnosis:

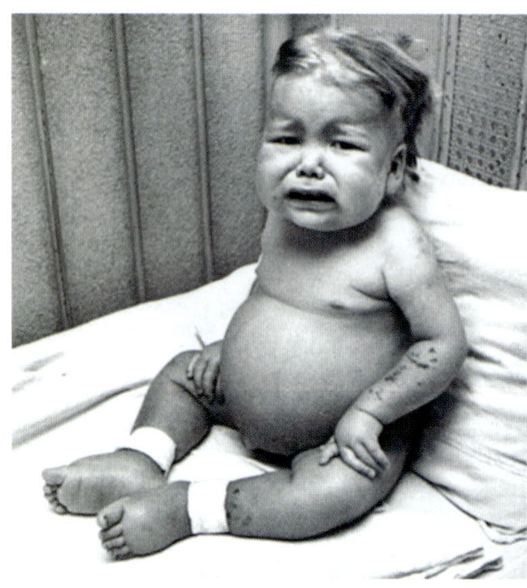

a. Marasmus
b. Scurvy
c. Kwashiorkor
d. Osteogenesis imperfecta

A classical case of kwashiorkor is dull, apathetic and miserable, evincing hardly any interest in the surroundings. His growth is stunted and there is marked muscle wasting with some retention of subcutaneous fat. He has pitting edema over the legs and feet and perhaps over certain other parts of the body.

2. Hair changes are suggestive of:

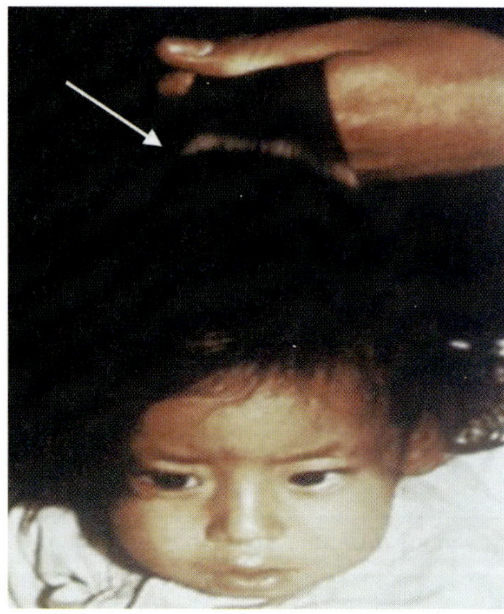

a. Marasmus
b. Rickets
c. Cretinism
d. Kwashiorkor

Hair changes of kwashiorkor are seen in the form of hypochromotrichia (light-colored hair), sparseness (areas of alopecia), change in texture (coarseness, silkiness) and easy pluckability. Alternate bands of light and dark color have earned the name "flag sign", which signifies periods of inadequate, adequate and inadequate nutrition over a prolonged period. This fascinating sign is only occasionally encountered.

3. Spot diagnosis:

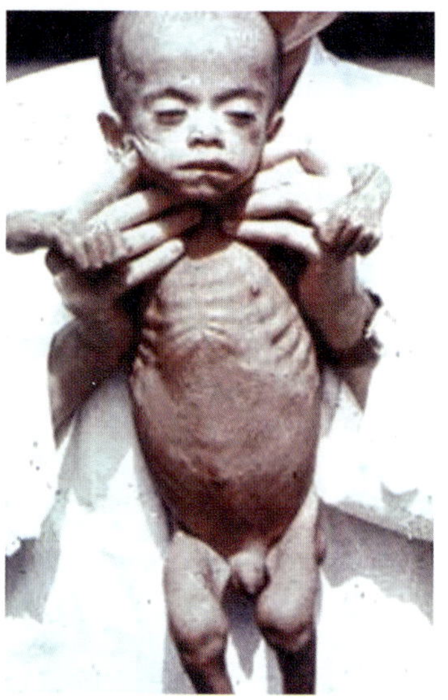

a. Kwashiorkor
b. Marasmus
c. Scurvy
d. von Willebrand disease

A characteristic feature of the clinical feature is remarkable wasting of both muscles and subcutaneous fat. The face is wizened and shrivelled—just as in the case of a monkey.

4. X-ray of such a patient will show:

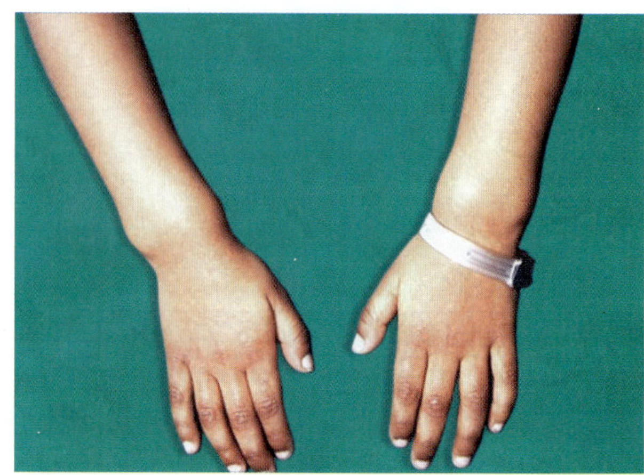

a. Epiphyseal dysgenesis
b. Cupping and splaying of metaphyses
c. Subperiosteal hemorrhages
d. Multiple fractures

X-ray findings in rickets are best seen at the wrist. These include cupping (saucer-like depression), flaring (widening) and fraying (rarefaction) of the lower ends of radius and ulna. There is an increase in the distance between the epiphyseal center and shaft of long bones due to radiotranslucency of the osteoid.

5. Spot diagnosis:

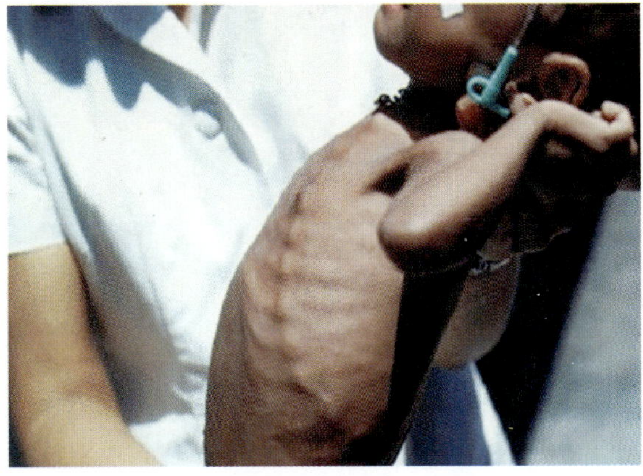

a. Rickets
b. Scurvy
c. Neonatal emphysema
d. Subcutaneous emphysema

Thorax in rickets: Rachitic rosary (smooth rounded, nontender, costochondral beading), pigeon-chest deformity (pectus carinatum), Harrison sulcus or groove (a depression along the insertion of diaphragm into the ribs), flaring of the lower ribs. "Violin-shaped" deformed chest is characteristic. Infrequently, sternum is unusually depressed, the so-called pectus excavatum.

6. Step to prevent such a condition:

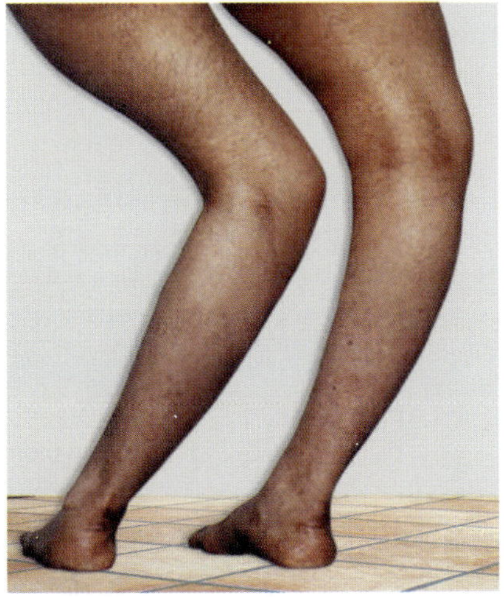

a. 100 IU of vitamin D
b. 200 IU of vitamin D
c. 300 IU of vitamin D
d. 400 IU of vitamin D

Wind-swept deformity is seen in rickets. To prevent rickets, availability of at least 400 IU of vitamin D through sun shine, diet or supplements must be ensured.

7. Which of the following is used for managing condition shown in figure:

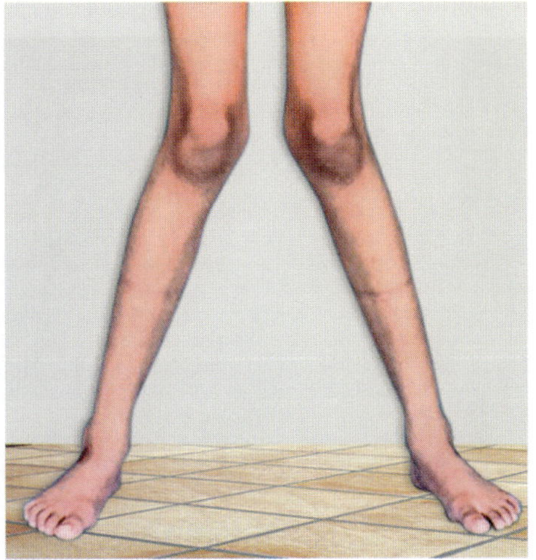

a. Pulse therapy
b. Stoss therapy
c. PUVA
d. Immunotherapy

Specific therapy (stoss therapy) for managing rickets, consists of administering a single massive dose of vitamin D_3 (3,00,000 units up to 1 year of age; 6,00,000 units for later ages) orally or intramuscularly together with supplementary calcium and phosphorous.

8. Spot diagnosis:

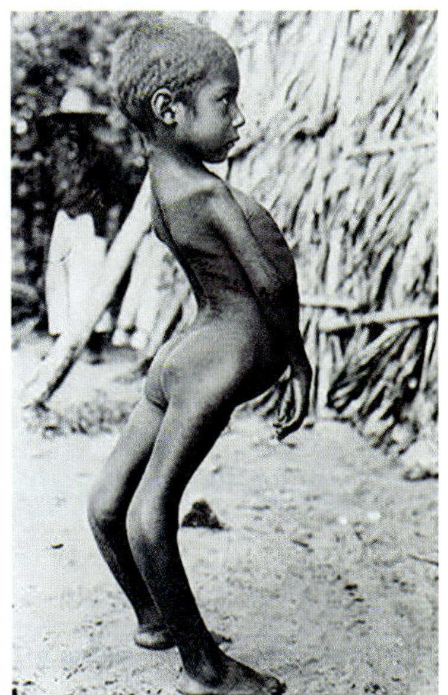

a. Genu varum
b. Genu valgum
c. Wind swept deformity
d. Genu recurvatum

Genu recurvatum is a deformity in the knee joint, so that the knee bends backwards. In this deformity, excessive extension occurs in the tibiofemoral joint.

9. Spot diagnosis:

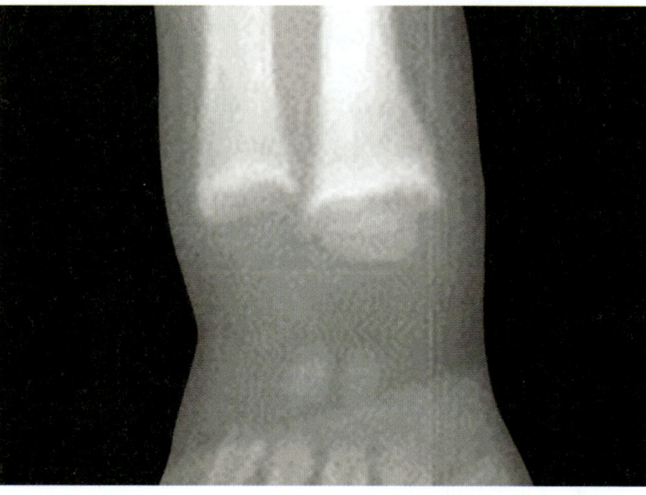

a. Scurvy
b. Rickets
c. Normal
d. Cretinism

X-ray findings in rickets are best seen at the wrist. These include cupping (saucer-like depression), flaring (widening) and fraying (rarefaction) of the lower ends of radius and ulna. There is an increase in the distance between the epiphyseal center and shaft of long bones due to radio-translucency of the osteoid.

10. Spot diagnosis:

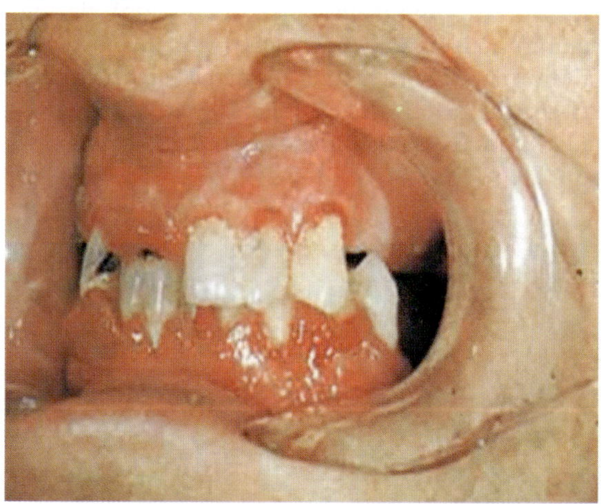

a. Marfan syndrome
b. Ehler Danlos syndrome
c. Scurvy
d. Rickets

In scurvy, hemorrhages may occur into the skin and mucous membranes. Hemorrhages into the gums may result in spongy, swollen, bluish purple gums, especially about the erupted teeth.

MCQ POINTS

S. No.	Question statements	Answers
1.	Height of a child is double the birth height at the age of	***4 years***
2.	Pincer grasp is attained at the age of:	***9 months***
3.	Child is able to build blocks of 5 cubes. Developmental age is	***16-24 months***
4.	First permanent teeth to appear is	***Lower 1st molar***
5.	Total number of milk teeth in human being	***20***
6.	Pica refers to	***Foreign body being put in mouth***
7.	Flaky paint dermatosis of skin is seen in	***Kwashiorkar***
8.	Breast milk is stored at room temperature for	***8 hours***
9.	Wind swept deformity is seen in	***Rickets***
10.	Keshan disease is caused by deficiency of	***Selenium***
11.	Neonatal period extends up to	***28 days of life***
12.	Organ NOT affected in asymmetrical IUGR	***Brain***
13.	Fetal lung maturity is assessed by	***L/S ratio***
14.	One gram of hemoglobin liberates how many mg of bilirubin	***34***
15.	MC type of congenital heart disease is	***MC type of congenital cyanotic heart disease: TOF***
16.	In patent ductus arteriosus, the connection is between	***Aorta and pulmonary artery***
17.	MC cause of acute intestinal obstruction in neonates	***Duodenal atresia***
18.	Commonest cause of intestinal obstruction in children	***Intussusception***
19.	Commonest site of regional enteritis	***Distal ileum and colon***
20.	MC cause of cholestatic jaundice in newborn is	***Neonatal hepatitis***
21.	MC cause of portal hypertension in children is	***Extrahepatic compression***
22.	Profuse watery diarrhea in an immunocompromised child is due to infestation by:	***Giardia***
23.	MC cause of convulsion on the first day of life in a newborn	***Anoxia***
24.	Initial drug of choice in a child with status epilepticus	***Lorazepam***
25.	MC intracranial tumor in children	***Glioma***
26.	Preventable cause of mental retardation	***Cretinism***
27.	Enzyme deficient in phenylketonuria	***Phenyl-Alanine-Hydroxylase***
28.	MC presentation of a child with Wilm's tumor	***Asymptomatic abdominal mass***
29.	Edema of hands and feet in infants is characteristic of which syndrome	***Turner's syndrome***
30.	Measles virus belongs to which group	***Paramyxovirus***
31.	Child draws a triangle at the age of	***5 years***
32.	MC cause of bronchiolitis is	***Respiratory synctial virus***
33.	Diagnosis of toxoplasmosis in newborn is best done by demonstrating which antibodies (to toxoplasma)	***IgM***
34.	MC enzyme deficiency leading to childhood hypertension	***21 alpha hydroxylase***
35.	Compression to ventilation ratio in neonates	***3:1***
36.	MC cause of neonatal meningitis	***Group B streptococci, E coli***
37.	MC cause of aseptic meningitis in children is	***Enterovirus***

S. No.	Question statements	Answers
38.	Management of a newborn of HBsAg positive mother	***Active (HBV) and passive (HBIG) immunization***
39.	MC cause of 1st day jaundice in a newborn	***Rh incompatibility***
40.	MC bacteria cause of diarrhea in children	***E. Coli***
41.	Which congenital heart defect is commoner in Down syndrome	***ASD (endocardial cushion defect)***
42.	Breathing and swallowing action develops in fetus at which week	***12-14 weeks***
43.	Moro's reflex is abnormal after how many weeks	***12 weeks***
44.	Best method of diagnosing childhood HIV	***HIV PCR***
45.	Epiphyseal dysgenesis is associated with	***Hypothyroidism***
46.	Most important cause of under 5 mortality is	***Respiratory tract infection***
47.	Commonest hematological malignancy in children is	***ALL***
48.	Commonest cause of death in diphtheric child	***Myocarditis***
49.	Vertical transmission of toxoplasmosis causes more severe disease in which trimester	***First trimester***
50.	% increase in length of infant in first year of life	***50% (25 cm)***
51.	Deletion of chromosome 11 leads to which disease	***Wilm's tumor***
52.	Which vessel carries highly oxygenated blood toward fetal heart	***Umbilical vein***
53.	Umbilical cord usually falls after how many days	***10-14 days***
54.	Alpha-1 antitrypsin is synthesized in which organ	***Liver***
55.	Weight of low birth baby	***Less than 2.5 kg***
56.	Boy who refuses to eat fruit comes with knee swelling and hematoma. Deficiency of which vitamin can be suspected	***Vitamin C***
57.	MC cause of UTI in children less than 5 years of age	***E. Coli***
58.	Normal value of fetal scalp pH is	***7.33***
59.	MC cause of pneumonia in children	***Streptococcus pneumoniae***
60.	Apnea in prematurity last for how many seconds	***20 seconds***
61.	MC cause of acute infantile gastroenteritis	***Rotavirus***
62.	MC cause of death in Klinefelter's syndrome	***Infections***
63.	MC thyroid tumor in children	***Papillary***
64.	What to give first in a severely malnourished child	***Dextrose***
65.	Fast breathing in a 3 year old child is breathing rate more than	***40/ minutes***
66.	Large doses of vitamin K in a newborn causes	***Hemolytic anemia***
67.	Iron and folic acid requirement of 6 months to 10 year old children is	***20 mg elemental iron and 100 microgram folic acid***
68.	A female presented with hypertension, hyperpigmentation and virilization. She is most likely to be suffering from deficiency of which enzyme	***11 beta hydroxylase***
69.	As per immunization schedule, Hepatitis A vaccine is recommended at the minimum age of	***2 year***
70.	MC cause of acute epiglottitis in children	***H. Influenzae type B***
71.	Non-immune hydrops is seen in	***Alpha thalassemia major***
72.	Severe hypothermia in a neonate is temperature below	***32 °C***
73.	PEM with marked muscle wasting:	***Marasmus***
74.	Harrison's sulcus is a feature of	***Rickets***
75.	Increased nuchal skin fold thickness (a indicator of Down syndrome) is seen on which imaging modality:	***USG***

S. No.	Question statements	Answers
76.	Short 4th metacarpal is a feature of:	***Turner syndrome***
77.	Notched incisors can be seen in which congenital infection:	***Late congenital syphilis***
78.	Physiological jaundice in a term baby lasts for:	***7-10 days***
79.	Chest radiography appearance in ARDS:	***Ground glass appearance***
80.	DOC for bronchiolitis	***Ribavirin***
81.	X-ray finding of TAPVC:	***Snowman/ figure of 8***
82.	MC type of anemia in children	***Iron deficiency anemia***
83.	Hair on end appearance (radiograph) is seen in	***Thalassemia***
84.	Vesicourethral reflux/ VUR is diagnosed by	***Micturating CystoUrethroGraphy***
85.	MC cause of nephrotic syndrome in children	***Minimal change disease/ lipoid nephrosis***
86.	MC malignant neoplasm in infancy	***Neuroblastoma***
87.	MC presentation of neuroblastoma	***Abdominal mass***
88.	MC soft tissue sarcoma is	***Rhabdomyosarcoma***
89.	Enzyme deficient in phenylketonuria	***Phenylalanine hydroxylase***
90.	Which amino acid becomes essential in Phenylketonuria	***Tyrosine***
91.	Urine turns/ dark on exposure to atmosphere in	***Alkaptonuria***
92.	MC type of seizure in newborn	***Subtle***
93.	DMD is a defect of	***Sarcolemmal protein defect***
94.	Andersen disease is due to deficiency of	***Branching enzyme***
95.	Condition in which unconjugated bilirubin gets deposited in basal ganglia	***Kernicterus***
96.	The height of a child is double the birth height at the age of ...... years	***4 years***
97.	Infant body weight is tripled by the age of .... years	***1 year***
98.	Pincer grasp is attained at the age of ...... months	***9 months***
99.	First permanent teeth to appear in a child is	***1st lower molar***
100.	In kwashiorkar, which Ig is most affected:	***IgA***
101.	Flaky paint appearance of skin is seen in:	***Kwashiorkar***
102.	Breast milk can be stored at room temperature for .... hours	***8 hours***
103.	Deficient mineralization in epiphyseal growth cartilage is seen in:	***Rickets***
104.	Windswept deformity is seen in which condition	***Rickets***
105.	A 30 year old female has high alkaline phosphatase, low calcium and phosphate. Diagnosis is:	***Osteomalacia***
106.	Keshan disease is deficiency of which micronutrient:	***Selenium***
107.	Neonatal period extends up to:	***First 28 days of life***
108.	Persistence of Moro's reflex is abnormal beyond the age of .... months:	***3 months***
109.	Which organ is not affected in asymmetrical IUGR:	***Brain***
110.	MC cause of sepsis in India, within 2 months of life:	***E. coli***
111.	Hyaline membrane seen in lungs composed of:	***Fibrin***
112.	Fetal lung maturity is assessed by:	***Lecithin/ sphingomyelin ratio***
113.	1 gm of hemoglobin liberates how many mg of bilirubin:	***34 mg***
114.	Jaundice within 24 hours of birth is commonly due to:	***Rh incompatibility***
115.	A 2 year old child is classified as having pneumonia, if the respiratory rate is more than:	***40/ minute***
116.	Oxygenated blood to fetus is carried out by which vessel:	***Umbilical vein***

S. No.	Question statements	Answers
117.	In patent ductus arteriosus, the connection is between which vessels	***Aorta and pulmonary artery***
118.	Coarctation of aorta is commoner in which syndrome:	***Turner syndrome***
119.	Egg on side appearance is seen in which condition:	***Transposition of great arteries***
120.	MC cause of stridor shortly after birth:	***Laryngomalacia***
121.	Croup syndrome is usually caused by which organism:	***Parainfluenza virus***
122.	6 year old child with palpable abdominal mass in epigastrium. There is no bile in vomitus. Diagnosis is:	***Pyloric stenosis***
123.	MC cause of acute intestinal obstruction in neonates is:	***Duodenal atresia***
124.	MC cause of intestinal obstruction in children is:	***Intussusception***
125.	Common site of regional enteritis is:	***Ileum***
126.	MC cause of cholestatic jaundice in newborn is:	***Neonatal hepatitis***
127.	Profuse watery diarrhea in an immunocompromised child is due to which parasite:	***Giardia***
128.	MC organism associated with hemolytic uremic syndrome:	***E. Coli***
129.	MC cause of convulsion on the first day of life in a newborn is:	***Hypoxic ischemic encephalopathy***
130.	Initial DOC for status epilepticus in a child is:	***Lorazepam***
131.	DOC for absence seizures:	***Valproate***
132.	MC causative agent of meningitis in the age group of 6 months to 3 years:	***H. Influenzae type B***
133.	MC intracranial tumor in children is:	***Glioma***
134.	Preventable cause of mental retardation is:	***Cretinism***
135.	In phenylketonuria, $FeCl_3$ test with urine gives which color:	***Green***
136.	Mousy odor of urine is seen in:	***Phenylketonuria***
137.	4 year old child having palpable abdominal mass and hypertension with sweating and diarrhea. Diagnosis:	***Neuroblastoma***
138.	MC presentation of a child with Wilm's tumor	***Asympatomatic abdominal mass***
139.	Baby presented with recurrent infections of ear and discharge, seborrheic dermatitis, hepatosplenomegaly and cystic skull lesions. Diagnosis:	***Histocytosis X***
140.	Which hemoglobin estimation will be diagnostically helpful in a case of beta thalassemia trait:	***HbA_2***
141.	Salmonellosis is commoner in which type of anemia:	***Sickle cell anemia***
142.	Gonads to testes differentiation is by which gene:	***SRY gene***
143.	Edema of hands and feet in infants is characteristic of which syndrome:	***Turner syndrome***
144.	Trisomy 13 is which syndrome:	***Patau syndrome***
145.	Measles virus belongs to which group:	***Paramyxovirus***
146.	Treatment of Kawasaki disease in children:	***I/V Ig***
147.	Congenital syphilis can be best diagnosed by which test:	***IgM FTA-ABS***
148.	A neonate born to infected hepatitis B mother, should be treated with:	***Active and passive immunization***
149.	Which drug is given to prevent HIV transmission from mother to child:	***Nevirapine***
150.	Giant cell (Hecht's) pneumonia is due to:	***Measle virus***
151.	Measles is infectious during ...... days before the rash and ..... days after the rash	***4 days, 5 days***
152.	In Down syndrome, the shape of the head is:	***Brachycephaly***
153.	Atavism means child resembles his:	***Grandparents***

S. No.	Question statements	Answers
154.	HIV detection in a 2 year old is done by:	***HIV PCR***
155.	MC cause of adrenogenital syndrome (congenital adrenal hyperplasia) is deficiency of which enzyme:	***21 alpha hydroxylase***
156.	Normal value of fetal scalp pH is:	***7.33***
157.	First sign of puberty in females:	***Thelarche***
158.	MC cardiac lesion in Down syndrome is:	***ASD***
159.	According to WHO, cut off level for hemoglobin in child for anemia is ... gm%:	***11 gm%***
160.	MC cause of acute infantile gastroenteritis is:	***Rotavirus***
161.	Large doses of vitamin K in a newborn will lead to ..... anemia:	***Hemolytic***
162.	Iron and folic acid requirement of 6 months to 10 years old children is:	***20 mg, 100 mcg***
163.	MC cause of acute epiglottitis in children is:	***H. Influenzae type B***
164.	MC gastrointestinal malignancy of childhood is:	***Lymphoma***
165.	The breathing and swallowing action develops in fetus at the age of .... weeks:	***12-14 weeks***
166.	Epiphyseal dysgenesis is a pathognomic feature of:	***Hypothyroidism***
167.	MC type of leukemia in children:	***ALL***
168.	Steroids are most useful in which type of nephropathy:	***Minimal change disease***
169.	Umbilical cord usually falls after how many days of birth:	***5-10 days***
170.	Alpha-1-antitrypsin is synthesized in which organ:	***Liver***
171.	Child can copy a triangle at the age of	***5 years***
172.	Body weight of a 4 year old child	***16 kg***

CHAPTER

7

OBSTETRICS

KEY POINTS

Amniotic Fluid Colour and Conditions

- Straw: Normal
- Golden colour: Rh incompatibility
- Greenish yellow (saffron): Post-maturity
- Dark coloured: Concealed accidental hemorrhage
- Dark brown (tobacco juice): Intrauterine death
- Meconium stained (green): Fetal distress
- Thick with flakes (pea-soup): Chronic fetal distress
- Purulent: Chorioamnionitis

Polyhydramnios

- Liquor amnii exceeds 2000 ml. OR,
- AFI > 20 cm/> 90th percentile for the gestational age

Oligohydramnios

- Liquor amnii is less than 100 ml. OR,
- AFI < 5 cm/< 10th percentile for gestational age

Procedure and Preferred Time

- Chorionic villous sampling: 10-12 weeks
- Placental villi sampling: > 12 weeks
- Amniocentesis: 14-16 weeks
- Cordocentesis: After 18 weeks

Weight Gain

- 1 kg in first trimester
- 5 kg each in second and third trimester

Pelvis

- Naegele's pelvis: Ala on one side is absent
- Robert's pelvis: Ala on both sides is absent

Diameter of Fetal Skull

- Bimastoid: 7.5 cm
- Bitemporal: 8 cm
- Submentobregmatic: 9.5 cm
- Biparietal: 9.5 cm
- Suboccipitobregmatic: 9.5 cm
- Suboccipitofrontal: 10 cm
- Occipitofrontal: 11.5 cm
- Submentovertical: 11.5 cm
- Mentovertical: 14 cm

Manning's Score

- Non-stress test
- Breathing movement – At least 1 in 30 minutes for 30 seconds duration
- At least 3 fetal movements in 30 minutes
- Fetal tone: At least 1 in 30 minutes
- Adequacy of amniotic fluid
- Maximum score – 10
  - 10-8 is Normal
  - 6 is Equivocal
  - 4 or less is Abnormal.

Prolonged Latent Phase of Labor

- Latent phase exceeds:
  - 20 hours in primigravidae and
  - 14 hours in multigravida.

Prolonged Labor

- Combined duration of first and second stage is more than 18 hours
- Labour is considered to be prolonged when:
  - Cervical dilatation rate is less than 1 cm/hr;
  - Descent is less than 1 cm/hr for a period of more than 4 hours.

Precipitate Labor

- Combined duration of the first and second stage is less than 2 hours.

Premature Rupture of Membranes

- Spontaneous rupture of membranes:
  - Any time beyond 28th week, of pregnancy
  - But before the onset of labour.

Inevitable Abortion

- It's a clinical type of abortion where the changes have progressed from where continuation of pregnancy is impossible.
- Increased vaginal bleeding
- Dilated internal os, through which products of conception are felt.

Incomplete Abortion

- Entire products of conception are not expelled but a part of it is left inside the uterine cavity.
- Persistence of vaginal bleeding.
- Patulous cervical os.

Threatened Abortion

- Process of abortion has started but has not reached stage, form where recovery is impossible.
- External os is closed.
- Slight vaginal bleeding.
- USG indicates a healthy fetus.
- Fetal cardiac movements are present SS.

Complete Abortion

- Products of conception are expelled en masse.
- Vaginal bleeding is absent /trace, following expulsion.
- Cervical os is closed.

Missed Abortion/Silent Miscarriage

- When the fetus is dead and retained inside the uterus for a vaginal discharge.
- Absent fetal heart sounds.
- Cervix firm.
- Empty gestational sac.

Hydatidiform Mole/Vesicular Mole

- Incomplete H. mole: Focal affection of the chorionic villi
- Complete H. mole: Have only placental parts, as sperm fertilizes an empty ovum
- Complete H. moles have 46 XX karyotype (molar chromosomes derived entirely from the father)
- MC presentation: Vaginal bleeding
- White currant in red currant juice: Blood may be mixed with fluid from the ruptured cysts.
- USG findings: Snow storm appearance and bunch of grapes appearance
- High HCG titre
- Routine follow-up must be done for at least 1 year (by regularly checking beta-HCG levels, and chest X-rays).

Risk Factors for Development of Choriocarcinoma

- Risk of development of choriocarcinoma: 2-10%
- Initial HCG level in urine > 1 lac IU/hour
- Histologically proven infiltrative mole
- Previous history of molar pregnancy
- Age > 35 years
- Parity >3

Indications of Medical Management in Ectopic Pregnancy

- Hemodynamically stable patient
- Unruptured pregnancy
- Gestational sac size < 3.5 cm in diameter
- HCG < 2500 IU/ml

Constriction Ring

- Eponym: Schroeder's ring
- Cause: Undue irritability of uterus
- Location: Usually at the junction of Upper and lower segment; May occur at other places; Position doesn't alter
- Tenderness: Absent
- Palpation: Fetal parts felt; Ring not felt; Round ligament not felt
- Fetal Heart Sounds present
- Vaginal Examination: Ring is felt
- Management: To relax ring after delivery of body

Effects of Pregnancy on Diabetes

- More insulin is required
- Progression and worsening of diabetic nephropathy

Effects of Diabetes on Mother

- Chorioamnionitis
- Endometritis
- Postpartum bleeding
- Increased risk of death in patients with diabetic Cardiomyopathy.

WHO Criteria for Diagnosis of Gestational Diabetes Mellitus

- Fasting:
  - Normal values: Less than 105
  - Impaired glucose tolerance: 105-139
  - Diabetes: More than 140

- 2 hours post glucose administration:
  - Normal values: Less than 160
  - Impaired glucose tolerance: 160-199
  - Diabetes: More than 200

Diagnostic Criteria of PIH

- Hypertension:
  - An absolute rise of blood pressure of at least 140/90 mm Hg, OR
  - A rise in systolic blood pressure of atleast 30 mm Hg, over the previously known blood pressure
  - A rise of 20 mm Hg MAP (mean arterial pressure) over the previous reading, OR
  - When the MAP is 105 mm Hg, of more.
  - The rise of blood pressure should be evident at least on two occasions, at least 4 hours apart.
- Edema:
  - Pitting edema over the ankles, after 12 hours of bed rest, OR
  - Rapid gain of weight of more than 1 pound/ week, or more than 5 pound a month.
- Proteinuria:
  - Protein in 24 hours urine, of more than 0.3 gm OR
  - More than 1 gm per litre,
  - In 2 or more midstream specimens,
  - Obtained 6 hours apart,
  - In the absence of UTI.

HELLP Syndrome

- **H**emolysis
- **E**levated **L**iver enzymes
- **L**ow **P**latelet count
- A complication of PIH.

Pritchard's Regime

- Magnesium sulphate—4 gm IV and 10 gm deep IM, 5 gm in alternate buttocks 4 hourly.
- Repeat injection only after ensuring
  - Urine output is more than 30 ml/ hour
  - Respiration rate is > 12/ minute
  - Knee jerk is present
- Therapeutic level of serum magnesium is 4-7 meq/l.

Placenta Previa

- Painless, causeless, recurrent bleeding
- Fetal heart sounds usually present
- Placenta is present in lower segment, so malpresentation is common
- Bleeding is always revealed
- Uterus is soft and relaxed.

Amniotic Fluid Indicators of Fetal Maturity

- Creatinine > 2mg/ 100 ml
- Orange colored cells > 50% when stained with 0.1 percent Nile blue sulphate
- Osmolarity of 250 mosmol/litre
- L:S ratio of >2,
- Identification of phosphatidylglycerol
- Optical density difference (at 650 m) greater than 0.15.

MSAFP (Maternal Serum Alpha Feto-Protein) Raised in

- Wrong gestational age
- Anterior abdominal wall defects
- Open neural defects
- Multiple pregnancy
- Renal anomalies
- IUFD.

MSAFP Lowered in

- Trisomies

Triple Test

- Used in detection of Down's syndrome
- Low MSAFP
- High HCG
- Low Estriol

Organisms Crossing Placenta

- Syphilis
- Parvovirus
- Hepatitis B and C
- Toxoplasma
- Rubella
- HIV
- CMV

Toxoplasmosis Transplacental Transmission

- First trimester:
  - Low incidence of transplacental infection,
  - But disease is more severe
- Third trimester:
  - High incidence of transmission,
  - But severity is less.

External Version

- Conversion is done by External manipulation only
- Done for Breech presentation and Transverse lie.

Internal Version

- Done in Transverse lie in case of second baby of twins.
- Conversion is done by one hand introduced into the uterus and the other on the abdomen.

Advantages of Forceps Over Ventouse

- Useful in suspected pelvic contraction
- Quicker, hence more useful in fetal distress
- Safer in premature babies
- Can be used in face presentation and after coming head of breech
- Incidence of hemorrhages in fetus is less.

Advantages of Ventouse Over Forceps

- It can be applied through incompletely dilated cervix (atleast 6 cm)
- Not space occupying
- Can be used in unrotated and malrotated Occipito-posterior position
- Lesser traction force required
- Can be applied at higher station.

Indications of Caesarean Section

Absolute indications	Relative
Central placenta previa	Cephalopelvic disproportion
Severe degree of CPD	Previous uterine scar
Cervical or broad	Fetal distress during first
ligament fibroid	stage of labour
Advanced carcinoma cervix	Abnormal uterine contraction
	In severe degree of placenta previa.
	In lesser degree of placenta previa when bleeding continues despite low rupture of membranes.
	Abruptio placentae
	Malpresentation –transverse lie brow, mentoposterior position.
	Bad obstetric history
	Hypertensive disorders—acute fulminating pre-eclampsia not responding to treatment. Uncontrolled eclampsia
	Failed surgical induction
	Elderly primigravidae
	Medical gynaecological disorders—chronic hypertension or chronic nephritis.
	Uncontrolled diabetes
	Uncorrected heart disease
	Pelvic tumours
	Vaginal atresia

Naegele's Formula

- If the periods are regular.
- Add 9 months and 7 days to the first day of the last menstrual cycle.
- If the cycle length is more than 28 days, then extra days are to be added, if less, then they should be subtracted.

Intrauterine Fetal Death

Blair Hartley's sign	Attitude of hyperextension or hyperflexion of fetal body. Seen after 3-4 weeks
Robert's sign	Gas translucencies are seen in fetal heart and great vessels. Seen after 12 hours
Halo sign of Deuel	Radiolucent halo around fetal cranium, due to edema of pericranial fat. Seen after 2 days
Helix sign	Presence of gas in umbilical cord

Terms

Superfecundation	Fertilization of two ova released in same menstrual cycles, by separate acts of coitus, within a short period of time.
Superfetation	Fertilization of two ova related in different menstrual cycles

Physiological Causes of Hyperprolactinemia

- Early morning/sleep
- High protein meal
- Stress, physical or psychological
- Late follicular phase of menstrual cycle
- Pregnancy, suckling
- Prolonged breast manipulation
- Coitus
- Exercise

MCQs WITH SHORT EXPLANATIONS

OBSTETRICS ANATOMY

1. **Shortest diameter of pelvic outlet:**
   a. Anteroposterior b. Intertuberous
   c. Bispinous d. All are equal

   Diameters of pelvic outlet
   - Antero-posterior diameters:
     - Anatomical antero-posterior diameter = 13 cm; from the tip of the coccyx to the lower border of symphysis pubis.
     - Obstetric antero-posterior diameter = 11 cm; from the tip of the sacrum to the lower border of symphysis pubis as the coccyx moves backwards during the second stage of labour.
   - Transverse diameters:
     - Bituberous diameter = 11 cm; between the inner aspects of the ischial tuberosities.
     - Bispinous diameter = 10.5 cm; between the tips of ischial spines.

2. **Largest diameter of the pelvic inlet:**
   a. Anatomical conjugate b. True conjugate
   c. Obstetric conjugate d. Diagonal conjugate

   Antero -posterior diameters
   - Anatomical/ antero-posterior diameter (true conjugate) = 11 cm; from the tip of the sacral promontory to the upper border of the symphysis pubis.
   - Obstetric conjugate = 10 cm; from the tip of the sacral promontory to the most bulging point on the back of symphysis pubis which is about 1 cm below its upper border. It is the shortest antero-posterior diameter.
   - Diagonal conjugate = 12 cm (1.5 – 2 cm longer than the true conjugate); From the tip of sacral promontory to the lower border of symphysis pubis.

3. **After how many days of ovulation, embryo implantation occurs?**
   a. 3–5 days
   b. 7–9 days
   c. 10–12 days
   d. 13–15 days

   Implantation/nidation occurs in the endometrium of the anterior or posterior wall of the body near the fundus on the 6th day which corresponds to the 20th day of a regular menstrual cycle.

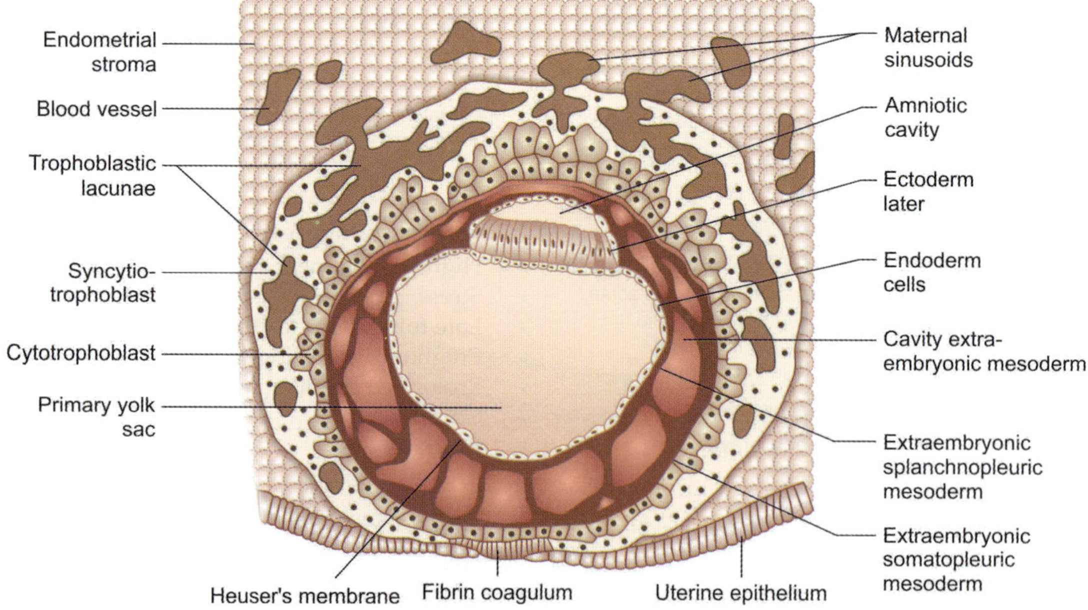

Schematic representation showing interstitial implantation of the blastocyst in stratum compactum of the decidua

4. **The distance from the upper end of sacrum to lower border of pubis corresponds to:**
   a. Transverse conjugate b. True conjugate
   c. Diagonal conjugate d. Obstetric conjugate

   Diagonal conjugate is the distance between the lower border of symphysis pubis to the midpoint on the sacral promontory. It measures 12 cm.

Ans. 1. **c.** Bispinous 2. **d.** Diagonal conjugate 3. **b.** 7-9 days 4. **c.** Diagonal conjugate

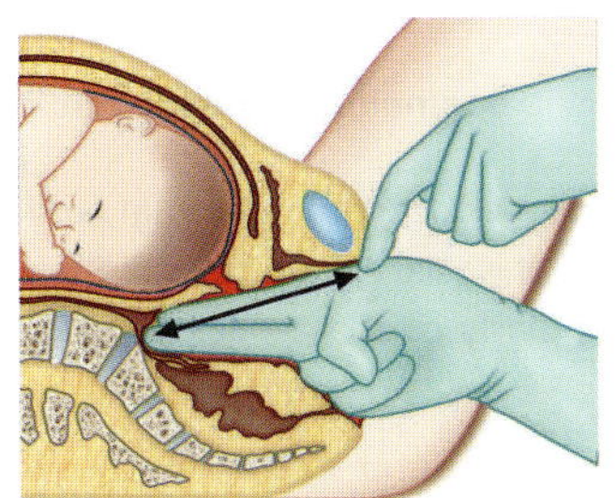

Measurement of diagonal conjugate

5. Smallest pelvic diameter in anteroposterior plane of inlet:

a. Obstetric conjugate b. Diagonal conjugate
c. True conjugate d. Transverse conjugate

Obstetric conjugate is the distance between the midpoint of the sacral promontory to prominent bony projection in the midline on the inner surface of the symphysis pubis. It measures 10 cm.

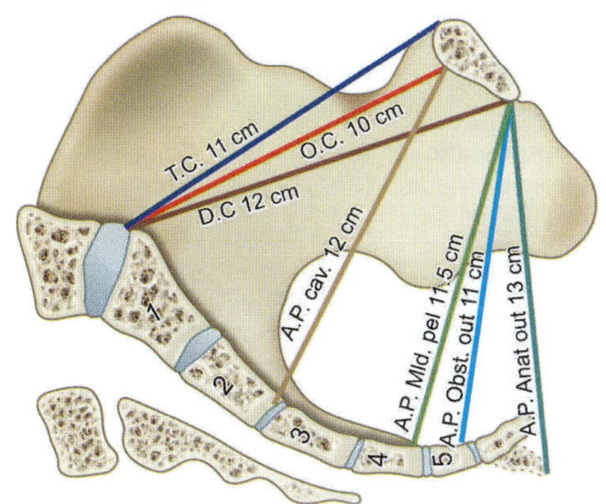

Sagittal section of the pelvis showing anteroposterior diameters in different planes

6. Largest fetal head diameter:

a. Occipitofrontal
b. Suboccipito-frontal
c. Mentovertical
d. Submentovertical

Mentovertical diameter extends from the midpoint of the chin to the highest point on the sagittal suture. It measures 14 cm.

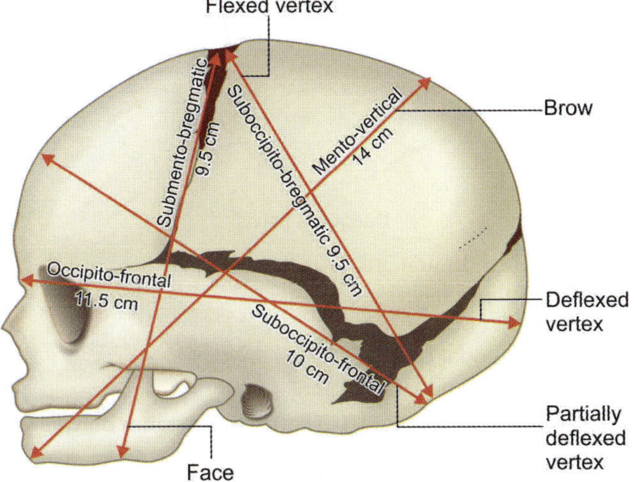

The important landmarks of fetal skull

7. MC type of female pelvis:

a. Platypelloid b. Android
c. Anthropoid d. Gynecoid

Gynecoid type of pelvis is the most common accounting for 50% of all types.

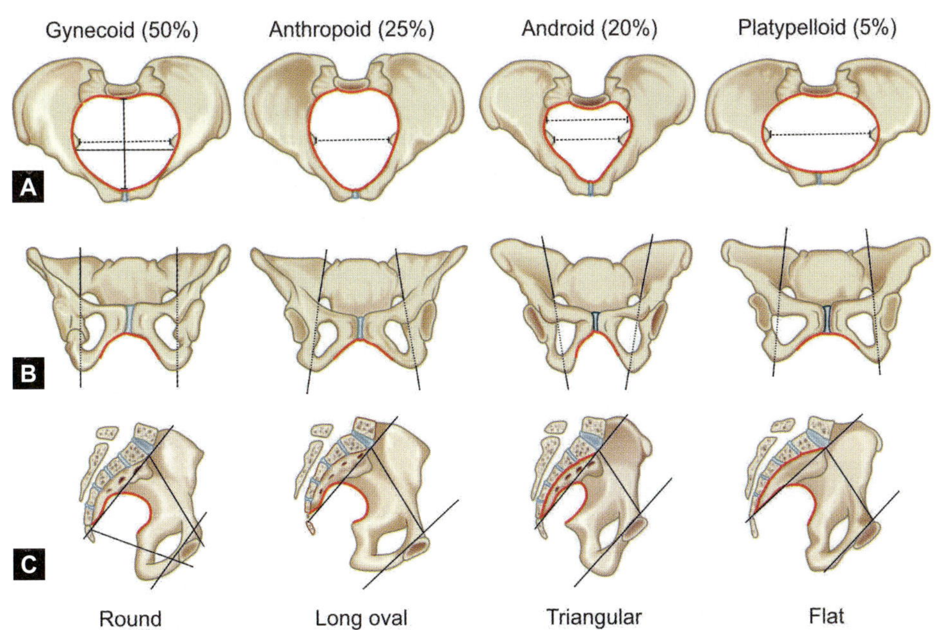

Anatomical features of parent pelvic types: (A) Inlet; (B) Cavity; (C) Outlet

Ans. 5. **a.** Obstetric conjugate 6. **c.** Mentovertical 7. **d.** Gynecoid

8. Pelvis with only one ala is known as:

a. Rachitic pelvis
b. Naegele's pelvis
c. Scoliotic pelvis
d. Robert's pelvis

Naegele's pelvis is produced due to arrested development of one ala of the sacrum.

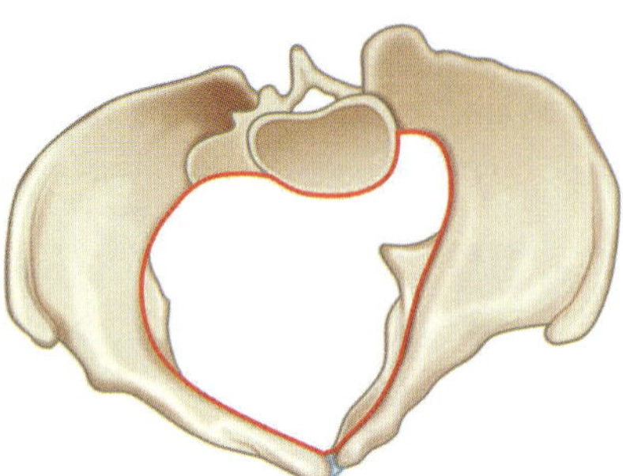

Naegele's pelvis

9. Smallest diameter of true pelvis:

a. Anteroposterior diameter
b. Left oblique
c. Diagonal conjugate
d. Interspinous diameter

Bispinous diameter (10.5 cm) is the distance between the tip of two ischial spines.

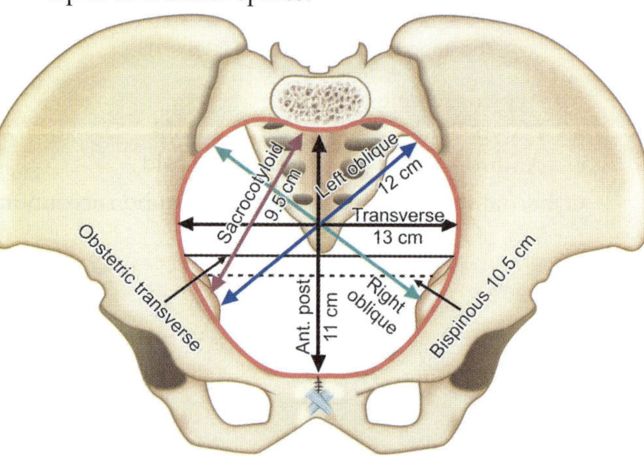

Different diameters of the inlet of obstetrical significance. Bispinous diameter is also demonstrated

10. Transverse diameter of the obstetrical outlet is:

a. 9.5
b. 10.5
c. 11.5
d. 12.5

Transverse/bispinous diameter of obstetrical outlet (plane of least pelvic dimension or narrow pelvic plane) measures 10.5 cm.

Obstetric significance of plane of least pelvic dimension
❑ It is the **narrowest** plane in the pelvis
❑ This plane corresponds roughly to the **origin of levator ani muscles**
❑ It is at this plane that the **internal rotation** of the fetal head occurs
❑ It marks the **beginning of the forward curve** of the pelvic axis
❑ It is a landmark used for **pudendal nerve block** analgesia
❑ This level of ischial spines indicate **Station 'O'**
❑ It is **irregularly oval** and notched on each side by ischial spine.

11. The shortest diameter in the fetal head is:

a. Biparietal diameter
b. Suboccipito-frontal diameter
c. Occipito-frontal diameter
d. Bitemporal diameter

Bitemporal diameter measures 8 cm and is calculated as the distance between the anteroinferior ends of the coronal suture.

Important diameters of the skull

Diameters	*Measurement in cm (inches)*	*Attitude of the head*	*Presentation*
Suboccipitobregmatic — extends from the nape of the neck to the center of the bregma	9.5 cm (3¾")	Complete flexion	Vertex
Suboccipito-frontal — extends from the nape of the neck to the anterior end of the anterior fontanel or center of the sinciput	10 cm (4")	Incomplete flexion	Vertex
Occipitofrontal — extends from the occipital eminence to the root of the nose (Glabella)	11.5 cm (4½")	Marked deflexion	Vertex
Mento-vertical — extends from the midpoint of the chin to the highest point on the sagittal suture	14 cm (5½")	Partial extension	Brow
Submentovertical — extends from junction of floor of the mouth and neck to the highest point on the sagittal suture	11.5 cm (4½")	Incomplete extension	Face
Submentobregmatic — extends from junction of floor of the mouth and neck to the center of the bregma	9.5 cm (3 ¾")	Complete extension	Face

ANTENATAL PERIOD

12. Which of the clotting factor is reduced in pregnancy:

a. XI
b. II
c. X
d. IX

Clotting factors in pregnancy

- Increased: I, VII, VIII, IX, X
- Unchanged/ mildly increased: II, V, XII
- Slightly decreased: XI, XIII

Ans. 8. **b.** Naegele's pelvis 9. **d.** Interspinous diameter 10. **b.** 10.5 11. **d.** Bitemporal diameter 12. **a.** XI

13. Which of the presentation is found in complete flexed head:

a. Vertex b. Brow
c. Face d. Occiput

Attitude of head in complete flexion

- Diameter of engagement: Sub-occipito-bregmatic (extends from the nape of neck to the centre of bregma)
- Measurement: 9.5 cm (sub-occipito-bregmatic)
- Presentation: Vertex

14. Fetal cardiac activity can by documented on transvaginal USG by:

a. 6th week b. 7th week
c. 8th week d. 9th week

Transvaginal Ultrasound

- Days 35-37: Gestational Sac of 5 mm (bHCG 1500-2000)
- Days 37-40: Yolk Sac (Gestation sac>9-10 mm, confirms intrauterine pregnancy)
- Day 40: Fetal Pole (Gestational Sac>16-18 mm, bHCG 5000)
- Day 45: Fetal Heart Activity (Crown rump length >5 mm, bHCG 17,000)

15. True for inevitable abortion:

a. Process of labor has not progressed to irreversible state
b. Cervical os dilated
c. Pregnancy can be continued
d. Fetal age more than 22 weeks

An inevitable miscarriage describes a condition in which the cervix has already dilated open, but the fetus has yet to be expelled. This usually will progress to a complete miscarriage. The heartbeat may have been shown to have stopped, but this is not part of the criteria.

16. A pregnant lady developed rapid gain in weight, hypertension & proteinuria. Such a picture suggests the diagnosis of:

a. Eclampsia b. Pre-eclampsia
c. Gestational hypertension
d. None of the above

Pre-eclampsia or preeclampsia (PE) is a disorder of pregnancy characterized by high blood pressure and a large amount of protein in the urine. The disorder usually occurs in the third trimester of pregnancy and gets worse over time. In severe disease there may be red blood cell breakdown, a low blood platelet count, impaired liver function, kidney dysfunction, swelling (gain in weight), shortness of breath due to fluid in the lungs, or visual disturbances.

17. Intrauterine fetal demise is suggested by:

a. Von Braun Fernwald's sign
b. Robert's sign
c. Goodell's sign d. Osiander's sign

Fetal death (sonographic features)

- Absent fetal heart beat
- Absent fetal movements
- Occasional finding
  - Overlapping of skull bones (Spalding sign)
  - Gross distortion of fetal anatomy (maceration)
  - Soft tissue oedema: skin >5 mm
- Uncommon findings
  - Thrombus in fetal heart
  - Gas shadow in fetal heart (Robert's sign)

18. Most useful investigation in suspected pregnancy:

a. MRI b. Culdocentesis
c. Serial beta-HCG estimation
d. USG

On USG, intradecidual gestational sac (GS) is identified as early as 29 to 35 days of gestation.

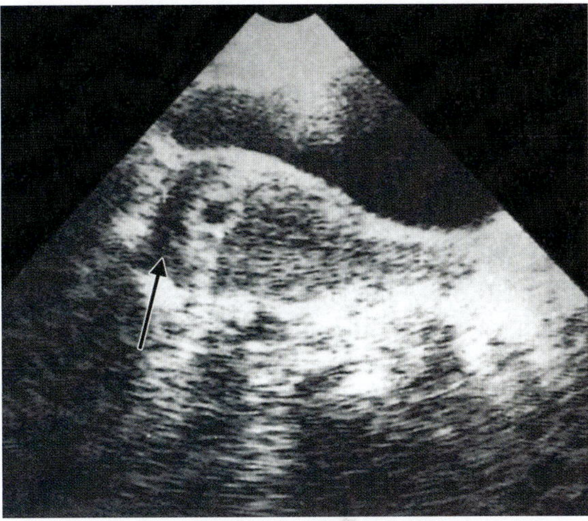

Gestational ring at 5th week

19. In Rh incompatibility, prognosis depends upon:

a. Serum bilirubin b. Coombs test
c. Blood smear d. Serum albumin

As soon as the umbilical cord is clamped, with continuing hemolysis in HDN (hemolytic disease of the newborn), the bilirubin concentration is increased. If the bilirubin rises to the critical level of 20 mg per 100 mL (340 micromol/L – normal 30 micromol/L), the bilirubin crosses the blood brain barrier to damage the basal nuclei of the brain permanently producing the clinical manifestations of kernicterus.

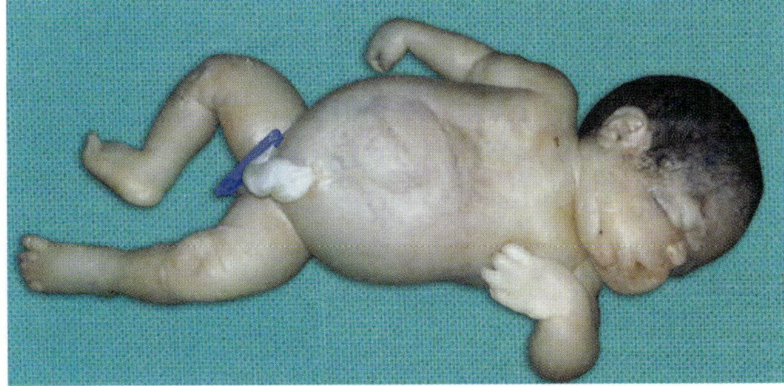

Hydrops fetalis – stillborn edematous infant due to Rhesus alloimmunization (HDFN)

Ans. 13. **a.** Vertex 14. **a.** 6th week 15. **b.** Cervical os dilated 16. **b.** Pre-eclampsia
17. **b.** Robert's sign 18. **d.** USG 19. **a.** Serum bilirubin

20. Most definitive clinical sign of pregnancy is:

a. Ballottement
b. Fetal heart sounds
c. Braxton Hicks contraction
d. Enlarged uterus

Positive or absolute signs of pregnancy are: (1) Palpation of fetal parts and perception of active fetal movements by the examiner at about 20th week (2) Auscultation of fetal heart sounds (3) Ultrasound evidence of embryo as early as 6th week and later on the fetus (4) Radiological demonstration of the fetal skeleton at 16th week and onwards.

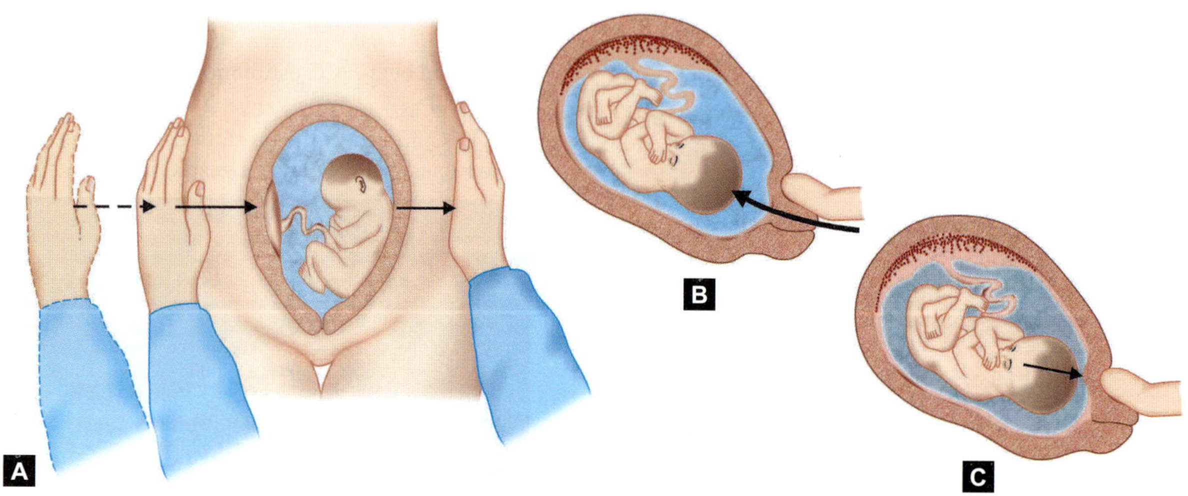

(A) External ballottement; (B and C) Steps showing how to elicit internal ballottement

21. Oligohydramnios is NOT associated with:

a. Renal agenesis
b. Polycystic kidney disease
c. Cleft palate
d. Obstructed uropathy

Facial clefts and neck masses are associated with polyhydramnios as they interfere with normal swallowing.

Production	Removal
❑ **Transudation** of maternal serum across the placental membranes	❑ **Fetus swallows** about 500–1,000 mL of liquor every day.
❑ **Transudation** from fetal circulation across the umbilical cord or placental membranes	❑ **Intramembranous absorption** of water and solutes (200–500 mL/day) from the amniotic compartment to fetal circulation through the fetal surface of the placenta.
❑ **Secretion** from amniotic epithelium	
❑ **Transudation** of fetal plasma through the highly permeable fetal skin before it is keratinized at 20th week	
❑ **Fetal urine** — Daily output at term is about 400–1,200 mL	
❑ **Fetal lung** that enters the amniotic cavity add to its volume.	

22. The best time to carry out chorion villous sampling for prenatal diagnosis is:

a. 8-10 weeks
b. 10-12 weeks
c. 12-14 weeks
d. 14-16 weeks

Chorionic villous sampling (CVS) is performed for prenatal diagnosis of genetic disorders. It is carried out transcervically between 10 weeks and 13 weeks and transabdominally from 10 weeks to term.

Prenatal diagnosis: CVS, Amniocentesis and Cordocentesis			
	Chorionic villus sampling	*Amniocentesis*	*Cordocentesis*
Time	Transcervical 10–13 weeks, Transabdominal 10 weeks to term	After 15 weeks (early 12–14 weeks)	18–20 weeks
Materials for study	Trophoblast cells	❑ Fetal fibroblasts ❑ Fluid for biochemical study	❑ Fetal white blood cells (others—infection and biochemical study)
Karyotype result	❑ Direct preparation: 24–48 hours. ❑ Culture: 10–14 days	❑ Culture: 3–4 weeks	❑ Culture: 24–48 hours

Contd...

Ans. 20. **b.** Fetal heart... 21. **c.** Cleft palate 22. **b.** 10-12 weeks

Contd...

	Chorionic villus sampling	*Amniocentesis*	*Cordocentesis*
Fetal loss	0.5–1%	0.5%	1–2%
Accuracy	Accurate; may need amniocentesis for confirmation	Highly accurate	Highly accurate
Termination of pregnancy when indicated	1st trimester—safe	2nd trimester—risky	2nd trimester—risky
Maternal effects following termination of pregnancy	Very little	More traumatic; physically and psychologically	Same as amniocentesis

23. Which of the following test is most sensitive for the detection of iron depletion in pregnancy?

a. Serum iron
b. Serum ferritin
c. Serum transferrin
d. Serum total iron binding capacity

Serum ferritin denote iron stores of the body and are the earliest to be depleted in IDA.

Blood values in iron deficiency anemia
❑ Serum iron is <30 µg/100 mL.
❑ Total iron binding capacity is raised (>400 mcg/dl)
❑ Percentage saturation is 10% or less
❑ Serum ferritin below 30 µg/l (confirms iron deficiency anemia)
❑ Serum bilirubin is not raised

24. Vaccine routinely administered in pregnancy:

a. Rabies
b. Oral polio
c. Influenza
d. Tetanus

In the developing countries, immunization in pregnancy is a routine for tetanus; others are given when epidemic occurs or travelling to an epidemic zone or for travelling overseas.

25. NOT a definitive sign of pregnancy:

a. Fetal skeleton on X-ray
b. Fetal heart sounds
c. Ultrasound examination
d. Amenorrhea

Presumptive symptoms and signs of pregnancy includes the features mainly appreciated by the women. (1) Amenorrhea (2) Frequency of micturition (3) Morning sickness (4) Fatigue (5) Breast changes (6) Skin changes (7) Quickening.

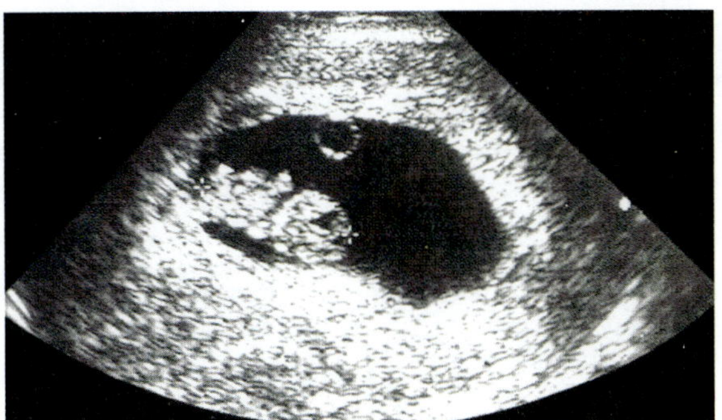

Sonogram demonstrating crown-rump length (between crosses) of an 8-week fetus. Yolk sac is in the near field

26. Most common type of vertex presentation:

a. Right Occipito Posterior
b. Left Occipito Posterior
c. Right Occipito Anterior
d. Left Occipito Anterior

Vertex occupying the left anterior quadrant of the maternal pelvis is the more common position and is called left occipito anterior (LOA). This is the first vertex position.

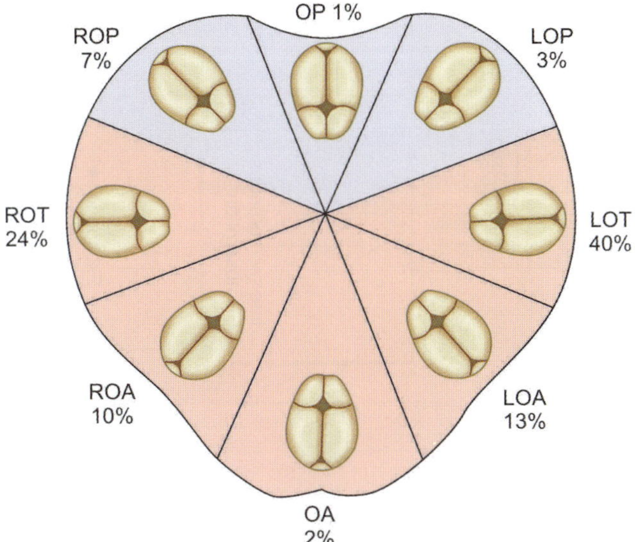

The position and relative frequency of the vertex position. However, some have retained the at the onset of labor

27. Pregnant lady presents with fulminant hepatitis. Most common cause:

a. Hepatitis D
b. Hepatitis E
c. Hepatitis B
d. Hepatitis A

Hepatitis E (HEV) behaves similar to hepatitis A virus infection. It is observed in Asia (Kashmir) and South America. It may lead to fulminant hepatitis.

Ans. 23. b. Serum ferritin 24. d. Tetanus 25. d. Amenorrhea 26. d. Left Occipito Anterior 27. b. Hepatitis E

Jaundice peculiar to the pregnant state	*Jaundice unrelated to pregnant state*	*Jaundice when pregnancy is superimposed on chronic liver disease*
❑ Intrahepatic cholestasis (obstetric hepatosis)—may be recurrent ❑ Severe preeclampsia, eclampsia, HELLP syndrome ❑ Acute fatty liver (acute yellow atrophy of the liver) ❑ Severe hyperemesis gravidarum ❑ Endotoxic shock—disseminated intravascular coagulation (DIC)	❑ Viral hepatitis: virus A – E, G ❑ Gall stone—obstructive jaundice ❑ Drug induced—isoniazid, phenothiazines ❑ Hemolytic jaundice—mismatched blood transfusion, malaria, *Clostridium welchii* infection, etc.	❑ Chronic hepatitis ❑ Cirrhosis, tumors

28. Polyhydramnios is seen in all of the following *except*:
a. DM
b. Renal agenesis
c. Esophageal atresia
d. Hydronephrosis

Renal agenesis results in oligohydramnios.

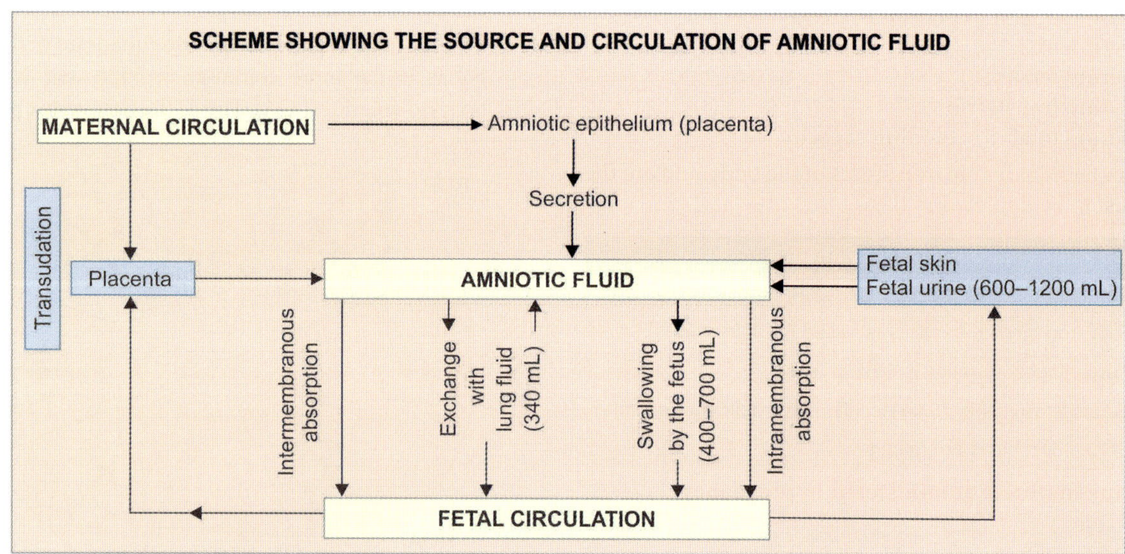

29. Ectopic pregnancy is MC in:
a. Previous H/O recurrent PID
b. Previous H/O abortion
c. Previous H/O twin pregnancy
d. Endometriosis

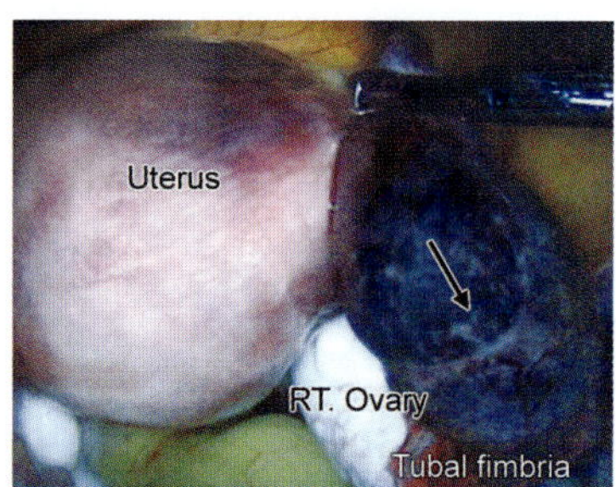

Laparoscopic view of an unruptured tubal ectopic pregnancy (Rt). Hugely dilated ampulla is seen (arrow)

Salpingitis and pelvic inflammatory disease (PID) increases the risk of ectopic pregnancy by sixfold to tenfold. Chlamydia infection is the most common risk factor.

30. Persistent occipito-posterior is common in:
a. Platypelloid pelvis
b. Gynecoid pelvis
c. Anthropoid pelvis
d. Android pelvis

Occiput-posterior is an abnormal position of the vertex rather than an abnormal presentation. In majority of cases (90%), anterior rotation of the occiput occurs and follows the course like that of an occipito-anterior and moreover, in certain type of pelvis (anthropoid), it is a favorable position.

Ans. **28. b.** Renal agenesis **29. a.** Previous H/O... **30. c.** Anthropoid pelvis

Anatomical Features of Parent Pelvic Types

		Gynecoid	*Anthropoid*	*Android*	*Platypelloid*
Inlet	❑ Shape	Round	Anteroposteriorly oval	Triangular	Transversely oval
	❑ Anterior and posterior segment	Almost equal and spacious	Both increased with slight anterior narrowing	Posterior segment short and anterior segment narrow	Both reduced-flat
	❑ Sacrum	Sacral angle (SA) more than 90°. Inclined backwards. Well curved from above down and side to side	SA more than 90°. Inclined posteriorly. Long and narrow. Usual curve	Sacral angle less than 90°. Inclined forwards and straight	SA more than 90°. Inclined posteriorly. Short and straight
Cavity	❑ Sacrosciatic notch	Wide and shallow	More wide and shallow	Narrow and deep	Slightly narrow and small
	❑ Sidewalls	Straight or slightly divergent	Straight or divergent	Convergent	Divergent
Outlet	❑ Ischial spines	Not prominent	Not prominent	Prominent	Not prominent
	❑ Pubic arch	Curved	Long and curved	Long and straight	Short and curved
	❑ Subpubic angle	Wide (85°)	Slightly narrow	Narrow	Very wide (more than 90°)
	❑ Bituberous diameter	Normal	Normal or short	Short	Wide

31. Placenta takes over function of corpus luteum for production of hormone at:

a. 6 weeks b. 12 weeks
c. 18 weeks d. 24 weeks

At 6-8 weeks, there is transfer of functions of corpus luteum to the placenta (luteal-placental shift) – which acts temporarily as a new endocrine organ or powerhouse of hormone production.

HORMONES OF PLACENTA AND THEIR CYTOCHEMICAL ORIGIN

Hypothalamic-like (releasing) hormones	Cytochemical origin
❑ Corticotropin-releasing hormone (CRH)	Cytotrophoblast and syncytiotrophoblast
❑ Gonadotropin-releasing hormone (GnRH)	+
❑ Thyrotropin-releasing hormone (TRH)	+
❑ Growth hormone releasing hormone (GHRH)	+

Pituitary-like hormones	Cytochemical origin
❑ Adrenocorticotropic hormone (ACTH)	Syncytiotrophoblast
❑ Human chorionic gonadotropin (hCG)	+
❑ Human chorionic thyrotropin (hCT)	+
❑ Human placental lactogen (hPL)	+

Other pregnancy proteins	Cytochemical origin
PSβG, PAPP – A	Syncytiotrophoblast
Relaxin	Corpus luteum, Decidua, Placenta
Prolactin	Decidua
Atrial natriuretic peptide (ANP)	Atrial myocyte
Early pregnancy factor (EPF)	Activated platelets ovaries

Growth factors	Cytochemical origin
❑ Inhibin, activin, transforming growth factor β (TGF-β)	Syncytiotrophoblast
IGF-1 and 2, Epidermal growth factor (EGF)	+

Steroid hormones	Cytochemical origin
❑ Estrogens (estriol)	Fetoplacental unit
❑ Progesterone	Before 6 weeks — corpus luteum thereafter placenta
❑ Cortisol	Decidua, adrenal

Ans. **31. a.** 6 weeks

32. MC presentation in case of twins:

a. Vertex-vertex b. Vertex-breech
c. Vertex-face d. Vertex-brow

The most common lie of the fetuses in multiple pregnancies is longitudinal (90%) but malpresentations are quite common. The combination of presentation of the fetuses are – (1) both vertex (50%), (2) first vertex and second breech (30%), (3) first breech and second vertex (10%), (4) both breech (10%), (5) first vertex and second transverse and so on, but rarest one, being both transverse when the possibility of conjoined twins should be ruled out.

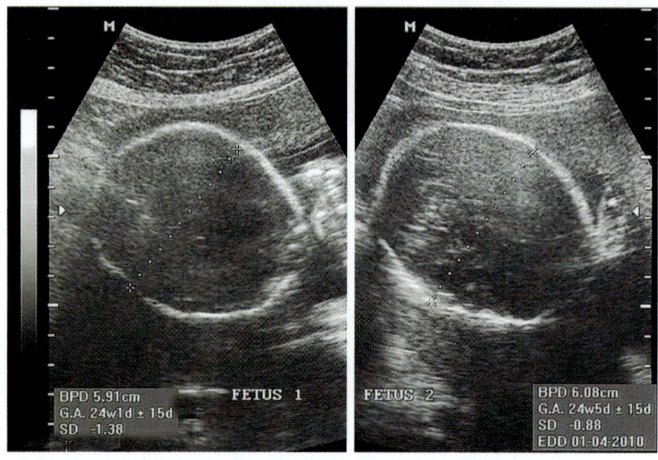

Ultrasonogram showing two fetal heads. BPDs are measured

33. Use of which vaccine is absolutely contraindicated in pregnancy?

a. Hepatitis B b. Cholera
c. Rabies d. Yellow fever

Live virus vaccines (rubella, mumps, measles, varicella, yellow fever) are contraindicated in pregnancy. Rabies, hepatitis A and B vaccines, toxoids can be given as in nonpregnant states.

34. IOC in a pregnant lady at 16 weeks of pregnancy with past H/O delivering a baby with Down syndrome:

a. Triple screen test
b. Amniocentesis
c. Chorionic villous sampling
d. USG

Genetic amniocentesis is an invasive procedure. It is performed after 15 weeks under ultrasonographic guidance. The fetal cells obtained in this procedure are subjected for cytogenetic analysis.

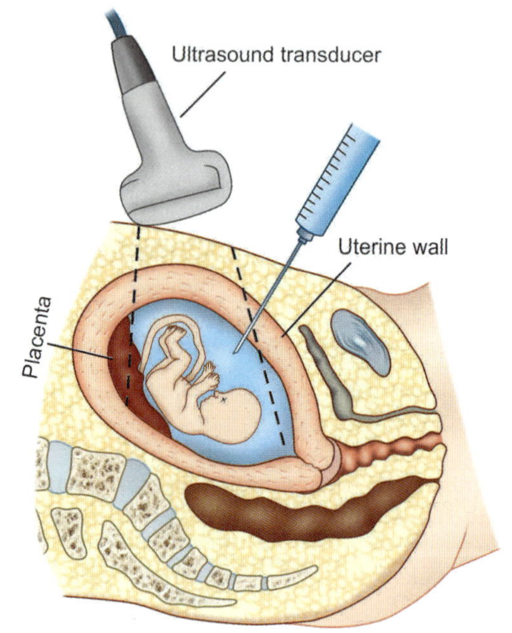

Amniocentesis—direct ultrasound control

35. MC type of ectopic pregnancy to rupture:

a. Infundibular b. Interstitial
c. Ampulla d. Isthmic

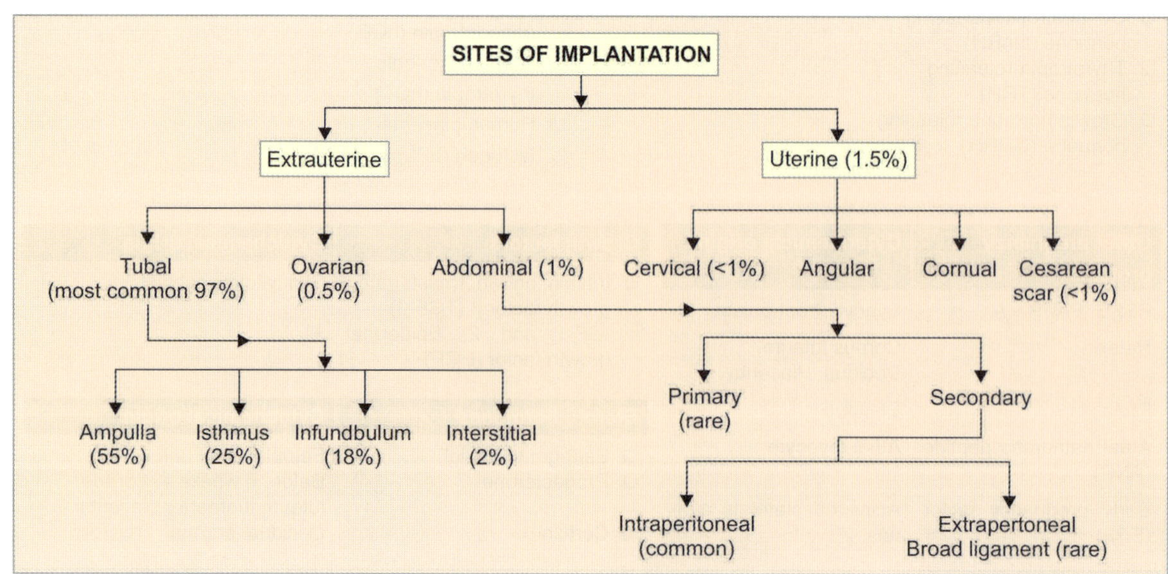

Ans. 32. **a.** Vertex-vertex 33. **d.** Yellow fever 34. **b.** Amniocentesis 35. **d.** Isthmic

Tubal rupture is predominantly common in isthmic and interstitial implantation. As the isthmic portion is narrow and the wall is less distensible, the wall may be easily eroded by the chorionic villi. Isthmic rupture usually occurs at 6-8 weeks, the ampullary one at 8-12 weeks and the interstitial one at about 4 months.

36. MC site of fertilization:

a. Infundibular b. Interstitial
c. Ampulla d. Isthmic

Almost always, fertilization occurs in the ampullary part of the fallopian tube.

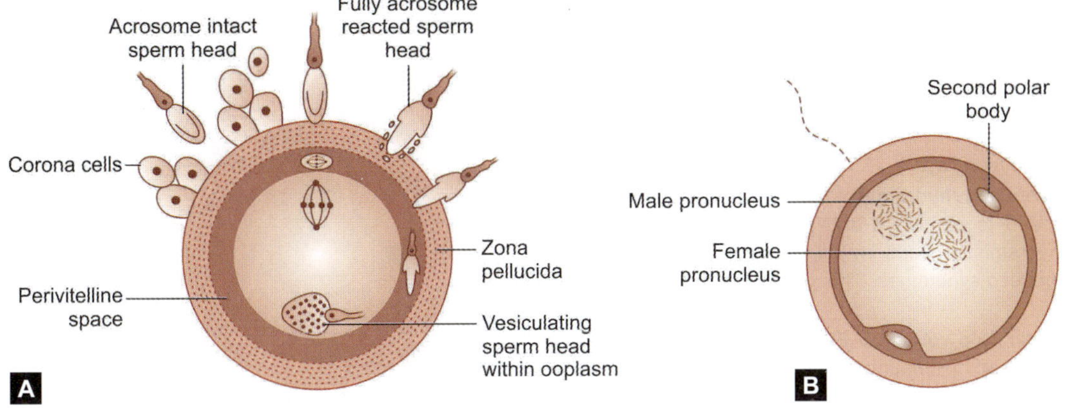

Schematic diagram showing sequence of changes during fertilization : (A) Sperm (acrosome intact) in between the corona radiata cells → attachment with zona → acrosome reacted sperm penetrating the zona → acrosome reacted sperm in the perivitelline space → incorporated sperm with vesiculating head. (B) Formation of male and female pronuclei with completion of second polar body

37. MC site of ectopic pregnancy:

a. Uterus
b. Cervix
c. Tubes
d. Abdomen

The incidence of tubal pregnancy varies from 1 in 300 to 1 in 150 deliveries.

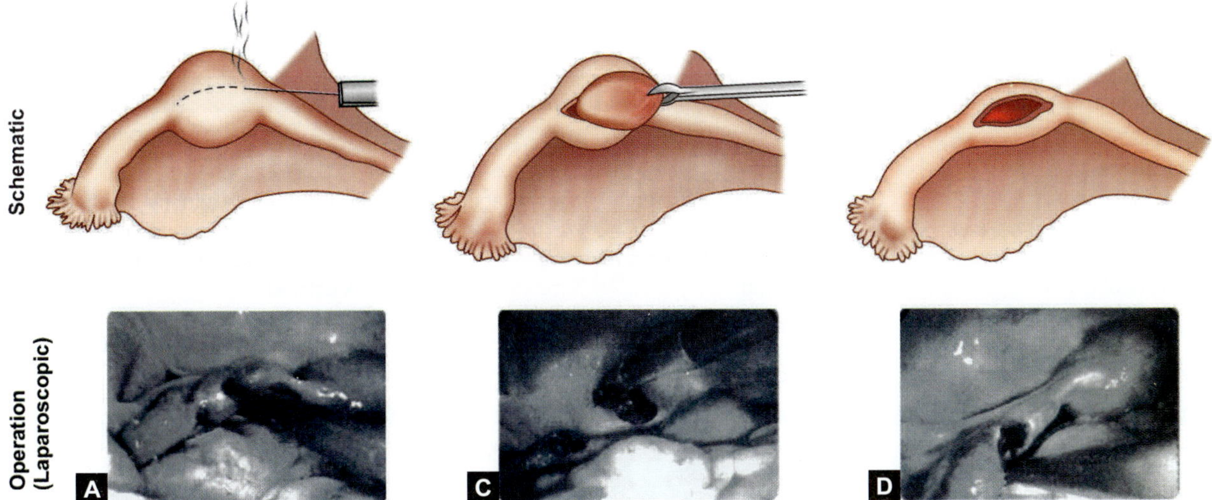

Laparoscopic linear salpingostomy for unruptured tubal pregnancy—(A) Linear incision on the antimesenteric border (B) Gestation sac is removed (C) Incision margins left unsutured. *Above: Schematic and Below: operation.*

38. Oligohydramnios is seen in:

a. Renal agenesis b. Cholangioma of placenta
c. *Spina bifida* d. *Esophageal atresia*

Fetal conditions causing oligohydramnios are: (i) Fetal chromosomal or structural anomalies (ii) Renal agenesis (iii) Obstructed uropathy (iv) spontaneous rupture of the membrane (v) Intrauterine infection (vi) Drugs: PG inhibitors, ACE inhibitors (vii) Postmaturity (viii) IUGR (ix) Amnion nodosum (failure of secretion by the cells of amnion covering the placenta).

Ans. **36. c.** Ampulla **37. c.** Tubes **38. a.** Renal agenesis

Key Points

- **Amniotic fluid volume** is related to gestational age. Amniotic fluid is dynamic and is replaced every 3 hours
- **Causes of polyhydramnios** and oligohydramnios are many.
- **Oligohydramnios** may be due to pregnancy complications with hypertensive disorders, placental insufficiency or idiopathic.
- **Amniotic fluid volume is estimated** clinically and through ultrasound measurements of AFI and DVP.
- **Polyhydramnios** (LVP > 8 cm) and **oligohydramnios** (LVP < 2 cm) is associated with significant perinatal morbidity and mortality.
- **Transient polyhydramnios** has got favorable outcome compared to persistent or worsened group. Persistent polyhydramnios needs investigations for fetal anomalies and genetic syndromes. This group need close monitoring.
- **Amniotic fluid volume (AFV) and AFI** can be increased or decreased by amount of maternal water intake.
- **Complications** of polyhydramnios are grouped into (a) Maternal and (b) Fetal
- **Complications** of oligohydramnios are mainly fetal
- **Important management issue** in both the groups is to detect any fetal congenital malformation. Referral to a fetal medicine unit should ideally be done when it is present and delivery is planned specially when associated with major structural anomaly or genetic syndromes.

39. Hydramnios is complicated by all *except*:

a. Placental abruption b. Pre-eclampsia
c. Post dated pregnancy d. Atonic hemorrhage

Premature rupture of membranes and preterm labor either spontaneous or induced is a common complication of hydramnios.

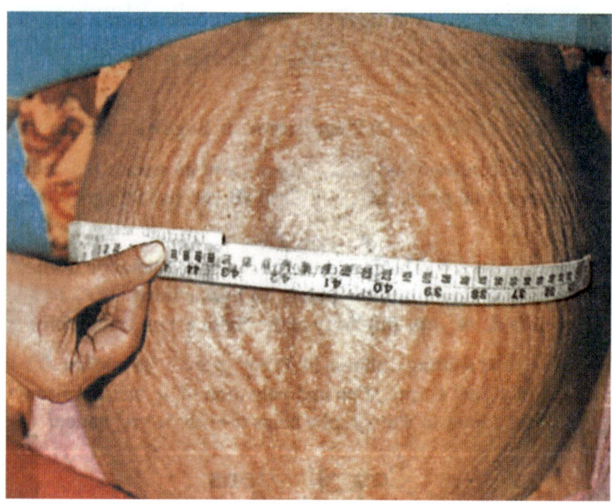

Abdominal girth round the umbilicus is more than normal

40. Painless, heavy and recurrent bleeding of sudden onset is seen in:

a. Cervical carcinoma
b. Circumvallate placenta
c. Placenta previa
d. Abruptio placentae

The only symptom of placenta previa is vaginal bleeding. The classical features of bleeding in placenta previa are sudden onset, painless, apparently causeless and recurrent.

Distinguishing features of placenta previa and abruptio placentae

Parameters	*Placenta previa*	*Abruptio placentae*
Clinical features:		
– Nature of bleeding	(a) Painless, apparently causeless and recurrent (b) Bleeding is always revealed	(a) Painful, often attributed to preeclampsia or trauma and continuous (b) Revealed, concealed or usually mixed
– Character of blood	Bright red	Dark colored
– General condition and anemia	Proportionate to visible blood loss	Out of proportion to the visible blood loss in concealed or mixed variety
– Features of preeclampsia	Not relevant	Present in one-third cases
Abdominal examination:		
– Height of uterus	Proportionate height to gestational age	May be disproportionately enlarged in concealed type
– Feel of uterus	Soft and relaxed	May be tense, tender and rigid
– Malpresentation	Malpresentation is common. The head is high floating	Unrelated, the head may be engaged
– FHS	Usually present	Usually absent especially in concealed type
Placentography (USG)	Placenta in lower segment	Placenta in upper segment
Vaginal examination	Placenta is felt on the lower segment	Placenta is not felt on lower segment. Blood clots should not be confused with placenta

Ans. 39. **c.** Post dated... 40. **c.** Placenta previa

41. Polyhydramnios is increase in amniotic fluid more than:

a. 1000 ml
b. 2000 ml
c. 3000 ml
d. 4000 ml

Anatomically, polyhydramnios is defined as a state where liquor amnii exceeds 2,000 mL. Sonographic diagnosis is made when amniotic fluid index (AFI) is more than 24 cm (more than 95th centile for gestational age) and a deepest vertical pocket (DVP) is more than 8 cm.

42. The consequences of RH incompatibility are NOT serious during first pregnancy because:

a. Antibodies are not able to cross placenta
b. Antibody titre is very low during primary immune response
c. IgG generated is ineffective against fetal RBC
d. Massive hemolysis is compensated by increased erythropoiesis

IgM type of antibody is the first to appear in the maternal circulation and agglutinates red cells containing D when suspended in saline. IgM being larger molecules cannot pass through the placental barrier and is not harmful to the fetus.

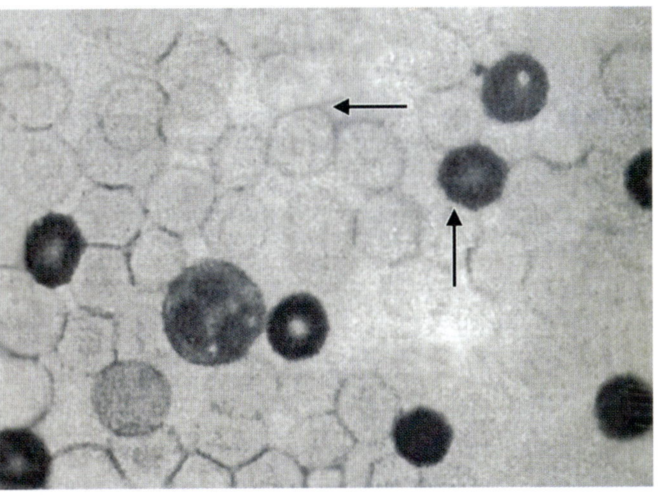

Peripheral smear showing dark fetal red cells and light-colored maternal cells. (Modified Kleihauer and Betke acid elution test)

43. All of the following may be used in pregnancy associated hypertension *except*:

a. Nifedipine
b. Captopril
c. Methyldopa
d. Hydralazine

ACE inhibitors should be avoided in pregnancy.

Antihypertensive drugs

Drugs	*Mechanism of action*	*Dose*	*Side effects*	*Contraindications and precautions*
METHYL-DOPA	Drug of first choice. Central and peripheral anti-adrenergic action. Effective and safe for both the mother and the fetus	❑ Orally – 250 mg bid – may be increased to 1 g qid depending upon the response ❑ IV infusion—250–500 mg	Maternal – Postural hypotension, hemolytic anemia, sodium retention, excessive sedation. Coombs' test may be positive ❑ Fetal – Intestinal ileus	Hepatic disorders, psychic patients, congestive cardiac failure Postpartum (risk of depression)
Hydralazine	Acts by peripheral vasodilatation as it relaxes the arterial smooth muscle. Orally it is weak and should be combined with methyldopa or β blockers. It increases the cardiac output and renal blood flow	❑ Orally – 100 mg/day in four divided doses ❑ IV 5–10 mg every 20 min maximum 20 mg	❑ Maternal hypotension, tachycardia, arrhythmia, palpitation, lupus like syndrome, fluid retention ❑ Fetal – reasonably safe ❑ Neonatal — thrombocytopenia	Because of variable sodium retention, diuretics should be used. To control arrhythmias, propranolol may be administered intravenously
LABETALOL	Combined α and β adrenergic blocking agent	❑ Orally – 100 mg tid may be increased up to 2,400 mg daily ❑ IV infusion (Hypertensive crisis) 20–40 mg IV every 10–15 min until desired effect, maximum up to 220 mg	❑ Tremors, headache, asthma, congestive cardiac failure ❑ Efficacy and safety with short-term use appear equal to methyldopa	❑ Hepatic disorders ❑ Asthma, congestive cardiac failure
NIFEDI-PINE	Direct arteriolar vasodilatation by inhibition of slow inward calcium channels in vascular smooth muscle	Orally 5–10 mg tid maximum dose 60–120 mg/day	Flushing, hypotension, headache, tachycardia, inhibition of labor	Simultaneous use of magnesium sulfate could be hazardous due to synergistic effect
SODIUM NITRO-PRUSSIDE	Direct vasodilator (arterial and venous)	IV infusion 0.25–8 μg/kg/min	❑ Maternal: Nausea, vomiting, severe hypotension ❑ Fetal toxicity due to metabolites — cyanide and thiocynate	**Drug of last resort** for acute hypertension. Should be used in critical care unit for very short time (10 minutes)

Contd...

Ans. **41. b.** 2000 ml **42. a.** Antibodies are not able to cross placenta **43. b.** Captopril

Contd...

Drugs	*Mechanism of action*	*Dose*	*Side effects*	*Contraindications and precautions*
NITROGLYCERINE	Relaxes mainly the venous but also arterial smooth muscle	Given as IV infusion 5 μg/min to be increased at every 3–5 min up to 100 μg/min	Tachycardia, headache, Methemoglobinemia	**Used in hypertensive crisis for short time only.** Contraindicated in hypertensive encephalopathy as it increases blood flow and intracranial pressure
ACE inhibitors/ Angiotensin-II receptor blockers (AARB)	ACE inhibitors: Inhibit formation of angiotensin II from angiotensin I. ARB–Blocks Angiotensin-II receptors	❑ Captopril Orally 6.25 mg bid ❑ Telmisartan orally 20–40 mg a day	❑ Maternal: Hypotension, headache, asthenia, arrhythmias ❑ Fetal: Oligohydramnios, IUGR, fetal renal tubular dysgenesis, neonatal renal failure, pulmonary hypoplasia	**Should be avoided in pregnancy.** Suitable for chronic hypertension in nonpregnant state or postpartum

44. Which infection has the highest risk of fetal infection in first trimester?

a. Hepatitis B virus
b. Syphilis
c. Toxoplasmosis
d. Rubella

Risk of major anomalies are more in rubella, if the infection occurs in first, second and third month, the incidence being 60%, 25% and 10% respectively.

45. Syphilis is maximally transmitted to fetus if:

a. Primary syphilis
b. Secondary syphilis
c. Both
d. None

Overall frequency of vertical transmission (congenital syphilis) is high in primary (50%) and secondary (50%) syphilis. In tertiary syphilis it is about 10%.

46. Supine hypotension is characteristic of:

a. Twin pregnancy
b. 3rd trimester of pregnancy
c. 2nd trimester of pregnancy
d. 1st trimester of pregnancy

During late pregnancy, the gravid uterus produces a compression effect on the inferior vena cava when the patient is in supine position. This is known as supine hypotension syndrome (Postural hypotension).This, however results in opening up of the collateral circulation by means of paravertebral and azygos veins.

47. Amount of amniotic fluid at 12 weeks of pregnancy:

a. 50 ml
b. 100 ml
c. 200 ml
d. 400 ml

Amniotic fluid is related to gestational age. It measures about 50 mL at 12 weeks, 400 mL at 20 weeks and reaches its peak of 1 liter at 36-38 weeks.

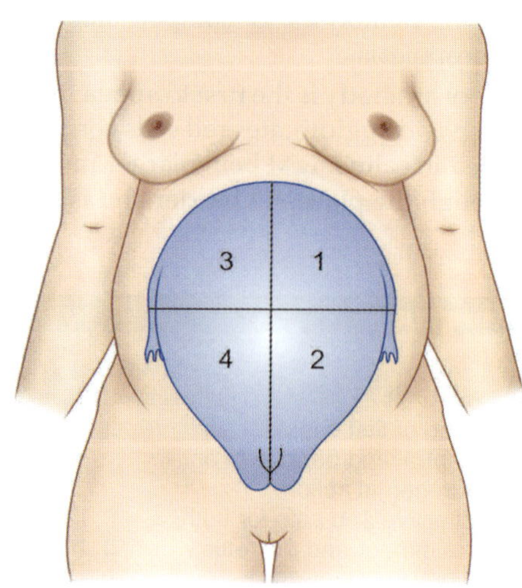

Amniotic fluid volume is measured to determine AFI

48. Accurate diagnosis of anencephaly in ultrasound can be done:

a. 5 weeks of gestation
b. 8 weeks of gestation
c. 10 weeks of gestation
d. 14 weeks of gestation

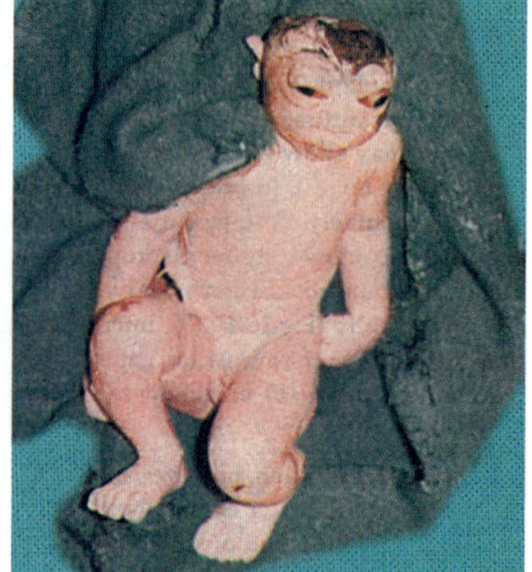
Anencephaly (*By courtesy*: Dr Mahesh Bharpilania)

Ans. **44. d.** Rubella **45. c.** Both **46. b.** 3rd trimester... **47. a.** 50 ml **48. d.** 14 weeks of gestation

Anencephaly is diagnosed by the absence of cranial vault (calvarium) and telencephalon. Brain tissue is angiomatous. Early diagnosis is possible at about 13 weeks.

49. Placenta prveia is characterized by all of the following *except*:

a. Painless bleeding
b. Causeless bleeding
c. Presents in first trimester
d. Recurrent bleeding

Painless and recurrent vaginal bleeding in the second half of pregnancy should be taken as placenta previa unless proved otherwise.

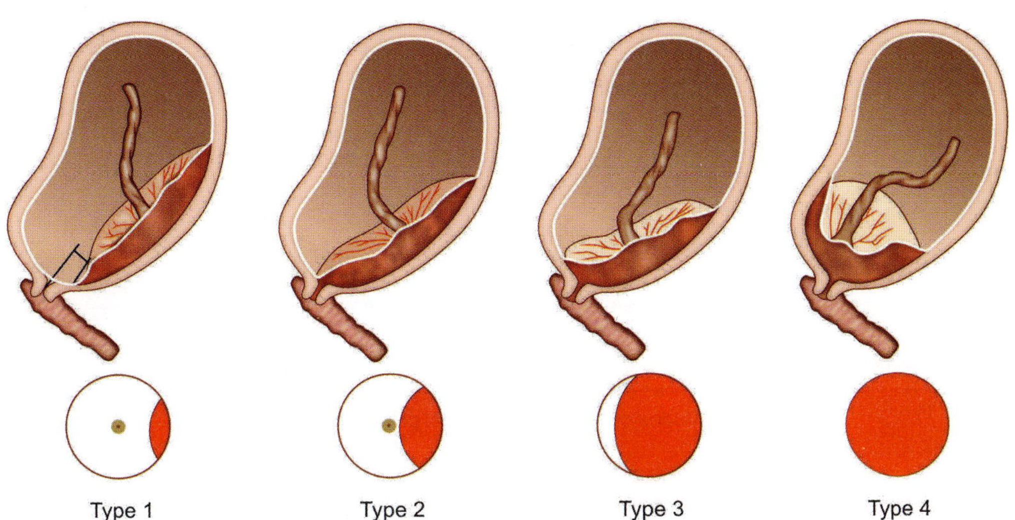

Degrees of placenta previa with findings on ultrasound examination

50. MC cause of 1st trimester abortion is:

a. Chromosomal abnormalities
b. Syphilis
c. Rhesus isoimmunization
d. Cervical immunocompetence

Parental chromosomal abnormalities are a proven cause of recurrent abortion in first trimester. The most common abnormality is a balanced translocation. Risk of miscarriage in couples with a balanced translocation is greater than 25%.

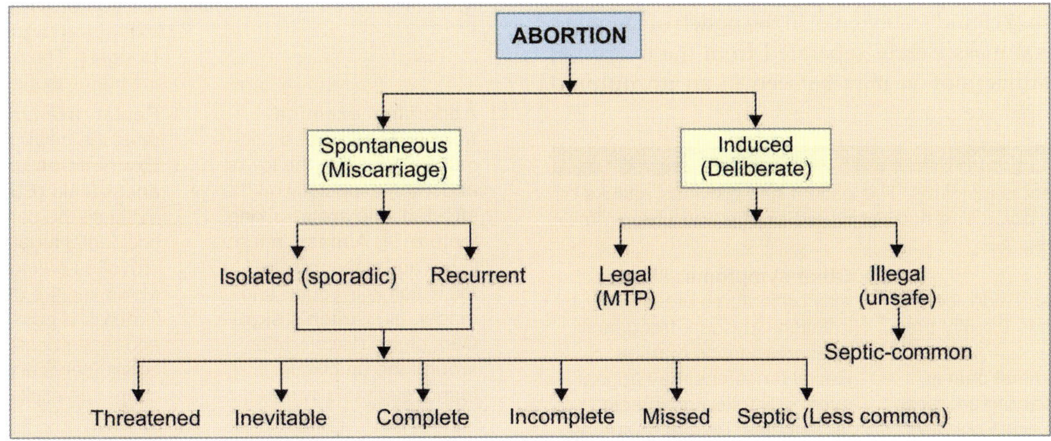

51. A woman presents with amenorrhea of 2 months duration, lower abdominal pain, facial pallor, fainting and shock. The diagnosis is:

a. Ruptured ovarian cyst
b. Ruptured ectopic pregnancy
c. Threatened abortion
d. Septic abortion

The classic triad of symptom of disturbed tubal pregnancy is abdominal pain (100%), preceded by amenorrhea (75%) and lastly, appearance of vaginal bleeding (70%). Syncopal attack (10%) is due to reflex vasomotor disturbances following peritoneal irritation from hemoperitoneum.

Ans. **49. c.** Presents in first... **50. a.** Chromosomal... **51. b.** Ruptured ectopic pregnancy

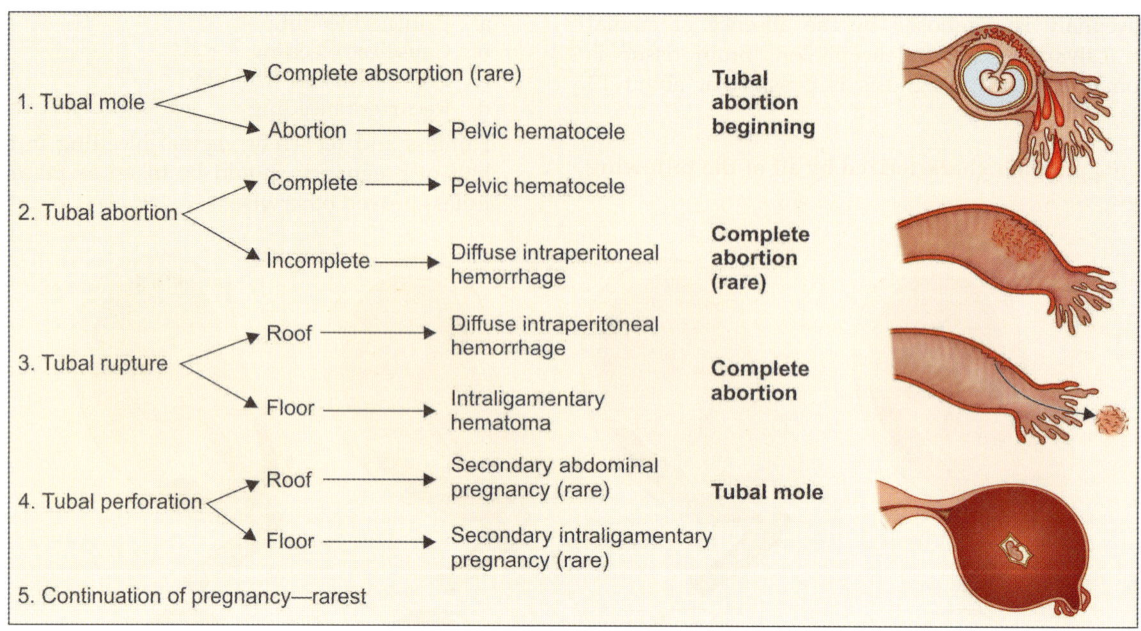

Modes of termination of tubal pregnancy

52. A young woman with 6 weeks amenorrhea presents with mass in abdomen. USG shows an empty uterus. Likely diagnosis is:

a. Ovarian cyst
b. Ectopic pregnancy
c. Complete abortion
d. None of the above

Transvaginal sonography/TVS is more informative for ectopic pregnancy. The diagnostic features are: (1) Absence of intrauterine pregnancy with a positive pregnancy test. (2) Fluid (echogenic) in the pouch of Douglas. (3) Adnexal mass clearly separated from the ovary. (4) Rarely cardiac motion may be seen in an unruptured tubal ectopic pregnancy.

Chronic or old ectopic	
Onset: The onset is insidious. The patient had previous attacks of acute pain from which she had recovered or she had chronic features from the beginning.	
Symptoms: ❑ **Amenorrhea:** Short period of 6-8 weeks is usually present. ❑ **Lower abdominal pain** is present with varying degrees. It starts as an acute one and gradually becomes dull or colicky in nature. ❑ **Vaginal bleeding** appears sooner or later following the pain. It is scanty, sanguinous or dark-colored and continuous in nature. Expulsion of decidual cast may be present	❑ **Other symptoms:** There may be features of bladder irritation—dysuria, frequency or even retention of urine. Rectal tenesmus may appear especially following infected hematocele. Rise of temperature may be due to infection or due to absorption of the products of degenerated blood accumulated in the abdomen.

Contd...

Contd...

On examination (signs): ❑ **The patient looks ill.** ❑ **Pallor** varying degree is present. ❑ Pulse persistently high even during rest—a conspicuous finding. ❑ **Features of shock** are absent. ❑ **Temperature** may be slightly elevated to 38°C.	❑ **Bimanual examination is painful and reveals:** (i) Vaginal mucosa—pale. (ii) Uterus seems to be normal in size or bulky, often incorporated in the mass occupying the pelvis. (iii) Extreme tenderness on movement of the cervix. (iv) **An ill-defined, boggy and extremely tender mass is felt through the posterolateral fornix extending to the pouch of Douglas.** The mass may push the uterus to the opposite side.
❑ **Abdominal examination:** (i) **Tenderness** and muscle guard on the lower abdomen especially on the affected side are a striking feature. (ii) **A mass** in the lower abdomen may be felt which is irregular and tender. (iii) **Cullen's sign**—Dark bluish discoloration around the umbilicus, if found, suggests intraperitoneal hemorrhage.	❑ **Rectal examination** corroborates the pelvic findings. ❑ **Examination under anesthesia (EUA)** is helpful to evaluate the pelvic findings but accidental tubal rupture may be provoked during manipulation. Moreover, the diagnostic features of pain on examination and tenderness on moving the cervix (cervical excitation pain) cannot be elicited.

53. Alpha-fetoprotein levels are lowered in:

a. Down's syndrome
b. Renal anomalies
c. Anterior abdominal wall defects
d. Anencephaly

Lower levels of MSAFP (maternal serum alpha fetoprotein) are found in trisomies (Down's syndrome), gestational trophoblastic disease.

Ans. 52. **b.** Ectopic pregnancy 53. **a.** Down's syndrome

Procedures for early detection of fetal (I) Genetic; (II) Chromosomal and (III) Structural Abnormalities	
❑ Triple test (combined test): MSAFP, unconjugated estriol (uE3) and hCG ❑ Quadruple test: (MSAFP, uE3, hCG, inhibin A) ❑ Integrated test: NT, PAPP-A + hCG ❑ Cell-free fetal DNA from maternal plasma/blood ❑ Maternal serum alpha fetoprotein (MSAFP) ❑ Chorionic villus biopsy ❑ Cordocentesis ❑ Amniocentesis	❑ Fetal cell isolation from maternal blood—(from isolated fetal nucleated red blood cells or trophoblast cells) ❑ High resolution ultrasonography for (nuchal thickening, nasal bone) ❑ Peri-implantation genetic diagnosis ❑ 3D or 4D ultrasound with increased resolution ❑ Fetoscopy

54. Source of HCG is:

a. Chorionic villi
b. Langhan's layer
c. Cytotrophoblast
d. Syncytiotrophoblast

hCG is produced by the synctiotrophoblast of the placenta and secreted into the blood of the both mother and fetus.

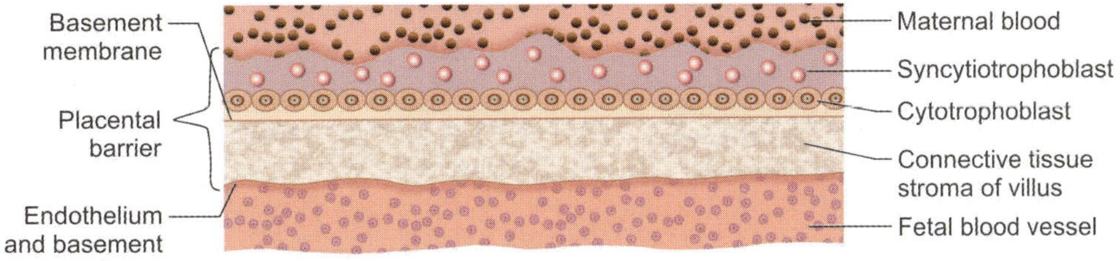

Schematic diagram showing layers of placental barrier

55. A pregnant lady in her first trimester presents with vaginal bleeding. On examination the os is closed and uterine size corresponds to the period of amenorrhoea. The condition could be:

a. Septic abortion
b. Complete abortion
c. Inevitable abortion
d. Threatened abortion

Threatened abortion is a clinical entity where the process of miscarriage has started but has not progressed to a state from where recovery is impossible.

Types of miscarriages and the diagnostic features

Type	Symptoms	Uterine size	Cervix (Ext. Os)	Ultrasonography
Threatened	❑ Vaginal bleeding present ❑ Pelvic pain	❑ Corresponds to gestational age	❑ Closed	❑ Fetus alive ❑ Retroplacental hemorrhage +
Inevitable	❑ Vaginal bleeding present ❑ Pelvic pain	❑ Same or smaller	❑ Open with palpable conceptus	❑ Fetus often dead ❑ Retroplacental hemorrhage +
Incomplete	❑ Vaginal bleeding (may be heavy)	❑ Smaller	❑ Open	❑ Products of conception partly retained
Complete	❑ Vaginal bleeding—trace or absent	❑ Smaller	❑ Closed	❑ Uterine cavity empty
Missed	❑ Vaginal bleeding—trace, brownish in color	❑ Smaller	❑ Closed	❑ Blighted ovum or fetus without cardiac activity
Septic	❑ Vaginal discharge: purulent, foul smelling with features of sepsis)	❑ Variable, may be larger	❑ Open	❑ Products of conception retained, presence of foreign body (±), free fluid in the peritoneal cavity/ POD

56. Post term pregnancy is the pregnancy which continues beyond:

a. 274 days
b. 284 days
c. 294 days
d. 304 days

For clinical purposes, a pregnancy continuing beyond 2 weeks of the expected date of delivery (>294 days) is called postmaturity or post-term pregnancy.

Ans. **54. d.** Syncytiotroph... **55. d.** Threatened abortion **56. c.** 294 days

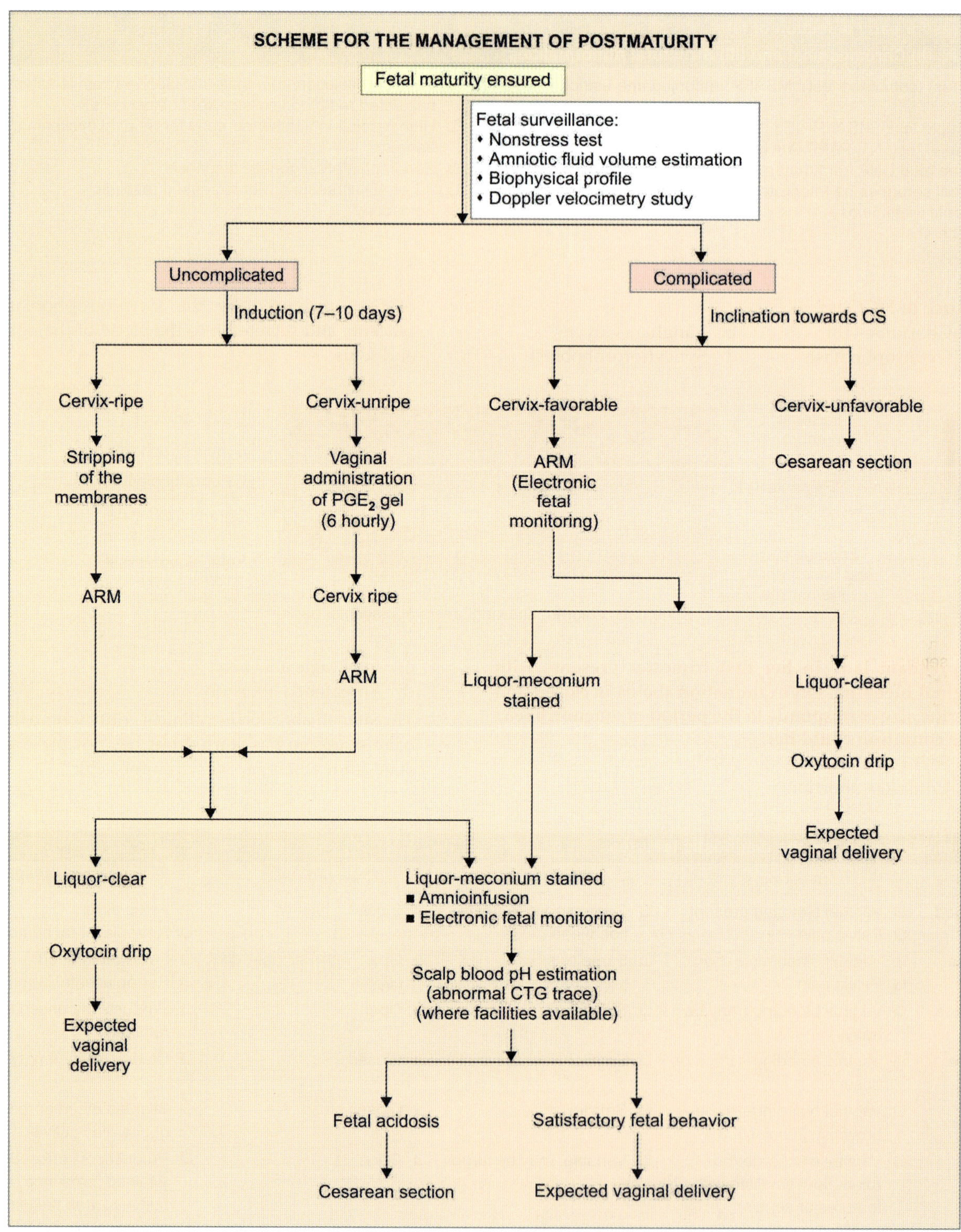

57. Ideal time for screening of blood sugar for diabetes in a pregnant female is:

a. 16-20 weeks b. 20-24 weeks
c. 24-28 weeks d. 12-16 weeks

The method employed for screening of gestational diabetes is by using 50 gm oral glucose challenge test without regard to time of the day or last meal, between 24 weeks and 28 weeks of pregnancy.

Ans. **57. c.** 24-28 weeks

Criteria for diagnosis of impaired glucose tolerance and diabetes with 75 gm oral glucose (american diabetic assocation)			
Time	*Normal Tolerance*	*Impaired Glucose Tolerance*	*Diabetes*
Fasting	<100	≥100 and <126	≥126
2 hour post glucose	<140	≥140 and <200	≥200

- Venous whole blood values are 15% less than the plasma
- m mol/l = mg% × 0.0555

International association of diabetes and pregnancy study groups (IADPSG) (75 gm Oral Glucose) (mg/ dL)	
Time	*Value*
Fasting	92
1-hour	180
2-hour	153

Based on IADPSG, diagnosis of GDM is made if one or more thresholds are met or exceeded.

58. A 28-year-old female presented with history of 6 weeks amenorrhea and pain in abdomen. USG showed fluid in pouch of Douglas. Aspiration revealed a dark coloured blood that failed to clot. Most likely diagnosis is:

a. Ruptured ovarian cyst
b. Ruptured ectopic pregnancy
c. Red degeneration of fibroid
d. Pelvic abscess

Through an 18-gauze lumbar puncture needle fitted with a syringe, the posterior fornix is punctured to gain access to the pouch of Douglas (culdocentesis). Aspiration of nonclotting blood with hematocrit greater than 15% signifies ruptured ectopic pregnancy.

Fate of secondary abdominal pregnancy

- **Death of the blastocyst** → complete absorption
- **Massive intraperitoneal hemorrhage** due to placental separation
- **Infection** → fistulous communication with intestine, bladder, umbilicus
- **Fetal death** → mummification, suppuration, adipocere formation, calcification (*lithopedion*)
- **Continue to term pregnancy** (rare—1.0%) (risk of fetal malformation and deformation)

59. FALSE statement about HCG:

a. It is secreted by cytotrophoblasts
b. It acts on the same receptor as that of LH
c. It has a luteotrophic action
d. It is a glycoprotein

hCG is secreted by syncytiotrophoblast.

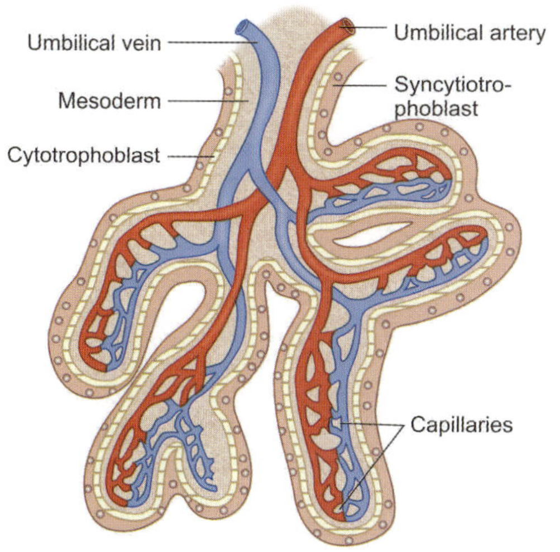

Schematic diagram showing terminal capillary networks in the villi

60. Snowstorm appearance on USG is seen in:

a. Hydatidiform mole
b. Ectopic pregnancy
c. Anencephaly
d. None of the above

Characteristic feature of molar pregnancy on USG is "snowstorm" appearance. Sometimes confusion arises with the missed abortion, partial mole or the degenerated fibroid.

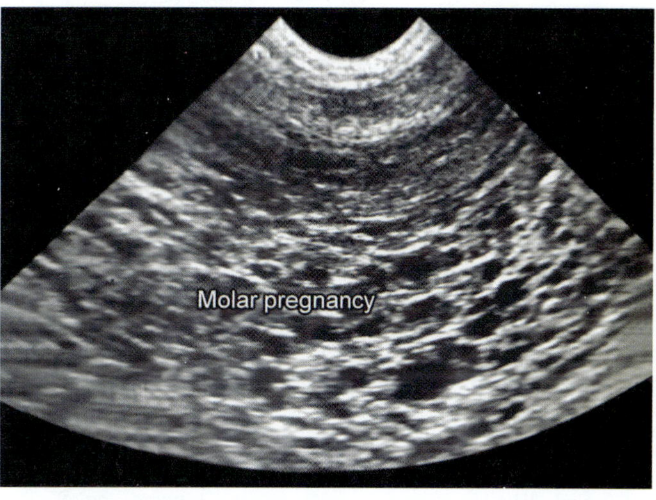

USG showing snow storm appearance of hydatidiform mole

61. NOT a product of placental synthesis or production:

a. Estriol
b. Prolactin
c. HPL
d. HCG

Prolactin is secreted by anterior pituitary gland. During normal pregnancy, the pituitary increases in weight by 30-50% and is enlarged to about twice its normal size. This is principally due to hyperplasia of acidophilic prolactin secreting cells.

(See Diagram on next page)

62. During pregnancy, maximum urinary HCG level is reached in:

a. 30 days
b. 50 days
c. 70 days
d. 90 days

Ans. 58. **b.** Ruptured... 59. **a.** It is secreted... 60. **a.** Hydatidiform mole 61. **b.** Prolactin 62. **c.** 70 days

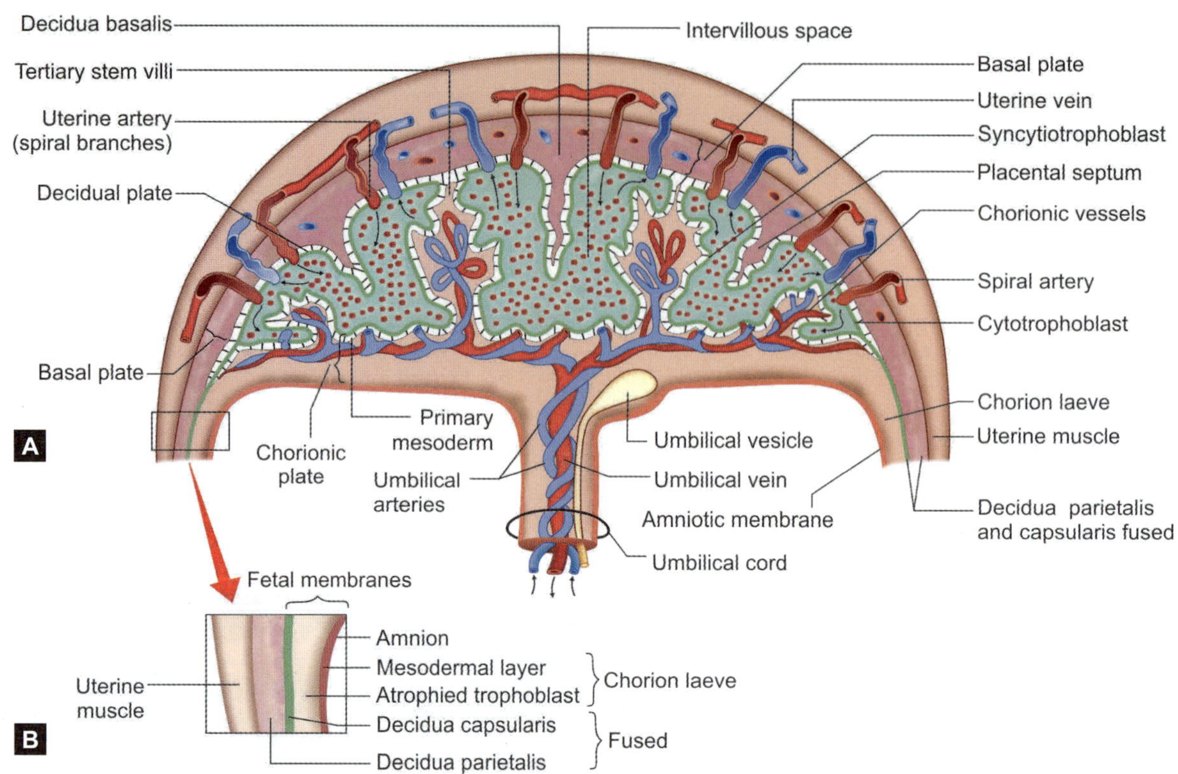

Schematic view of (A) Structure of placenta at term; (B) Structure of the membranes in relation to decidua

The blood and urine levels of hCG reach maximum levels ranging 60 to 70 days of pregnancy. The concentration falls slowly reaching a low level of 10-20 IU/mL, between 100-130 days. Thereafter, the levels remain constant throughout pregnancy with a slight secondary peak at 32 weeks.

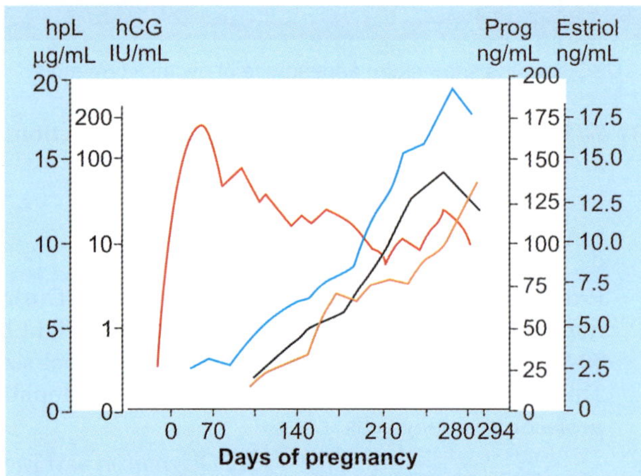

Mean serum levels of placental hormones during pregnancy as measured by radioimmunoassay

63. Drug for managing PIH are all except:

a. Labetalol
b. Hydralazine
c. Methyldopa
d. ACE inhibitors

ACE inhibitors are contraindicated in pregnancy.

Commonly used drugs in the management of preeclampsia

Drug	*Mode of action*	*Dose*
Methyl-dopa	Central and peripheral antiadrenergic action	250–500 mg tid or qid
Labetalol	Adrenoceptor antagonist (α and β blockers)	100 mg tid or qid
Nifedipine	Calcium channel blocker	10–20 mg bid
Hydralazine	Vascular smooth muscle relaxant	10–25 mg bid

64. A 32-week-pregnant lady presents in emergency room with continuous bleeding per vaginam. The uterus is painful and tender. Most likely diagnosis is:

a. Circumvallate placenta
b. Rupture of membranes
c. Placenta previa
d. Accidental hemorrhage

Abruptio placentae/accidental hemorrhage/premature separation of placenta is one form of antepartum hemorrhage where the bleeding occurs due to premature separation of normally situated placenta. Uterine tenderness may vary depending upon the grade of separation.

Ans. **63. d.** ACE inhibitors **64. d.** Accidental hemorrhage

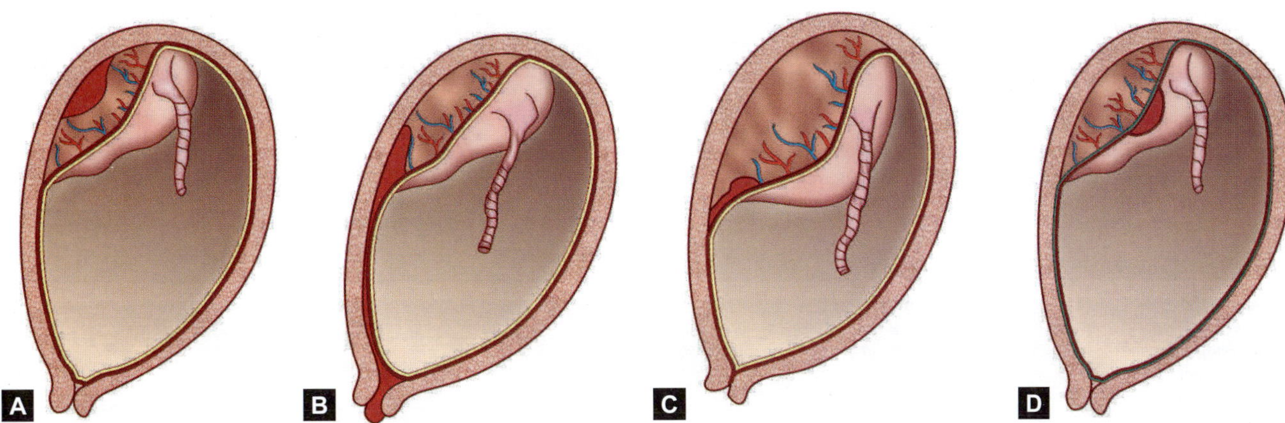

Varieties of abruptio placentae: (A) Concealed; (B) Revealed; (C) Marginal (subchorionic) and; (D) Preplacental (subamniotic)

65. Most useful investigation in the first trimester to identify risk of fetal malformation in a fetus of a diabetic mother:

a. Glycosylated Hb b. USG
c. Maternal serum AFP d. Amniocentesis

Estimation of glycosylated hemoglobin A (HbA1c) before 14 weeks of pregnancy, reflect the quality of diabetic control over the previous 3 months. Overall risk of fetal malformations are increased when the level of HbA1c is high (normal <6%).

Major birth defects in infants of diabetic mothers (6–10%)				
CNS and skeletal	*Cardiovascular*	*Renal*	*Gastrointestinal*	*Others*
❑ Neural tube defects	❑ VSD, ASD	❑ Renal agenesis	❑ Duodenal atresia	❑ Single umbilical artery
❑ Anencephaly	❑ Coarctation of aorta	❑ Hydronephrosis	❑ Anorectal atresia	
❑ Microcephaly	❑ Transposition of great vessels	❑ Double ureter	❑ Omphalocele	
❑ Caudal regression syndrome	❑ Situs inversus	❑ Polycystic kidneys	❑ Tracheoesophageal fistula	
❑ Sacral agenesis	❑ Fallot's tetralogy			

Good glycemic control with preconceptional counseling can reduce the incidence to 0.8–2%

66. Late deceleration indicates:

a. Head compression b. Cord compression
c. Fetal hypoxia d. Breech presentation

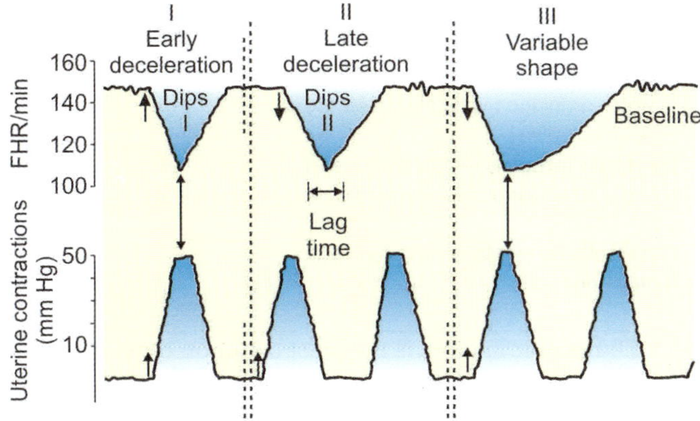

Graphic representation showing various types of decelerations in relation to uterine contractions

Late deceleration (Type II dips), uniform, repetitive periodic slowing of fetal heart rate. It suggests uteroplacental insufficiency and fetal hypoxia.

67. Doppler USG in pregnancy detects:

a. Cardiovascular malformation
b. Neural tube defect
c. Abdominal mass
d. IUGR

Doppler Ultrasound Velocimetry

Venous Doppler (Ductus venosus, Umbilical vein) parameters provide information about cardiac forward function (cardiac compliance, contractility and afterload)

Arterial Doppler (umbilical artery) waveforms are helpful to assess the downstream vascular resistance. The arterial Doppler waveform is used to measure the peak systolic (S), peak diastolic (D) and mean (M) volumes.

Ans. **65. a.** Glycosylated Hb **66. c.** Fetal hypoxia **67. a.** Cardiovascular malformation

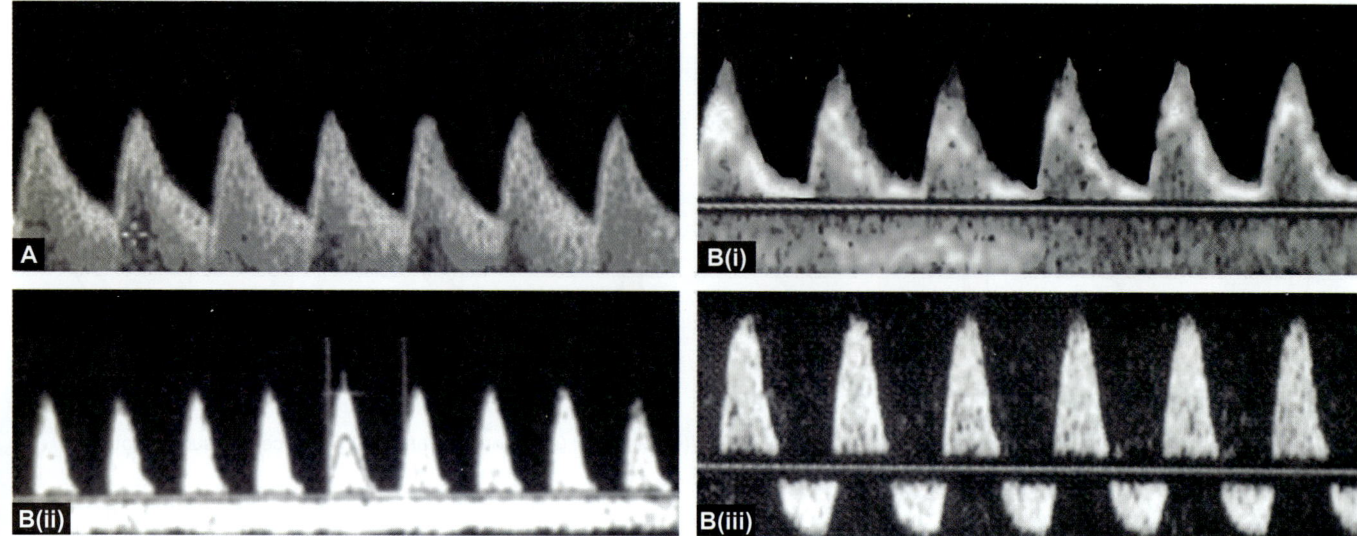

Umbilical artery flow velocity waveform: (A) Normal; (B) Abnormal—(i) Reduced end-diastolic flow; (ii) Absent end-diastolic flow; (iii) Reversed end-diastolic flow

68. NOT used for first trimester MTP:

a. Ethacridine (extra-amniotic)
b. Suction and evacuation
c. RU-486
d. Dilatation and evacuation

Extra-amniotic instillation of 0.1% ethacridine lactate (estimated amount is 10 mL/week) is done transcervically through a No. 16 Foley's catheter for termination of pregnancy between 16-20 weeks.

Methods of termination of pregnancy	
First trimester (Up to 12 weeks)	*Second trimester (13–20 weeks)*
Medical ❑ Mifepristone ❑ Mifepristone and misoprostol (PGE_1) ❑ Methotrexate and misoprostol ❑ Tamoxifen and misoprostol **Surgical** ❑ Menstrual regulation ❑ Vacuum aspiration (MVA/EVA) ❑ Suction evacuation and/or curettage ❑ Dilatation and evacuation: – Rapid method – Slow method	❑ **Prostaglandins** PGE_1 (misoprostol), 15 methyl $PGF_2\alpha$ (Carboprost), PGE_2 (Dinoprostone) and their analogs (used—intravaginally, intramuscularly or intraamniotically) ❑ **Dilation and evacuation** (13–14 weeks) ❑ **Intrauterine instillation of hyperosmotic solutions** – Extra-amniotic—ethacridine lactate, Prostaglandins (PGE_2, $PGF_2\alpha$) – Extra-amniotic saline infusion (isotonic) with a transcervical catheter balloon – Intra-amniotic hypertonic urea (30%), saline (20%) ❑ **Oxytocin infusion**—high dose used along with either of the above two methods ❑ **Hysterotomy** (abdominal)—less commonly done

69. Type of anemia in pregnancy is:

a. Megaloblastic
b. Microcytic hypochromic
c. Dimorphic
d. Normochromic normocytic

Dimorphic anemia is the most common type of anemia met with in the tropics. It is related to dietary inadequacy or intestinal malabsorption. As such, anemia results from deficiency of both iron and folic acid or vitamin B12.

Ans. **68. a.** Ethacridine... **69. c.** Dimorphic

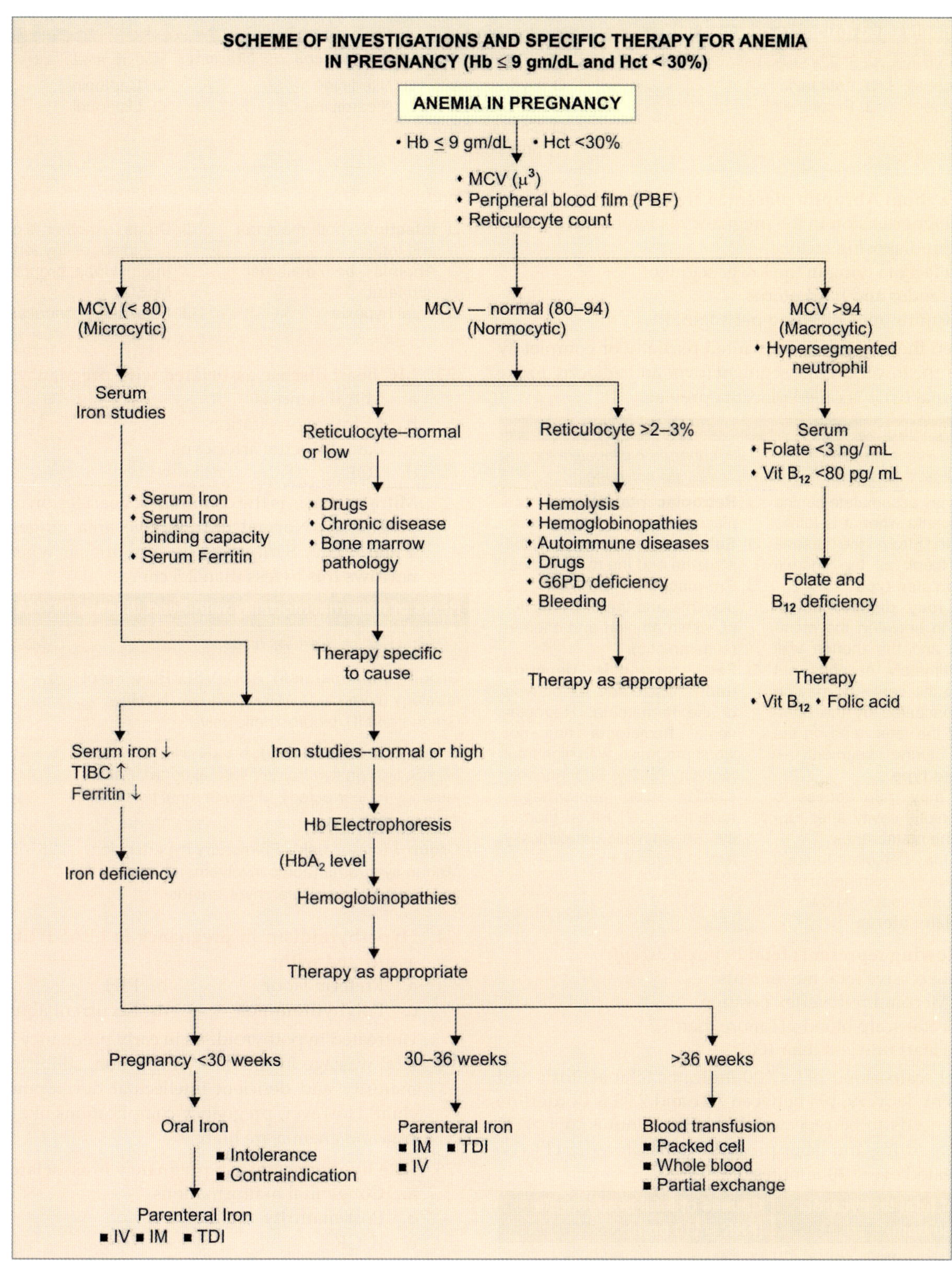

70. Drug of choice in chronically hypertensive pregnant women requiring long term antihypertensive therapy:

a. Nifedipine b. Metaprolol
c. Methyldopa d. Hydralazine

Antihypertensive agents are essential when the BP is 160/110 mm Hg to protect the mother from eclampsia, cerebral hemorrhage, cardiac failure and placental abruption. Methyldopa is the drug of first choice.

Ans. **70. c.** Methyldopa

The commonly used drugs are grouped into:				
I. Sympatholytics	*II. Andrenergic receptor blocking agents*	*III. Vasodilators*	*IV. Calcium channel blockers*	*V. ACE inhibitors*
❑ Methyldopa ❑ Reserpine	❑ Labetalol ❑ Propranolol	❑ Hydralazine ❑ Nitroglycerin ❑ Sodium nitroprusside	❑ Nifedipine ❑ Nicardipine	❑ Captopiril ❑ Lisinopril

71. True about Abruptio placentae are all *except*:

a. Hypertension in the pregnancy is important predisposing factor
b. Placenta lying in the lower segment
c. Tender and hard uterus
d. Continuous bleeding per vaginal

When the placenta is implanted partially or completely over the lower uterine segment (over and adjacent to the internal os) it is called placenta previa.

Abruptio placentae	
Clinical manifestations of hemorrhage	*Ultrasonographic localization of hemorrhage*
❑ Blood may accumulate behind the placenta when it is totally separated from the uterine wall except at the margin — **concealed type**. ❑ **Blood may dissect downwards** in between the membranes and the uterine wall and ultimately escapes out through the cervix or may be kept concealed by the pressure of the fetal head on the lower uterine segment — **revealed type**. ❑ **Blood may gain access** to the amniotic cavity after rupturing the membranes ❑ **Blood** may percolate through the layers of myometrium upto the serous coat – known as **Couvelaire uterus**	❑ **Retroplacental**: Between the placenta and the myometrium ❑ **Subchorionic:** Between the placenta and the membranes. ❑ **Pre-placental**: Between the placenta and the amniotic fluid, within amnion and chorion (subamniotic). ❑ **Fetal prognosis depends upon**: (i) size and (ii) the type of the hematoma. Retroplacental hematoma has got worst prognosis with high fetal mortality (50%). Subchorionic smaller sized hemorrhages have less (10%) fetal mortality. Subamniotic is clinically less significant.

72. Following represents fetal hypoxia *except*:

a. Excessive fetal movements
b. Meconium in vertex position
c. Fetal scalp blood pH more than 7.3
d. Heart rate less than 100

Fetal scalp blood pH <7.20 indicates fetal acidosis and urgent delivery, pH between 7.21 and 7.25 is borderline and needs to be repeated within 30 minutes. pH >7.25 is reassuring and labor progress is monitored. pH to be repeated every 30 minutes.

Causes of fetal tachycardia (FHR > 160 bpm)	Causes of fetal bradycardia (FHR < 110 bpm)
❑ **Drugs to mother:** (i) β-sympathomimetic agents used to inhibit preterm labor (isoxsuprine, ritodrine); (ii) Vagolytic : atropine ❑ **Infection**—both maternal and fetal ❑ **Anemia**—both maternal and fetal ❑ Fetal hypoxia	❑ Fetal hypoxia, acidosis ❑ Fetal sepsis, anomalies ❑ Use of local anesthetic drugs, epidural analgesia ❑ Drugs to mother, e.g. pethidine, antihypertensives (methyldopa, propranolol), $MgSO_4$ ❑ Fetal heart conduction defect (SLE)

73. MC heart disease associated with pregnancy:

a. Mitral stenosis
b. Mitral regurgitation
c. Patent ductus arteriosus
d. TOF

Mitral stenosis is the commonest heart lesion met during pregnancy. Normal mitral valve area ranges between 4 and 6 cm^2. Symptoms usually appear when stenosis narrows this to less than 2.5 cm^2.

Risks of maternal mortality with heart disease (NYHA, 1992)	
Cardiac disease	*Mortality (%)*
Group 1 (minimal risk): ASD, VSD, PDA, Fallot tetralogy (corrected), Mitral stenosis (NYHA–Grade I and II), bioprosthetic valve	0 – 1
Group 2 (moderate risk): MS (NYHA – III and IV) AS, Marfan syndrome (Normal aorta), Fallot tetralogy (uncorrected), M S with atrial fibrillation, artificial valve	5 – 15
Group 3 (major risk): Pulmonary hypertension, Marfan syndrome (aortic involvement), aortic coarctation with valvular involvement	25 – 50

74. Hypothyroidism in pregnancy is LEAST likely to be associated with:

a. Preterm labor
b. PIH
c. Polyhydramnios
d. Recurrent abortions

Untreated hypothyroidism in early pregnancy has a high fetal wastage in the form of abortion, stillbirth and prematurity and deficient intellectual development of the child. However, pregnancy complications like preeclampsia and anemia are high.

75. Late hyperglycemia in pregnancy is associated with:

a. Congenital malformations
b. Post-maturity
c. IUGR
d. Macrosomia

Fetal macrosomia (40-50%) with birth weight >4 kg (>90th percentile) probably results from: (a) Maternal hyperglycemia → hypertrophy and hyperplasia of fetal islets of Langerhans → increased secretion of fetal in-

Ans. 71. **b.** Placenta lying... 72. **c.** Fetal scalp blood... 73. **a.** Mitral stenosis 74. **c.** Polyhydramnios 75. **d.** Macrosomia

sulin → stimulates carbohydrate utilization and accumulation of fat. (b) Elevation of maternal free fatty acids (FFA) in diabetes leads to increased transfer to the fetus → acceleration of triglyceride synthesis → adiposity.

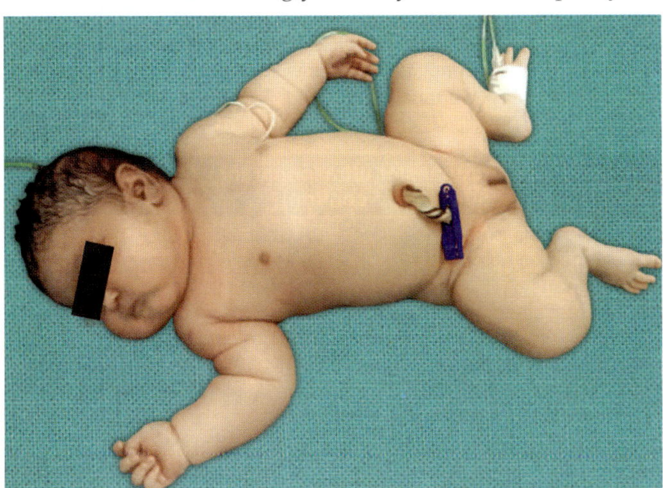

Macrosomic baby, weighing 5.3 kg, of a diabetic mother, looked plethoric (due to polycythemia), with plumpy face, buried eyes and excessive buccal fat

76. MC cause of breech presentation is:

a. Prematurity b. Post maturity
c. DM d. Osteomalacia

Prematurity is the MC cause of breech presentation.

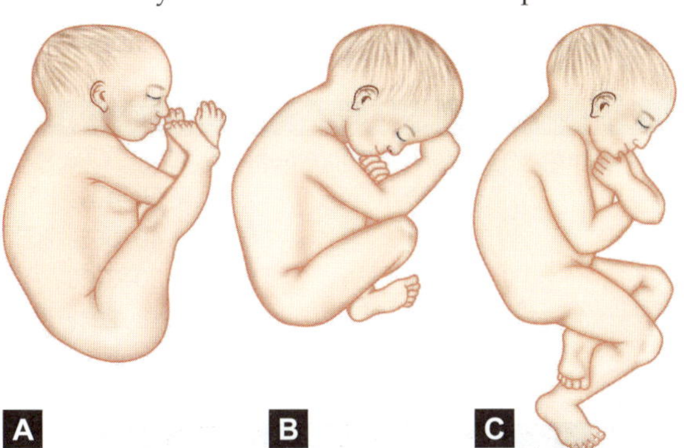

Varieties of breech presentation—(A) Breech with extended legs (frank breech); (B) FlexedJ breech (complete breech); (C) Footling presentation

77. Uterine blood flow at term:

a. More than 500 ml/min b. 350-400 ml/min
c. 150-200 ml/min d. 50-75 ml/min

Uterine blood flow is increased from 50 mL/min in nonpregnant state to about 750 mL near term. Nonpregnant uterus receives 2% of cardiac output and breast 1%. Increase in blood flow going to the organs is about 50% due to overall increase in CO. The increase is due to the combined effect of uteroplacental and fetoplacental vasodilatation.

Hemodynamic changes during pregnancy

Parameters	*Nonpregnant*	*Pregnancy near term*	*Change*
Cardiac output (L/min)	4.5	6.26	+ 40%
Stroke volume (mL)	65	75	+ 27%
Heart rate (per minute)	70	85	+ 17%
Blood pressure	Unaffected or mid-pregnancy drop of diastolic pressure by 5–10 mm Hg		
Venous pressure	10 cm (femoral)	20–25 cm water	+ 100%
Colloid oncotic pressure (mm Hg)	20	18	– 14%
Systemic vascular resistance (SVR)	—	—	– 21%
Pulmonary vascular resistance (PVR)	—	—	– 34%

78. Heparin is re-introduced to a cardiac patient with pregnancy at:

a. 32 weeks b. 36 weeks
c. 40 weeks d. At the time of labor

Anticoagulants for heart diseases

- The patient taking warfarin should discontinue it as soon as pregnancy is diagnosed and to replace it by heparin 5,000 units twice daily subcutaneously up to 12th week. Low molecular weight heparin (LMWH) can also be used.
- This is then replaced by warfarin tablet 3 mg. daily to be taken at the same time each day and continued up to 36 weeks.
- Thereafter it is replaced by heparin up to 7 days postpartum.
- Warfarin is then to be continued.

Anticoagulants

Drug	*Mode of action*	*Dose*	*Side effects*
Heparin ❑ (unfractionated heparin) ❑ **Low-molecular-weight heparin (LMWH)**	Inhibits action of thrombin, it also enhances the activity of antithrombin III, increases factor Xa inhibitor **Antidote:** Protamine sulfate	5,000–10,000 IU to be administered parenterally. **DVT and pulmonary embolism**: loading dose 5,000 units IV followed by continuous infusion of 18 units/kg/hr. **Pregnancy**: 5,000-10,000 SC every 12 hrs (with monitoring). **LMWH**: Enoxaparin 1 mg/kg twice daily SC, less antithrombotic effect	**Maternal**: Hemorrhage, urticaria with long-term use thrombocytopenia and osteopenia, hyperkalemia **Fetal**: It does not cross the placenta, not teratogenic **Low-molecular-weight heparins**—as effective and safe as unfractionated heparin. Longer half-life and once daily dose is convenient. Standard dose does not require monitoring

Contd...

Ans. **76. a.** Prematurity **77. a.** More than 500 ml/min **78. b.** 36 weeks

Contd...

Drug	*Mode of action*	*Dose*	*Side effects*
Warfarin	**Interferes with synthesis of vitamin K dependent factors** (II, VII, IX, X)	5–10 mg orally daily for initial 2 days then 3–9 mg daily (taken at the same time each day) depending upon the prothrombin time (INR) (INR – 2.5–3.5)	**Maternal**: Hemorrhage **Fetal**: Warfarin embryopathy (5%), nasal hypoplasia, bone stiplings, optic atrophy, mental retardation, microcephaly, chondrodysplasia punctata. Women with mechanical heart valves, warfarin is preferred. To avoid first trimester.

79. Treatment of genital warts in pregnancy:

a. Cryotherapy
b. Podophyllotoxin
c. Imiquimod
d. Salicylic acid with lactic acid solution

Cryotherapy for external genital warts can be used safely during pregnancy. Treating genital warts may not cure a human papillomavirus (HPV) infection. The virus may remain in the body in an inactive state after warts are removed.

80. Ultrasound is done in 1st trimester for all *except*:

a. Multiple pregnancy
b. Fetal anomalies
c. To estimate gestational age
d. To know the position of the placenta

The relationship of placenta to the internal cervical os is important to define low lying placenta and placenta previa. This best evaluated in second trimester USG. Only 5% of placenta previa identified in the second trimester will persist to term.

Indication of first trimester ultrasonography (ACR 2007) (To evaluate, estimate or to confirm)	
❑ Intrauterine pregnancy ❑ Suspected ectopic pregnancy ❑ Vaginal bleeding (in all trimesters) ❑ Fetal anomalies (anencephaly) ❑ Suspected molar pregnancy	❑ Gestational age ❑ Multiple pregnancy (chorionicity) ❑ To confirm cardiac activity ❑ Screening of aneuploidy ❑ Evaluation of pelvic/adnexal masses (all trimesters)

81. Maximal level of cardiac output is seen at:

a. 22-26 weeks of pregnancy
b. 26-30 weeks of pregnancy
c. 30-34 weeks of pregnancy
d. 34-38 weeks of pregnancy

The CO starts to increase from 5th week of pregnancy and reaches its peak 40-50% at about 30-34 weeks. Thereafter the CO remains static till term when the observation is made at lateral recumbent position. CO increases further during labor (+50%) and immediately following delivery (+70%) over the pre-labor values.

Principal blood changes during pregnancy

Parameters	*Nonpregnant*	*Pregnancy near term*	*Total increment*	*Change*
Blood volume (mL)	4000	5500	1500	+ 30–40%
Plasma volume (mL)	2500	3750	1250	+ 40–50%
Red Cell volume (mL)	1400	1750	350	+ 20–30%
Total Hb (g)	475	560	85	+ 18–20%
Hematocrit (whole body)	38%	32%		Diminished

82. Congenital anomalies that can be easily identified by USG are all *except*:

a. Hydrops fetalis
b. Esophageal atresia
c. Anencephaly
d. Cystic hygroma

Fetal anomalies detection on USG

- Hydrops fetalis is detected by edema in skin, scalp and pleural or pericardial effusion and echogenic bowel.
- Esophageal atresia is suspected when stomach bubble is absent (normally seen at 20 weeks of gestational age).
- Anencephaly is diagnosed by the absence of cranial vault (calvarium) and telencephalon. Brain tissue is angiomatous.

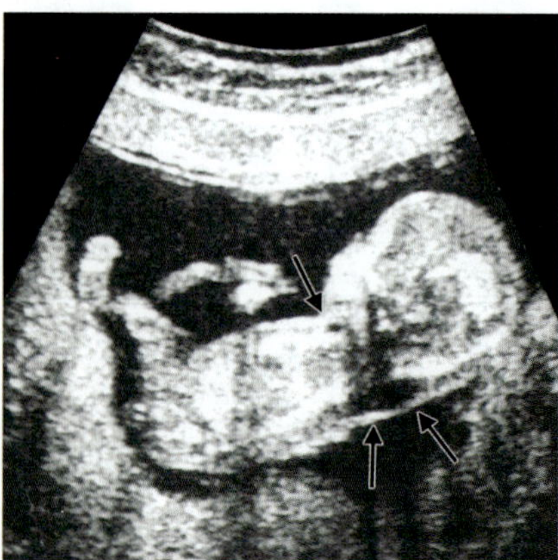

Longitudinal view of a 12-week fetus with a thickened nuchal translucency (arrows). This is due to dilatation of the lymphatic capillaries and edema. Fetuses with nuchal abnormalities need amniocentesis

Ans. 79. **a.** Cryotherapy 80. **d.** To know the position... 81. **c.** 30-34 weeks of pregnancy 82. **d.** Cystic hygroma

83. Embryonic structure, identified earliest on USG, for confirmation of pregnancy is:

a. Fetal pole   b. Fetal Heart activity
c. Gestation sac   d. Fetal skeleton

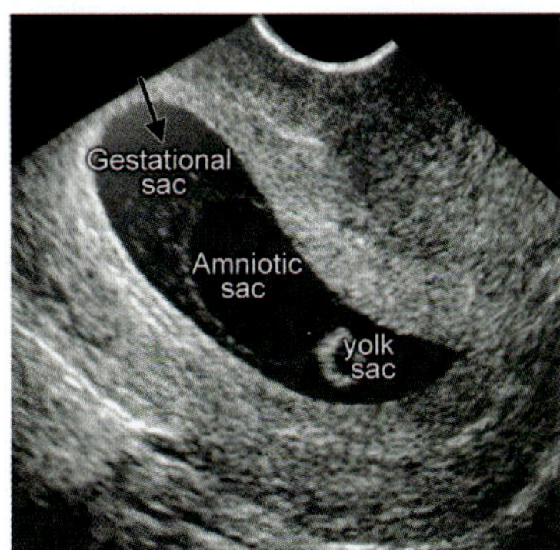

Ultrasonogram: gestational sac

Presence of an intrauterine gestational sac is a reliable evidence of intrauterine pregnancy. The sac is eccentrically located. The gestational sac could be seen as early as 4.5 to 5 weeks with the use of TVS (transvaginal sonography).

84. Which of the following (in maternal serum) indicate open neural tube defect?

a. Increased folic acid levels
b. Increased Alpha fetoprotein levels
c. Decreased Alpha fetoprotein levels
d. Decreased beta-HCG

MSAFP is elevated in a number of conditions: (a) wrong gestational age, (b) open neural tube defects (NTDs), (c) multiple pregnancy, Rh isoimmunization, (d) IUFD, (e) anterior abdominal wall defects and (f) renal anomalies.

Prenatal diagnosis: biochemical and biophysical screening tests

	β-hCG + PAPP-A + NT	*MSAFP*	*MSAFP, hCG, uE$_3$ (Triple test)*	*MSAFP, uE$_3$, hCG, Inhibin A*	*Soft tissue marker (Nuchal translucency; nasal bone)*
Time (weeks)	11–14	15–20	15–18	15–20	11–14
Observation	β-hCG (↑), PAPP-A (↓)	MSAFP (↑)	MSAFP (↓); uE$_3$ ↓; hCG (↑)	MSAFP (↓); uE$_3$ ↓; hCG (↑); Inhibin (↑)	Nuchal thickness (NT) > 3 mm, Nasal bone absent
Anomaly to detect	**Down's syndrome**	**Open neural tube defects**	**Down's syndrome**	**Down's syndrome**	**Down's syndrome, Turner's syndrome and others**
Comment	A cut off value 1 in 300 is screen positive	Cut-off level of 2.5 MOM can detect 90% of anencephaly, 80% open spina bifida	A cut-off value of 1 in 200 is screen positive	Detection rate is high	Detection rate of Down's syndrome is high (92%), when NT and NB are combined
Detection rate	85–92%	85%	73%	85–92%	85–92%
False-positive rate	5%	3–5%	5%	0.9%	3–5%

Women who are screen positive should be offered fetal karyotyping by invasive methods

85. Melasma, during pregnancy is seen on:

a. Breast   b. Face
c. Abdomen   d. Limbs

Chloasma gravidarum or pregnancy mask is an extreme form of pigmentation around the cheek, forehead and around the eyes. It may be patchy or diffuse; disappears spontaneously after delivery.

86. Best time to do USG in pregnancy, if it is to be done once in entire pregnancy, would be:

a. 6-8 weeks   b. 10-12 weeks
c. 18-22 weeks   d. 34-36 weeks

Routine USG at 18-22 weeks gestation has the following effects: (i) Reduces the incidence of post-term pregnancy (39%) and rates of induction of labor for post-term pregnancy. (ii) Increases detection of multiple pregnancy (92%). (iii) Increases detection of major fetal anomalies when termination is possible. (iv) No significant differences in the clinical outcomes such as perinatal mortality. (v) Reduce neonatal admission to special care baby unit (14%).

Ultrasound markers of chromosomal abnormalities (genetic sonography)

Observation	*Chromosomal abnormality*	*Observation*	*Chromosomal abnormality*
(a) **Head** ❑ Choroid plexus cyst ❑ Strawberry skull ❑ Hydrocephalus ❑ Holoprosencephaly	Trisomy 18, 13, triploidy	(f) **Hands/feet** ❑ Flexed overlapping fingers ❑ Rockerbottom/club foot ❑ Polydactyly ❑ Wide gap between 1st and 2nd toes	Trisomy 18 Trisomy 13

Ans. 83. **c.** Gestation sac   84. **b.** Increased Alpha...   85. **b.** Face   86. **c.** 18-22 weeks

Contd...

Observation	*Chromosomal abnormality*
(b) **Face**	
❑ Cleft lip/palate	Trisomy 13, 18, Meckel-Gruber syndrome
❑ Micrognathia	Triploidy
❑ Low set ears	Trisomy 21, 18, 13,
(c) **Nuchal translucency** >3 mm	Turner syndrome Trisomy 13, 18, 21
(d) **Cardiac defects**	
(e) **Renal anomalies**	
❑ Horseshoe kidney	Trisomy 13, 18, 21
❑ Bilateral dilatation of renal pelvis	Triploidy
❑ Cystic dysplasia	
❑ Clinodactyly	Trisomy 21
❑ Short femur	
(g) **GI system**	
❑ Echogenic bowel	Trisomy 13, 18
❑ Omphalocele	Trisomy 21
❑ Duodenal atresia	
(h) **General**	
❑ Early IUGR	Trisomy 13, 18, 21
❑ Hydrops	Triploidy, 45XO

87. MTP is done before the age of:

a. 10 weeks b. 20 weeks
c. 30 weeks d. Anytime

Termination of pregnancy is permitted up to 20 weeks of pregnancy. When the pregnancy exceeds 12 weeks, opinion of two medical practitioners is required.

88. Increased calories required during mid-pregnancy:

a. 300 b. 400
c. 550 d. 800

The increased calorie requirement is to the extent of 300 over the nonpregnancy state during second half of pregnancy.

Daily dietary allowances for a woman of reproductive age, pregnancy and lactation

Dietary components	*Nonpregnant*	*Pregnancy second half*	*Lactation*	*Sources*
Energy (kcal)	2,200 kcal	2,500 kcal	2,600 kcal	Protein, fat, carbohydrate
Protein (g)	50 g	60 g	65 g	Meat, fish, poultry, dairy product
Iron (mg)	18 mg	40 mg*	30 mg*	Meat, egg, grains [*to be supplemented]
Calcium (mg)	500 mg	1,000 mg	1,500 mg	Dairy products
Zinc (mg)	12 mg	15 mg	19 mg	Meat, egg, seafood
Iodine (μg)	150 μg	175 μg	200 μg	Iodized salt, seafood
Vitamin A (IU)	5,000 IU	6,000 IU	8,000 IU	Vegetables, liver, fruits
Vitamin D (IU)	200 IU	400 IU	400 IU	Dairy products
Thiamine (mg)	1.1 mg	1.5 mg		Grains, cereals
Riboflavin (mg)	1.1 mg	1.6 mg		Meat, liver, grains
Nicotinic acid (mg)	15 mg	17 mg	Almost same	Meat, nuts, cereals
Ascorbic acid (mg)	60 mg	70 mg	as in pregnancy	Citrus fruits, tomato
Folic acid (μg)	200 μg	400 μg		Leafy vegetables, liver
Vitamin B_{12} (μg)	2 μg	2.2 μg		Animal proteins

89. Triple test for Down syndrome is by using all *except*:

a. Maternal HCG
b. Maternal estriol
c. Maternal alphafetoprotein
d. Maternal HPL

Triple test is a combined biochemical test which includes MSAFP, hCG and uE3 (unconjugated estriol). Maternal age in relation to confirmed gestation age is also taken into account. It is used for detection of Down's syndrome. In affected pregnancy, levels of MSAFP and uE3 tend to be low while that of hCG is high.

Risk factors for prenatal genetic screening

Maternal risk factors	*Prenatal risk factors*
❑ Maternal age > 35 years ❑ Family history of neural tube defects ❑ Previous baby born with neural tube defect	❑ Oligohydramnios ❑ Polyhydramnios ❑ Severe symmetrical fetal growth restriction
❑ Previous child with chromosomal anomaly ❑ One or both parents—carriers of sex-linked or autosomal traits	❑ Abnormal ultrasound findings (structural anomalies) ❑ Uncontrolled diabetes mellitus in the periconceptional period

Contd...

Ans. 87. **b.** 20 weeks 88. **a.** 300 89. **d.** Maternal HPL

Contd...

Maternal risk factors	*Prenatal risk factors*
❑ One parent is known to carry a balanced translocation ❑ History of recurrent miscarriage	Contact with infection (teratogenic), e.g. rubella, cytomegalovirus or intake of teratogenic drugs ❑ Presence of soft tissue markers of chromosomal anomaly on ultrasonography ❑ Abnormal maternal serum screening

90. One of the following antihypertensives is NOT used in pregnancy:

a. Enalapril
b. Labetalol
c. Hydralazine
d. Nifedipine

ACE inhibitors are contraindicated in pregnancy.

Commonly used drugs in the management of hypertensive crisis

Drug	*Onset of action*	*Dose schedule*	*Maximum dose*	*Maintenance dose*
Labetalol *	5 min	10–20 mg IV every 10 minute	300 mg IV	40 mg/h
Hydralazine	10 min	5 mg IV every 30 minute	30 mg IV	10 mg/h
Nifedipine	10 min	10–20 mg oral, can be repeated in 30 minute	240 mg/24 hr	4–6 hours interval
Nitroglycerin	0.5–5 min	5 µg/minute IV	Short-term therapy only when the other drugs have failed	
Sodium nitroprusside		0.25–5 µg/kg/minute IV		

* To avoid labetalol in women having asthma or cardiac failure.

91. Blood is of fetal origin in:

a. Placenta previa
b. Abruptio placentae
c. Vasa previa
d. Placenta accrete

In velamentous placenta, the cord is attached to the membranes. If the leash of blood vessels happens to traverse through the membranes overlying the internal os, in front of the presenting part, the condition is called vasa previa.Rupture of the membranes involving the overlying vessels leads to vaginal bleeding. As it is entirely fetal blood, this may result in fetal exsanguinations and even death.

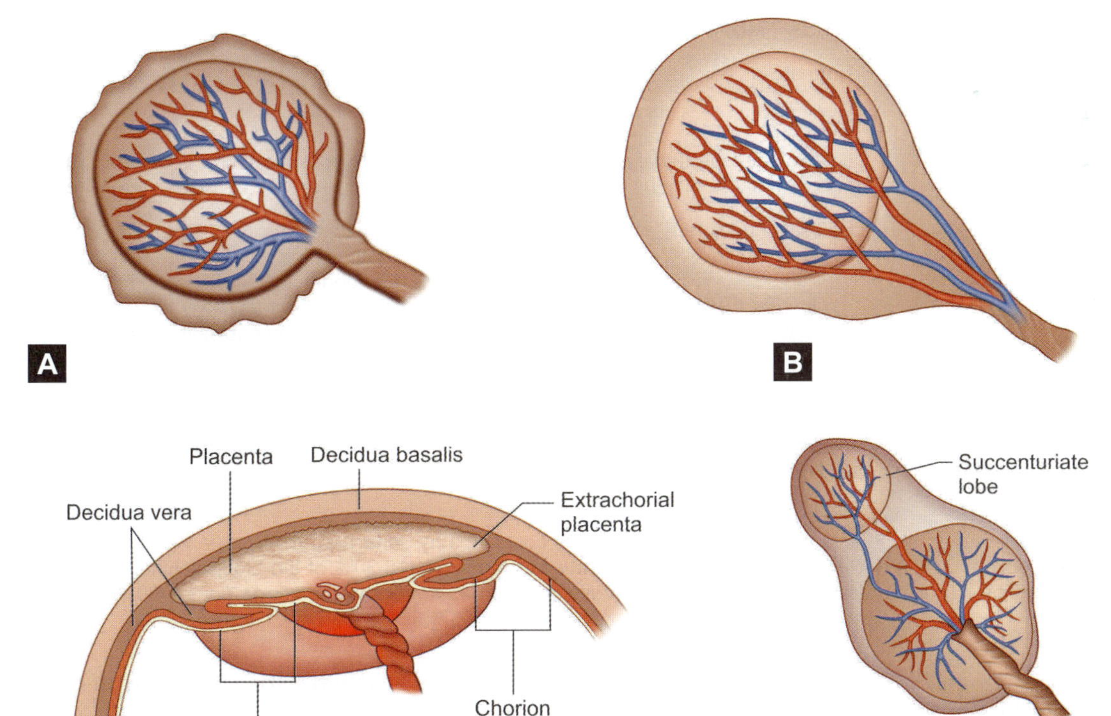

Common types of abnormal placentae of obstetric significance (A, B, C and D)

Ans. 90. a. Enalapril 91. c. Vasa previa 92. b. Accidental hemorrhage

92. **The most important cause of the coagulation failure in obstetrics is:**
   a. Intrauterine fetal death
   b. Accidental hemorrhage
   c. Placenta previa
   d. Rupture of the uterus

Blood coagulopathy is abruptio placentae is due to excess consumption of plasma fibrinogen due to disseminated intravascular coagulation and retroplacental bleeding. There is overt hypofibrinogenemia (<150 mg/dL) and elevated levels of fibrin degradation products and D-dimer.

Clinical features of revealed and mixed variety of abruptio placentae

Parameters	*Revealed*	*Mixed (Concealed features predominate)*
Symptoms	Abdominal discomfort or pain followed by vaginal bleeding (usually slight)	Abdominal acute intenses pain followed by slight vaginal bleeding. The pain becomes continuous
Character of bleeding	Continuous dark color (slight to moderate)	Continuous, dark color (usually slight) or blood stained serous discharge
General condition	Proportionate to the visible blood loss, shock is usually absent.	* Shock may be pronounced which is out of proportion to the visible blood loss.
Pallor	Related with the visible blood loss	Pallor is usually severe and out of proportion to the visible bleeding
Features of preeclampsia	May be absent	Frequent association
Uterine height	Proportionate to the period of gestation.	May be disproportionately enlarged and globular.
Uterine feel	Normal feel with localized tenderness, contractions frequent and local amplitude.	Uterus is tense, tender and rigid
Fetal parts	Can be identified easily	Difficult to make out
FHS	Usually present	Usually absent
Urine output	Normal	Usually diminished
Laboratory Tests:		
Blood: Hb%	Low value proportionate to the blood loss	Markedly lower, out of proportion to the visible blood loss
Coagulation profile	Usually unchanged	Variable changes: ❑ Clotting time increased (> 6 min) ❑ Fibrinogen level-low (< 150 mg/dL) ❑ Platelet count-low ❑ ↑ partial thromboplastin time ❑ ↑ FDP and D-dimer
Urine for protein	May be absent	Usually present
Confusion in diagnosis	With placenta previa. As such vaginal examination is withheld unless certain in the diagnosis	With acute obstetrical-gynecological-surgical complications

***Shock**: Shock is often due to blood loss and hypovolemia or due to coagulopathy. **Mild hemorrhage** (< 15% of the blood volume loss) is generally not associated with any change of vital signs. **Moderate hemorrhage** (15-30% of the blood volume loss) is associated with tachycardia, hypotension, ↓ pulse pressure and mean arterial pressure whereas **severe hemorrhage** (loss > 30-40%) is associated with features of shock.

93. **True about HCG:**
   a. Produced by cytotrophoblast
   b. Prevent involution of corpus luteum
   c. Value reaches maximum level at 20 week of pregnancy
   d. Its secretion starts after 2 days of ovulation

hCG acts as a stimulus for the secretion of progesterone by the corpus luteum of pregnancy. Rescue and maintenance of corpus luteum till 6 weeks of pregnancy is the major biological function of hCG.

Ans. **93. b.** Prevent involution of corpus luteum

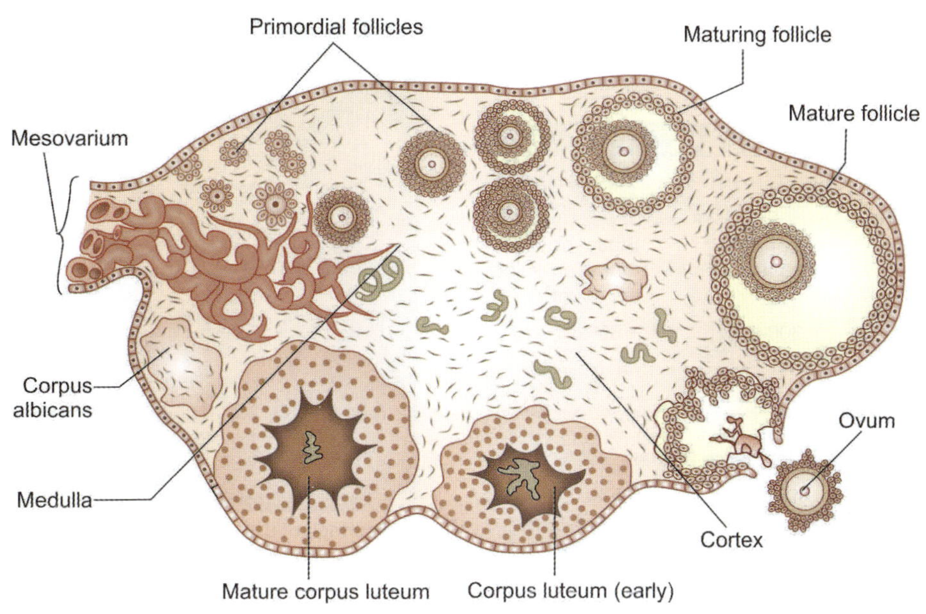

Histological structure of the ovary

94. Best investigation to diagnose fetal age is:

a. Serial ultrasound
b. Amniocentesis
c. Fundal height measurement
d. X-ray

USG examination is the best method to estimate the gestational age dating. The error with LMP is due to late ovulation (>14 days after LMP). CRL is the most accurate with an error of 2.1 days in the first trimester. BPD, FL, HC and AC are commonly used for dating thereafter.

Fetal features on transvaginal sonography (TVS) for dating in pregnancy	
Mean sac diameter (MSD)	*Findings*
5–8 mm	Yolk sac
12 mm	Embryo
15–18 mm	Cardiac activity
Embryo CRL ≥ 4 mm	Cardiac activity

GS should increase by 1.1 mm in diameter per day

Gestational age and embryonic structures identified by transvaginal sonography (TVS)	
Menstrual age (weeks)	*Fetal structures*
4	Choriodecidual thickness, chorionic sac
5	Gestation sac, embryo yolk sac
6	Fetal pole, cardiac activity
7	Lower limb buds, midgut herniation (physiological)
8	Upper limb buds, stomach
9	Spine, choroid plexus

95. Which of the following is the earliest sign of magnesium toxicity in a patient with eclampsia on treatment with magnesium sulphate?

a. Loss of deep tendon reflexes
b. Respiratory depression
c. Cardiac arrest
d. Decreased urine output

Magnesium toxicity and serum Mg levels

- Loss of deep tendon reflexes (>7 mEq/L)
- Respiratory depression (more than 10 mEq/L)
- Cardiac arrest (more than 25 mEq/L)

Monitoring of magnesium toxicity	Management for magnesium toxicity
❑ Loss of deep tendon reflexes ❑ Decreased respiratory rate (<12 per minute) ❑ Urine output (< 30 mL/h) ❑ Chest pain, heart block	❑ Stop magnesium therapy ❑ Estimation of serum magnesium and creatinine levels ❑ Injection calcium gluconate 10 mL (10% solution), IV

96. Blood coagulation profile in pregnancy:

a. Increase in fibrinogen level
b. Decrease in factor X, XI, XII
c. Decrease in plasminogen activity
d. Increase in platelet count

Ans. **94. a.** Serial ultrasound **95. a.** Loss of deep... **96. a.** Increase in fibrinogen level

Pregnancy is a hypercoagulable state. Fibrinogen level is raised by 50% from 200-400 mg/dL in nonpregnant to 300-600 mg/dL in pregnancy.

Changes in blood coagulation factors

Parameters	*Nonpregnant*	*Pregnancy near term*	*Change*
Platelets (mm³)	1,60,000–2,00,000	Conflicting observation	Static or 15% reduction of the count
Fibrinogen (mg%)	200–400	300–600	+ 50%
Fibrinolytic activity	—	Depressed	—
Clotting time	—	Unaffected	—
ESR	10 mm/h	40 mm/h	Marked increase (4 times)

97. The maximum chances of HIV infection being transmitted to the fetus/infant in an HIV infected mother are during:

a. First trimester
b. Third trimester
c. During labor
d. During breastfeeding

Vertical transmission of HIV to the neonates is about 14-25%. Transmission of HIV2 is less frequent (1-4%) than the HIV1 (15-40%). Transplacental transmission occurs: 20% before 36 weeks, over 80% of transmission occur around the time of labor and delivery.

98. Placenta with umbilical cord attached to its margin is called:

a. Battledore placenta
b. Circumvallate placenta
c. Succenturiate placenta
d. Velamentous placenta

In Battledore placenta, the cord is attached to the margin of the placenta. If associated with low implantation of the placenta, there is chance of cord compression in vaginal delivery leading to fetal anoxia or even death; otherwise, it has got little clinical significance.

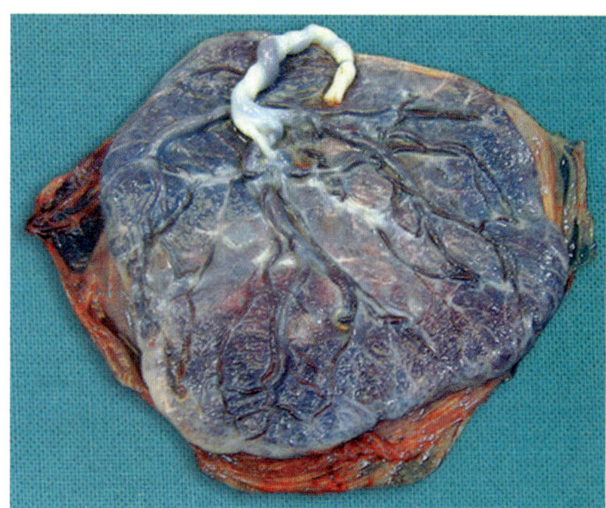

Fetal surface of the placenta showing attachment of the umbilical cord with ramification of the umbilical vessels

99. Most severely affected child in Rh-isoimmunization patients if:

a. Rh negative mother with Rh positive in 2nd child
b. Rh positive mother with Rh negative in 2nd child
c. Rh positive mother with Rh negative in 1st child
d. Rh negative mother with Rh negative in 2nd child

Red cell alloimmunization occurs if an Rh-negative woman bears an Rh-positive fetus. If the ABO compatible (mother and fetus have the same ABO group or when the fetus is group 'O'), Rh-positive fetal red cells enter the mother's blood, they remain in the circulation for their remaining lifespan. Thereafter, they are removed from the circulation by the reticuloendothelial tissues and are broken down with liberation of the antigen. The antibody production is related not only to the responsiveness of the reticuloendothelial system but also to the amount of Rh antigen liberated, therefore to the number of red cells that have entered the maternal blood. Because this takes a long time, immunization in a first pregnancy is unlikely.

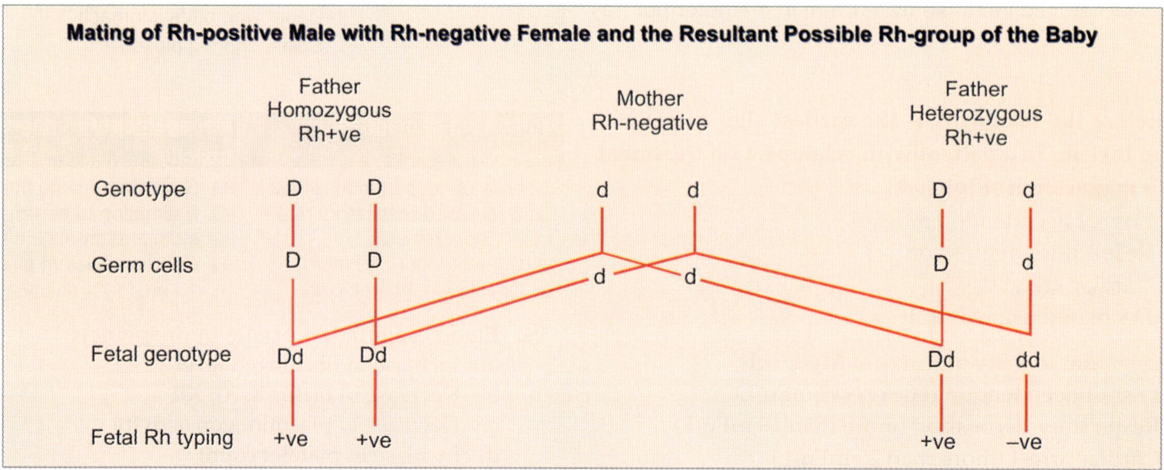

Ans. **97. c.** During labor **98. a.** Battledore placenta **99. a.** Rh negative mother with Rh positive in 2nd child

100. Amniotic fluid at 38 weeks in normal pregnancy is:

a. 800 cc
b. 1100 cc
c. 1500 cc
d. 1800 cc

At term, amniotic fluid measures 600-800 mL.

101. Ideal time to perform screening test for gestational diabetes (in weeks) is:

a. 6-8
b. 12-14
c. 24-28
d. 36-38

Screening of GDM is done by using 50 gm oral glucose challenge test without regard to time of day or last meal, between 24 weeks and 28 weeks of pregnancy.

Criteria for diagnosis of GDM with 100 gm oral glucose (O'Sullivan and Mahan modified by carpenter and coustan) and national diabetes data group

GTT: Venous Plasma (mg/dL)

Time	Carpenter and coustan	NDDG
Fasting	95	105
1 hour	180	190
2 hours	155	165
3 hours	140	145

GDM is diagnosed when any two values are met or elevated

102. Amniocentesis is best diagnostic if done in:

a. 8-10 weeks
b. 12-14 weeks
c. 16-18 weeks
d. 20-22 weeks

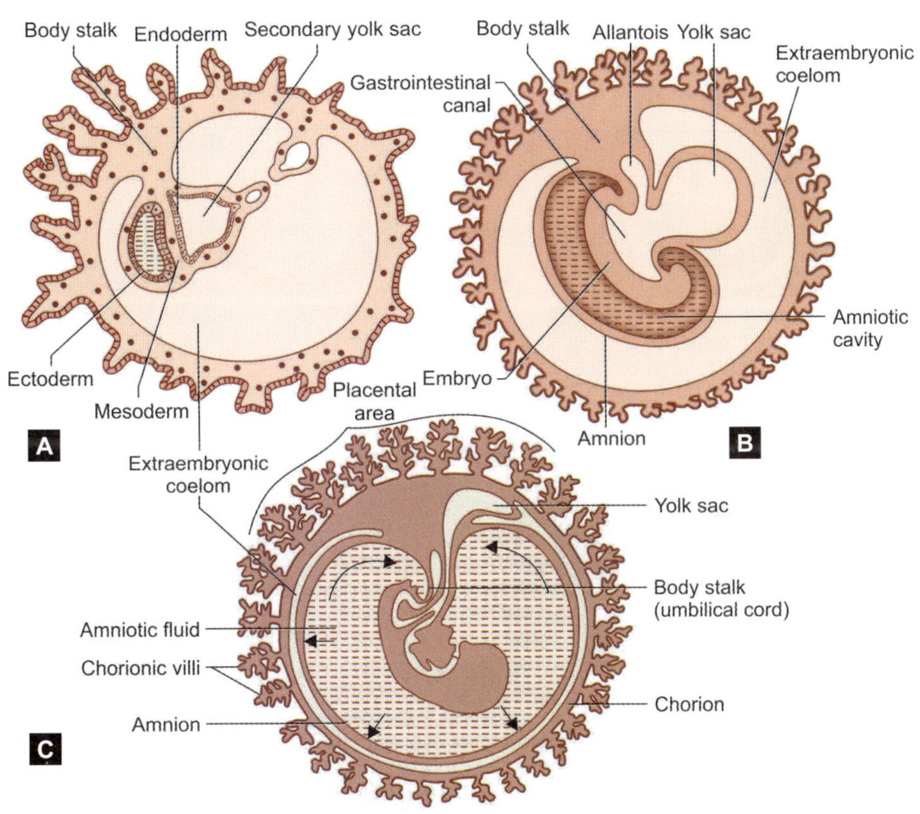

Schematic representation of formation of amniotic cavity, secondary yolk sac, extraembryonic coelom and body stalk: (A) Enlargement of extraembryonic coelomic cavity (B) The amniotic sac enlarges and begins to occupy the extraembryonic coelom (C) The amniotic sac has surrounded the embryo with almost completely obliterating the extraembryonic coelom; formation of body stalk completed

Genetic amniocentesis is an invasive procedure. It is performed after 15 weeks under ultrasonographic guidance. The fetal cells obtained in this procedure are subjected for cytogenetic analysis. Early amniocentesis (11-14 weeks) not to be done for genetic indications as the cell culture failure rate is high. Less fluid is withdrawn. Rates of complications are high.

103. Incidence of breech presentation at term:

a. 21%
b. 15%
c. 9%
d. 3%

The incidence of breech presentation is about 20% at 28 week and drops to 5% at 34 week and to 3-4% at term.

Ans. **100. a.** 800 cc **101. c.** 24-28 **102. c.** 16-18 weeks **103. d.** 3%

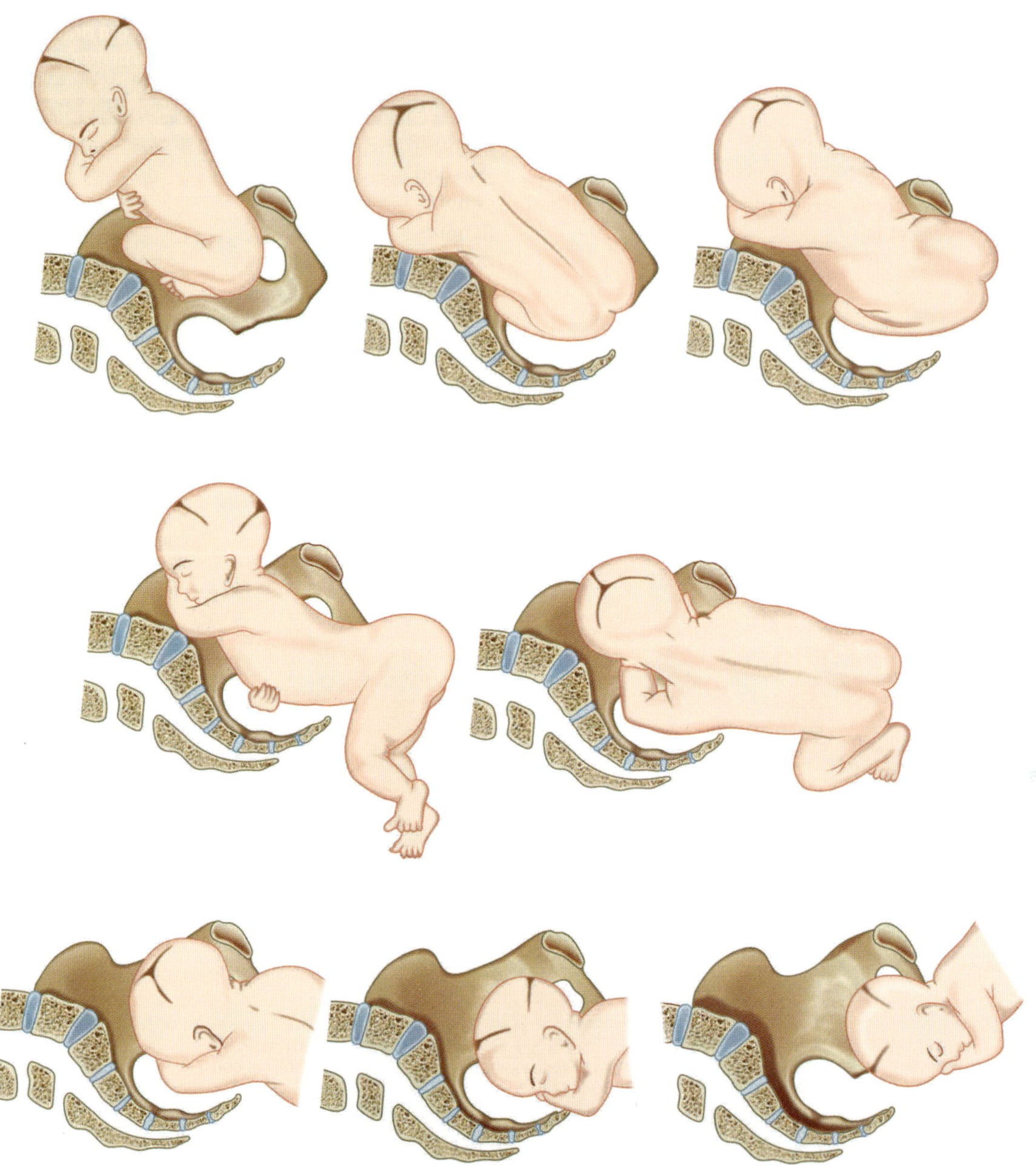

Mechanism of labor in breech (RSA)

104. The drug of choice for prevention of seizures in a patient with severe preeclampsia is:

a. Phenytoin
b. Magnesium sulphate
c. Diazepam
d. Nifedipine

Magnesium sulfate is the drug of choice for controlling seizures in pre-eclampsia. It acts as membrane stabilizer and neuroprotector. It reduces motor endplate sensitivity to acetylcholine. Magnesium also blocks neuronal calcium influx. It induces cerebral vasodilatation, dilates uterine arteries, increases production of endothelial prostacyclin and inhibits platelet activation.

Regimens of $MgSO_4$ for the management of severe preeclampsia and eclampsia

Regimen	*Loading dose*	*Maintenance dose*
Intramuscular (Pritchard)	4 g (20% solution) IV over 3–5 minute followed by 10 g (50%), deep IM (5 gm in each buttock)	5 g (50%) IM 4 hourly in alternate buttock
Intravenous (Zuspan or Sibai)	4–6 g IV slow over 15–20 minute	1–2 g/h IV infusion

Ans. 104. b. Magnesium sulphate

105. In the Manning scoring system of biophysical profile for foetal monitoring, which parameter is NOT included?

a. Fetal tone
b. Fetal gross body movements
c. Oxytocin challenge test
d. Non-stress test

Oxytocin challenge test/contraction stress test is an invasive method to assess the fetal well being during pregnancy. Where there is alteration in FHR in response to uterine contractions, it suggests fetal hypoxia. The test is based on determination of the respiratory function of the fetoplacental unit during induced contractions when the blood flow through the unit is curtailed.

Biophysical profile scoring (Manning—1992)		
Observation for 30 minutes Normal score = 2; Abnormal = 0		
Parameters	*Minimal normal criteria*	*Score*
Non-stress test (NST)	Reactive pattern	2
Fetal breathing movements	≥ 1 episode lasting > 30 second	2
Gross body movements	≥ 3 discrete body/limb movements	2
Fetal muscle tone	≥ 1 episode of active extension (limb or trunk) with return of flexion; opening and closing of hand, considered normal	2
Amniotic fluid	≥ 1 pocket measuring 2 cm in two perpendicular planes (2 × 2 cm pocket)	2

106. Which is NOT transmitted to the baby during delivery?

a. Toxoplasmosis
b. Gonococcus
c. Herpes simplex type II
d. Hepatitis B

The fetal risk of toxoplasmosis infection increases with duration of pregnancy and is approximately 15%, 30% and 60% in the first, second and third trimesters respectively. The fetus is only at risk if the mother is seronegative. The risk of fetal damage (severity) decreases from 60% in first trimester to almost zero percent at the end of pregnancy.

107. The commonest pathogen responsible for acute pyelonephritis in pregnancy is:

a. Escherichia coli
b. Klebsiella pneumoniae
c. Proteus mirabilis
d. Pseudomonas aeruginosa

The organisms responsible for pyelonephritis in pregnancy are E. coli (70%), Klebsiella pneumoniae (10%), Enterobacter, Proteus, Pseudomonas and Staphylococcus aureus group.

108. Most common cause of Placenta previa:

a. Myomectomy
b. Primigravida
c. Multigravida
d. Previous cesarean section

The high risk factors for Placenta previa are – (a) Multiparity (b) Increased maternal age (>35 years) (c) History of previous cesarean section or any other scar in the uterus (myomectomy or hysterectomy) (d) Placental size and abnormality (succenturiate lobes) (e) Smoking – causes placental hypertrophy to compensate carbon monoxide induced hypoxemia (f) Prior curettage.

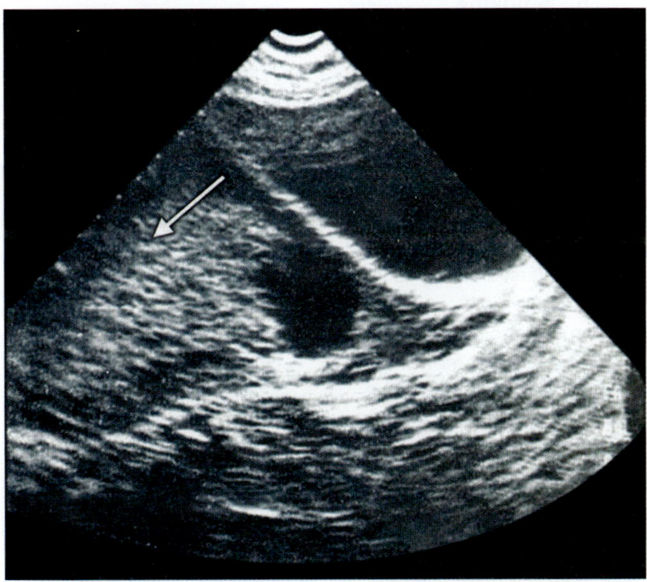

Ultrasonography showing central placenta previa (see arrow)

109. Monoamniotic-monochorionic twin results if division occurs:

a. Before 24 hours
b. 1-4 days
c. 4-8 days
d. More than 8 days

If the division occurs after eight day of fertilization, when the amniotic cavity has already formed, a monoamniotic-monochorionic twin develops (M/M: 1-2%).

Ans. **105. c.** Oxytocin chall... **106. a.** Toxoplasmosis **107. a.** Escherichia coli **108. c.** Multigravida **109. d.** More than...

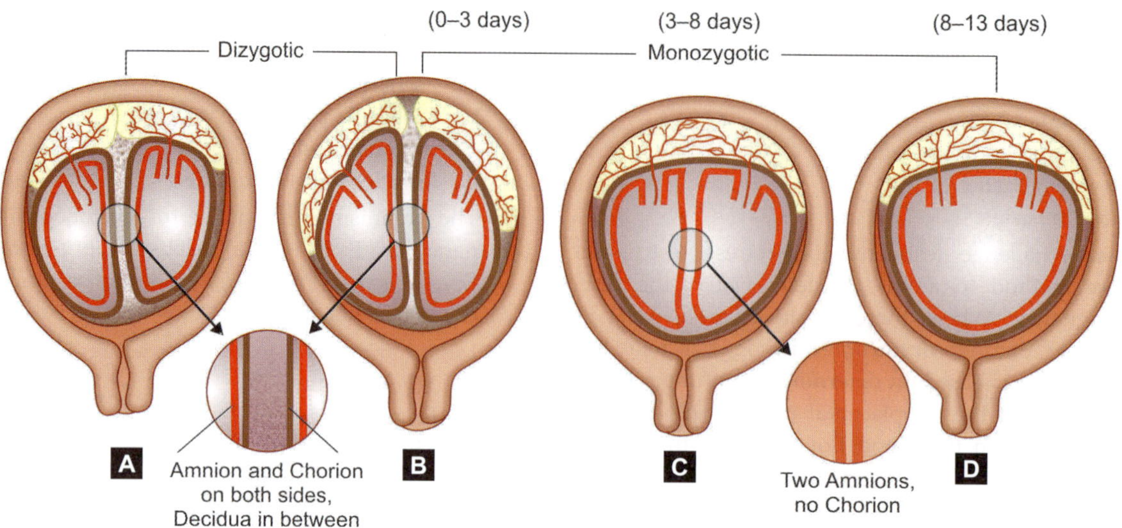

Twin placenta. **Dizygotic twins** (A, B) have two placentae (D/D): (A) separated and (B) fused without any vascular communications; intervening membranes consist of 4 layers (D/D). **Monozygotic twins**; (B) two placentae (D/D); (C) one placenta with free internal vascular anastomosis; the intervening membranes consist of 2 layers (D/M); (D) same as (C) but without any intervening membranes (M/M)

110. Risk factor for preeclampsia:

a. Chronic hypertension
b. Smoking
c. Nullipara
d. Placenta previa

Family history of hypertension or preeclampsia is a risk factor for development of preeclampsia.

Risk factors for preeclampsia	Etiopathological factors for preeclaampsia
❑ **Primigravida**: Young or elderly (first time exposure to chorionic villi) ❑ **Family history**: Hypertension, preeclampsia	❑ Failure of trophoblast invasion (abnormal placentation) ❑ Vascular endothelial damage ❑ Inflammatory mediators (cytokines)
❑ **Placental abnormalities**: – Hyperplacentosis: Excessive exposure to chorionic villi—(molar pregnancy twins, diabetes) – Placental ischemia. ❑ **Obesity**: BMI >35 kg/m^2, Insulin resistance. ❑ **Pre-existing vascular disease** ❑ **New paternity** ❑ **Thrombophilias** [antiphospholipid syndrome, protein C, S deficiency, Factor V Leiden].	❑ Immunological intolerance between maternal and fetal tissues – Coagulation abnormalities ❑ Increased oxygen free radicals ❑ Imbalance of angiogenic and antiangiogenic proteins) ❑ Genetic predisposition (polygenic disorder) ❑ Dietary deficiency or excess

111. In an epidemic of Hepatitis E infection in which of the following carries a poor prognosis?

a. Malnourished male
b. Pregnant women
c. Anaemic male
d. Postmenopausal women

Maternal mortality following acute HEV infection is high (15-20%).

112. Weight gain during pregnancy is:

a. 10 kg
b. 12 kg
c. 15 kg
d. 20 kg

The total weight gain during the course of a singleton pregnancy for a healthy woman averages 11 kg (24 lb). This has been distributed to 1 kg in first trimester and 5 kg each in second and third trimester.

I. Reproductive weight gain: 6 kg	II. Net maternal weight gain: 6 kg
Fetus—3.3 kg, placenta—0.6 kg and liquor—0.8 kg	Increase in blood volume—1.3 kg
Uterus—0.9 kg and breasts—0.4 kg	Increase in extracellular fluid—1.2 kg
Accumulation of fat (mainly) and protein—3.5 kg	

113. Fetal nuchal skin thickness is useful in detecting:

a. Fetal infection
b. Down syndrome
c. Anencephaly
d. Hydrops fetalis

Increased fetal nuchal skin thickness (in the first trimester) >3 mm by TVS is a strong marker for chromosomal anomalies (trisomy 21 [Down's syndrome], 18, 13, triploidy and Turner's syndrome).

Ans. **110. a.** Chronic... **111. b.** Pregnant women **112. b.** 12 kg **113. b.** Down syndrome

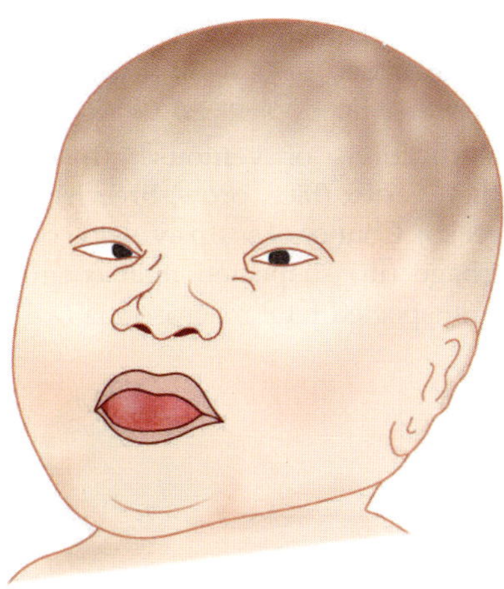
Baby with Down's syndrome

114. True about herpes simplex genitalis are all *except*:
a. Caused due to herpes simplex virus-2
b. Risk of fetal infection is high at term
c. May lead to malignancy
d. Treated by acyclovir

Genital tract infection is due to HSV-2. Infection may be primary, nonprimary, first episode and recurrent. It is transmitted by sexual contact. Primary infection may occur during pregnancy. If the primary infection is acquired in the last trimester there is chance of premature labor or IUGR.

115. Most common type of monozygotic twin pregnancy is:
a. Conjoined twins
b. Monoamniotic-monochorionic twins
c. Diamniotic-monochorionic twins
d. Diamniotic-dichorionic twins

If the division takes place within 72 hours after fertilization (prior to morula stage) the resulting embryos will have two separate placenta, chorions and amnions (diamniotic-dichorionic or D/D: 30%)

Summary of determination of zygosity

Zygosity	*Placenta*	*Communicating vessels*	*Intervening membranes*	*Sex*	*Genetic features (dominant blood group) DNA fingerprinting*	*Skin grafting (Reciprocal)*	*Follow-up*
Monozygotic	One	Present	2 (amnions)	Always identical	Same	Acceptance	Usually identical
Dizygotic	Two (most often fused)	Absent	4 (2 amnions 2 chorions)	May differ	Differ	Rejection	Not identical

116. Lecithin: Sphingomyelin ratio is measured for assessing maturity of:
a. Brain
b. Liver
c. Kidney
d. Lung

Estimation of pulmonary surfactant by lecithin/ sphingomyelin (L/S) ratio is done to assess fetal pulmonary maturity. Amniotic fluid L/S ratio at 31-32 weeks is 1; at 35 weeks L/S ratio is 2. L/S ratio ≥ indicates pulmonary maturity.

117. Parameter (biophysical profile) affected last in a state of fetal compromise:
a. Gross body movement
b. Fetal tone
c. Breathing movement
d. Liquor pocket

Earliest diagnosis of IUFD is possible with sonography. The evidences are: (a) Lack of all fetal motions (including cardiac) during a 10-minute period of careful observation with a real-time sonar is a strong presumptive evidence of fetal death and (b) oligohydramnios and collapsed cranial bones are evident.

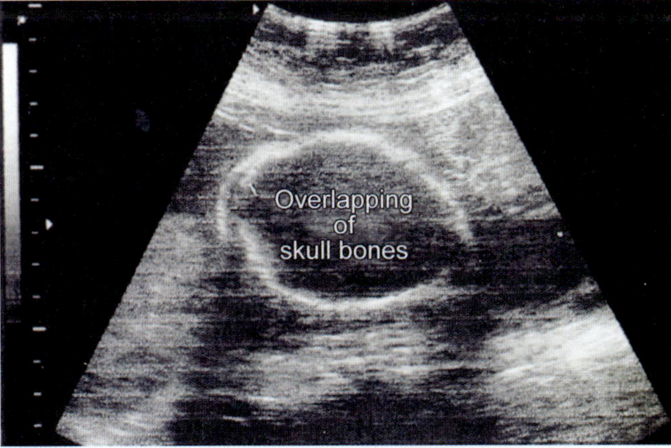

Sonographic plate showing collapsed cranial bones—a late feature of IUD

LABOR

118. During 3rd stage of labor (in mm Hg), intrauterine pressure is:
a. 30–40
b. 100–120
c. 80–100
d. 40–60

Intrauterine pressure
- First stage: 40–50 mm Hg
- Second & third stage: 100-200 mm Hg

Ans. 114. **c.** May lead... 115. **d.** Diamniotic... 116. **d.** Lung 117. **b.** Fetal tone 118. **b.** 100–120

119. Amniotic fluid at term (in ml):

a. 1000–1200
b. 800–1000
c. 900–1000
d. 700–800

By term, a fetus produces on average from 600 to 800 ml/day with a slight decline in hourly fetal urine production after 40 weeks gestation.

120. NOT a CONTRAINDICATION to ventouse:

a. Fetal distress
b. Anemia
c. Transverse lie
d. Face presentation

Contraindications of ventouse: (i) Any presentation other than vertex (face, brow, breech) (ii) preterm fetus (<34 weeks). Chance of scalp avulsion or subaponeurotic hemorrhage (iii) suspected fetal coagulation disorder and (iv) suspected fetal macrosomia ($\geq$ 4 kg).

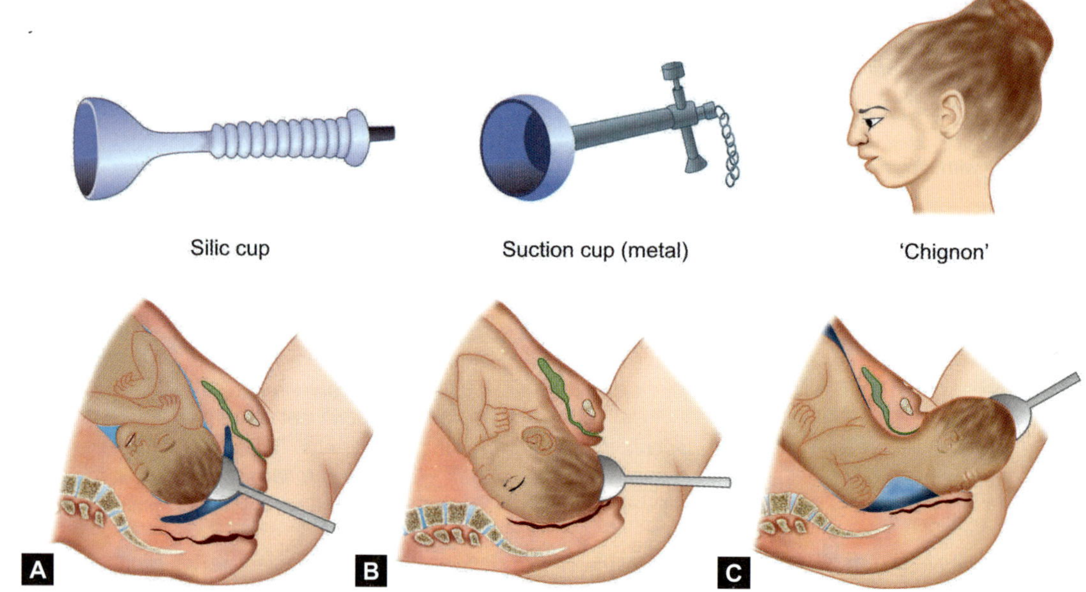

Application of vacuum extractor; (A to C) indicating the directions of traction at different stations of the fetal head. Traction over this flexion or pivot point either by ventouse or forceps promotes flexion and presents smaller diameter to the pelvis

121. Contraindication to artificial rupture of membranes:

a. Intrauterine death
b. Pregnancy induced hypertension
c. Diabetes
d. Heart disease

ARM is contraindicated in intrauterine fetal death, maternal AIDS, genital active herpes infection.

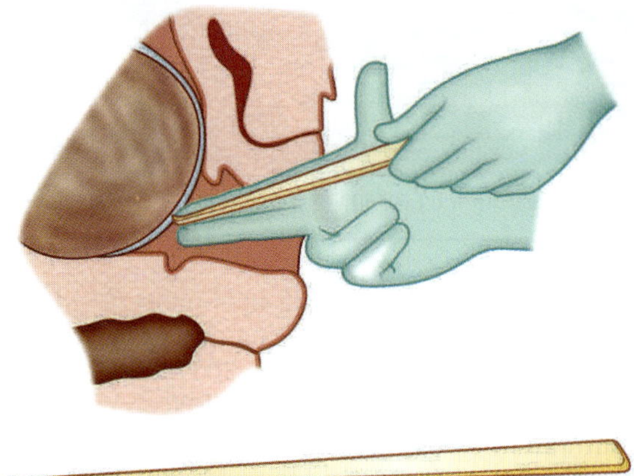

Artificial rupture of the membranes (ARM) using amni-hook

122. Advantages of median episiotomy over mediolateral episiotomy are all except:

a. Less blood loss
b. Easy repair
c. Extension of the incision is easy
d. Muscles are not cut

One of the disadvantages of median episiotomy is that extension, if occurs, may involve rectum.

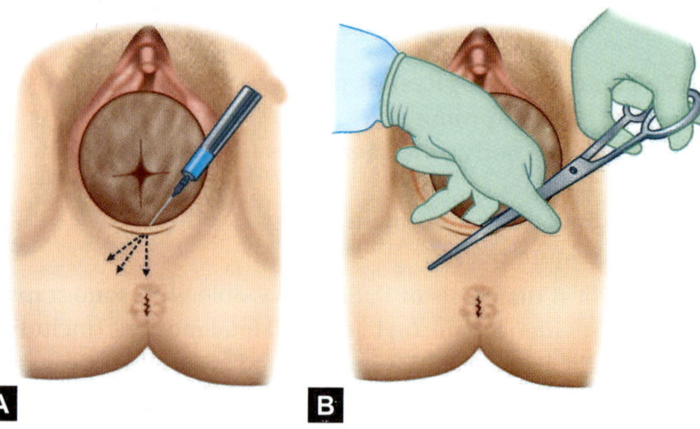

Steps of mediolateral episiotomy—(A) Perineal infiltration; (B) Cutting the perineum

Ans. 119. d. 700–800 **120. b.** Anemia **121. a.** Intrauterine death **122. c.** Extension of the incision...

123. Progress of the labour is assessed with the help of:

a. Cervicograph
b. Partogram
c. Dilatation chart
d. Growth curve

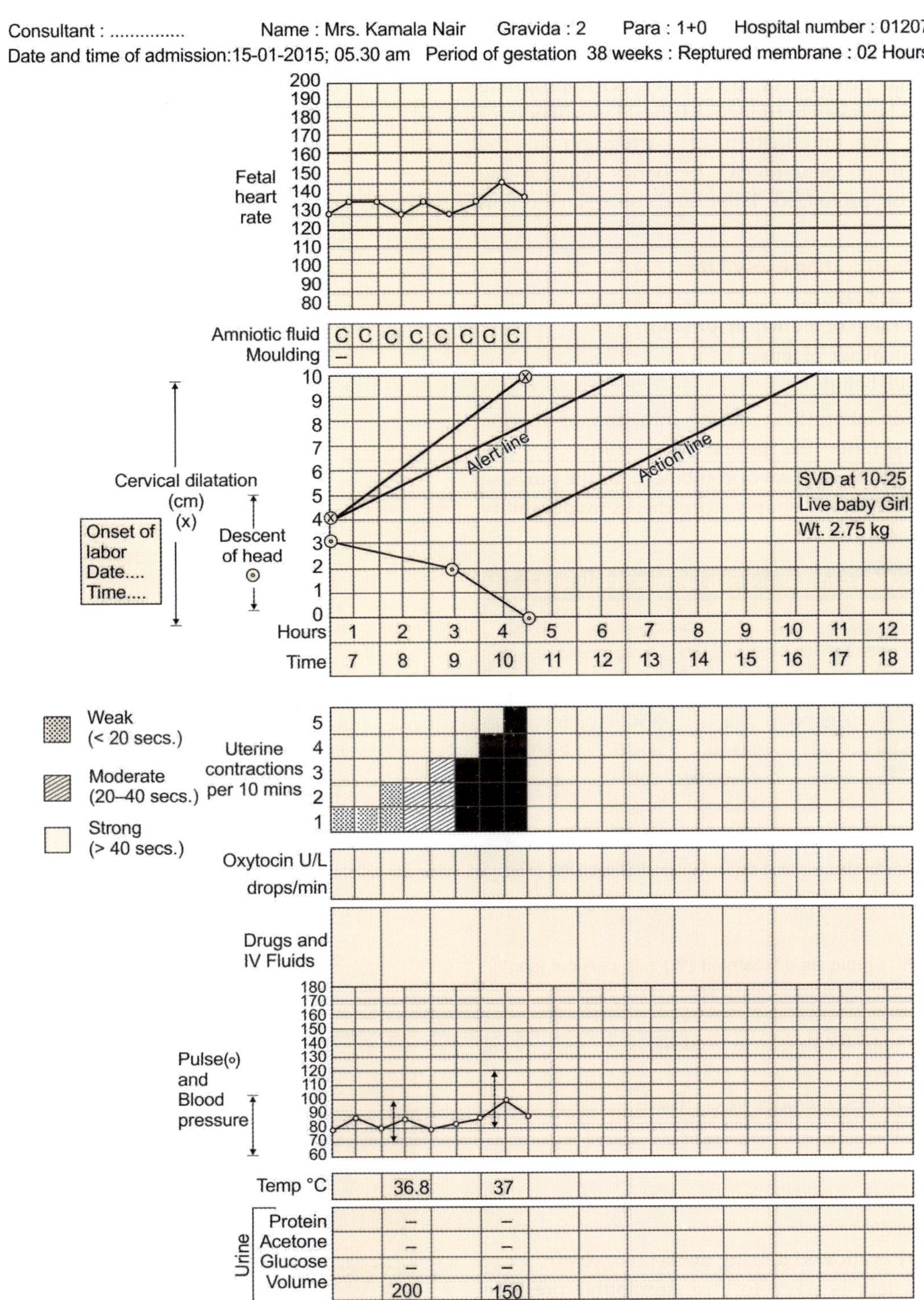

Partograph (modified WHO) representing graphically the important observations in labor. The cervical dilatation and descent of head are shown in relation to alert and action lines. Intensity and duration of uterine contraction are shown with shades

Ans. 123. **b.** Partogram

Partograph is a composite graphical record of key data (maternal and fetal) during labor, entered against time on a single sheet of paper. Advantages of a partograph: (i) A single sheet of paper can provide details of necessary information at a glance; (ii) No need to record labor events repeatedly; (iii) It can predict deviation from normal progress of labor early. So appropriate steps could be taken in time; (iv) It facilitates handover procedure; (v) Introduction of partograph in the management of labor (WHO 1994) has reduced the incidence of prolonged labor and cesarean section rate.

124. Bishop's classification is used for:

a. Progress of labor
b. Requirement of induction for labor
c. Gestational age of fetus
d. Fetal well being

Induction of labor (IOL) means initiation of uterine contractions (after the period of viability) by any method (medical, surgical or combined) for the purpose of vaginal delivery. Bishop's score checks favourability for induction.

Bishop's preinduction cervical scoring system (modified)

Parameters	Score			
	0	1	2	3
Cervix				
❑ Dilatation (cm)	Closed	1–2	3–4	5 +
❑ *Effacement (%)	0-30	40-50	60-70	≥ 80
❑ Consistency	Firm	Medium	Soft	–
❑ Position	Posterior	Midline	Anterior	–
Head: Station	–3	–2	–1,0	+ 1, + 2
Total score = 13; Favorable score = 6-13; Unfavorable score = 0-5				
* Cervical length (cm)	> 4	2-4	1-2	< 1

* Modification (1991) replaces effacement (%) with cervical length in cm.

125. Burns-Marshall technique is used to:

a. Deliver head
b. Deliver after-coming head of breech
c. Deliver leg
d. Deliver placenta

Burns-Marshall method for delivering aftercoming head of breech

- The baby is allowed to hang by its own weight
- The assistant is asked to give suprapubic pressure with a flat of the hand in a downward and backward direction, the pressure is to be exerted more toward the sinciput.
- When the nape of the neck is visible under the pubic arch, the baby is grasped by the ankles with finger in between the two.
- Maintaining a steady traction and forming a wide arc of a circle, the trunk is swung in upward and forward direction.

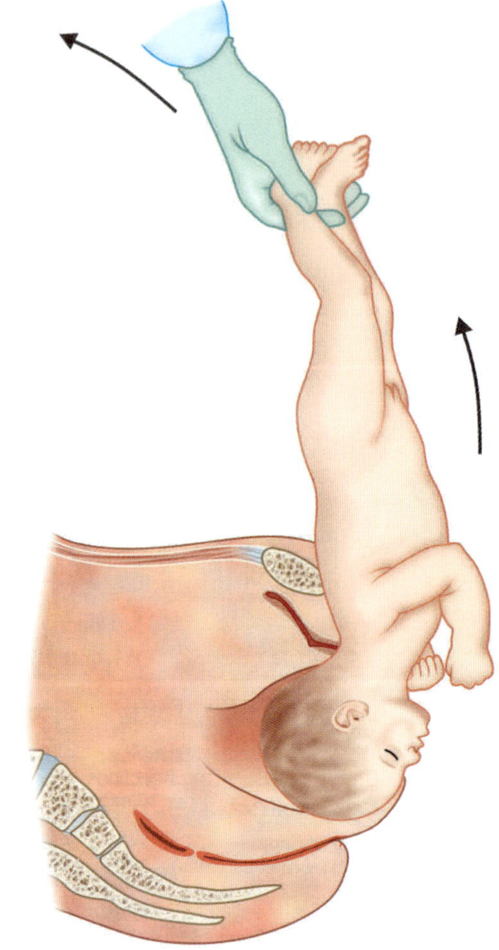

Continuation of the Burns–Marshall method

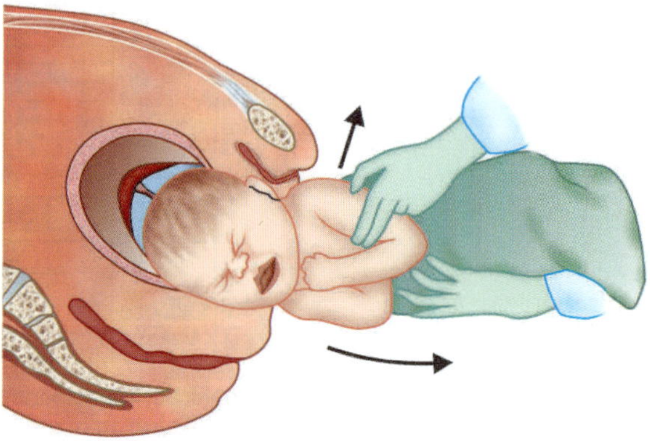

Delivery of the anterior arm

Ans. 124. b. Requirement... 125. b. Deliver after-coming head of breech

126. In second stage of labor, on per-vaginam examination, anterior fontanelle and supra-orbital ridge can be felt. The likely presentation is:

a. Face b. Flexed head
c. Deflexed head d. Brow

Brow is the rarest variety of cephalic presentation where the presenting part is the brow and the attitude of the head is short that of degree of extension necessary to produce face presentation, i.e. the head lies in between full extension and full flexion. The position is to be confirmed on vaginal examination by palpating supraorbital ridges and anterior fontanel.

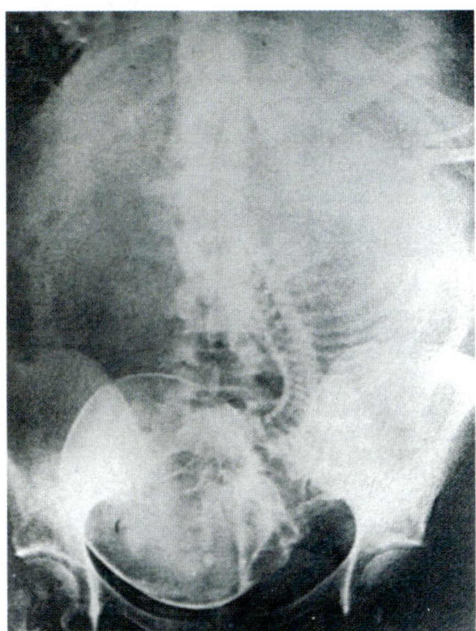

Straight X-ray abdomen showing brow presentation. The head feels very big. Patient was delivered by cesarean section

127. Vaginal delivery is contraindicated in:

a. Mento-posterior
b. Twins with one vertex and other breech
c. Mento-anterior
d. Extended breech

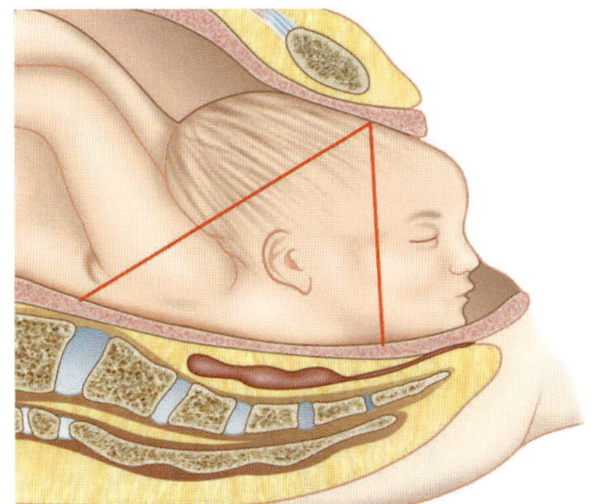

Head cannot extend further, nor flexion is possible. Bregmaticsternal diameter (18 cm or 7") cannot be accommodated in the pelvis resulting in obstructed labor

Unlike persistent occipito-posterior, where occasional face-to-pubis delivery occurs, there is no possibility of spontaneous delivery in persistent mento-posterior. This is because the relatively short neck cannot clear off the total length of the sacrum (12 cm). As such the thorax is thrust in, resulting bregmaticosternal diameter (18 cm or 7") to occupy the pelvis. As a result, the labor becomes inevitably obstructed.

128. Bandl's ring is seen in:

a. Injudicious use of oxytocic
b. Obstructed labor
c. Premature rupture of membrane
d. Undilated cervix

In obstructed labor, there is gradual increase in intensity, duration and frequency of uterine contraction. The relaxation phase becomes less and less; ultimately a state of tonic contraction develops. Retraction, however, continues. As the labor advances, the lower segment elongates and becomes progressively thinner to accommodate the fetus driven from the upper segment. A circular groove encircling the uterus is formed between the active upper segment and the distended lower segment, called pathological retraction ring (Bandl's ring).

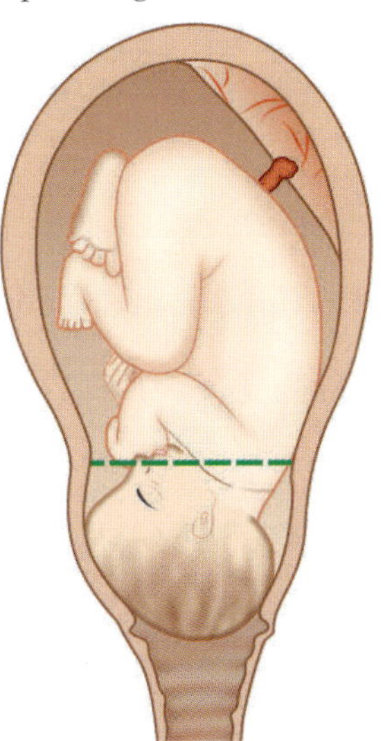

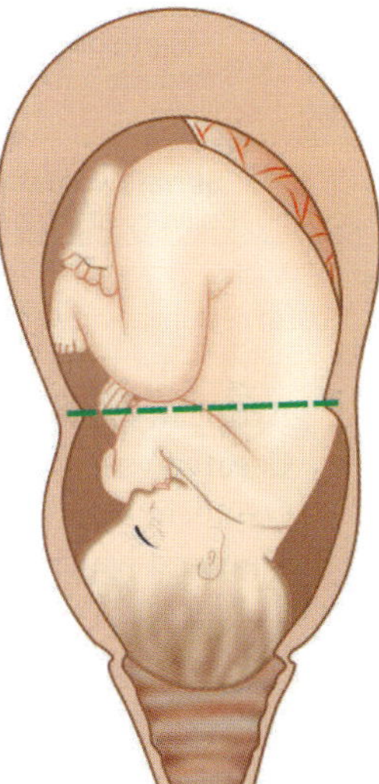

Pathogenesis of retraction ring (Bandl's ring). (A) Normal labor; (B) Late obstruction. Note the circumferential dilatation and progressive stretching of the lower segment with corresponding thickening of the upper segment and rise in the level of retraction ring following obstruction

129. Rupture of membrane is said to be premature if:

a. It occurs at 38 weeks of pregnancy
b. It occurs at 32 weeks of pregnancy
c. It occurs prior to 1st stage of labor
d. It occurs at IInd stage of labor

Spontaneous rupture of the membranes any time beyond 28th week of pregnancy, but before the onset of labor is called prelabor rupture of membranes/premature rupture of membranes (PROM).

Ans. 126. **d.** Brow 127. **b.** Twins with one... 128. **b.** Obstructed labor 129. **c.** It occurs prior to 1st...

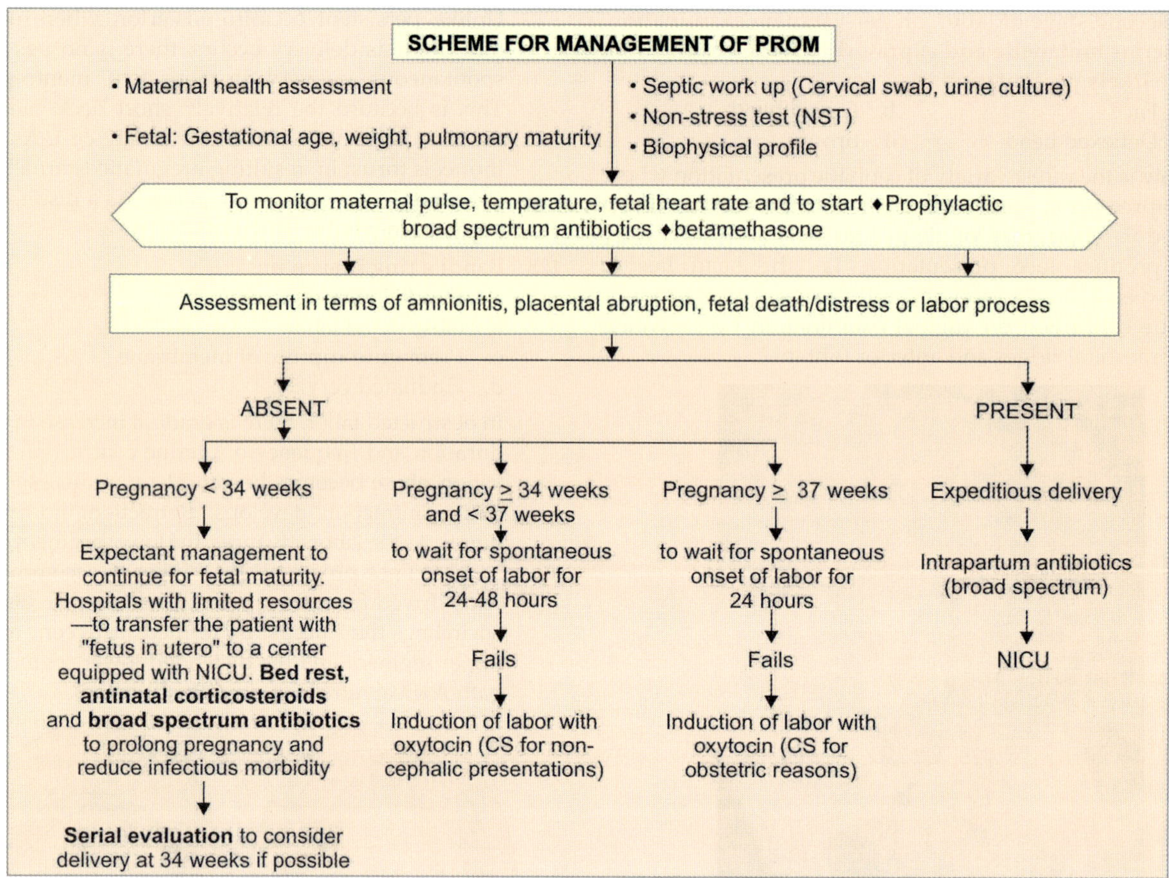

130. Preferred management of occipito-posterior position during labor:

a. Artificial rupture of membranes
b. Cesarean section
c. Oxytocin drip
d. Wait and watch

In occipito-posterior position there is increased maternal morbidity, incidental to prolonged labor and increased incidence of operative delivery (1 in 5). There is also increased perinatal morbidity and mortality (10%) due to asphyxia or trauma during vaginal operative delivery. However, it is to be morbidity and remembered that in 4 out of 5 cases, there is usually no trouble and the fetus is delivered spontaneously.

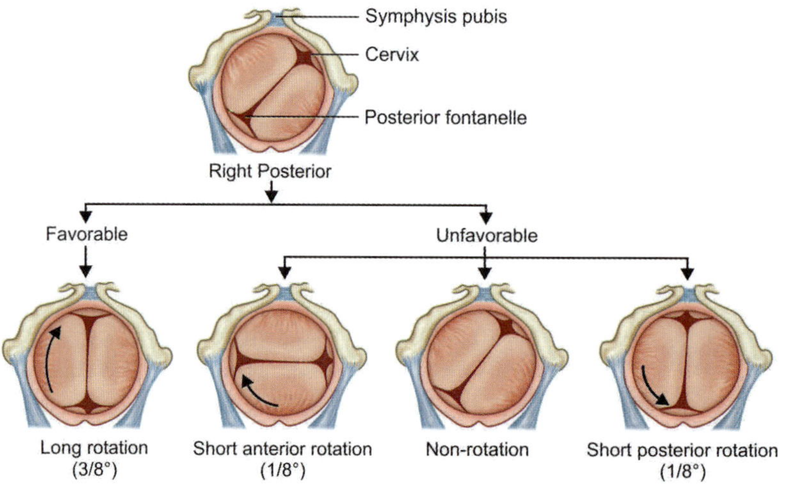

Diagrammatic representation showing favorable and unfavorable rotation of occipitoposterior position

Ans. **130. d.** Wait and watch

131. Partogram is used for:

a. Determining pattern of fetal heart rate
b. Determining position of cervix
c. Assessing integrity of utero-placental unit
d. Recording progress of labor

Partograph can diagnose any dysfunctional labor early and help to initiate correct management.

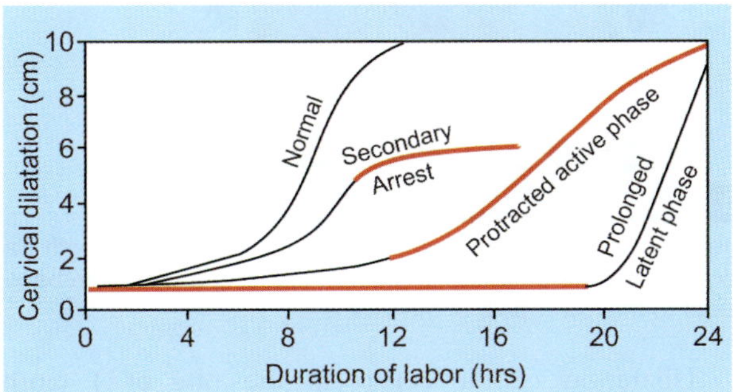

Partographic analysis of labor to detect types of prolonged labor—protracted latent phase, protracted active phase and secondary arrest

132. Which of the following types of placenta complicate third stage of labour and is associated with a past history of caesarean section?

a. Placenta succenturia
b. Placenta extracholis
c. Placenta membranacea
d. Placenta accreta

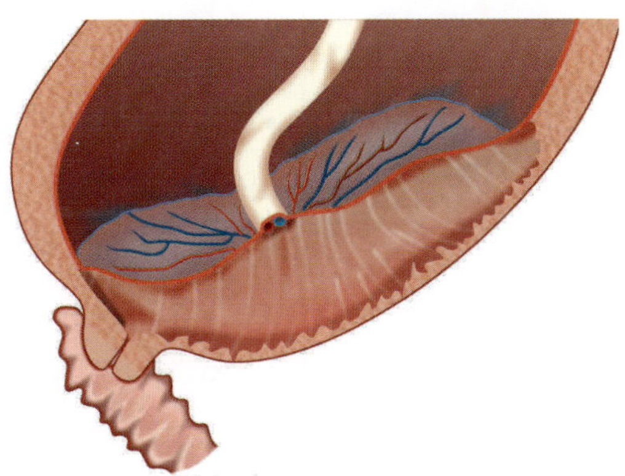

Placenta accreta

Placenta accreta (morbid adherent placenta) is an extremely rare form in which the placenta is directly anchored to the myometrium partially or completely without any intervening deciduas. The probable cause is due to absence of decidua basalis and poor development of fibrinoid layer. The most important risk factors are the placenta previa and previous cesarean section.

133. Inversion of the uterus, a complication is noticed in:

a. Ist stage of labor
b. IInd stage of labor
c. IIIrd stage of labor
d. Post partum period

Inversion of uterus is an extremely rare but a life-threatening complication in third stage in which uterus is turned inside out partially or completely. The incidence is about 1 in 20,000 deliveries.

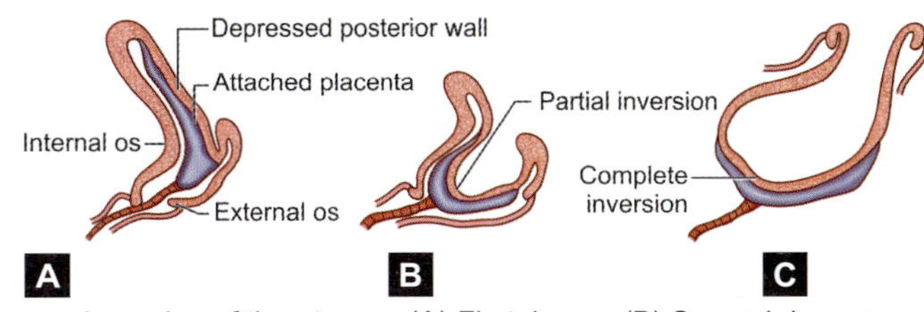

Inversion of the uterus—(A) First degree (B) Second degree (C) Third degree

134. External cephalic version (ECV) is contraindicated in:

a. Primigravida
b. Flexed breech
c. Anemia
d. PIH

C/I of ECV

- Antepartum hemorrhage
- Fetal causes–hyperextension of the head, large fetus (>3.5 kg), major congenital abnormalities, dead fetus, IUGR
- Multiple pregnancy
- Rupture membranes – with drainage of liquor
- Abnormal cardiotocography
- Contracted pelvis
- Previous cesarean section
- Obstetrics complications: Severe pre-eclampsia, obesity, elderly primigravida, bad obstetric history
- Oligohydramnios
- Rhesus isoimmunization

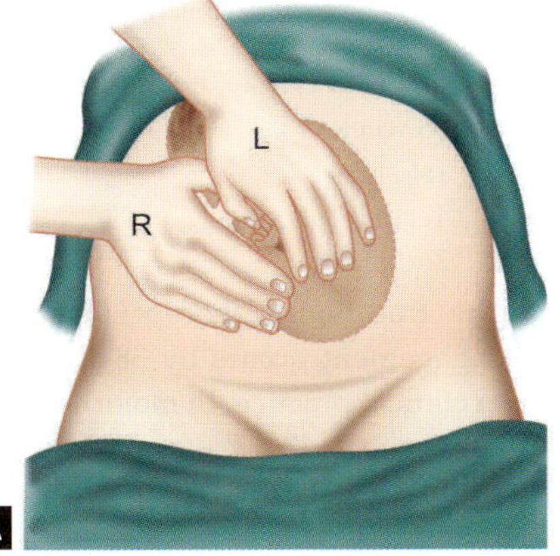

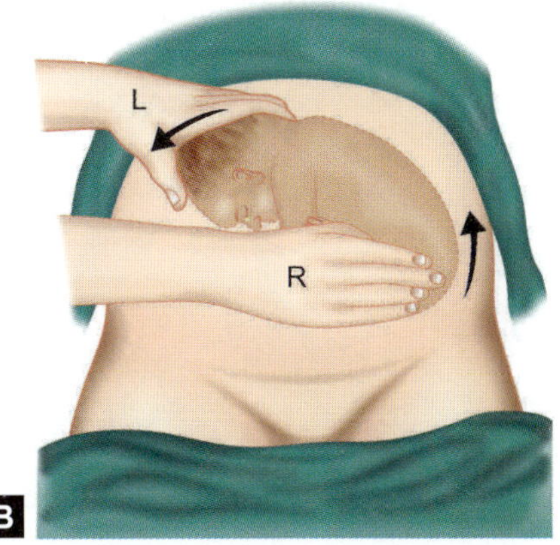

Ans. 131. **d.** Recording... 132. **d.** Placenta accreta 133. **c.** IIIrd stage of labor 134. **d.** PIH

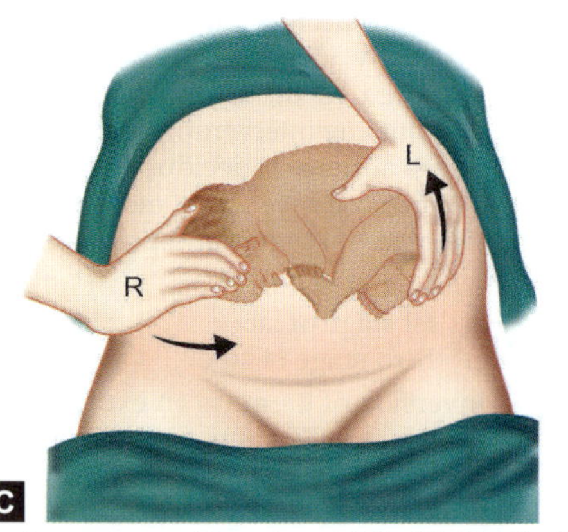

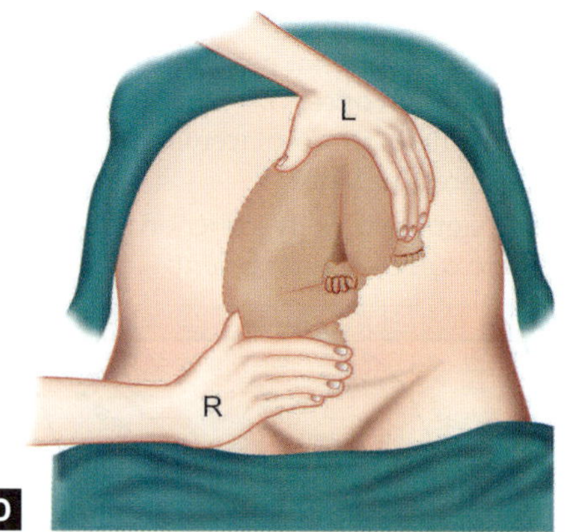

Steps of external cephalic version — (Breech — LSA): (A) Mobilization of the buttocks to the iliac fossa towards the back using both hands; (B) Rotation of the trunk holding the poles and maintaining flexion of the trunk; (C) Change of hands to prevent crossing after the lie becomes transverse; (D) The lie becomes longitudinal with the cephalic pole being brought to the lower pole of the uterus

135. During active labor, cervical dilatation per hour in primi is:

a. 1 cm
b. 1.5 cm
c. 2 cm
d. 2.5 cm

Dilatation of the cervix at the rate of 1 cm/h in primigravidae and 1.5 cm in multigravidae beyond 4 cm dilatation (active phase of labor) is considered satisfactory.

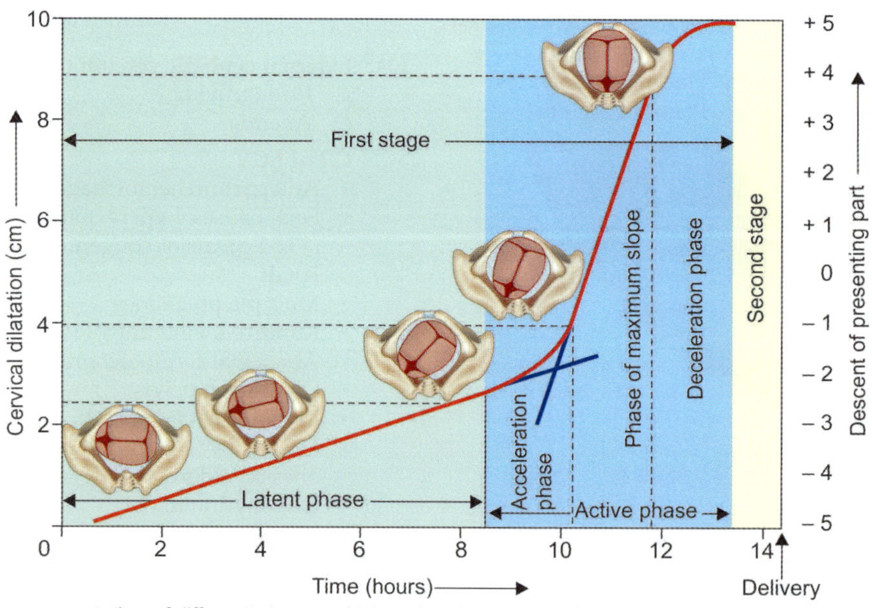

Composite partographic representation of different phases of labor showing progressive cervical dilatation, descent and rotation of the head

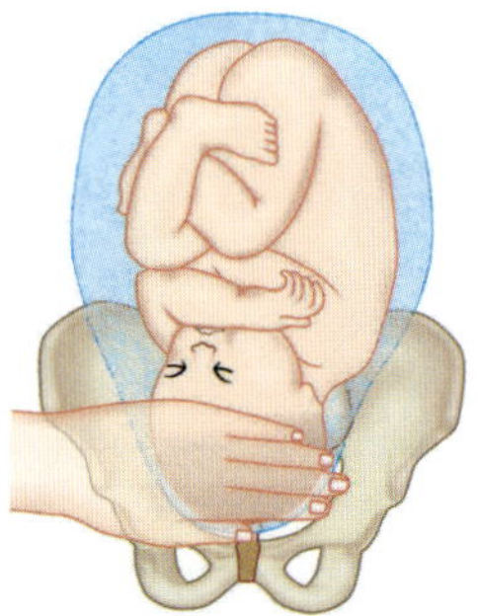

Head is palpable five-fifths above the symphysis pubis. Head is mobile, free and not engaged

136. In a primigravidae, head engages at:

a. 36 weeks
b. 1st stage
c. Term
d. 2nd stage

The traditional concept that in primigravidae, the engagement occurs by 38 weeks is not corroborative in clinical practice. In majority, the engagement occurs between 38-42 weeks or even during first stage of labor.

Ans. **135. a.** 1 cm **136. c.** Term

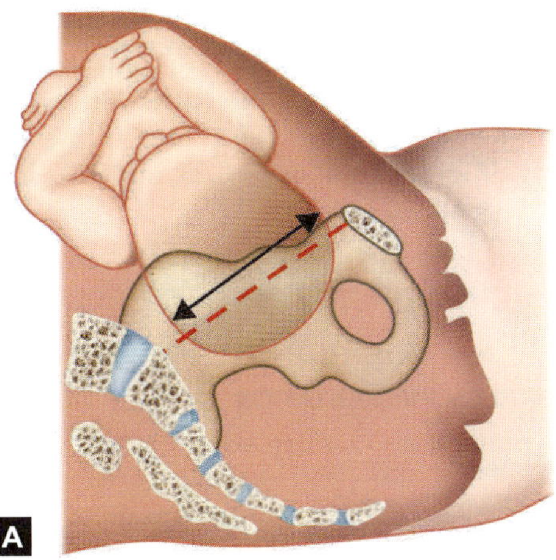

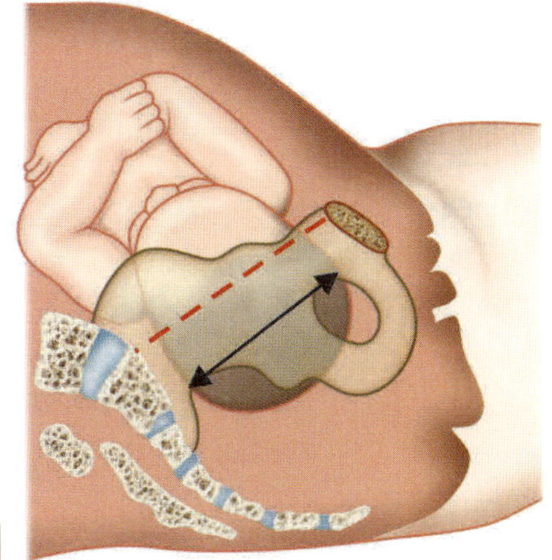

The relationship of the biparietal diameter to the pelvic brim and that of lower pole of the head to the ischial spines in: (A) Non-engaged head; (B) Engaged head

137. Bishop's score include all *except*:

a. Dilatation of cervix
b. Effacement of cervix
c. Contraction of uterus
d. Station of head

Bishop's score also include consistency and position of cervix.

Predictive factors for successful induction of labor	
Period of gestation	Pregnancy nearer the term or post-term—more the success
Preinduction score	Bishop score ≥ 6 is favorable. Dilatation of the cervix is most important.
Sensitivity of the uterus	Positive oxytocin sensitivity test is favorable for IOL
Cervical ripening	Favorable in multiparous and in cases with PROM. Less responsive in elderly primigravidae or cases with prolonged retention of dead fetus.
Presence of fetal fibronectin (fFN) in vaginal swab (> 50 ng/mL)	Favorable for successful IOL
Other positive factors	Maternal height > 5'; Normal BMI, EFW < 3 kg

138. The commonest cause of occipito-posterior position of fetal head during labor is:

a. Maternal obesity
b. Deflexion of fetal head
c. Multiparity
d. Android pelvis

The shape of the pelvic inlet significantly determines the position of the head at the onset of labor. In more than 50%, the occipito-posterior position is associated with either an anthropoid or android pelvis. The wide occiput can comfortably be placed in the wider posterior segment of the pelvis.

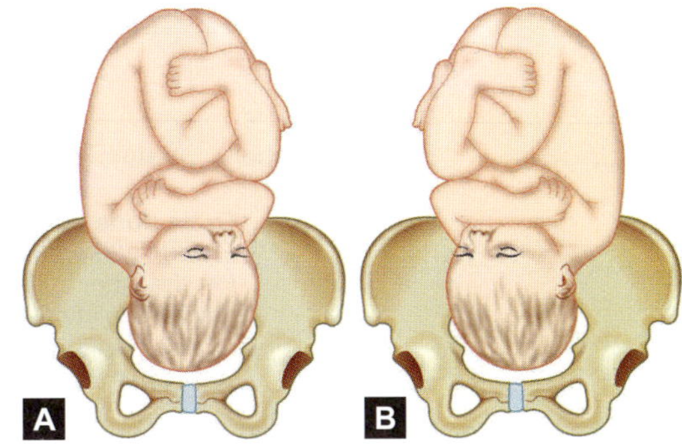

(A) Right occipito-posterior position, (B) Left occipito-posterior position

139. Engagement of fetal head is:

a. When the occiput has gone below the pelvic inlet
b. When the widest diameter of the presenting part has passed through the pelvic inlet
c. When the presenting part can be pushed into the pelvic cavity
d. Synonymous with fixation of head

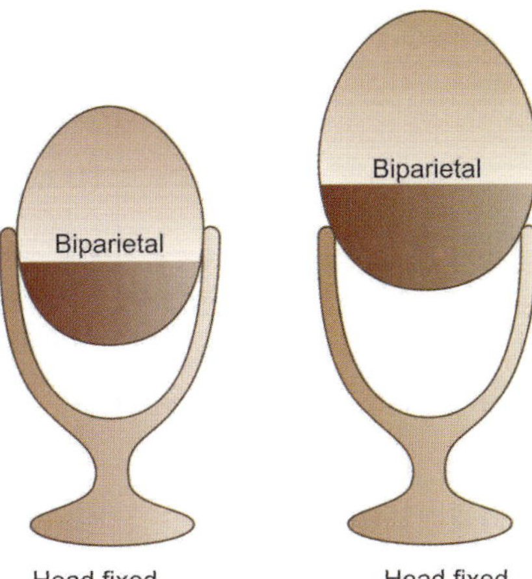

Diagrammatic representation showing the difference between an engaged and a fixed head by use of egg cups and eggs

Ans. **137. c.** Contraction... **138. d.** Android pelvis **139. b.** When the widest...

When the greatest horizontal plane of the fetal skull, the biparietal, has passed the plane of pelvic brim, the fetal head is said to be engaged.

140. External cephalic version is contraindicated in all *except*:

a. Antepartum haemorrhage
b. Multiple pregnancy
c. Contracted pelvis
d. Breech presentation

ECV is carried out after 36 weeks in the labor delivery complex for breech presentation. Tocolytic drug (terbutaline – 0.25 mg SC), if required, can be administered.

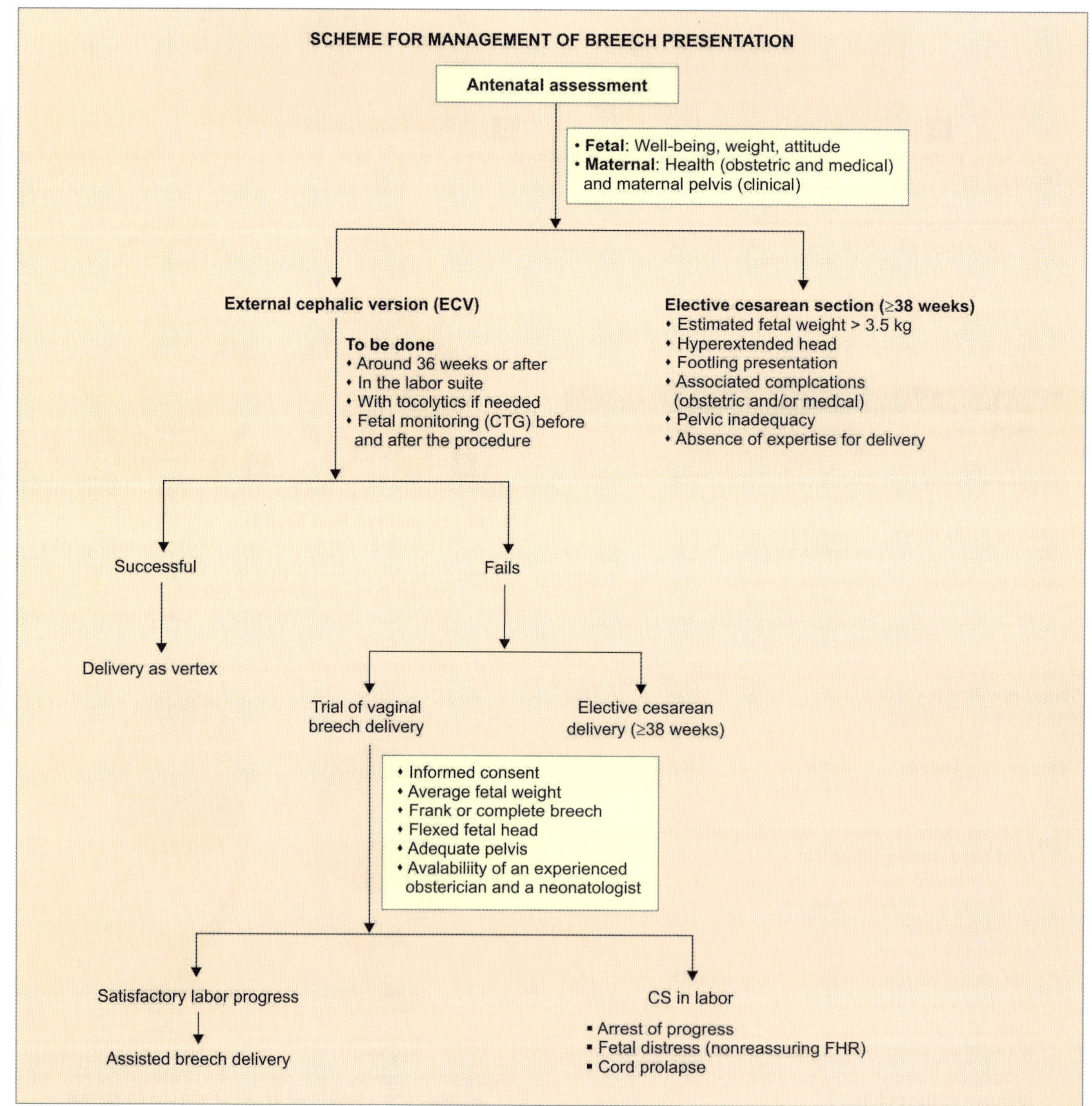

Ans. 140. d. Breech...

141. Value of critical obstetrics conjugate for trial of labor:

a. 8.5 cm b. 9 cm
c. 9.5 cm d. 10 cm

Degree of disproportion and contracted pelvis: Based on the clinical and supplemented by imaging pelvimetry, the following degrees of disproportion at the brim are evaluated:

(1) Severe disproportion: Where obstetric conjugate is <7.5 cm (3"). Such type is rare to see.

(2) Borderline: Where obstetric conjugate is between 9.5 cm and 10 cm.

POSTPARTUM PERIOD

142. True for Cephalhaematoma:

a. Tension varies on crying b. May cause jaundice
c. Edematous fluid d. Cross suture line

Cephalohematoma is a hemorrhage of blood between the skull and the periosteum of a newborn baby secondary to rupture of blood vessels crossing the periosteum. Because the swelling is subperiosteal its boundaries are limited by the individual bones (does not cross suture line), in contrast to a Caput succedaneum. If severe the child may develop jaundice, anemia or hypotension.

143. Involution of uterus is completed by:

a. 6 weeks b. 8 weeks
c. 12 weeks d. 16 weeks

At the end of 6 weeks, the measurement of uterus is similar to that of the nonpregnant state and weighs about 60 g. The decrease in size of the uterus and cervix has been shown with serial MRI.

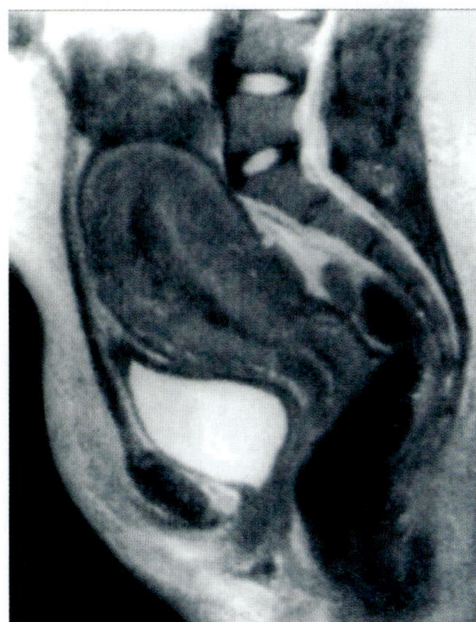

MRI — sagittal view of the uterus and cervix showing large size and thick walls after 6 days of delivery

144. NOT a useful drug in controlling PPH:

a. Prostaglandins
b. Progesterone
c. Methergine
d. Oxytocin

Progesterone in conjunction with estrogen stimulates growth of the uterus, causes decidual changes of the endometrium required for implantation and inhibits myometrial contraction.

(See Flow Chart on next page)

145. Commonest cause of PPH:

a. Uterine atony
b. Coagulopathy
c. Cervical tear
d. Vaginal laceration

Atonicity of the uterus is the commonest cause of PPH (80%). With separation of the placenta, the uterine sinuses, which are torn, cannot be compressed effectively due to imperfect contraction and retraction of the uterine musculature and bleeding continues.

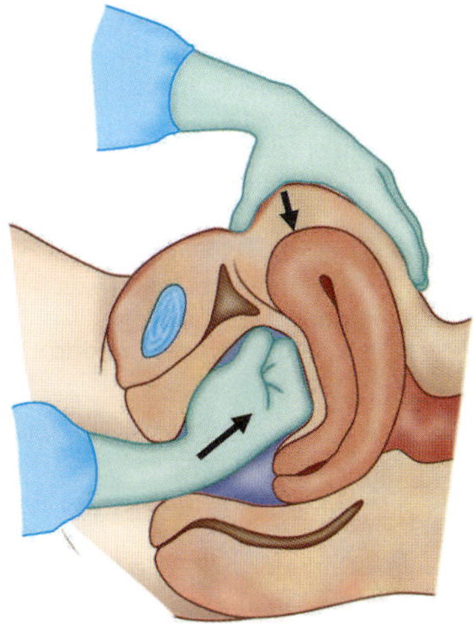

Bimanual compression of the uterus

146. Vesicovaginal fistula as a result of obstructed labor, manifests:

a. Within 24 hours of delivery
b. Within 72 hours of delivery
c. Within 1st week of delivery
d. After 1st week of delivery

In sloughing fistula, there is a history of prolonged labor and dribbling of urine occurs after varying interval following delivery (5-7 days).

147. Cause of lactational amenorrhea:

a. Oxytocin induced inhibition of FSH
b. Oxytocin induced inhibition of GnRH
c. Prolactin induced inhibition of FSH
d. Prolactin induced inhibition of GnRH

The physiological basis of anovulation and amenorrhea is due to elevated levels of serum prolactin associated with suckling. If a woman does not breastfeed her baby, menstruation returns by 12th week following delivery in 80% of cases. The meantime for onset of first menstruation is 7-9 weeks.

Ans. 141. **c.** 9.5 cm 142. **b.** May cause jaundice 143. **a.** 6 weeks 144. **b.** Progesterone
145. **a.** Uterine atony 146. **c.** Within 1st week... 147. **d.** Prolactin induced inhibition of GnRH

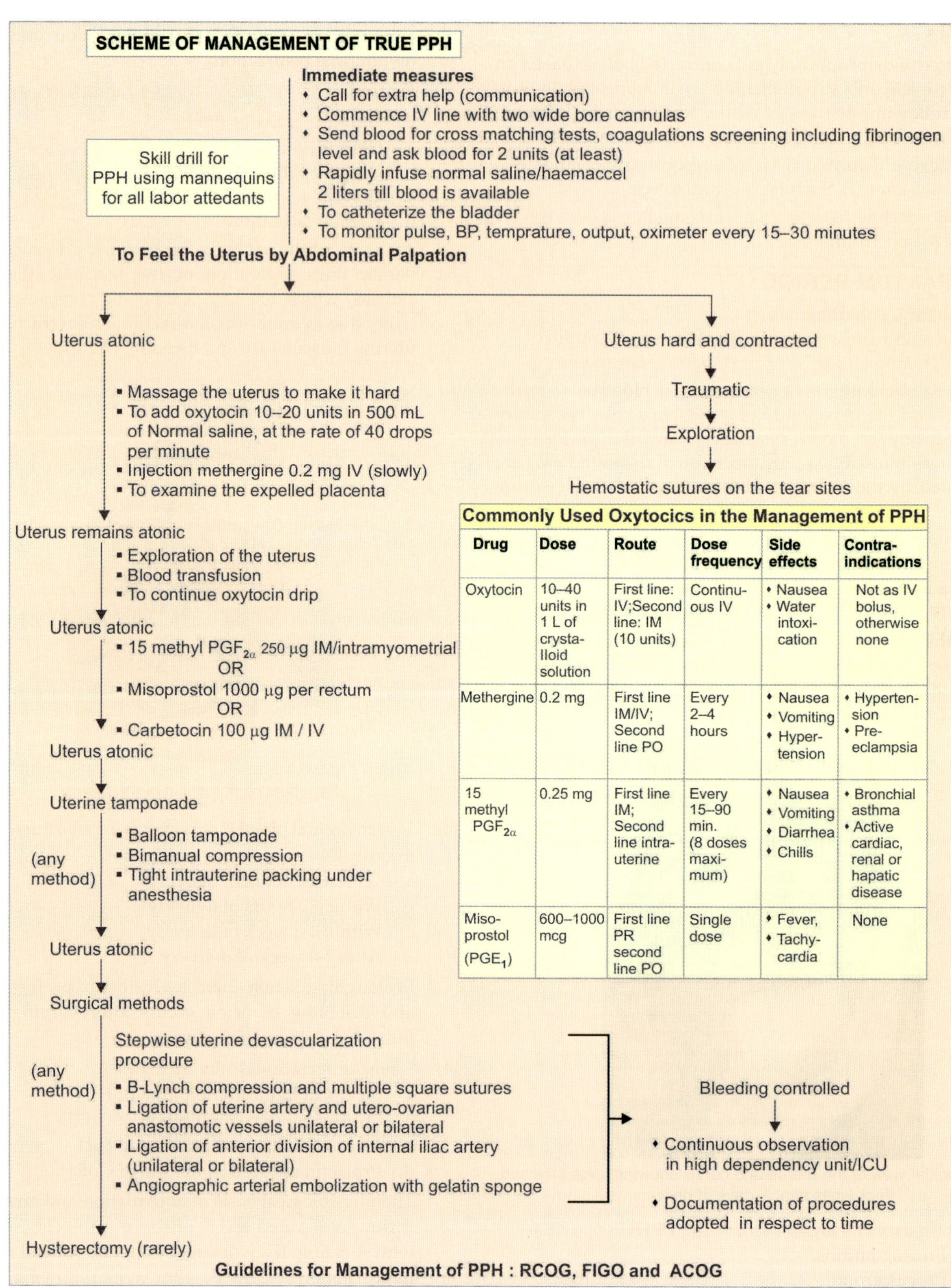

Commonly Used Oxytocics in the Management of PPH

Drug	Dose	Route	Dose frequency	Side effects	Contra-indications
Oxytocin	10–40 units in 1 L of crystalloid solution	First line: IV;Second line: IM (10 units)	Continuous IV	• Nausea • Water intoxication	Not as IV bolus, otherwise none
Methergine	0.2 mg	First line IM/IV; Second line PO	Every 2–4 hours	• Nausea • Vomiting • Hypertension	• Hypertension • Pre-eclampsia
15 methyl $PGF_{2\alpha}$	0.25 mg	First line IM; Second line intra-uterine	Every 15–90 min. (8 doses maximum)	• Nausea • Vomiting • Diarrhea • Chills	• Bronchial asthma • Active cardiac, renal or hapatic disease
Misoprostol (PGE_1)	600–1000 mcg	First line PR second line PO	Single dose	• Fever, • Tachycardia	None

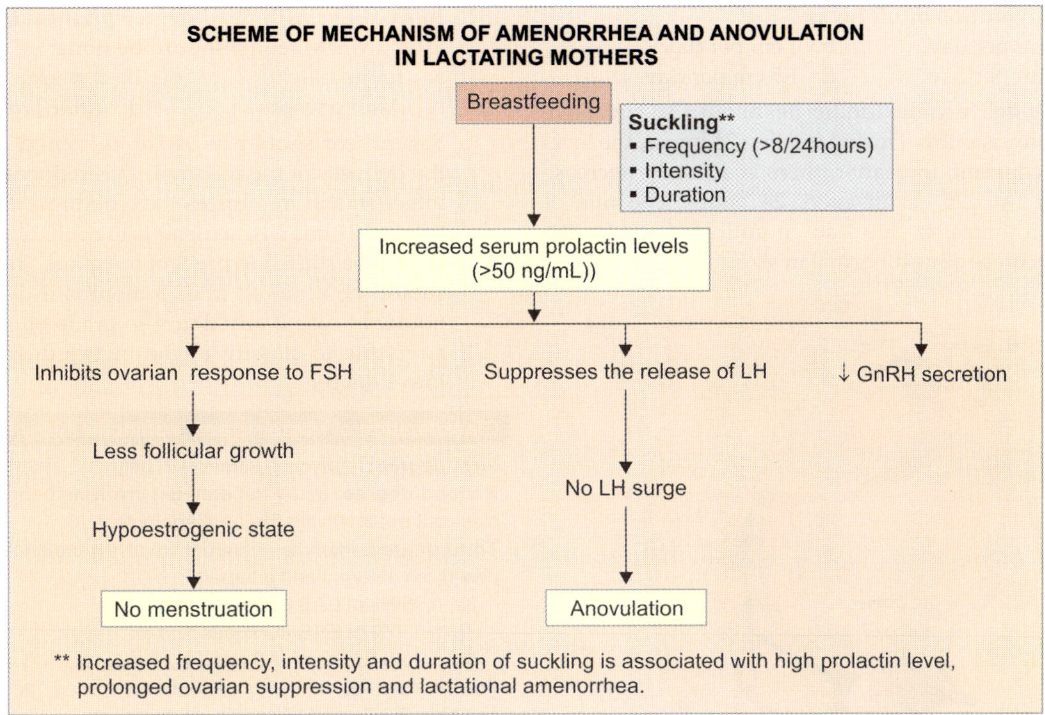

148. Postpartum decidual secretions are known as:

a. Lochia
b. Bleeding per vaginam
c. Vasa previa
d. Decidua capsularis

Lochia is the vaginal discharge for the first fortnight during puerperium. The discharge originates from the uterine body, cervix and vagina.

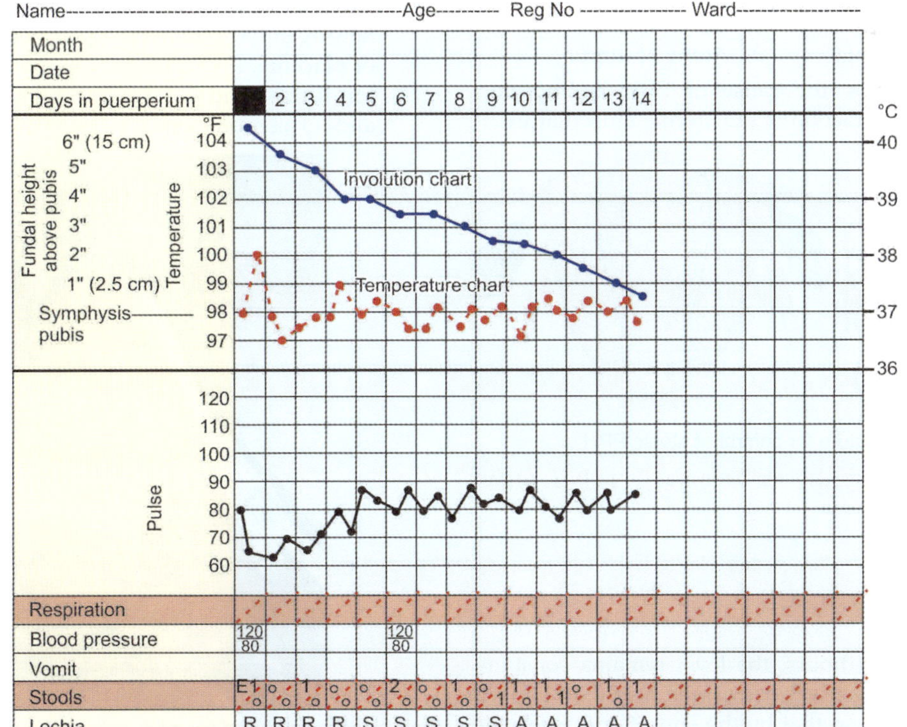

A composite chart to note the important clinical events in the puerperium

Ans. 148. a. Lochia

149. Rate of involution of uterus is:

a. 0.75 cm per day b. 1 cm per day
c. 1.25 cm per day d. 1.5 cm per day

Following delivery, the fundus lies about 13.5 cm above the symphysis pubis. During the first 24 hours, the level remains constant; thereafter, there is a steady decrease in height by 1.25 cm in every 24 hours. The rate of involution thereafter slows down until by 6 weeks, the uterus becomes almost normal in size.

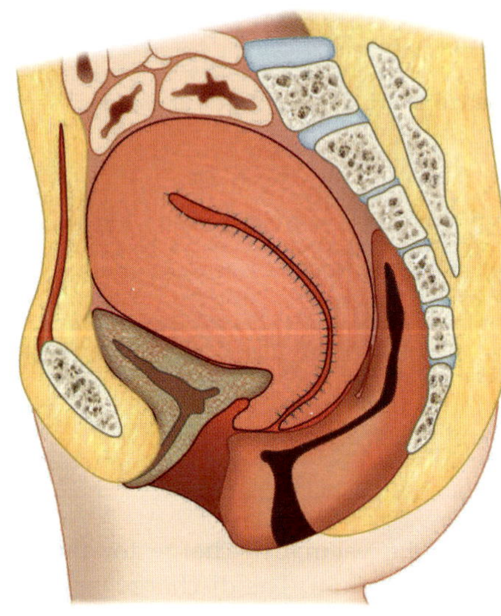

Sagittal section showing uterus 5 days after delivery

150. NOT a cause of post-partum hemorrhage in a retracted uterus:

a. Vaginal tear b. Cervical laceration
c. Retained placenta d. Atony of uterus

In atony of uterus, the cause of PPH is imperfect contraction and retraction of the uterine musculature.

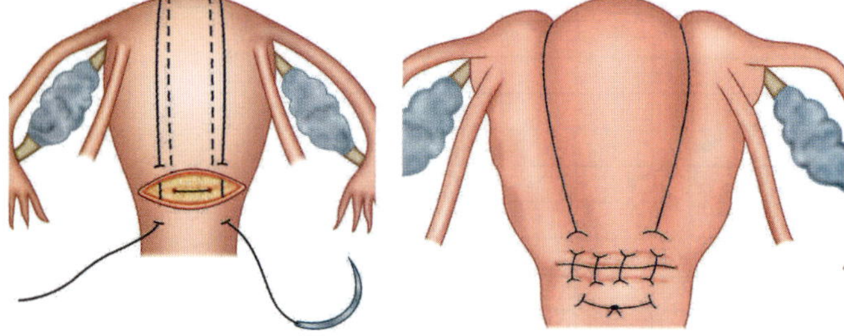

B-Lynch brace suture for control of atonic PPH

151. Following delivery, uterus becomes a pelvic organ after:

a. 2 weeks
b. 4 weeks
c. 6 weeks
d. 8 weeks

During the first 24 hours, the level remains constant; thereafter, there is a steady decrease in height by 1.25 cm in every 24 hours, so that by the end of 2nd week the uterus becomes a pelvic organ.

152. In a patient with third degree perineal tear, presenting after 1 week, repair should be done:

a. Immediately b. 2 weeks
c. After 6 weeks d. After 12 weeks

Recent tear should be repaired immediately following the delivery of the placenta. This reduces the chances of infection and minimizes the blood loss. In case of delay beyond 24 hours, the repair is to be withheld. Antibiotics should be started to prevent infection. The complete tear should be repaired after 3 months if delay beyond 24 hours. In case if any doubt to grade of 3rd degree, it is advisable to classify to the higher degree rather than lower degree.

Classification of obstetric anal sphincter injury (RCOG–2007)

First degree: Injury to perineal skin only
Second degree: Injury to perineum involving perineal body (muscles) but not involving the anal sphincter
Third degree: Injury to perineum, involving the anal sphincter complex (both external and internal)
3a : <50% of EAS thickness torn
3b : >50% of EAS thickness torn
3c : Both EAS and IAS torn
Fourth degree: Injury to perineum involving the anal sphincter complex (EAS and IAS) and anal epithelium

153. Uncommon cause of death in inversion of uterus:

a. Neurogenic shock
b. Hemorrhage
c. Pulmonary embolism
d. Infection

Dangers of inversion of the uterus: (1) Shock, mainly neurogenic, (2) Hemorrhage, especially after detachment of placenta, (3) Pulmonary embolism (4) If left uncared for, it may lead to – (a) infection, (b) uterine sloughing and (c) a chronic one.

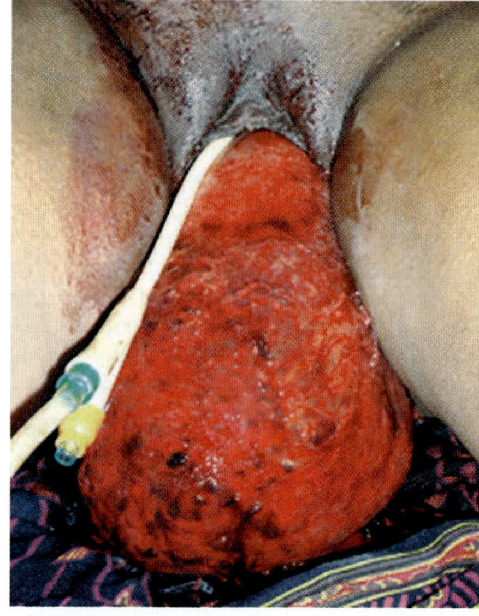

Spontaneous acute and complete uterine inversion. *By courtesy*: department of obstetrics and gynecology, NRS medical college, Calcutta

Ans. **149. c.** 1.25 cm per day **150. d.** Atony of uterus **151. a.** 2 weeks **152. d.** After 12 weeks **153. d.** Infection

154. Post-partum hemorrhage is present when blood loss exceeds:

a. 200 cc b. 400 cc
c. 500 cc d. 700 cc

Quantitative definition of PPH is arbitrary and is related to the amount of blood loss in excess of 500 mL following birth of the baby (WHO). The average blood loss following vaginal delivery, cesarean delivery and cesarean hysterectomy is 500 mL, 1000 mL and 1500 mL respectively.

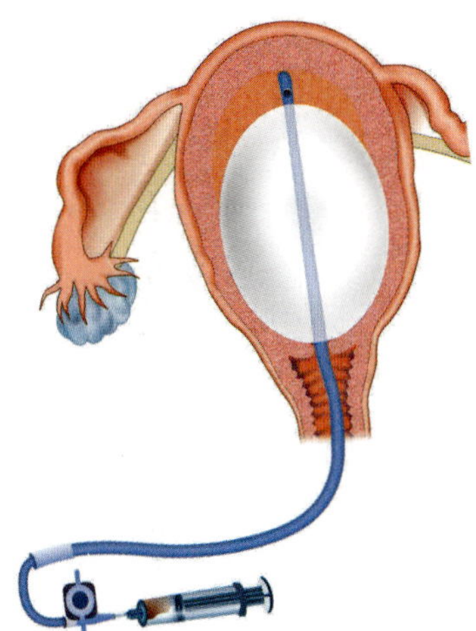

Uterine tamponade using Bakri balloon

155. Sequence of lochia during puerperium is:

a. Serosa → alba → rubra b. Rubra → alba → serosa
c. Rubra → serosa → alba d. Alba → serosa → rubra

Depending upon the variation of the color of the discharge, it is named as: (1) lochia rubra (red) 1-4 days, (2) lochia serosa (5-9 days) – the color is yellowish or pink or pale brownish, (3) lochia alba (pale white) – 10 to 15 days.

MISCELLANEOUS

156. Number of oogonia in body:

a. 6 million b. 4 million
c. 5 million d. 7 million

Oogonia proliferate via mitosis during the 9th to 22nd week of embryonic development. There can be up to 600,000 oogonia by the 8th week of development and up to 7,000,000 by the 5th month.

157. Which of the following is the most common cause of neonatal sepsis in the community?

a. *Streptococcus pneumoniae*
b. *Streptococcus pyogenes*
c. *E. coli*
d. *H. influenzae*

Group B streptococcus (GBS; Streptococcus agalactiae) and gram-negative enteric organisms (predominantly Escherichia coli) account for most cases of early-onset sepsis.

158. A 40-year-old lady with complete family has been diagnosed to have H. mole. The treatment would be:

a. Radiotherapy b. Chemotherapy
c. Total hysterectomy d. Radio + Chemotherapy

Hysterectomy is justified in H. mole in: (i) Women approaching 40 years. (ii) Patient completed her family irrespective of age. (iii) Uncontrolled hemorrhage or perforation during surgical evacuation. Hysterectomy reduces the risk of GTN (gestational trophoblastic neoplasia) by fivefold. *(See Diagram on next page)*

159. MC side effect of IUD insertion:

a. Bleeding b. Pain
c. Pelvic infection d. Ectopic pregnancy

The excessive bleeding because of IUD insertion, involves increased menstrual blood loss, prolongation of duration of period and intermenstrual bleeding. The patient may become anemic and is of concern in one who is already anemic.

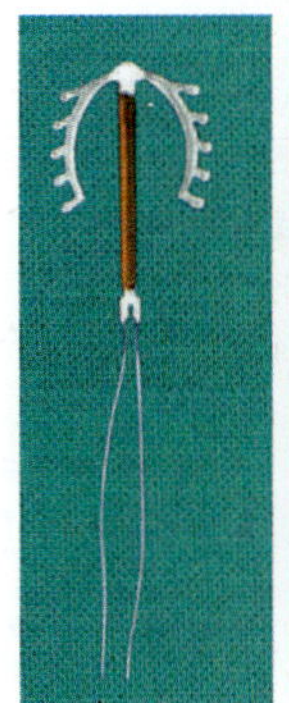

Multiload 375

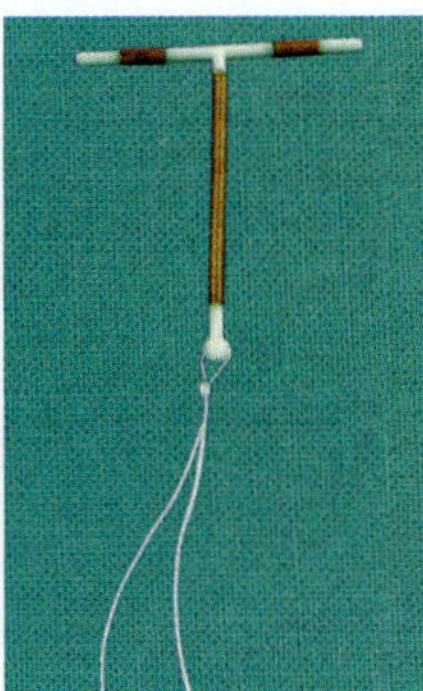

Cu T 380A

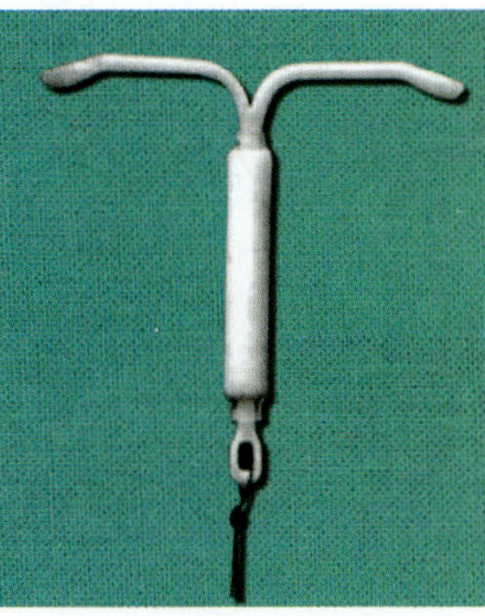

Levonorgestrel containing IUD (LNG-IUS)

Commonly used IUD

160. True regarding tetanus immunization are all *except*:

a. If already immunized, a booster in the last trimester is advocated
b. Vaccine is given intramuscularly
c. Tetanus immunoglobulin is injected to the mother
d. 2 doses are recommended

Immunization against tetanus not only protects the mother but also the neonates. In unprotected women, 0.5 mL tetanus toxoid is given intramuscularly at 6 weeks interval for 2 such, the first one to be given between 16 and 24 weeks. Women who are immunized in the past, a booster dose of 0.5 mL IM is given in the last trimester.

161. Commonest presentation of hydatidiform mole is:

a. Hyperemesis gravidarum
b. Bleeding
c. Pre-eclampsia d. Choriocarcinoma

Vaginal bleeding is the commonest presentation (90%) of H. mole. Often the symptom may mimic an incomplete or threatened abortion. The blood may be mixed with a gelatinous fluid from ruptured cysts giving the appearance of discharge "white currant in red currant juice".

Ans. **154. c.** 500 cc **155. c.** Rubra → serosa alba **156. d.** 7 million **157. c.** *E. coli*
158. c. Total hysterect... **159. a.** Bleeding **160. c.** Tetanus immun... **161. b.** Bleeding

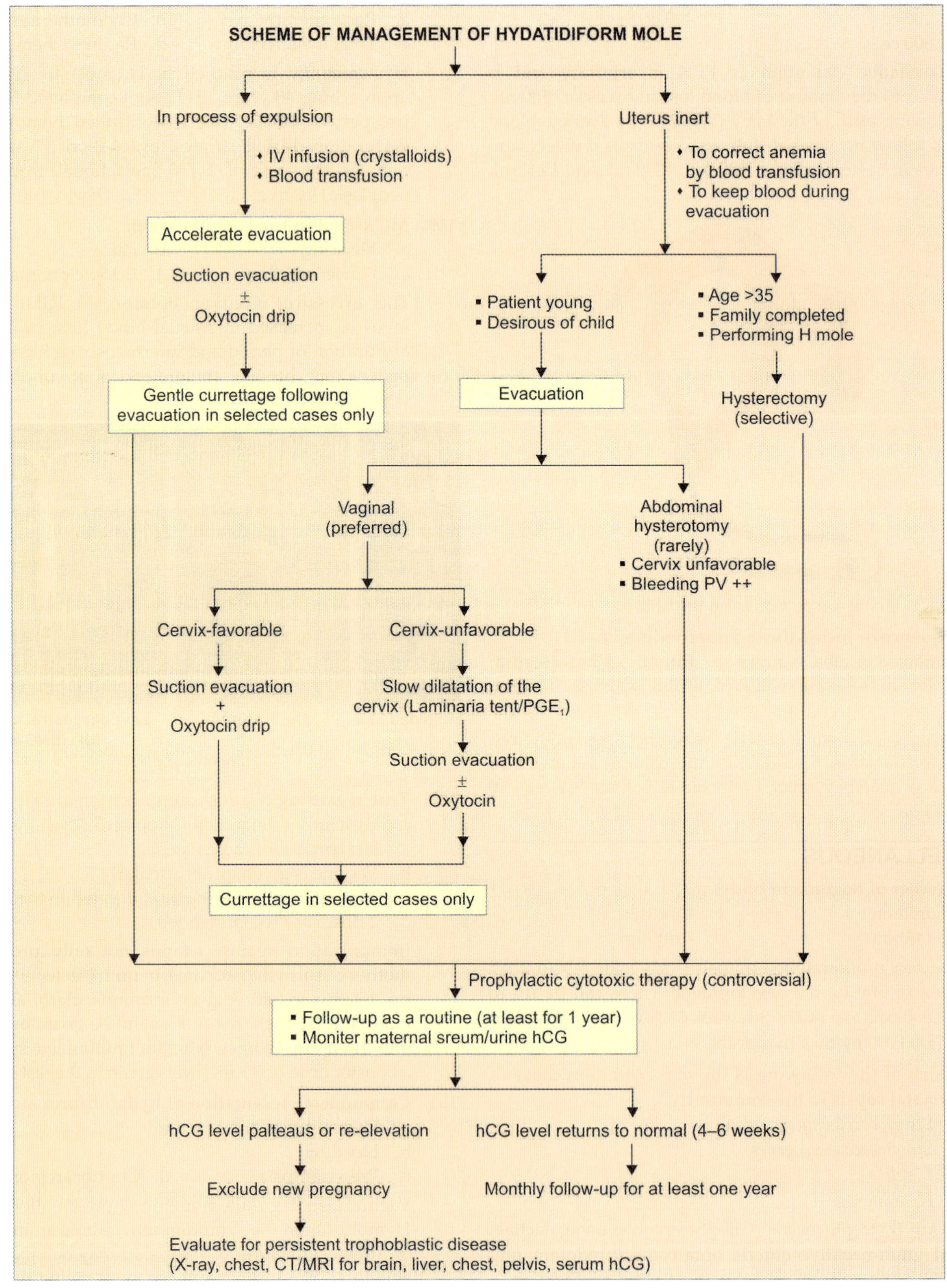
SCHEME OF MANAGEMENT OF HYDATIDIFORM MOLE
In process of expulsion
• IV infusion (crystalloids)
• Blood transfusion
Accelerate evacuation
Suction evacuation
±
Oxytocin drip
Gentle currettage following evacuation in selected cases only
Uterus inert
• To correct anemia by blood transfusion
• To keep blood during evacuation
• Patient young
• Desirous of child
Evacuation
• Age >35
• Family completed
• Performing H mole
Hysterectomy (selective)
Vaginal (preferred)
Abdominal hysterotomy (rarely)
• Cervix unfavorable
• Bleeding PV ++
Cervix-favorable
Suction evacuation
+
Oxytocin drip
Cervix-unfavorable
Slow dilatation of the cervix (Laminaria tent/PGE$_1$)
Suction evacuation
±
Oxytocin
Currettage in selected cases only
Prophylactic cytotoxic therapy (controversial)
• Follow-up as a routine (at least for 1 year)
• Moniter maternal sreum/urine hCG
hCG level palteaus or re-elevation
Exclude new pregnancy
Evaluate for persistent trophoblastic disease
(X-ray, chest, CT/MRI for brain, liver, chest, pelvis, serum hCG)
hCG level returns to normal (4–6 weeks)
Monthly follow-up for at least one year

Important features of complete and partial moles		
Features	*Complete mole*	*Partial mole*
Embryo/Fetus	Absent	Present
Hydropic degeneration of villi	Pronounced and diffused	Variable and focal
Trophoblast hyperplasia	Diffuse	Focal
Uterine size	More than the date (30–60%)	Less than the date
Theca lutein cysts	Common (25–50%)	Uncommon
Karyotype	46, XX (85%), paternal in origin	Triploid (90%), diploid (10%)
β-hCG	High (>50,000)	Slight elevation (<50,000)
Classic clinical symptoms	Common	Rare
Risk of persistent GTN	20%	<5%
Immunostaining ($p57^{KIP2}$)	Negative	Positive

162. Breast feeding is known to transmit:

a. Tuberculosis b. CMV
c. Varicella d. Rubella

In mothers with active TB lesion, not only is breastfeeding contraindicated but the baby is to be isolated from the mother following delivery.

Contraindications of breastfeeding		
	Temporary	*Permanent*
Maternal	1. Acute puerperal illness	1. Chronic medical illness such as decompensated organic heart lesion, active untreated pulmonary tuberculosis
	2. Acute breast complications such as cracked nipples, mastitis or breast abscess	2. Puerperal psychosis
	3. Herpes simplex lesion of the breast	3. Mother having high doses of antiepileptic, antithyroid, antipsychotic or anticancer drugs
Neonatal	1. Very low birth weight baby	1. Severe degree of cleft palate
	2. Asphyxia and intracranial stress	2. Galactosemia
	3. Acute illness	

163. The essential investigation to be included in follow-up of hydatidiform mole is:

a. Ultrasound abdomen b. Chest X-ray
c. Serum levels of HCG d. Serum levels of TSH

Routine follow-up of H. mole is mandatory for all cases for at least 1 year. The occurrence of choriocarcinoma is mostly confined to this period. The prime objective is to diagnose persistent trophoblastic disease (20-30%) that is considered malignant. However, hCG levels following evacuation should regress to normal within 3 months time.

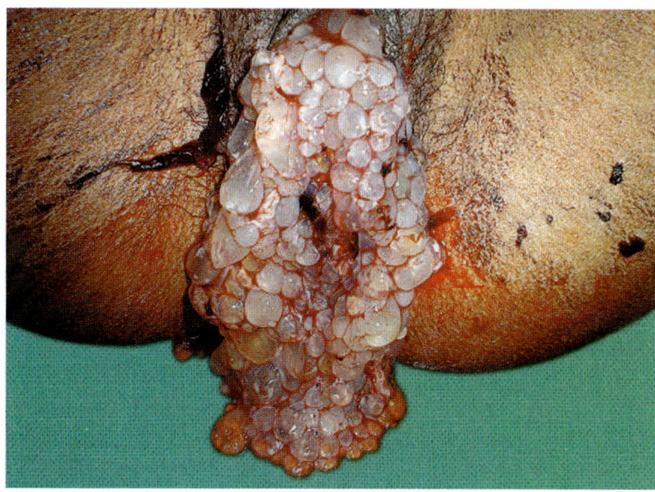

Hydatidiform mole in the process of expulsion showing clusters of vesicles of varying sizes. *By courtesy*: *Dr Subrata Bhattacharya, Silchar*

164. Deep transverse arrest is seen in all *except*:

a. Android pelvis
b. Epidural analgesia
c. Transverse lie
d. Uterine inertia

In DTA, the head is deep into the cavity; the sagittal suture is placed in the transverse bispinous diameter and there is no progress in descent of the head even after half-one hour following full dilatation of the cervix. The arrest in occipitotransverse position may be the result of incomplete anterior rotation (1/8th of circle) of oblique occipitoposterior position, or it may be due to nonrotation of the commonly primary occipitotransverse position of normal mechanism of labor. This is seen in faulty pelvic architecture or weak uterine contractions.

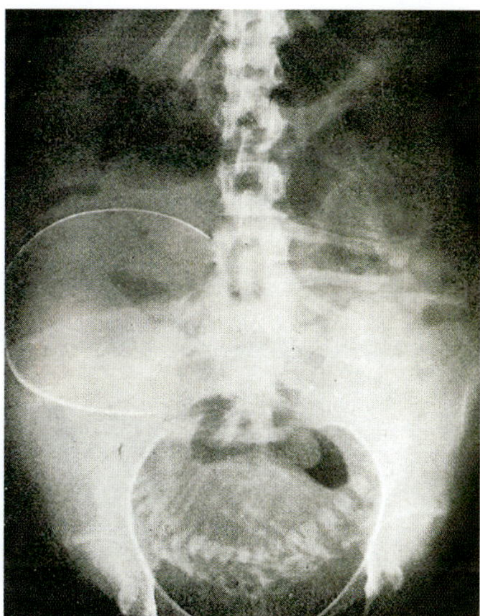

Straight X-ray abdomen showing single fetus with transverse lie [*Courtesy: G & O Dept. Patna MCH*]

Ans. **162. a.** Tuberculosis **163. c.** Serum levels... **164. c.** Transverse lie

165. Most common cause of direct obstetric deaths:
a. Anaemia
b. Hemorrhage
c. Obstructed labour
d. Infection

Whereas in the organized sector (developed countries) – hypertensive disorders, hemorrhage and pulmonary embolism are the main causes, in the developing countries – hemorrhage, sepsis and preeclampsia-eclampsia and unsafe abortion are the main causes.

Important causes of maternal deaths and main interventions

Causes	*Percentage*	*Proven Interventions*
Hemorrhage: Mostly due to postpartum hemorrhage. Other causes are : (i) Antepartum hemorrhage (abruptio placenta, placenta previa) (ii) Retained placenta (iii) Abortion complications and ectopic pregnancy. Hemorrhage is more dangerous when the woman is anemic.	20–25	❑ Treat anemia in pregnancy ❑ Skilled attendant at birth ❑ Prevent/treat hemorrhage ❑ Use oxytocics in time ❑ Replace fluid loss ❑ Transfusion of blood, if severe hemorrhage
Infection is associated with labor and puerperium. Infections from premature rupture of membranes, prolonged and obstructed labor are still frequent in the developing world.	15–20	❑ Skilled attendant at birth ❑ Clean practices (three cleans) during delivery ❑ Antibiotics — if infection is evident
Hypertension during pregnancy preeclampsia, eclampsia	12–15	❑ Early detection ❑ Appropriate referral ❑ Antiseizure prophylaxis/treatment with $MgSO_4$
Unsafe abortion	10–13	❑ Skilled attendant ❑ Access to family planning and safe abortion services ❑ Antibiotics after evacuation ❑ Postabortion cares
Obstructed labor—due to cephalopelvic disproportion, abnormal lie or malpresentation.	**8**	❑ Use of partograph ❑ Detection in time ❑ Refer for operative delivery
Anemia is an indirect cause of death. About 50% of pregnant women worldwide suffer from anemia. Anemia is commonly due to dietary deficiency (nutrition, iron, folic acid, iodine and other micronutrients) or infections.	15–20	❑ Routine Iron-folic acid supplementation ❑ Treat hookworm, malaria, HIV, etc. ❑ Admit when Hb ≤ 7 g/dL
Other indirect causes: Viral hepatitis is endemic in India with high mortality. Death is mostly in the last trimester due to hepatic coma and coagulation failure and postpartum hemorrhage.	5–10	❑ Safe drinking water ❑ Immunization ❑ Appropriate referral and supportive care

80% of these deaths can be prevented through actions that are effective and affordable in developing country settings (WHO, UNICEF and UNFPA-2001).

166. Most common cause of maternal mortality in India:
a. Infection
b. Anaemia
c. Obstructed labour
d. Hemorrhage

Hemorrhage is the MC direct cause of maternal deaths in India.

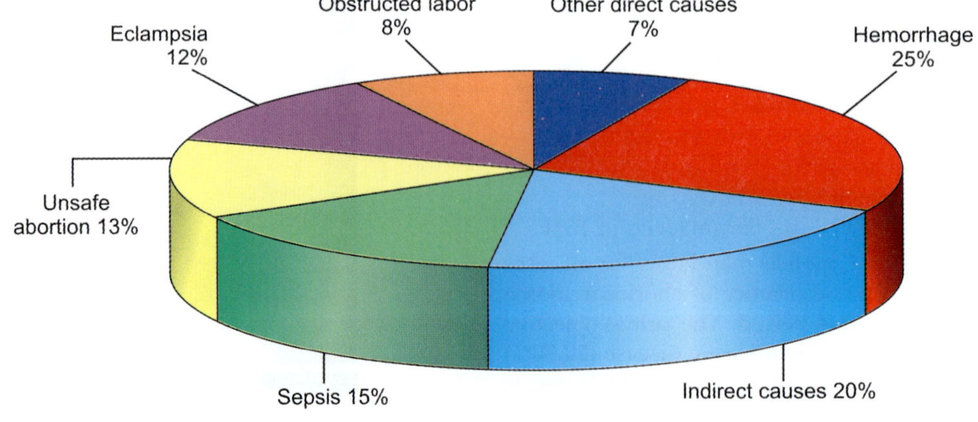

Important causes of maternal deaths

Ans. **165. b.** Hemorrhage **166. d.** Hemorrhage

167. Incidence of scar rupture in previous lower segment caesarean section:

a. 1% b. 5%
c. 6% d. 7%

The risk of lower segment scar-rupture is low (0.2-1.5%) and even if it does occur, maternal death is much less and the perinatal mortality is about one in eight.

Differences between lower segment scar and classical or hysterotomy scar

	Lower segment scar	*Classical or hysterotomy scar*
Apposition	Thin cut margins facilitate perfect apposition without leaving any pocket	Difficult to appose the thick muscle layer. Pockets are formed that contain blood, which is subsequently replaced by fibrous tissue. Formation of gutter on the inner surface is likely, as the decidua is more often than not excluded during suture
State of uterus during healing	The part of the uterus remains inert while healing process is going on	The part of the uterus contracts and retracts so that the sutures become loose leading to imperfect healing
Stretching effect	The scar is made to stretch during future pregnancy and normal labor more along the line of scar	The stretch is at right angles to the scar
Placental implantation in future pregnancy	Chance of weakening the scar by placental attachment is unlikely	The placenta is more likely to implant on the scar and weakens it by trophoblastic penetration or herniation of the amniotic sac through the gutter
Net effect	(a) Scar is sound; (b) rupture may occur only during labor (0.2–1.5%)	(a) Scar is weak; (b) rupture may occur both during pregnancy and labor (4–9%)
	Following rupture: Maternal death—less perinatal death—1 in 8	Following rupture: Maternal death—5% Perinatal death—6 in 8

168. Fetal adrenals release which hormone predominantly:

a. Estrogen b. Testosterone
c. Aldosterone d. Cortisone

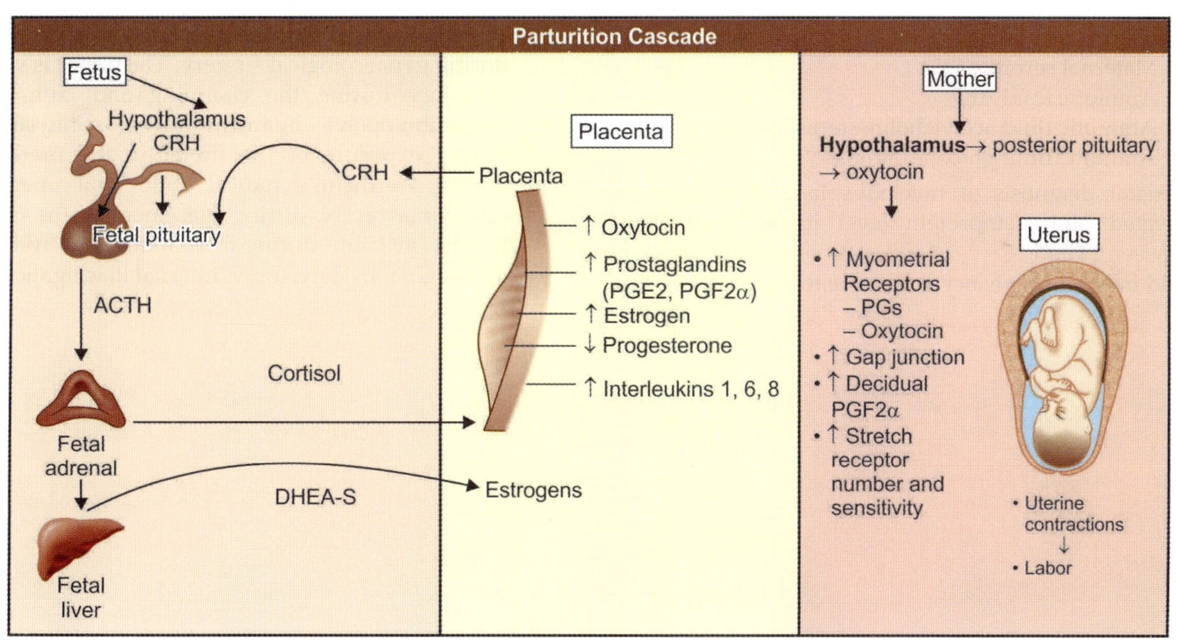

Initiation of parturition

Fetoplacental contribution in the onset of labor: Cascade of events activate fetal hypothalamic-pituitary-adrenal axis prior to onset of labor → increased CRH → increased release of ACTH → fetal adrenals → increased cortisol secretion → accelerated production of estrogen and prostaglandins from the placenta.

169. Which structure will remain intact in a lady with 3rd degree tear as a result of midline episiotomy and delivering a 9 lb baby?

a. Rectal mucosa
b. Perineal muscles
c. Perineal body
d. Anal sphincter

Risk factors for third degree perineal tears

- Big baby (weight ≥ 3 kg)
- Nulliparity
- Outlet contraction with narrow pubic arch
- Shoulder dystocia

Ans. 167. **a.** 1% 168. **d.** Cortisone 169. **a.** Rectal mucosa

- Forceps delivery
- Scar in the perineum (perineorrhaphy, episiotomy)
- Face to pubis delivery
- Midline episiotomy
- Precipitate labor

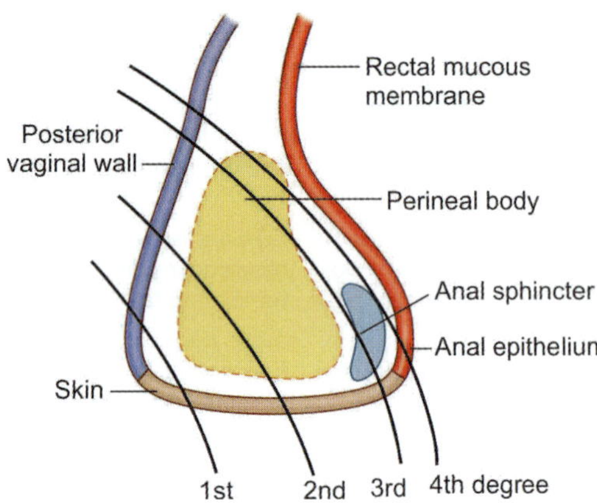

Diagrammatic representation showing different degrees of perineal tear

170. Which one of the following is NOT sensitive to detect open spina bifida?

a. Maternal serum AFP
b. Amniotic fluid AFP
c. Amniotic fluid acetylcholinesterase
d. Amniotic fluid glucohexaminase

Prenatal diagnosis of myelodysplasia is possible by elevated alpha-fetoprotein level in maternal blood between 14 and 16 weeks of gestation, or in the amniotic fluid in early pregnancy where the test is more specific. Additional test in amniotic fluid includes acetyl cholinesterase estimation.

171. Use of mifepristone is in:

a. Habitual abortion
b. Molar pregnancy
c. Ectopic pregnancy
d. All of the above

Mifepristone injected into the unruptured ectopic pregnancy cause its resolution.

172. MC site for metastasis in choriocarcinoma is:

a. Lungs
b. Brain
c. Liver
d. Spine

The general metastases probably develop early in choriocarcinoma, the growth disseminating by way of the blood stream. Multiple metastases may form in the lungs and cause hemoptysis.

173. What is the most common complication after radical hysterectomy?

a. Ureteral injury
b. Bladder atony
c. Prolapse of vaginal vault
d. Bowel dysfunction

The hollow pelvic viscera are vulnerable to injury during gynaecological surgery. The ureter is vulnerable to injury during the clamping and cutting of the infundibulopelvic ligament during panhysterectomy, during exposure of the ureter in the ureteric canal during Wertheim's radical abdominal operation for carcinoma cervix, during placement of the clamps on the parametrium during total abdominal hysterectomy and vaginal hysterectomy, internal iliac ligation.

Ans. **170. d.** Amniotic... **171. c.** Ectopic pregnancy **172. a.** Lungs **173. a.** Ureteral injury

ANSWERS WITH REFERENCES

OBSTETRICS ANATOMY

1. **Ans. (c)** Bispinous
Ref: Dutta's Obstetrics, 7/e p91

2. **Ans. (d)** Diagonal conjugate
Ref: Dutta's Obstetrics, 7/e p88

3. **Ans. (b)** 7-9 days
Ref: Dutta's Obstetrics 8/e p26

4. **Ans. (c)** Diagonal conjugate
Ref: Dutta's Obstetrics 8/e p100

5. **Ans. (a)** Obstetric conjugate
Ref: Dutta's Obstetrics 8/e p100

6. **Ans. (c)** Mentovertical
Ref: Dutta's Obstetrics 8/e p96

7. **Ans. (d)** Gynecoid
Ref: Dutta's Obstetrics 8/e p403

8. **Ans. (b)** Naegele's pelvis
Ref: Dutta's Obstetrics 8/e p405

9. **Ans. (d)** Interspinous diameter
Ref: Dutta's Obstetrics 8/e p101

10. **Ans. (b)** 10.5
Ref: Dutta's Obstetrics 8/e p102

11. **Ans. (d)** Bitemporal diameter
Ref: Dutta's Obstetrics 8/e p96

ANTENATAL PERIOD

12. **Ans. (a)** XI
Ref: Dutta's Obstetrics 7/e p52

13. **Ans. (a)** Vertex
Ref: Dutta's Obstetrics 7/e p85t

14. **Ans. (a)** 6th week
Ref: Dutta's Obstetrics 7/e p642

15. **Ans. (b)** Cervical os dilated
Ref: Dutta's Obstetrics 7/e p162

16. **Ans. (b)** Pre-eclampsia
Ref: Dutta's Obstetrics 7/e p225

17. **Ans. (b)** Robert's sign
Ref: Dutta's Obstetrics 7/e p324

18. **Ans. (d)** USG
Ref: Dutta's Obstetrics 8/e p77

19. **Ans. (a)** Serum bilirubin
Ref: Dutta's Obstetrics 8/e p389

20. **Ans. (b)** Fetal heart sounds
Ref: Dutta's Obstetrics 8/e p79

21. **Ans. (c)** Cleft palate
Ref: Dutta's Obstetrics 8/e p42

22. **Ans. (b)** 10-12 weeks
Ref: Dutta's Obstetrics 8/e p130

23. **Ans. (b)** Serum ferritin
Ref: Dutta's Obstetrics 8/e p307

24. **Ans. (d)** Tetanus
Ref: Dutta's Obstetrics 8/e p113

25. **Ans. (d)** Amenorrhea
Ref: Dutta's Obstetrics 8/e p733

26. **Ans. (d)** Left Occipito Anterior
Ref: Dutta's Obstetrics 8/e p87

27. **Ans. (b)** Hepatitis E
Ref: Dutta's Obstetrics 8/e p335

28. **Ans. (b)** Renal agenesis
Ref: Dutta's Obstetrics 8/e p42

29. **Ans. (a)** Previous H/O recurrent PID
Ref: Dutta's Obstetrics 8/e p211

30. **Ans. (c)** Anthropoid pelvis
Ref: Dutta's Obstetrics 8/e p403

31. **Ans. (a)** 6 weeks
Ref: Dutta's Obstetrics 8/e p66

32. **Ans. (a)** Vertex-vertex
Ref: Dutta's Obstetrics 8/e p238

33. **Ans. (d)** Yellow fever
Ref: Dutta's Obstetrics 8/e p113

34. **Ans. (b)** Amniocentesis
Ref: Dutta's Obstetrics 8/e p742

35. **Ans. (d)** Isthmic
Ref: Dutta's Obstetrics 8/e p207

36. **Ans. (c)** Ampulla
Ref: Dutta's Obstetrics 8/e p23

37. **Ans. (c)** Tubes
Ref: Dutta's Obstetrics 8/e p218

38. **Ans. (a)** **Renal agenesis**
Ref: Dutta's Obstetrics 8/e p251

39. **Ans. (c)** **Post dated pregnancy**
Ref: Dutta's Obstetrics 8/e p247

40. **Ans. (c)** **Placenta previa**
Ref: Dutta's Obstetrics 8/e p287

41. **Ans. (b)** **2000 ml**
Ref: Dutta's Obstetrics 8/e p246

42. **Ans. (a)** **Antibodies are not able to cross placenta**
Ref: Dutta's Obstetrics 8/e p396

43. **Ans. (b)** **Captopril**
Ref: Dutta's Obstetrics 8/e p581

44. **Ans. (d)** **Rubella**
Ref: Dutta's Obstetrics 8/e p348

45. **Ans. (c)** **Both**
Ref: Dutta's Obstetrics 8/e p342

46. **Ans. (b)** **3rd trimester of pregnancy**
Ref: Dutta's Obstetrics 8/e p61

47. **Ans. (a)** **50 ml**
Ref: Dutta's Obstetrics 8/e p44

48. **Ans. (d)** **14 weeks of gestation**
Ref: Dutta's Obstetrics 8/e p471

49. **Ans. (c)** **Presents in first trimester**
Ref: Dutta's Obstetrics 8/e p283

50. **Ans. (a)** **Chromosomal abnormalities**
Ref: Dutta's Obstetrics 8/e p185

51. **Ans. (b)** **Ruptured ectopic pregnancy**
Ref: Dutta's Obstetrics 8/e p210

52. **Ans. (b)** **Ectopic pregnancy**
Ref: Dutta's Obstetrics 8/e p212

53. **Ans. (a)** **Down's syndrome**
Ref: Dutta's Obstetrics 8/e p128

54. **Ans. (d)** **Syncytiotrophoblast**
Ref: Dutta's Obstetrics 8/e p38

55. **Ans. (d)** **Threatened abortion**
Ref: Dutta's Obstetrics 8/e p195

56. **Ans. (c)** **294 days**
Ref: Dutta's Obstetrics 8/e p373

57. **Ans. (c)** **24-28 weeks**
Ref: Dutta's Obstetrics 8/e p328

58. **Ans. (b)** **Ruptured ectopic pregnancy**
Ref: Dutta's Obstetrics 8/e p210

59. **Ans. (a)** **It is secreted by cytotrophoblasts**
Ref: Dutta's Obstetrics 8/e p38

60. **Ans. (a)** **Hydatidiform mole**
Ref: Dutta's Obstetrics 8/e p225

61. **Ans. (b)** **Prolactin**
Ref: Dutta's Obstetrics 8/e p34

62. **Ans. (c)** **70 days**
Ref: Dutta's Obstetrics 8/e p67

63. **Ans. (d)** **ACE inhibitors**
Ref: Dutta's Obstetrics 8/e p265

64. **Ans. (d)** **Accidental hemorrhage**
Ref: Dutta's Obstetrics 8/e p294

65. **Ans. (a)** **Glycosylated Hb**
Ref: Dutta's Obstetrics 8/e p330

66. **Ans. (c)** **Fetal hypoxia**
Ref: Dutta's Obstetrics 8/e p694

67. **Ans. (a)** **Cardiovascular malformation**
Ref: Dutta's Obstetrics 8/e p123

68. **Ans. (a)** **Ethacridine (extra-amniotic)**
Ref: Dutta's Obstetrics 8/e p203

69. **Ans. (c)** **Dimorphic**
Ref: Dutta's Obstetrics 8/e p315

70. **Ans. (c)** **Methyldopa**
Ref: Dutta's Obstetrics 8/e p581

71. **Ans. (b)** **Placenta lying in the lower segment**
Ref: Dutta's Obstetrics 8/e p296

72. **Ans. (c)** **Fetal scalp blood pH more than 7.3**
Ref: Dutta's Obstetrics 8/e p693

73. **Ans. (a)** **Mitral stenosis**
Ref: Dutta's Obstetrics 8/e p321

74. **Ans. (c)** **Polyhydramnios**
Ref: Dutta's Obstetrics 8/e p335

75. **Ans. (d)** **Macrosomia**
Ref: Dutta's Obstetrics 8/e p329

76. **Ans. (a)** **Prematurity**
Ref: Dutta's Obstetrics 8/e p434

77. **Ans. (a)** **More than 500 ml/ min**
Ref: Dutta's Obstetrics 8/e p60

78. **Ans. (b)** **36 weeks**
Ref: Dutta's Obstetrics 8/e p585

79. **Ans. (a)** Cryotherapy
Ref: Internet resources

80. **Ans. (d)** To know the position of the placenta
Ref: Dutta's Obstetrics 8/e p734

81. **Ans. (c)** 30-34 weeks of pregnancy
Ref: Dutta's Obstetrics 8/e p58

82. **Ans. (d)** Cystic hygroma
Ref: Dutta's Obstetrics 8/e p738

83. **Ans. (c)** Gestation sac
Ref: Dutta's Obstetrics 8/e p761

84. **Ans. (b)** Increased Alpha fetoprotein levels
Ref: Dutta's Obstetrics 8/e p132

85. **Ans. (b)** Face
Ref: Dutta's Obstetrics 8/e p56

86. **Ans. (c)** 18-22 weeks
Ref: Dutta's Obstetrics 8/e p738

87. **Ans. (b)** 20 weeks
Ref: Dutta's Obstetrics 8/e p203

88. **Ans. (a)** 300
Ref: Dutta's Obstetrics 8/e p112

89. **Ans. (d)** Maternal HPL
Ref: Dutta's Obstetrics 8/e p128

90. **Ans. (a)** Enalapril
Ref: Dutta's Obstetrics 8/e p265

91. **Ans. (c)** Vasa previa
Ref: Dutta's Obstetrics 8/e p252

92. **Ans. (b)** Accidental hemorrhage
Ref: Dutta's Obstetrics 8/e p298

93. **Ans. (b)** Prevent involution of corpus luteum
Ref: Dutta's Obstetrics 8/e p10

94. **Ans. (a)** Serial ultrasound
Ref: Dutta's Obstetrics 8/e p734

95. **Ans. (a)** Loss of deep tendon reflexes
Ref: Dutta's Obstetrics 8/e p273

96. **Ans. (a)** Increase in fibrinogen level
Ref: Dutta's Obstetrics 8/e p59

97. **Ans. (c)** During labor
Ref: Dutta's Obstetrics 8/e p351

98. **Ans. (a)** Battledore placenta
Ref: Dutta's Obstetrics 8/e p33

99. **Ans. (a)** Rh negative mother with Rh positive in 2nd child
Ref: Dutta's Obstetrics 8/e p386

100. **Ans. (a)** 800 cc
Ref: Dutta's Obstetrics 8/e p43

101. **Ans. (c)** 24-28
Ref: Dutta's Obstetrics 8/e p327

102. **Ans. (c)** 16-18 weeks
Ref: Dutta's Obstetrics 8/e p30

103. **Ans. (d)** 3%
Ref: Dutta's Obstetrics 8/e p437

104. **Ans. (b)** Magnesium sulphate
Ref: Dutta's Obstetrics 8/e p273

105. **Ans. (c)** Oxytocin challenge test
Ref: Dutta's Obstetrics 8/e p122

106. **Ans. (a)** Toxoplasmosis
Ref: Dutta's Obstetrics 8/e p345

107. **Ans. (a)** Escherichia coli
Ref: Dutta's Obstetrics 8/e p346

108. **Ans. (c)** Multigravida
Ref: Dutta's Obstetrics 8/e p286

109. **Ans. (d)** More than 8 days
Ref: Dutta's Obstetrics 8/e p234

110. **Ans. (a)** Chronic hypertension
Ref: Dutta's Obstetrics 8/e p256

111. **Ans. (b)** Pregnant women
Ref: Dutta's Obstetrics 8/e p337

112. **Ans. (b)** 12 kg
Ref: Dutta's Obstetrics 8/e p57

113. **Ans. (b)** Down syndrome
Ref: Dutta's Obstetrics 8/e p569

114. **Ans. (c)** May lead to malignancy
Ref: Dutta's Obstetrics 8/e p350

115. **Ans. (d)** Diamniotic-dichorionic twins
Ref: Dutta's Obstetrics 8/e p235

116. **Ans. (d)** Lung
Ref: Dutta's Obstetrics 8/e p124

117. **Ans. (b)** Fetal tone
Ref: Dutta's Obstetrics 8/e p377

LABOR

118. **Ans. (b)** 100–120
Ref: Dutta's Obstetrics, 7/e p117

119. **Ans. (d)** 700–800
Ref: Dutta's Obstetrics, 7/e p38

120. **Ans. (b) Anemia**
Ref: Dutta's Obstetrics 8/e p662

121. **Ans. (a) Intrauterine death**
Ref: Dutta's Obstetrics 8/e p601

122. **Ans. (c) Extension of the incision is easy**
Ref: Dutta's Obstetrics 8/e p649

123. **Ans. (b) Partogram**
Ref: Dutta's Obstetrics 8/e p606

124. **Ans. (b) Requirement of induction for labor**
Ref: Dutta's Obstetrics 8/e p600

125. **Ans. (b) Deliver after-coming head of breech**
Ref: Dutta's Obstetrics 8/e p445

126. **Ans. (d) Brow**
Ref: Dutta's Obstetrics 8/e p454

127. **Ans. (b) Twins with one vertex and other breech**
Ref: Dutta's Obstetrics 8/e p450

128. **Ans. (b) Obstructed labor**
Ref: Dutta's Obstetrics 8/e p421

129. **Ans. (c) It occurs prior to 1st stage of labor**
Ref: Dutta's Obstetrics 8/e p370

130. **Ans. (d) Wait and watch**
Ref: Dutta's Obstetrics 8/e p427

131. **Ans. (d) Recording progress of labor**
Ref: Dutta's Obstetrics 8/e p464

132. **Ans. (d) Placenta accreta**
Ref: Dutta's Obstetrics 8/e p486

133. **Ans. (c) IIIrd stage of labor**
Ref: Dutta's Obstetrics 8/e p487

134. **Ans. (d) PIH**
Ref: Dutta's Obstetrics 8/e p664

135. **Ans. (a) 1 cm**
Ref: Dutta's Obstetrics 8/e p151

136. **Ans. (c) Term**
Ref: Dutta's Obstetrics 8/e p92

137. **Ans. (c) Contraction of uterus**
Ref: Dutta's Obstetrics 8/e p599

138. **Ans. (d) Android pelvis**
Ref: Dutta's Obstetrics 8/e p424

139. **Ans. (b) When the widest diameter of the presenting part has passed through the pelvic inlet**
Ref: Dutta's Obstetrics 8/e p93

140. **Ans. (d) Breech presentation**
Ref: Dutta's Obstetrics 8/e p442

141. **Ans. (c) 9.5 cm**
Ref: Dutta's Obstetrics 8/e p412

POSTPARTUM PERIOD

142. **Ans. (b) May cause jaundice**
Ref: Dutta's Obstetrics, 7/e p483

143. **Ans. (a) 6 weeks**
Ref: Dutta's Obstetrics 8/e p169

144. **Ans. (b) Progesterone**
Ref: Dutta's Obstetrics 8/e p481

145. **Ans. (a) Uterine atony**
Ref: Dutta's Obstetrics 8/e p480

146. **Ans. (c) Within 1st week of delivery**
Ref: Dutta's Obstetrics 8/e p499

147. **Ans. (d) Prolactin induced inhibition of GnRH**
Ref: Dutta's Obstetrics 8/e p172

148. **Ans. (a) Lochia**
Ref: Dutta's Obstetrics 8/e p177

149. **Ans. (c) 1.25 cm per day**
Ref: Dutta's Obstetrics 8/e p168

150. **Ans. (d) Atony of uterus**
Ref: Dutta's Obstetrics 8/e p482

151. **Ans. (a) 2 weeks**
Ref: Dutta's Obstetrics 8/e p170

152. **Ans. (d) After 12 weeks**
Ref: Dutta's Obstetrics 8/e p490

153. **Ans. (d) Infection**
Ref: Dutta's Obstetrics 8/e p488

154. **Ans. (c) 500 cc**
Ref: Dutta's Obstetrics 8/e p482

155. **Ans. (c) Rubra → serosa → alba**
Ref: Dutta's Obstetrics 8/e p170

MISCELLANEOUS

156. **Ans. (d) 7 million**
Ref: Dutta's Obstetrics, 7/e p17

157. **Ans. (c) *E. coli***
Ref: Ghai's Paediatrics, 6/e p161

158. **Ans. (c) Total hysterectomy**
Ref: Dutta's Obstetrics 8/e p229

159. **Ans. (a) Bleeding**
Ref: Dutta's Obstetrics 8/e p616

160. **Ans. (c) Tetanus immunoglobulin is injected to the mother**
Ref: Dutta's Obstetrics 8/e p114

161. **Ans. (b) Bleeding**
Ref: Dutta's Obstetrics 8/e p230

162. **Ans. (a) Tuberculosis**
Ref: Dutta's Obstetrics 8/e p523

163. **Ans. (c) Serum levels of HCG**
Ref: Dutta's Obstetrics 8/e p226

164. **Ans. (c) Transverse lie**
Ref: Dutta's Obstetrics 8/e p455

165. **Ans. (b) Hemorrhage**
Ref: Dutta's Obstetrics 8/e p685

166. **Ans. (d) Hemorrhage**
Ref: Dutta's Obstetrics 8/e p684

167. **Ans. (a) 1%**
Ref: Dutta's Obstetrics 8/e p382

168. **Ans. (d) Cortisone**
Ref: Dutta's Obstetrics 8/e p135

169. **Ans. (a) Rectal mucosa**
Ref: Dutta's Obstetrics 8/e p489

170. **Ans. (d) Amniotic fluid glucohexaminase**
Ref: Ghai's Pediatrics 8/e p576

171. **Ans. (c) Ectopic pregnancy**
Ref: Shaw's Gynecology 13/e p307

172. **Ans. (a) Lungs**
Ref: Shaw's Gynecology 13/e p256

173. **Ans. (a) Ureteral injury**
Ref: Shaw's Gynecology 13/e p180

PRACTICE QUESTIONS

OBSTETRICS ANATOMY

1. Pelvis with prominent ischial spines:
a. Gynaecoid
b. Platypelloid
c. Android
d. Anthropoid

2. Pelvis in which AP diameter is more than transverse diameter?
a. Anthropoid
b. Android
c. Gynaecoid
d. Platypelloid

3. MC type of pelvis:
a. Platypelloid
b. Gynaecoid
c. Android
d. Anthropoid

ANTENATAL PERIOD

4. One of the common complication of dichorionic diamniotic twins:
a. Cord compression
b. Intrauterine growth retardation
c. Intrauterine fetal death
d. Preterm labor

5. Earliest time, when twin pregnancy can be diagnosed on USG:
a. 6th week
b. 8th week
c. 10th week
d. 12th week

6. Doubling time of beta-HCG:
a. 1 day
b. 2 days
c. 3 days
d. 4 days

7. Length of uterus at term:
a. 35 cm
b. 40 cm
c. 45 cm
d. 50 cm

8. MC site of ectopic pregnancy:
a. Isthmus
b. Ampulla
c. Infundibulum
d. Interstitial

9. Placenta succenturiate is defined as:
a. Smaller placenta
b. Placenta having two different lobes
c. Irregular surfaces of placenta
d. Thin fibrous ring at the margin of placenta

10. Maternal contribution in the formation of placenta:
a. Decidua capsularis
b. Decidua basalis
c. Decidua parietalis
d. Decidua superficialis

11. HELLP syndrome consists of all *except*:
a. Hyperglycemia
b. Hemolysis
c. Raised liver enzymes
d. Decreased platelet count

12. What is seen in HELLP syndrome?
a. Sickle cell anemia
b. Iron deficiency like picture
c. Increased RBC destruction
d. Increased RBC production

13. Treatment of idiopathic cholestasis of pregnancy:
a. Cholic acid
b. Chenodeoxycholic acid
c. Ursodeoxycholic acid
d. Elaidic acid

14. Cord compression shows which type of deceleration in fetal heart rate/FHR monitoring?
a. Early deceleration
b. Middle deceleration
c. Late deceleration
d. Variable deceleration

15. Agent of choice to treat hyperthyroidism in pregnancy:
a. Iodine
b. Propylthiouracil
c. Radioactive iodine
d. All of the above

16. $MgSO_4$ toxicity is monitored by:
a. Heart rate
b. Knee jerk
c. Pupillary reflex
d. Gait

17. Which murmur can be normally heard during pregnancy?
a. Systolic
b. Pansystolic
c. Diastolic
d. All of the above

18. Condition in which pregnancy should be terminated:
a. ASD
b. Pulmonary hypertension
c. VSD
d. Tetralogy of Fallot

19. Which of the following measures the amount of fetal blood entering maternal circulation?
a. Kleihauer-Betke test
b. Serum bilirubin
c. Renal function test
d. Liver function test

Ans.
1. c. Android **2. a.** Anthropoid **3. b.** Gynaecoid **4. d.** Preterm labor
5. c. 10th week **6. b.** 2 days **7. a.** 35 cm **8. b.** Ampulla
9. b. Placenta having... **10. b.** Decidua basalis **11. a.** Hyperglycemia **12. c.** Increased RBC...
13. c. Ursodeoxycholic... **14. d.** Variable deceleration **15. b.** Propyl thiouracil **16. b.** Knee jerk
17. a. Systolic **18. b.** Pulmonary hypertension **19. a.** Kleihauer-Betke test

20. Immune hydrops is associated with:
a. Thalassemia
b. Rh incompatibility
c. Hereditary spherocytosis
d. Sickle cell anemia

21. Karyotype of complete mole:
a. 46XX b. 69XXY
c. 69XYY d. 47XXY

22. MC complication of succenturiate lobe:
a. Antepartum hemorrhage
b. Placenta previa
c. Postpartum hemorrhage
d. Preterm labor

23. Oligohydramnios associated with:
a. Twin pregnancy b. Anencephaly
c. Open spina bifida d. Renal agenesis

24. A female with recurrent abortions and isolated prolonged aPTT is most likely associated with:
a. Lupus anticoagulant
b. DIC
c. Von Willebrand disease
d. Hemophilia

25. Which of the following is NOT associated with HELLP syndrome?
a. Increased lactate dehydrogenase
b. Low platelet count
c. Raised liver enzymes
d. Liver rupture

26. Volume of amniotic fluid is maximum at which gestational weeks?
a. 24-28 b. 28-32
c. 32-36 d. 36-38

27. Which is done to screen the presence of fetus at the earliest?
a. Transvaginal USG b. Transabdominal USG
c. MRI scan d. CT scan

28. Last menstrual period of a patient is 30 June 2014. Expected date of delivery would be:
a. 23 March 2015 b. 30 March 2015
c. 7 April 2015 d. 14 April 2015

29. Which of the following is NOT a component of triad of ectopic pregnancy?
a. Vomiting
b. Bleeding
c. Abdominal pain
d. Amenorrhoea

30. All of the following drugs are NOT useful in pregnancy with hypertension *except*:
a. Propranolol b. Acebutolol
c. Lisinopril d. Labetalol

31. What would be the best line of management for a 32 weeks pregnant female with antepartum hemorrhage but no active bleeding?
a. Emergency Caesarean section
b. Wait and watch
c. Hospitalization
d. Induction of labor

32. A pregnant lady in 2nd trimester of pregnancy presented with bleeding per vaginam. Ultrasound examination revealed a uterine fibroid. Best line of management:
a. Conservative
b. Laparoscopic myomectomy
c. Curettage
d. Hysterectomy

33. Theca lutein cysts are associated with which of the following?
a. Complete mole b. Partial mole
c. Tubal ectopic d. Threatened abortion

34. Which of the following is the best indicator of successfully medically terminated ectopic pregnancy?
a. Beta HCG values less than 5
b. Size of uterus
c. Gestational sac
d. Duration of pregnancy

35. Which of the following is used in managing severe pre-eclamptic patient?
a. Diuretics
b. Anti-hypertensive medicines
c. $MgSO_4$
d. Admission and observation

36. Which of the following is LEASTLY associated with twin pregnancy?
a. Multigravida
b. Genetics
c. Young age
d. Patient treated for fertility

37. Which layer give rise to fetal placenta?
a. Zona basalis b. Zona capsularis
c. Zona parietalis d. Inner cell mass

Ans. **20. b.** Rh incompatibility **21. a.** 46XX **22. c.** Postpartum hemorrhage **23. d.** Renal agenesis
24. a. Lupus anti... **25. a.** Increased lactate... **26. d.** 36-38 **27. a.** Transvaginal USG
28. c. 7 April 2015 **29. a.** Vomiting **30. d.** Labetalol **31. b.** Wait and watch
32. a. Conservative **33. a.** Complete mole **34. a.** Beta HCG values... **35. b.** Anti-hypertensive...
36. c. Young age **37. a.** Zona basalis

38. All of the following are FALSE statements *except*:
- a. Placenta is formed when the fertilized egg is in morula stage
- b. Implantation occurs post 10th post-fertilization day
- c. During initial days of pregnancy, LH maintains corpus luteum
- d. Fertilization occurs in ampulla

39. All of the following are true regarding fertilization *except*:
- a. Sperm penetrates corona radiata
- b. Implantation occurs post 6th day of fertilization
- c. Digestion of zona pellucida occurs due to hyaluronidase
- d. Zona reaction attracts sperms

40. Chadwick's sign is:
- a. Pelvis congestion causing bluish/purplish hue to vagina
- b. Pelvis congestion causing bluish/purplish hue to cervix
- c. Pelvis congestion causing bluish/purplish hue to uterus
- d. Pelvis congestion causing bluish/purplish hue to fallopian tube

41. Chadwick's sign time:
- a. 6 weeks b. 8 weeks
- c. 10 weeks d. 12 weeks

42. Timing for performing amniocentesis:
- a. 8-11 weeks b. 12-20 weeks
- c. 20-25 weeks d. 26-30 weeks

43. Tobacco juice/dark brown colour amniotic fluid is seen in:
- a. Post maturity b. Intra uterine death
- c. Rh incompatibility d. Fetal distress

44. Pea soup coloured amniotic fluid:
- a. Post maturity b. IUD
- c. Rh incompatibility d. Fetal distress

45. What will occur if, chorionic villous sampling/CVS is done before 10 weeks of gestation?
- a. IUGR b. Oligohydramnios
- c. Orofacial limb defects d. Polyhydramnios

46. MC type of compound presentation:
- a. Head with leg
- b. Head with hand
- c. Head with leg and hand
- d. None

47. Spalding sign is defined as:
- a. Gas in great vessels
- b. Hyper flexion of spine
- c. Overlapping of skull bones
- d. Crowding of ribs

48. Hegar's sign is seen at:
- a. 2-6 weeks b. 6-10 weeks
- c. 10-14 weeks d. 14-18 weeks

49. Insulin status in pregnancy:
- a. No change b. Decrease
- c. Increase d. None

50. MC site of ectopic pregnancy:
- a. Ovary b. Fallopian tube
- c. Cervix d. Vagina

51. A lady presented with 24 weeks molar pregnancy. Management of choice:
- a. Suction evacuation b. Dilatation & curettage
- c. Caesarean section d. Wait & watch

52. A pregnant lady in 2nd trimester presented with vaginal bleeding. USG showed snowstorm appearance. What levels of beta-HCG would correlate with a diagnosis of molar pregnancy?
- a. >2500 b. >10,000
- c. >100,000 d. >1,00,000

53. True statement regarding physiological changes in alimentary system in pregnancy:
- a. Increased risk of peptic ulcer
- b. Decreased tone & motility
- c. Increased cardiac sphincter tone
- d. Diarrhoea

54. Synytiotrophoblast is:
- a. Uninucleated b. Multinucleated
- c. Non-nucleated d. Variable

55. Steroid & protein synthesized from:
- a. Cytotrophoblast b. Corpus luteum
- c. Decidua d. Synytiotrophoblast

56. Decidua forms after:
- a. Ovulation b. Fertilization
- c. Implantation d. Oogenesis

57. Most chances of death are seen in which type of twin pregnancy?
- a. Monoamniotic monochorionic
- b. Monoamniotic dichorionic
- c. Diamniotic dichorionic
- d. Dizygotic twins

Ans.
38. d. Fertilization... **39. d.** Zona reaction... **40. a.** Pelvis congestion... **41. b.** 8 weeks
42. b. 12-20 weeks **43. b.** Intra uterine death **44. d.** Fetal distress **45. c.** Orofacial limb defects
46. b. Head with hand **47. c.** Overlapping of... **48. b.** 6-10 weeks **49. c.** Increase
50. b. Fallopian tube **51. a.** Suction evacuation **52. c.** >100,000 **53. b.** Decreased tone & motility
54. b. Multinucleated **55. d.** Synytiotrophoblast **56. c.** Implantation **57. a.** Monoamniotic monoch...

58. MC cause of intrauterine death in twin pregnancy:
a. Infections b. Hemorrhage
c. Preterm birth d. Cord compression

59. MC tubal pregnancy to rupture:
a. Isthmus b. Interstitium
c. Ampullary d. Fimbria

60. Target to maintain systolic BP in severe pre-eclampsia patient by drug therapy:
a. <160 b. <150
c. <140 d. <130

61. MC symptom of HELLP syndrome:
a. Epigastric pain b. Headache
c. Hematuria d. Bleeding

62. First sign to appear indicating toxicity of $MgSO_4$:
a. Diminished plantar response
b. Respiratory depression
c. Cardiac arrest
d. None of the above

LABOR

63. Face to pubis delivery is common in which type of pelvis?
a. Anthropoid b. Android
c. Gynaecoid d. Platypelloid

64. A 38 weeks pregnant lady presented with breech presentation with footling. Such case is best managed by:
a. Trial of vaginal delivery
b. Caesarean section
c. Forceps
d. Internal podalic version

65. NOT a component of Bishop score:
a. Cervical consistency
b. Dilatation of cervix
c. Position of cervix
d. Length of cervix

66. Which of the following is the best parameter to decide for continuation of pregnancy in a lady presenting with pregnancy induced hypertension & bleeding P/V?
a. Presence of fetal cardiac activity
b. Arrangement of blood transfusion
c. Normal Blood pressure
d. ICU facilities

67. Which of the following is comparatively the best position of twins to conduct normal vaginal delivery?
a. First non-vertex, second vertex
b. Both vertex
c. Both non-vertex
d. Any position

68. Which of the following is the best line of treatment of a pregnant lady of 37 weeks gestational age with centrally located placenta previa and bleeding P/V?
a. Caesarean section b. Observation
c. Vacuum delivery d. Forceps application

POSTPARTUM PERIOD

69. Which of the following is a severe complication in a newborn?
a. Intracranial hemorrhage
b. Cephalhematoma
c. Caput succedaneum
d. Subconjunctival hemorrhage

70. All of the following closes after birth *except*:
a. Ductus arteriosus b. Ductus venosus
c. Cardinal vein d. Umbilical vein

MISCELLANEOUS

71. Which of the following is NOT an effect of oxytocin?
a. Milk production
b. Milk let down reflex
c. Milk ejection
d. Contraction of myoepithelial cells

Ans. **58. d.** Cord compression **59. a.** Isthmus **60. c.** <140 **61. a.** Epigastric pain
62. a. Diminished plan... **63. a.** Anthropoid **64. b.** Caesarean section **65. d.** Length of cervix
66. a. Presence of fetal... **67. b.** Both vertex **68. a.** Caesarean section **69. a.** Intracranial hemorrhage
70. c. Cardinal vein **71. a.** Milk production

IMAGE-BASED QUESTIONS

1. Which sign?

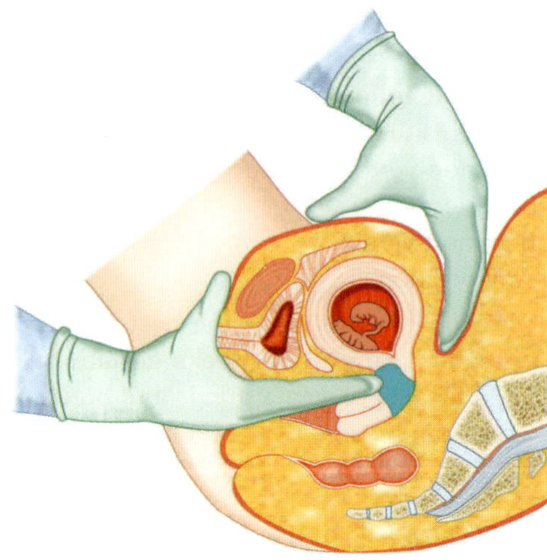

a. Palmer's sign
b. Chadwick's sign
c. Hegar's sign
d. Osiander's sign

Because of variation in consistency, on bimanual examination (two fingers in the anterior fornix and the abdominal fingers behind the uterus), the abdominal and vaginal fingers seem to appose below the body of the uterus. This is Hegar's sign.

2. Which type of pelvis?

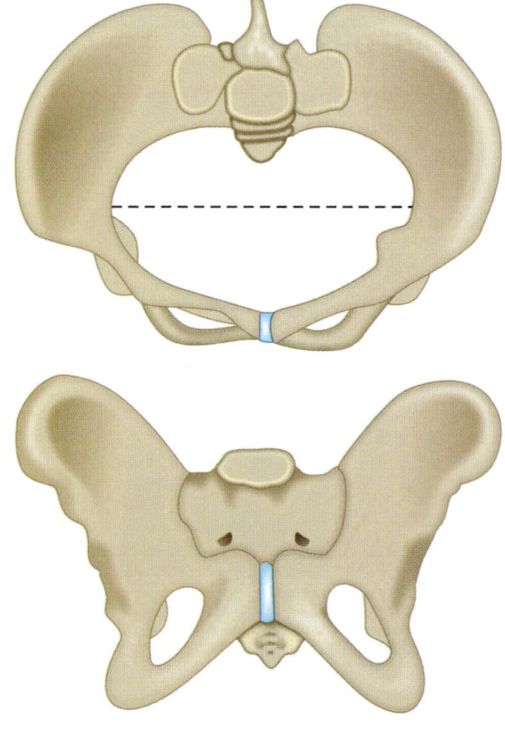

a. Android
b. Anthropoid
c. Gynecoid
d. Platypelloid

Platypelloid pelvis is transversely oval. Subpubic angle is very wide (more than 90 degree).

3. Presentation, if engaging diameter is 4:

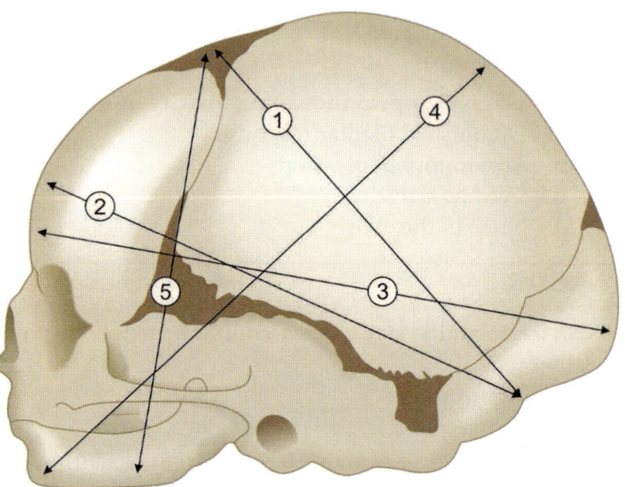

a. Vertex
b. Brow
c. Face
d. Chin

Brow is the presentation if the engaging diameter is mento-vertical, which extends from the midpoint of the chin to the highest point on the sagittal suture.

4. Duration of the stage of labor shown below, in primigravida is:

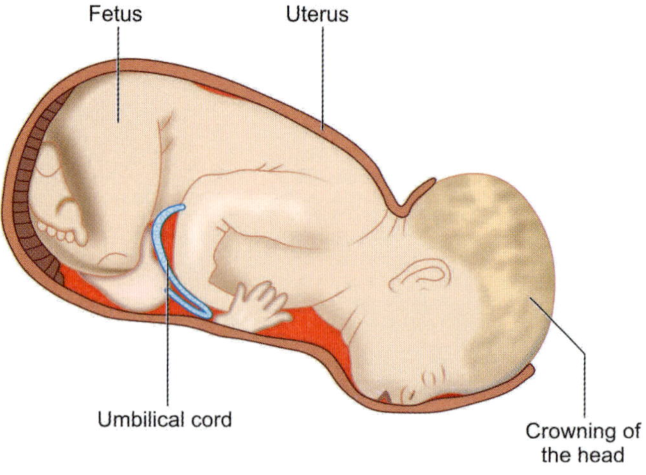

a. 12 hours
b. 6 hours
c. 2 hours
d. 30 minutes

The second stage of labor starts from full dilatation of the cervix and ends with expulsion of the fetus. Its average duration is 2 hours in primigravida and 30 minutes in multiparae.

5. Intrauterine pressure in the stage of labor shown below:

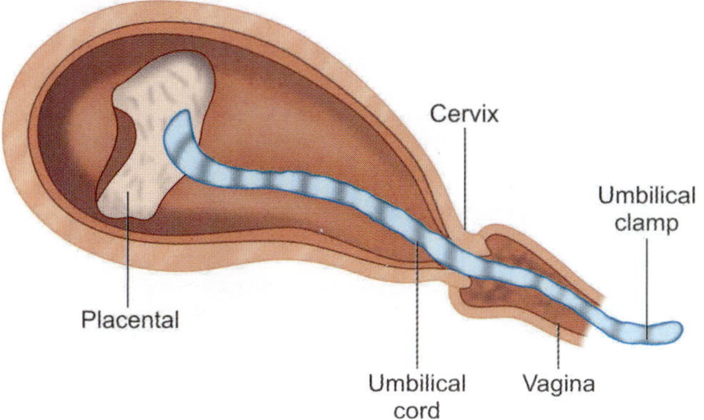

a. 10-40 mm Hg
b. 40-50 mm Hg
c. 100-200 mm Hg
d. 200-400 mm Hg

The intensity of uterine contraction gradually increases with advancement of labor until it becomes maximum in the second stage during delivery of the baby. Intrauterine pressure is raised to 40-50 mm Hg during the first stage and about 100-200 mm Hg in second stage of labor during contractions. In spite of diminished pain in third stage, the intrauterine pressure is probably the same as that in the second stage.

6. The surgery shown below is done for:

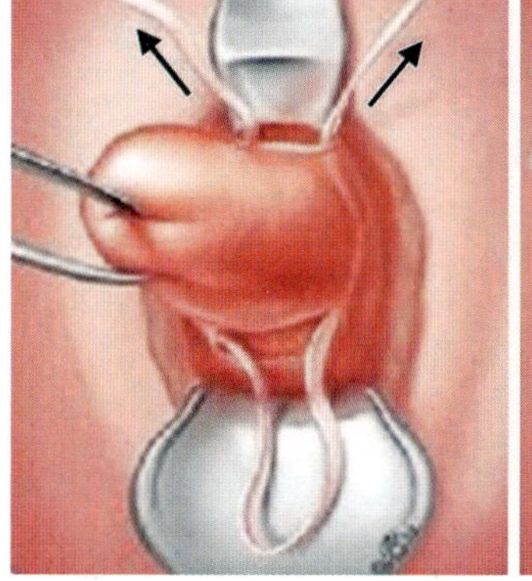
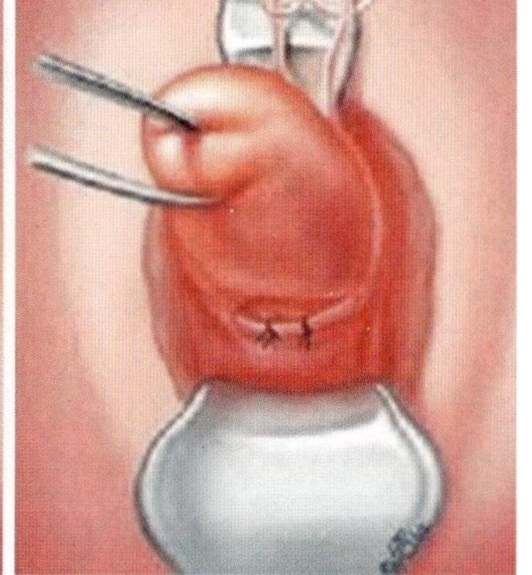

a. Cervical laceration
b. Cervical carcinoma
c. Cervical incompetence
d. Cervicitis

Shirodkar's procedure is done for cervical incompetence. The procedure reinforces the weak cervix by a nonabsorbable suture material – Mersilene (Dacron) or Ethibond tape, placed around the cervix at the level of internal os.

7. USG is suggestive of:

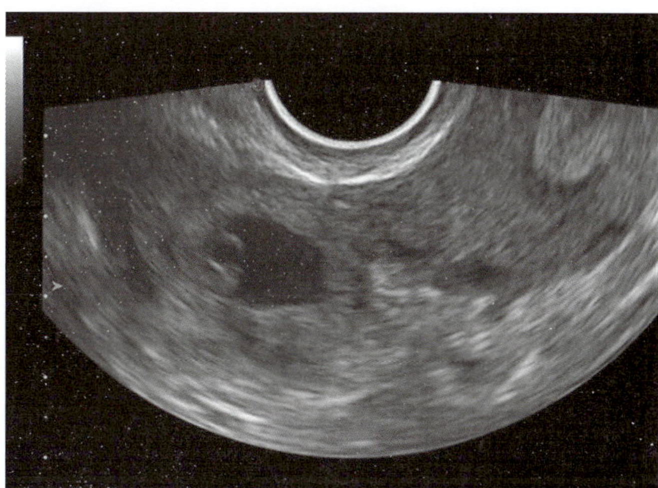

a. Normal pregnancy
b. H. mole
c. Ectopic pregnancy
d. Multiple pregnancy

Transvaginal sonography/TVS is more informative for diagnosing ectopic pregnancy: The diagnostic features are: (1) Absence of intrauterine pregnancy with a positive pregnancy test (2) Adnexal mass clearly separated from the ovary (3) Rarely cardiac motion may be seen in an unruptured tubal ectopic pregnancy.

8. USG is suggestive of:

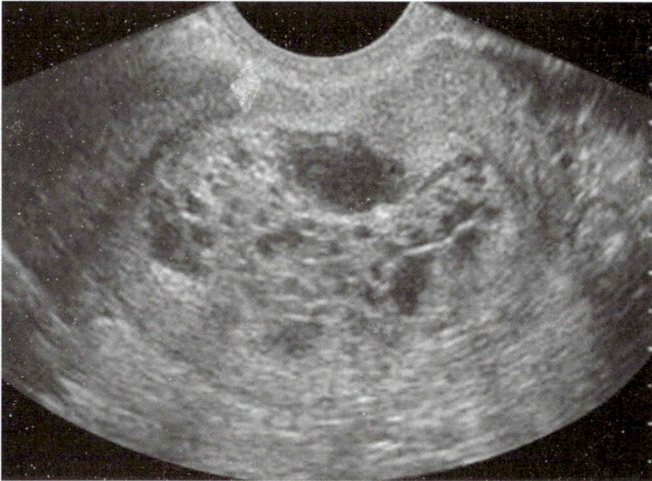

a. Fibroma uterus
b. Uterine malignancy
c. H. mole
d. PCOD

Characteristic feature of molar pregnancy is "snow-storm" appearance.

9. Which manoeuvre?

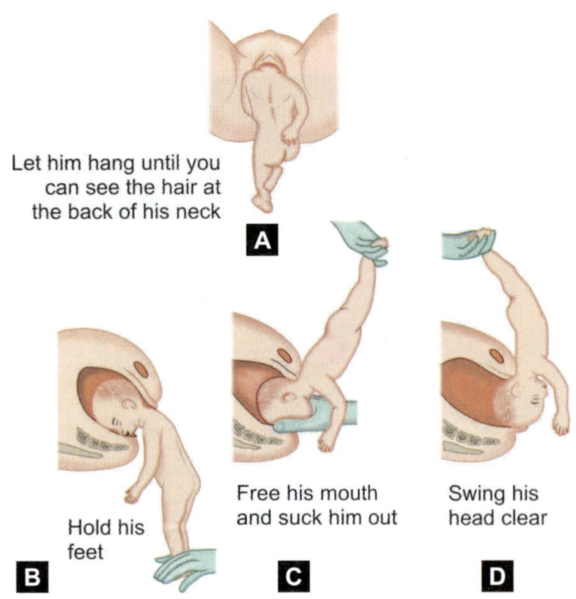

a. Mauriceau-Smellie-Veit technique
b. Modified Mauriceau-Smellie-Veit technique
c. Burns-Marshall method
d. Pinard's manoeuvre

Burns-Marshall method is used for delivering after-coming head of breech.

10. USG is suggestive of:

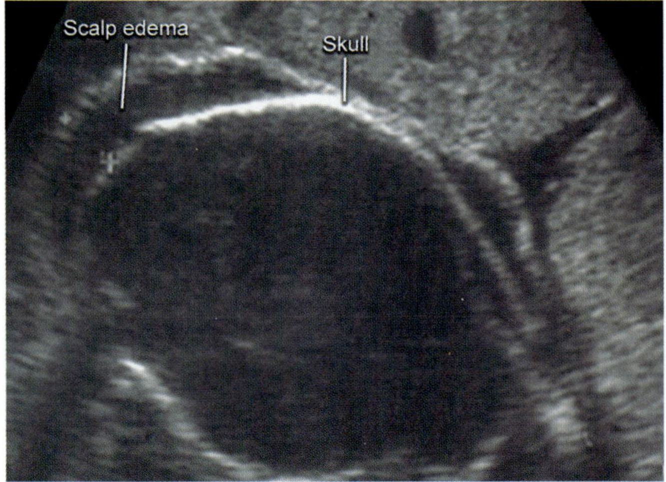

a. IUFD
b. Maceration
c. Rh isoimmunization
d. Gestational diabetes

Sonography (real time combined with pulse Doppler) is done in Rh isoimmunization to detect edema in the skin, scalp and pleural or pericardial effusion and echogenic bowel.

MCQ POINTS

S. No.	Question statements	Answers
1.	Epithelium of fallopian tube	***Ciliated columnar***
2.	Function of umbilical vein	***Carries oxygenated blood towards fetus***
3.	Poly-hydramnios is associated with	***Esophageal atresia, duodenal atresia***
4.	A lady giving birth to a baby. She will be called as:	***Parturient***
5.	Earliest detection of pregnancy by USG can be done by demonstrating	***Gestational sac***
6.	Longest diameter of fetal skull	***Mentovertical***
7.	Graphical representation of stages of labor is done in	***Partogram***
8.	Involution of uterus occurs at the rate of	***1.25 cm/day***
9.	A young girl with 6 weeks of amenorrhea with abdominal mass and empty uterus on USG is having	***Ectopic pregnancy***
10.	Investigation of choice for diagnosing H. mole	***USG***
11.	Earliest sign of immune hydrops on USG	***Scalp edema***
12.	MC heart disease associated with pregnancy	***Mitral stenosis***
13.	Heart disease carrying highest mortality in pregnancy	***Eisenmenger's syndrome***
14.	Magnesium sulphate is indicated in management of:	***Eclampsia***
15.	MC cause of PPH	***Uterine atony***
16.	Variable deceleration in fetal heart monitoring is suggestive of	***Cord compression***
17.	Maternal serum AFP is lowered in	***Down syndrome***
18.	Very severe disease, in case of transplacental transfer of toxoplasmosis is in … trimester	***First***
19.	Stage of labor lasting from full dilatation of cervix to complete birth of baby is …. stage	***2nd***
20.	Chorionic villous sampling, if done before 10 weeks result in	***Oromandibular limb defect***
21.	Maximum levels of HCG are reached on	***70 days***
22.	MC type of compound presentation	***Head and hand***
23.	Complication of succenturiate placenta	***Postpartum hemorrhage***
24.	HCG is secreted by	***Synytiotrophoblast***
25.	MC organism responsible for puerperal pyrexia	***Streptococcus***
26.	Smallest pelvic diameter in anteroposterior plane of inlet	***Obstetric conjugate***
27.	Largest fetal head diameter	***Mentovertical***
28.	Most common type of vertex presentation	***Left occiput anterior/left occiput transverse***
29.	Most common cause of a pregnant lady presenting with fulminant hepatitis	***Hepatitis E virus***
30.	Immunoglobulin crossing placenta	***IgG***
31.	Best time to diagnose fetal anomalies by USG	***18 weeks***
32.	MC presentation of H. mole	***Bleeding per vaginam***
33.	Bishops classification is used for	***Need of induction of labor***
34.	Average blood loss in normal delivery	***500 cc***
35.	Most common cause of uterovesical fistula in India is	***Obstructed labor***
36.	% of scar dehiscence in lower segment caesaren section	***0.5-1%***
37.	Involution of the uterus occurs at the rate of	***1.25 cm/day***
38.	MC cause of ectopic pregnancy	***Previous tubal disease***

S. No.	Question statements	Answers
39.	Ovulation returns in non-lactating women occurs after	***4 weeks***
40.	Low birth weight baby is defined as	***Less than 2.5 kg***
41.	Embryonic structure identified earliest on USG to confirm pregnancy	***Gestation sac***
42.	Increase in cardiac output in pregnancy is by	***40%***
43.	Relation of different parts of the fetus to each other is known as	***Fetal attitude***
44.	Uterus reaches upto umbilical level at	***24 weeks***
45.	Ideal time for screening of blood sugar to rule out diabetes in a pregnant female	***24-28 weeks***
46.	MC type of anemia in pregnancy	***Iron deficiency anemia***
47.	DOC for chronically hypertensive pregnant lady requiring long term anti-hypertensive therapy	***Methyldopa***
48.	Polyhydramnios is defined as amniotic fluid volume of more than	***2000 ml***
49.	HCG is secreted by	***Syncytiotrophoblast***
50.	MC site of ectopic pregnancy in fallopian tube	***Ampulla***

CHAPTER

8

GYNECOLOGY

KEY POINTS

Development of Vagina

- Upper 4/5th , above the hymen is developed from: Mucus membrane from endoderm of the canalized sinovaginal bulbs
- Musculature: From the mesoderm of two fused Mullerian ducts
- Lower 1/5th , below the Hymen is developed from: Endoderm of the urogenital sinus.

Rokitansky-Küster-Hauser Syndrome

- Congenital hypoplasia/absence of vagina in combination with an abnormal or absent uterus
- Second most common cause of primary amenorrhoea
- Gonadal dysgenesis is the most common cause of primary amenorrhoea

Fallopian Tube

- Lined by: Ciliated columnar epithelium
- Length: 10 cm

Female Urethra

- Length: 4 cm/40 mm (diameter: 6 mm)
- Lining: Transitional epithelium

Fallopian tube has four parts

- Interstitial (narrowest part)
- Isthmus
- Ampullary (fertilization takens place here)
- Infundibulum

Female Genital Tract

- Uterus measures 8 cm and weighs 50-80 gm
- Female urethra measures 4 cm.
- Gland of Cloquet or Rosenmuller—upper most deep femoral gland

Uterine Position

Anteversion	Long axis of the uterus is bent forward on the long axis of vagina, making an angle of 90 degree
Anteflexion	Long axis of the body of uterus is bent forward at the level of internal os with the long axis of the cervix, making an angle of 120 degrees

Doderlein's Bacillus

- It appears on vagina after birth, then disappears by 10-14 days; to reappear at puberty and then disappears at menopause
- It converts glycogen present in vaginal mucosa into lactic acid, to maintain acidic vaginal pH which protects against infection by pathogenic organisms

Fern Test

- Cervical mucus shows characteristic fern pattern on microscopic examination, during the estrogenic phase of cycle
- It is due to sodium chloride in mucus
- It disappears after 21 days

OCP	Progestin	Oestrogen
Mala N	Norgestrel 30 µg	Ethinyl estradiol 30 µg
Ovral L	Levonorgestrel µg	Ethinyl estradiol 30 µg
Mala D	D Norgestrel 30 µg	Ethinyl estradiol 30 µg
Femilon	Desonorgestrel µg	Ethinyl estradiol 20 µg

Contraindications to use of OCP

Absolute	Relative
Thromboembolism	Hypertension
Active liver disease	Diabetes
Liver adenoma	Epilepsy
Gall bladder disease	Smokers over 35

Contd...

Contd...

Absolute	Relative
Cholestatic jaundice	Age over 45
During pregnancy	Obesity
Surgery within 1 month	Lactation
General/breast carcinoma	Past liver disease
Focal migraine	Recent history of depression
	Adolescence
	Sickle cell disease
	Hyperlipidemia

OC Pills

Tumors associated	Provides protection
Cervical cancer	Ovarian tumors
Hepatic adenoma	Uterine tumors
Pituitary adenoma	Benign breast disease

Centchroman/Saheli

- Nonhormonal OCP
- Dose 30 mg twice weekly for 3 months then once a week
- Weak estrogenic and potent antiestrogenic effect
- Suppresses endometrial proliferation
- Interferes endometrial with nidation of embryo
- Can be used in DUB and emergency contraception

Half Lives

Cu-T 200/Cu-T 200B/ Multiload Cu 250	3 years
Cu T-380 A	10 years
Nova T	5 years
Progestasert	1 years
LNG- IUS	5 years

Timing for IUCD Insertion

- Postmenstrual day 4/5
- Postabortal after MTP

Indications of MTP

- S-Social
- H-Humanitarian
- E-Eugenic fetal anomalies
- L-Life saving
- F-Failure of contraception

Indications of Therapeutic Termination of Pregnancy

- Primary pulmonary hypertension
- Eisenmenger's syndrome
- Pulmonary veno-occlusive disease

Degrees of Retroversion

- First degree: Fundus is vertical and pointing towards the sacral promontory
- Second degree: Fundus lies in the sacral hollow but not below the internal os
- Third degree: Fundus lies below the level of internal os

Degrees of Uterine Prolapse

- First degree: Uterus descends from the normal position
- Second degree: External os protrudes outside the vaginal introitus but the uterine body still remains inside the vagina
- Third degree procidentia/complete prolapsed: Uterine body descends to lie outside the introitus

Indications of Pessary Treatment

- Early pregnancy, up to 18 weeks
- Patients unfit for surgery
- Puerperium
- Patients unwilling of surgery
- Patients waiting to complete family

Metropathia Hemorrhagica/Schroeder's Disease

- Cystic glandular hyperplasia
- Swiss cheese appearance of endometrium on microscopy

Terms

- Menorrhagia (Hypermenorrhoea): Excess and/or prolonged bleeding
- Epimenorrhoea (polymenorrhoea): <21 days
- Oligomenorrhoea: >35 days
- Hypomenorrhoea: Scant bleeding
- Metrorrhagia: Irregular, acyclic bleeding

Mittelschmerz

- Lower abdominal pain cyclically 2 weeks before menstruation (in mid menstrual period)

Swellings

- Cystic swelling at junction of lower1/3rd and upper 2 /3rd of vaginal wall should be Gartner's duct
- Cystic swelling at the junction of posterior 1/3rd and anterior 2/3rd of labium majus should be Bartholin's cyst

Follicular Ovarian Cyst

- Arises due to failure of rupture of follicle
- Usually unilateral
- Spontaneously disappear within 2 months

Remember

- Corpus luteal cyst appears due to failure of regression of corpus luteam in 14 days. It can cause delayed mense
- LH surge precedes ovulation by 24-36 horus.
- Subnuclear vacuole seen on day 16 is the first sign of ovulation

Pap Smear is used to Diagnose

- HPV
- Herpes infection
- Trichomoniasis
- Cervical cancer
- It is taken from posterior part of vaginal wall
- For hormonal cytological evaluation, it is taken form lateral part of vaginal wall

Histological Findings

Call Exner bodies	Granulosa cell tumor
Reinke's crystal	Hilus cell tumor
Signet ring	Krukenberg tumor
Schiller-Duval bodies	Endodermal sinus tumor
Psammoma bodies	Serouscystadenocarcinoma

Remember

- Meigs syndrome—Fibroma
- Pseudo-Meigs syndrome—Brenner tumor
- Clue cells – diagnostic of bacterial vaginosis
- Strawberry appearance of vagina is seen in Trichomoniasis
- Endometrial biopsy is done between 21st – 23rd days of menstrual cycle; If cycle is irregular then, it is done within 24 hours period.
- Fibroid is the most common pelvic tumour
- Mucinous cystadenoma—is the largest benign ovarian tumour
- Commonest site of endometriosis is ovary
- Premature ovarian failure, when before 40 years

Normal Sperm Values

- Volume: > 2 ml
- Sperm: > 20 million/ml
- Motility: > 50 percent
- Morphology: > 30 percent normal forms

Terms

- Infertility is inability of a couple to achieve conception after 1 year of unprotected sex
- Oligospermia/Oligozoospermia: Count is less than 20 million spermatozoa per ml
- Polyzoospermia: When the count is more than 350 million per ml
- Azoospermia: No spermatozoa in the semen
- Asthenospermia: Means reduction in the vitality of spermatozoa
- Necrospermia/Necrozoospermia: Condition in which the spermatozoa are dead or motionless
- Teratospermia/teratozoospermia: Presence of high number of malformed spermatozoa in the semen

Semen

- Normal pH 7.5
- Seminal vesicle contributes to the bulk of volume.
- Also contributes fructose, which is source of energy.
- Prostate alkalinizes semen, contributes clotting enzyme and fibrinolysin.

Clomiphene

Indicated in	Contraindicated in
Anovulatory infertility	Ovarian cyst
Polycystic ovarian disease associated with infertility	Chronic liver disease
In in vitro fertilization,	Scotoma
GIFT technique and ART	

Tamoxifen

- Nonsteroidal antiestrogenic

Danazol

- Androgen derivative,
- Gonadotropin inhibitor
- Used in:
  - Endometriosis
  - Cyclic and non-cyclic mastalgia
  - Primary menorrhagia
  - Precocious puberty, etc.

Other Drugs

- Antitubercular C/I in pregnancy:
  - Streptomycin
  - Pyrazinamide

Precocious and Delayed

- Precocious menstruation: If menstruation starts before the child reaches the age of 10
- Precocious puberty: Appearance of appropriate secondary characters before the age of 8 years in girls
- Delayed puberty: Breast tissue and/ or pubic hair have not appeared by 13-14 years or menarche has not occurred by 16 years.

Turner Syndrome

- 16 years old female with amenorrhea
- Webbed neck
- Low hair line and
- Widely spaced nipples
- USG showing streaky gonads (ovaries)

Turner's Syndrome

- 45 X
- Gonads are streaky
- Sex chromatin study is negative
- Hypergonadotropic hypogonadism
- Presents with primary amenorrhoea with delayed appearance of secondary sexual characteristics

McCune-Albright Syndrome

- Sexual precocity
- Multiple cystic bone lesions
- Endocrinopathies
- Café-au-lait spots on the skin

Klinefelter's Syndrome

- Sex chromatin is positive
- Karyotype is XXY or XXXY
- Small and underdeveloped male genitalia
- Eunuchoid appearance
- Gynecomastia
- Azoospermia

Androgen Insensitivity Syndrome/Testicular Feminization

- X-linked recessive inheritance
- Testicular feminization syndrome is the most common from of male intersex
- Primary amenorrhoea phenotypically and psychologically females with adequate breast development
- Absence of axillary and pubic hair. Normal external genitalia
- Short and blind vagina
- Testes are placed in labia, inguinal canal or abdomen
- Sex chromatin is negative
- Karyotype is 46,XY
- Normal testosterone level

Endometrial Ca

- 60 years old female
- Hypertensive and DM with
- Vaginal bleeding

Sheehan Syndrome

- 24 years old female
- 2 weeks after delivery with
- Inability to breast feed her baby
- Weakness and fatigability with
- Low ACTH, LH, FSH

Condyloma Acuminata (HPV)

- 28 years old female with
- Soft, pinkish, cauliflower like lesions
- H/O multiple partners
- Responding to Imiquimod

Toxic Shock Syndrome

- Female with fever
- Hypotension
- Skin rash
- Headache and
- Diarrhea and altered mental status
- H/O using vaginal tampon

Adenomyosis

- 35 year female with
- Dysmenorrhea
- Menorrhagia
- Chronic pelvic pain
- Symmetrically enlarged uterus
- Smooth and tender on palpation

Endometriosis

- 36 years old female,
- Dysmenorrhea
- Dyspareunia with
- Fixed retroverted uterus and

Nodularity of Uterosacral Ligaments—Premenstrual Syndrome

- 20 years female with irritability
- Breast tenderness
- Headache and bloating before menstrual cycles

Ovarian Ca

- 60 years old female with
- Abdominal and pelvic swelling
- Increased CA 125 level

Bacterial Vaginosis

- 28 years old female, with
- Profuse watery

- Dirty grey discharge
- Positive Whiff test

Herpes Simplex II/Herpes Genitalis

- 24 years old female with
- Paraesthesia,
- Burning pain in perineal area and
- Vesicles showing Cowdry inclusions
- Painful inguinal lympho-adenopathy

Trichomonas Vaginalis

- 28 years female with
- Foul smelling
- Frothy
- Light green colored vaginal discharge
- Strawberry cervix and
- Vaginal erythema

Diagnostic Criteria of PCOS

Major

- Chronic anovulation
- Hyperandrogenism
- Clinical signs of hyperandrogenism
- Exclusion of other etiologies

Minor

- Insulin resistance
- Perimenarchal onest of Hirsutism and obesity
- Elevated LH to FSH ratio
- Intermittent anovulation associated with hyperandroenism

Ultrasound criteria

- Increased ovatian area/volume
- 10-15 microcytes organized in a peripheral rosary pattern
- Increased echogenicity of ovarian stroma

Stein-Leventhal syndrome

- Increased androgens
- Increased estrogens
- Increased LH
- Increased GNRH
- Decreased FSH
- Hirsutism and amenorrhoea
- Decreased ovarian follicular maturation
- HAIR-AN syndrome – hyperandrogenism, insulin resistance, acanthosis nigricans
- LH:FSH ratio is > than 3:1
- Treatment:
  - Clomiphene
  - Surgical resection

Incontinence

- Stress incontinence: Leakage of urine coincides with stress. No prior urge to void. Small amount. Patient aware Micturition is normal
- Urge incontinence: Unable to control escape of urine once there is urge to void. Large amount. Patient aware. Urgency and frequency
- Detrusor instability: Incompetence may occur abruptly without a full bladder. Large amount. Patient of aware. Frequency and nocturia

Triple Swab Test for Fistulas

- Uppermost swab: Placed in vaginal vault
- Second in middle part
- Third: Placed in the lower part, just above introitus
- Methylene blue dye is instilled in the bladder

Results

- Ureterovaginal fistula: Upper most swab soaked with urine but unstained with dye, lower two swabs remain dry
- Vesicovaginal fistula: Upper and lower swabs remain dry but the middle swab stained with dye
- Urethrovaginal fistula: Upper two swabs remain dry but the lower swab stained with dye

Fistula	Symptoms
Ureterovaginal	Urge present. Can pass urine normally
Vesicovaginal	Urge absent
Urethrovaginal	Urge present. Cannot pass urine normally

Remember

- Vesicovaginal fistula is the commonest genitourinary fistula
- Most commonly caused by obstructed labour in developing countries and following operative injury in developed countries.

MCQs WITH SHORT EXPLANATIONS

GYNECOLOGICAL ANATOMY

1. 'Peg cells' are seen in:

a. Tubes b. Ovary
c. Vulva d. Vagina

The mucous membrane of the fallopian tube is thrown into folds. It is lined by columnar epithelium, partly ciliated, others secretory nonciliated and "peg cells'.

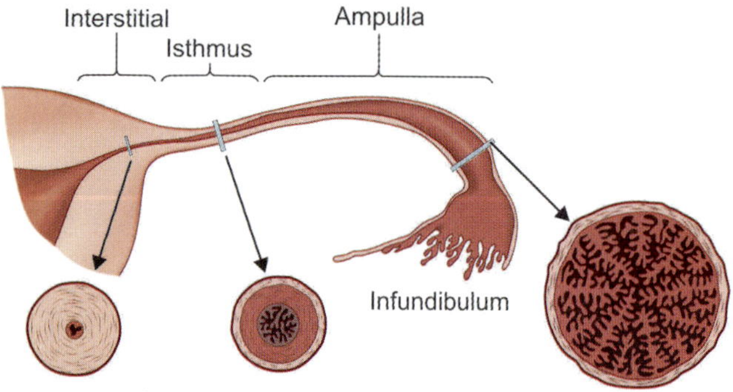

Cut section of the tube showing complex mucosal pattern

2. The mucosal lining in vagina is:

a. Transitional
b. Ciliated columnar
c. Stratified squamous nonkeratinized
d. Pseudostratified columnar

Mucous coat of vagina is lined by stratified squamous epithelium without any secreting glands.

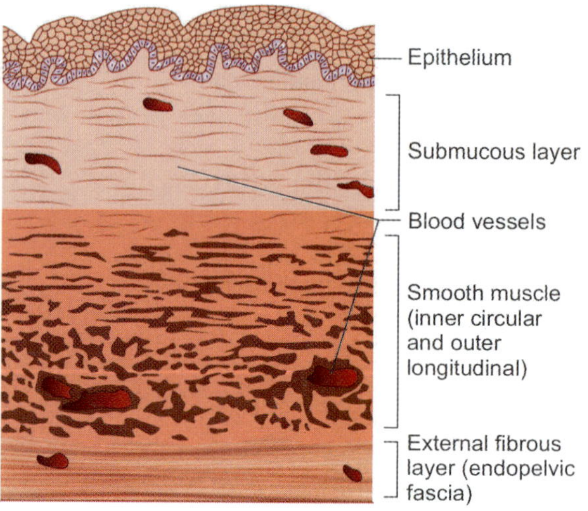

Structure of vaginal wall

3. All are true for vagina EXCEPT:

a. Partly or wholly derived from urogenital sinus
b. Rich in glands
c. Lined by stratified squamous glands
d. Posterior fornix lengthier than anterior fornix

From puberty till menopause, the vaginal epithelium is stratified squamous and devoid of any gland.

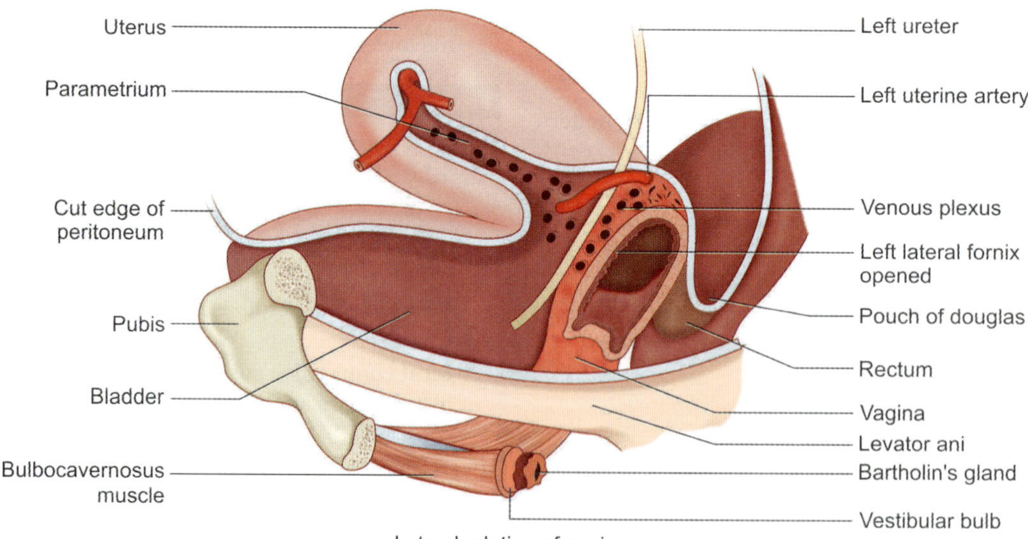

Lateral relation of vagina

4. Main support to uterus is from:

a. Pubocervical ligaments b. Cardinal ligaments
c. Round ligaments d. Broad ligaments

Cardinal ligament/ Mackenrodt's ligament/ Transverse cervical ligament is the lateral stabilizer of the cervix at the level of ischial spine.

Ans. 1. **a.** Tubes 2. **c.** Stratified squamous... 3. **b.** Rich in glands 4. **b.** Cardinal ligaments

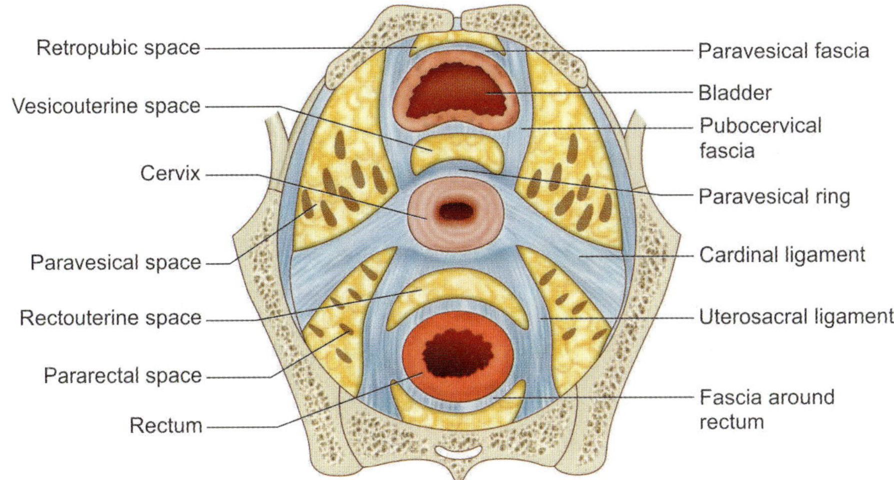

The main supporting ligaments of the uterus viewed from above

5. Size of uterus (in inch):

a. 4 × 2 × 1 b. 3 × 2 × 1
c. 4 × 3 × 1 d. 5 × 4 × 2

The uterus measures about 8 cm, 5 cm wide at the fundus and its walls are about 1.25 cm thick.

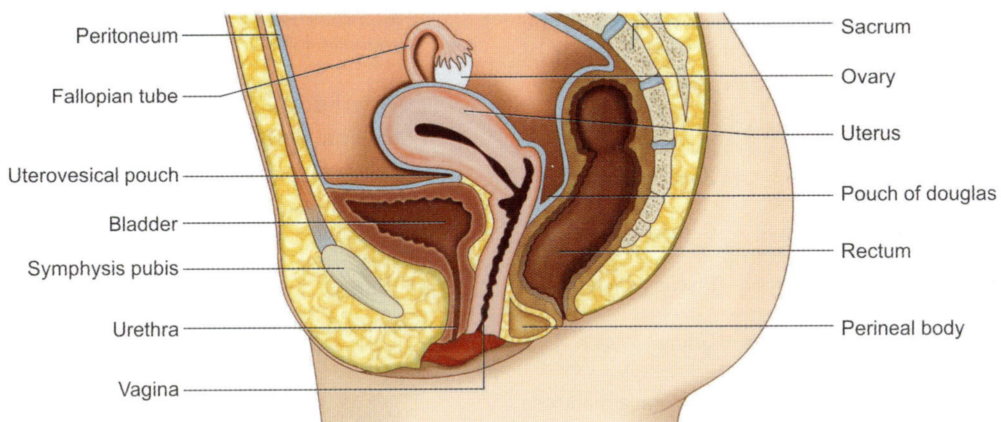

Mid-sagittal section of the female pelvis showing relative position of the pelvic organs

6. Before puberty, what is the ratio between the cervical length and uterine body:

a. 1:2 b. 2:1
c. 1:3 d. 1:4

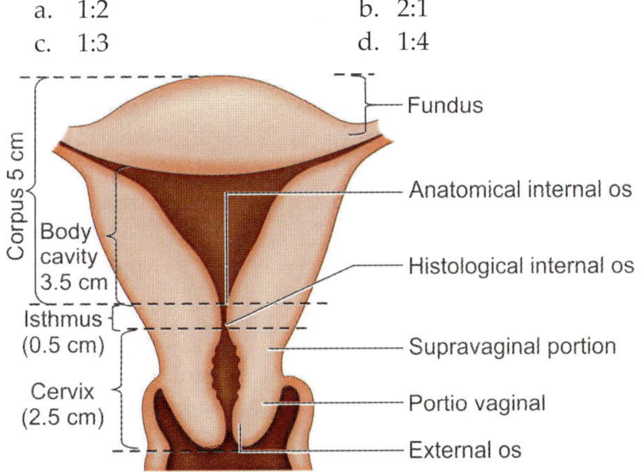

Coronal section showing different parts of uterus

At birth, the uterus lies in the false pelvis; the cervix is much longer than the body. In childhood, the proportion is maintained but reduced to 2:1.

7. Ovary is formed from:

a. Genital ridge
b. Wolffian duct
c. Genital ridge
d. Genital tubercle

The ovary is developed on either side from the genital or gonadal ridge. This ridge is formed in a four-week embryo between the dorsal mesentery (medially) and the mesonephric ridge (laterally) by the multiplication of the coelomic epithelium along with condensation of the underlying mesenchyme.

Ans. 5. **b.** 3 × 2 × 1 6. **b.** 2:1 7. **c.** Genital ridge

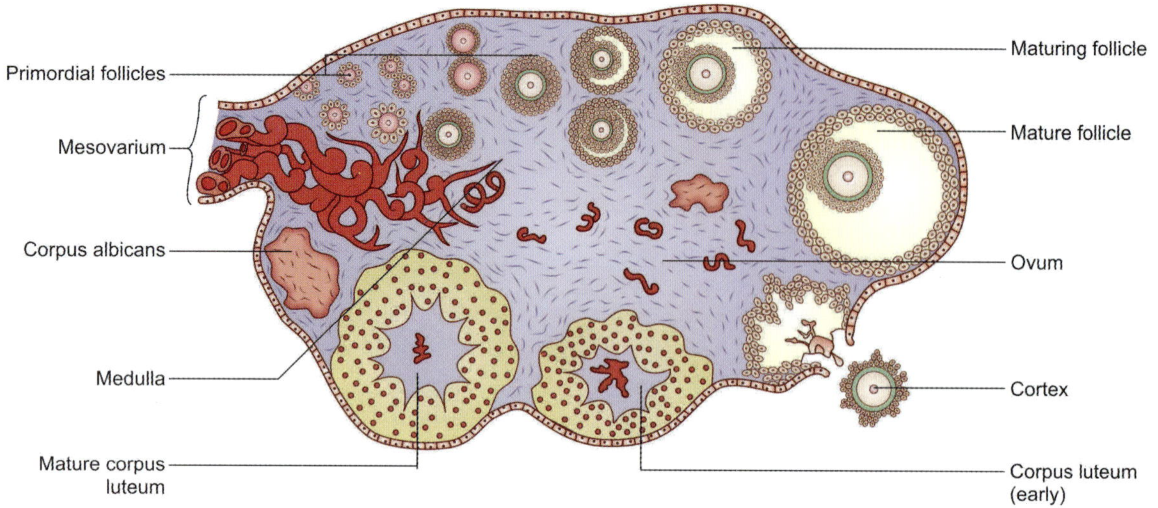

Histological structures of the ovary

8. Primordial follicles present at birth:

a. 2000 b. 20,000
c. 2 lakhs d. 2 millions

Total number of oocytes at 20 weeks of intrauterine life is about 6-7 million. At birth, the total number of primordial follicles is estimated to be about 2 million.

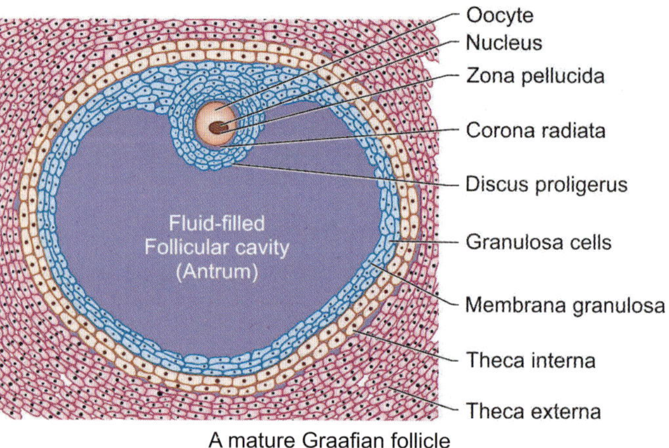

A mature Graafian follicle

9. Uterus develops from:

a. Mesonephric duct b. Paramesonephric duct
c. Genital ridge d. Genital tubercle

Uterus is developed by the fusion of the intermediate horizontal and the adjoining vertical part of the Mullerian ducts, which begins at 7-8 weeks (22 cm CR length) and completes at 12th week.

Male and Female Derivatives of Embryonic Urogenital Structures

Embryonic structure	*Derivatives*	
	Male	*Female*
labioscrotal swelling	Scrotum	Labia majora
Urogenital folds	Ventral aspect of penis	Labia minora
Genital tubercle	Penis	Clitoris
Urogenital sinus	Urinary bladder Urethra except navicular fossa Prostate gland Prostatic utricle Bulbourethral glands	Urinary bladder, urethra Urethral and paraurethral glands Vagina Bartholin's glands
Paramesonephric duct	Appendix of testes	Hydatid of Morgagni, uterus, cervix fallopian tubes, vagina (muscular wall)
Mesonephric duct	Ductus epididymis Ductus differens and seminal vesicles	Duct of epoophoron Gartner's duct
Mesonephric tubules	Ductuli efferentes Paradidymis	Epoophoron Paroophoron
Undifferentiated gonad Cortex Medulla	Testis Seminiferous tubules Rete testis	Ovary Ovarian follicles Rete ovarii
Gubernaculum	Gubernaculum testis	Ovarian ligament Round ligament
Müllerian tubercle	Seminal colliculus	Hymen

10. Shortest and narrowest part of fallopian tube:

a. Interstitial b. Isthmus
c. Ampulla d. Infundibulum

There are four parts of the fallopian tube, from medial to lateral, they are – (1) intramural/interstitial lying in the

Ans. 8. **d.** 2 millions 9. **b.** Paramesonephric duct

uterine wall and measures 1.25 cm in length and 1 mm in diameter; (2) isthmus almost straight and measures about 2.5 cm in length and 2.5 mm in diameter; (3) ampulla – tortuous part and measures about 5 cm in length which ends in wide; (4) infundibulum measuring about 1.25 cm long with a maximum diameter of 6 mm.

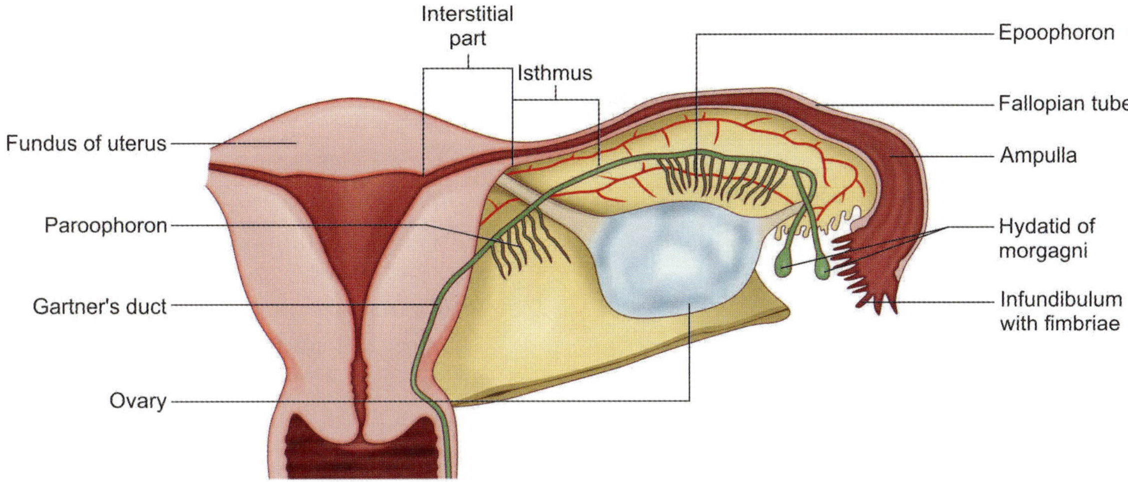

Half of uterine cavity and Fallopian tube of one side are cut open to show different parts of the tube. The vestigial structures in the broad ligament are shown

CONTRACEPTIVES

11. A couple presented after 4 days of unprotected coitus. What would you advise?

a. OCPs
b. Cu-T 380A
c. Yuzpe method
d. Low dose POP with norgesterol

The copper IUD is the most effective form of emergency contraception. It is more effective than the hormonal EC pills currently available. The pregnancy rate among those using the copper IUD for EC is 0.09%. It can be used for EC up to 5 days after the act of unprotected sex and does not decrease in effectiveness during the 5 days. An additional advantage of using the copper IUD for emergency contraception is that it can be used as a form of birth control for 10–12 years after insertion.

12. All are beneficial effects of OCP's EXCEPT:

a. Protection from endometrial carcinoma
b. Protection from breast malignancy
c. Improvement in menstrual abnormalities
d. Reduction of premenstrual syndrome

There is a slight increase in breast cancer risk among current users, which disappears 5–10 years after use of OCP has stopped

13. Contraceptive which is supplied by government free of cost:

a. Minipill
b. Norplant
c. Mala-N
d. Centchroman

New users should normally start their pill packet on day one of theory cycle. One tablet is to be taken daily preferably at bed time for consecutive 21 days. It is continued for 21 days and then have a 7 days break, with this routine there is contraceptive protection from the first pill. Next pack should be started on the eighth day, irrespective of bleeding (same day of the week, the pill finished).

Some of the Oral Contraceptives and their Composition

Commercial names	*Composition*		*No. of tablets*
	Progestins (mg)	*Estrogen (μg)*	
1. Mala N (Govt of india)	Levonorgestrel 0.15	Ethinyl estradiol 30	21 + 7 iron tablets
2. Mala-D	Levonorgestrel 0.15	—do—	21 + 7 iron tablets
3. Loette (Wyeth)	Desogestrel 0.15	Ethinyl estradiol 20	21
4. Yasmin (schering)	Drospirenone 3 mg (p. 531)	Ethinyl estradiol 30	21

Depending on the amount of ethinyl estradiol (E) and the types of progestin (P) used, pills are defined as: **1st generation** — with E 50 μg or more; **2nd generation** — with E 20–35 μg and P as levonorgestrel or norgestimate; **3rd generation** — with E 20–30 μg and P as desogestrel or gestodene; **4th generation** — E as third generation, with P as drospirenone, dienogest or nomegestrol. low dose pills have E less than 50 μg.

Ans. **10. a.** Interstitial **11. b.** Cu-T 380A **12. b.** Protection... **13. c.** Mala-N

14. RU-486 is NOT used for:

a. MTP
b. Induction of labor
c. Cervical ripening
d. Post-coital contraception

Anti-progesterone (RU-486-Mifepristone) binds competitively to progesterone receptors and nullifies the effect of endogenous progesterone.

Emergency Contraceptives		
Drug	*Dose*	*Pregnancy rate (%)*
Levonorgestrel	0.75 mg stat and after 12 hours	0–1
Ethinyl estradiol 50 µg + norgestrel 0.25 mg	2 tab stat and 2 after 12 hours	0–2
Ethinyl estradiol	2.5 mg BD × 5 days	0–0.6
Mifepristone	100 mg single dose	0–0.6
Copper IUDS (Gold standard)	Insertion within 5 days	0–0.1
Ulipristal acetate	30 mg PO	0–1

15. Pearl index is used to calculate:

a. Accidental pregnancies
b. Population
c. Fertility rate
d. Abortions

The pearl index, also called the Pear rate, is the most common technique used in clinical trials for reporting the effectiveness of a birth control method.

Failure Rate of Contraceptive Methods in First 12 Months of Use	
Methods	*Pregnancy rate per 100 women years (approx.)*
No method	85
Natural (calender, temperature, mucus)	25
Withdrawal	27
Lactational amenorrhea	2
Condom (male)	15
Condom (female)	21
Diaphragm	16
IuCd:	
CuT 380A	0.8
InG 20	0.1
Combined oral pill	0.1
Progestin only pill	1
DMPA and NET injectables	0.3
Norplant	0.05
Implanon	0.01
Vasectomy	0.15
Tubectomy	0.15
Failure rate is further less when methods are used correctly and consistently	

16. Levonorgestrel containing IUCD prevents pregnancy primarily due to:

a. Making endometrium unreceptive
b. Suppressing ovulation
c. Initiating inflammatory changes within the endometrium
d. Making cervical mucus thin

LNG-IUS (Mirena) induces strong and uniform suppression of endometrium. Cervical mucus becomes very scanty. Anovulation and insufficient luteal phase activity has also been mentioned.

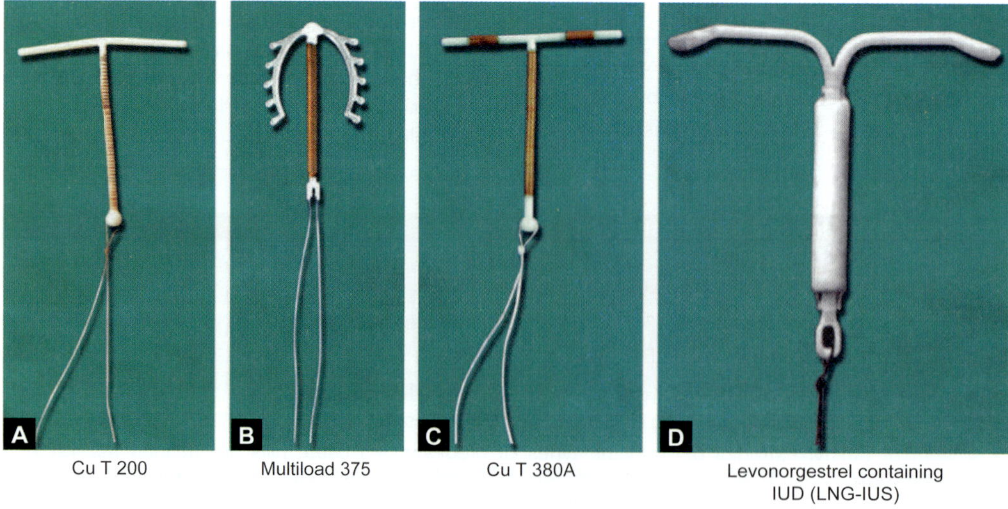

A: Cu T 200; B: Multiload 375; C: Cu T 380A; D: Levonorgestrel containing IUD (LNG-IUS)

Commonly used IUD

Ans. **14. c.** Cervical ripening **15. a.** Accidental pregnancies **16. a.** Making endometrium unreceptive

17. Technique of Cu-T insertion:

a. Surgery under local anaesthesia
b. Surgery under general anaesthesia
c. Withdrawal technique
d. Laparotomy

The inserter with the device placed inside is introduced through the cervical canal right up to the fundus and after positioning it by the guard, the inserter is withdrawn keeping the plunger in position. Thus, the device is not pushed out of the tube but held in place by the plunger while the inserter is withdrawn (withdrawal technique).

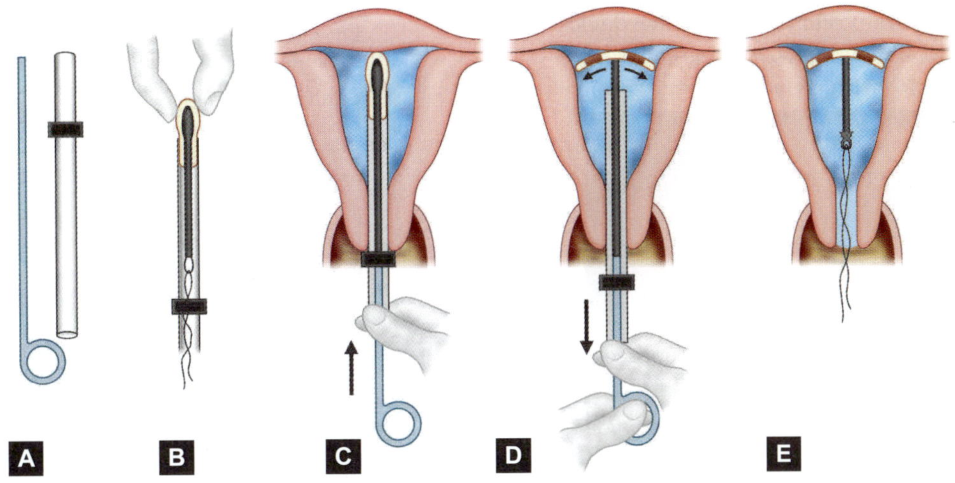

Withdrawal technique of insertion of Cu T

18. Which of the following IUCD has a life span of 10 years:

a. Cu 380 A
b. Cu 200
c. NOVA-T
d. Multiload

Cu-T 380A frame contains barium sulfate and is radio-opaque. Replacement is every 10 years.

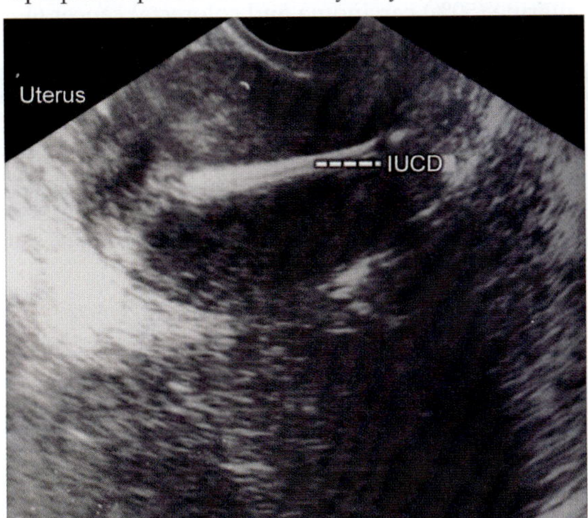

Ultrasonogram showing the Cu T inside the uterine cavity. Thread was missing in this case

19. MC site of ligation by clip in female sterilization:

a. Fimbrial
b. Cornual
c. Ampullary
d. Isthmus

Laparoscopic sterilization by Fallope or Filshie clip is carried out after creating pneumoperitoneum and then ring load applicator approaches one side of the tube and grasps at the junction of the proximal and middle third of tube. A loop of the tube (2.5 cm) is lifted up, drawn into the cylinder of the applicator and the ring is slipped into the base of the loop under direct vision.

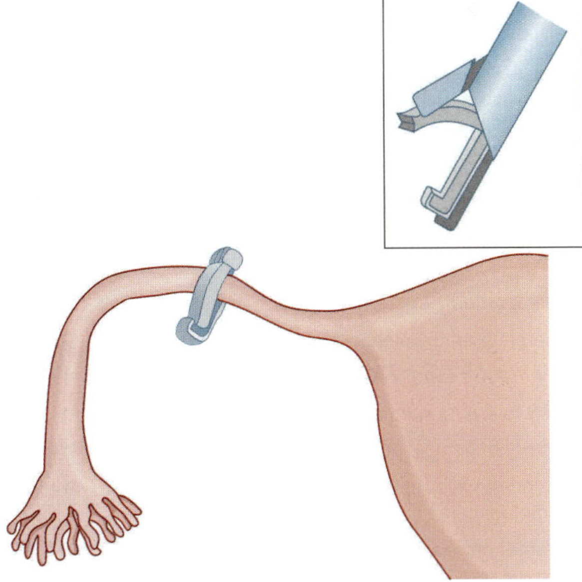

Laparoscopic tubal sterilization by Filshie clip. Filshie (GM Filshie) clip is made of titanium and the inner surfaces are lined with silicon. It is easier to apply and damage to the tube is less

Ans. 17. **c.** Withdrawal tech... 18. **a.** Cu 380 A 19. **d.** Isthmus

20. Intrauterine Cu-T 200 is called Cu 200 because:
a. Contains 200 mg of Cu
b. Contains 200 sq. mm. of Cu
c. Has 200 turns of Cu
d. Can be retained for 200 days

The widely used medicated device is Copper T-200B. It carries 215 sq mm surface area of fine copper wire wounded round the vertical stem of the device. The copper is lost at the rate of 50 microgram per 24 hours during a period of one year.

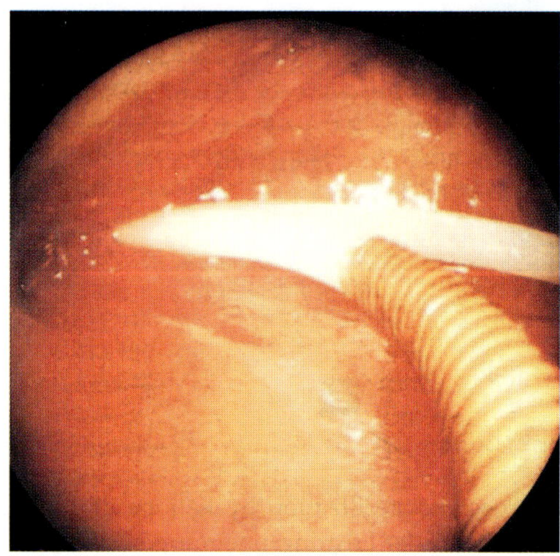

Hysteroscopic view of IUCD in uterine cavity. The threads are coiled inside

21. Mechanism of action of IUCD are all EXCEPT:
a. Ovulation inhibition
b. Chronic endometritis
c. Uterine endometrial atrophy
d. Tubal dysmotility

Mechanism of anti-fertility effect of all the IUDs is not yet clear. They act predominantly in the uterine cavity and do not inhibit ovulation.

IUD (Cu Devices and Hormone Releasing IUDS)	
Advantages	*Disadvantages*
1. Inexpensive: cu T-distributed free of cost through Government channel	1. Require motivation
2. Simplicity in techniques of insertion and most cost effective of all methods	2. Limitation in its use
3. Prolonged contraceptive protection after insertion (5–10 years) and suitable for the rural population of developing countries	3. Adverse local reactions manifested by menstrual abnormalities, PiD, pelvic pain and heavy periods. beside effects are less with third generation of IUDs
4. systemic side effects are nil. Suitable for hypertensives, breastfeeding women and epileptics	4. Risk of ectopic pregnancy.
5. Reversibility to fertility is prompt after removal	Failure rate — 0.1–2 (HWY)

22. OCP may cause all EXCEPT:
a. Ca in situ cervix
b. Breast Ca
c. Endometrial Ca
d. Thromboembolic episodes

OCPs are protective for ovarian (50%), endometrial/ uterine (50%) carcinoma and colorectal cancer (40%).

Medical Eligibility Criteria for Contraceptive Use (WHO/FRM/FPP—1996)		
Combined Oral Contraceptives (COCs)		
Indications of COCs	*Contraindications of COCs*	
No restriction of use (WHO Category–1)	*Relative (WHO Category–2 and 3)*	*Absolute (WHO Category–4)*
❑ Age: menarche to 40 years	A. WHO Category–2: (Advantages outweigh the risks)	(A) Circulatory diseases (past or present)
❑ Postabortion	❑ Age ≥ 40 years	❑ Arterial or venous thrombosis
❑ Anemia (iron deficiency, malaria)	❑ Smoker < 35 years	❑ Severe hypertension
❑ HIV or AIDs (additional to condom use)	❑ History of jaundice	❑ History of stroke
❑ GTN following normal hCG level	❑ Mild hypertension	❑ Heart disease: valvular, ischemic
❑ History of ectopic pregnancy	❑ Gallbladder disease	❑ Diabetes with vascular complications
❑ Endometriosis, uterine fibroid, ovarian or endometrial cancer	❑ Diabetes	❑ Migraine with focal neurologic symptoms
❑ Dysmenorrhea, DUB	❑ Sickle cell disease	(B) diseases of the liver
❑ PID	❑ Headache	❑ Active liver disease
❑ Epilepsy	❑ Cancer cervix or CIN	❑ Liver adenoma, carcinoma

Contd...

Ans. **20. b.** Contains 200... **21. a.** Ovulation inhibition **22. c.** Endometrial Ca

Contd...

Combined Oral Contraceptives (COCs)		
Indications of COCs	*Contraindications of COCs*	
No restriction of use (WHO Category–1)	*Relative (WHO Category–2 and 3)*	*Absolute (WHO Category–4)*
❑ Thyroid disease	B. WhO Category–3: (Risks outweigh the advantages)	(C) Others
❑ Varicose veins	❑ Unexplained vaginal bleeding	❑ Pregnancy
❑ Tuberculosis	❑ Hyperlipidemia	❑ Breastfeeding (postpartum 6 weeks)
❑ Benign breast disease	❑ Liver tumors (benign)	❑ Major surgery or prolonged immobilization
	❑ Breastfeeding (postpartum 6 weeks to 6 months)	❑ Estrogen dependent neoplasms, e.g. breast cancer
	❑ Heavy smoker (> 20 cigarettes/day)	
	❑ Past breast cancer	

23. Progesterone of choice in emergency contraception:

a. Micronized progesterone
b. Norgesterone
c. Levonorgestrel
d. DMPA

Levonorgestrel (E. Pills) 0.75 mg, two doses given at 12 hours interval, is very successful and without any side effects. The two tablets (1.50 mg) can be taken as a single dose also. The first dose should be taken within 72 hours.

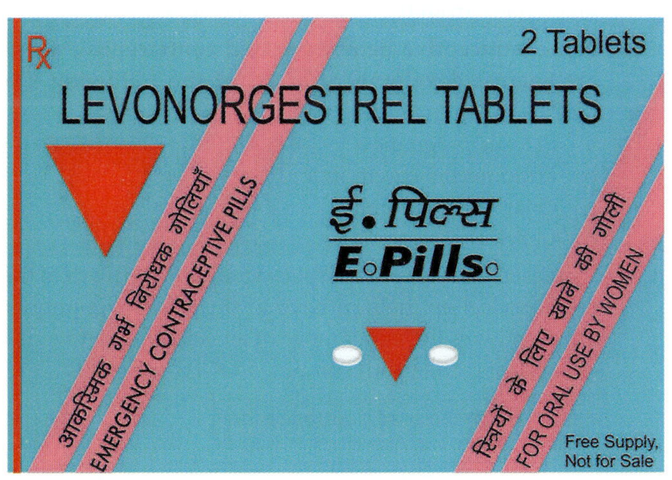

Levonorgestrel pill

24. OCP protects against all EXCEPT:

a. Hepatic adenoma
b. Fibroadenoma breast
c. Carcinoma ovary
d. Uterine malignancy

Diseases of the liver like active liver disease, liver adenomas and liver carcinoma are absolute contraindications to use of combined OCPs.

Combined Preparations	
Advantages	*Disadvantages*
1. Highly effective	1. Requires education and motivation
2. Good cycle control	2. Limitation in its use (see above)
3. Well-tolerated in majority	3. Requires initial check up and periodic supervision
4. Additional non-contraceptive — benefits are many (see above)	4. Inconvenience caused in its use due to daily schedule
5. Low dose pill with 'lipid friendly' progestins further reduces the risk	5. Risk of drug interactions
6. Reversibility rate is prompt	6. Costly but free supply through government channel (Mala-N)
	Failure rate—0.1 (HWY)

25. The following are the contraindications to the use of combined oral contraceptive pills EXCEPT:

a. Breastfeeding
b. History of deep venous thrombosis
c. Active viral hepatitis
d. Menstrual irregularities

OCPs causes an improvement of menstrual abnormalities – (1) Regulation of menstrual cycle, (2) Reduction of dysmenorrhoea – 40%, (3) Reduction of menorrhagia – 50%, (4) Reduction of premenstrual tension syndrome/PMS, (5) Reduction of Mittelschmerz's syndrome.

Ans. 23. **c.** Levonorgestrel 24. **a.** Hepatic adenoma 25. **d.** Menstrual irregularities

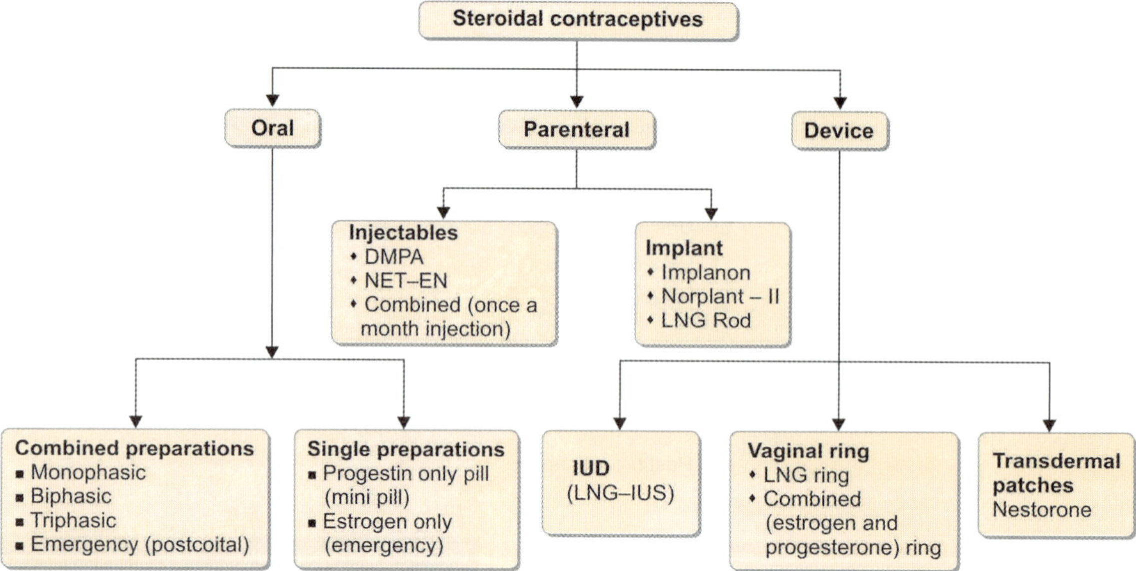

26. Which of the following has the highest risk of ectopic pregnancy:

a. Cu-T
b. Mini pill
c. OCP
d. LGN

Should pregnancy occur with a device (IUCD) in situ, there is risk of ectopic pregnancy (0.02%). IUD can prevent an uterine pregnancy but not an ectopic pregnancy. Third generation of IUDs like Cu T 380A and LNG-IUS give some amount of protection against an ectopic pregnancy.

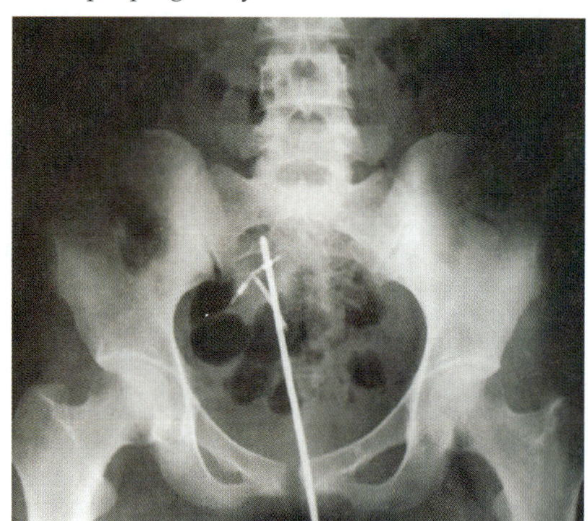

Straight X-ray of the pelvis with an uterine sound placed inside the uterine cavity — (a) the displaced IUCD seems inside the uterine cavity with AP view. Lateral view is needed for confirmation [*By courtesy:* Dr Swati Shirodkar, HOD, Dept of Obst Gyn, MGM Medical College, Aurangabad]

27. Levonorgesticeol content of Mini pill is:

a. 10 microgram
b. 20 microgram
c. 30 microgram
d. 40 microgram

POP is devoid of any estrogen compound. It contains very low dose of progestin in any one of the following form – Levonorgestrel 75 microgram, norethisterone 350 microgram, desogestrel 75 microgram, lynestrenol 500 microgram or norgestrel 30 microgram. It has to be taken daily from the first day of the cycle.

28. Noncontraceptive benefits of oral contraceptive agent are against development of all of the following EXCEPT:

a. Ectopic pregnancy
b. Endometrial carcinoma
c. Ovarian carcinoma
d. Cervical carcinoma

Increased glandular hyperplasia and downgrowth of the endocervical epithelium beyond the squamo-columnar junction gives the appearance of an ectopy. Relative risk of cervical cancer with combined OCPS use is 1:1.

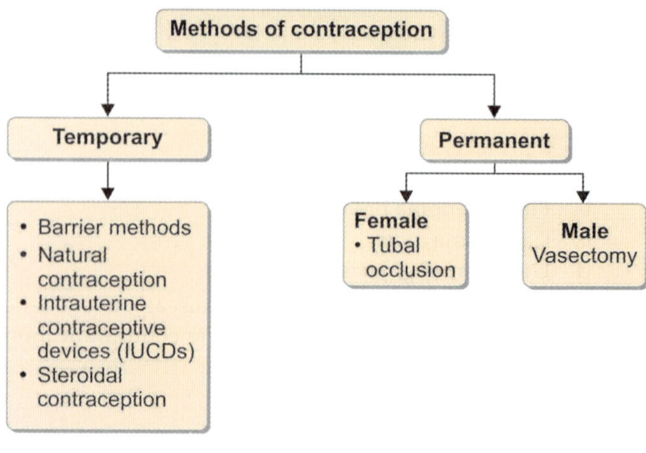

Ans. **26. a.** Cu-T **27. c.** 30 microgram **28. d.** Cervical carcinoma

GYNECOLOGICAL INFECTION

29. Which of the following statement regarding bacterial vaginosis is NOT true?

a. Not an STD
b. pH less than 4.5
c. Fishy odour
d. Gardenella vaginalis is responsible

To control bacterial growth, the vagina is normally slightly acidic with a pH of 3.8–4.2. A swab of the discharge is put onto litmus paper to check its acidity. A pH greater than 4.5 is considered alkaline and is suggestive of bacterial vaginosis.

30. On hysterosalpingography, Golf club appearance of fallopian tube suggest the diagnosis of:

a. TB
b. Gonorrhoea
c. Chlamydial infection
d. None of the above

Hysterosalpingographic presentation of tubal TB vary from non-specific changes such as hydrosalpinx to specific pattern such as "beaded tube", "golf club tube", "pipestem tube", "cobble stone tube" and the "leopard skin tube"

31. Gold standard investigation in diagnosing PID is:

a. Anti chlamydial Ab
b. Laparoscopy
c. USG
d. Blood leucocyte count

Laparoscopy is considered the "gold standard" procedure for diagnosing PID. While it is the most reliable aid to support the clinical diagnosis but it may not be feasible to do in all cases.

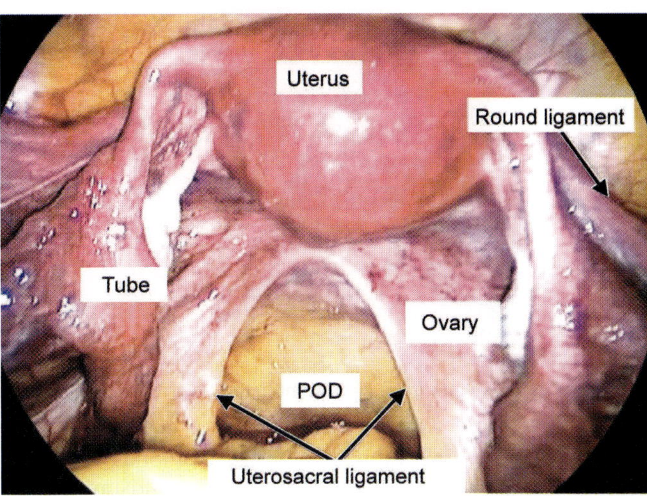

Laparoscopic view of a normal pelvis showing uterus tubes, ovaries, round ligament (Rt), uterosacral ligaments and the pouch of Douglas *(Courtesy: Prof. Alka Kriplani, Dept. Ob-Gyn., AIIMS, New Delhi)*

32. Most likely to be associated with vaginal pH of 4:

a. Atrophic vaginitis
b. Trichomanas vaginatis
c. Candidal vaginitis
d. Gardenella vaginitis

Vaginal pH in candidiasis is <4.5

Differential Diagnosis of Vaginal Discharge

Characteristics	*Trichomoniasis*	*Candidiasis*	*Bacterial vaginosis*	*Chlamydia*	*Normal vaginal discharge*
Color	Greenish yellow	Curdy white	Gray white to green yellow white	Mucopurulent	White
Consistency	Thin, frothy	Thick	Thin	Thick	Thin
Whiff test	Negative	Negative	Positive (fishy amine)	Negative	Negative
pH	≥ 5	< 4.5	≥ 5	< 4.5	< 4.5
Pruritus	+++	++	Non-irritating	—	—
Diagnosis (Wet mount microscopy)	Motile *Trichomonas*	hyphae or spores	Clue cells (> 20%)	Chlamydia NAAT	—
Treatment	Metronidazole 2 gm single dose or 200 mg. TID × 7 days	Imidazole fluconazole 150 mg P.O. weekly for 6 weeks	Metronidazole 200 mg. TID × 7 days	Azithromycin 1 gm orally single dose	—

33. A female presented with thick white discharge and pruritus. Aetiological agent is:

a. Gardnerella
b. Trichomonas vaginalis
c. Candida albicans
d. Gonococci

The patient with candida vaginitis/moniliasis complains of vaginal discharge with intense vulvovaginal pruritus. The pruritus is out of proportion to the discharge. The discharge is thick, curdy white and in flakes (cottage cheese type) often adherent to the vaginal wall.

Ans. **29.** b. pH less... **30.** a. TB **31.** b. Laparoscopy **32.** c. Candidal vaginitis **33.** c. Candida albicans

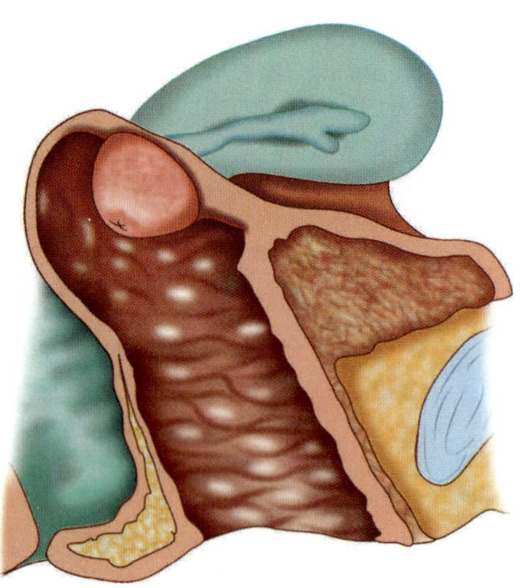

Curdy white flakes adherent to the vaginal wall

34. Clue cells are seen on a vaginal smear in ...... infection:

a. Hemophilus vaginalis b. Trichomonas vaginalis
c. Herpes simplex type I d. Hemophilus influenza

A smear of vaginal discharge is prepared with drops of normal saline on a glass slide and is seen under a microscope. Vaginal epithelial cells are seen covered with the coccobacilli and the cells appear as stippled or granular. At times, the cells are so heavily stippled that the cell borders are obscured. These stippled epithelial cells are called "clue cells". Presence of clue cells (>20% of cells) are diagnostic of BV, which is caused by Gardnerella vaginalis (haemophilus vaginalis).

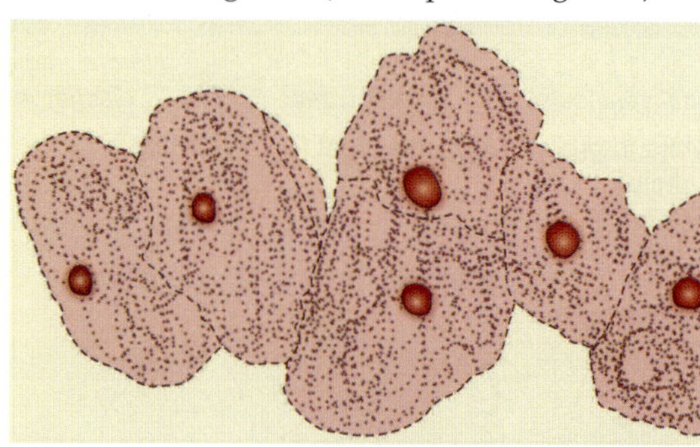

Clue cells

35. Strawberry vagina is seen with:

a. Trichomonas vaginalis
b. Hemophilus vaginalis
c. Candida
d. Herpes simplex

In trichomoniasis, the vaginal wall becomes red and inflammed with multiple punctate hemorrhagic spots. Similar spots are also found over the mucosa of the portio vaginalis part of the cervix on speculum examination giving the appearance of 'strawberry'.

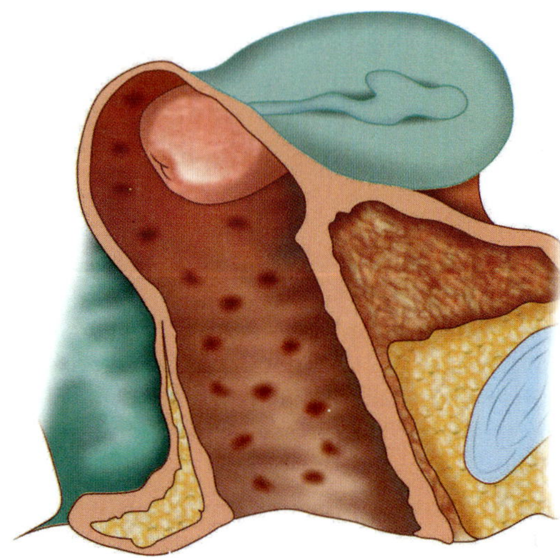

Punctate hemorrhagic spots and 'strawberry' appearance on cervix

36. A 40 years old woman presented to the gynaecologist with complaints of profuse vaginal discharge. There was no discharge from the cervix on the speculum examination. The diagnosis of bacterial vaginosis was made based upon all of the following findings on microscopy EXCEPT:

a. Abundance of gram variable coccobacilli
b. Absence of lactobacilli
c. Abundance of polymorphis
d. Presence of clue cells

Bacterial vaginois is characterized by malodorous vaginal discharge. Ther term vaginosis is preferred as there is no vaginal inflammation.

Sexually Transmitted Infections (STIs)

Disease	*Agent*	*Prevention of STIs and RTIs*
Gonorrhoea Non-gonococcal urethritis Syphilis Lymphogranuloma venereum Chancroid Granuloma inguinale Non-Specific Vaginitis Mycoplasma infection	❑ Bacterial *Neisseria gonorrhoeae* *Chlamydia trachomatis (D-K serotypes)* *Treponema pallidum* *Chlamydia trachomatis (L serotypes)* *Hemophilus ducreyi* *Donovania granulomatis* *Hemophilus vaginalis* *Mycoplasma hominis*	❑ Safe sex as STIs are entirely preventable. ❑ Use of barrier contraception: Condom, diaphragm, spermicides.

Contd...

Ans. **34. a.** Hemophilus vaginalis **35. a.** Trichomonas vaginalis **36.c.** Abundance of polymorphs

Contd...

Disease	*Agent*	*Prevention of STIs and RTIs*
AIDs Genital herpes Condyloma acuminata Molluscum contagiosum Viral hepatitis CIN	❑ Viral *Human immunodeficiency virus* (HIV 1 or HIV 2) *Herpes simplex virus* (HSV 2) *Human papilloma virus* (HPV) *HPV – 16, 18 or 31* *Pox virus* *Hepatitis B and C virus*	❑ Reducing the number of sexual partners — monogamous relationship reduces the risk of STIs and RTIs. ❑ Contact tracing and effective treatment.
Bacterial vaginosis (BV) Trichomonas vaginitis	❑ Protozoal *Gardnerella vaginalis* *Trichomonas vaginalis*	❑ Screening in asymptomatic or symptomatic cases for STIs and RTIs.
Monilial vaginitis	❑ Fungal *Candida albicans*	
Scabies Pediculosis pubis	❑ Ectoparasites Sarcoptes scabiei Crab louse (Phthirus pubis)	❑ Aseptic procedures in delivery, MTP procedures and IUCD insertion.

37. Which one of the following is NOT a characteristic feature of bacterial vaginosis:

a. Presence of clue cells
b. Thick white discharge
c. Vaginal pH > 4.5
d. Fishy odour

Thick, curdy white discharge in flakes is suggestive of candidiasis.

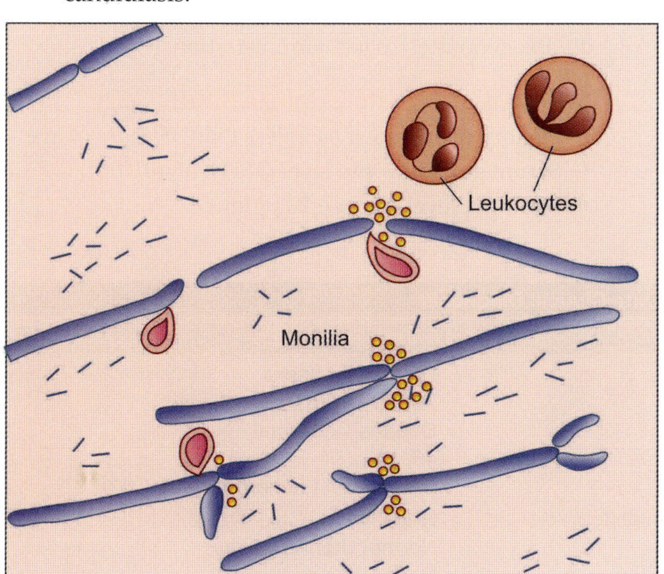

Physical appearance of *Candida albicans*

38. The commonest complication of pregnancy after complete treatment of genital TB is:

a. Abortion
b. Ectopic pregnancy
c. Malpresentation
d. Intrauterine death

In terms of future reproduction the prognosis of genital TB is most unfavorable. Pregnancy is rare (5-10%), and is occurs, chance of ectopic pregnancy is more (40%). In uterine pregnancy, abortion is likely and a pregnancy going upto term is a rare event.

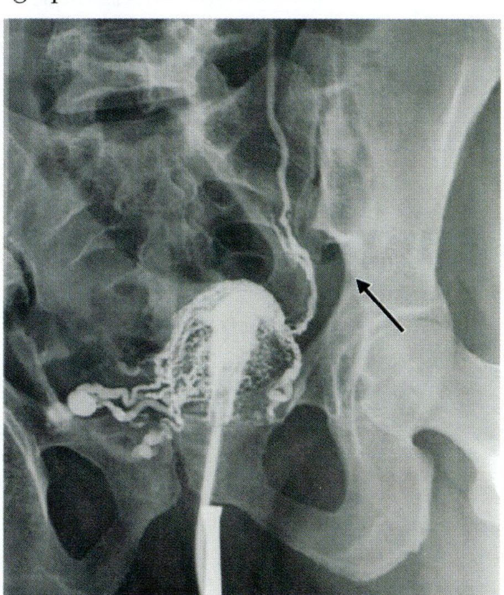

Hysterosalpingogram showing marked extravasation of dye in venous and lymphatic channels. It was proved to be a case of tubercular endometritis [*By courtesy Dr. H. Roy, Patna*]

39. True about genital infection in bacterial vaginosis are all EXCEPT:

a. Clue cells present
b. Gardnerella is the causative agent
c. Pruritus seen
d. Grey and foul smelling discharge

Clinically, BV is characterised by creamy vaginal discharge with fishy smell without extensive evidence of inflammation.

Ans. 37. **b.** Thick white discharge 38. **b.** Ectopic pregnancy 39. **c.** Pruritus seen

40. Most common symptom of acute pelvic inflammatory disease:

a. Bleeding per vaginum
b. Abdominal pain
c. Vomiting
d. Amenorrhoea

Patients with acute PID present with a wide range of non-specific clinical symptoms. Symptoms usually appear at the time and immediately after the menstruation. Bilateral lower abdominal and pelvic pain which is dull in nature. The onset of pain is more rapid and acute in gonococcal infection (3 days) than in chlamydial infection (5-7 days).

Clinical Features of Acute Salpingitis, Acute Appendicitis and Disturbed Ectopic

Symptoms and signs	*Acute salpingitis*	*Acute appendicitis*	*Disturbed ectopic*
❑ Pain	Acute lower abdominal on both sides	Starts near umbilicus but settles to right iliac fossa	Acute lower abdomen on one side
❑ Amenorrhea and bleeding PV	Unrelated	Unrelated	Usually Present
❑ GI symptoms such as nausea, vomiting	Inconsistently present	Usual	Absent
❑ General look	Face-flushed	Toxic	Pale
❑ Tongue	No significant change	Furred	Pale
❑ Pulse	Rapid but proportionate with temperature	Rapid, out of proportion to temperature	Persistent rise even with normal temperature
❑ Temperature	More raised	Slightly raised	Not raised
❑ Tenderness	Lower abdomen on both sides	On McBurney's point may have muscle guard	Lower abdomen more on one side
❑ Per vaginum	Tenderness on both fornices. A mass may be felt	Tenderness on right fornix and high up	Mass may be felt through one fornix extending up to pouch of Douglas

MENSTRUAL DISTURBANCES

41. A 36 years old woman has absence of menses for the last 4 months. Pregnancy test is negative. Serum levels of LH and FSH are raised. Serum estradiol level is low. These findings suggest:

a. Bilateral tubal obstruction
b. PCOD
c. Premature menopause
d. Exogenous estrogen administration

Diagnosis of premature ovarian insufficiency

- History of amenorrhea in less than 35 years of age
- Serum gonadotropin level (FSH >40 mIU/ml) is high
- Serum E_2 level is low (<20 pg/ml)

Special Investigations in a Case of Primary Amenorrhea to Corroborate Clinical Diagnosis

Probable diagnosis	*Investigations*	*Findings*
Müllerian agenesis (Mayer-Rokitansky–Küster-Hauser syndrome)	❑ Ultrasonography ❑ Laparoscopy ❑ Karyotype ❑ IVP	Uterus — absent Tubes — present Ovaries — normal 46, XX Urinary tract abnormalities (30%)
Unresponsive endometrium	❑ *Progesterone challenge test ❑ HSG/hysteroscopy ❑ Hormonal studies	Negative Normal Uterine Cavity Normal
Uterine synechiae	❑ Progesterone challenge test ❑ HSG ❑ Hysteroscopy	Negative Honeycomb appearance Direct visualization
Tubercular	❑ Blood — ESR ❑ X-Ray — Chest ❑ Mantoux test ❑ Endometrial biopsy	Raised May have positive finding Positive (usually) Positive lesion may be detected

Contd...

Ans. **40. b.** Abdominal pain **41. c.** Premature menopause

Contd...

Probable diagnosis	*Investigations*	*Findings*
Hypogonadotropic–hypogonadism	– Progesterone challenge test – Serum gonadotropins – Serum estradiol	Negative Low < 5 mIU/mL Low (< 20 pg/mL)
Primary ovarian failure (see p. 444)	❑ Karyotype ❑ Serum estradiol ❑ Serum gonadotropins ❑ Ovarian biopsy (ovaries — small/ ❑ Streak) ovarian biopsy is not essential for diagnosis	46, XX Low (< 20 pg/mL) Elevated > 40 mIU/mL (i) Afollicular (common), (ii) follicular or (iii) autoimmune (lymphocytic infiltration) type. Follicles are present in resistant ovarian syndrome
Turner (p. 422)	❑ Laparoscopy ❑ Serum gonadotropins ❑ Karyotype	'Streak' gonads High 45, XO or 45, XO/46, XX
Androgen insensitivity syndrome (p. 424)	❑ Laparoscopy ❑ Serum testosterone ❑ Karyotype ❑ Gonadal biopsy	Uterus — absent Tubes — absent Equal to normal males 46, XY Testicular structure
Adrenogenital syndrome (p. 421)	❑ Karyotype ❑ Serum 17 hydroxy-progesterone ❑ Urinary pregnanetriol	46, XX Elevated (> 8 ng/mL) Elevated
Thyroid dysfunction (Hypo)	❑ Serum TSH ❑ T_3, T_4	Elevated Lowered
Diabetes	❑ Blood sugar	Elevated

* The test is performed by administrating injection progesterone in oil 75 mg IM or Tablet medroxyprogesterone 10 mg daily or micronized progesterone 200 mg daily for 10 days. Withdrawal bleeding usually occurs within 10 days, if the test is positive

42. Increased LH: FSH ratio is seen in:

a. Premature menopause
b. Sheehan syndrome
c. PCOD
d. Turners syndrome

Hypothalamic-pituitary compartment in PCOS

- Increased pulse frequency of GnRH leads to increased pulse frequency of LH
- Increased pulse frequency and amplitude of LH results in tonically elevated level of LH
- FSH level is not increased. This is mainly due to the negative feedback of chronically elevated estrogen and the follicular inhibin

Scheme–1

Hypothalamus→Increased pulse frequency of GnRH→Pituitary sensitivity to GnRH↓ →Increased pulse frequency of LH (preferential) compared to FSH→LH (↑): FSH (↓)

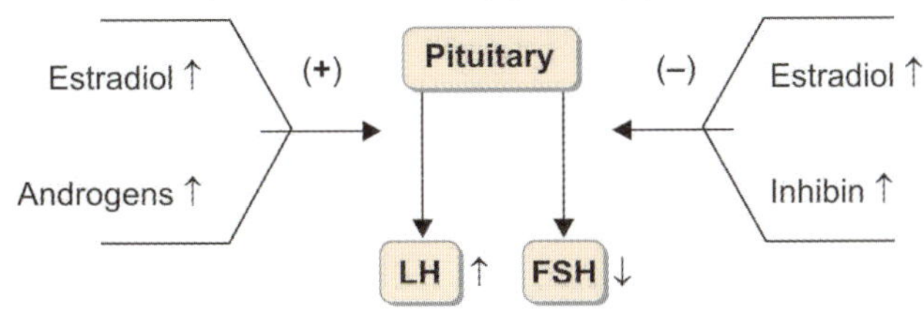

43. Menstrual blood in menorrhagia is:

a. More than 20 ml
b. More than 40 ml
c. More than 60 ml
d. More than 80 ml

Menorrhagia/hypermenorrhea is defined as cyclic bleeding at normal intervals; the bleeding is either excessive in amount (>80 mL) or duration (>7 days) or both. The term menotaxis is often used to denote prolonged bleeding.

Common Causes of Menorrhagia
❑ Dysfunctional uterine bleeding
❑ Fibroid uterus
❑ Adenomyosis
❑ Chronic tubo-ovarian mass

44. The most common cause secondary amenorrhea in India is:

a. Endometrial TB
b. Premature ovarian failure
c. Polycystic ovarian syndrome
d. Sheehan's syndrome

Secondary amenorrhea is more common menstrual abnormality noted in endometrial TB. It may be the only presenting symptom that makes the patient to seek medical advice.

Ans. 42. c. PCOD 43. d. More than 80 ml 44. a. Endometrial TB

Etiopathogenesis of Secondary Amenorrhea	
Etiology	*Mechanism*
Uterine factors ❑ Tubercular endometritis ❑ Postradiation ❑ Synechiae ❑ Surgical removal	❑ Destruction of the endometrium or inhibition of ovarian function by tubercular toxin ❑ Destruction of the endometrium ❑ Intrauterine adhesions → viscerocortical reflex → amenorrhea ❑ Ablation of endometrium by laser, resectoscope
Ovarian factors ❑ Polycystic ovarian syndrome ❑ Premature ovarian failure ❑ Resistant ovarian syndrome (Savage's syndrome)	❑ Tonically elevated LH → Increased androgen production from the theca (PCOS) cells and stroma of the ovaries → Decrease SHBG → increased unbound estrogens and androgens → Pituitary sensitivity to GnRH is increased → Preferential increased production of LH, decreased production of FSH due to inhibin. Disturbed adrenal function is also implicated in androgen excess. A state of hyperandrogenism produces amenorrhea by its antiestrogenic action ❑ Absence of follicle or accelerated rate of depletion of follicles in the ovaries ❑ Follicles are present but are resistant to gonadotropins (defect in FSH receptor)
❑ Hyperestrogenic state – Persistent follicles in metropathia – Feminizing tumor of the ovary (Granulosa cell tumor)	❑ The estrogen level remains high and there is no fluctuation As such, so long as endometrial support is not lost, amenorrhea continues
❑ Masculinizing tumor of the ovary (Sertoli-Leydig cell tumor) ❑ Hypo-estrogenic state – Ablation of the ovaries – Pelvic radiation	❑ Androgen excess opposes the effect of estrogen on the endometrium ❑ Removal of the site of production of estrogens ❑ Makes the ovaries unresponsive to gonadotropins
Pituitary factors ❑ Adenoma (prolactinoma) ❑ Cushing's disease ❑ Acromegaly ❑ Sheehan's syndrome ❑ Simmond's disease (unrelated to pregnancy)	❑ Microadenoma usually associated with hyperprolactinemia ❑ It either inhibits ovarian steroidogenesis directly or inhibits pituitary gonadotropin release. ❑ There is partial or complete destruction of the pituitary by ischemia caused by venous thrombosis following severe postpartum hemorrhage and shock. The principal hormones affected are growth hormone, gonadotropins, TSH, adrenocorticotropins and prolactin
Hypothalamic factors ❑ Psychogenic shock, stress, anorexia nervosa, strenuous exercise, pseudocyesis, etc. ❑ Congenital malformation ❑ Trauma: Accidents, surgery or radiotherapy ❑ Infection: Tubercular or sarcoid granulomas ❑ Tumors: Craniopharyngioma, meningioma	❑ Inhibit the release of GnRH or affect dopamine metabolism There is low level of estrogen and LH but FSH level remains normal (see below) Lead to hypogonadotropic hypogonadism. There may be hyperprolactinemia due to altered dopamine inhibition. Tumors of the hypothalamus or pituitary need surgical excision or radiotherapy. Management needs a team approach including a neurosurgeon, a radiotherapist and an endocrinologist
Adrenal factors ❑ Adrenal tumor or hyperplasia ❑ Cushing syndrome	❑ Androgen excess opposes the effect of estrogen on the endometrium ❑ —do— —do—
Thyroid factors ❑ Hypothyroid state	❑ Raised TSH and hyperprolactinemia by direct action of TRH on the galactophore cells in the pituitary
General disease ❑ Malnutrition, tuberculosis, chronic nephritis, diabetes, etc.	❑ Probably affecting the hypothalamopituitary ovarian axis
Iatrogenic ❑ Contraceptive pills (post pill amenorrhea) ❑ Psychotrophic phenothiazine derivative drugs ❑ Antihypertensive drugs like reserpine or dopamine antagonists	❑ Suppression of GnRH release ❑ Dopamine receptor blocking agents raise the prolactin level ❑ Dopamine depleting agents raise the prolactin level

45. NOT a feature of Polycystic ovarian syndrome:

a. Infertility b. Obesity
c. Polymenorrhea d. Hirsutism

PCOS was originally described in 1935 by Stein and Leventhal as a syndrome manifested by amenorrhea, hirsutism and obesity associated with enlarged polycystic ovaries.

Common Causes of Secondary Amenorrhea

Hypothalamus	Pituitary	Ovary	Uterine	Systemic
❑ Stress				
❑ Post pill	❑ Adenoma	❑ PCOS		❑ Malnutrition
❑ Sudden change in weight—either too much loss or too much gain	❑ Sheehan's	❑ Premature ovarian failure	❑ Synechiae	❑ Hypothyroid state
❑ Psychotropic and antihypertensive drugs				❑ Diabetes

46. In case of dysfunctional uterine bleeding, the hormone which is DEFICIENT:

a. Estrogen b. Progesterone
c. ACTH d. Cortisone

Anovular bleeding in DUB is usually excessive. In the absence of growth limiting progesterone due to anovulation, the endometrial growth is under the influence of estrogen throughout the cycle. There is inadequate structural stromal support and the endometrium remains fragile. Thus, with the withdrawal of estrogen due to negative feedback action of FSH, the endometrial shedding continues for a longer period in asynchronous sequences because of lack of compactness.

Medical Management of Dub
A. Hormones – Norethisterone acetate – Medroxyprogesterone acetate – Dydrogesterone – Equine conjugated estrogen – Combined estrogens and progestogens (contraceptive pills) – 19 norsteroid derivative (Gestrinone) – Danazol (17 α-ethinyl testosterone) – Progestin releasing IUCD LNG – ius – Mifepristone (RU 486) – GNRH analogues – Desmopressin
B. Prostaglandin synthetase inhibitors (PSI) – Fenamates (Mefenamic acid)
C. Antifibrinolytic agents – Tranexamic acid (TA)
For side effects of each drug used

47. In a woman presenting with amenorrhea, headache, blurred vision and galactorrhea, the appropriate investigation is:

a. Prolactin level b. LH
c. FSH d. HCG

Hyperprolactinemia inhibits ovarian steroidogenesis. Hyperprolactinemia causes secondary amenorrhea in about 30% of women. Hyperprolactinemia is commonly due to pituitary adenomas (microadenoma or macroadenoma). Visual field examination is essential to detect any compression effect on the optic nerves.

(See diagram on next page)

48. Hot flushes in postmenopausal women are best treated with which of the following:

a. Estrogen b. Danazol
c. OCP d. Tamoxifen

The characteristic symptom of menopause is "hot flush" (vasomotor symptoms). Hot flush is characterized by sudden feeling of heat followed by profuse sweating.

Benefits of Hormone Replacement Therapy (Hrt)
❑ Improvement of vasomotor symptoms (70– 80%)
❑ Improvement urogenital atrophy
❑ Increase in bone mineral density (2–5%)
❑ Decreased risk in vertebral and hip fractures (25–50%)
❑ Reduction in colorectal cancer (20%)
❑ Possibly cardioprotection

49. Cystoglandular hyperplasia is a feature of:

a. Metropathia hemorrhagica
b. Oligomenorrhea
c. Polymenorrhea
d. Menorrhagia

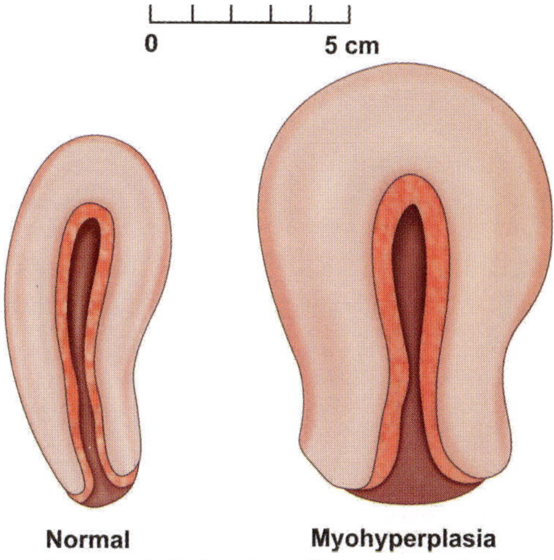

Increased uterine size with myohyperplasia

Ans. 45. c. Polymenorrhea 46. b. Progesterone 47. a. Prolactin level 48. a. Estrogen
49. a. Metropathia hemorrhagica

Scheme B

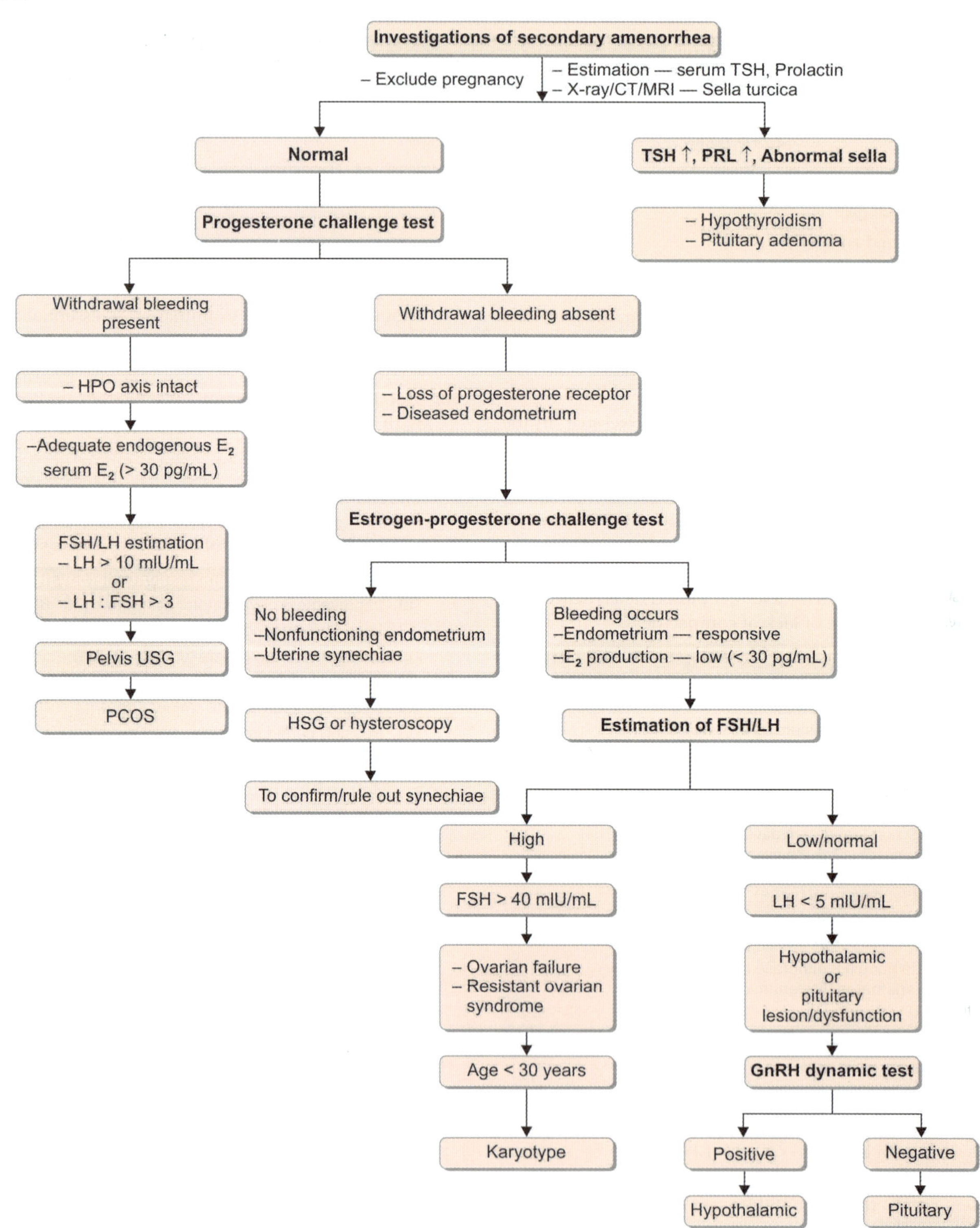

Volume II Clinical Subjects

Cystic glandular hyperplasia/Metropathia hem-orrhagica/ Schroeder's disease is a type of abnormal bleeding usually met in premenopausal women. Bleeding is prolonged until the endometrium and blood vessels regenerate to control it.

50. A 10 years old girl presented with primary amenorrhea, absent breasts, malformed uterus. The most likely diagnosis is:

a. Mayer Rokitansky Kuster Hauser syndrome
b. Turner's syndrome
c. Swyers syndrome
d. Mixed gonadal dysgenesis

Turner's syndrome cases usually present as primary amenorrhea with delayed secondary sex characters. Vagina, uterus and fallopian tubes are present. The uterus is small but is responsive to exogenous estrogen.

Diagnosis of Primary Amenorrhea based on Clinical Examinations

Physical appearance	*External genitalia*	*Internal genitalia*	*Probable diagnosis*
❑ Secondary sex characters ❑ Stature			
❑ Normal breast development ❑ Normal sexual hair ❑ Average stature	❑ Normal	❑ Absence of vagina ❑ Absent uterus	❑ Müllerian agenesis (Mayer-Rokitansky–Küster-Hauser syndrome)
—do—	—do—	❑ Normal	❑ Unresponsive endometrium — receptor defect (Rare) ❑ Uterine synechiae (Rare)
❑ Poor breast development ❑ Scanty pubic hair ❑ Average stature	❑ Underdeveloped	❑ Underdeveloped (vaginal rugosity absent)	❑ Hypogonadotropic – hypogonadism
❑ Tall and lanky	—do—	—do—	❑ Primary ovarian failure
❑ Poor secondary sex characters ❑ Stature — short ❑ Webbing of the neck and cubitus valgus present ❑ Congenital malformations of cardiac, renal or great vessels (coarctation of aorta)	—do—	—do— 'Streak' gonads	❑ ❑ Turner's syndrome ❑ ❑ ❑ ❑ ❑
❑ Phenotypically female ❑ Average height ❑ Delayed secondary sex characters	Normal	Bilateral 'streak' gonads	❑ ❑ Pure gonadal dysgenesis
❑ Normal breast development without areolar pigmentation ❑ Scanty pubic and axillary hair ❑ Average stature	❑ Labial or inguinal gonads	❑ Short blind vagina ❑ Absence of uterus	❑ ❑ Androgen insensitivity syndrome
❑ Normal phenotypically female ❑ Average stature	❑ Labial fusion ❑ Enlargement of clitoris	❑ Normal	❑ Adrenogenital syndrome (Late onset)
❑ Features of (Hypogonadotropic hypogonadism) – Short stature – Mental retardation – Obesity, retinitis pigmentosa	❑ Underdeveloped	❑ Underdeveloped	❑ Cretinism due to hypothyroidism ❑ ❑ Hypothalamo-pituitary dysfunction (rare) – Kallmann syndrome – Prader–Labhardt – Willi syndrome – Laurence – Moon – Bardet–Biedl syndrome (rare)

Ans. 50. **b.** Turners syndrome

51. LH/FSH ratio is increased in:

a. Turners syndrome b. Sheehans syndrome
c. Premature menopause d. Polycystic ovarian disease

In PCOS, LH level is elevated and/or the ratio LH:FSH is >2:1.

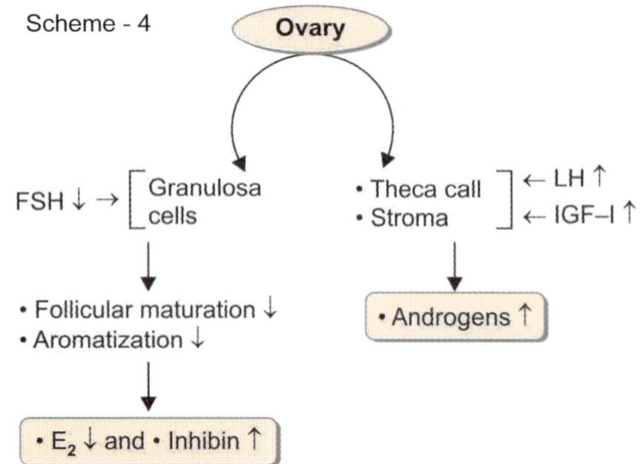

52. NOT classified as primary amenorrhea:

a. Mayer Rokitansky Kuster Hauser syndrome
b. Kaftan's syndrome
c. Sheehan' syndrome
d. All of the above

In Sheehan's syndrome there is history of severe post-partum hemorrhage, shock or even infection. The common manifestations are failing lactation, loss of pubic and axillary hair, lethargy, hypotension, secondary amenorrhea and atrophy of the breasts and genitalia.

(See Diagram on next page)

53. A patient presented with primary amenorrhoea with developed secondary characters and a bulging at hymen. Most probable diagnosis is:

a. PCOS
b. Rokitansky-Kuster-Hauser syndrome
c. Imperforate hymen
d. Kallmann's syndrome

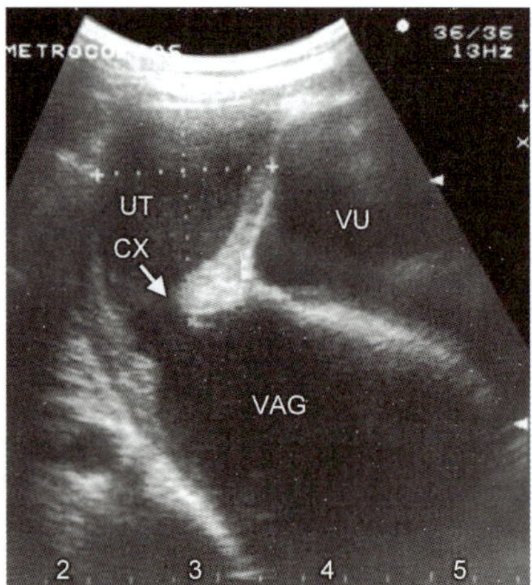

Ultrasonographic view of hematometra and hematocolpos in a girl with imperforate hymen

The chief complains of imperforate hymen are periodic lower abdominal pain, which may be continuous, primary amenorrhoea and urinary symptoms, such as frquency, dysuria or even retention of urine. Vulval inspection reveals a tense bulging membrane of bluish coloration.

54. True for Mayer-Rokitansky-Kuster-Hauser syndrome:

a. Uterus present; tubes and ovaries absent
b. Uterus absent; tubes and ovaries present
c. All are absent
d. All are present

Findings in Mullerian agenesis/MRKH syndrome: Uterus – absent; tubes – present and ovaries – normal.

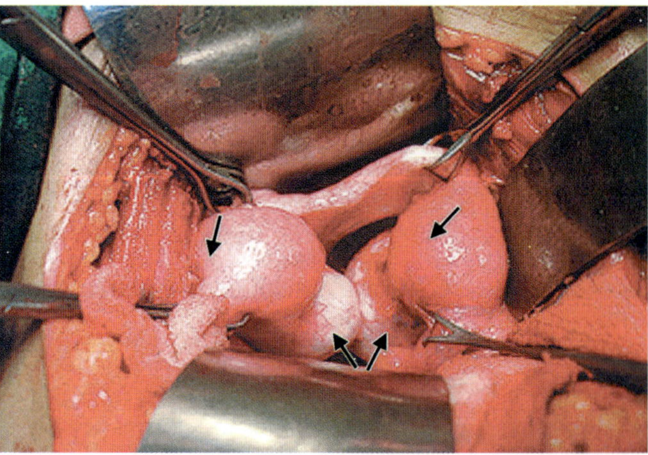

Müllerian agenesis with small uterine knobs one on either side (down arrow). Normal ovaries are seen (up arrow). Cervix and vagina were absent in this case [*By courtesy*: Dr PK Biswas, Professor, Department of Obstetrics and Gynecology, CNMCH, Kolkata]

55. A female presented with primary amenorrhea, normal breast development but scanty pubic hair. Most probably she is having:

a. Turner syndrome
b. Mullerin agenesis
c. Testicular feminizing syndrome
d. Gonadal dysgenesis

TFS/androgen insensitivity syndrome

- Usually presents with primary amenorrhea and or infertility
- Breast development is adequate
- Absent or sparse axillary and pubic hair

Differentiation of a normal looking girl presenting with primary amenorrhea having normal breast development but absent uterus

Characters	*Androgen insensitivity syndrome*	*Müllerian agenesis (m-RK-H syndrome)*
1. sexual hair (pubic and axillary)	Absent or sparce	Normal female

Contd...

Ans. **51. d.** Polycystic... **52. c.** Sheehan's syndrome **53. c.** Imperforate hymen **54. b.** Uterus absent; tubes... **55. c.** Testicular...

Scheme A

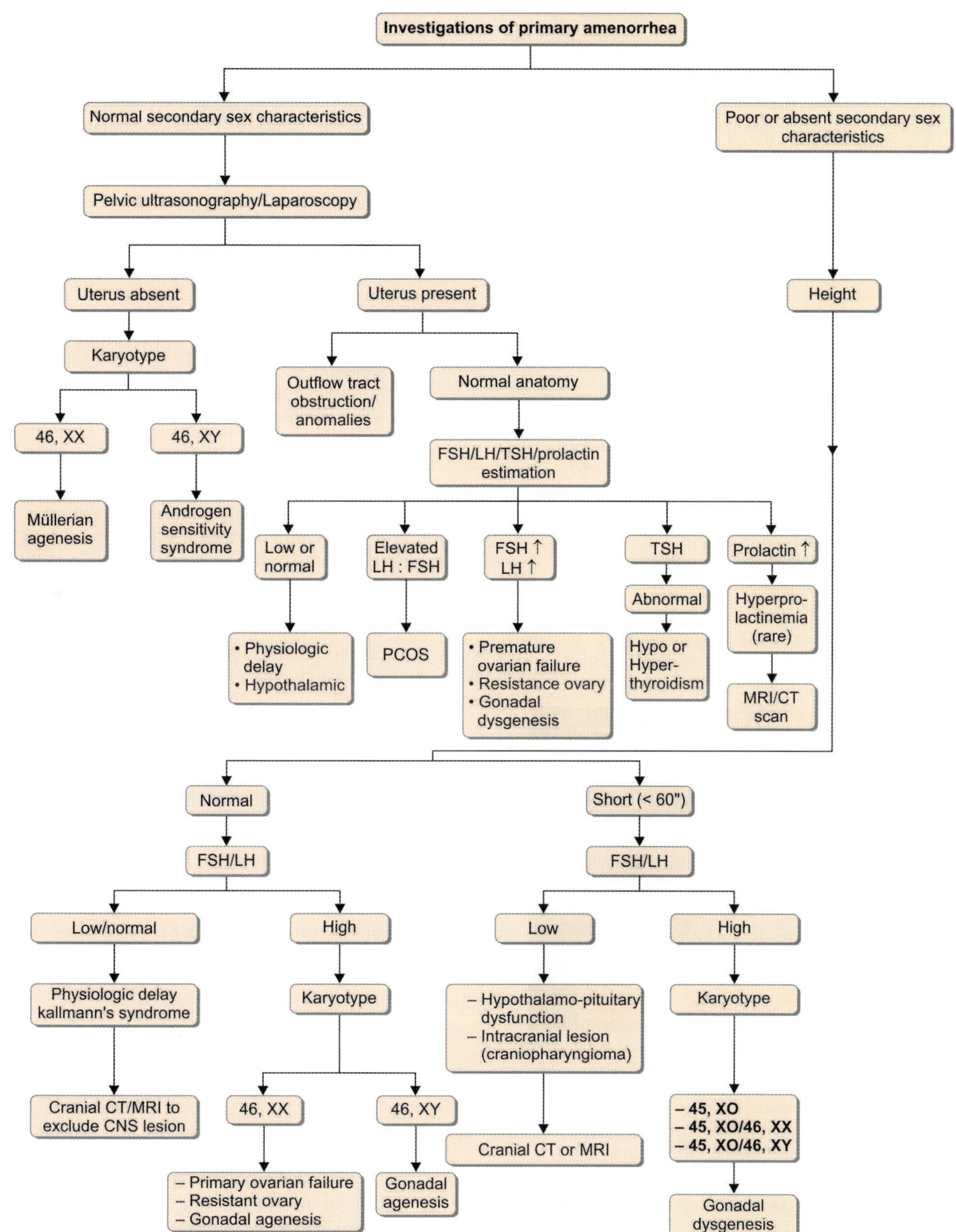
Investigations of primary amenorrhea
Normal secondary sex characteristics
Poor or absent secondary sex characteristics
Pelvic ultrasonography/Laparoscopy
Uterus absent
Uterus present
Height
Karyotype
Outflow tract obstruction/ anomalies
Normal anatomy
46, XX
46, XY
FSH/LH/TSH/prolactin estimation
Müllerian agenesis
Androgen sensitivity syndrome
Low or normal
Elevated LH : FSH
FSH ↑ LH ↑
TSH
Prolactin ↑
Abnormal
Hyperpro-lactinemia (rare)
• Physiologic delay
• Hypothalamic
PCOS
• Premature ovarian failure
• Resistance ovary
• Gonadal dysgenesis
Hypo or Hyper-thyroidism
MRI/CT scan
Normal
Short (< 60")
FSH/LH
FSH/LH
Low/normal
High
Low
High
Physiologic delay kallmann's syndrome
Karyotype
– Hypothalamo-pituitary dysfunction
– Intracranial lesion (craniopharyngioma)
Karyotype
Cranial CT/MRI to exclude CNS lesion
46, XX
46, XY
Cranial CT or MRI
– 45, XO
– 45, XO/46, XX
– 45, XO/46, XY
– Primary ovarian failure
– Resistant ovary
– Gonadal agenesis
Gonadal agenesis
Gonadal dysgenesis

Contd...

Characters	*Androgen insensitivity syndrome*	*Müllerian agenesis (m-RK-H syndrome)*
2. Primary amenorrhea	Present	Present
3. Vagina	Short and blind	Absent
4. Clitoris	Enlarged	Normal female
5. Gonads: – Structure – Location	Testes inguinal, labial or abdominal	Ovary Abdominal
6. Breasts	Developed	Developed
7. Serum testosterone level	Slightly elevated	Normal female
8. Müllerian system	Absent	Absent or rudimentary
9. Wolffian system	Absent	Absent
10. Karyotype	46, XY	46, XX
11. Associated anomalies	Rare	Skeletal 12% and urological (renal) 47%

56. Primary amenorrhoea is a feature of all EXCEPT:

a. Turner's syndrome
b. Stein-Leventhal syndrome
c. Rokitansky-Kustner-Hauser syndrome
d. Kallman syndrome

Patient with PCOS/ Stein Leventhal syndrome complains of increasing obesity (abdominal – 50%), menstrual abnormalities (70%) in the form of oligomenorrhea, secondary amenorrhhea or DUB and infertility.

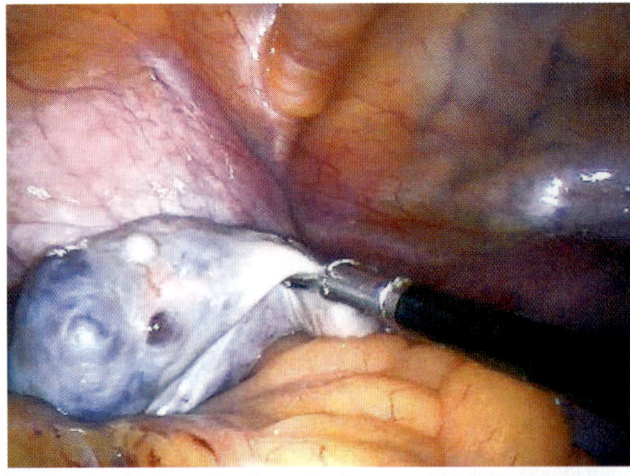

Laparoscopic view of polycystic changes (PCOS) of the ovary. Multiple small peripheral cysts are seen on the ovarian surface

57. Irregular and infrequent menstruation is known as:

a. Amenorrhoea b. Oligomenorrhoea
c. Polymenorrhoea d. Menorrhagia

Menstrual bleeding occurring more than 35 days apart and which remains constant at that frequency is called oligomenorrhea.

Common Causes of Oligomenorrhea
❑ Age-related—during adolescence and preceding menopause
❑ Weight-related—obesity
❑ Stress and exercise related
❑ Endocrine disorders—PCOS (commonest), hyperprolactinemia, hyperthyroidism
❑ Androgen producing tumors—ovarian, adrenal
❑ Tubercular endometritis—late cases
❑ **Drugs:** – Phenothiazines • Cimetidine • Methyldopa

GYNECOLOGICAL ONCOLOGY

58. All are germ cell tumours EXCEPT:

a. Teratoma b. Clear cell tumour
c. Endodermal sinus tumour
d. Dysgerminoma

Germ cell tumors

- The **germinomatous** or **seminomatous** germ cell tumors (GGCT, SGCT) include only germinoma and its synonyms dysgerminoma and seminoma.
- The **nongerminomatous** or **nonseminomatous** germ cell tumors (NGGCT, NSGCT) include embryonal carcinoma, endodermal sinus tumour/ yolk sac tumour, choriocarcinoma, teratoma, polyembryoma & gonadoblastoma

59. All are associated with trophoblast EXCEPT:

a. Choriocarcinoma
b. H. mole
c. Placental site trophoblast tumour
d. Chorioangioma

Chorioangiomas generally thought to arise as a malformation of the primitive angioblastic tissue of the placenta. The angiomas are perfused by the fetal circulation and thus, when they are large, may represent a significant impediment to fetal cardiac activity. They may also sequester platelets and can in turn give a fetal thrombocytopenia.

60. Endometrial carcinoma stage I is best managed by:

a. Wait & watch
b. Chemotherapy followed by radiotherapy
c. Simple hysterectomy
d. Bilateral salpingo-oophorectomy

Treatment options for stage I endometrial carcinoma

- Surgery (total hysterectomy and bilateral salpingo-oophorectomy). Lymph nodes in the pelvis and abdomen may also be removed and sent for histological examination.
- Surgery (total hysterectomy and bilateral salpingo-oophorectomy, with or without removal of lymph nodes in the pelvis and abdomen) followed by internal or external radiation therapy to the pelvis.

Ans. 56. **b.** Stein-Leventhal... 57. **b.** Oligomenorrhoea 58. **b.** Clear cell... 59. **d.** Chorioangioma 60. **c.** Simple hysterectomy

- Radiation therapy alone for patients who cannot have surgery.
- Surgery followed by adjuvant chemotherapy with or without radiation therapy in stage I endometrial cancer that is likely to recur

61. MC cause of postmenopausal bleeding in women is:

a. Ca cervix   b. Ca endometrium
c. Hormone replacement therapy
d. Senile endometritis

Symptoms of carcinoma endometrium include postmenopausal bleeding (75%) which may be slight, irregular or continuous. The bleeding at times may be excessive. A case of postmenopausal bleeding is considered to be due to endometrial carcinoma unless proved otherwise.

Common Causes of Postmenopausal Bleeding	
❑ Genital malignancy	❑ Decubitus ulcer
❑ DUB	❑ Urethral caruncle
❑ Senile endometritis	❑ Retained pessary or IUCD

62. MC cause of pyometra:

a. Uterine myoma   b. Carcinoma vagina
c. Carcinoma cervix   d. Carcinoma endometrium

The gynecological conditions which are associated with pyometra are: (a) Carcinoma in the lower part of the body of uterus, (b) Endocervical carcinoma, (c) Senile endometritis, (d) Infected hematometra following amputation, conization or deep cauterization of cervix, (e) Tubercular endometritis.

63. Best management of a 40 years old lady with CIN-III:

a. Punch biopsy
b. Total abdominal hysterectomy
c. Wertheim's hysterectomy
d. Conization

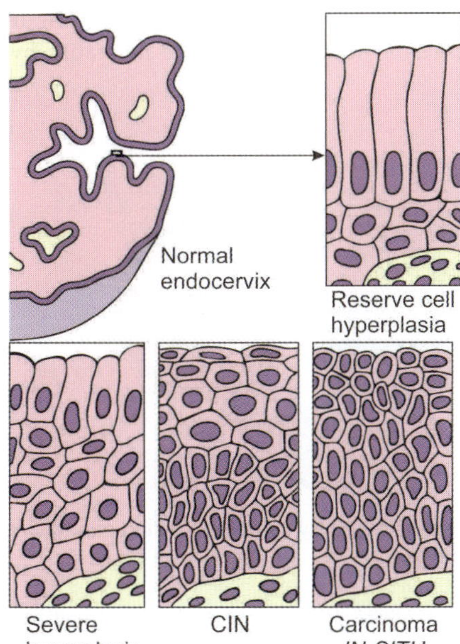

Continuum of changes from reserve cell hyperplasia to carcinoma *in situ* through severe hyperplasia, CIN and CIS

Hysterectomy is done in patients with CIN grade III, CIN associated with other gynecologic problems (prolapse, fibroid, PID or endometriosis), CIN extended into vagina, high grade CGIN in elderly patients, etc.

64. MC degenerative change in uterine myoma:

a. Hemorrhage
b. Malignant change
c. Hyaline degeneration
d. Red degeneration

Hyaline degeneration is the MC (65%) type of degeneration affecting all sizes of fibroids except the tiny one. It is more common specially in tumors having more connective tissue.

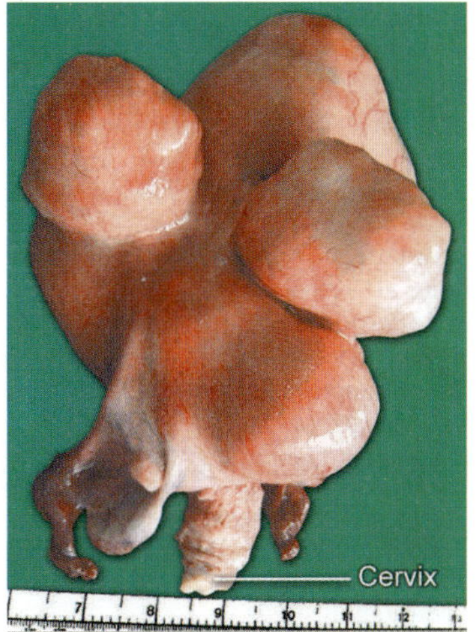

Multiple fibroids causing marked distortion of the uterus. The uterine corpus is almost completely replaced by multiple myomas in subserous, intramural and submucous positions.

65. MC malignancy of ovary:

a. Granulosa cell tumour
b. Dermoid cyst
c. Mucinous
d. Serous cyst adenoma

Serous cyst arises from the totipotent surface epithelium of the ovary. It is quite common and accounts for about 40% of ovarian tumors. It is bilateral in about 40% and chance of malignancy is about 40%.

Classification of Ovarian Tumor

I. **Epithelial tumor (60–70%)**
These tumors may be benign, borderline malignant or malignant.
a. Serous tumor
b. Mucinous cyst adenoma
c. Endometrioid tumors
d. Mesonephroid or clear cell tumors
e. Brenner tumors
f. Mixed epithelial tumors
g. Undiff erentiated carcinoma
h. Unclassified epithelial tumors

Contd...

Ans. 61. b. Ca endometrium 62. c. Carcinoma cervix 63. b. Total abdominal... 64. c. Hyaline degeneration 65. d. Serous cyst adenoma

Contd...

Classification of Ovarian Tumor
II. Sex cord stromal tumors (6–10%) a. Granulosa cell tumors b. Tumors of thecoma-fibroma group ❑ Thecoma ❑ Fibroma ❑ Unclassified c. Androblastoma ❑ Sertoli cell tumor ❑ Sertoli leydig cell tumor ❑ Hilus cell tumor d. Gynandroblastoma e. Unclassified
III. Lipid cell tumor
IV. Germ cell tumors of the ovary (20–25% of all primary ovarian neoplasms) i. *Germ cell tumors* a. Dysgerminoma b. Endodermal sinus tumor c. Embryonal cell carcinoma d. Polyembryoma e. Choriocarcinoma f. Teratoma:
i. Immature; ii. Mature (Dermoid cyst); iii. Monodermal: ❑ Struma ovarii ❑ Carcinoid g) Mixed forms (combinations of types A to F) iv. Tumors composed of germ cells and sex cord stromal derivatives a. Gonadoblastoma b. Mixed germ cell — sex cord stromal tumor
V. Gonadoblastoma
VI. Unclassified
VII. Secondary metastasis

66. The risk of endometrial carcinoma is highest with the following histological pattern of endometrial hyperplasia:

a. Simple hyperplasia with atypia
b. Simple hyperplasia without atypia
c. Complex hyperplasia with atypia
d. Complex hyperplasia without atypia

Complex hyperplasia (adenomatous with atypia) progresses to endometrial cancer in about 29% of cases.

Effects of prolonged unopposed estrogen stimulation on endometrium

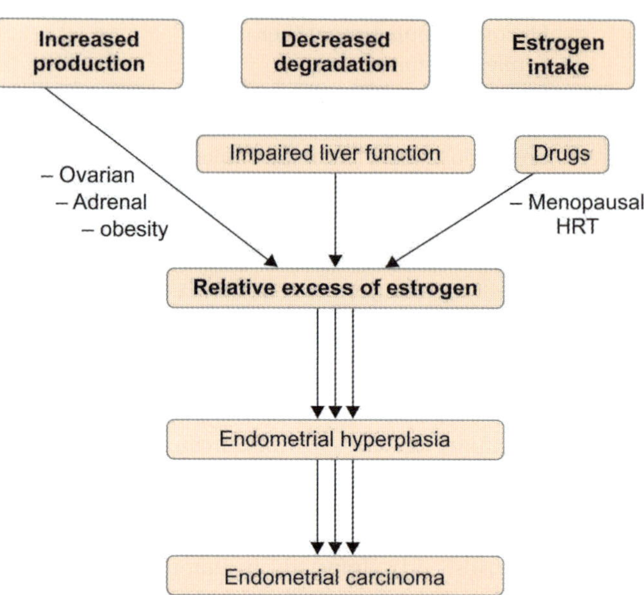

67. Sensitivity of conventional PAP smear in picking up cervical cancer is:

a. 70% b. 80%
c. 90% d. 100%

A single Pap smear has a diagnostic sensitivity of about 60%. False negative results may be up to 25%. Pap smear test has been effective reducing the incidence of cervical cancer by 80% and the mortality by 70%.

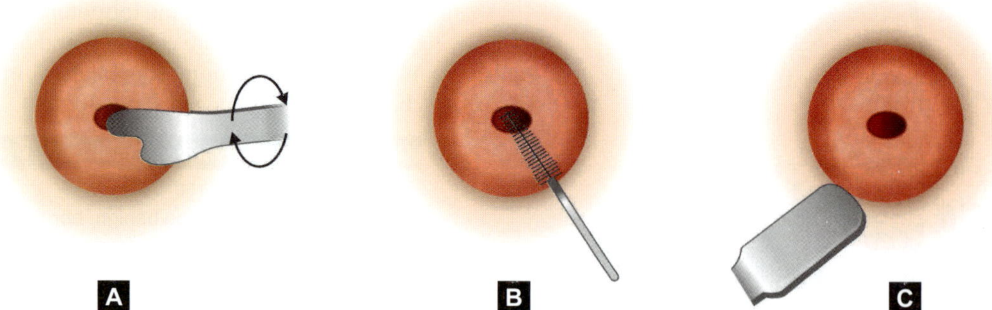

Collection of smear: (A) Using Ayre's spatula from the squamocolumnar junction for screening; (B) By cytobrush taking endocervical sampling for screening; and (C) By wooden spatula from the lateral vaginal fornix for cytohormonal study

68. NOT useful for diagnosis, in a female of 55 years presenting with postmenopausal bleeding:

a. Transvaginal USG b. Postcoital test
c. Pap smear d. Endometrial biopsy

Postcoital test/ PCT is a test for infertility. It is the examination of the cervical mucus to evaluate the presence of progressively motile sperm in it. This test is done several hours after (within 8-12 hours) sexual intercourse.

Ans. **66. c.** Complex hyper... **67. a.** 70% **68. b.** Postcoital test

Infertility Work up Calendar

Identification of factor	*Methods employed*	*Day of cycle*	*Observation*	
Ovulation	❑ BBT	Throughout cycle	Biphasic pattern	
	❑ Endometrial biopsy	D 21–23	Secretory endometrium	
	❑ Cervical mucus	D 12–14 and D 21–23	D 12–14	D 21–23
	Nature		Clear, watery	Thick, viscid
	Threadability		+	–
	Fern pattern		+	–
	❑ Vaginal cytology	D 12–14 and D 21–23	D 12–14	D 21–23
			Discrete cells	Folded edges.
			Pyknotic nuclei,	In clumps
			background	background
			clear	dirty
	❑ Serum progesterone	D 8 and D 21	D-8 < 1 ng/mL	D-21 > 6 ng/mL
	❑ Serum LH ❑ Urinary LH	Midcycle daily (D 12–14)	Ovulation: About 10–12 hours after LH surge	
	❑ Serial transvaginal sonography	D 12–14	Follicular measurements-approaching 20 mm	
	❑ Laparoscopy	Secretory phase	Recent corpus luteum	
Tubal factor	❑ Insufflation test	Proliferative phase - 2 days after the bleeding stops	i. Drop in pressure when raised to 120 mm Hg ii. Hissing sound on iliac fossa iii. Shoulder pain	
	❑ Hysterosalpingography	As above	Spillage of dye into the peritoneal cavity	
	❑ Laparoscopy and dye test	Proliferative phase (7th-10th day of cycle) RCOG	❑ Peritubal pathology ❑ Pelvic pathology (endometriosis) ❑ Ovulation ❑ Tubal patency by dye spillage from both the tubes	
	❑ Sonohysterosalpingography	Proliferative phase	Better than HSG for detection of intra-uterine pathology.	
	❑ Falloposcopy	Proliferative phase	Tubal luminal pathology	
Cervical	❑ Postcoital test (PCT)	Around ovulation (D 12–14)	Presence of progressive motile sperm (10 per high power field)	
	❑ Sperm cervical mucus contact test (SCMCT)	As above	Sperm antibodies	

69. HCG is a tumour marker for:

a. Teratoma b. Serous cystadenoma

c. Colonic carcinoma d. Choriocarcinoma

Choriocarcinoma is a highly malignant tumour arising from the chorionic epithelium. It should be remembered that it is not a tumour of the uterus which is secondarily involved.

Diagnostic criteria for post-molar GTN (FIGO)
Levels of serum βhCG are followed up.
1. ≥ Four values of plateaued hCG (±10%) over at least 3 weeks time.
2. A rise of hCG of > 10% for > 3 values over at least 2 weeks time.
3. Histologic diagnosis of choriocarcinoma.
4. Persistence of hCG beyond 6 months of mole evacuation.

70. Colposcopy used to visualize all EXCEPT:

a. Upper 2/3rd endocervix b. Lower 1/3rd endocervix

c. Lateral fornix d. Vault of vagina

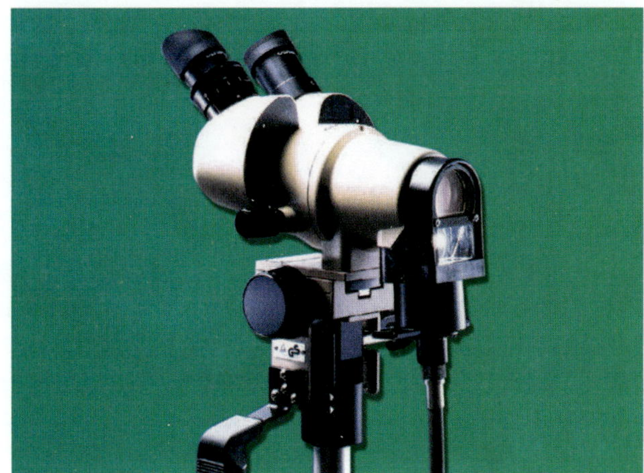

Colposcope

Technique of colposcopy needs ease of maneuver (frontal distance of 225 to 250 mm), magnification (6–16 times), adequate light source (30,000 lux), the stand to permit mobility and the examination table for patient's comfort

Ans. 69. **d.** Choriocarcinoma 70. **a.** Upper 2/3rd endocervix

Colposcope is designed to magnify the surface epithelium of the vaginal part of the cervix including entire transformation zone.

71. Pressure symptoms are commoner with:

a. Submucous fibroid b. Subserous fibroid
c. Both d. None

Pressure symptoms are rare in body fibroids. The fibroids in the posterior wall may be impacted in the pelvis producing constipation, dysuria or even retention of urine. A broad ligament fibroid may produce ureteric compression.

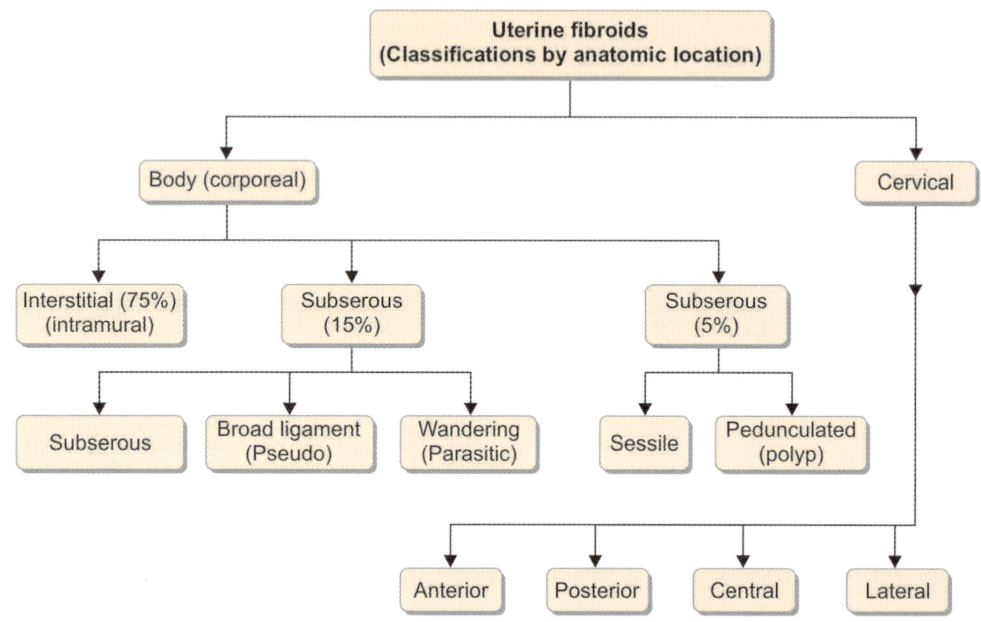

72. Retention of urine may be a feature of:

a. Anterior cervical fibroid
b. Posterior cervical fibroid
c. Central cervical fibroid
d. Lateral cervical fibroid

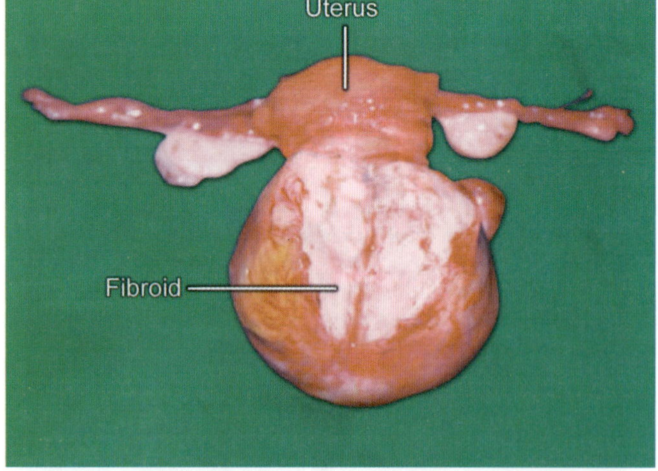

Central cervical fibroid (huge) [*Courtesy: Dr Biswajit Ghosh, Burnpur*]

Anterior cervical fibroid causes bladder symptoms like frequency or even retention of urine. The retention is more due to pressure than elongation of urethra.

Posterior cervical fibroids causes rectal symptoms in the form of constipation.

73. Endometrial carcinoma with vaginal metastasis. This is FIGO stage:

a. Stage III a b. Stage III b
c. Stage III c d. Stage IV a

Stage IIIB is endometrial tumour with vaginal and/or parametrial involvement.

FIGO Surgical Staging of Endometrial Carcinoma (2009)

Stage		*Description*
Stage	I*	Tumor confined to the corpus uteri
	IA*	No or less than half myometrial invasion
	IB*	Invasion equal to or more than half of the myometrium
Stage	II*	Tumor invades cervical stroma, but does not extend beyond the uterus**
Stage	III*	Local and/or regional spread of the tumor
	IIIA*	Tumor invades the serosa of the corpus uteri and/or adnexae*
	IIIB*	Vaginal and/or parametrial involvement*
	IIIC*	Metastases to pelvic and/or paraaortic lymph nodes*
	IIIC1*	Positive pelvic nodes

Contd...

Ans. **71. b.** Subserous fibroid **72. a.** Anterior cervical... **73. b.** Stage III b

Contd...

Stage		*Description*
	IIIC2*	Positive paraaortic lymph nodes with or without positive pelvic lymph nodes
Stage	IV*	Tumor involves bladder and/or bowel mucosa, and/or distant metastases.
	IVA*	Tumor invasion of bladder and/or bowel mucosa
	IVB*	Distant metastases, including intraabdominal metastases and/or inguinal lymph nodes
*Either G_1, G_2 or G_3. Depending upon the percentage of solid nonsquamous component, G_1 has ≤ 5%, G_2 has 6–50% and G_3 has > 50% of solid component. **Endocervical glandular involvement only is considered as stage i and no longer as stage II. *Positive cytology has to be reported separately without changing the stage.		

74. Therapeutic conisation is indicated in:

a. CIN III
b. Cervical metaplasia
c. Microinvasive carcinoma
d. Unsatisfactory colposcopy with cervical dysplasia

Conization/Cone biopsy can be done as a OPD procedure under local anesthesia with colposcopic guidance. Blood loss is less. Conization for CIN is as effective as hysterectomy provided the cone margins are free of disease.

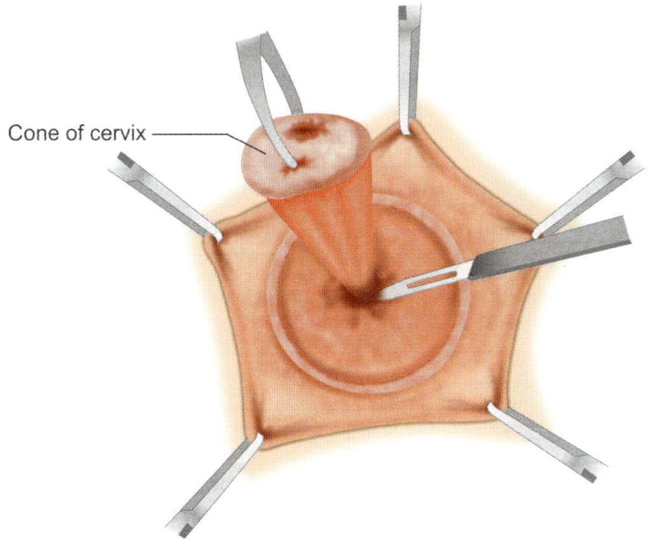

Cone biopsy (knife)

75. Treatment of choice for choriocarcinoma:

a. Observation b. Hysterectomy
c. Chemotherapy with methotrexate
d. Radiotherapy

In general, patients with non-metastatic (low-risk) and good prognosis disease are treated effectively with single agent therapy (methotrexate or actinomycin). The patients with poor prognosis metastatic disease should be treated with combination drug regimen (EMACO regimen).

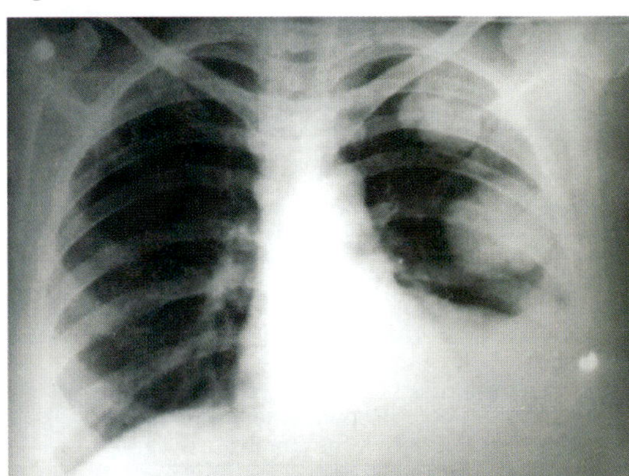

Cannon ball shadow in the left apical and mid region of the lung with pleural effusion in choriocarcinoma [*By courtesy* — Eden Hospital, MCH, Kolkata]

76. Pap smear shows carcinoma-in situ. Next logical procedure:

a. HPV-DNA viral testing b. Hysterectomy
c. Colposcopy and biopsy d. Conization

Colposcopy detects an abnormal area → biopsy is taken under its guidance (targeted biopsy).

(See diagram on next page)

77. Schiller Duval bodies are a feature of:

a. Arrhenoblastoma b. Granulosa cell tumour
c. Choriocarcinoma d. Endodermal sinus tumour

Characteristic histological feature of EST/yolk sac tumor is the presence of cystic spaces lined by flattened epithelium. Within this space a tuft of vascular tissue is often seen. This is called Schiller-Duval body.

Types of malignant germ cell tumor

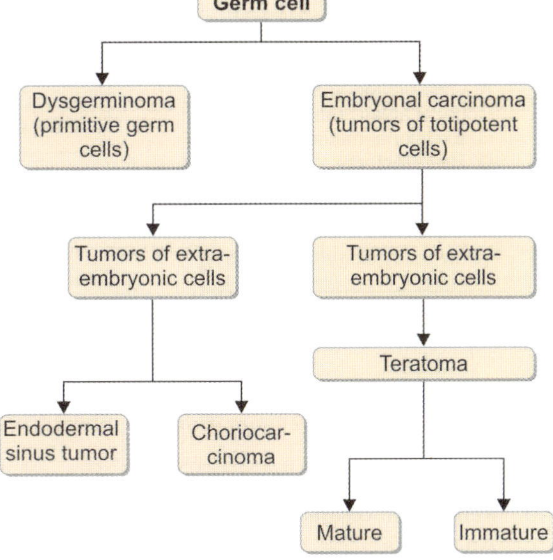

Ans. 74. a. CIN III 75. c. Chemotherapy... 76. c. Colposcopy and... 77. d. Endodermal sinus tumour

Scheme — 3: Evaluation of cervical cytology screening

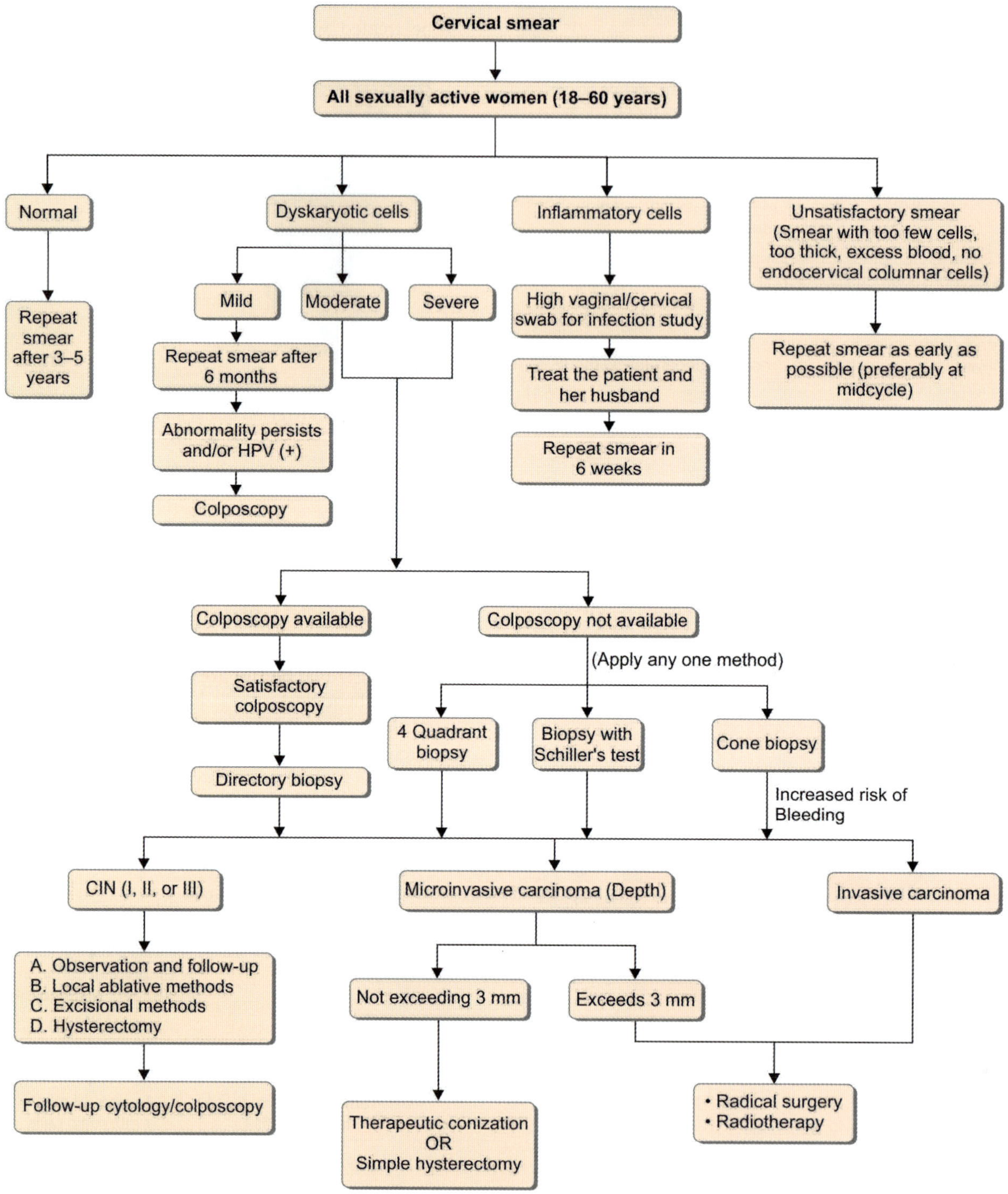

78. Treatment of red degeneration of fibroid during pregnancy is:

a. Termination of pregnancy
b. Removal at cesarean section
c. Analgesics
d. Laparotomy

Red degeneration (carneous degeneration) occurs in a large fibroid mainly during second half of pregnancy and puerperium. The cause is not known but is probably vascular in origin. Infection does not play any part.

Ans. 78. **c.** Analgesics

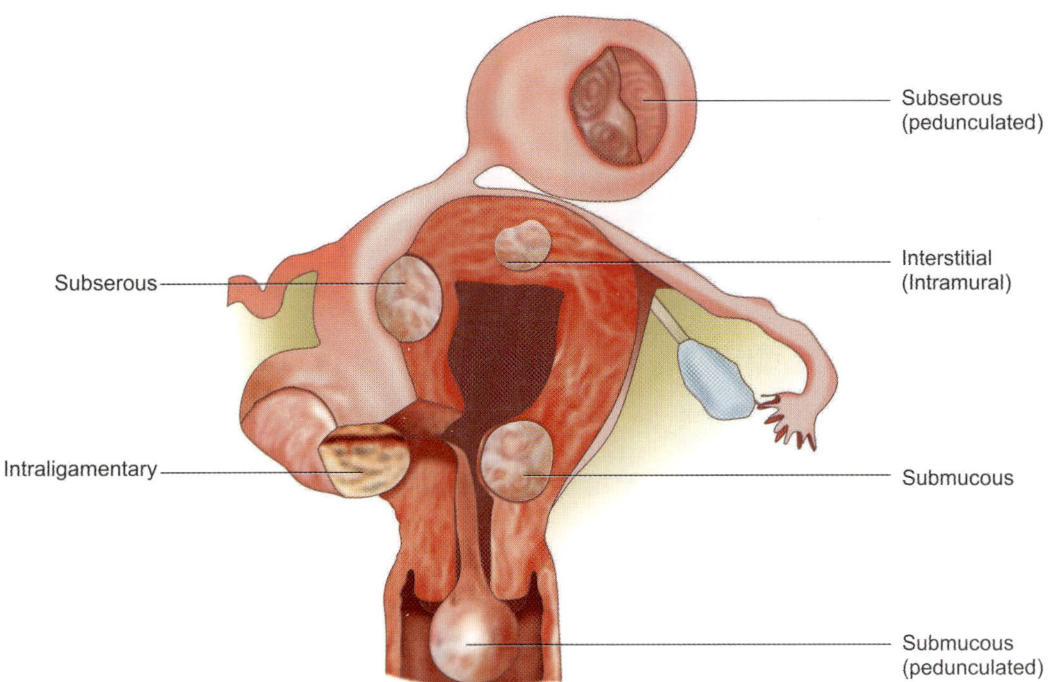

Various types of uterine fibroids

79. Bilateral ovarian tumour:

a. Embryonal cell carcinoma b. Immature teratoma
c. Endodermal sinus tumour d. Dysgerminoma

Dysgerminoma may be bilateral in 10% of cases. It is the commonest (30-40%) malignant germ cell tumor.

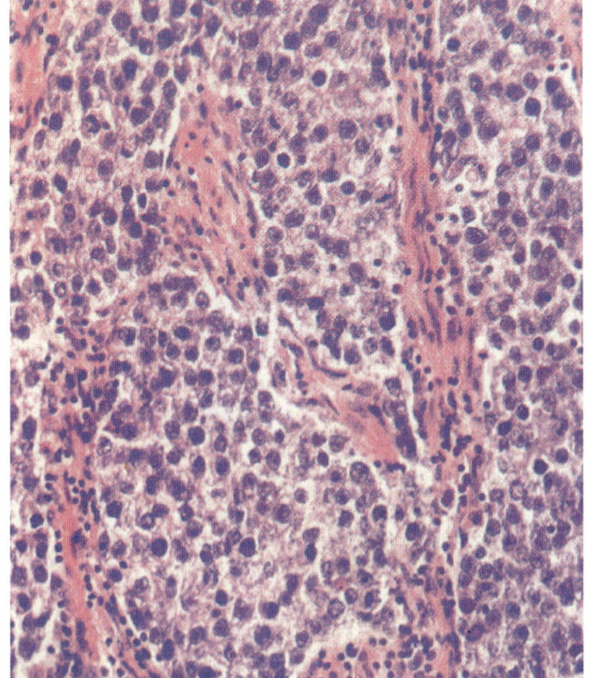
Histologic picture of dysgerminoma cells are mostly uniform (monotonous pattern) in size. The stroma is dense with lymphocytic infiltrate

80. Marker for granulosa cell tumour:

a. CA-50 b. CA 19-9
c. Inhibin d. All of the above

The granulosa tumour cells secrete inhibin and it is an useful marker for the disease.

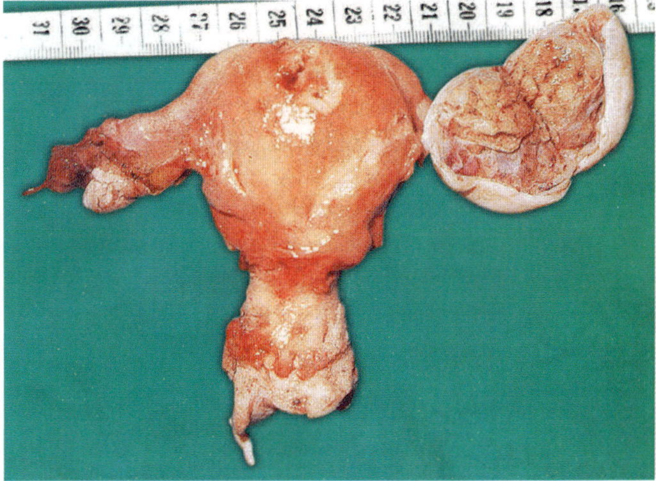
Cut section of granulosa cell tumor

81. NOT associated with fibroid:

a. Pelvic mass
b. Amenorrhoea
c. Infertility
d. Menstrual irregularity

Menorrhagia (30%) is the classical symptom of symptomatic fibroid.

Ans. 79. **d.** Dysgerminoma 80. **c.** Inhibin 81. **b.** Amenorrhoea

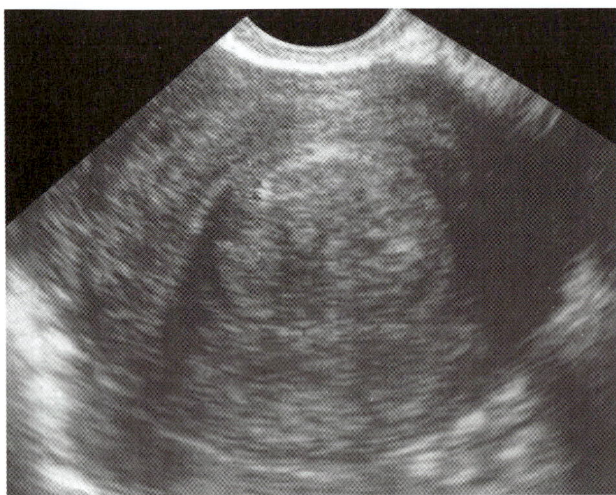
Ultrasonographic view of a uterine fibroid

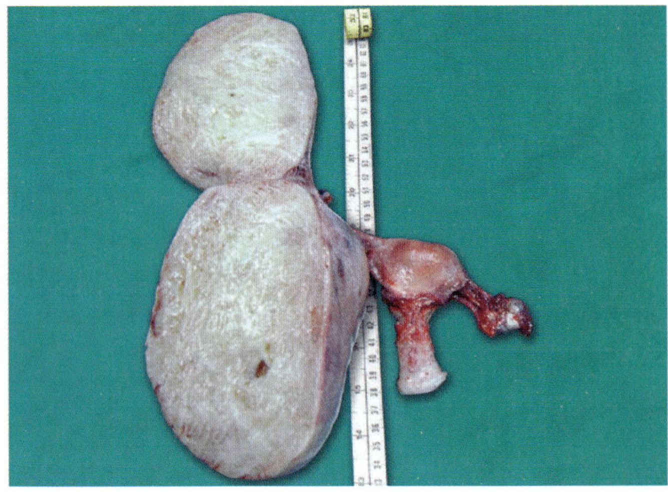
Cut section of a theca cell tumour of the ovary

82. A 46 years old lady has abnormal uterine bleeding with simple hyperplasia of endometrium. The treatment of choice would be:

a. Total Hysterectomy b. Progesterone
c. Estrogen + progestogen d. Estrogen

In perimenopausal and postmenopausal women with hyperplasia without atypia, continuous progestin therapy may be considered. However, hysterectomy with bilateral salpingo-oophorectomy is done as an alternative as the risk of carcinoma increases with age.

'High Risk' Factors for Endometrial Cancer
❑ Late menopause
❑ Nulliparity
❑ Unopposed estrogen therapy
❑ History of persistent anovulation (PCOS)
❑ History of irregular and excessive premenopausal bleeding
❑ Obesity, diabetes, hypertension
❑ Personal or family history of breast, ovary, colon or endometrial cancer
❑ Atypical endometrial hyperplasia
❑ Tamoxifen therapy
❑ Radiation menopause

83. Meigs syndrome is commonly associated with:

a. Teratoma b. Brenner tumour
c. Fibroma d. Theca cell tumour

Ascites and right-sided hydrothorax in association with fibroma of the ovary, Brenner, thecoma and granulosa cell tumor is called Meigs syndrome. There is spontaneous remission of ascites and hydrothorax on removal of the tumor. Ascites and hydrothorax when present in conditions other than those mentioned above, are called pseudo-Meigs syndrome.

84. Most common cervical carcinoma:

a. Adenocarcinoma
b. Sarcoma
c. Squamous cell carcinoma
d. Small cell carcinoma

The commonest variety of the cervical carcinoma is squamous cell carcinoma (85-90%) either well differentiated or moderately or poorly differentiated. These arise from the ectocervix. The source of the squamous epithelium which turn into malignancy are – squamocolumnar junction, squamous metaplasia of the columnar epithelium.

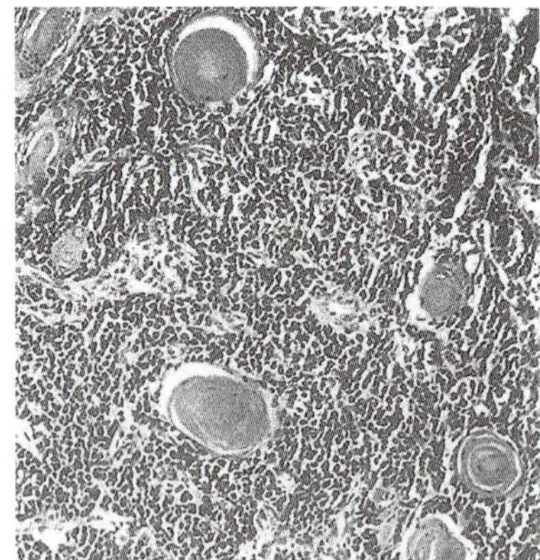
Histology of squamous cell carcinoma of the cervix (small cell type). Keratin pearls are seen

85. Pain in fibroid is due to all EXCEPT:

a. Hyaline changes
b. Torsion
c. Sarcomatous degeneration
d. Red degeneration

The fibroids are usually painless. Pain may be due to some complications of the tumor (degeneration, torsion of subserous pedunculated fibroid or extrusion of polyp) or due to associated pelvic pathology (endometriosis, PID).

Ans. 82. **a.** Total hysterect... 83. **c.** Fibroma 84. **c.** Squamous cell car... 85. **a.** Hyaline changes

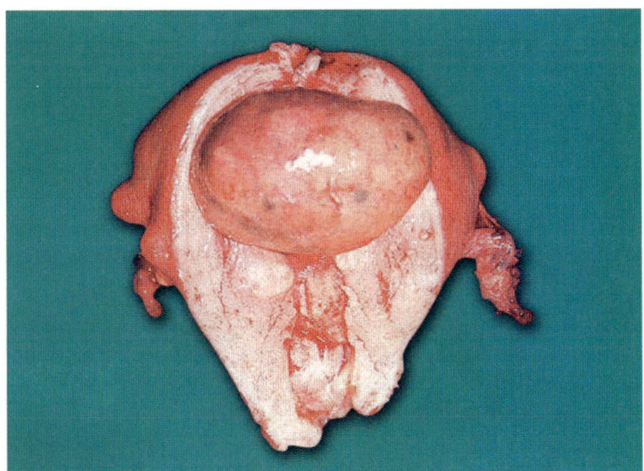

Cut section of a uterus showing a submucous fibroid

86. Endometrial cancer is associated with all EXCEPT:

a. Dysgerminoma b. Granulosa cell tumour
c. Endometrial hyperplasia d. Fibromyoma

Endometrial carcinoma is associated with unopposed estrogen stimulation. Conditions such as functioning ovarian tumors (granulosa cell) or polycystic ovarian syndrome (PCOS) are associated with increased risk of endometrial cancer. Fibroid is associated in about 30% cases of endometrial cancer.

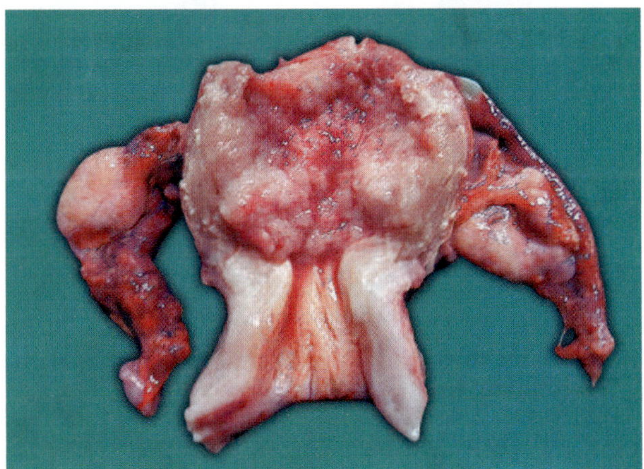

Diffuse type of endometrial carcinoma

87. Which one of the following is NOT an epithelial tumour of the ovary:

a. Serous cystadenoma
b. Brenner tumour
c. Clear cell tumour
d. Endodermal sinus tumour

EST/YST is the second MC (20%) malignant germ cell tumor of the ovary. EST are unilateral and are usually solid, more than 10 cm in diameter.

Pathology of Ovarian Malignancy

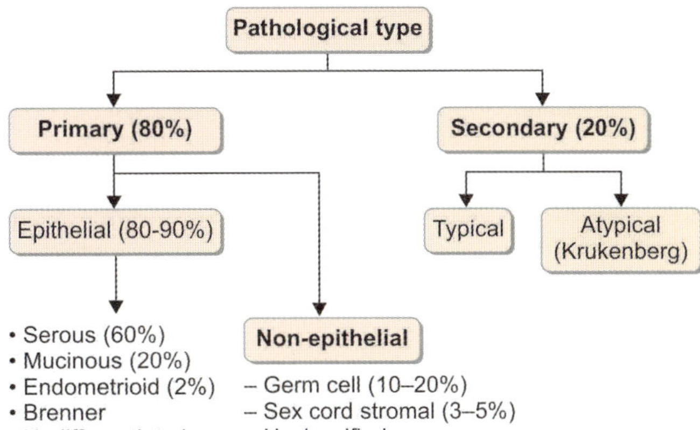

- Serous (60%)
- Mucinous (20%)
- Endometrioid (2%)
- Brenner
- Undifferentiated

– Germ cell (10–20%)
– Sex cord stromal (3–5%)
– Unclassified

88. Chemotherapy for dysgerminoma is:

a. Cisplatin, etoposide, bleomycin
b. Cyclophosphamide, vincristine, prednisolone
c. Adriamycin, cyclophosphamide, cisplatin
d. Methotrexate, oncovin, procarbacine

Systemic chemotherapy is the treatment of choice for dysgerminoma, where fertility is to be preserved, even in the presence of metastatic disease.

Recommended Drugs and Doses of Chemotherapy (Bep, Vbp)

Drugs	*Dose*	*Schedule*
Bleomycin (B)	15 units/m^2	Every week
Etoposide (E)	100 mg/m^2	On days 1-3, every 4 weeks
Cisplatin (P)	100 mg/m^2	Every 3 weeks
Vinblastin (V)	12 mg/m^2	Every 3 weeks
Drugs are given IV for 3–4 cycles, combinations used are BEP and VBP.		

89. Management of CIN II includes:

a. Yearly follow-up b. LLETZ
c. Radiotherapy d. Chemotherapy

The fact that over a prolonged follow-up, about 10-15% of CIN I and II progress to CIS, it is quite impossible to predict which one will remain stationary and which one will progress to severe dysplasia or CIS. A such, CIN II is commonly treated with LLETZ (large loop excision of transformation zone).

Scheme—2: Life cycle of unstable cervical epithelium

Cervical epithelium	*CIN I*	*CIN II*	*CIN III/CIS*
Regression to normal (%)	60	40	30
Persistence (%)	30	35	50

Contd...

Ans. **86. a.** Dysgerminoma **87. d.** Endodermal sinus... **88. a.** Cisplatin, etoposide... **89. b.** LLETZ

Contd...

Cervical epithelium	*CIN I*	*CIN II*	*CIN III/CIS*
Progression to CIN III/CIS (%)	10	20	—
Progression to invasion (%)	< 1	5	20

Duration of disease progression (years)	Normal	CIN I, II	CIN III/CIS	Invasion	
	0	5		10	20
Age of the patient (year)		25–30	30–35	40–45	

90. Most common site of metastasis in choriocarcinoma is:

a. Liver b. Lungs
c. Brain d. Ovaries

The common sites of metastases from choriocarcinoma are lungs (80%), anterior vaginal wall (30%), brain (10%), liver (10%) and others.

Figo Anatomic Staging for GTT	
Stage I	The lesion is confined to the uterus.
Stage II	The lesion spreads outside the uterus but is confined to the genital organs.
Stage III	The lesion metastasizes to the lungs.
Stage IV	The lesion metastasizes to sites such as brain, liver or gastrointestinal tract.

91. Most of the carcinoma cervix presents as:

a. Abdominal pain b. Amenorrhoea
c. Post coital bleeding d. Features of metastasis

Patients with carcinoma cervix are usually multiparous, in pre-menopausal age group. They have previous history of postcoital or intermenstrual bleeding which they ignored.

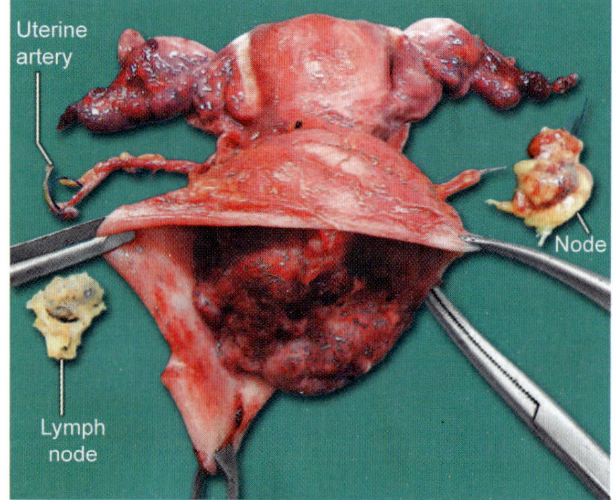

A specimen of carcinoma (squamous cell) of the cervix showing marked exophytic growth. Radical hysterectomy had been done. Uterine arteries are ligated at their origin from the internal iliac artery. Both the ovaries and upper third of vagina had been removed. Pelvic lymph adenectomy done (one enlarged node on either side is seen)

92. Condyloma acuminata is caused by:

a. HSV b. HSV
c. HPV d. HIV

Condylomata acuminata/ genital warts are papillary lesions caused by Human Papilloma Virus (HPV) usually type 6 and 11. Anatomic distribution of anogenital HPV infection is: Cervix 70%, Vulva 25%, Vagina 10% and Anus 20%.

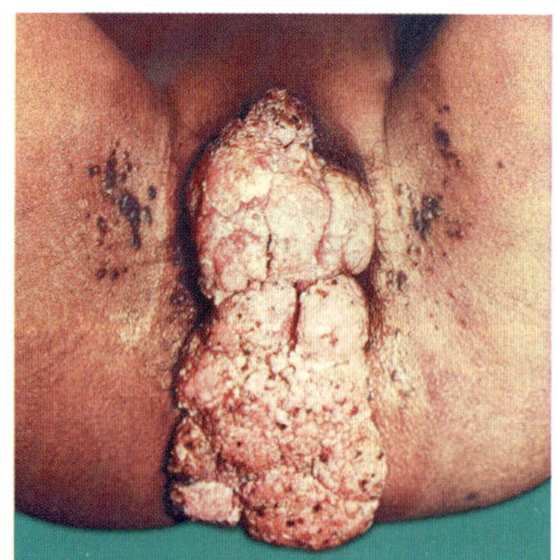

Giant condyloma acuminata of vulva

93. NOT included in WHO prognosis scoring system for gestational trophoblastic disease:

a. Antecedent pregnancy
b. Age
c. Post treatment HCG levels
d. Site of metastasis

WHO prognostic scoring system of gestational trophoblastic disease include pretreatment hCG levels.

Who Prognostic Scoring System of Gestational Trophoplastic Disease as Modified by FIGO (2000)

	Score			
Parameter	*0*	*1*	*2*	*4*
Age (years)	< 40	> 40	—	—
Antecedent pregnancy	Mole	Abortion	Term	—

Contd...

Ans. 90. **b.** Lungs 91. **c.** Post coital bleeding 92. **c.** HPV 93. **c.** Post treatment...

Contd...

Parameter	Score			
	0	*1*	*2*	*4*
Interval (month)‡	< 4	4–6	7–12	≥ 13
Pretreatment hCG (iu/l)	< 10^3	10^3–10^4	10^4–10^5	> 10^5
Largest tumor (cm)	< 3	3 – 5	> 5	—
Site of metastases	Lung Pelvis	Spleen kidney	GI tract liver	Brain
No. of metastases detected	—	1–4	5–8	> 8
Prior chemotherapy	—	—	Single drug	Multiple drugs

Total score: < 6 is low risk and a total score ≥ 7 is high risk.
‡ Interval: Time between antecedent pregnancy and start of chemotherapy.

94. High risk gestational trophoblastic disease (according to WHO) has:

a. Score of less than 4
b. 4-8
c. Score of more than 8
d. None of the above

If the score (WHO prognostic scoring system of gestational trophoblastic disease) is less than 6, it is low risk and ≥7 is considered as high risk.

Management of GTN	
A. Stage I Low risk GTn	❑ Single agent chemotherapy.
High risk or Resistant	❑ Combination therapy ❑ Family completed → hysterectomy.
B. Stage II and III Low risk GTN	❑ Single agent chemotherapy. ❑ Hysterectomy (family completed) to reduce tumor mass.
High risk or resistant	❑ Combination therapy ❑ Hysterectomy — to reduce (trophoblastic) tumor mass.
C. Stage IV	❑ Combination chemotherapy. ❑ Surgery (hepatic resection, craniotomy). ❑ Radiation (cerebral metastasis).

95. Treatment of choice for choriocarcinoma is:

a. Hysterectomy
b. Radiotherapy
c. Conservative
d. Chemotherapy

The advent of chemotherapy has revolutionized the treatment of both the non-metastastic and metastatic lesion of choriocarcinoma. Chemotherapy is now the mainstay in the treatment.

Formalities to be Followed During Therapy	
Blood counts Liver function Kidney function	Daily
X-ray chest	To repeat only if hCG titer plateaus or rises
Serum/urine hCG	Weekly

❑ Treatment course should not be repeated if :
- WBC < 3000 cu mm
- Polymorphonuclear leucocytes < 1500 cu mm
- Platelet counts < 100,000 cu mm
- Significant elevation of BUN, SGPT

❑ Continue treatment at 1–3 weekly interval until three consecutive negative weekly hCG titers.

96. What should be done to reduce blood loss during myomectomy for fibroid uterus:

a. Preoperative oral contraceptive pills administration
b. Postoperative control of hypertension
c. Tourniquet use
d. Intraoperative blood transfusion

Measures to control blood loss during myomectomy

- Preoperative treatment with GnRH analogue
- Use of vasoconstrictive agents (vasopressin)
- Use of Victor Bonney's specially designed clamp
- Use of tourniquets – to occlude the uterine vessels and also the ovarian vessels at the infundibulopelvic ligament.

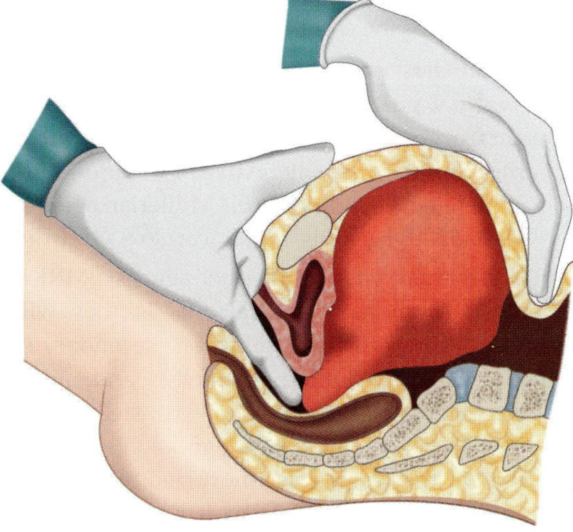

Bimanual examination in a case of uterine fibroid

MISCELLANEOUS

97. NOT used for hirsutism in PCOD:

a. OCPs
b. Spironolactone
c. Flutamide
d. Norgestrel

When appropriate (e.g., in women of child-bearing age who require contraception), a standard contraceptive pill is frequently effective in reducing hirsutism.

Ans. 94. c. Score of more than 8 95. d. Chemotherapy 96. c. Tourniquet use 97. d. Norgestrel

Progestogens such as norgestrel and levonorgestrel should be avoided due to their androgenic effects. Other drugs with anti-androgen effects include flutamide, and spironolactone, which can give some improvement in hirsutism.

98. Most common cause of hirsutism in females:

a. Metropathia haemorrhagica
b. PCOS
c. Endometriosis
d. Chronic PID

Common causes of hirsutism

- Polycystic ovary syndrome (PCOS), the most common cause
- Congenital adrenal hyperplasia, in turn mostly caused by 21-α hydroxylase deficiency
- Cushing's disease
- Growth hormone excess (acromegaly)
- Tumors in the ovaries

99. FALSE for Turner syndrome:

a. 45XO
b. Primary amenorrhoea
c. Patent ductus arteriosus
d. Short stature

The most commonly observed cardiac lesions in TS are congenital obstructive lesions of the left side of the heart, leading to reduced flow on this side of the heart. This includes bicuspid aortic valve and coarctation (narrowing) of the aorta.

100. A female has primary amenorrhoea, normal breast and normal pubic hairs. USG showed absent uterus, absent cervix and short vaginal pouch but normal ovaries. Findings are suggestive of diagnosis of:

a. Klinefelter's syndrome b. Mullerian agenesis
c. Gonadal dysgenesis d. Turner's syndrome

An individual with Mullerian agenesis/MRKH syndrome is hormonally normal; that is, they will enter puberty with development of secondary sexual characteristics including thelarche and adrenarche (pubic hair). Their chromosome constellation will be 46,XX. Ovaries are intact and ovulation usually occurs. Typically, the vagina is shortened and intercourse may, in some cases, be difficult and painful. Medical examination supported by gynecologic ultrasonography demonstrates a complete or partial absence of the cervix, uterus, and vagina.

101. Hormone responsible for ferning pattern of cervical mucus:

a. Progesterone
b. Estrogen
c. LH
d. Prolactin

Ferning of cervical mucus is due to high sodium chloride and low protein content in the mucus due to high estrogen in the midmenstrual phase prior to ovulation.

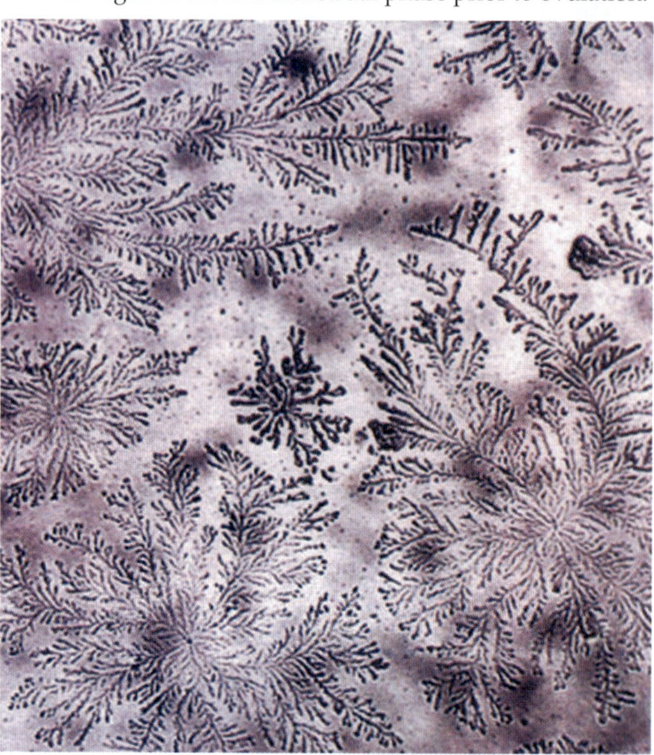

Typical fern pattern appearance of cervical mucus

102. Onset of LH surge precedes ovulation by:

a. 12 hours
b. 24 hours
c. 36 hours
d. 48 hours

Ovulation occurs approximately 10-12 hours after the LH peak or 32-36 hours after the onset of LH surge.

Approximate Time Interval of Events in Menstrual Cycle Prior to Ovulation

Events	Hours
Estradiol rise	83
Onset of LH surge	34–36
Estradiol peak	24–36
LH peak	10–12
Progesterone rise	8

103. Effect of progesterone on lipids:

a. Increased LDL and lowered HDL
b. Increased LDL and increased HDL
c. Lowered LDL and lowered HDL
d. Lowered LDL and increased HDL

Progestins decrease HDL cholesterol and increase LDL cholesterol thereby promote heart disease.

Ans. 98. **b.** PCOS 99. **c.** Patent ductus... 100. **b.** Mullerian... 101. **b.** Estrogen 102. **c.** 36 hours 103. **a.** Increased LDL and lowered HDL

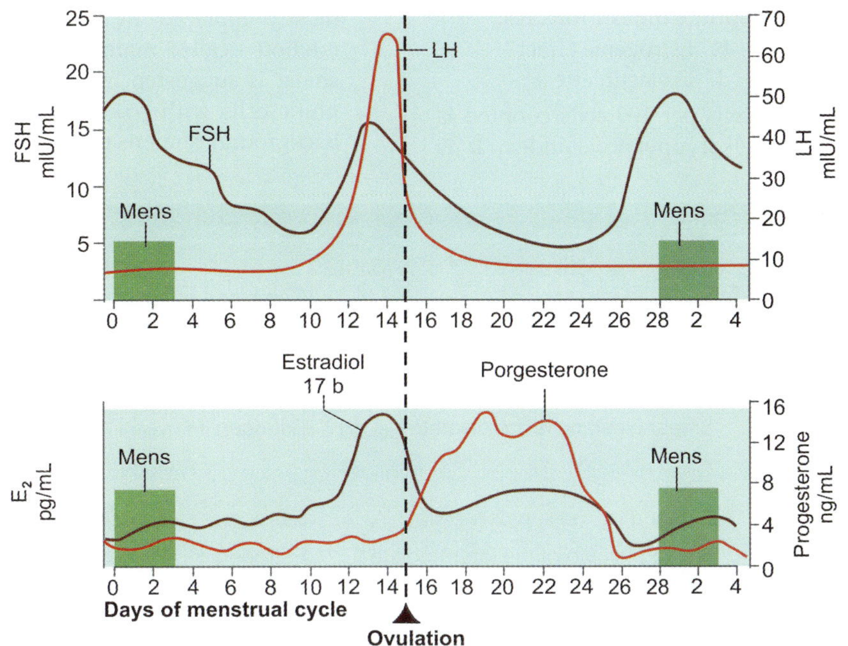

Fluctuation of different hormone levels during menstrual cycle (ovulatory)

104. In a young female of reproductive age group with regular menstrual cycle of 28 days. Ovulation occurs around 14th day of periods. When is the first polar body extruded:

a. 24 hours prior to ovulation
b. Accompanied by ovulation
c. 48 hours after the ovulation
d. At the time of fertilization

The combined LH/FSH midcycle surge is responsible for the final stage of maturation of the follicle, completion of the first meiotic division of the oocyte with extrusion of the first polar body and expulsion of the oocyte (ovulation).

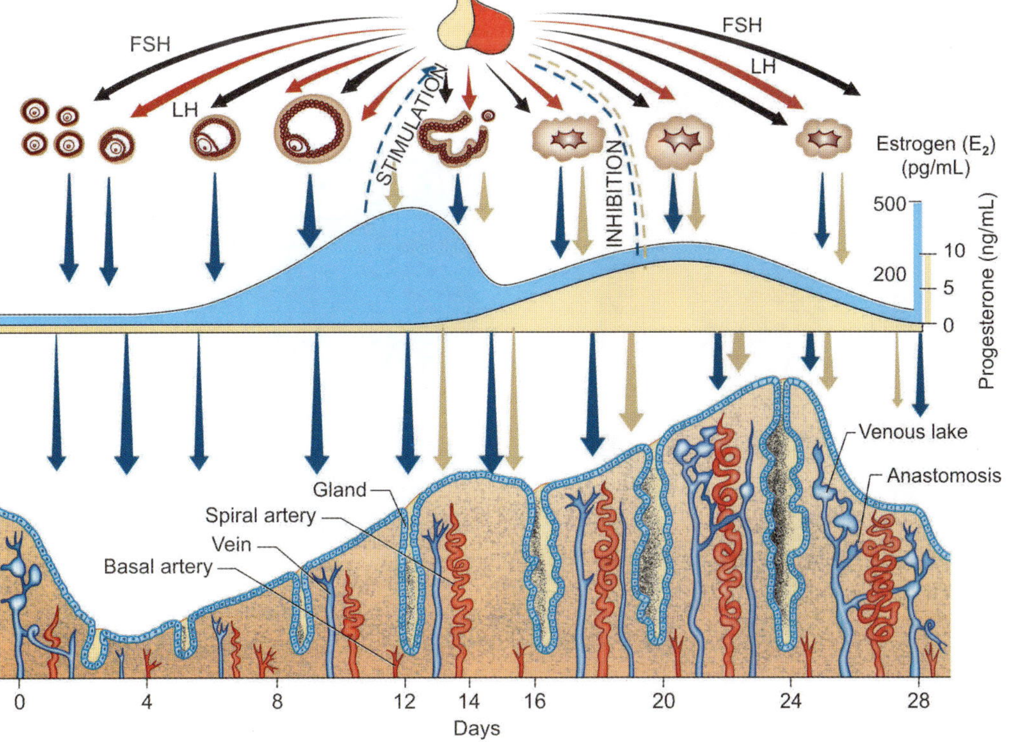

Hormones controlling the ovarian and endometrial cycles

Ans. **104. b.** Accompanied...

105. Cornification index/eosinophilic index indicates:

a. Effect of LH
b. Estrogenic effect
c. Progesterone effect
d. Prolactin effect

The number of cornified cells per 100 cells counted is expressed as cornification/karyopyknotic index. It is mostly replaced by a more appropriate expressive method – called maturation index (MI). The estrogenic smear is suggested by preponderance of large eosinophilic cells with pyknotic nuclei (cornified cells). The background remains clear.

Maturation Index from Birth to Menopause

	MI	*Smear features*	*Inference*
At birth	0/95/5	—	Combined effect of circulating maternal hormones—estrogen, progesterone and corticoids
Childhood	80/20/0	—	MI shifting to left because of diminished steroid hormones
Reproductive period: ❑ Preovulatory	0/40/60	Smear clear, cells are discrete	Estrogen ++
❑ Mild secretory	0/70/30	Smear dirty, cells in clusters	Estrogen +; Progesterone ++
❑ During pregnancy	0/95/5	Marked folding of the intermediate cells — 'navicular cells'	Estrogen ++; Progesterone ++; Corticosteroids +
❑ Postpartum	100/0/0	—	Parabasal maturation
Postmenopausal	0/100/0 or 100/0/0	—	Lack of estrogen

106. Post-coital test is employed to assess:

a. Uterine factor
b. Cervical factor
c. Vaginal factor
d. Tubal factor

PCT is to assess the quality of cervical mucus and the ability of the sperm to survive in it.

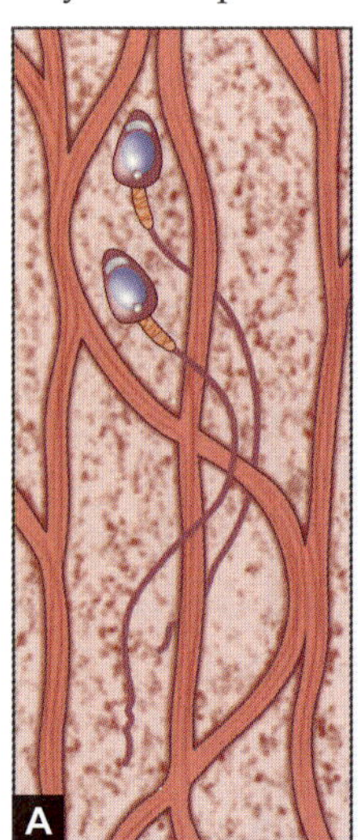

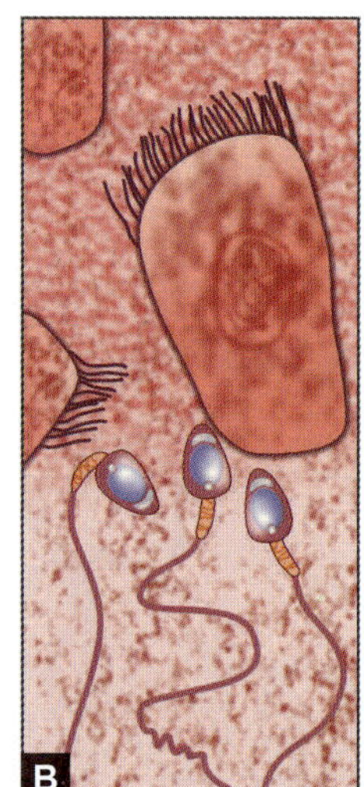

(A) Estrogenic effect on cervical mucus facilitates sperm penetration. (B) Progesterone effect hinders the penetration

107. Corpus luteum secretes:

a. Estrogen
b. Progesterone
c. Both
d. None

Hormones – predominantly progesterone is secreted by the corpus luteum to support the endometrium of the luteal phase. There is also secretion of estrogen, inhibin and relaxin. Progesterone along with estrogen from corpus luteum maintain the growth of the fertilized ovum. This is essential till the luteal function is taken over by placenta.

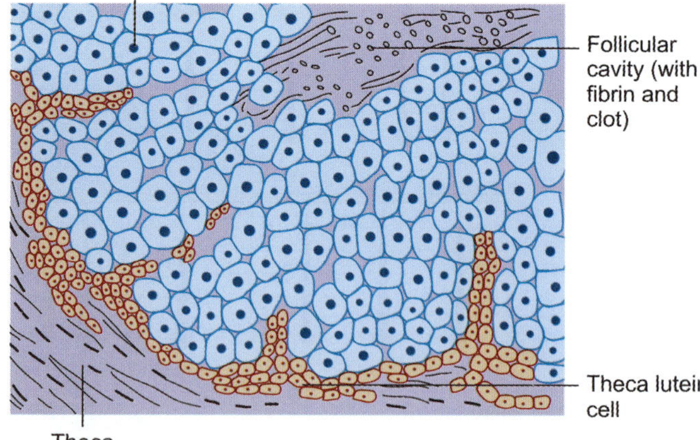

Histologic appearance of a section of corpus luteum

108. Hematocolpos is seen in:

a. Septate uterus
b. Bicornuate uterus
c. Unicornuate uterus
d. Imperforate hymen

Ans. 105. b. Estrogenic effect **106. b.** Cervical factor **107. c.** Both **108. d.** Imperforate hymen

Vulval inspection in a case of imperforate hymen reveals a tense bulging membrane of bluish discoloration. In majority, however, it is not the true hymen but the obstructing membrane is a transverse vaginal septum close to the inner aspect of the hymen.

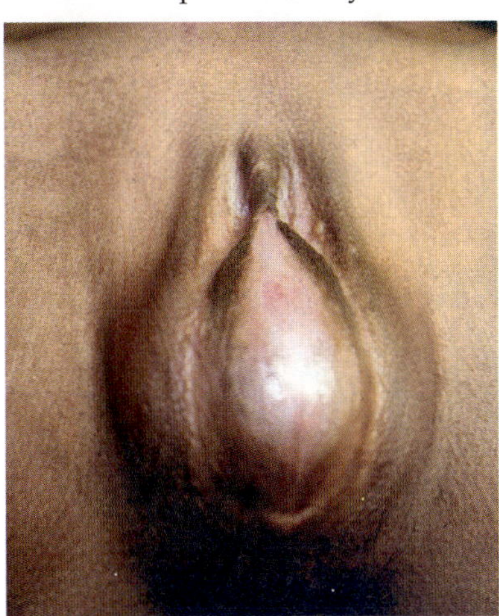

Tense bulging of the hymen in hematocolpos

109. Estrogen deficiency leads to:

a. Postmenopausal bleeding
b. Decreased risk of cardiovascular diseases
c. Osteoporosis
d. Dysmenorrhea

Following menopause there is decline in collagenous bone matrix resulting in osteoporotic changes. Osteoporosis may be primary (Type 1) due to estrogen loss, age, deficient nutrition (calcium, vit. D) or hereditary. It may be secondary (Type 2) to endocrine abnormalities (parathyroid, diabetes) or medication.

Risk factors for osteoporosis in a woman
❑ Family history
❑ Age—Elderly
❑ Race—Asian, White race
❑ Lack of estrogen
❑ Body weight—Low BMI
❑ Early menopause—Surgical, radiation
❑ Dietary—↓ Calcium and ↓ Vitamin D, ↑ Caffeine, ↑ Smoking
❑ Sedentary habit
❑ Drugs—Heparin, corticosteroids, GnRH analogue
❑ Diseases—Thyroid disorders, hyperparathyroidism malabsorption, multiple myeloma.

110. Source of progesterone during normal menstrual cycle:

a. Corpus luteum
b. Stroma
c. Surface epithelium of ovary
d. None of the above

Hormones—predominantly progesterone is secreted by the corpus luteum to support the endometrium of the luteal phase. There is also secretion of estrogen, inhibin and relaxin.

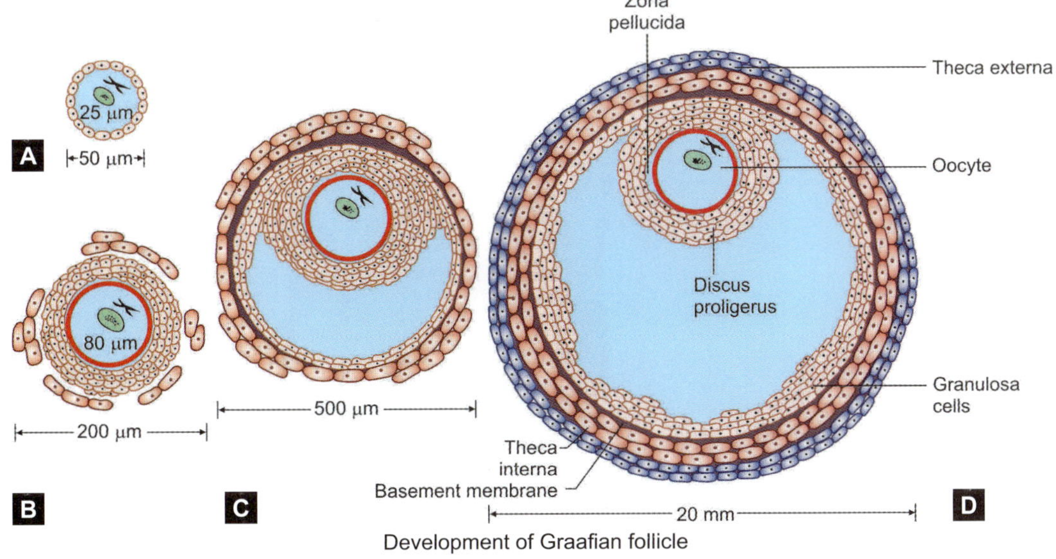

Development of Graafian follicle

111. Vaginal cytology for hormonal changes is best taken from:

a. Posterior wall
b. Anterior wall
c. Lateral wall
d. Any wall

The lateral wall of the upper-third of the vagina (most sensitive to hormonal influence) is lightly scrapped with a wooden spatula after taking due precautions. The material so collected is to be fixed and stained.

Ans. **109. c.** Osteoporosis **110. a.** Corpus luteum **111. c.** Lateral wall

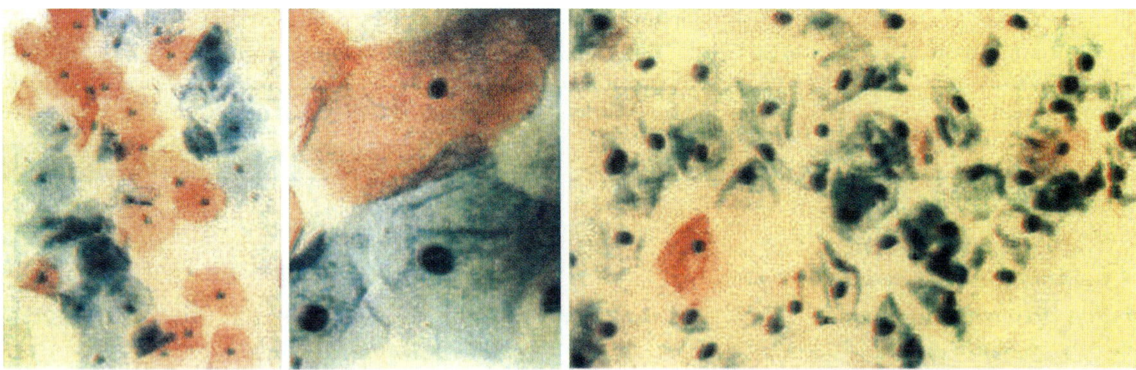

Vaginal cytology—In the late proliferative phase, there are preponderance of superficial large cornified cells with pyknotic nuclei. The background is clear. In the premenstrual phase, there is preponderance of navicular cells. The background is dirty

112. Barr body is seen in:

a. Turners syndrome b. Klinefelter's syndrome
c. Testicular feminization d. 46XY

Sex chromatin study reveals positive Barr body. Sex chromatin is positive in Klinefelter's syndrome.

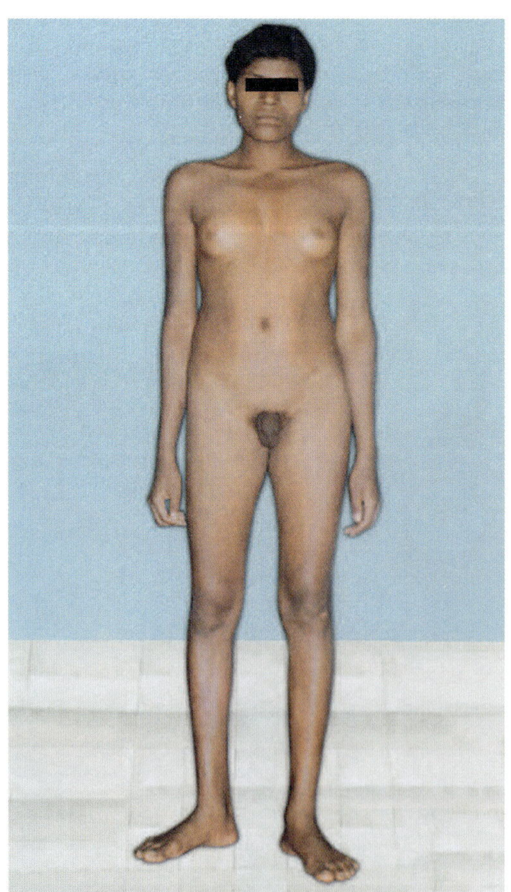

A case of Klinefelter's syndrome having gynecomastias [By courtesy: Dr B Ghosh, Burnpur]

113. Best diagnosis of ovulation is by:

a. Chromotubation b. Endometrial biopsy
c. Laparoscopy d. USG

Ans. 112. b. Klinefelter's... **113. b.** Endometrial biopsy

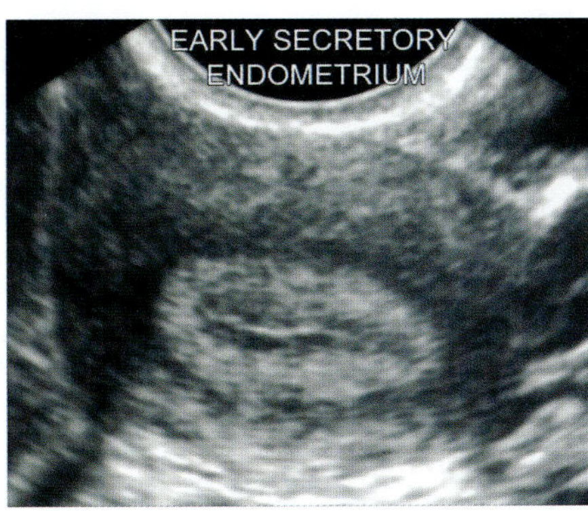

Transvaginal scan demonstrating thickened, triple line endometrium (preovulatory phase)

Endometrial sample biopsy and histology can precisely determine the date of menstrual cycle. Any discrepancy of more than two days when examined in the post-ovulatory phase is called luteal phase defect.

114. NOT a operative procedure for genital prolapse:

a. LeForte's
b. Ward Mayo's
c. Fenton's
d. Fothergill's

In Fenton's method, a transverse incision is made along the fourchette for doing perineoplasty. Perineoplasty is the reconstruction of the narrow vaginal introitus to make it adequate for sexual function.

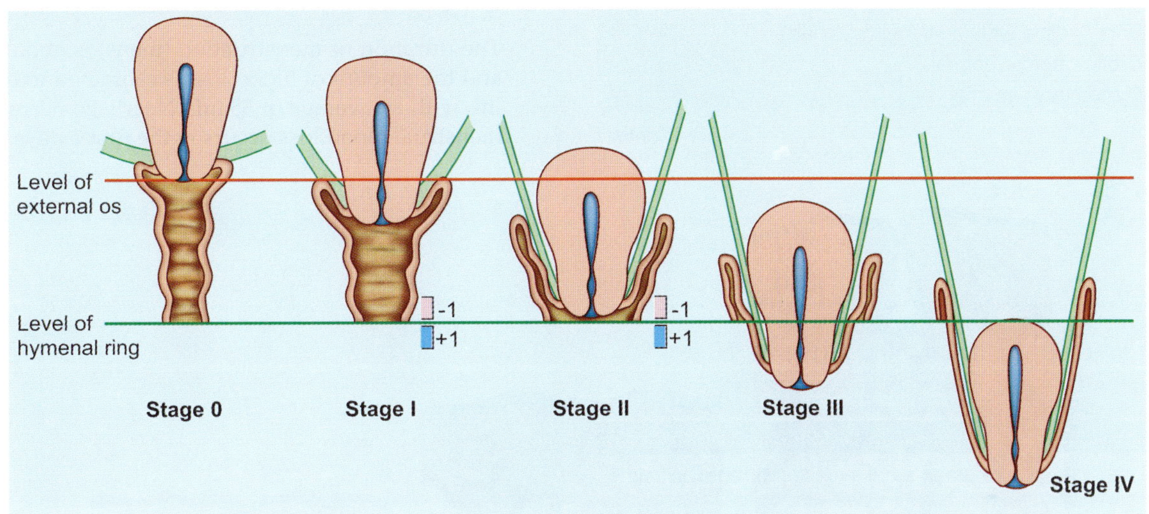

Quanti tati ve gradings of Pelvic Organ Prolapse [ICS, AUGS, SGS – 1996]

115. Corpus luteum of menstrual cycle persists for:

a. 5 days
b. 10 days
c. 14 days
d. 30 days

Soon following the LH surge, the level of estrogen drops down within an hour and the LH peak after 24 hours. LH initiates and maintains the corpus luteum from which both progesterone and estrogen are secreted. The life span of corpus luteum is about 12-14 days.

Cervical Cycle, Vaginal Cycle and General Changes in Follicular and Luteal Phase		
Cervical Cycle		
Follicular phase		*Luteal phase*
❑ Internal os — funnel-shaped ❑ Mucus — thin and watery ❑ Stretchability — increased to beyond 10 cm ❑ Fern tree pattern present ❑ Glycoprotein network — parallel, thus facilitating sperm penetration ❑ Glandular epithelium — taller		❑ Tightly closed ❑ Thick and viscid ❑ Lost ❑ Lost ❑ Interlacing bridges, preventing sperm penetration ❑ Glands — more branched
Follicular phase		Luteal phase
❑ Cytology — showing preponderance of superficial large cornified cells with pyknotic nuclei ❑ Background of the smear — clear		❑ Preponderance of intermediate cells with folded edges (navicular cells) ❑ Dirty due to presence of leucocytes and bacilli
❑ No symptom	❑ Pain abdomen on either iliac fossa ❑ Slight vaginal bleeding ❑ Mucoid vaginal discharge	❑ Irritability, lethargy, constipation ❑ Acne ❑ Pelvic discomfort ❑ Abnormal gain in weight ❑ Mastalgia

Ans. **114. c.** Fenton's **115. c.** 14 days

116. Bonney's test is employed for:

a. Utero-vesical fistula
b. Vesico-vaginal fistula
c. Urge incontinence
d. Stress incontinence

Marshall-Boney test tries to anticipate the clinical efforts of a suspension operation in relation to cure urinary incontinence: using the index and middle fingers, the paraurethral tissue is lifted and the patient is asked for coughing or valsalva provocation with a full bladder.

Diagnosis of GSI
❑ Clinical stress test—positive.
❑ Pad test—positive.
❑ Midstream urine analysis—normal.
❑ Urinary diary (volume frequency chart).
❑ Uroflowmetry—normal.
❑ Cystometry—normal.
❑ Significant lowering of urethral closure pressure during strain.
❑ Leak-point pressure (Valsalva) test—positive.
❑ Cystourethroscopy—negative finding.
❑ Videocystourethrography—bladder neck funneling.
❑ Transvaginal endosonography—altered anatomical relationship (descent) of urethrovesical junction and bladder base.

Contd...

117. Amount of blood loss in normal menstrual cycle:

a. 10 cc
b. 35 cc
c. 50 cc
d. 75 cc

The duration of menstruation (mens) is about 4-5 days and the amount of blood loss is estimated to be 20 to 80 mL with an average of 35 mL. Nearly 70 percent of total menstrual blood loss occurs in the first 2 days.

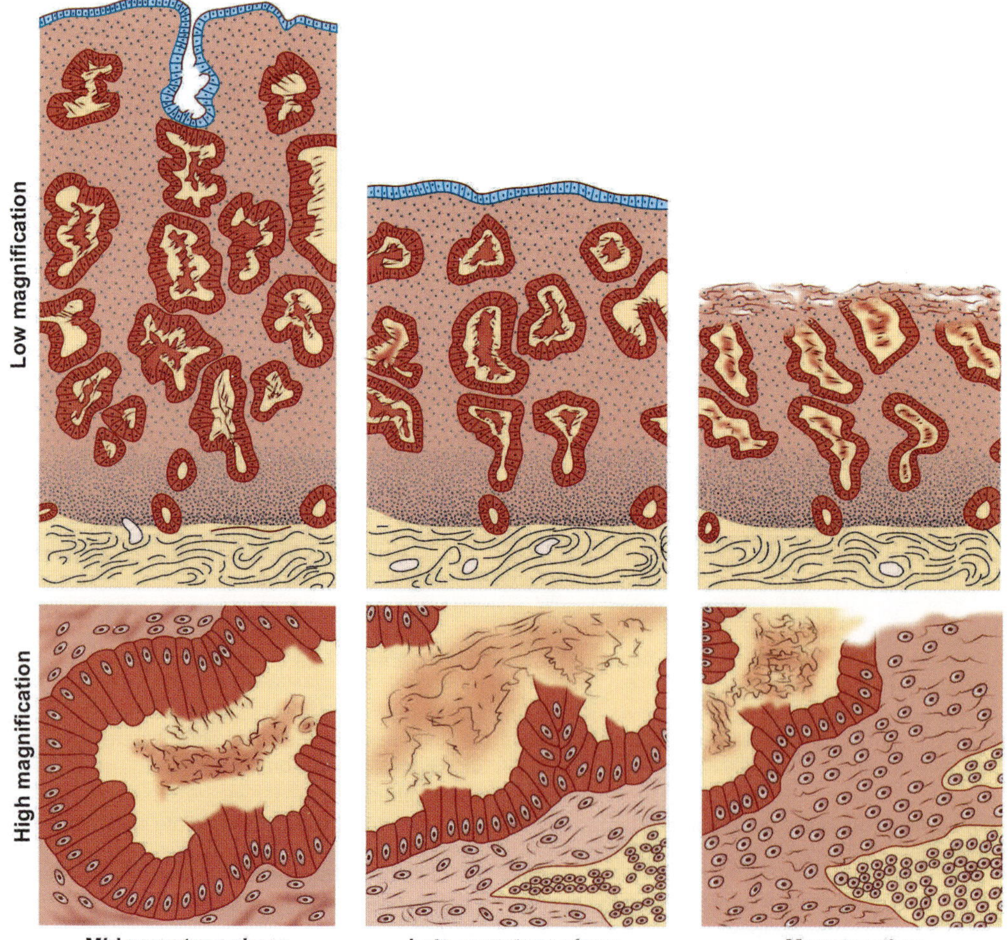

Endometrium in secretory and menstrual phase. Note the marked tortuosity of the glands with secretion in the lumen in the midsecretory phase. The nucleus is pushed to the base

Ans. **116. d.** Stress incont... **117. b.** 35 cc

118. pH of normal adult vagina:

a. 4.5 b. 6.5
c. 7 d. 7.5

The pH of vagina is acidic and varies during different phases of life and menstrual cycle. Conversion of glycogen in the exfoliated squamous cells to lactic acid by the Doderlein's bacilli is dependent on estrogen. As such, the pH is more towards acidic during child-bearing period and ranges between 4 and 5.5 with average of 4.5. The pH is highest in upper vagina because of contaminated cervical secretions (alkaline).

	ESTROGEN	EPITHELIUM	GLYCOGEN	pH	FLORA
BIRTH TO 2 WEEKS	+		+	ACID 4 - 5	STERILE ↓ DODERLEIN'S BACILLI SECRETION ABUNDANT
2 WEEKS TO PREPUBERTY	–		–	ALKALINE > 7	DODERLEIN'S BACILLI ABSENT SECRETION SCANT
PREPUBERTY	APPEARS		– → +	ALKALINE ↓ ACID	SPARSE, COCCAL ↓ RICH BACILLARY
REPRODUCTIVE PERIOD	++		+	ACID 4 - 5	DODERLEIN'S BACILLI APPEAR SECRETION ABUNDANT
POST MENOPAUSE	+ → –		–	NEUTRAL OR ALKALINE 6 - > 7	DODERLEIN'S BACILLI ABSENT SECRETION SCANT

Estrogenic effect on vaginal epithelium and flora at different ages

119. Investigations to be done in a girl presenting with delayed puberty are:

a. FSH and LH b. X-rays
c. Karyotyping d. All

Puberty is said to be delayed when the breast tissue and/or pubic hair have not appeared by 13-14 years or menarche appears as late as 16 years. The normal upper age limit of menarche is 15 years.

Causes of delayed puberty

- ❑ Hypergonadotropic hypogonadism
  - Gonadal dysgenesis, 45 XO
  - Pure gonadal dysgenesis 46 XX, 46 XY
  - Ovarian failure 46 XX
- ❑ Hypogonadotropic hypogonadism
  - Constitutional delay

Contd...

Contd...

Causes of delayed puberty

  - Chronic illness, malnutrition
  - Primary hypothyroidism
  - Isolated gonadotropin deficiency (Kallmann's syndrome)
  - Intracranial lesions—tumors: craniopharyngioma, pituitary adenomas
- ❑ Eugonadism
  - Anatomical causes
    - Müllerian agenesis
    - Imperforate hymen
    - Transverse vaginal septum
  - Androgen insensitivity syndrome

120. A woman presents with fluctuant NON tender swelling at the introitus. The best treatment is:

a. Marsupialization b. Incision and drainage
c. Surgical resection d. Aspiration

Ans. 118. a. 4.5 **119. d.** All **120. a.** Marsupialization

Marsupialization is the gratifying surgery for Bartholin's cyst. An incision is made on the inner aspect of the labium minus just outside the hymenal ring. The incision includes the vaginal wall and the cyst wall.

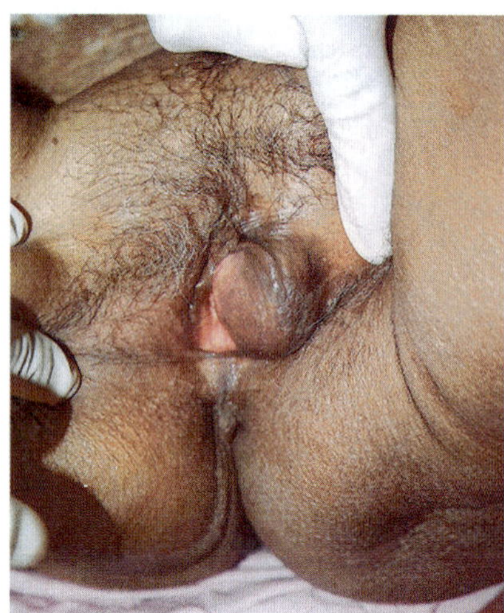

Bartholin's cyst (left)

121. B-lynch suture is applied on:

a. Ovaries b. Tubes
c. Uterus d. Cervix

The B-lynch suture or B-lynch procedure is a form of compression suture. It is used to mechanically compress an atonic uterus in the face of severe postpartum hemorrhage.

122. Polycystic kidney is associated with:

a. Thyroid dysfunction b. Pancreatic overactivity
c. Adrenal hyperplasia d. Phaeochromocytoma

Young women with adrenal hyperplasia may present with symptoms of polycystic ovarian syndrome (oligomenorrhea, polycystic ovaries, hirsutism).

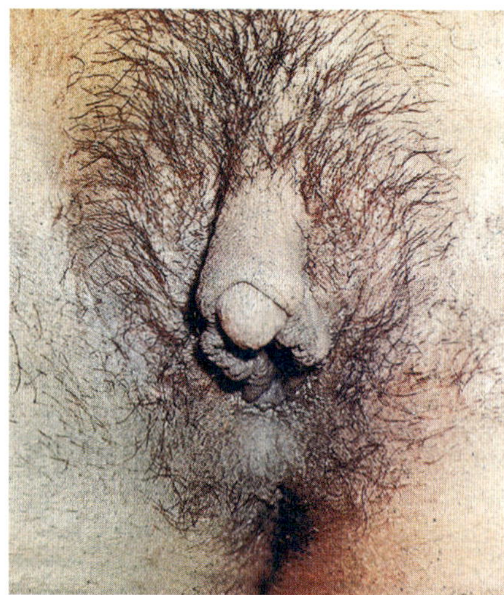

Enlarged clitoris, fused labia minora in adrenogenital syndrome (*By courtesy*: Prof BN Chakravorty, IRM, Kolkata)

123. A lady underwent vaginal hysterectomy and lymph node dissection. Now she presents with incontinence of urine and passing some amount of urine, which is under her control. Most likely diagnosis is:

a. Vesicovaginal fistula
b. Ureterovaginal fistula
c. Stress incontinence
d. Urge incontinence

Operative injury likely to produce fistula includes operations like anterior colporrhaphy, abdominal hysterectomy for benign or malignant lesions or removal of Gartner's cyst.

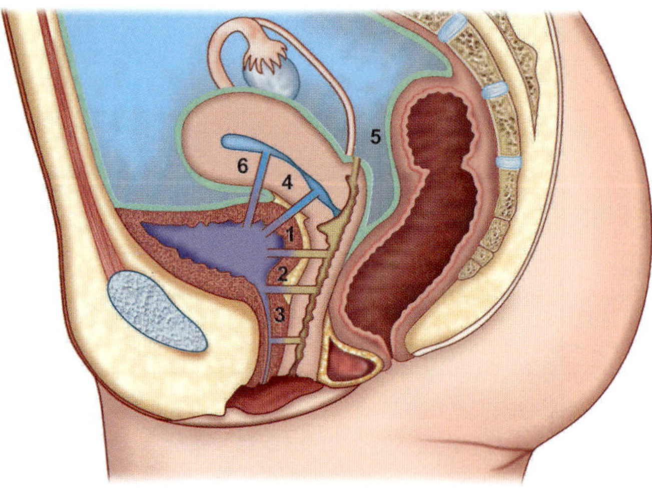

Types of genitourinary fistula—
(1) Vesicovaginal (2) Vesicourethrovaginal (3) Urethrovaginal (4) Vesicocervical (5) Ureterovaginal (6) Vesicouterine

124. Ferning pattern of drying cervical mucus suggests the action of:

a. Estrogen
b. Progesterone
c. Prolactin
d. 17-ketosteroids

Ferning of cervical mucus is due to high sodium chloride and low protein content in the mucus due to high estrogen in the mid menstrual phase prior to ovulation. After ovulation with increasing progesterone, the ferning disappears completely after 21st day. Thus, the presence of ferning even after 21st days suggests anovulation and its disappearance is presumptive evidence of ovulation.

125. Best investigation to assess tubal patency is:

a. Rubin's test
b. Hysterosalpingogram
c. Laparotomy
d. Laparoscopic chromotubation

Laparoscopy is the gold standard (definitive method) for evaluation of tubal factors of infertility. It is done after male factor and ovulatory functions have been found normal or corrected.

Ans. **121. c.** Uterus **122. c.** Adrenal hyperplasia **123. b.** Ureterovaginal... **124. a.** Estrogen
125. d. Laparoscopic chromotubation

Indications of laparoscopy in infertility	
Diagnostic	❑ Age > 35 years ❑ Abnormal HSG ❑ Failure to conceive after reasonable period (6 months) with normal HSG ❑ Women with comorbid pelvic pathology (PID, endometriosis). ❑ Unexplained infertility
Operative	❑ Ovarian drilling ❑ Reconstructive tubal surgery ❑ Adhesiolysis ❑ Fulguration of endometriotic implants ❑ GIFT and ZIFT procedures

126. In azoospermia, the diagnostic test which can distinguish between testicular failure and obstruction in the vas deferens is:

a. Estimation of FSH level
b. Estimation of testosterone level
c. Karyotyping
d. FNAC of testes

Testicular biopsy is done to differentiate primary testicular failure from obstruction as a cause of azoospermia or severe oligospermia. The biopsy materials is to be sent in Bouin's solution and not in formol saline. Testicular tissues may be cryopreserved for future use in IVF/ ICSI.

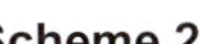

Scheme 2

ABNORMAL SEMEN ANALYSIS (APPARENTLY UNEXPLAINED)

- Azoospermia
- Oligospermia (extreme)

- Hormonal study
  - Serum TSH → High → Hypothyroid state
  - Testosterone → Low → Dysfunction
    - Hypothalamo-pituitary
    - Leydig cell
    - → Injection hCG 5000 units or Injection hCG + pure FSH 3 times weekly or GnRH SC/infusion pump
      - Unresponsive → Klinefelter's → Confirmed by Karyotyping (XXY)
      - Responsive → Hypogonadotrophic-hypogonadism
  - Prolactin → High → Dopamine agonist
  - FSH
    - High → Testicular failure (small testicular volume)
      - Klinefelter's syndrome
      - Sertoli cell only syndrome
      - Testicular atrophy
      - → • Adoption • AID
    - Normal (normal testicular volume) → Testicular biopsy
      - Spermatogenesis normal → Obstruction to efferent ducts → • Vasovasostomy • Vasoepididymostomy • TESE/PESA → I C S I
      - Spermatogenesis absent → Destruction of tubular epithelium → Donor sperm (AID)
    - Low/undetectable → Hypogonadotropism → Kallmann's syndrome → Injection hCG 5000 IU 3 times weekly
- Fructose content of seminal fluid → Absent
  - Congenital absence of seminal vesicle
  - Partial duct obstruction
  - Both
  - → PESA → ICSI
- Microscopic study Pus cells++ Leukocytospermia → Prostatic massage → Smear and culture → Appropriate antibiotics

Ans. 126. **a.** Estimation...

127. Which is NOT an essential criteria (according to WHO) for normal semen analysis:

a. Sperm count > 20 million/ml
b. Volume of 1 ml
c. Sperm with normal morphology (strict criteria) > 15%
d. Motility > 25% with rapidly progressive motility

Volume of semen should be 2.0 mL or more (1.5 mL).

Semen analysis (WHO–2010)	
Semen analysis	Normal reference value and lower reference (within parenthesis) limit
Volume	2.0 ml or more (1.5 ml)
pH	7.2–7.8
Viscosity	< 3 (scale 0–4)
Sperm concentration	20 million/ml (15 million/ml)
Total sperm count	> 40 million/ejaculate (39 million/ejaculate)
Motility	> 50% progressive forward motility (Progressive motility = 32%)
Morphology	> 14% normal form (4%)
Viability	75% or more living (58%)
Leucocytes	Less than 1 million/ml
Round cells	< 5 million/ml
Sperm agglutination	< 10% spermatozoa with adherent particles

128. HRT is NOT useful in:

a. Coronary heart disease
b. Vaginal atrophy
c. Osteoporosis
d. Flushing

Combined HRT therapy shows a relative hazard (RR, 1.29) of coronary heart disease. Hypertension has not been observed to be a risk of HRT.

Monitoring prior to and during HRT
A base level parameter of the following and their subsequent check up (at least annually) are mandatory.
❑ Physical examination including pelvic examination.
❑ Blood pressure recording.
❑ Breast examination and Mammography.
❑ Cervical cytology.
❑ Pelvic ultrasonography (TVS) to measure endometrial thickness (normal <5 mm).
Any irregular bleeding should be investigated thoroughly (endometrial biopsy, hysteroscopy).
Ideal serum level of estradiol should be 100 pg/mL during HRT therapy. Serum level of estradiol is useful to monitor the HRT therapy rather than that of serum FSH.

129. Most common genital fistula in India is:

a. Ureterovaginal fistula
b. Ureteroabdominal fistula
c. Urethrovaginal fistula
d. Vesicovaginal fistula

In vesicovaginal fistula/VVF, there is communication between the bladder and the vagina and the urine escapes into the vagina causing true incontinence. This is the commonest type of genitourinary fistula.

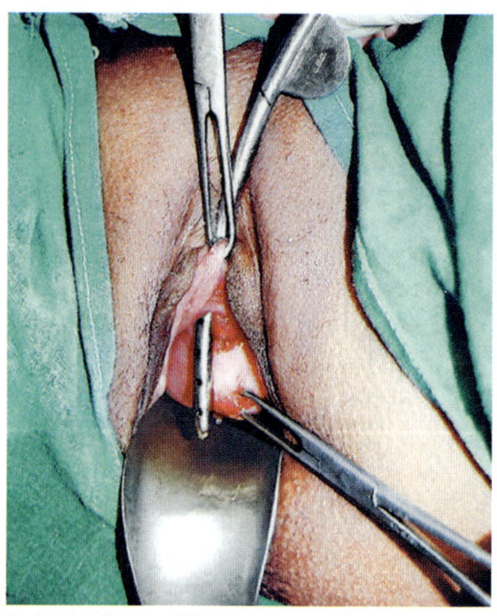

Midvaginal obstetric fistula (VVF). It was of moderate size to allow a metal catheter which is clearly visible [By *courtesy Dr. P. Mukherjee, Professor, Dept of G&O, IPGME&R, Kolkata*]

130. Media commonly used for distension in hysteroscopy is:

a. Oxygen
b. Carbon dioxide
c. Nitrous oxide
d. Hydrogen

Carbon dioxide is commonly used distending media, for diagnostic purposes. It is soluble in blood and is safe.

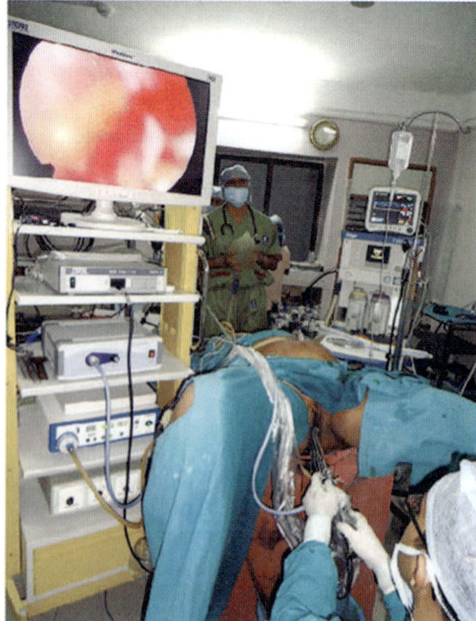

Hysteroscopic procedures in progress

Ans. 127. b. Volume of 1 ml 128. a. Coronary heart... 129. d. Vesicovaginal fistula 130. b. Carbon dioxide

131. Alpha fetoprotein levels are elevated in all EXCEPT:
a. Intrauterine death
b. Twin pregnancy
c. Down syndrome
d. Open neural tube defects

AFP levels are low in Down syndrome.

132. In recurrent abortions, all tests are to be done EXCEPT:
a. TORCH infection screening
b. Thyroid profile
c. Parental cytogenetics
d. Antiphospholipid antibodies

TORCH, which includes Toxoplasmosis, other (Syphilis, Varicella-zoster, Parvovirus B19), Rubella, Cytomegalovirus (CMV), and Herpes infections, are some of the most common infections associated with congenital anomalies.

133. Absolute CONTRAINDICATION of HRT is:
a. Breast carcinoma b. Heart disease
c. Osteoarthritis d. Endometriosis

Combined estrogen and progestins replacement therapy, increases the risk of breast cancer slightly (RR 1.26). Adverse effects of hormone therapy are related to the dose and duration of therapy.

Contraindications to HRT
❑ Undiagnosed genital tract bleeding
❑ Estrogen dependent neoplasm in the body
❑ History of venous thromboembolism
❑ Active liver disease
❑ Gallbladder disease

134. In azoospermia, the diagnostic test which can distinguish between testicular failure and obstruction in the vas deferens is:
a. Estimation of FSH level
b. Estimation of testosterone level
c. Karyotyping
d. FNAC of testes

135. Time of ovulation is detected by all EXCEPT:
a. Urine LH b. Urine FSH
c. Serum estradiol d. Basal body temperature

The function of FSH is predominantly morphogenic, related to the growth and maturation of the Graafian follicle.

Diagnosis of Ovulation

Indirect
- ❑ Menstrual history
- ❑ Evaluation of peripheral or endorgan changes
  - BBT
  - Cervical mucus study
  - Vaginal cytology
  - Hormone estimation
    - Serum progesterone
    - Serum LH
    - Serum estradiol
    - Urine LH
  - Endometrial biopsy
- ❑ Sonography (TVS)

Direct
Laparoscopy

Conclusive
Pregnancy

136. Protective bacterium in normal vagina is:
a. Peptostreptococcus b. Lactobacillus
c. Gardnerella vaginalis d. E. coli

Doderlein's bacillus is a rod-shaped gram-positive bacillus which grows anaerobically on acid media. It appears in vagina 3-4 days after birth and disappears after 10-14 days. It appears again at puberty and disappears after menopause.

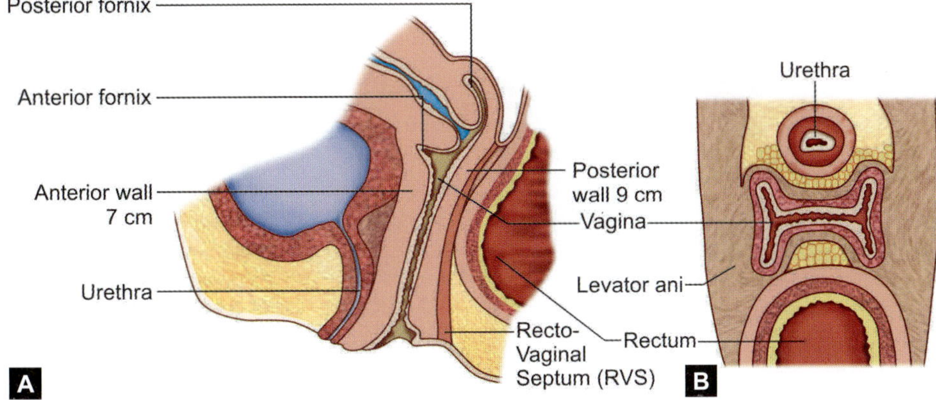

(A) Relation of the anterior and posterior vaginal wall; (B) 'H' shaped on cross-section

137. FSH is secreted by:
a. Anterior pituitary gland
b. Intermediate pituitary gland
c. Posterior pituitary gland
d. Hypothalamus

There are two gonadotropic hormones secreted from the anterior pituitary—(a) Follicle stimulating hormone (FSH) and (b) Luteinizing hormone (LH).

Ans. **131. c.** Down syndrome **132. a.** TORCH infection... **133. a.** Breast carcinoma **134. a.** Estimation of FSH level **135. b.** Urine FSH **136. b.** Lactobacillus **137. a.** Anterior pituitary gland

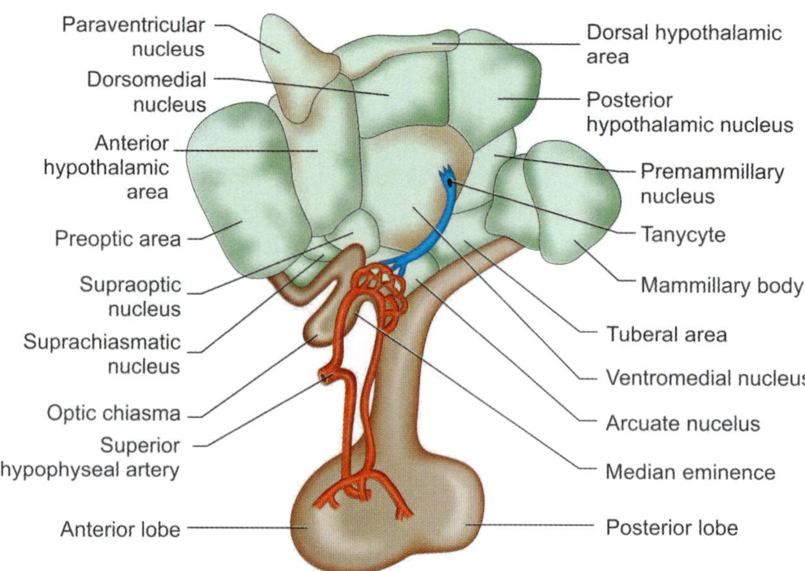

Anatomy of the hypothalamus and pituitary

138. Purandare operation is indicated in:

a. Multiparous prolapse b. Nulliparous prolapse
c. Both of the above d. None of the above

Cervicopexy/sling operation (Purandare's operation) is indicated in congenital or nulliparous prolapsed without cystocele where the cervix is pulled up mechanically through abdominal route.

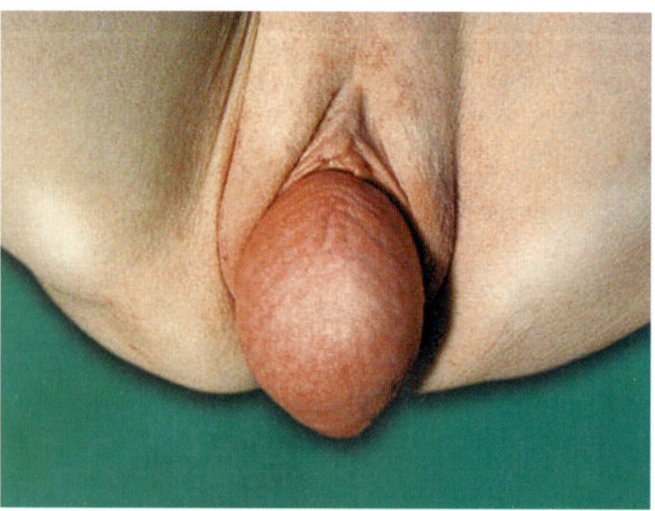
Second degree uterine prolapse. Marked cystocele and there is decubitus ulcer

139. First sign of puberty in girls:

a. Menstruation
b. Growth spurt
c. Appearance of breast buds
d. Pubic and axillary hair growth

The most common order is beginning of the growth spurt → breast budding (thelarche) → pubic and axillary hair growth (adrenarche) → peak growth in height → menstruation (menarche). All these changes are usually between the age of 10 and 16 years.

Tanner stages of pubertal development in girls

Stage	*Breast*	*Pubic hair*
Stage I	Prepubertal state, elevation of papilla only	No pubic hair present
Stage II	Breast buds and papilla slightly elevated, and side of labia areola begins to enlarge. (Median age: 9.8 years)	Sparse, long hair on either majora. (Median age: 10.5 years)
Stage III	Further enlargement of entire breast tissue	Darker, coarser and curly hair over the mons pubis
Stage IV	Secondary mound of areola and papilla projecting above the breast tissue. (Median age: 12.1 years)	Adult type hair covering the mons only. (Median age: 12.0 years)
Stage V	Areola recessed to general contour of breast. (Median age : 14.6 years)	Adult hair with an inverse triangle distribution (female escutcheon) covering the medial thighs. (Median age: 13.7 years)

140. XO is seen in:

a. Down syndrome b. Klinefelter's syndrome
c. Turner syndrome d. Down syndrome

Karyotype of Turner's syndrome is 45, XO and sex chromatin study is negative.

Ans. 138. **b.** Nulliparous... 139. **c.** Appearance of breast... 140. **c.** Turner syndrome

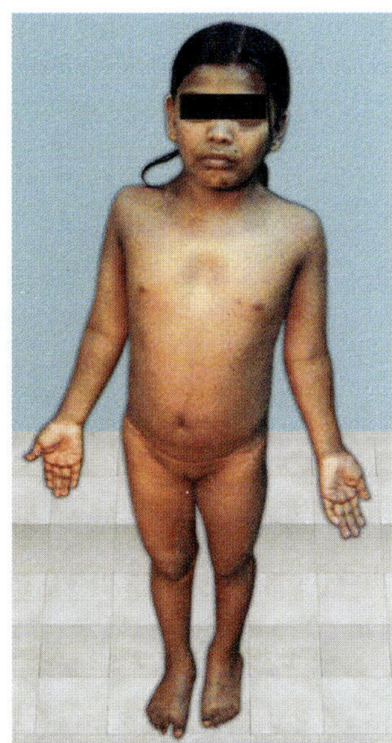

17 Years old girl with Turner's syndrome (45, X). Characteristic somatic abnormalities seen are: short stature (130 cm), shield chest, widely apart nipples, cubitus vulgus, short neck and absent secondary sex characters.

141. Secretion of estrogen is maximum at:

a. At time of ovulation
b. Just before ovulation
c. 14 days prior to menstruation
d. At puberty

Duration the follicular phase, under the influence of LH, androgens (androstenedione and testosterone) are produced in the theca cells. These androgens diffuse into the granulosa cells where they are aromatized under the influence of FSH to estrogens—estradiol predominantly and to lesser extent estrone.

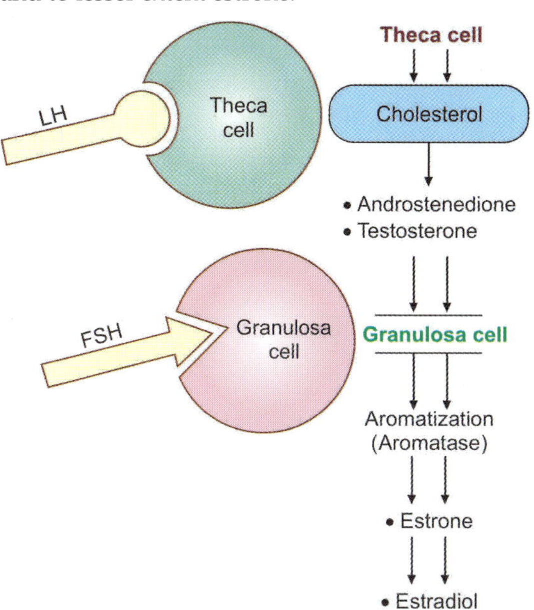

Two cell two gonadotropin theory of ovarian steroidogenesis

142. Most common presentation of uterus didelphys:

a. Oligomenorrhoea
b. Amenorrhoea
c. Dyspareunia
d. Recurrent abortion

In uterus didelphys, there is complete lack of fusion of the Müllerian ducts with a double uterus, double cervix and a double vagina. Infertility and dyspareunia are often related in association with vaginal septum.

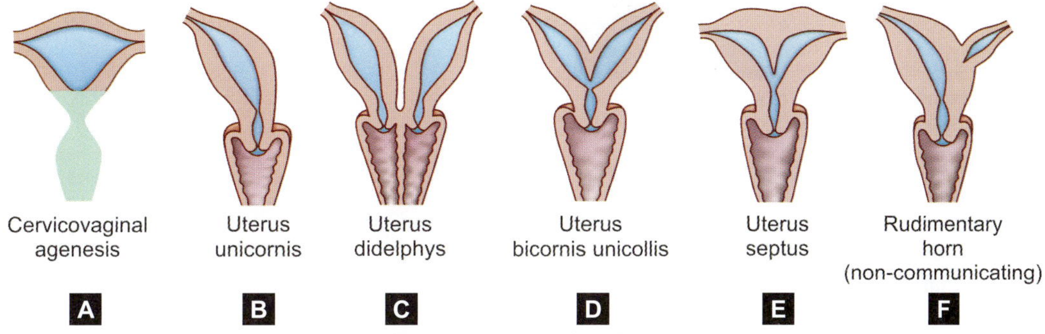

A to F: Malformations of the Müllerian ducts

143. LH surge occurs:

a. 48-72 hours before ovulation
b. 24-36 hours before ovulation
c. 24-36 hours after ovulation
d. 48-72 hours after ovulation

LH levels remain almost static throughout the cycle except at least 12 hours prior to ovulation, when it attains its peak, called LH surge.

Daily production, serum values and urinary excretion of hormones

Hormones	*Follicular phase*	*At ovulation*	*Luteal phase*
Daily production			
Estradiol (μg)	50	150–300	100
Progesterone (mg)	2–3		20–30

Contd...

Ans. **141. b.** Just before... **142. c.** Dyspareunia **143. b.** 24-36 hours before ovulation

Contd...

Hormones	*Follicular phase*	*At ovulation*	*Luteal phase*
Serum values			
Estradiol (pg/mL)	50	300–600	150–200
Progesterone (ng/mL)	< 1		> 5
FSH (mIU/mL)	10	15–20	10
LH (mIU/mL)	5	60	5
Daily excretion			
Total estrogen (µg)	10–25	35–100	25–75
Pregnanediol (mg)	< 1		3–6

144. For uterine anomalies, investigation of choice is:

a. Hysterosalpingography
b. Laparoscopy
c. Hysteroscopy
d. Hystero and laparoscopy both

Müllerian anomalies like arcuate, subseptate, septate, bicornuate uterus or uterus didelphys can be diagnosed with hysteroscopy. The procedure is combined with laparoscopy for confirmation.

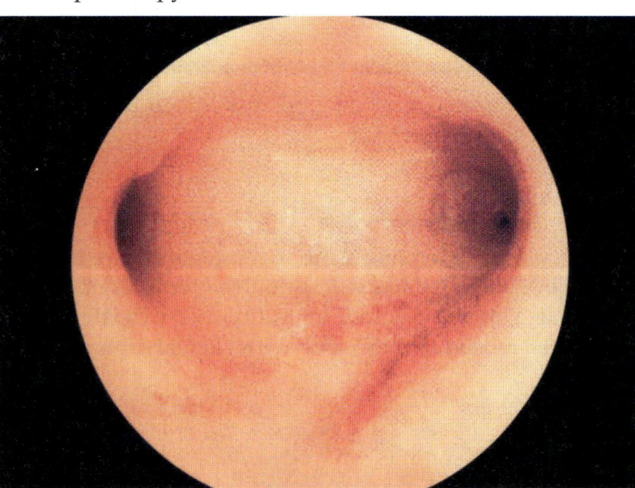

Panoramic view of the uterine cavity with a hysteroscope. Tubal ostium is seen one on either side

145. True regarding karyopyknotic index/KPI levels:

a. Highest in proliferative phase
b. Highest in secretory phase
c. Highest on the day of ovulation
d. Highest in pregnancy

Karyopyknotic index is an index used to monitor the hormonal status of the patient as reflected by exfoliated vaginal cells and their morphology, an expression of the percentage of immediate and superficial cells from squamous cells of vaginal epithelium which have pyknotic nuclei.

146. Corpus luteum is maintained by:

a. Progesterone
b. Estrogen
c. FSH
d. LH

LH initiates and maintains the corpus luteum from which progesterone and estrogen are secreted.

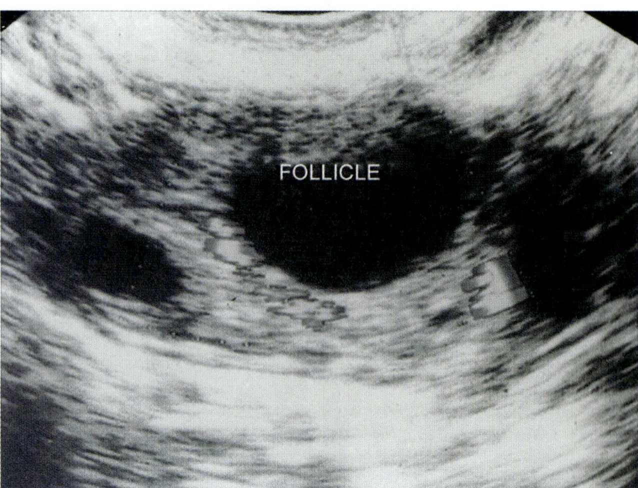

Color Doppler (TV) sonogram showing a mature Graafian follicle prior to ovulation

147. Estrogen level in premature ovarian failure:

a. Normal
b. Raised
c. Less
d. Variable

Premature ovarian failure/insufficiency is defined when the ovarian failure occurs before the age of forty. Serum gonadotropin level (FSH >40 mIU/ mL) is high whereas serum E2 level is low (<20 pg/ mL).

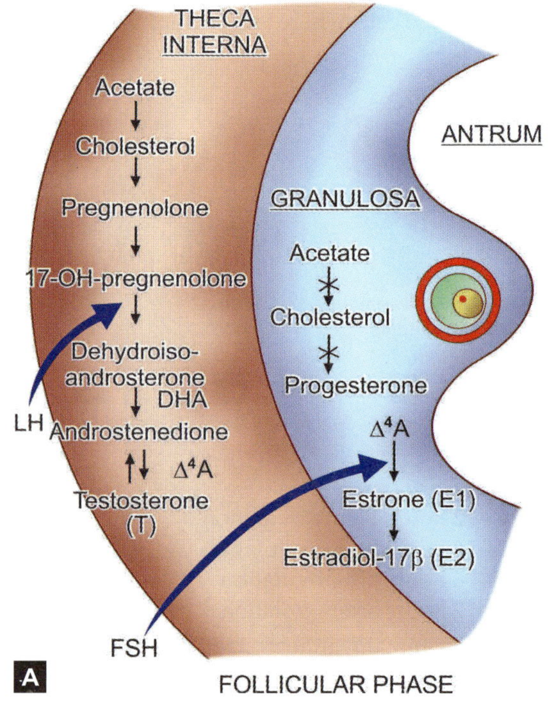

Ans. **144. c.** Hysteroscopy **145. c.** Highest on the day... **146. d.** LH **147. c.** Less

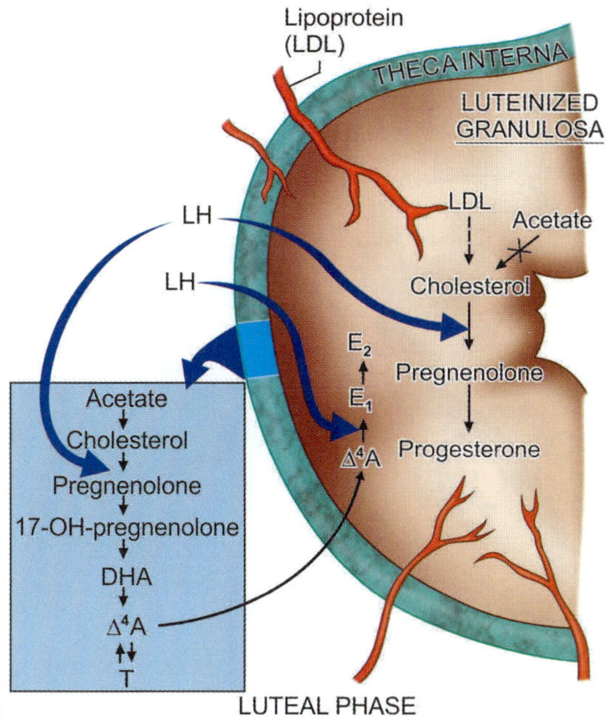

Schematic representation of the ovarian steroidogenesis (Two cell, two gonadotropin A and two cell, one gonadotropin B concept)

148. Hormone responsible for ovulation:

a. FSH
b. LH
c. Estrogen
d. Progesterone

The main function of LH is steroidogenic but along with FSH, it is responsible for full maturation of the Graafian follicle and oocyte and ovulation.

(See Diagram on Next Page)

149. Teratospermia is defined as:

a. No motile sperm
b. Dead sperms
c. Abnormal morphology of sperms
d. Low sperm count

Teratospermia is >70% spermatozoa with abnormal morphology.

Nomenclature
❑ *Aspermia:* Failure of emission of semen (no ejaculate).
❑ *Oligospermia/Oligozoospermia:* Sperm count is less than 20 million per ml.
❑ *Polyzoospermia:* Count is more than 350 million/ml.
❑ *Azoospermia:* No spermatozoan in the semen.
❑ *Asthenozoospermia:* Reduced sperm motility. Leucocytospermia: Increased white cells in semen.
❑ *Necrozoospermia:* Spermatozoa are dead or motionless.
❑ *Teratozoospermia:* > 70% spermatozoa with abnormal morphology.
❑ *Oligoasthenoteratozoospermia:* Disturbance of all 3 variables.

150. Treatment of choice for Asherman's syndrome:

a. Hormones
b. Hysteroscopy and adhesiolysis
c. IUCD
d. All of the above

In uterine synechiae/Asherman's syndrome, there is formation of adhesions following post-abortion and puerperal curettage and also following diagnostic curettage in dysfunctional uterine bleeding. Rarely, it follows tubercular endometritis.

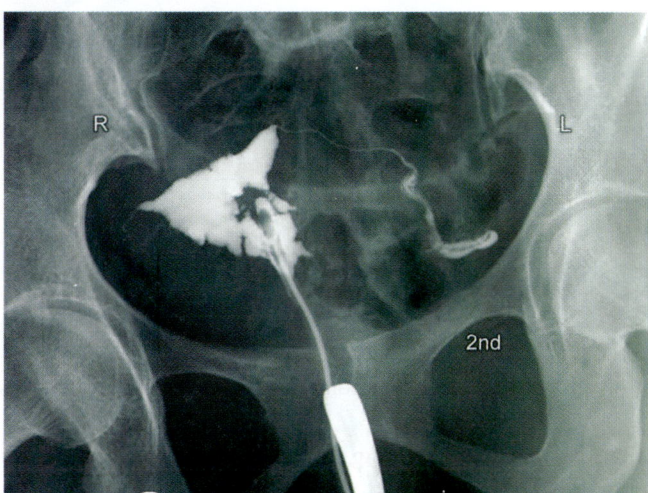

Hysterosalpingogram showing intrauterine adhesion. A case of tuberculous endometritis.
[*Courtesy by* Dr H Roy, Patna]

Ans. **148. b.** LH **149. c.** Abnormal morphology...**150.d.** All of the above

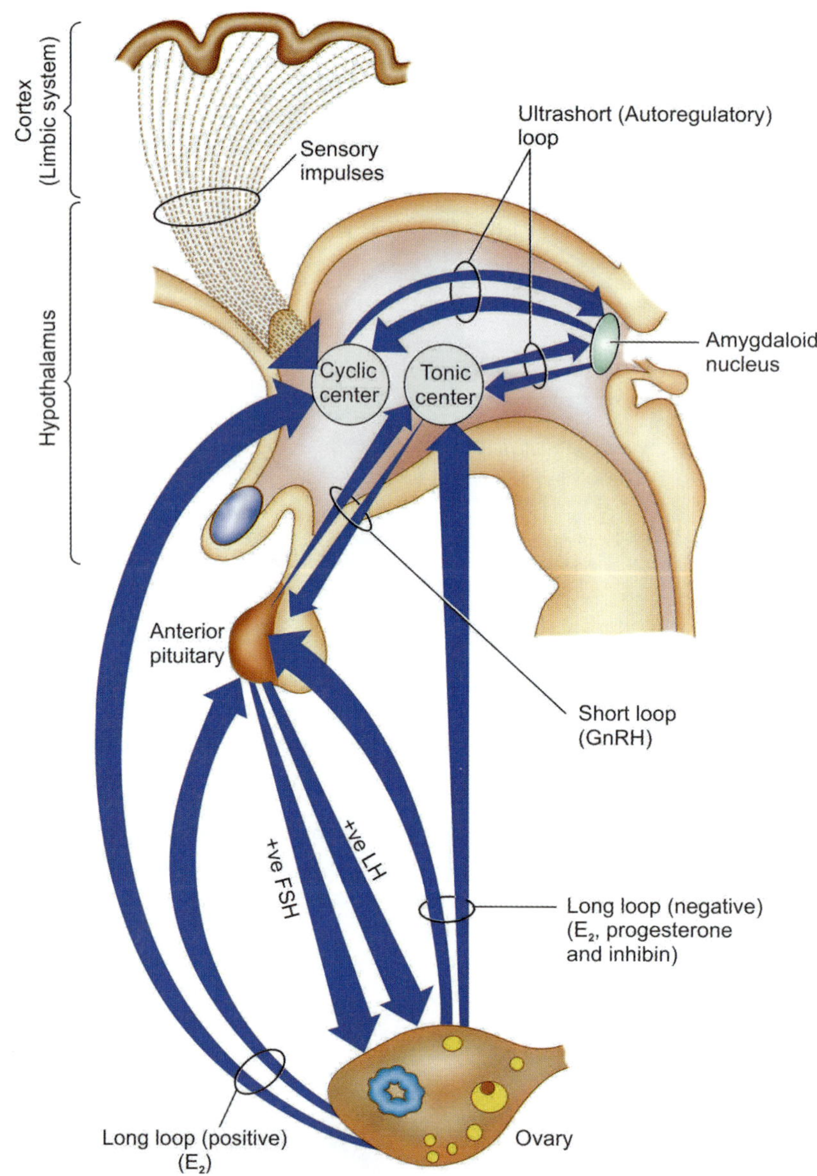

Interplay of hormones along the hypothalamo-pituitary-ovarian axis through feedback mechanism

151. While doing suction and evacuation, there is perforation of uterus. Next step is:

a. Laparoscopy
b. Hysterotomy
c. Laparotomy
d. Hysterectomy

Perforation of uterus is associated with varying degrees of internal hemorrhage. As such laparotomy is justified.

152. All of the following are true for anorexia nervosa EXCEPT:

a. Menorrhagia
b. Decreased FSH levels
c. Bulimia
d. Hypothermia

Anorexia nervosa is a state of self-imposed starvation. Patient denies food and is markedly under weight. Amenorrhea is the rule.

153. Serum progesterone estimation for luteal phase defect/ LPD should be done on:

a. 7th day of menstrual cycle
b. 14st day of menstrual cycle
c. 21st day of menstrual cycle
d. 28th day of menstrual cycle

Serum progesterone estimated on 8th day following ovulation is less than 10 ng/ml in LPD.

Ans. **151. c.** Laparotomy **152. a.** Menorrhagia **153. c.** 21st day of menstrual cycle

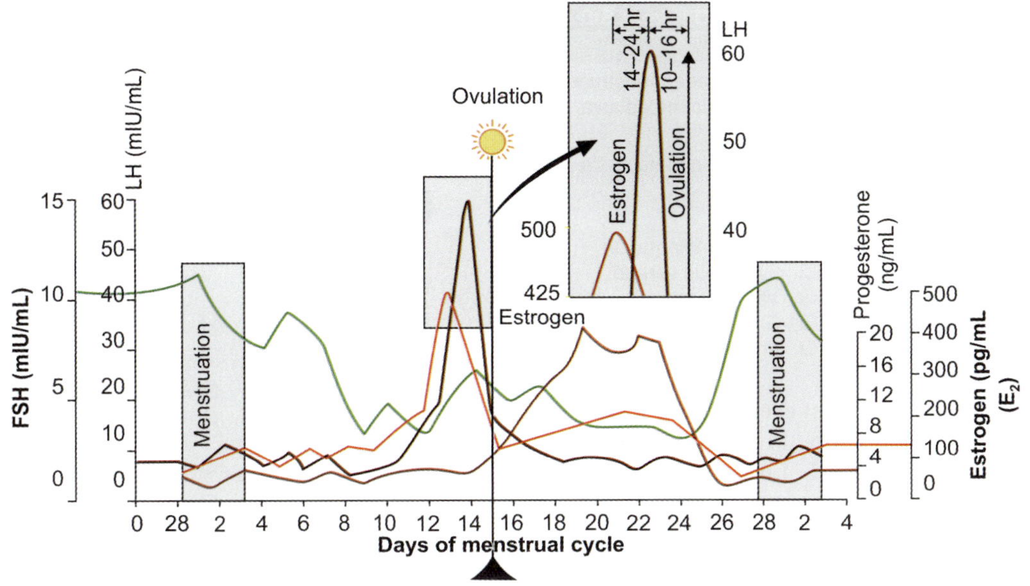

Fluctuation of serum levels of ovarian steroids and gonadotropins in a normal ovulatory cycle

154. MC site of endometriosis:

a. Peritoneal cavity b. Urinary bladder
c. Ovary d. Vagina

Presence of functioning endometrium (glands and stroma) in sites other than uterine mucosa is called endometriosis. It can occur at any sites but is usually confined to the abdominal structures below the level of umbilicus. Common sites include ovaries, pelvic peritoneum, Pouch of Douglas, Uterosacral ligaments, etc.

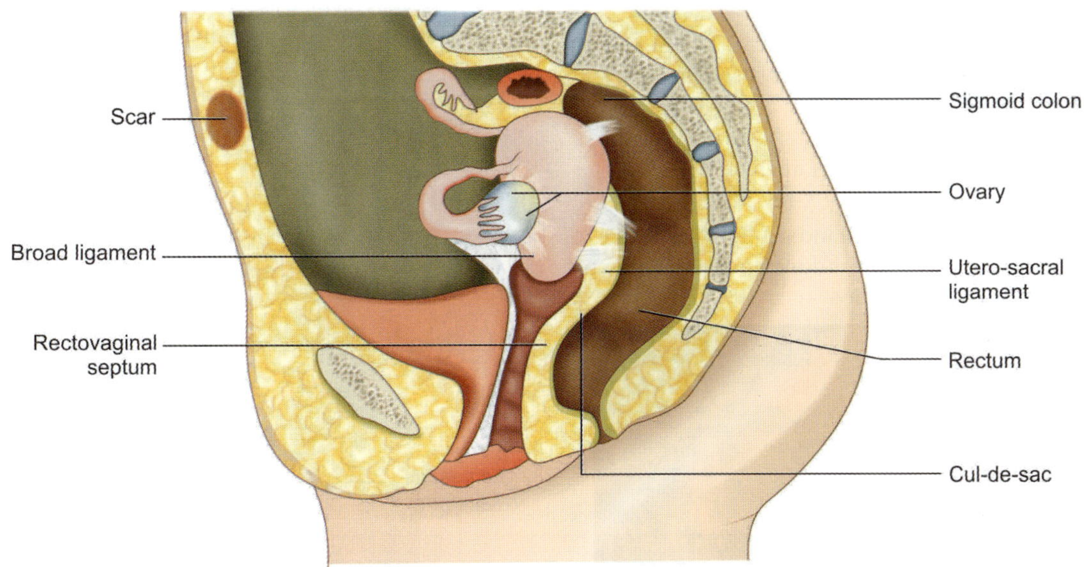

Common sites of endometriosis

155. Sampson's theory for endometriosis:

a. Metastatic theory
b. Implantation theory
c. Histogenesis by induction
d. Coelomic metaplasia theory

Retrograde menstruation (Sampson's theory): There is retrograde flow of menstrual blood through the uterine tubes during menstruation. The endometrial fragments get implanted in the peritoneal surface of the pelvic organs (dependent sites, e.g. ovaries, uterosacral ligaments).

Ans. **154. c.** Ovary **155. b.** Implantation theory

Theories to Explain Endometriosis at Different Sites	
Sites	*Theory*
❑ Pelvic endometriosis ❑ Pelvic peritoneum	❑ Retrograde menstruation ❑ Coelomic metaplasia
❑ Abdominal viscera ❑ Rectovaginal septum ❑ Umbilicus	❑ Coelomic metaplasia
❑ Abdominal scar ❑ Episiotomy scar ❑ Vagina, cervix ❑ Lymph nodes ❑ Distant sites (lungs, ❑ Pleura, skin, lymph nodes, nerves)	❑ Direct implantation ❑ Lymphatic spread ❑ Vascular spread ❑ Genetic ❑ Immunologic

156. Endometriosis can be present everywhere EXCEPT:

a. Ovary b. Broad ligaments
c. Uterosacral ligaments d. Liver

The common extra-abdominal sites are abdominal scar of hysterectomy, cesarean section, tubectomy and myomectomy, umbilicus, episiotomy scar, vagina and cervix.

Sites of Endometriosis		
Common sites	*Rare and remote sites*	
❑ Ovaries	❑ Umbilicus	
❑ Pelvic peritoneum	❑ Abdominal scar	
❑ Pouch of Douglas	❑ Episiotomy scar	
❑ Uterosacral ligaments	❑ Lungs	
❑ Rectovaginal septum	❑ Pleura	
❑ Sigmoid colon	❑ Ureter	
❑ Appendix	❑ Kidney	
❑ Pelvic lymph nodes	❑ Arms	❑ Legs
❑ Fallopian tubes	❑ Nasal mucosa	

157. Best investigation to establish the diagnosis of endometriosis is:

a. USG b. Laparoscopy
c. CT scan d. X-ray pelvis

Laparoscopy is the gold standard for diagnosis of endometriosis. Confirmation is done by double puncture laparoscopy or by laparotomy.

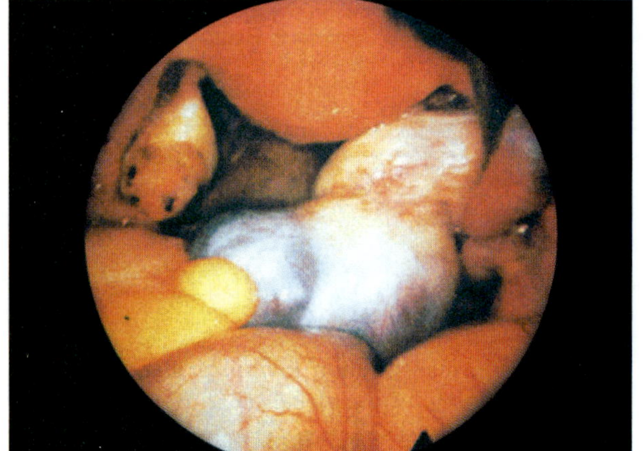

Laparoscopic view of pelvic endometriosis: Left ovary-endometriotic implants, right ovary-chocolate cyst

158. Following are used for the treatment of endometriosis EXCEPT:

a. OCP b. D and C
c. Progestins d. Surgical procedure

D and C is an operative procedure whereby dilatation of the cervical canal followed by uterine curettage is done.

Indications of D and C	
Diagnostic	❑ Infertility
	❑ DUB
	❑ Pathologic amenorrhea
	❑ Endometrial tuberculosis
	❑ Endometrial carcinoma
	❑ Postm enopausal bleeding
	❑ Chorionepithelioma
Therapeutic	❑ DUB
	❑ Endometrial polyp
	❑ Removal of IUD
	❑ Incomplete abortion
Combined	❑ DUB
	❑ Endometrial polyp

159. Most common symptom of endometriosis is:

a. Dysmenorrhoea b. Dyspareunia
c. Infertility d. Abdominal pain

Dysmenorrhea is present in 70% of the patients of endometriosis, which is progressively increasing secondary dysmenorrheal. The pain starts a few days prior to menstruation; gets worsened during menstruation and takes time, even after cessation of period, to get relief of pain (comenstrual dysmenorrhea).

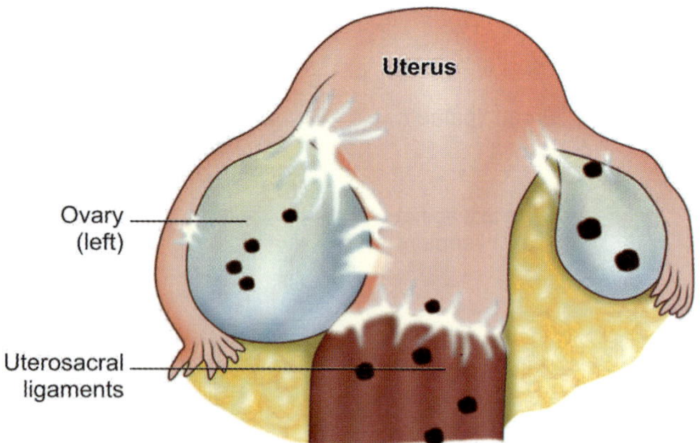

The appearance of pelvic endometriosis. Note the black dots and puckered peritoneum. Sites of involvement are: ovaries, uterosacral ligaments and pelvic peritoneum

160. Best investigation to assess tubal patency is:

a. Rubin's test
b. Hysterosalpingogram
c. Laparotomy
d. Laparoscopic chromotubation

Ans. 156. **d.** Liver 157. **b.** Laparoscopy 158. **b.** D and C 159. **a.** Dysmenorrhoea
160. **d.** Laparoscopic chromotubation

Laparoscopy is the gold standard (definitive method) for evaluation of tubal factors of infertility. It is done after male factor and ovulatory functions have been found normal or corrected.

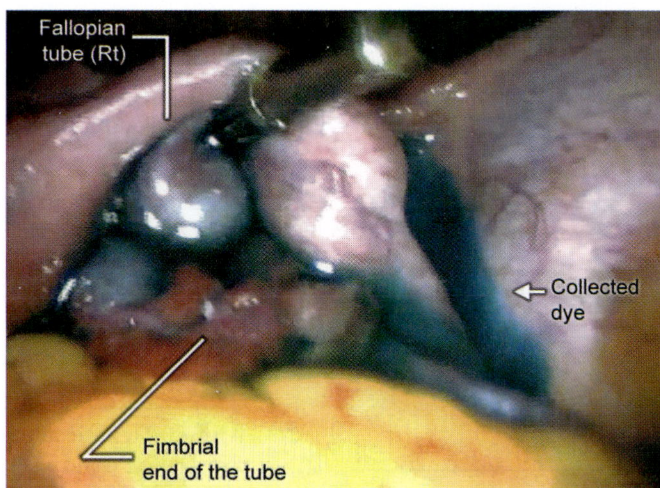

Chromopertubation shows the patency of the tubes with spillage of dye (methylene blue) in the peritoneal cavity *(Courtesy: Dr. Manoj Samanta)*

ANSWERS WITH REFERENCES

GYNECOLOGICAL ANATOMY

1. **Ans. (a)** Tubes
Ref: Dutta's Gynecology 6/e p11

2. **Ans. (c)** Stratified squamous nonkeratinized
Ref: Dutta's Gynecology 6/e p6

3. **Ans. (b)** Rich in glands
Ref: Dutta's Gynecology 6/e p5

4. **Ans. (b)** Cardinal ligaments
Ref: Dutta's Gynecology 6/e p22

5. **Ans. (b)** 3 × 2 × 1
Ref: Dutta's Gynecology 6/e p4

6. **Ans. (b)** 2:1
Ref: Dutta's Gynecology 6/e p7

7. **Ans. (c)** Genital ridge
Ref: Dutta's Gynecology 6/e p13

8. **Ans. (d)** 2 millions
Ref: Dutta's Gynecology 6/e p86

9. **Ans. (b)** Paramesonephric duct
Ref: Dutta's Gynecology 6/e p39

10. **Ans. (a)** Interstitial
Ref: Dutta's Gynecology 6/e p10

CONTRACEPTIVES

11. **Ans. (b)** Cu-T 380A
Ref: Shaw's Gynaecology, 13th/ed p229

12. **Ans. (b)** Protection from breast malignancy
Ref: Shaw's Gynaecology, 13th/ed p227

13. **Ans. (c)** Mala-N
Ref: Dutta's Gynecology 6/e p486

14. **Ans. (c)** Cervical ripening
Ref: Dutta's Gynecology 6/e p492

15. **Ans. (a)** Accidental pregnancies
Ref: Dutta's Gynecology 6/e p476

16. **Ans. (a)** Making endometrium unreceptive
Ref: Dutta's Gynecology 6/e p479

17. **Ans. (c)** Withdrawal technique
Ref: Dutta's Gynecology 6/e p481

18. **Ans. (a)** Cu 380 A
Ref: Dutta's Gynecology 6/e p482

19. **Ans. (d)** Isthmus
Ref: Dutta's Gynecology 6/e p497

20. **Ans. (b)** Contains 200 sq. mm. of Cu
Ref: Dutta's Gynecology 6/e p482

21. **Ans. (a)** Ovulation inhibition
Ref: Dutta's Gynecology 6/e p483

22. **Ans. (c)** Endometrial Ca
Ref: Dutta's Gynecology 6/e p487

23. **Ans. (c)** Levonorgestrel
Ref: Dutta's Gynecology 6/e p493

24. **Ans. (a)** Hepatic adenoma
Ref: Dutta's Gynecology 6/e p488

25. **Ans. (d)** Menstrual irregularities
Ref: Dutta's Gynecology 6/e p485

26. **Ans. (a)** Cu-T
Ref: Dutta's Gynecology 6/e p483

27. **Ans. (c)** 30 microgram
Ref: Dutta's Gynecology 6/e p491

28. **Ans. (d)** Cervical carcinoma
Ref: Dutta's Gynecology 6/e p475

GYNECOLOGICAL INFECTION

29. **Ans. (b)** pH less than 4.5
Ref: Shaw's Gynaecology, 13th/ed p129

30. **Ans. (a)** TB
Ref: Internet resources

31. **Ans. (b)** Laparoscopy
Ref: Dutta's Gynecology 6/e p611

32. **Ans. (c)** Candidal vaginitis
Ref: Dutta's Gynecology 6/e p166

33. **Ans. (c)** Candida albicans
Ref: Dutta's Gynecology 6/e p165

34. **Ans. (a)** Hemophilus vaginalis
Ref: Dutta's Gynecology 6/e p152

35. **Ans. (a)** Trichomonas vaginalis
Ref: Dutta's Gynecology 6/e p164

36. **Ans. (c)** Abundance of polymorphs
Ref: Dutta's Gynecology 6/e p146

37. **Ans. (b)** Thick white discharge
Ref: Dutta's Gynecology 6/e p165

38. **Ans. (b) Ectopic pregnancy**
Ref: Dutta's Gynecology 6/e p141

39. **Ans. (c) Pruritis seen**
Ref: Dutta's Gynecology 6/e p152

40. **Ans. (b) Abdominal pain**
Ref: Dutta's Gynecology 6/e p131

MENSTRUAL DISTURBANCES

41. **Ans. (c) Premature menopause**
Ref: Dutta's Gynecology 6/e p454

42. **Ans. (c) PCOD**
Ref: Dutta's Gynecology 6/e p460

43. **Ans. (d) More than 80 ml**
Ref: Dutta's Gynecology 6/e p185

44. **Ans. (a) Endometrial TB**
Ref: Dutta's Gynecology 6/e p457

45. **Ans. (c) Polymenorrhea**
Ref: Dutta's Gynecology 6/e p458

46. **Ans. (b) Progesterone**
Ref: Dutta's Gynecology 6/e p191

47. **Ans. (a) Prolactin level**
Ref: Dutta's Gynecology 6/e p467

48. **Ans. (a) Estrogen**
Ref: Dutta's Gynecology 6/e p62

49. **Ans. (a) Metropathia hemorrhagica**
Ref: Dutta's Gynecology 6/e p188

50. **Ans. (b) Turners syndrome**
Ref: Dutta's Gynecology 6/e p453

51. **Ans. (d) Polycystic ovarian disease**
Ref: Dutta's Gynecology 6/e p461

52. **Ans. (c) Sheehan's syndrome**
Ref: Dutta's Gynecology 6/e p455

53. **Ans. (c) Imperforate hymen**
Ref: Dutta's Gynecology 6/e p42

54. **Ans. (b) Uterus absent; tubes and ovaries present**
Ref: Dutta's Gynecology 6/e p451

55. **Ans. (c) Testicular feminizing syndrome**
Ref: Dutta's Gynecology 6/e p445

56. **Ans. (b) Stein-Leventhal syndrome**
Ref: Dutta's Gynecology 6/e p459

57. **Ans. (b) Oligomenorrhoea**
Ref: Dutta's Gynecology 6/e p186

GYNECOLOGICAL ONCOLOGY

58. **Ans. (b) Clear cell tumour**
Ref: Shaw's Gynaecology, 13th/ed p356t

59. **Ans. (d) Chorioangioma**
Ref: Internet resources

60. **Ans. (c) Simple hysterectomy**
Ref: Shaw's Gynaecology, 13th/ed., p-

61. **Ans. (b) Ca endometrium**
Ref: Dutta's Gynecology 6/e p559

62. **Ans. (c) Carcinoma cervix**
Ref: Dutta's Gynecology 6/e p169

63. **Ans. (b) Total abdominal hysterectomy**
Ref: Dutta's Gynecology 6/e p321

64. **Ans. (c) Hyaline degeneration**
Ref: Dutta's Gynecology 6/e p274

65. **Ans. (d) Serous cyst adenoma**
Ref: Dutta's Gynecology 6/e p291

66. **Ans. (c) Complex hyperplasia with atypia**
Ref: Dutta's Gynecology 6/e p330

67. **Ans. (a) 70%**
Ref: Dutta's Gynecology 6/e p110

68. **Ans. (b) Postcoital test**
Ref: Dutta's Gynecology 6/e p240

69. **Ans. (d) Choriocarcinoma**
Ref: Dutta's Gynecology 6/e p363

70. **Ans. (a) Upper 2/3rd endocervix**
Ref: Dutta's Gynecology 6/e p116

71. **Ans. (b) Subserous fibroid**
Ref: Dutta's Gynecology 6/e p273

72. **Ans. (a) Anterior cervical fibroid**
Ref: Dutta's Gynecology 6/e p284

73. **Ans. (b) Stage III b**
Ref: Dutta's Gynecology 6/e p357

74. **Ans. (a) CIN III**
Ref: Dutta's Gynecology 6/e p590

75. **Ans. (c) Chemotherapy with methotrexate**
Ref: Dutta's Gynecology 6/e p364

76. **Ans. (c) Colposcopy and biopsy**
Ref: Dutta's Gynecology 6/e p328

77. **Ans. (d) Endodermal sinus tumour**
Ref: Dutta's Gynecology 6/e p382

78. **Ans. (c) Analgesics**
Ref: Dutta's Gynecology 6/e p272

79. **Ans. (d) Dysgerminoma**
Ref: Dutta's Gynecology 6/e p382

80. **Ans. (c) Inhibin**
Ref: Dutta's Gynecology 6/e p384

81. **Ans. (b) Amenorrhoea**
Ref: Dutta's Gynecology 6/e p279

82. **Ans. (a) Total hysterectomy**
Ref: Dutta's Gynecology 6/e p358

83. **Ans. (c) Fibroma**
Ref: Dutta's Gynecology 6/e p385

84. **Ans. (c) Squamous cell carcinoma**
Ref: Dutta's Gynecology 6/e p340

85. **Ans. (a) Hyaline changes**
Ref: Dutta's Gynecology 6/e p274

86. **Ans. (a) Dysgerminoma**
Ref: Dutta's Gynecology 6/e p355

87. **Ans. (d) Endodermal sinus tumour**
Ref: Dutta's Gynecology 6/e p371

88. **Ans. (a) Cisplatin, etoposide, bleomycin**
Ref: Dutta's Gynecology 6/e p382

89. **Ans. (b) LLETZ**
Ref: Dutta's Gynecology 6/e p323

90. **Ans. (b) Lungs**
Ref: Dutta's Gynecology 6/e p364

91. **Ans. (c) Post coital bleeding**
Ref: Dutta's Gynecology 6/e p655

92. **Ans. (c) HPV**
Ref: Dutta's Gynecology 6/e p157

93. **Ans. (c) Post treatment HCG levels**
Ref: Dutta's Gynecology 6/e p364

94. **Ans. (c) Score of more than 8**
Ref: Dutta's Gynecology 6/e p366

95. **Ans. (d) Chemotherapy**
Ref: Dutta's Gynecology 6/e p365

96. **Ans. (c) Tourniquet use**
Ref: Dutta's Gynecology 6/e p278

MISCELLANEOUS

97. **Ans. (d) Norgestrel**
Ref: Shaw's Gynaecology, 13th/ed p108

98. **Ans. (b) PCOS**
Ref: Shaw's Gynaecology, 13th/ed p354

99. **Ans. (c) Patent ductus arteriosus**
Ref: Shaw's Gynaecology, 13th/ed p100

100. **Ans. (b) Mullerian agenesis**
Ref: Shaw's Gynaecology, 13th/ed p280

101. **Ans. (b) Estrogen**
Ref: Dutta's Gynecology 6/e p115

102. **Ans. (c) 36 hours**
Ref: Dutta's Gynecology 6/e p93

103. **Ans. (a) Increased LDL and lowered HDL**
Ref: Dutta's Gynecology 6/e p74

104. **Ans. (b) Accompanied by ovulation**
Ref: Dutta's Gynecology 6/e p94

105. **Ans. (b) Estrogenic effect**
Ref: Dutta's Gynecology 6/e p114

106. **Ans. (b) Cervical factor**
Ref: Dutta's Gynecology 6/e p241

107. **Ans. (c) Both**
Ref: Dutta's Gynecology 6/e p87

108. **Ans. (d) Imperforate hymen**
Ref: Dutta's Gynecology 6/e p43

109. **Ans. (c) Osteoporosis**
Ref: Dutta's Gynecology 6/e p62

110. **Ans. (a) Corpus luteum**
Ref: Dutta's Gynecology 6/e p84

111. **Ans. (c) Lateral wall**
Ref: Dutta's Gynecology 6/e p95

112. **Ans. (b) Klinefelter's syndrome**
Ref: Dutta's Gynecology 6/e p443

113. **Ans. (b) Endometrial biopsy**
Ref: Dutta's Gynecology 6/e p91

114. **Ans. (c) Fenton's**
Ref: Dutta's Gynecology 6/e p206

115. **Ans. (c) 14 days**
Ref: Dutta's Gynecology 6/e p96

116. **Ans. (d) Stress incontinence**
Ref: Dutta's Gynecology 6/e p401

117. **Ans. (b) 35 cc**
Ref: Dutta's Gynecology 6/e p 89

118. **Ans. (a) 4.5**
Ref: Dutta's Gynecology 6/e p6

119. **Ans. (d) All**
Ref: Dutta's Gynecology 6/e p 54

120. **Ans. (a) Marsupialization**
Ref: Dutta's Gynecology 6/e p162

121. **Ans. (c) Uterus**
Ref: Internet resources

122. **Ans. (c) Adrenal hyperplasia**
Ref: Dutta's Gynecology 6/e p440

123. **Ans. (b) Ureterovaginal fistula**
Ref: Dutta's Gynecology 6/e p417

124. **Ans. (a) Estrogen**
Ref: Dutta's Gynecology 6/e p115

125. **Ans. (d) Laparoscopic chromotubation**
Ref: Dutta's Gynecology 6/e p238

126. **Ans. (a) Estimation of FSH level**
Ref: Dutta's Gynecology 6/e p233

127. **Ans. (b) Volume of 1 ml**
Ref: Dutta's Gynecology 6/e p232

128. **Ans. (a) Coronary heart disease**
Ref: Dutta's Gynecology 6/e p63

129. **Ans. (d) Vesicovaginal fistula**
Ref: Dutta's Gynecology 6/e p418

130. **Ans. (b) Carbon dioxide**
Ref: Dutta's Gynecology 6/e p621

131. **Ans. (c) Down syndrome**
Ref: Internet resources

132. **Ans. (a) TORCH infection screening**
Ref: Internet resources

133. **Ans. (a) Breast carcinoma**
Ref: Dutta's Gynecology 6/e p62

134. **Ans. (a) Estimation of FSH level**
Ref: Dutta's Gynecology 6/e p

135. **Ans. (b) Urine FSH**
Ref: Dutta's Gynecology 6/e p235

136. **Ans. (b) Lactobacillus**
Ref: Dutta's Gynecology 6/e p4

137. **Ans. (a) Anterior pituitary gland**
Ref: Dutta's Gynecology 6/e p7.1

138. **Ans. (b) Nulliparous prolapse**
Ref: Dutta's Gynecology 6/e p206

139. **Ans. (c) Appearance of breast buds**
Ref: Dutta's Gynecology 6/e p50

140. **Ans. (c) Turner syndrome**
Ref: Dutta's Gynecology 6/e p441

141. **Ans. (b) Just before ovulation**
Ref: Dutta's Gynecology 6/e p73

142. **Ans. (c) Dyspareunia**
Ref: Dutta's Gynecology 6/e p45

143. **Ans. (b) 24-36 hours before ovulation**
Ref: Dutta's Gynecology 6/e p79

144. **Ans. (c) Hysteroscopy**
Ref: Dutta's Gynecology 6/e p619

145. **Ans. (c) Highest on the day of ovulation**
Ref: Internet resources

146. **Ans. (d) LH**
Ref: Dutta's Gynecology 6/e p85

147. **Ans. (c) Less**
Ref: Dutta's Gynecology 6/e p72

148. **Ans. (b) LH**
Ref: Dutta's Gynecology 6/e p78

149. **Ans. (c) Abnormal morphology of sperms**
Ref: Dutta's Gynecology 6/e p232

150. **Ans. (d) All of the above**
Ref: Dutta's Gynecology 6/e p659

151. **Ans. (c) Laparotomy**
Ref: Internet resources

152. **Ans. (a) Menorrhagia**
Ref: Dutta's Gynecology 6/e p464

153. **Ans. (c) 21st day of menstrual cycle**
Ref: Dutta's Gynecology 6/e p94

154. **Ans. (c) Ovary**
Ref: Dutta's Gynecology 6/e p304

155. **Ans. (b) Implantation theory**
Ref: Dutta's Gynecology 6/e p305

156. **Ans. (d) Liver**
Ref: Dutta's Gynecology 6/e p305

157. **Ans. (b) Laparoscopy**
Ref: Dutta's Gynecology 6/e p308

158. **Ans. (b) D and C**
Ref: Dutta's Gynecology 6/e p585

159. **Ans. (a) Dysmenorrhoea**
Ref: Dutta's Gynecology 6/e p306

160. **Ans. (d) Laparoscopic chromotubation**
Ref: Dutta's Gynecology 6/e p239

PRACTICE QUESTIONS

GYNECOLOGICAL ANATOMY

1. FALSE statement regarding vagina:
- a. Excretory channel for uterine secretions
- b. Forms 45 degree angle with horizontal in erect posture
- c. Long axis parallel to plane of pelvic inlet
- d. Length of anterior wall is 9 cm

CONTRACEPTIVES

2. Contraceptive of choice after abortion of molar pregnancy:
- a. IUCD
- b. Barrier methods
- c. Abstinence methods
- d. OCPs

3. OCP reduces the risk of:
- a. Breast carcinoma
- b. Endometrial carcinoma
- c. Hepatocellular carcinoma
- d. Biliary carcinoma

4. All of the following are attributed to the estrogenic component of OCPs EXCEPT:
- a. Increased hepatic secretion of proteins
- b. Hyperglycemia
- c. Increased HDL cholesterol
- d. Decreased LDL cholesterol

GYNECOLOGICAL INFECTIONS

5. Investigation of choice in PID:
- a. Blood culture
- b. Gram staining
- c. Biopsy
- d. Laparoscopy

MENSTRUAL DISTURBANCES

6. A lady presented with menstrual bleeding for >7 days and the amount is >100 ml. This pattern of bleeding is:
- a. Normal menstruation
- b. Hypermenorrhoea
- c. Oligomenorrhoea
- d. Polymenorrhoea

7. MC cause of postmenopausal bleeding:
- a. Carcinoma endometrium
- b. Carcinoma cervix
- c. Hormone replacement therapy
- d. Carcinoma vulva

8. DUB is commonly associated with:
- a. Hypomenorrhoea
- b. Oligomenorrhoea
- c. Metropathia hemorrhagica
- d. Postmenopausal bleeding

9. A young lady presented with irregular bleeding. On work-up, no pathology could be detected. Microscopically 'Swiss cheese' pattern of endometrium was seen. Most probable diagnosis :
- a. Carcinoma cervix
- b. Cystic glandular hyperplasia
- c. Bacterial vaginosis
- d. Androgen producing tumours

GYNECOLOGICAL ONCOLOGY

10. MC causative agent of carcinoma cervix:
- a. EBV
- b. HPV 16,18
- c. HIV
- d. HHV

11. Inhibin is secreted by which tumour:
- a. Hilus cell tumour
- b. Arrhenoblastoma
- c. Granulosa cell tumour
- d. Leydig cell tumour

12. Best confirmatory test for cervical carcinoma:
- a. Speculum examination
- b. Bimanual examination
- c. CT scan
- d. Cervicography

13. Primary group of lymph nodes affected in cervical carcinoma:
- a. Common iliac group
- b. Inguinal nodes
- c. Obturator nodes
- d. Para aortic nodes

14. Side effect of tamoxifen:
- a. Ovarian carcinoma
- b. Vulval carcinoma
- c. Vaginal carcinoma
- d. Endometrial carcinoma

15. Which of the following ovarian neoplasm shows Rokitansky's protuberance:
- a. Androblastoma
- b. Mucinous cyst adenoma
- c. Dermoid cyst
- d. Papillary serous cyst adenoma

Ans. 1. **d.** Length of ant... 2. **d.** OCPs 3. **b.** Endometrial car... 4. **b.** Hyperglycemia 5. **d.** Laparoscopy 6. **b.** Hypermenorrhoea 7. **b.** Carcinoma cervix 8. **c.** Metropathia hemorrh... 9. **b.** Cystic glandular... 10. **b.** HPV 16,18 11. **c.** Granulosa cell tumour 12. **d.** Cervicography 13. **c.** Obturator nodes 14. **d.** Endometrial... 15. **c.** Dermoid cyst

16. **Management of cervical carcinoma stage III:**
   a. Chemotherapy
   b. Radiotherapy
   c. Chemo-radiotherapy
   d. Simple hysterectomy

17. **In staging of vulvar carcinoma, involvement of urethra is which stage:**
   a. I
   b. II
   c. III
   d. IV

18. **Vulvar ulcers caused by which of the following organism may convert to malignancy:**
   a. Herpes simplex virus 1
   b. Herpes simplex virus 2
   c. Treponema pallidum
   d. Human papilloma virus

19. **Common primary site of Krukenberg tumour:**
   a. Ovary
   b. Gall bladder
   c. Colon
   d. Breast

MISCELLANEOUS

20. **Management of senile vaginitis:**
   a. Progesterone cream
   b. Levonorgestrel
   c. Estrogen cream
   d. Prostaglandin cream

21. **Management of PCOD:**
   a. Tamoxifen
   b. Raloxifene
   c. Clomiphene citrate
   d. OCPs

22. **HAIR-AN syndrome, wrong statement:**
   a. Insulin resistance
   b. Hypoandrogenism
   c. Acanthosis nigricans
   d. PCOS

23. **A young lady presented with hyperandrogenism, high estrogen and raised testosterone levels. She is also having acne and hirsutism. Most likely diagnosis:**
   a. Osteoporosis
   b. Osteopetrosis
   c. Polycystic ovarian disease
   d. Granulosa cell tumour

24. **What with the degree of perineal tear in a patient of perineal tear involving the anal sphincter but uninvolved anal mucosa:**
   a. I b. II
   c. III d. IV

25. **Upper and lower swab were dry but middle swab was stained with dye:**
   a. Ureterovaginal fistula b. Urethrovaginal fistula
   c. Rectovaginal fistula d. Vesicovaginal fistula

26. **Urge present but the patient can NOT pass the urine normally:**
   a. Ureterovaginal fistula
   b. Vesicovaginal fistula
   c. Urethrovaginal fistula
   d. Vesicocervical fistula

27. **An infertile male with eunuchoid appearance and breast enlargement is possibly a case of:**
   a. Liver failure
   b. Klinefelter's syndrome
   c. Carcinoma prostate
   d. Testicular feminization syndrome

28. **A girl with a height of 130 cm has primary amenorrhoea and delayed secondary sexual characters. She also had webbing of neck, cubitus valgus and broad shield chest. Investigation shows hypergonadotropism:**
   a. Turner syndrome
   b. Klinefelter syndrome
   c. Down syndrome
   d. Felty syndrome

29. **Precocious puberty, Cafe-au-lait spots and multiple bone cysts hints towards the diagnosis of:**
   a. Prader-Willi syndrome
   b. PCOS
   c. Eosinophilic granuloma
   d. McCune Albright syndrome

30. **Fluctuant and non-tender swelling at the junction of posterior one third and anterior two-third of labia majora:**
   a. Gartner duct cyst
   b. Bartholin's cyst
   c. Vulval cyst
   d. Vaginal cyst

31. **Ferning pattern of cervical mucus is seen in:**
   a. Early proliferative phase
   b. Late proliferative phase
   c. Early secretory phase
   d. Late secretory phase

Ans.

16. c. Chemo-radio...	**17. d.** IV	**18. d.** Human papilloma...	**19. c.** Colon
20. c. Estrogen cream	**21. c.** Clomiphene citrate	**22. b.** Hypoandrogenism	**23. c.** Polycystic ovarian disease
24. c. III	**25. d.** Vesicovaginal fistula	**26. c.** Urethrovaginal fistula	**27. b.** Klinefelter's syndrome
28. a. Turner syndrome	**29. d.** McCune Albright...	**30. b.** Bartholin's cyst	**31. c.** Early secretory phase

IMAGE-BASED QUESTIONS

1. The causative organism for such a clinical presentation:

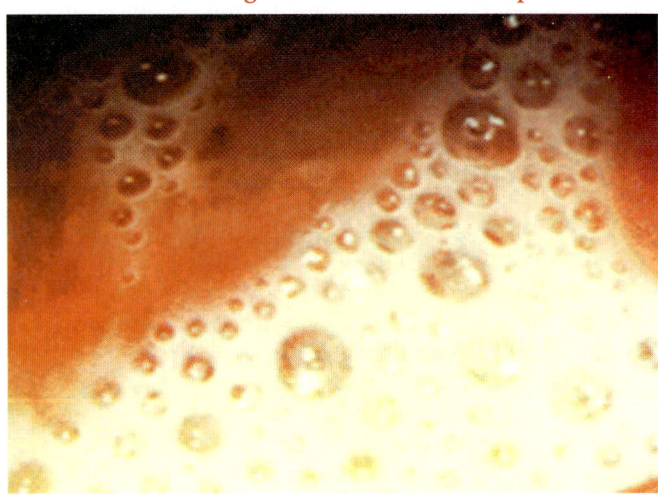

a. H. vaginalis
b. Trichomonas vaginalis
c. Candida albicans
d. Chlamydia trachomatis

In trichomoniasis, there is thin, greenish-yellow and frothy offensive discharge per vaginam.

2. The causative organism for such a clinical presentation:

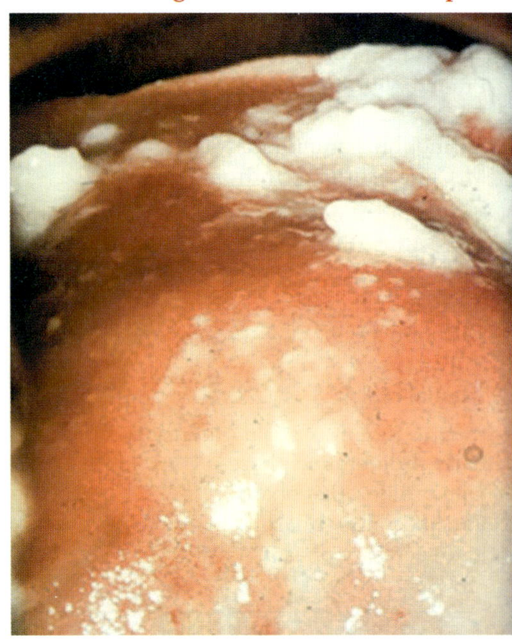

a. H. vaginalis
b. Trichomonas vaginalis
c. Candida albicans
d. Chlamydia trachomatis

In candidiasis, the discharge is thick, curdy white and in flakes, (cottage cheese type) often adherent to the vaginal wall.

3. The causative organism for such a clinical presentation:

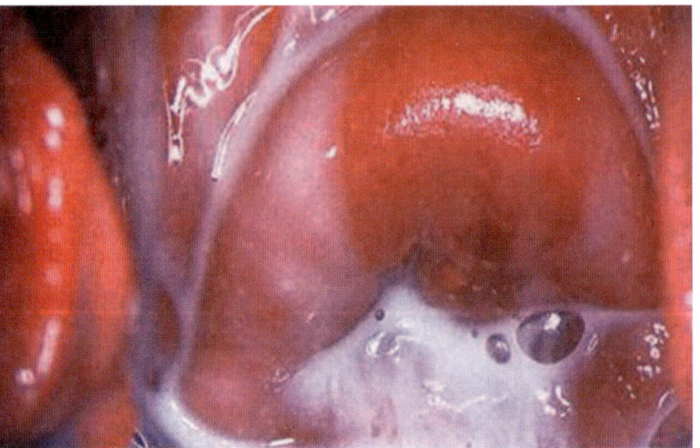

a. H. vaginalis
b. Trichomonas vaginalis
c. Candida albicans
d. Chlamydia trachomatis

In bacterial vaginosis, the discharge is homogenous, greyish-white and adherent to the vaginal wall.

4. The causative organism for such a clinical presentation:

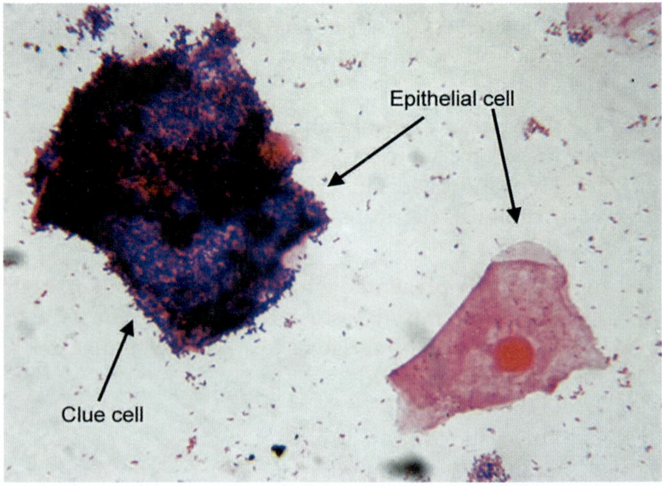

a. H. vaginalis
b. Trichomonas vaginalis
c. Candida albicans
d. Chlamydia trachomatis

Presence of clue cells (>20% of cells) are diagnostic of BV.

5. Identify the pathology:

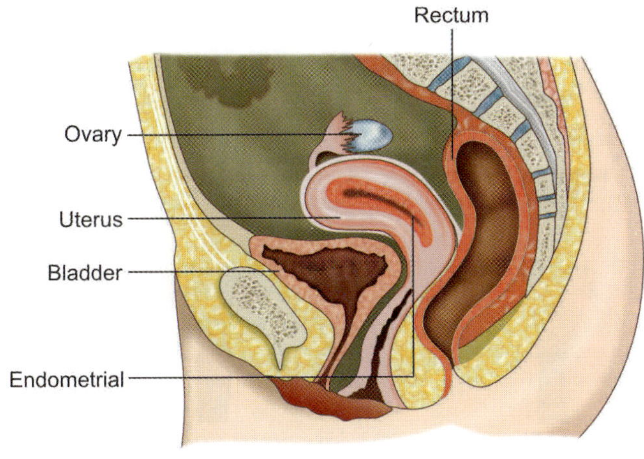

a. Adenomyosis
b. Endometriosis
c. Ectopic pregnancy
d. Normal pregnancy

Presence of functioning endometrium (glands and stroma) in sites other than uterine mucosa is called endometriosis.

6. Following image is suggestive of management of which condition:

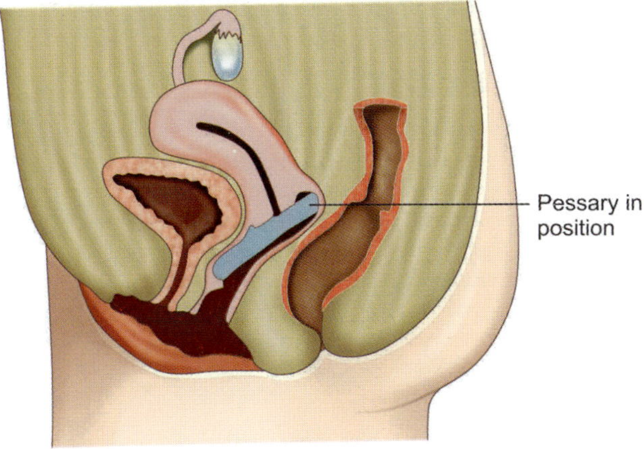

a. Genital fistula
b. Genital prolapse
c. Contraception
d. Rectal prolapse

Pessary treatment relieves the symptoms of prolapse by stretching the hiatus urogenitalis, thus preventing vaginal and uterine descent. It is indicated in early pregnancy (up to 18 weeks), puerperium or unfit/unwilling/waiting patients for surgery.

7. Which of the following would be normal in such a case:

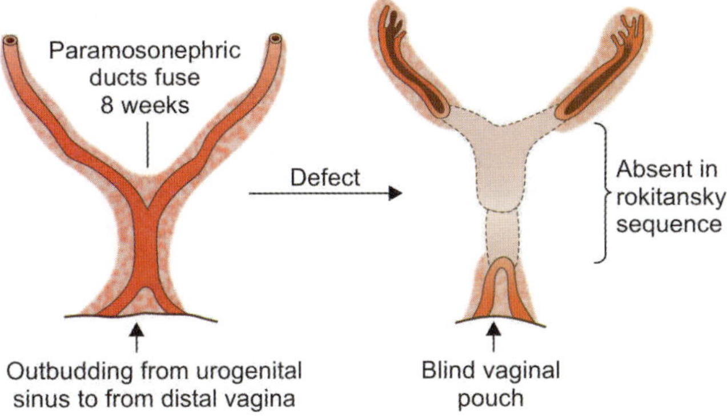

a. Uterus
b. Urinary tract
c. Ovaries
d. Cervix

In Müllerian agenesis/MRKH syndrome, uterus is absent, tubes are present, ovaries are normal and 30% cases may have urinary tract abnormalities.

8. Karyotype of such a patient:

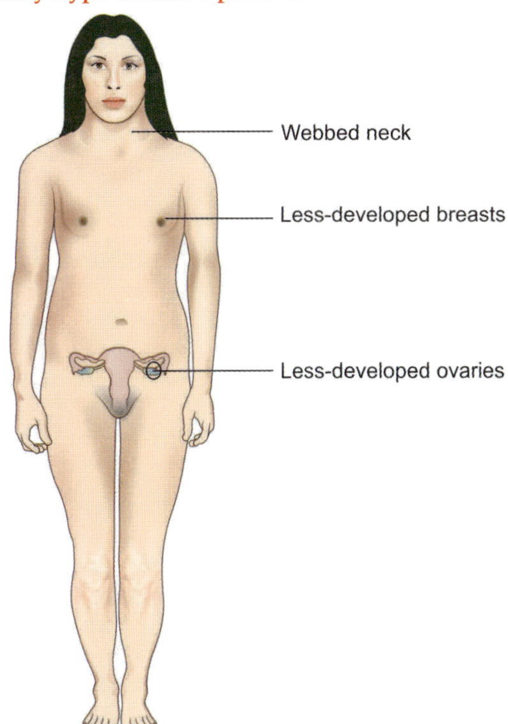

a. 46XX
b. 46XY
c. 45XO
d. 47XXY

Karyotype of Turner's syndrome is 45XO

9. Name the procedure:

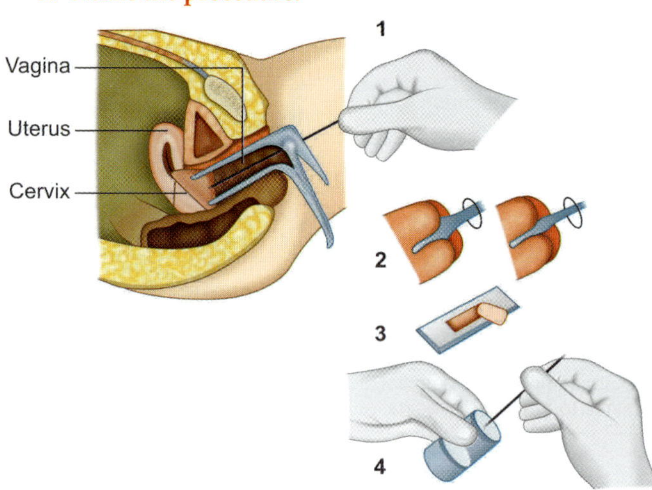

a. LEEP
b. LLETZ
c. Conization
d. Pap smear

In pap smear, the material from the cervix is best collected using Ayre's spatula made of wood or plastic. Whole of the squamocolumnar junction has to be scrapped to obtain good material. The material so collected should be immediately spread over a microscopic slide and at once put into the fixative ethyl alcohol (95%) before drying.

10. Which stage of carcinoma cervix:

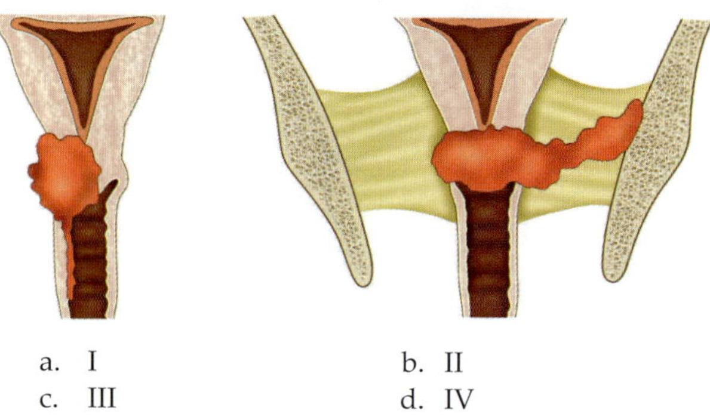

a. I
b. II
c. III
d. IV

In stage III of carcinoma cervix, the tumor extends to the pelvic wall and/or involves lower third of the vagina and/or causes hydronephrosis or non-functioning kidneys.

MCQ POINTS

S. No.	Question statements	Answers
1.	Genital ridge forms	***Ovary***
2.	MC site of genital TB	***Fallopian tube***
3.	Cervix develops from	***Mullerian duct***
4.	MC site of endometriosis	***Ovary***
5.	Strawberry vagina is seen in	***Trichomoniasis***
6.	MC cause of pyometra	***Ca cervix***
7.	Spasmodic dysmenorrhoea is seen in	***Endometriosis***
8.	MC cause of postmenopausal bleeding in India	***1. Hormone replacement therapy, 2. Ca endometrium***
9.	MC type of cervical carcinoma	***Squamous***
10.	Corpus luteum of menstruation persists for how many days	***14 days***
11.	MTP act was passed in which year	***1971***
12.	Most radiosensitive ovarian tumour	***Dysgerminoma***
13.	Call Exner bodies are seen in	***Granulosa cell tumour***
14.	Ferning of cervical mucus disappears on which day	***21st day***
15.	Splegelbereg's criteria is used for	***Ectopic pregnancy***
16.	Best test for tubal patency	***Laparoscopic chromotubation***
17.	CA 125 is a marker for	***Ovarian Ca***
18.	MC type of endometrial carcinoma	***Adenocarcinoma***
19.	Red degeneration of fibroid is seen in	***2nd trimester of pregnancy/puerperium***
20.	MC cause of death in carcinoma cervix	***Renal failure***
21.	Earliest presenting feature of carcinoma cervix	***Postcoital bleeding (Ca cervix: an entity of females in reproductive age group so should not be counted as a cause of post-menopausal bleeding)***
22.	MC site of laparoscopic sterilization in females	***Isthmus***
23.	OCP of choice in lactating females	***Minipill***
24.	DOC for bacterial vaginosis	***Metronidazole***
25.	White curdy discharge per vaginum, with intense itching is suggestive of	***Candida***
26.	Mucosal lining of vagina	***Stratified squamous, non-keratinized***
27.	Pearl index is used for calculating	***Failure rate of contraceptives***
28.	Life-span of Cu-T 380A	***10 years***
29.	Gold standard investigation for diagnosing PID	***Laparoscopy (should not be done in acute PID)***
30.	Infection associated with vaginal ph of 4.0	***Candida***
31.	DOC for bacterial vaginosis	***Metronidazole***
32.	MC histological type of cervical carcinoma	***Squamous***
33.	Endometrial carcinoma with vaginal metastasis is which stage	***Stage IIIb***
34.	Treatment of choice for choriocarcinoma	***Methotrexate***
35.	FIGO stage IIa of cervical carcinoma is	***Tumour extends beyond cervix but not to lateral pelvic wall or lower third of vagina***
36.	Tumour marker for endodermal sinus tumour	***Alpha Fetoprotein***
37.	Investigation of choice for cervical neoplasm is	***Biopsy***

S. No.	Question statements	Answers
38.	18 year old girl presents with primary amenorrhea, normal breast development, absent pubic & axillary hair. Condition is	***Testicular feminization syndrome/ androgen insensitivity syndrome***
39.	MC complication of abdominal hysterectomy	***Ureteral injury***
40.	Cervix can be visualized by which instrument	***Colposcope***
41.	Treatment for Bartholin's cyst	***Marsupialization***
42.	Chromosome complement in patient with Klinefelter's syndrome	***47XXY***
43.	Trisomy 21 is known as .... syndrome	***Down syndrome***
44.	Gold standard investigation for female infertility	***Laparoscopy and hysteroscopy***
45.	MC symptom of endometriosis	***Dysmenorrhoea***
46.	MC genital fistula in India	***Vesicovaginal fistula***
47.	White thick curdy vaginal discharge with intense itching is suggestive of ...... infection	***Candida***
48.	Epithelial lining of fallopian tube	***Ciliated columnar***
49.	Cause of endometrial carcinoma	***Unopposed estrogen activity***
50.	Webbing of neck & streaky gonads is indicative of .... syndrome	***Turner syndrome***

CHAPTER

9

DERMATOLOGY

KEY POINTS

Skin

- Skin is stratified squamous keratinized epithelium
- Skin doubling time/normal turnover time of epidermis is: 4 weeks
- Correct sequence of cell cycle: G0-G1-S-G2-M

Layers of Skin

- Stratum germinativum/Malpighian layer
  - Basal cell layer: Melanocytes present
  - Prickle cell layer/stratum spinosum
- Stratum granulosum (granular cell layer)
- Stratum lucidum (clear cell layer) and
- Stratum corneum (horny cell layer): Most superficial layer

Keratin

- Keratinization causes dehydration of cells
- Keratin filaments are hallmark of epidermal cells

Melanocyte

- Melanocyte (and also merkel cells) is immigrant cells
- Melanocyte are present in: Stratum basale

Stratum Lucidum

- It is sandwiched between S. corneum and S. granulosum
- It contains degenerated cells
- It is underdeveloped in very low birth weight infants within first 7 days

Macule

- Skin lesion which is neither raised nor depressed
- Flat discoloration of skin of 1 cm

Acantholysis

- Loss of coherence between epidermal cells
- Seen in Pemphigus

Hair

- Anagen phase of hair indicates: Phase of activity and growth

Sweat Gland

- Sweat gland of palm can be differentiated from others by: Secretion stimulated by emotional stimuli
- Hypothalamic preoptic nuclei has key role in sweating
- Miliaria is due to disruption of: Eccrine sweat ductal integrity

Apocrine Gland

- Modified sweat gland
- Present in groin and axilla
- Infection of apocrine gland is known as: Hidradenitis suppurativa

Fordyce Spots

- Ectopic sebaceous gland
- Mainly involves: Lips and buccal mucosa
- Common in adult woman

Rhinophyma/Potato Nose

- Glandular form of acne rosacea
- Sebaceous gland hypertrophy

Phases of Growth of Hair

- Anagen: Growing
- Catagen: Transitional phase
- Telogen: Resting phase

Structure Blocked and Disease

- Eccrine sweat glands: Crystalline miliaria
- Apocrine sweat glands: Hidradenitis suppurativa (Fox-Fordyce disease)
- Sebaceous glands: Fordyce disease

Acne

- Causative factors for acne: Hypercornification of duct, androgen, lipophilic yeast, bacterial contamination
- Management of acne is by: 13-cis-retinol/isotretinoin, minocycline, erythromycin

Nodulocystic Acne (NA)

- Treatment of NA: Isotretinoin (synthetic retinoic acid)

Retinoids

- Drug used to treat recalcitrant acne: Retinoid
- Most common side effect of retinoid: Skin rashes

Cicatricial Alopecia (CA)/Pseudopelade

- Scarring alopecia
- Causes of CA: Lichen planus, discoid lupus erythematosus, lupus vulgaris, SLE

Alopecia Areata (AA)

- Noncicatricial/non scaring alopecia
- Thought to be autoimmune in origin
- Exclamation mark sign is characteristic
- Clinical presentation: Single or multiple circumscribed smooth patchy hair loss, most obviously on scalp but frequently involving any hair bearing skin like beard, eyebrows, eyelashes, with pathognomonic "exclamation marks" and "going gray overnight" phenomenon
- AA is treated by: Minoxidil

Types of Alopecia

- Alopecia universalis: When hair has been lost over the entire body
- Alopecia areata: Patches of smooth area with loss of hair. At the periphery of patches is exclamation hair.
- Alopecia totalis: Total loss of scalp hair

Special Form

- Kerion celsii: Is a boggy indurated area exuding pus.
- Black dot: Areas of alopecia studded with black dots representing hair broken off at surface of the scalp caused by endothrix fungi.
- Gray patch: Characterized by scaly patches with stubs of broken hair and easy puckability of hair. Caused by ectothrix fungi.

Pemphigus

- Nikolsky sign present
- Bullae are intrapidermal and flaccid
- Mucosa involved
- Acantholysis present
- Involves upper part of body
- Age-40–60
- Prognosis poor

Nikolsky Sign

- Sliding of superficial layers of skin on the deeper layer when a tangential force is applied with the pulp of thumb, especially over bony prominences
- Positive in
  - Pemphigus
  - Staphylococcal scalded skin syndrome
  - Toxic epidermal necrolysis
  - Epidermolysis bullosa congenital

Pemphigoid

- Nikolsky sign absent
- Bullae are subepidermal and tense
- Mucosae are Not involved
- Acantholysis Absent
- Involves lower part of body
- Age 60–80
- Prognosis good

Tinea and Regions

- Tinea capitis: Scalp
- Tinea cruris: Affects groin
- Tinea corporis: Affects trunk
- Tinea mannum: Affects only the palms with scaling

Special Tinea

- Tinea Pedis/athlete's foot: T. mentagrophytes causes vesicular or bullous lesions in web spaces
- Tinea imbricata/Jock itch/Crotch itch/Dhobi's itch: Concentric rings of scales forming extensive patches with polycyclic borders. Caused by tinea concentricum
- Trichophytic granuloma/Majocchi's granuloma: Perifollicular granuloma which is annular, raised and crusty, seen on wrists, and shin, caused by tinea rubrun and T. mentagrophytes

Signs of Atopy

- Extra crease line just below the lower eyelid, exceeding midline (pupil)
- Dennie Morgan folds (extra fold beneath the eyelid is called the Dennie Morgan fold)
- White dermographism
- Triple response is replaced by blanching of skin
- Keratosis pilaris
- Hertoghe's sign

Lepromatous Leprosy

- Features:
  - Gynaecomastia,
  - Madarosis,
  - Collapse of nasal bridge
- Histology: Dermis contains characteristic highly vacoulated cells (foam cells) (Absent/few non-caseating granuloma)

Lepra Reaction

- Type II (ENL):
  - Type III hypersensitivity reaction,
  - Thalidomide is effective
- Type I
  - Type IV hypersensitivity reaction
  - DOC for type I lepra reaction: Corticosteroids

Types of Leprosy and Features

- LL: Bilaterally symmetrical, small oily lesion. Sensations present
- BB: Inverted saucer appearance
- BT: Satellite lesions are seen
- TT: Sensations are absent

Wood's Lamp Examination (Disease and Appearance)

- Albinism: Bright-white/blue-white
- Tuberous sclerosis: Blue white
- T. versicolor: Golden yellow
- P.aeruginosa: Aqua green
- Leprosy: Blue- white
- Vitiligo: Bright- white/blue -white
- Tinea capitis: Green fluorescence

Features of Ulcers

- Syphilitic ulcer: Wash leather slough
- Tuberculous ulcer: Apple jelly granulation tissue, pale scanty granulation tissue base
- Spreading ulcer: Necrotic tissue with slough

MCQs WITH SHORT EXPLANATIONS

BACTERIAL INFECTION

1. Which of the following is NOT associated with lepromatous leprosy:

a. Hypopigmented plaque b. Facies leprosa

c. Iris pearls d. Madarosis

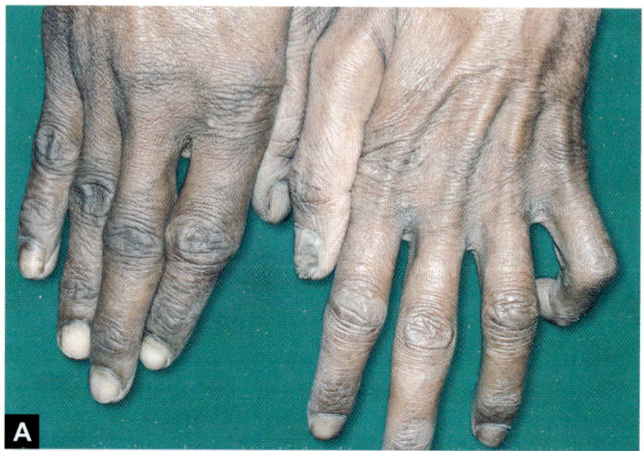

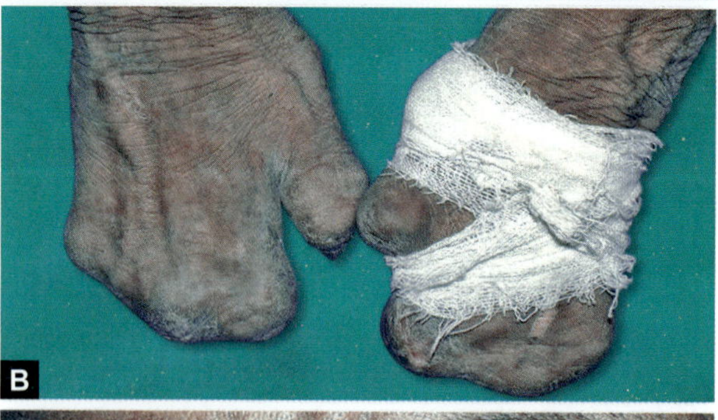

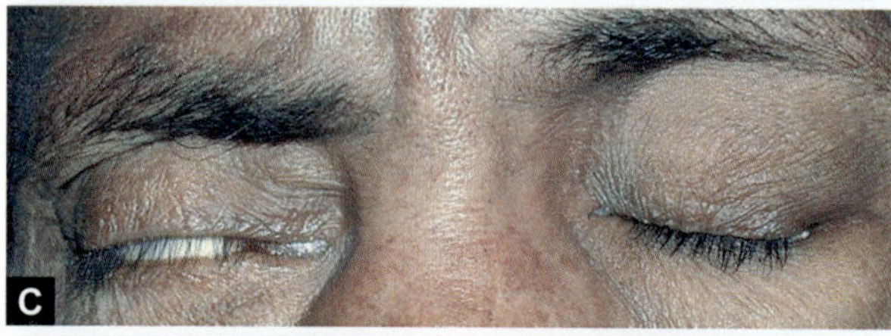

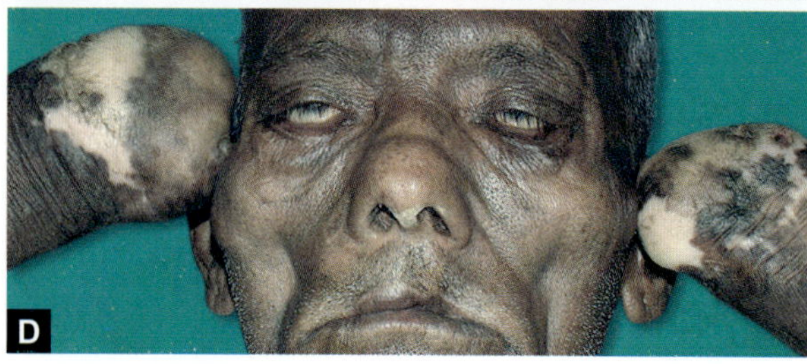

Deformities due to lepromatous leprosy. A. Claw hand deformity showing flexion deformity of little and ring fingers; B. Absorption of fingers; C. Lagopthalmos left eye; D. Lagophthalmos both eyes with absorption of fingers

Most commonly a patient with tuberculoid leprosy presents with a single hypopigmented or coppery red colored, well defined, dry, scaly plaque of variable size in the vicinity of cutaneous nerve or nerve trunk.

2. Treatment of type II lepra reaction are all EXCEPT:

a. Clofazimine

b. Thalidomide

c. Steroids

d. Cessation of antileprosy treatment

Management of type II lepra reaction/erythema nodosum leprosum/ENL

- Reassurance to the patient that disease is not worsening. It is a reaction against dead bacilli and it will be settled very soon
- Antileprotic treatment should remain continue
- Thalidomide is superior to steroids in controlling ENL
- Clofazimine in the dose of 300 mg/day has an anti-inflammatory effect in ENL and can be used for several months.

Features of type I and II lepra reactions

Type I	*Type II*
It is a delayed type of hypersensitivity and is a example of type IV hypersensitivity reaction	It is an immune complex syndrome and is an example of type III hypersensitivity reaction
Associated with rapid change of CMI	Not associated with change in CMI but is precipitated by certain factors (see below)
It is commonly seen in borderline (Bt, BB and BL) patients due to their unstable immunity	Exclusively seen in LL, ocasionally in BL
Most likely time is first 6 months of treatment. But may occur many years after stopping therapy	Unusual in first 6 months, seen later when most of the bacilli become granular
Fever and constitutional symptoms are uncommon	Usually have fever, arthritis, and malaise
1. New lesions may appear.	No change in existing lesions. But additional ENL lesions are seen
2 Existing skin lesions become purplish red, shiny and warm. Tenderness and edema of hands and feet. 3. Neuritis and nerve damage	
Lab findings: No changes seen	Anemia, rise in neutrophil count, ESR, platelets, IgG, and C2, C2

Abbreviations: ENS: Erythema nodosum leprosum ESR: Erythrocyte sedimentation rate; IgG: Immunoglobulin G.

Ans. 1. **c.** Iris pearls 2. **d.** Cessation...

3. LGV is caused by:

a. Chlamydia trachomatis b. H. ducreyi
c. Donovana granulomatis d. Trichomonas vaginalis

Most of the recent outbreaks of LGV are caused by type L2 chlamydia trachomatis.

Different types of serotypes causing various diseases	
Serotypes	*Diseases*
A, B, Ba, C	Hyperendemic blinding trachoma
D, E, F, G, H, I, J, K	Inclusion conjunctivitis Nongonococcal urethritis, cervicitis, salpingitis, epididymitis
L1, L2, L3	Lymphogranuloma venereum

4. Incubation period of syphilis is:

a. 2–5 days b. 21 days
c. 7–14 days d. 9–90 days

Incubation period of syphilis is 9–90 days (usually 14–21 days).

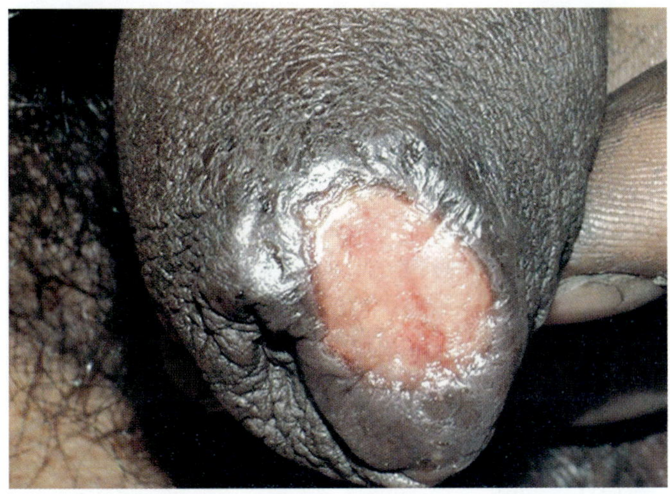

Syphilitic chancre

5. TB of skin is known as:

a. Lupus vulgaris b. Verruca vulgaris
c. Sclerema d. Scleroderma

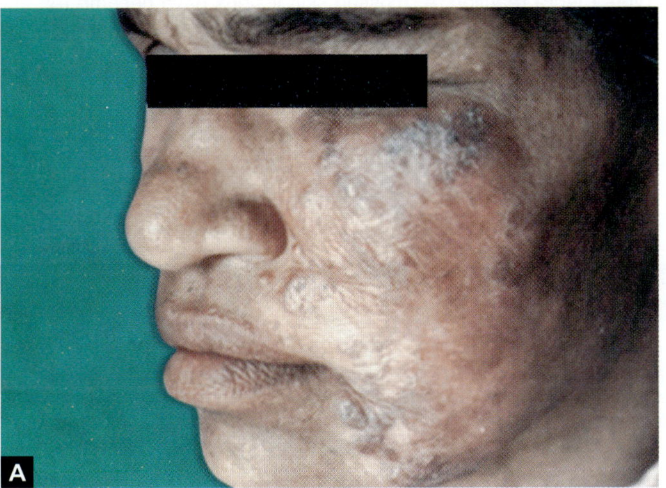

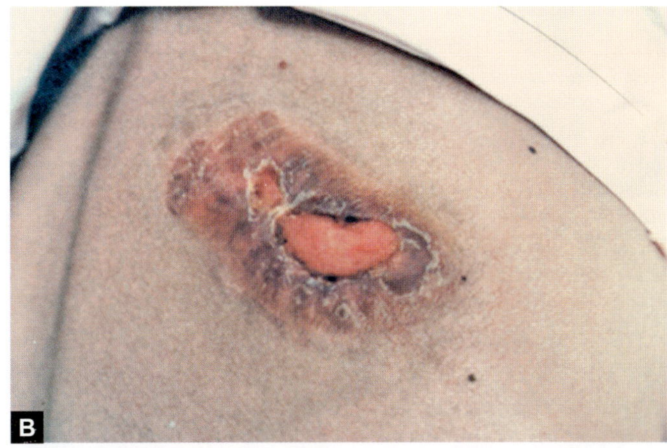

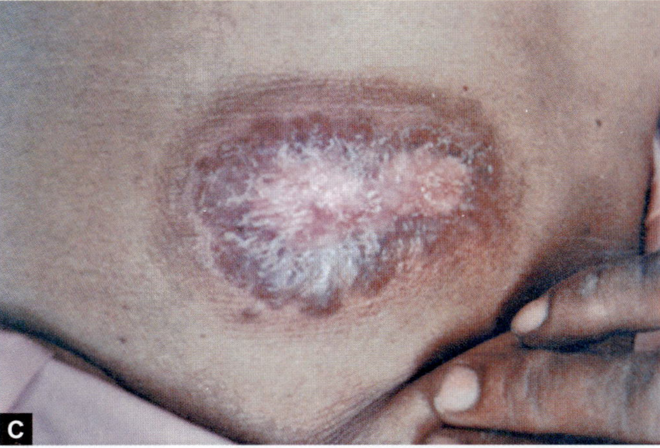

Lupus vulgaris. Involving three sites simultaneously and showing central atrophic scarring. A. On face; B. On upper back; C. On lower back

Lupus vulgaris is a chronic and progressive form of skin TB which is seen in previously infected (post-primary) persons.

6. MC nerve involved in leprosy:

a. Ulnar b. Median
c. Radial d. Musculocutaneous

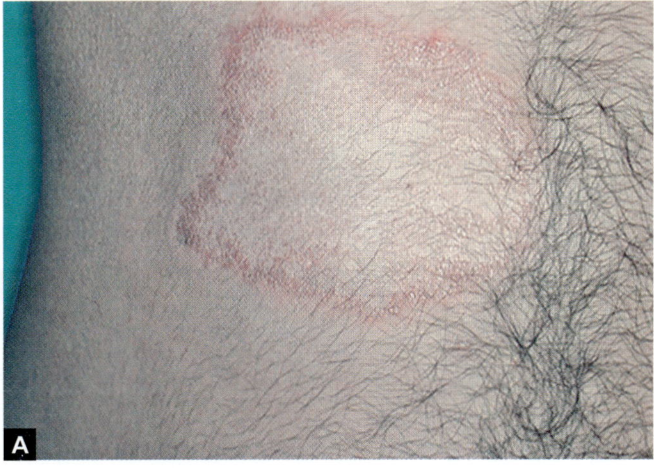

Contd...

Ans. 3. **a.** Chlamydia... 4. **d.** 9-90 days 5. **a.** Lupus vulgaris 6. **a.** Ulnar

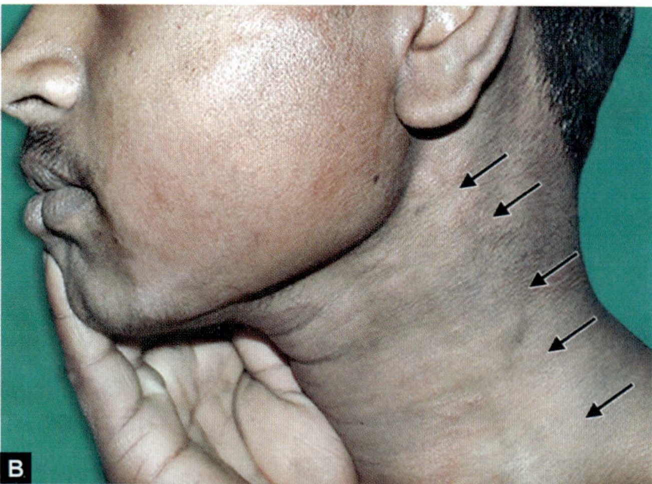

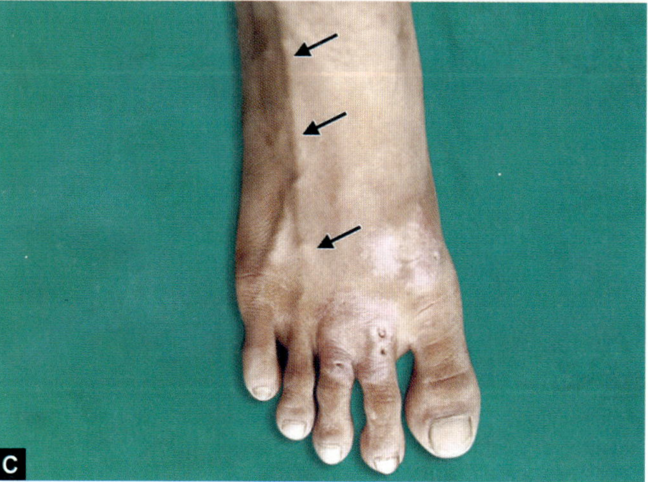

Tuberculoid leprosy. **A.** Single patch with central flattening and hair loss; **B.** Single large patch on face arrows showing enlargement of great auricular nerve; **C.** Arrows showing thickening of superficial cutaneous nerve

In lepromatous leprosy, decreasing order of frequency of involvement of motor nerve is posterior tibial, ulnar, median, lateral popliteal and facial nerves.

7. **DOC with type I lepra reaction with severe neuritis is:**
   a. Systemic steroids
   b. Clofazimine
   c. Thalidomide
   d. Chloroquine

Steroids in type I lepra reaction

- If NSAIDs are insufficient, then 40-60 mg prednisolone may be added. Dose may be reduced by 5 mg every 2–4 weeks. It may require 2–4 months to control the reaction.
- Steroids relieve the pressure on nerve fibers by dispersing intraneural edema
- Intraneural injection may be required to relieve a severe nerve pain.

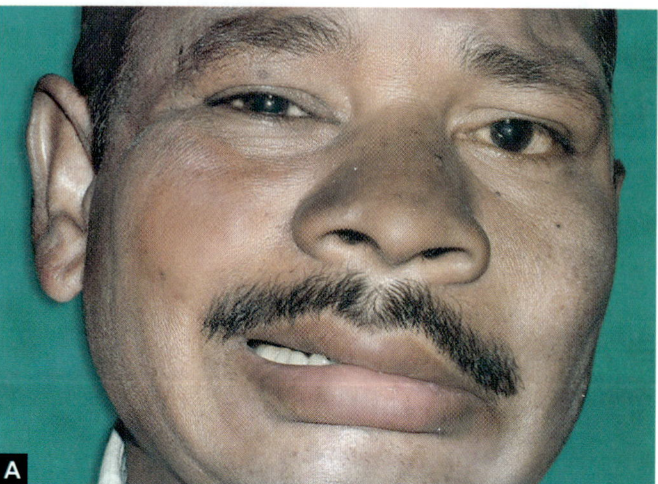

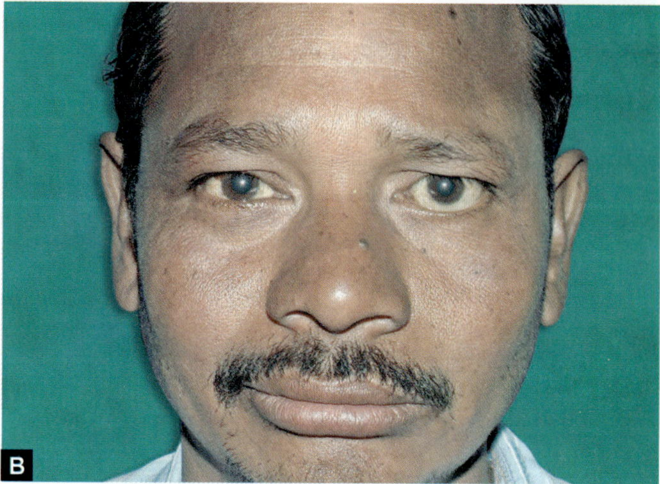

Type 1 lepra reaction. A. Existing skin lesions have become red and shiny. In addition, there is a left facial palsy. B. After treatment

8. **Nerve abscess in tuberculoid leprosy is best treated by:**
   a. Aspiration
   b. High dose clofazimine
   c. Steroids
   d. Thalidomide

Nerve abscess is managed by aspiration or neurolysis.

Salient features of various types of leprosy

	TT	BT	BB	BL	LL
Skin lesions					
Number, size, type and surface	Single, large sized well defined plaque with dry scaly surface	2-3 less well defined lesions Satellite lesion is an important feature	4-8 less well defined lesions. Punched out lesions are characteristic	Numerous but countable with ill defined margins with less scaly surface	Uncountable, small sized, ill defined macules, papules diffuse infiltrations, plaques or nodules with shiny surface

Contd...

Ans. 7. **a.** Systemic steroids 8. **a.** Aspiration

Contd...

	TT	*BT*	*BB*	*BL*	*LL*
Hair loss	Prominent loss	Less prominent loss	No significant loss	No loss	No loss
Sensation	Anesthetic	Hypoesthetic	Impaired	No significant loss	Lesions have no loss. Glove and stocking type in hands and feet
Symmetry	Asymmetrical	Asymmetrical	Asymmetrically bilateral	Tend to be symmetrical	Bilateral symmetrical
Nerves	A nerve may be thickened near the plaque	1-2 nerves may be thickened	Multiple nerves thickened asymmetrically	Tend to be symmetrical	Symmetrically involved
Lepra reactions	Type I	Type I	Type I	Type II	Type II
Immunity	Fairly high	Good	Weak	Poor	Very poor
Lepromin test	Strongly positive	Positive	Negative	Negative	Negative
Histopathology					
Granuloma	Compact granuloma around nerves and vessels Granuloma made of epitheloid cells, peripheral rim of lymphocytes	Epitheloid cell granuloma	Diffuse epitheloid cell granuloma Lymphocytes are scanty	Macrophage granuloma in which lymphocytes are prominent	Thin epidermis, flat rete redges Diffuse leproma in dermis made of foamy macrophages laden with AFB
Grenz zone	No grenz zone	Seen	Prominently seen	Prominently seen	Prominently seen
AFBs	Rarely seen	Very scanty	Many AFBs are seen	Large no AFBs are seen	Seen singly and in groups
Slit skin smear	No bacilli are found	Few AFB may be found	Scanty AFBs seen	BI 3+ or 4+	BI 5+ or 6+

Abbreviations: TT: Tuberculoid; BT: Borderline tuberculoid; BB: Borderline borderline; BL: Borderline lepromatous; AFB: Acid-fast bacilli

9. Moth eaten alopecia is seen in:

a. Black dot tinea b. Telogen effluvium
c. Alopecia areata d. Secondary syphilis

Scalp may show patchy or diffuse alopecia in secondary syphilis. The margins of patches of hair loss being not sharp are described as moth eaten.

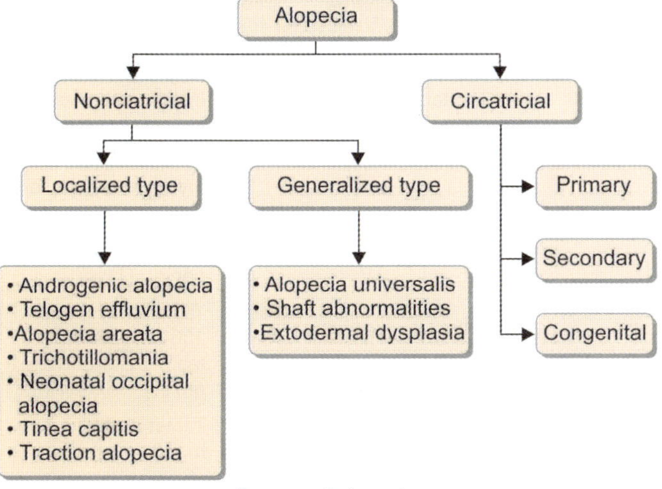

Causes of alopecia

10. Which of the following organism is responsible for vesicular eruptions and 'honey-coloured' crusts over face:

a. TB bacilli b. Staphylococcus aureus
c. Hansen's bacilli d. Herpes zoster

Nonbullous impetigo/impetigo contagiosa presents as thin walled vesicles, which ruptures rapidly. The exudates get dried to form yellowish, thick and dirty brown (honey colored crusts). In developing countries, staphylococcus aureus is the most common cause of NBI/IC.

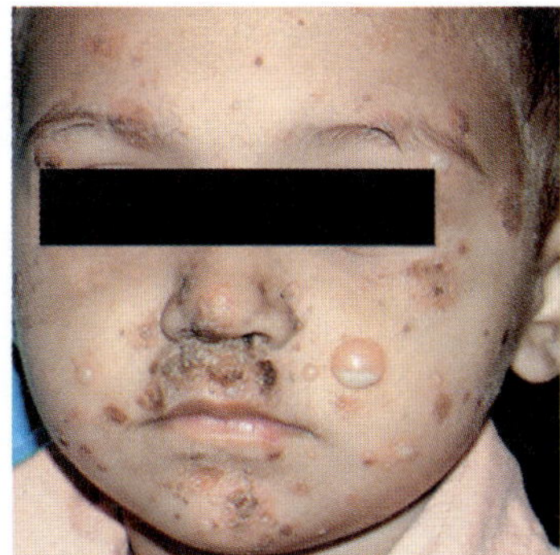

Impetigo contagiosa showing thick dirty brown crusts

Ans. 9. **d.** Secondary syphilis 10. **b.** Staphylococcus aureus

11. Apple jelly nodule on diascopy, is a feature of:

a. Aspergillosis
b. Rhinoscleroma
c. Erysipelas
d. Lupus vulgaris

On diascopy, plaque of lupus vulgaris may show apple jelly nodules which are seen in the active edge as pinhead sized, transparent, reddish brown or skin colored papules.

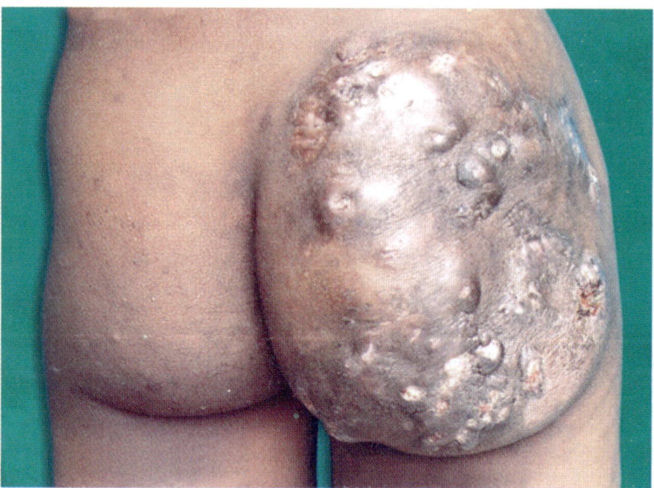

Lupus vulgaris on buttock. Annular gradually progressive plaque on buttock with crusting, induration at periphery and scarring in the central region

12. Which of the following condition present with purulent urethral discharge:

a. Syphilis
b. Chancroid
c. Gonorrhea
d. Lymphogranuloma venereum

Patient with gonorrhea complains of burning micturition, purulent urethral discharge and staining of underclothes.

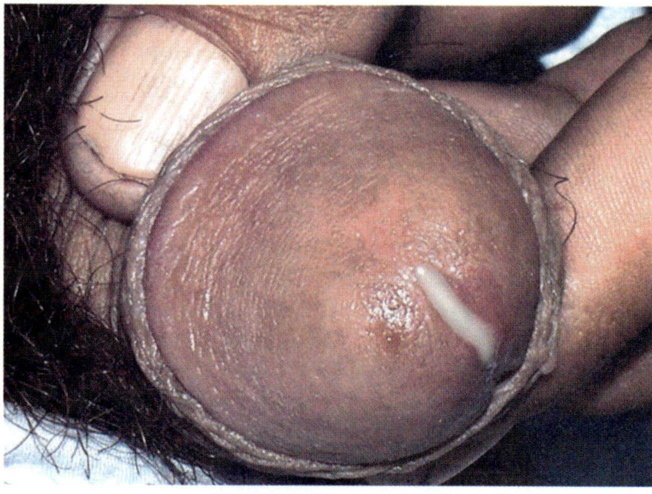

Acute gonorrhea in male

13. Which of the following is NOT a test for syphilis:

a. VDRL
b. Frei test
c. TPHA
d. FTA-Abs

Frei test is an obsolete intradermal test done for LGV.

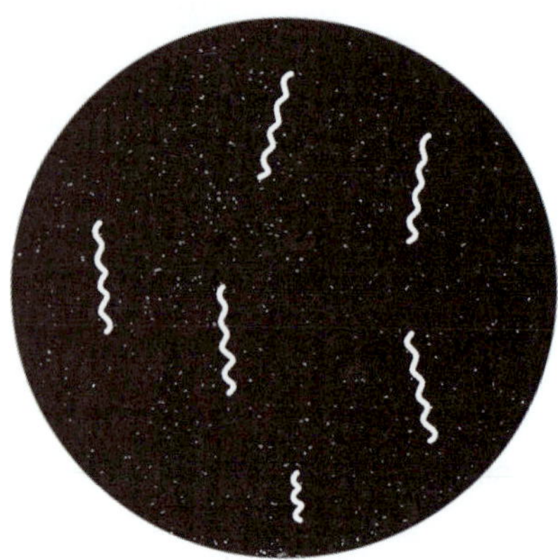

Dark ground illumination showing spirochetes (a diagrammatic representation)

14. 24-year-old male complains of mild urethral discharge after sexual contact with a sex-worker. Drug used to treat such a patient:

a. Azithromycin 1 mg single dose
b. Azithromycin 1 mg for 3 weeks
c. Azithromycin 500 mg single dose
d. Azithromycin 1 gram single dose

Chlamydia trachomatis nongonococcal urethritis is managed by Azithromycin 1 g single stat dose, which also take care of mycoplasma.

Color coded kits for syndromic management			
Kit no.	*Syndrome*	*Color*	*Contents*
1.	Urethral discharge, cervical discharge, Anorectal discharge, Painful scrotal swelling	Grey	Tablet azithromycin 1 g (1) and tablet cefixime 400 mg (1)
2.	Vaginal discharge	Green	Tablet secnidazole 2 g (1) and tablet fluconazole 150 mg (1)
3.	Genital Ulcer Disease – non herpetic	White	Injection benzathine penicillin 2.4 MU (1) and tablet azithromycin 1 gm (1) and disposable syringe 10 mL with 21 gauge needle (1)
4.	Genital ulcer disease—non herpetic for patients allergic to penicillin	Blue	Tablet doxycycline 100 mg (30) and tablet azithromycin 1 gm (1)
5.	Genital ulcer disease herpetic	Red	Tablet acyclovir 400 mg (21)

Contd...

Ans. **11. d.** Lupus vulgaris **12. c.** Gonorrhea **13. b.** Frei test **14. d.** Azithromycin 1 gram...

Contd...

Kit no.	Syndrome	Color	Contents
6.	Lower abdominal pain	Yellow	Tablet cefixime 400 mg (1) and tablet metronidazole 400 mg (28) and capsule doxycycline 100 mg (28)
7.	Inguinal bubo	Black	Tablet doxycycline 100 mg (42) and tablet azithromycin 1 gm (1)

15. All are true for Hutchinson triad EXCEPT:

a. Hutchinson teeth b. Eight nerve deafness
c. Posterior uveitis d. Interstitial keratitis

Hutchinson's triad of congenital syphilis comprises Hutchinson's teeth, interstitial keratitis and 8th nerve deafness.

16. Confirmation of congenital syphilis is done by:

a. VRDL b. FTA-abs
c. TPI d. Kahn's test

Fluorescent treponemal antibody absorption (FTA-ABS) test is the most sensitive and earliest (at third week) to become positive in primary syphilis. It can detect IgM antibodies which enables us to differentiate between congenital syphilis and passive transfer of antibodies.

17. Drug of choice for syphilis:

a. Ceftriaxone
b. Erythromycin
c. Tetracycline
d. Benzathine penicillin

Parenteral administration of penicillin is drug of choice at all stages of syphilis. Penicillin is easy to administer, less expensive and has few side effects. It is most effective treponemicide and no resistance has developed.

Treatment of various types of syphilis

Type	Treatment
Primary or secondary syphilis	❑ Two IM injections of benzathine penicillin (1.2 mega units in each buttock) after sensitivity test given stat one time. It maintains effective levels for 2 weeks
	❑ **Alternative drugs:** – Procaine penicillin, 0.6 million units IM OD for 10–12 days ❑ Doxycycline, 100 mg BD for 14 days ❑ Erythromycin, 500 mg QID for 14 days ❑ Azithromycin, 500 mg OD for 10 days ❑ Ceftriaxone, 500 mg IM daily for 10 days ❑ **Follow-up:** – If there is a four-fold increase in VDRL titer within 6 months, patient should be investigated for HIV infection – If reinfection is ruled out and CSF examination indicates neurosyphilis, treat the patient with intravenous penicillin – If there is no neurosyphilis, then treat with three doses of benzathine penicillin IM 1 week apart
Late syphilis	❑ It requires a longer duration of therapy because spirochetes are dividing more slowly ❑ It is treated by benzathine penicillin 2.4 mega units IM weekly for 3 weeks or doxycycline 100 mg BD for 28 days
Neurosyphilis	❑ The penetration into CSF by aqueous procaine benzyipenicillin, erythromycin and benzathine penicillin is poor, poorer and poorest respectively ❑ **Treatment of choice:** Crystalline benzylpenicillin G* in the dosage of 3.5–4 million units IV every 4 hours (18–24 million units/day) for 10–14 days ❑ **Alternative:** 2.4 million units of procaine penicillin G IM daily plus 500 mg QID probenecid daily for 10–14 days ❑ Re-examine CSF at 6 months intervals until it becomes normal. The cell counts decrease by 6 months, while CSF VDRL and protein levels take 2 years to become normal
Penicillin hypersensitivity	❑ Doxycycline
During pregnancy	❑ The penicillin regimen appropriate as per the stage of disease ❑ Alternative drugs are azithromycin or erythromycin
HIV seropositive syphilis	❑ They are treated by penicillin-based regimen appropriate for neurosyphilis irrespective of the stage of infection
Congenital syphilis	❑ **Neonatal period:** Crystalline benzylpenicillin G, 50,000 units/kg/dose IV BD for first 7 days and TDS for next 3 days. Alternatively, procaine penicillin G, 50,000 units/kg IM daily for 10–14 days ❑ **Postnatal period:** If CSF examination is normal, 50,000 units/kg of benzathine penicillin is used. If neurosyphilis is there, crystalline benzylpenicillin G, 50,000 units/kg/dose every 4–6 hours IV for 10–14 days is used ❑ **Follow-up:** Should be made every 3 months until test becomes nonreactive. VDRL titer disappears by the age of 6 months

*It is also known as aqueous penicillin G. It is very soluble in water and sparingly soluble in alcohol.

Abbreviations: IM: Intramuscular; VDRL: Venereal Disease Research Laboratory; HIV: Human immunodeficiency virus; CSF: Cerebrospinal fluid; IV, intravenous

Ans. **15. c.** Posterior uveitis **16. b.** FTA-abs **17. d.** Benzathine penicillin

18. RPR test is done for:

a. Syphilis b. HIV
c. TB d. Malaria

Rapid plasma reagin (RPR) test is one valuable test for syphilis in which VDRL antigen is suspended with fine carbon particles as marker. It is carried out on disposable cards on unheated serum or plasma. The clumping of carbon particles is visible with naked eyes is considered as positive test.

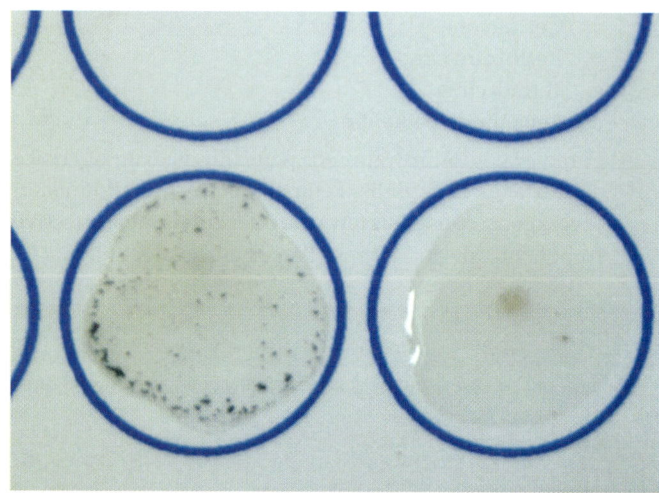

Positive rapid plasma reagin test showing clumping of carbon particles

FUNGAL INFECTION

19. Dhobi's itch is:

a. Tinea corporis b. Tinea cruris
c. Tinea barbae d. Tinea capitis

Tinea cruris/dhobie itch/jock itch/eczema marginatum is a very common dermatophyte infection. It involves groins, genitals, and skin of pubic, perineal, and perianal areas. Itching of groins is a predominant complaint.

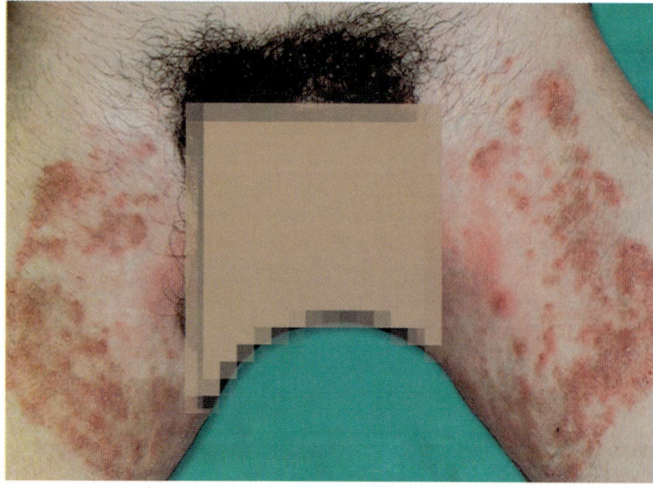

Tinea cruris

20. Tinea versicolor is caused by:

a. Malassezia furfur b. Candida
c. Trichophyton rubrum
d. Trichophyton mentagrophyte

Pityriasis versicolor is a mild chronic opportunistic infection of skin caused by yeast Malassezia. The previous name tinea versicolor is no longer used.

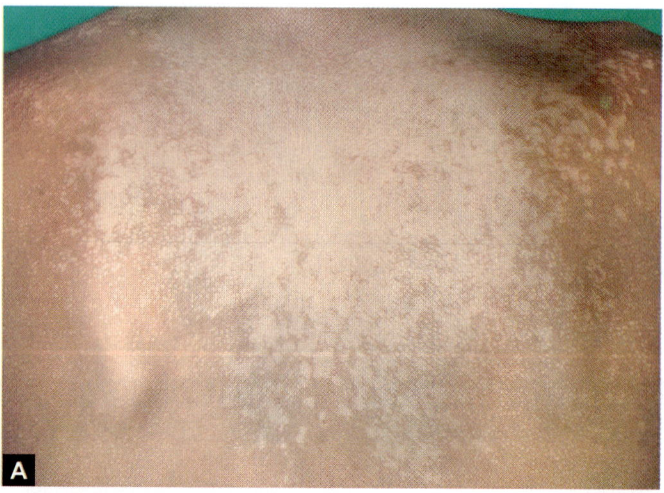

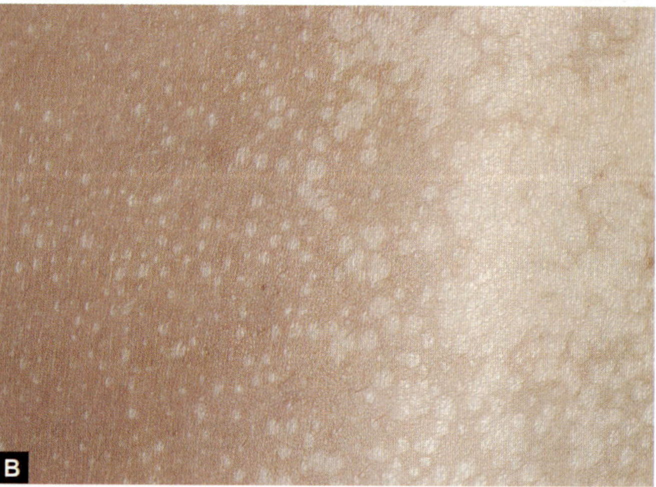

Pityriasis versicolor. A. Confluence of lesions in the central part; B. Discrete satellite lesions at the margin

21. Dermatophytes can affect:

a. Hair b. Nail
c. Scalp d. All of the above

Dermatophytes are keratinophilic, and infection is characteristically confined to dead keratinized tissue where it exists as mycelium and arthroconidia.

Site of infection of various dermatophytes

Dermatophytes	*Site of infection*		
	Skin	*Hair*	*Nails*
Epidermophyton	+	-	+
Microsporum	+	+	-
Trichophyton	+	+	+

Ans. **18. a.** Syphilis **19. b.** Tinea cruris **20. a.** Malassezia furfur **21. d.** All of the above

PIGMENTATION DISORDER

22. Rain drop pigmentation is seen in:

a. Chronic lead poisoning
b. Chronic arsenic poisoning
c. Chronic mercury poisoning
d. All of the above

Patients with arsenic poison may have hyperpigmentation on the trunk studded with small areas of hypopigmentation which appears as rain drops in the dust.

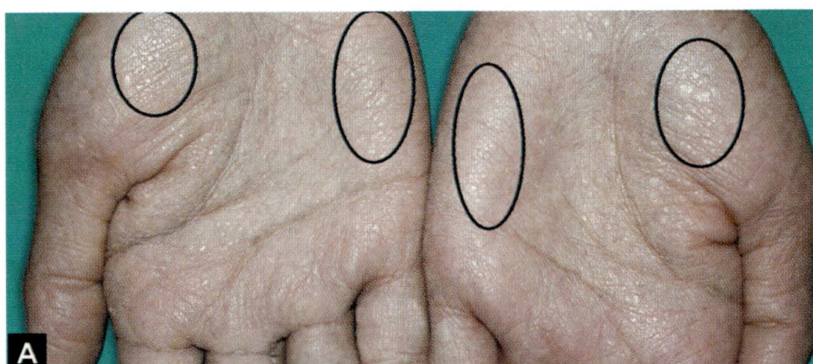
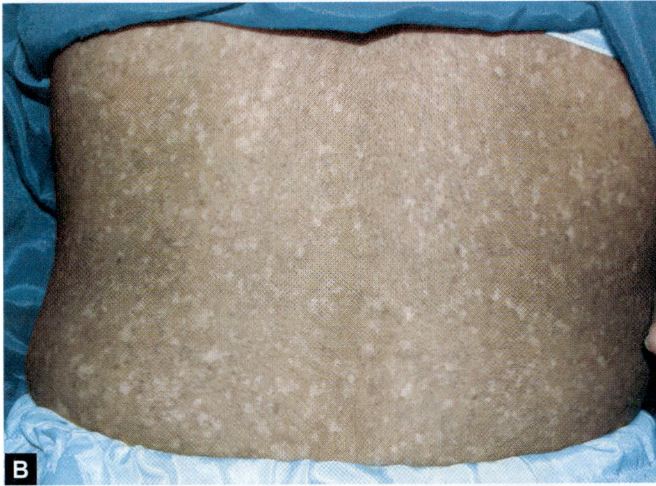
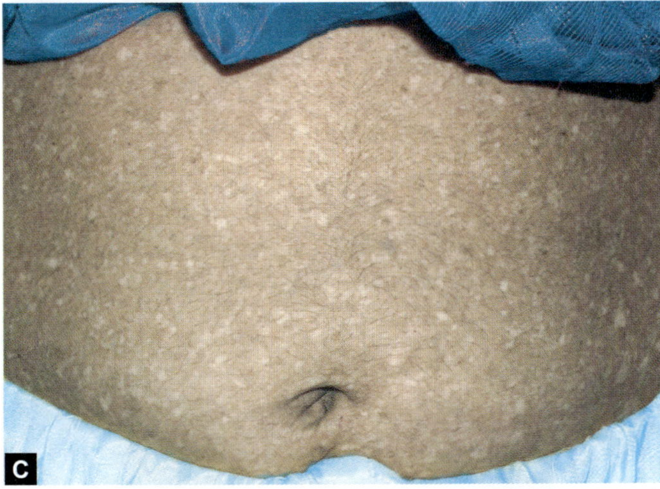

Arsenic keratosis. A. Keratotic papules on palms; B. Appearance of 'rain drops in the dust' on back; C. On abdomen

MISCELLANEOUS

23. A child presented to the skin OPD with rashes involving the flexures of elbows and knees. He is having intense pruritus. The clinical image is given below. There is a positive family history of asthma. Most likely diagnosis:

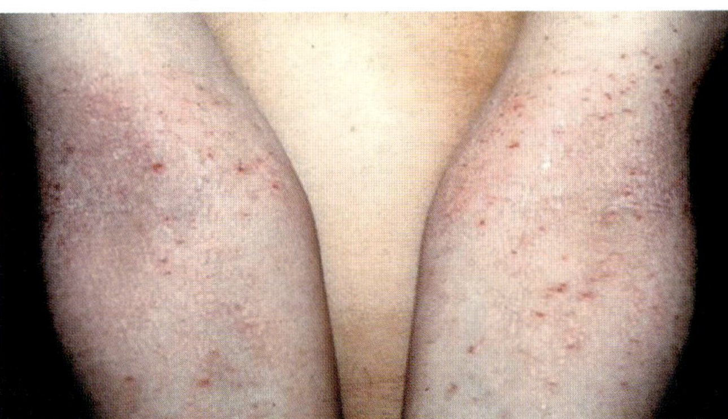

a. Erysipelas
b. Allergic contact dermatitis
c. Atopic dermatitis
d. Gluten sensitive enteropathy

Severe pruritus (severe and worse at evening), involvement of flexures of elbows and knees (also cervical regions, wrist and ankles) and a personal or family history of atopic disorders goes in favour of atopic disease.

Hanifin and Rajka diagnostic criteria for atopic dermatitis (AD)
Major criteria: (Must have three or more of)
❑ Pruritus ❑ Typical morphology and distribution – Flexural lichenification or linearity in adults – Facial and extensor involvement in infants and children ❑ Chronic or chronically-relapsing dermatitis ❑ Personal or family history of atopy (asthma, allergic rhinitis, and atopic dermatitis)
Minor criteria: (Should have three or more of)
On history
❑ Itch when sweating ❑ Intolerance to wool and lipid solvents ❑ Food intolerance ❑ Course influenced by environmental or emotional factors
On General Examination
❑ Xerosis ❑ Ichthyosis, palmar hyperlinearity or keratosis pilaris ❑ Early age of onset ❑ Tendency toward cutaneous infections (especially *Staphylococcus aureus* and herpes simplex) or impaired cell-medicated immunity ❑ Tendency toward nonspecific hand or foot dermatitis Nipple eczema ❑ Anterior neck folds ❑ Perifollicular accentuation

Contd...

MCQs with Short Explanations

Ans. 22. **b.** Chronic arsenic.... 23. **c.** Atopic dermatitis

Contd...

Hanifin and Rajka diagnostic criteria for atopic dermatitis (AD)
On face examination
❑ Cheilitis ❑ Dennie-Morgan infraorbital fold ❑ Orbital darkening ❑ Facial pallor or facial erythema ❑ Pityriasis alba
On eye examination
❑ Recurrent conjunctivitis ❑ Keratoconus ❑ Anterior subcapsular cataracts
On investigation
❑ Immediate (type 1) skin-test reactivity ❑ Raised serum IgE ❑ White dermographism or delayed branch

24. Which of the following is related to Malpighian layer:

a. Stratum basale & Stratum granulosum
b. Stratum spinosum & Stratum basale
c. Startum corenuam & Stratum spinosum
d. Stratum corenum & Stratum lucidium

The Malpighian layer of the skin is generally defined as both the stratum basale and stratum spinosum as a unit, although it is occasionally defined as the stratum basale specifically, or the stratum spinosum specifically. It is named after Marcello Malpighi.

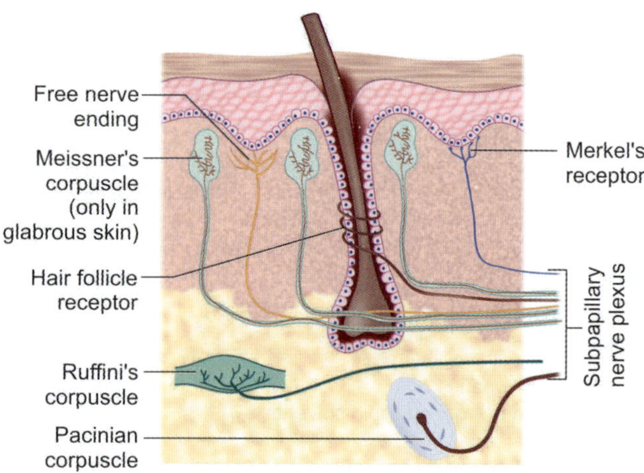

Cutaneous receptors

25. Which of the following is related to cutis marmorata:

a. Humidity b. Dust
c. Micro-organism d. Cold temperature

Cutis marmorata telangiectatica congenita (CMTC) is an uncommon, sporadic, congenital cutaneous vascular anomaly evident as persistent *cutis marmorata*, telangiectasia, and phlebectasia. *Cutis marmorata* telangiectatica congenita is most commonly localized in distribution, evident over the lower limbs. It appears in response to cold temperatures. It's usually temporary and benign.

26. Which of the following is NOT a risk factor for development of cutaneous lymphoma (mycosis fungoides):

a. Age more than 50 years b. Males
c. Normal immune system d. HIV

Mycosis fungoides (cutaneous lymphoma) are commonly seen in immune-compromised individuals.

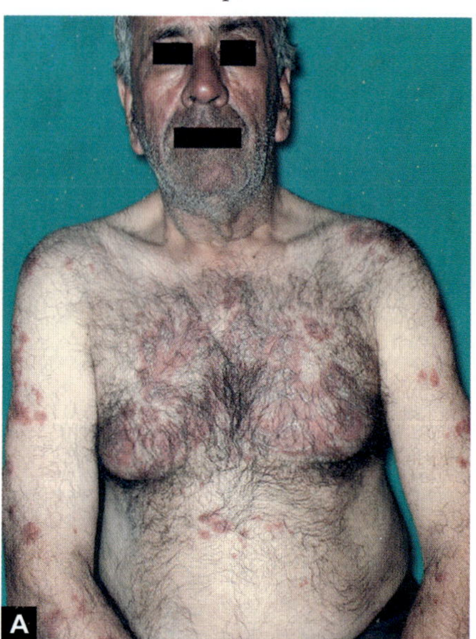

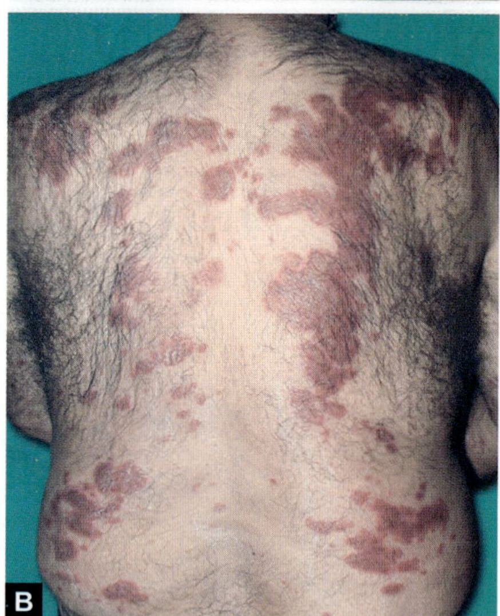

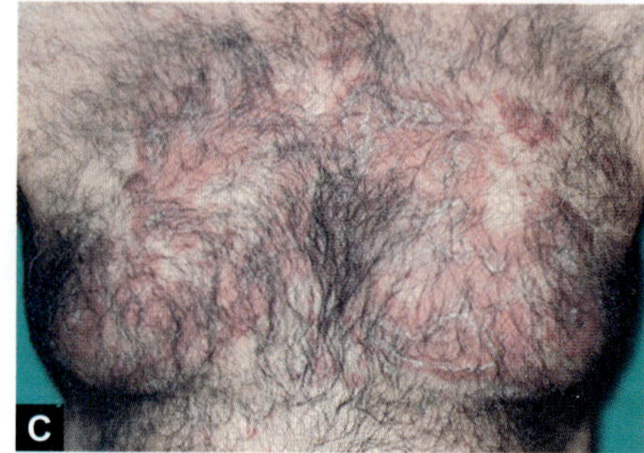

Patch stage mycosis fungoides

Ans. 24. **b.** Stratum spinos... 25. **d.** Cold temperature 26. **c.** Normal immune system

27. **Identify the image:**

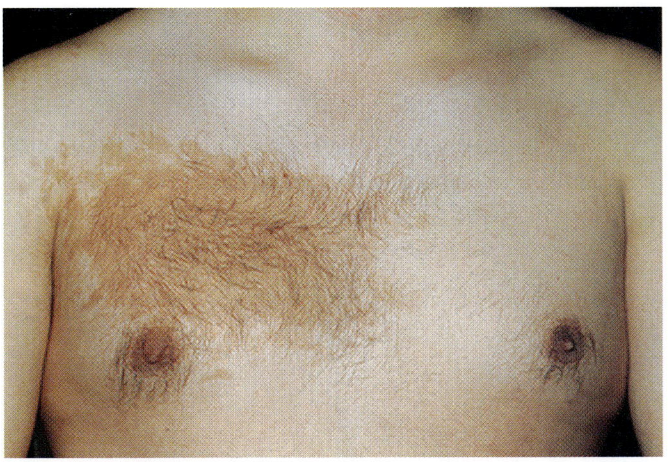

a. Epidermal nevus b. Spitz nevus
c. Hypopigmented macule d. Becker nevus

A *Becker's nevus* often becomes darker, and excessive hair growth (hypertrichosis) and acne may develop within the *nevus*. *Becker's nevus* is due to overgrowth of the epidermis (upper layer of the skin), pigment cells (melanocytes) and hair follicles.

Classification of nevi

Epidermal Nevi

- Verrucous epidermal nervus
- Inflammatory linear verrucous epidermal nevus
- Nevus sebaceous
- Nevus comedonicus
- Eccrine nevus
- Apocrine nevus
- Becker's nevus (see page no. 277)
- Benign hyperplasias of melanocytic nevi
  - Acquired melanocytic nevi, e.g., cellular nevus (mole), halo nevus
  - Spitz nevus
  - Congenital melanocytic nevi, e.g., giant congenital melanocytic nevus

Dermal Nevi

- Steatocystoma multiplex
- Dermal melanocytic nevi (see page no. 272)
  - Nevus of Ota
  - Nevus of Ito
  - Mongolian spots
- Vascular nevi
  - Vascular tumors, e.g., infantile hemangioma (IH)
  - Vascular malformations, e.g., port-wine stain and salmon patch
  - Angiokeratomas, e.g., angiokeratoma of the scrotum and vulva

28. **Delayed hypersensitivity in skin tests, is assessed by:**

a. Erythema b. Bulla
c. Necrosis d. Induration

Tuberculin test is observed at 48-72 hours and widest diameter of the area of induration (not erythema) in millimeters is recorded.

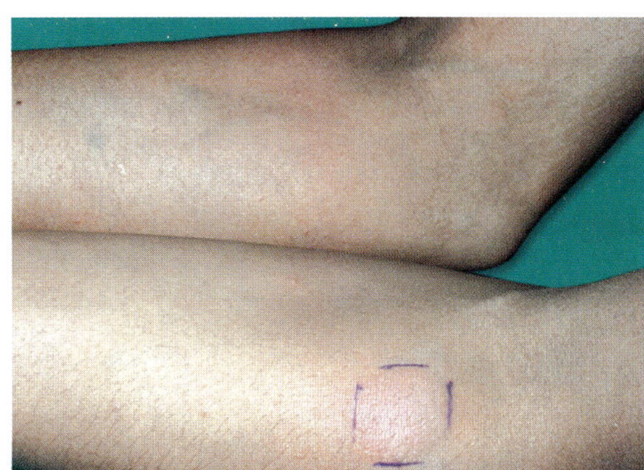

Positive tuberculin test showing erythema and induration on left forearm

29. **Wavelength of light produced by Wood's lamp:**

a. 320 nm b. 360 nm
c. 400 nm d. 480 nm

Wood's lamp provides invisible long wave ultraviolet (UV) radiation (365 nm) which is used to induce visible fluorescence for the diagnosis of certain disorders.

30. **Epidermal cells of normal tissue are replaced completely by:**

a. 4 days b. 12 days
c. 37 days d. 48 days

The amount of time taken by whole epidermal cell population to replace itself is called turnover time or epidermal turnover time. It is also called as regeneration time or replacement time. The mean turnover time of normal skin is 47-48 days.

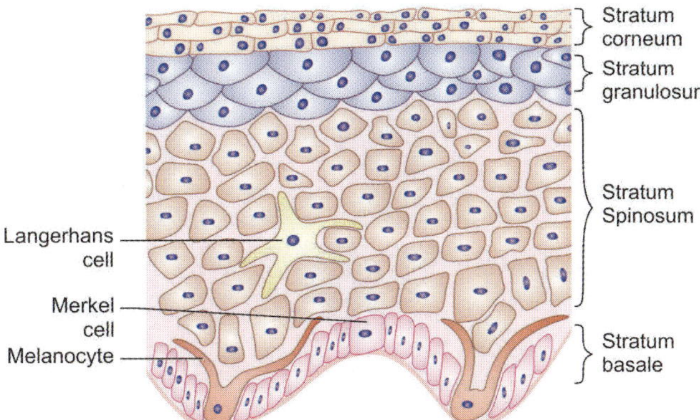

Diagrammatic representation of epidermal cell layers

31. **Wood's lamp filter is made of:**

a. Tin and chromium oxide
b. Nickel oxide and silica
c. Copper oxide and barium oxide
d. Zinc oxide

Source of light in Wood's lamp examination is a high pressure mercury lamp. From this light visible rays have been filtered by barium silicate glass (Wood's filter) containing 9% nickel oxide.

Ans. 27. **d.** Becker nevus 28. **d.** Induration 29. **b.** 360 nm 30. **d.** 48 days 31. **b.** Nickel oxide & silica

32. Most severe form of scabies:

a. Norwegian scabies
b. Neular scabies
c. Animal scabies
d. Genital scabies

Patient of crusted/norwegian scabies is highly infectious and more than a million mites populate the skin. These patients may have generalized erythema and scaling on face, neck, trunk and hands to the extent of erythroderma.

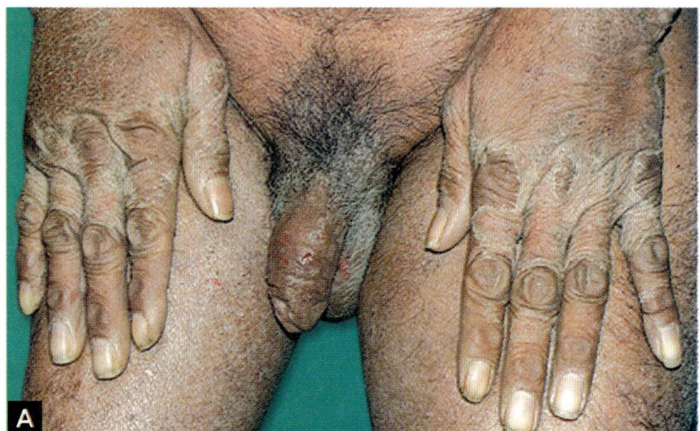

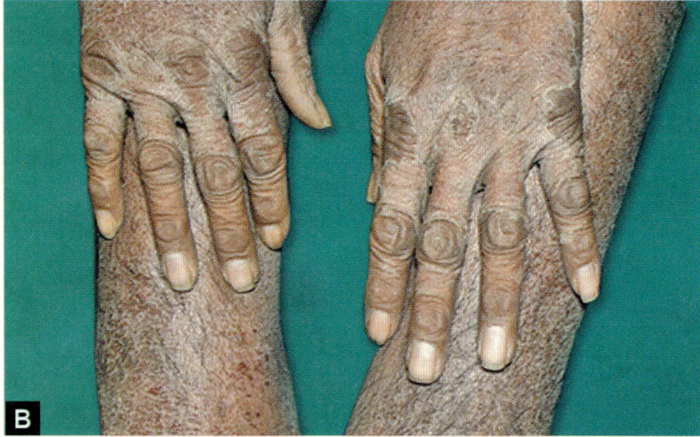

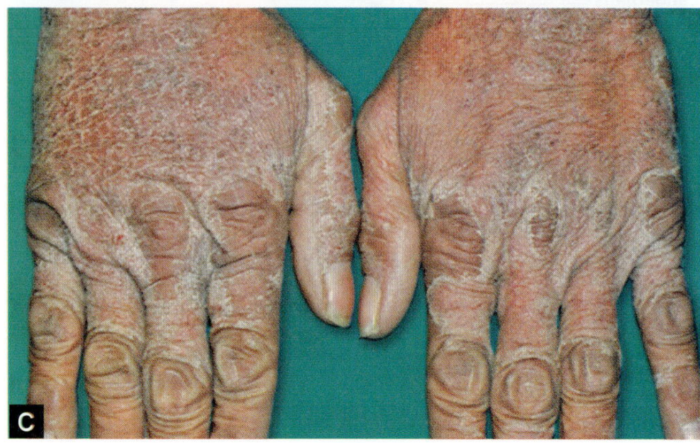

Norwegian scabies showing generalized erythema and scaling. A. On groin and hands; B. On hands and legs; C. On dorsa of hands

33. Characteristic lesion of scabies is:

a. Burrow
b. Fissure
c. Vesicle
d. Papule

The burrows are pathognomonic lesions of scabies. It is difficult to detect burrows in good hygienic patients. By careful observation, they are seen as slightly raised and brownish dark tortous lines 1–10 mm in length.

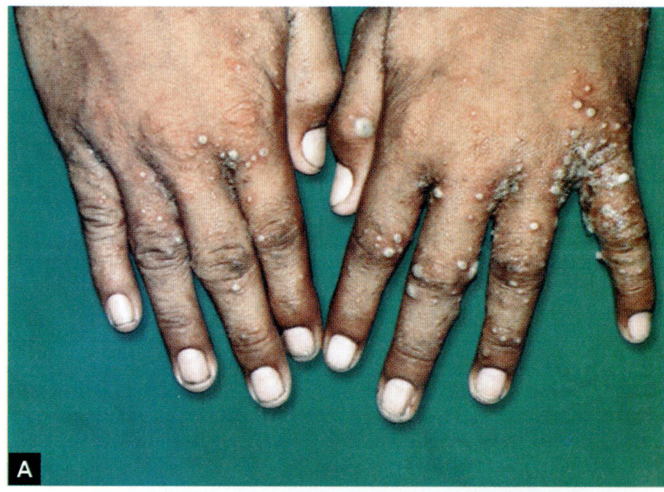

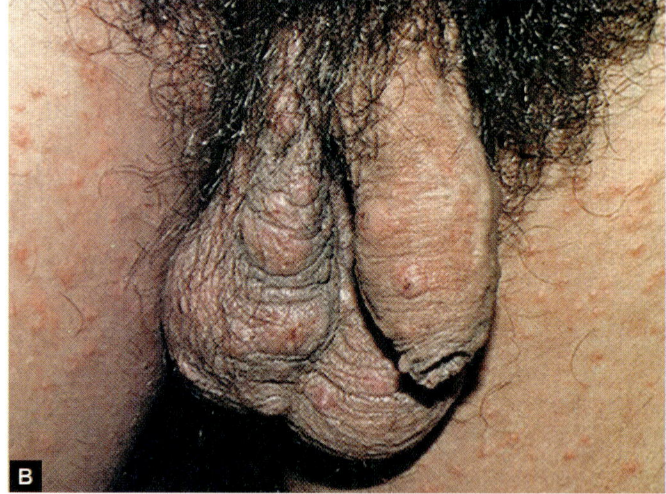

Scabies. A. Infected scabies; B. Genital involvement in adults

34. Scabies in children differ from that in adults in that it affects:

a. Webspace
b. Face
c. Genitalia
d. Axilla

In infants, the scalp, soles and trunk are common sites of involvement in scabies.

Ans. **32. a.** Norwegian... **33. a.** Burrow **34. b.** Face

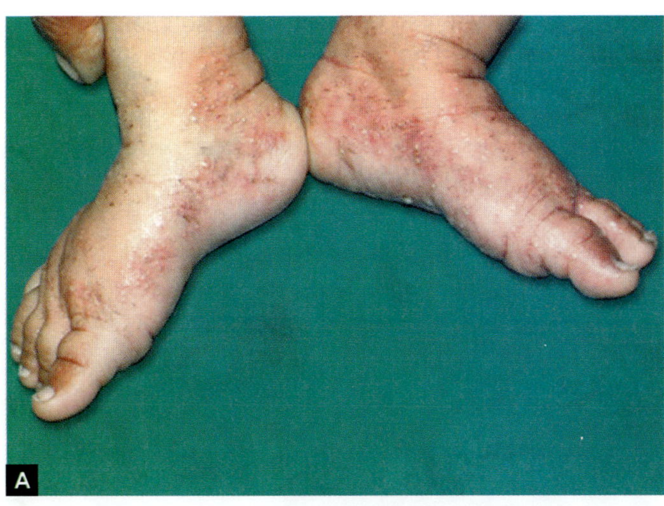
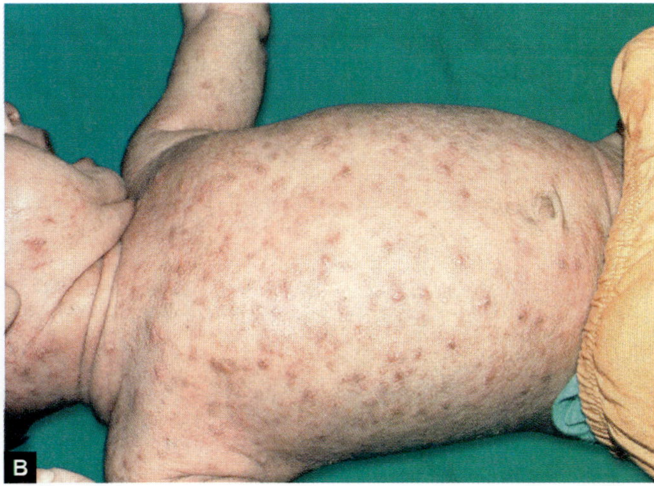

Scabies in infants. A. Involvement of soles; B. Trunk involvement

35. A 30-year-old male presented with pruritic, flat topped, polygonal, shiny violaceous papules with flexural distribution. The most likely diagnosis is:

a. Psoriasis
b. Pityriasis rosea
c. Lichen planus
d. Lichenoid dermatitis

Cutaneous lesions of lichen planus presents as purplish, plain topped, pruritic, polygonal, papules on peripheral parts of body with mild scaling in a bilateral symmetrical manner.

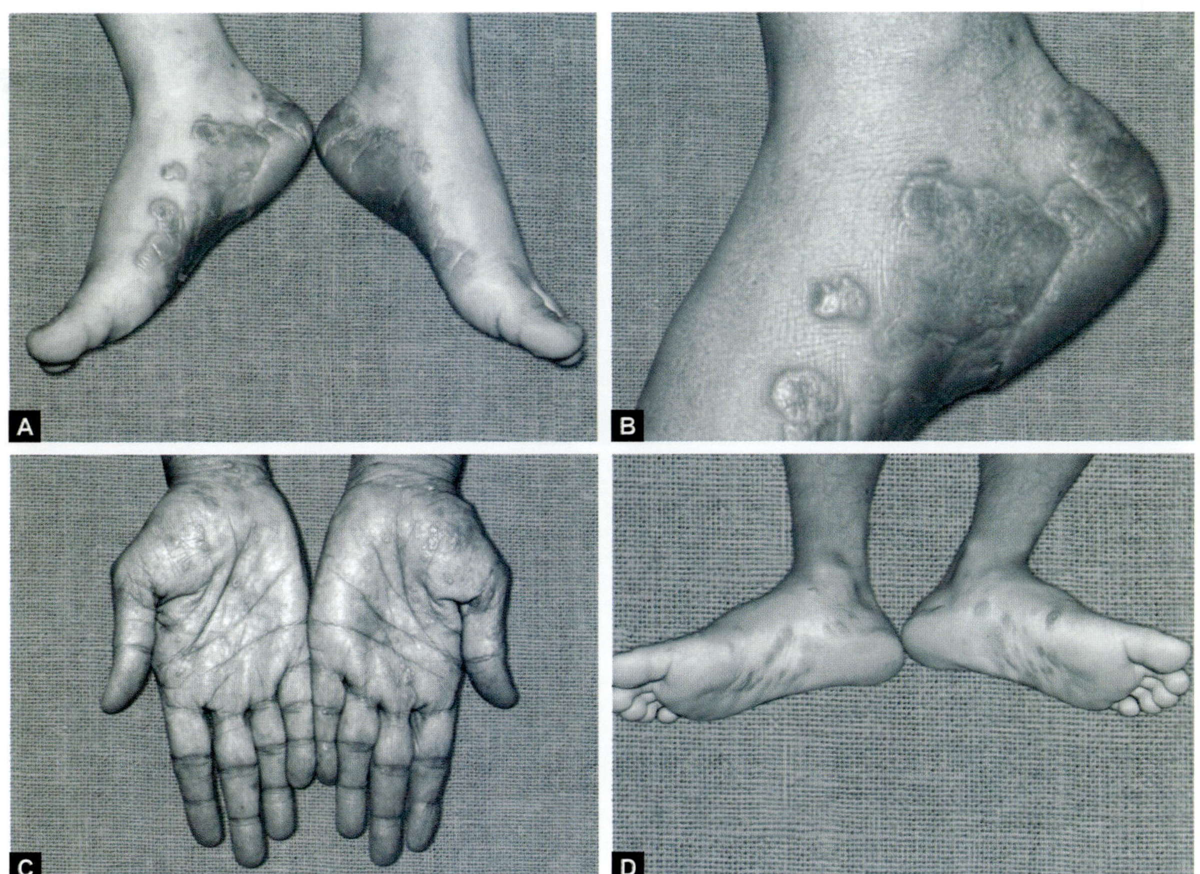

Lichen planus. A. On soles; B. Magnified view on soles; C. On palms; D. Another patient showing lesions on soles

Ans. **35. c.** Lichen planus

36. Important feature of psoriasis is:

a. Crusting
b. Scaling
c. Oozing
d. Erythema

Cutaneous lesions of psoriasis are well-defined, erythematous raised plaques with silvery white scaling.

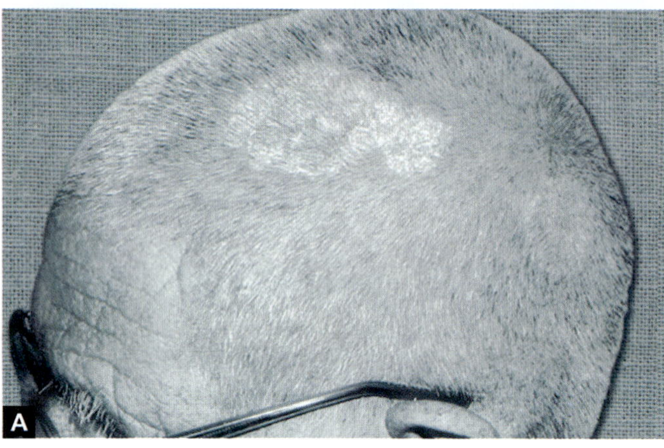

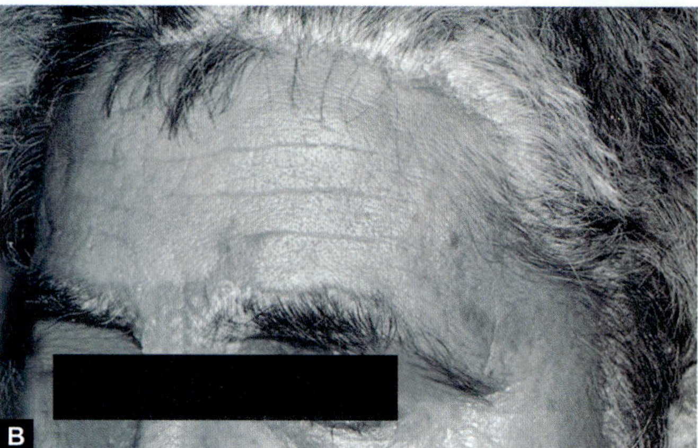

Scalp psoriasis. A. Multiple discrete plaques; B. Limitation to hairline

37. Herald patch is the 1st feature of:

a. Pityriasis rosea
b. Pemphigus
c. Psoriasis
d. Leprosy

The appearance of the herald patch (mother patch) is usually the first manifestation of pityriasis rosea, which is larger (2–5 cm) and more conspicuous than later lesions. It may be present on trunk, upper arm, thigh or neck.

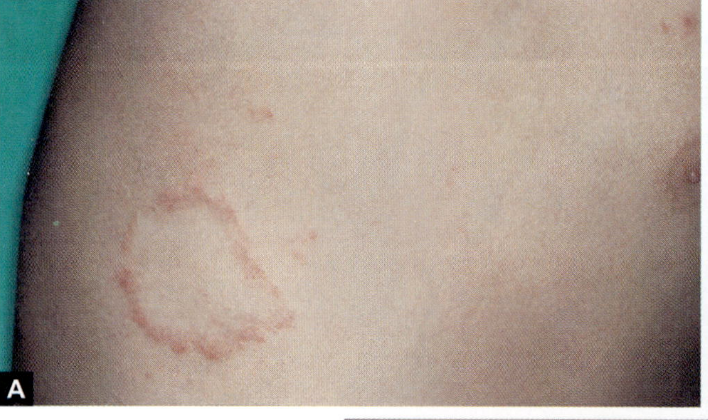

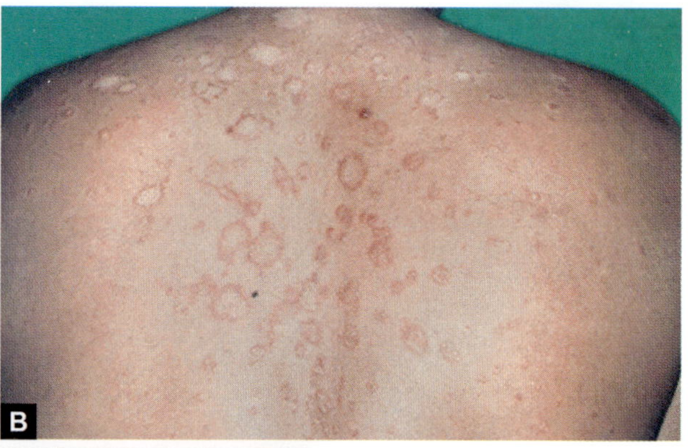

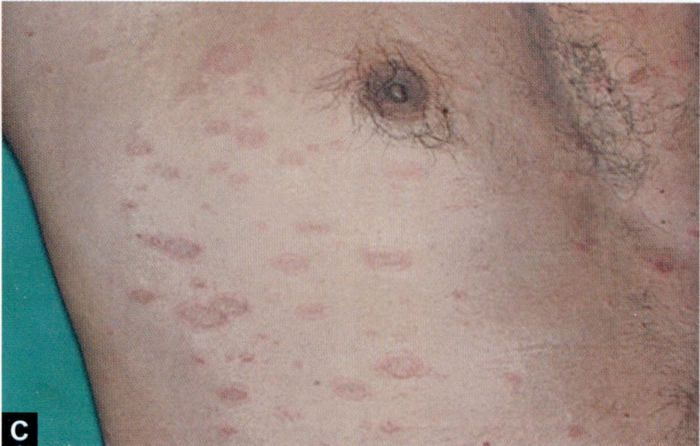

Pityriasis rosea. A. Herald patch and on trunk; B and C. Generalized eruptions on back and trunk; Pityriasis rosea. A. Herald patch and on trunk; B and C. Generalized eruptions on back and trunk

Ans. **36. b.** Scaling **37. a.** Pityriasis rosea

38. **DOC for a pregnant woman in 2nd trimester with pustular psoriasis is:**
   a. Prednisolone
   b. Dapsone
   c. Acitretin
   d. Methotrexate

Management of gestational pustular psoriasis

- If GPP is threatening the life of mother, termination or early delivery should be done.
- Otherwise, prednisolone which is least hazardous for fetus can be used.
- Cyclosporine has also been used safely.
- After delivery, MTX may be needed to wean off steroids or cyclosporine.

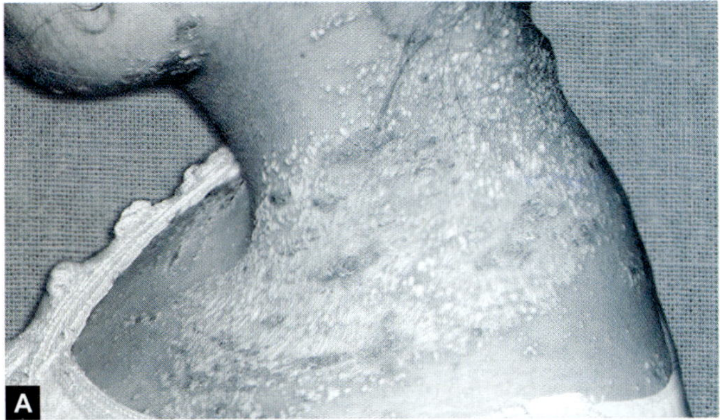

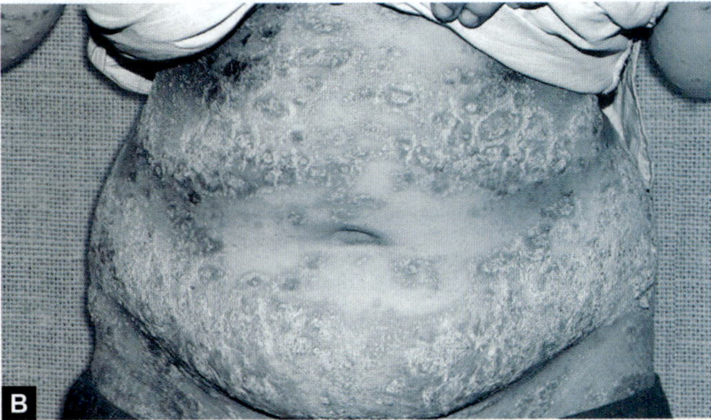

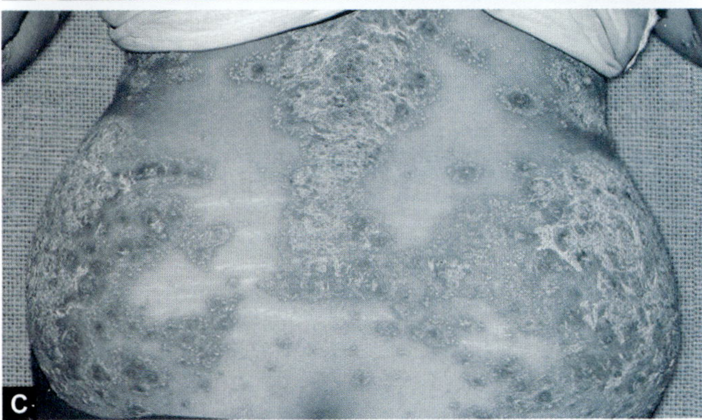

Generalized pustular psoriasis. Psoriatic plaques studded with macroscopic pustules. A. On neck; B. On trunk; C. On back

39. **Auspitz sign is seen in:**
   a. Pustular psoriasis
   b. Plaque type psoriasis
   c. Lichen planus
   d. Pityriasis rubra pilaris

Grattage test refers to the demonstration of easy removal of silvery white scales from cutaneous lesions with the edge of glass slide. On further removal of scales, a smooth glossy red membrane (Burkley's membrane) appears. On further scrapping, pinpoint bleeding spots (Auspitz's sign) are visible on the membrane. This sign has diagnostic value.

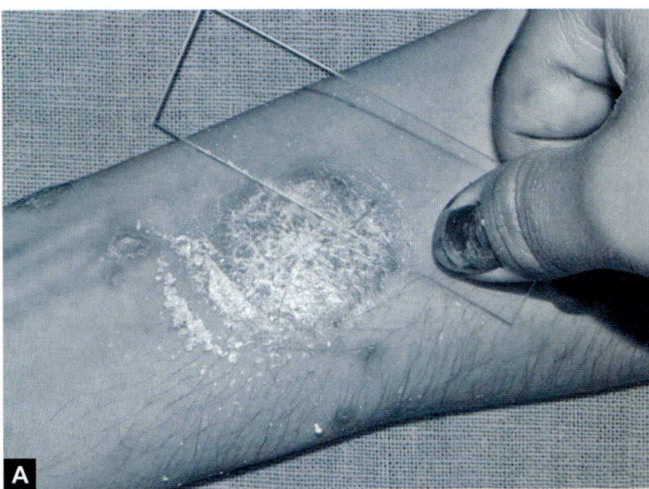

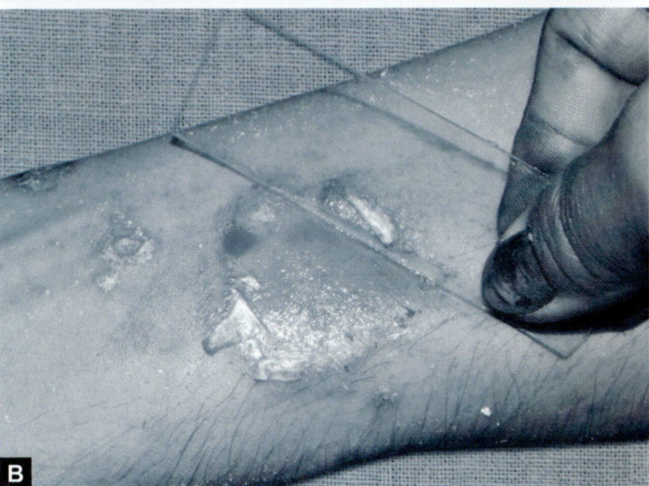

Psoriasis (grattage test). A. Burkley's membrane; B. Auspitz's sign

40. **Acne vulgaris involves:**
   a. Sweat glands
   b. Pilosebaceous glands
   c. Sebaceous glands
   d. Apocrine glands

Pathogenesis of acne vulgaris

- Increased sebum production
- Colonization of the duct by P. acne
- Hypercornification of pilosebaceous duct and occlusion of follicular orifice
- Inflammatory response

Ans. 38. **a.** Prednisolone 39. **b.** Plaque type psoriasis 40. **b.** Pilosebaceous glands

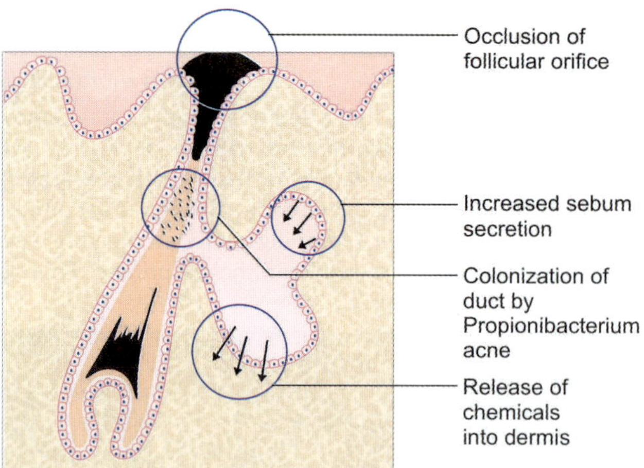

Pathogenesis of acne

41. Comedones are characteristic of:

a. Acne vulgaris
b. Acne rosacea
c. SLE
d. Adenoma sebaceum

The comedones are common and primary noninflammatory lesions of acne.

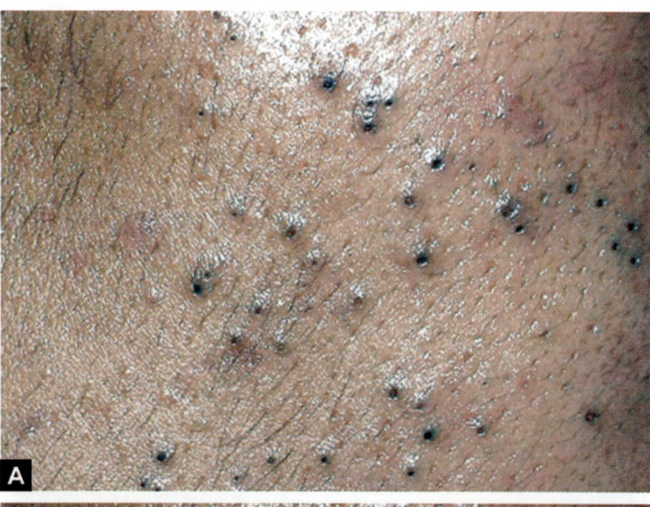

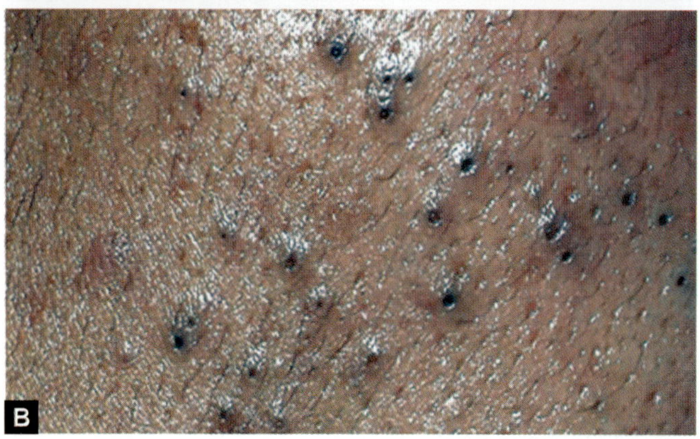

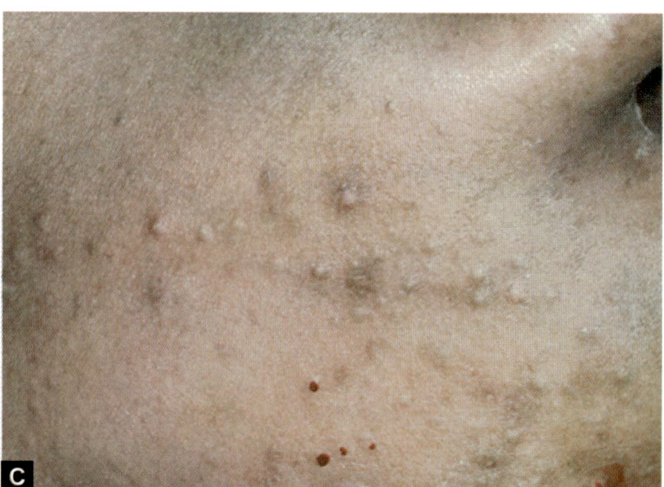

Acne comedones. A. Open comedones; B. Magnified view; C. Closed comedones

42. The treatment of dermatitis herpetiformis is:

a. Gluten free diet
b. Carbamazepine
c. Acyclovir
d. Systemic steroids

DH is associated with gluten sensitive enteropathy (GSE), which may be asymptomatic. Dietary antigens lead to formation of antibodies and immune complexes. The latter get deposited at dermal papillae and inflammation and dermoepidermal cleavage.

Sources of gluten and gluten free diet

Sources of gluten	*Gluten free diet*
Wheat, barley, and rye	Corn, rice, oats, potato, nuts, millet, Tapioca sorghum, flax, beans and legumes
Biscuits, breaded foods, buns, cakes, pies, donuts, hotdogs crackers and snacks	Fruits, vegetables, dry fruits, milk based items (ghee, butter, cream), egg, meat, poultry and fish
Pasta, pizza, gravy, pan cakes, wafers, soups, and beer	Pasta, pancakes, bread, pastries, cassava (made from alternative grains, e.g., rice or corn flour)

43. Nikolsky sign is seen in:

a. Pemphigus vulgaris
b. Herpes zoster
c. Herpes simplex
d. All of the above

Nikolsky's sign is positive in pemphigus vulgaris. On application of sliding pressure on the normal looking skin of bony prominences or on the skin surrounding the blisters there is a peeling of epidermis. This sign is positive in pemphigus and rarely in TEN (toxic epidermal necrolysis).

Ans. **41. a.** Acne vulgaris **42. a.** Gluten free diet **43. a.** Pemphigus vulgaris

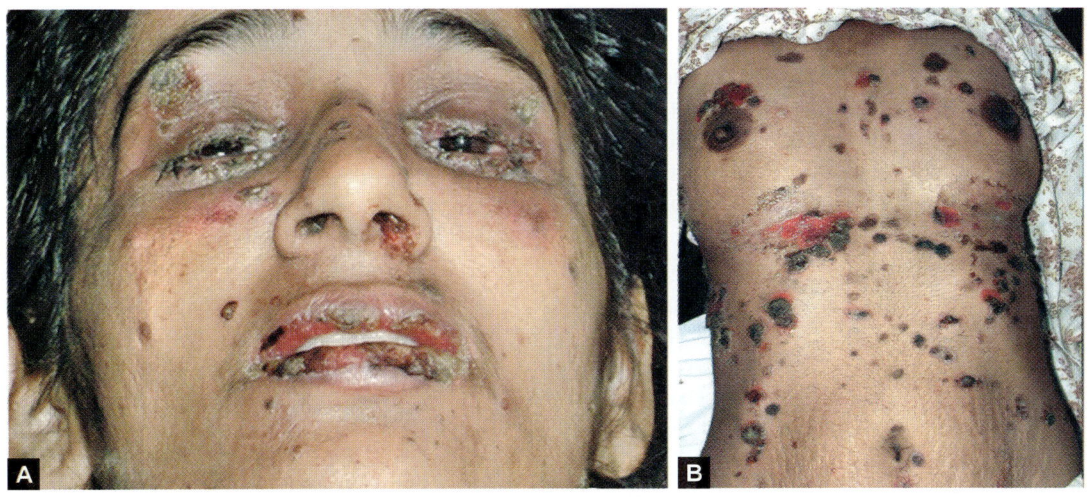

Pemphigus vulgaris. A. Involvement of oral mucosa;
B. Erosions and crusting on trunk

44. HLA associated with dermatitis herpetiformis:

a. HLA A5
b. HLA DR3
c. HLA B27
d. HLA A28

DH has strong associations with HLA-DR3 and DQW2.

Histopathological and immunofluorescence findings in common vesiculobullous disorders

Disease	*Epidermal changes*	*Dermal changes*	*Direct Immunofluorescence (detects antibodies deposited in skin)*	*Indirect Immunofluorescence (detects circulating antibodies)*
Pemphigus vulgaris	❑ Intercellular edema (spongiosis) ❑ Suprabasal cells shows loss of intercellular adhesions (acantholysis) ❑ Suprabasal cleft ❑ Basal cells separate from each other and remain attached to basement membrane, appear as "row of tomb stones"	❑ Dermal edema ❑ Mixed perivascular inflammatory infiltrate	❑ IgG on the surface of keratinocytes ❑ Found throughout epidermis ❑ Fishnet pattern ❑ Most sensitive for oral pemphigus	❑ Seen in > 80% of patients ❑ Titer correlates well with disease activity
Pemphigus foliaceus	Cleft forms in the granular layer or just below the corneal layer (subcorneal)	– do –	Immunofluorescence findings are similar in both pemphigus vulgaris and pemphigus foliaceus	
Bullous pemphigoid	❑ Intact epidermis forms roof of the blister. ❑ No epidermal necrosis or acanthosis	❑ Biopsy from erythematous area show infiltration by eosinophils and neutrophils ❑ Blister is subepidermal at the level of lamina lucida	❑ IgG and C3 or C3 alone along the basement membrane zone ❑ Performed on perilesional skin (within 2 cm) ❑ Linear band pattern	❑ IgG found in 75% of patients ❑ Titer do not correlate with disease activity
Dermatitis herpetiformis	Epidermis is normal. Note: Changes are best seen in the erythematous skin adjacent to early blisters	❑ Sub epidermal vesicle at the level of lamina lucida ❑ Dense accumulation of neutrophils and eosinophils within dermal papillae to form microabscesses	❑ IgA deposition in dermal papillae tips ❑ Preferred sites are normal skin of forearm and buttocks ❑ Granular pattern	Immune complexes in < 40% of patients
Linear IgA disease	Epidermis is normal	❑ Sub epidermal cleft ❑ Neutrophil collection along basement membrane	❑ IgA at dermoepidermal junction ❑ Linear	Low titer IgA

Ans. **44. b.** HLA DR3

45. DOC for dermatitis herpetiformis is:

a. Dapsone
b. Methotrexate
c. Clotrimazole
d. Thiabendazole

Dapsone is the most effective and widely used treatment for DH. It is used in 100–200 mg/day dose. It controls the disease very effectively in 2–3 days. Response to dapsone is considered as a therapeutic test for diagnosis of DH.

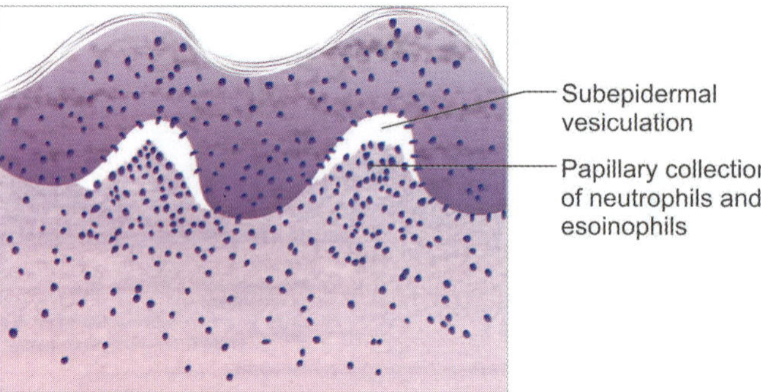

Dermatitis herpetiformis. Diagrammatic histopathological findings

46. Subepidermal bulla is seen in:

a. Pemphigoid
b. Pemphigus
c. Pityriasis rosea
d. Psoriasis

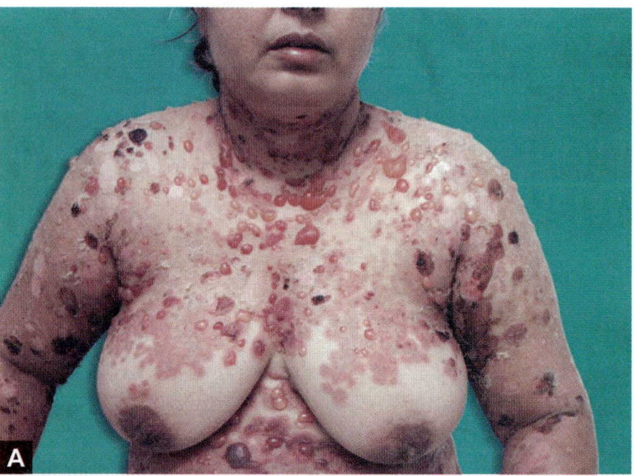

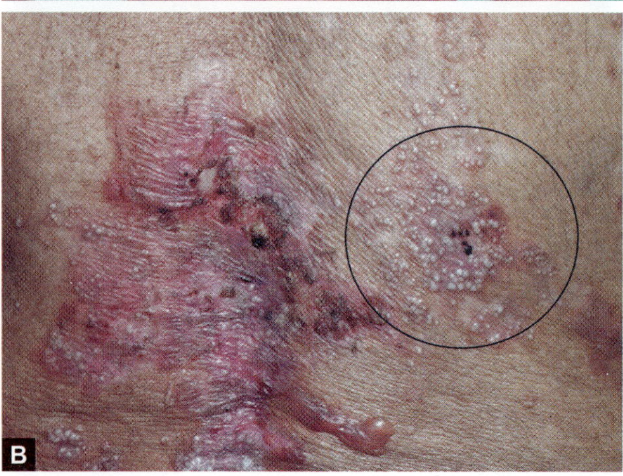

Bullous pemphigoid: A. Intact tense vesicle and bullae on erythematous skin; B. Healing by milia formation (round showing)

Being subepidermal, blisters of bullous pemphigoid are tense, dome-shaped of variable sizes on erythematous or normal skin.

47. Acantholysis is seen in:

a. Epidermis
b. Dermis
c. Dermoepidermal junction
d. Subcutaneous tissue

Acantholysis refers to loss of cohesion between epidermal or epithelial cells due to breakdown of intercellular bridges. It is typically seen in pemphigus vulgaris (lower epidermis) and pemphigus foliaceus (upper epidermis).

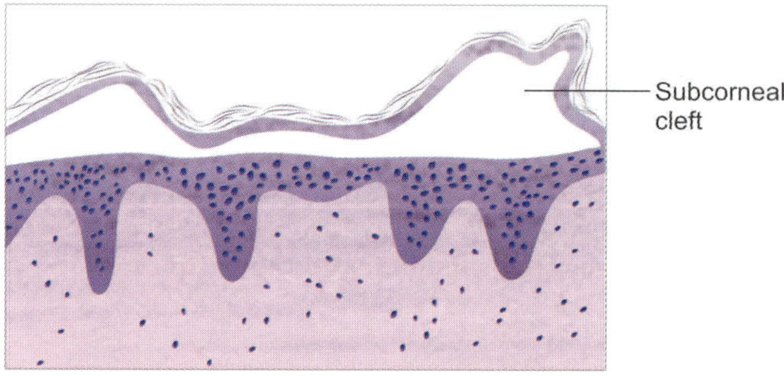

Pemphigus foliaceus. Diagrammatic histopathological findings

48. A 50-year-old man has a 2-year-old history of facial bullae and oral ulcers. Microscopic smear from skin lesions is most likely to disclose:

a. Tzanck cells
b. Acantholytic cells
c. Necrosis
d. Koilocytes

Tzanck smear is prepared in pemphigus vulgaris. The scrapings from floor of blister are smeared on a microscopic slide and examine under light microscope after staining with Leishman's stain. Acantholytic cells are seen as large round cells lying free with no attachment with other epidermal cells.

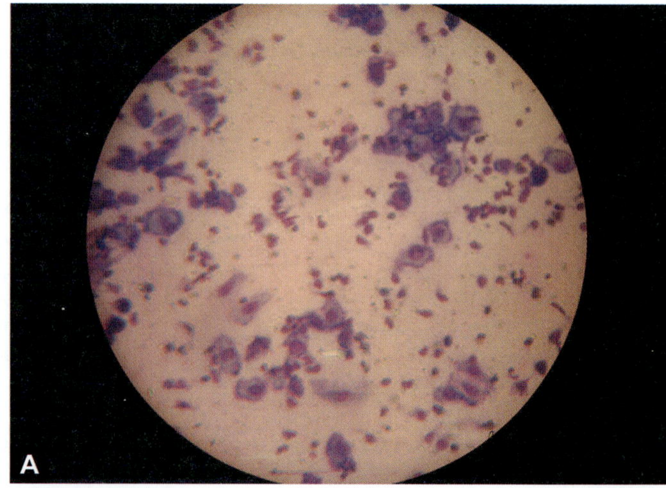

Contd...

Ans. 45. **a.** Dapsone 46. **a.** Pemphigoid 47. **a.** Epidermis 48. **b.** Acantholytic cells

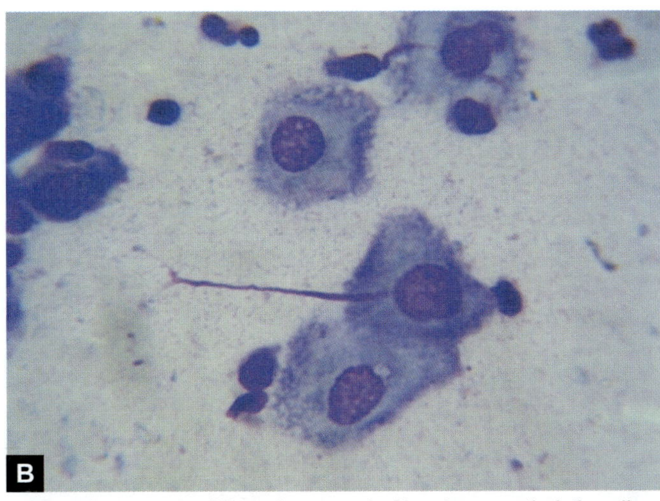

Microphotograph of Tzanck smear. A. Showing acantholytic cells under low power; B. Under high power

49. A 23-year-old lady presents with vesicular lesions in the buccal mucosa and flaccid blisters on the skin. The possible diagnosis is:

a. Pemphigus vulgaris
b. Pemphigus foliaceus
c. Pemphigoid
d. Dermatitis herpetiformis

Oral lesions are present in 50–70% of patients of pemphigus vulgaris. Cutaneous lesions erupt in crops and consists of flaccid blisters filled with fluid.

Difference between pemphigus vulgaris and bullous pemphigoid

Features	*Pemphigus vulgaris*	*Bullous pemphigoid*
Age	Middle age	Older age
Prodromal phase	None	May be preceded by urticaria or nonspecific eczema
Morphology	Crops of flaccid blisters that rupture easily	Tense, domeshaped blisters remain intact for several days
Sign	Nikolsky's and Bulla spread sign are positive	Negative
Surrounding skin	Normal	Urticarial or erythematous
Erosions	Less tendency to heal, painful and tend to spread peripher-ally	Rapid healing, don't expand peripherally
Healing by	Without scarring, but pigmentary changes are common	Minimum scarring or hyperpigmentation
Oral lesions	Almost seen in every patient	Less frequently seen

50. Adenoma sebaceum is a feature of:

a. Neurofibromatosis
b. Tuberous sclerosis
c. Xanthomatosis
d. Incontinentia pigmenti

Angiofibromas are diagnostic cutaneous lesions of tuberous sclerosis. Formerly misnamed as adenoma sebaceum and consists of hyperplastic blood vessels and sebaceous glands.

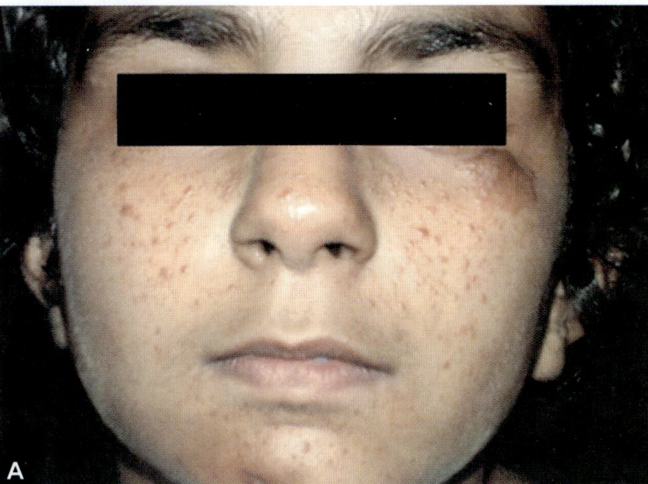

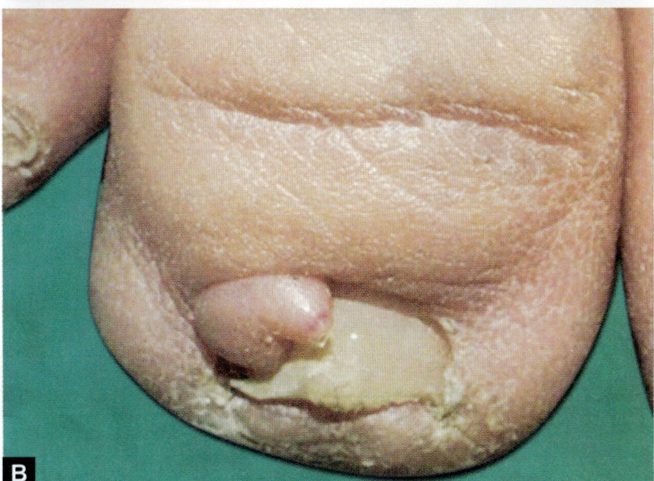

Tuberous sclerosis complex. A. Angiofibromas on cheeks; B. Koenen's tumor

51. Which of the following does NOT have a lymphatic spread:

a. Squamous cell Ca
b. Basal cell Ca
c. Malignant melanoma
d. Adeno Ca

BCC is most common neoplasm of skin. It is a locally invasive tumor showing slow progressive extension and cana result into extensive tissue damage, if left untreated. Metastasis is extremely rare.

Ans. **49. a.** Pemphigus... **50. b.** Tuberous sclerosis **51. b.** Basal cell Ca

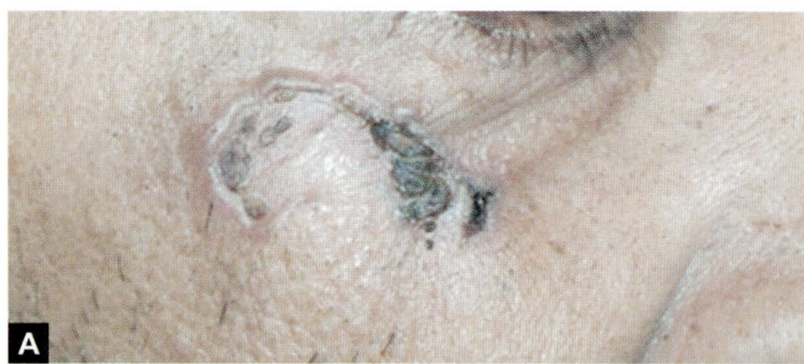

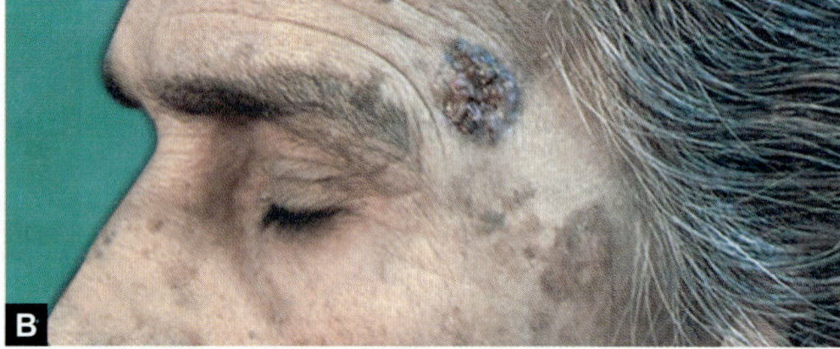

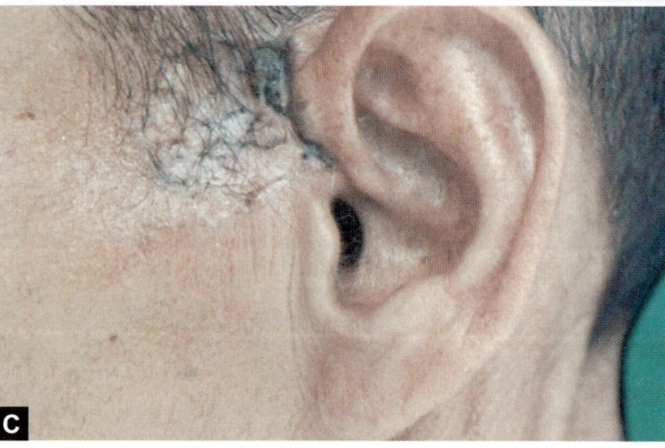

A. Nodular BCC with typical rolled borders;
B. Thickened plaque of BCC; C. Pigmented BCC

52. Mycosis cells are altered:

a. T lymphocytes b. Monocytes
c. B lymphocytes d. Eosinophils

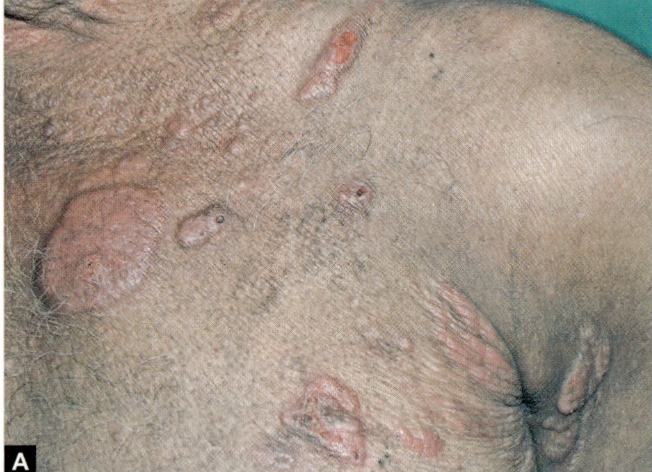

Contd...

Contd...

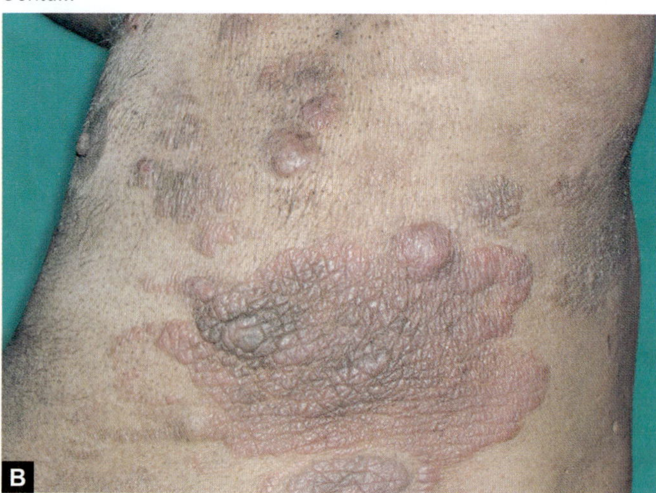

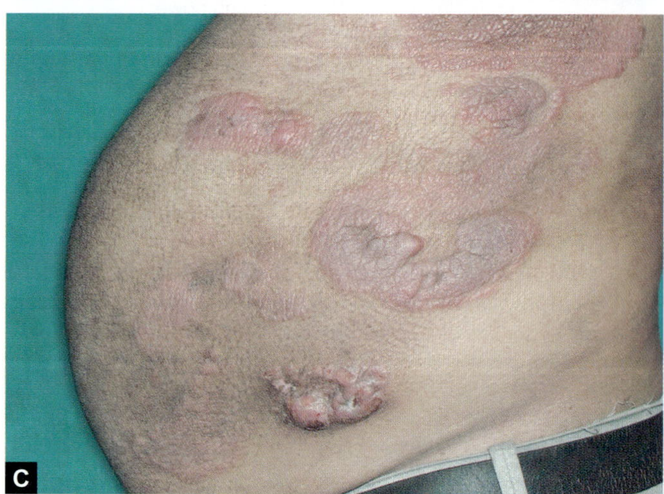

Mycosis fungoides tumor stages. A. On chest; B. On infra-axillary region; C. On Lower abdomen

Mycosis fungoides (MF) and Sezary syndrome (SS) are the most frequently seen cutaneous T-cell lymphoma (CTCL).

53. Darier's sign is seen in:

a. Xeroderma pigmentosum
b. Urticaria pigmentosa
c. Herpes zoster d. Glucagonoma

In urticaria pigmentosa, mild trauma, scratching, rubbing or stoking of lesions with a blunt object produces urtication and erythema within few minutes. This is known as Darier's sign.

Clinical classification of mastocytosis	
Indolent mastocytosis	❑ Cutaneous – Urticaria pigmentosa – Mastocytoma – Diffuse cutaneous mastocytosis
	❑ Systemic (involving at least one organ)

Contd...

Ans. 52. **a.** T lymphocytes 53. **b.** Urticaria pigmentosa

Contd...

Mastocytosis associated with hematological disorders	❑ Myeloproliferative disease ❑ Myelodysplastic disease
Aggressive mastocytosis	
Mast cell leukemia	

54. Koebner phenomenon is seen typically with:

a. Psoriasis
b. Eczema
c. Scabies
d. Lupus vulgaris

Psoriasis exhibits Koebner phenomenon (isomorphic phenomenon) in approximately 20% of patients. It refers to the appearance of psoriatic lesions in response to various types of trauma in previously uninvolved skin. It takes 7–14 days for the psoriatic lesions to appear after trauma.

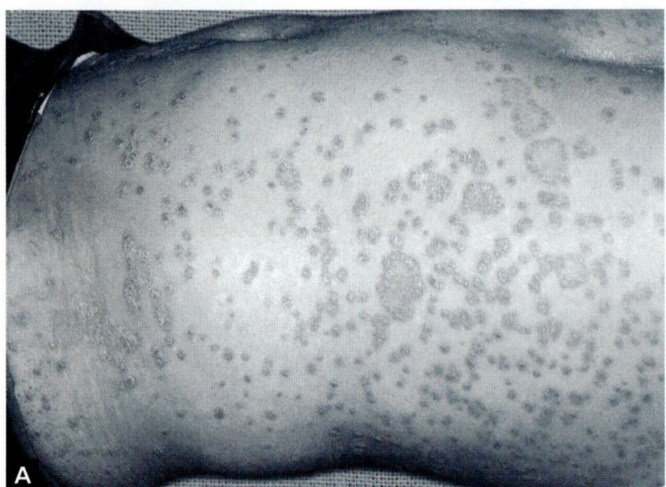

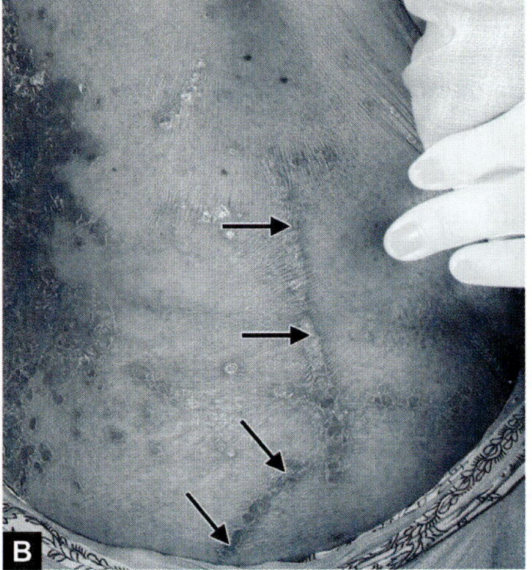

Contd...

Contd...

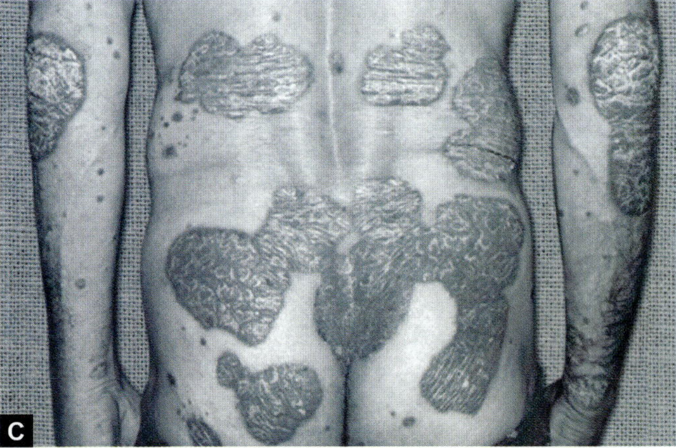

Psoriasis vulgaris. A. Rebound phenomenon exhibiting as appearance of more number of new skin lesions; B. Arrows showing Koebner phenomenon; C. On lower back and extensor surfaces

55. Wickham's striae are seen in:

a. Lichen nitidus
b. Lichen planus
c. Lichen scrufosum
d. DLE

Clinical diagnosis of lichen planus can be made by the presence of purple colored, pruritic, polygonal, plain topped papules showing Wickham's striae on peripheral parts of body (six Ps).

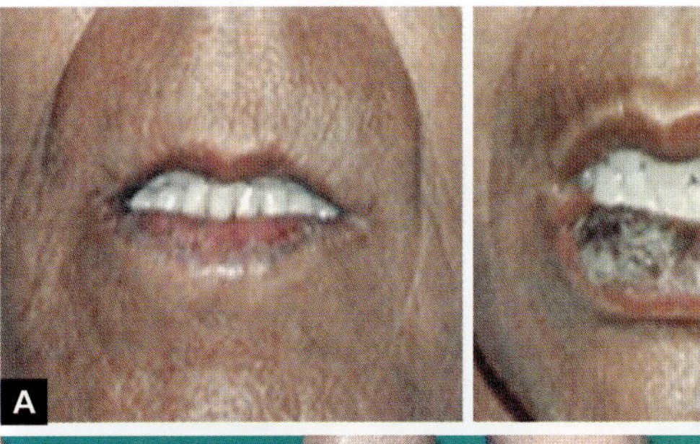

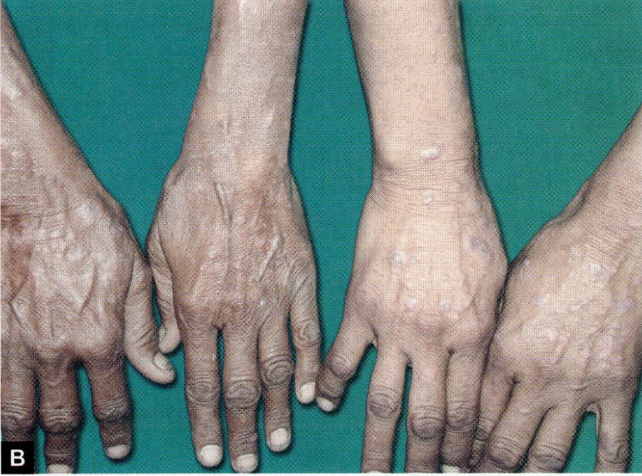

Familial lichen planus in two real sisters. A. On face; B. On dorsa of hands

Ans. 54. **a.** Psoriasis 55. **b.** Lichen planus

56. Lisch nodule is seen in:

a. von-Recklinghausen's disease
b. Motor disease
c. Myasthenia gravis
d. Drug induced myopathy

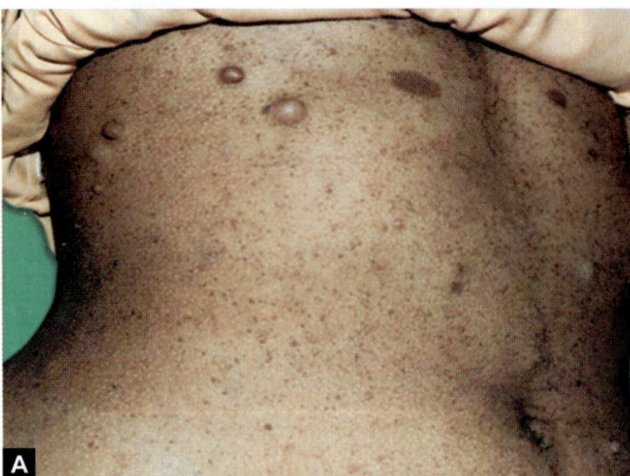

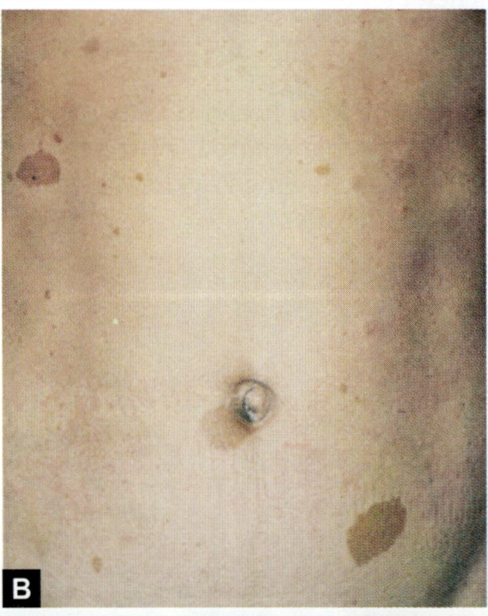

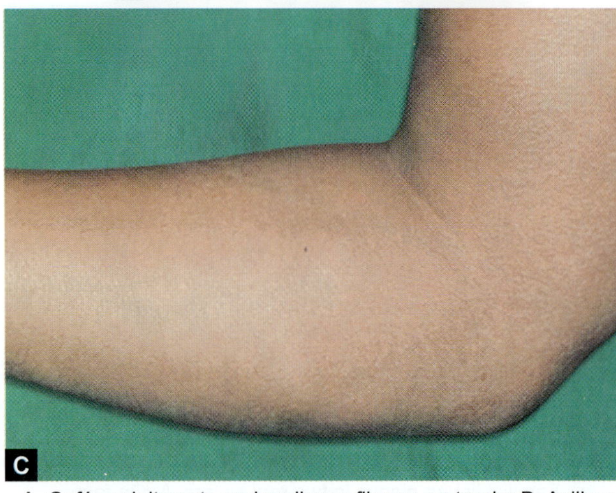

A. Café-au-lait spots and mollusca fibrosa on trunk ; B. Axillary freckling; C. Arrows showing subcutaneous neurofibromas

Lisch nodules are pigmented iris hamartomas, which are asymptomatic, dome-shaped and are present around iris. They are seen in neurofibromatosis-1 (von Recklinghausen's neurofibromatosis).

57. Butterfly rash is seen in:

a. Polyarteritis nodosa
b. SLE
c. Henoch-Schonlein purpura
d. Buerger's disease

Localized acute cutaneous lupus erythematosus present as malar or butterfly rash. Rash consists of erythema and edema symmetrically distributed on bridge of nose and malar eminences characteristically sparing nasolabial folds.

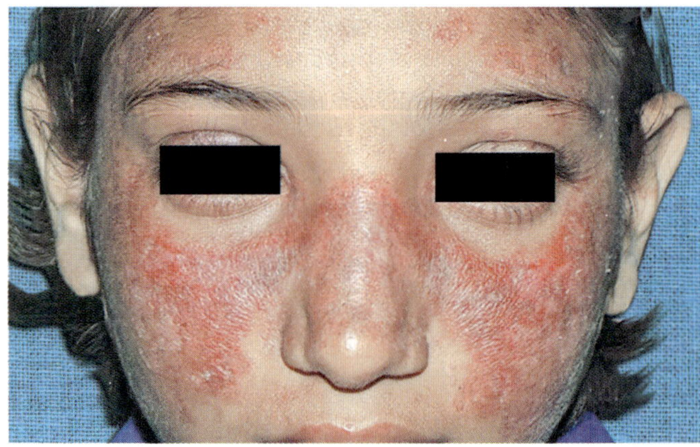

Localized acute cutaneous lupus erythematosus. (Butterfly rash sparing nasolabial folds)

58. NOT seen in tuberous sclerosis:

a. Angioma
b. Angiofibroma
c. Shagreen patch
d. Ash leaf macules

Diagnostic cutaneous lesions of tuberous sclerosis

- Angiofibromas
- Koenen's tumor (periungual fibromas)
- Shagreen's patch
- Ash leaf macules

59. Most common cause of airborne dermatitis:

a. Rubber
b. Medicines
c. Cosmetics
d. Parthenium

Airborne contact dermatitis/ABCD is a typical example of allergic contact dermatitis. It is caused by various types of air borne allergens which includes pollen grains, fungal spores, and other unknown particles from decorative plants and weeds, etc. Parthenium hysterophorus is a commonly noticed flowering weed causing ABCD in farmers and other field workers.

Ans. **56. a.** Von-Recklingh... **57. b.** SLE **58. a.** Angioma **59. d.** Parthenium

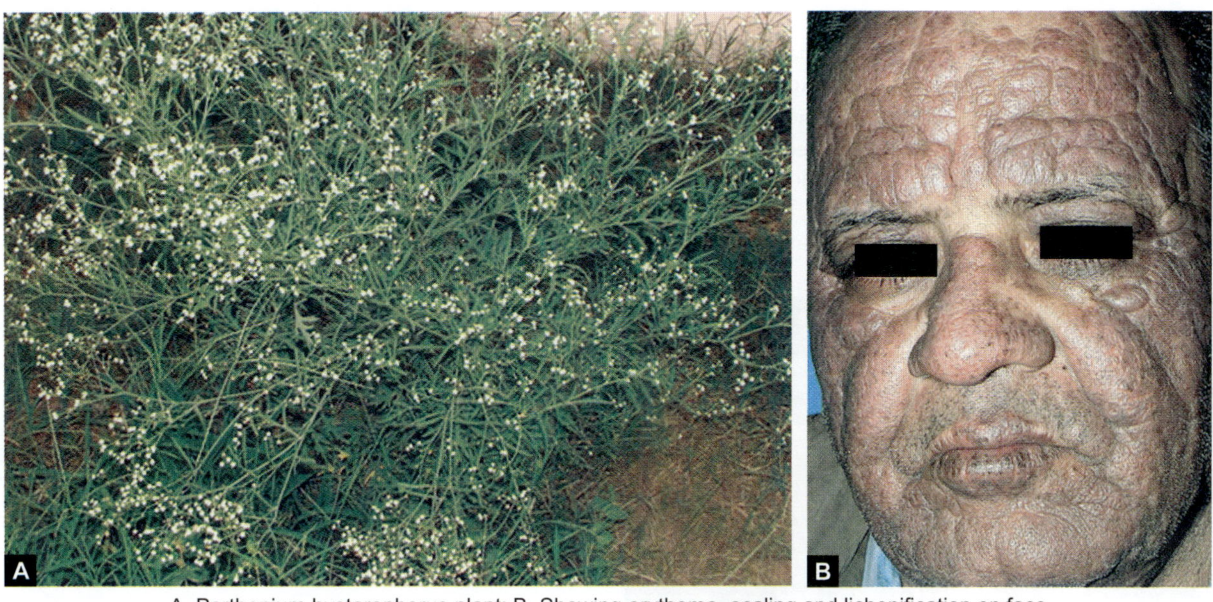
A. Parthenium hysterophorus plant; B. Showing erythema, scaling and lichenification on face

60. Gottron's papule is a feature of:

a. Dermatomyositis

b. Systemic lupus erythematosus

c. Discoid lupus erythematosus

d. Subacute cutaneous lupus erythematosus

Gottron's papules are small, reddish or violaceous papules or small plaques seen in dermatomyos-itis.

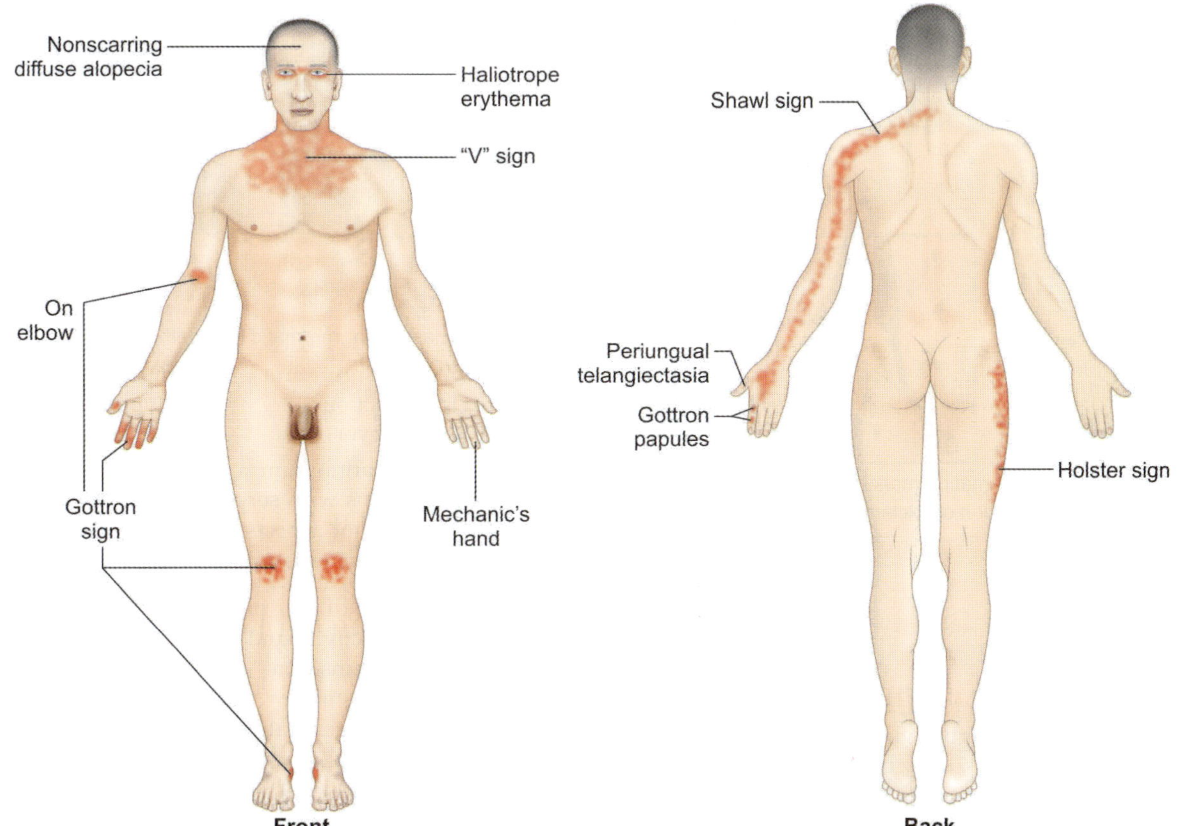

Cutaneous manifestations of dermatomyositis

Ans. **60. a.** Dermatomyositis

61. Exclamation mark hairs are seen in:

a. Syphilis
b. Alopecia areata
c. Psoriasis
d. Dermatophytosis

Alopecia areata presents typically as variable sized, well defined totally bald patch noticed by patient or by others. At the periphery of the lesion characteristic 'exclamation mark hairs' can be seen. These are short, broken, easily pluckable hairs where upper ends are broader than lower ends.

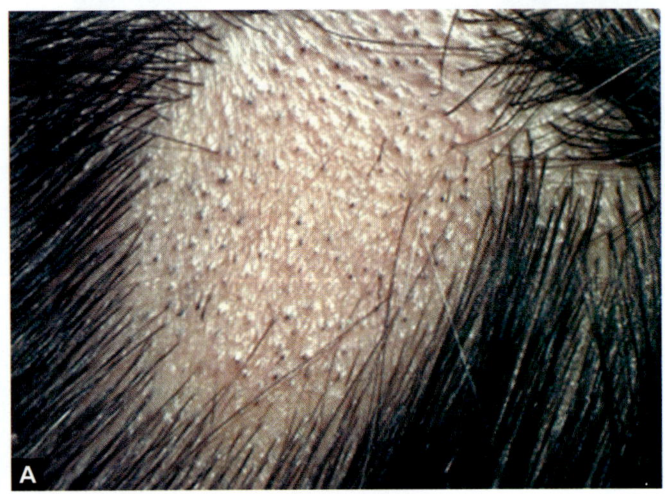

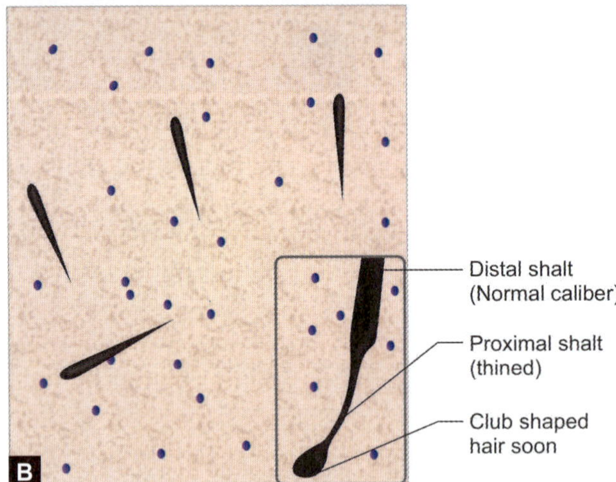

Alopecia areata. A. 'Exclamation mark hairs'; B. Diagrammatic representation of exclamation hair

62. Etiology of Pityriasis rosea is:

a. M. furfur
b. Herpes virus
c. Autoimmune
d. Staphylococcus

Etiology of pityriasis rosea is uncertain. Viral etiology is speculated. Two herpes viruses, human herpes virus 6 (HHV-6) and HHV-7 may be involved. Certain drugs can produce pityriasis rosea like eruptions, e.g. arsenic, captopril, isotretinoin, metronidazole, omeprazole, terbinafine, etc.

Difference between pityriasis rosea and secondary syphilis

Pityriasis rosea	*Secondary syphilis*
History of exposure: Absent	History of exposure and penile ulcer is usually found
Morphology: Annular lesions with collarette of scales. Extremities are infrequently involved sparing palms and soles	Papulosquamous lesions on trunk, extremities including palms and soles
Olendorf's sign: Negative	Positive
Mucosal involvement: Not involved	Oral mucosa and anal region may be involved
Lymph nodes: Not enlarged	Lymphadenopathy is frequent
Serological tests: Negative	Positive

63. Munro microabscesses are characteristically seen in:

a. Lichen planus
b. Lupus erythematosus
c. Psoriasis
d. Seborrhoeic dermatitis

Presence of aggregations of neutrophils in the parakeratotic layer (Munro's microabscesses) and in upper spinous layer (spongiform pustules of Kogoj) are considered as diagnostic features of psoriasis.

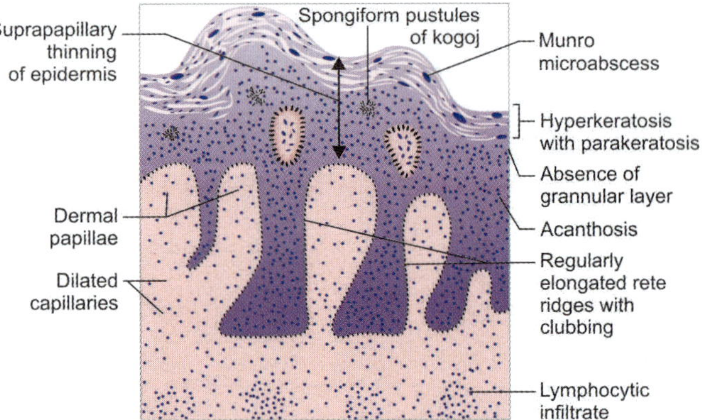

Psoriasis. Diagrammatic histopathological findings

64. Erythema marginatum is seen in:

a. Drug reactions
b. Typhus fever
c. Enteric fever
d. Rheumatic fever

Erythema marginatum are erythematous non-pruritic annular lesions with serpiginous borders, usually seen over the anterior aspects of the chest and abdomen and over the thighs in rheumatic fever.

65. Anagen phase of hair indicates:

a. Phase of activity and growth
b. Phase of transition
c. Phase of resting
d. Phase of degeneration

The growth of hair is cyclical and different phases of follicle are, growing phase (anagen) which lasts for 3–10 years, involuting phase (catagen) which lasts for 2–3 weeks and the resting phase (telogen) which lasts

Ans. 61. **b.** Alopecia areata 62. **b.** Herpes virus 63. **c.** Psoriasis 64. **d.** Rheumatic fever 65. **a.** Phase of activity...

for 3–4 months. At least 85% of hair follicles are in anagen phase at any one time.

66. Necrobiosis lipoidica is seen in:

a. Hypertension
b. Diabetes mellitus
c. Syphilis
d. Leprosy

Necrobiosis lipoidica is a very specific skin lesion associated with diabetes.

67. Necrobiosis lipoidica dibeticorum is MC in:

a. Back
b. Front of legs
c. Shoulder
d. Trunk

Patients of necrobiosis lipoidica presents with erythematous plaques on the shin which later becomes yellowish brown and undergoes central atrophy. The lesions have a glazed appearance and may ulcerate and then heal with scarring.

68. Acrodermatitis enteropathica, true is:

a. Abnormal mucosa on histology
b. Long treatment
c. Zinc will give partial relief
d. Autosomal dominant

The response to zinc, 1-2 mg/kg/day (elemental) in divided doses is dramatic with improvement in diarrhea and prompt healing of skin lesions. With the availability of zinc for therapeutic use, di-iodohydroxyquin which was supposed to yield good results but was likely to cause optic neuritis in infants is no longer recommended.

69. Acrodermatitis enteropathica, NOT true is:

a. Zinc deficiency syndrome
b. Autosomal dominant inheritance
c. May be associated with growth retardation
d. Periorificial region commonly involved

Acrodermatitis is a familial disorder with autosomal recessive inheritance and with unique cocktail of clinical manifestations.

Ans. 66. **b.** Diabetes mellitus 67. **b.** Front of legs 68. **b.** Long treatment 69. **b.** Autosomal dominant...

ANSWERS WITH REFERENCES

BACTERIAL INFECTION

1. **Ans. (c)** Iris pearls
Ref: Bansal's Dermatology, 1/e p466

2. **Ans. (d)** Cessation of antileprosy treatment
Ref: Bansal's Dermatology 1/e p479

3. **Ans. (a)** Chlamydia trachomatis
Ref: Bansal's Dermatology 1/e p441

4. **Ans. (d)** 9-90 days
Ref: Bansal's Dermatology 1/e p429

5. **Ans. (a)** Lupus vulgaris
Ref: Bansal's Dermatology 1/e p58

6. **Ans. (a)** Ulnar
Ref: Bansal's Dermatology 1/e p469

7. **Ans. (a)** Systemic steroids
Ref: Bansal's Dermatology 1/e p479

8. **Ans. (a)** Aspiration
Ref: Bansal's Dermatology 1/e p470

9. **Ans. (d)** Secondary syphilis
Ref: Bansal's Dermatology 1/e p241

10. **Ans. (b)** Staphylococcus aureus
Ref: Bansal's Dermatology 1/e p42

11. **Ans. (d)** Lupus vulgaris
Ref: Bansal's Dermatology 1/e p58

12. **Ans. (c)** Gonorrhea
Ref: Bansal's Dermatology 1/e p439

13. **Ans. (b)** Frei test
Ref: Bansal's Dermatology 1/e p435

14. **Ans. (d)** Azithromycin 1 gram single dose
Ref: Bansal's Dermatology 1/e p454

15. **Ans. (c)** Posterior uveitis
Ref: Bansal's Dermatology 1/e p434

16. **Ans. (b)** FTA-abs
Ref: Bansal's Dermatology 1/e p436

17. **Ans. (d)** Benzathine penicillin
Ref: Bansal's Dermatology 1/e p438

18. **Ans. (a)** Syphilis
Ref: Bansal's Dermatology 1/e p435

FUNGAL INFECTION

19. **Ans. (b)** Tinea cruris
Ref: Bansal's Dermatology 1/e p94

20. **Ans. (a)** Malassezia furfur
Ref: Bansal's Dermatology 1/e p104

21. **Ans. (d)** All of the above
Ref: Bansal's Dermatology 1/e p87

PIGMENTATION DISORDER

22. **Ans. (b)** Chronic arsenic poisoning
Ref: Bansal's Dermatology 1/e p344

MISCELLANEOUS

23. **Ans. (c)** Atopic dermatitis
Ref: Bansal's Dermatology, 1/e p118

24. **Ans. (b)** Stratum spinosum & Stratum basale
Ref: Bansal's Dermatology, 1/e p8

25. **Ans. (d)** Cold temperature
Ref: Internet resources

26. **Ans. (c)** Normal immune system
Ref: Bansal's Dermatology, 1/e p359

27. **Ans. (d)** Becker nevus
Ref: Bansal's Dermatology, 1/e p332

28. **Ans. (d)** Induration
Ref: Bansal's Dermatology 1/e p60

29. **Ans. (b)** 360 nm
Ref: Bansal's Dermatology 1/e p18

30. **Ans. (d)** 48 days
Ref: Bansal's Dermatology 1/e p4

31. **Ans. (b)** Nickel oxide & silica
Ref: Bansal's Dermatology 1/e p18

32. **Ans. (a)** Norwegian scabies
Ref: Bansal's Dermatology 1/e p35

33. **Ans. (a)** Burrow
Ref: Bansal's Dermatology 1/e p32

34. **Ans. (b)** Face
Ref: Bansal's Dermatology 1/e p33

35. **Ans. (c) Lichen planus**
Ref: Bansal's Dermatology 1/e p192

36. **Ans. (b) Scaling**
Ref: Bansal's Dermatology 1/e p178

37. **Ans. (a) Pityriasis rosea**
Ref: Bansal's Dermatology 1/e p199

38. **Ans. (a) Prednisolone**
Ref: Bansal's Dermatology 1/e p189

39. **Ans. (b) Plaque type psoriasis**
Ref: Bansal's Dermatology 1/e p177

40. **Ans. (b) Pilosebaceous glands**
Ref: Bansal's Dermatology 1/e p227

41. **Ans. (a) Acne vulgaris**
Ref: Bansal's Dermatology 1/e p228

42. **Ans. (a) Gluten free diet**
Ref: Bansal's Dermatology 1/e p160

43. **Ans. (a) Pemphigus vulgaris**
Ref: Bansal's Dermatology 1/e p150

44. **Ans. (b) HLA DR3**
Ref: Bansal's Dermatology 1/e p153

45. **Ans. (a) Dapsone**
Ref: Bansal's Dermatology 1/e p154

46. **Ans. (a) Pemphigoid**
Ref: Bansal's Dermatology 1/e p159

47. **Ans. (a) Epidermis**
Ref: Bansal's Dermatology 1/e p154

48. **Ans. (b) Acantholytic cells**
Ref: Bansal's Dermatology 1/e p152

49. **Ans. (a) Pemphigus vulgaris**
Ref: Bansal's Dermatology 1/e p151

50. **Ans. (b) Tuberous sclerosis**
Ref: Bansal's Dermatology 1/e p139

51. **Ans. (b) Basal cell Ca**
Ref: Bansal's Dermatology 1/e p347

52. **Ans. (a) T lymphocytes**
Ref: Bansal's Dermatology 1/e p362

53. **Ans. (b) Urticaria pigmentosa**
Ref: Bansal's Dermatology 1/e p305

54. **Ans. (a) Psoriasis**
Ref: Bansal's Dermatology 1/e p177

55. **Ans. (b) Lichen planus**
Ref: Bansal's Dermatology 1/e p191

56. **Ans. (a) Von-Recklinghausen's disease**
Ref: Bansal's Dermatology 1/e p136

57. **Ans. (b) SLE**
Ref: Bansal's Dermatology 1/e p206

58. **Ans. (a) Angioma**
Ref: Bansal's Dermatology 1/e p139

59. **Ans. (d) Parthenium**
Ref: Bansal's Dermatology 1/e p127

60. **Ans. (a) Dermatomyositis**
Ref: Bansal's Dermatology 1/e p224

61. **Ans. (b) Alopecia areata**
Ref: Bansal's Dermatology 1/e p245

62. **Ans. (b) Herpes virus**
Ref: Bansal's Dermatology 1/e p200

63. **Ans. (c) Psoriasis**
Ref: Bansal's Dermatology 1/e p182

64. **Ans. (d) Rheumatic fever**
Ref: KV Krishna Das's Medicine 5/e p193

65. **Ans. (a) Phase of activity and growth**
Ref: KV Krishna Das's Medicine 5/e p1346

66. **Ans. (b) Diabetes mellitus**
Ref: KV Krishna Das's Medicine 5/e p1391

67. **Ans. (b) Front of legs**
Ref: KV Krishna Das's Medicine 5/e p1391

68. **Ans. (b) Long treatment**
Ref: Gupte's Pediatricsis 11/e p471

69. **Ans. (b) Autosomal dominant inheritance**
Ref: Gupte's Pediatricsis 11/e p470

PRACTICE QUESTIONS

BACTERIAL INFECTION

1. All of the following conditions may present with genital ulceration EXCEPT:
- a. Gonorrhea
- b. Chancroid
- c. Syphilis
- d. Lymphogranuloma venereum

2. An adult went for a leisure trip. Now after 2 weeks, he presented with fever, rubbery genital ulcer, enlarged inguinal lymph nodes. Most probable causative organism:
- a. Chlamydia trachomatis
- b. Treponema pallidum
- c. H. ducreyi
- d. Neisseria gonorrhea

FUNGAL INFECTION

3. Which of the following is classified as dermatophyte:
- a. Tinea versicolor
- b. Trichophyton rubrum
- c. Sporothrix
- d. Histoplasmosis

PIGMENTATION DISORDER

4. A obese patient with type II diabetes mellitus & known case of adenocaricinoma of stomach, is having velvety skin especially in axilla. Likely diagnosis:
- a. Malignancy associated hyperpigmentation
- b. Follicular hyperkeratosis
- c. Acanthosis nigricans
- d. Dermatitis

MISCELLANEOUS

5. Scabies is caused by:
- a. Ixodes
- b. Sarcoptes scabiei
- c. Xenopsylla
- d. Phlebotomus

6. A young patient presented with silvery scales on extensor surface of knees. Most likely diagnosis:
- a. Pemphigus
- b. Pemphigoid
- c. Psoriasis
- d. Lichen planus

7. Toxic epidermal necrolysis is commonly associated with:
- a. HIV
- b. Drugs intake
- c. SLE
- d. TB

8. A patient had history of gluten sensitive enteropathy. Direct Immunofluorescence shows deposits of IgA in dermal papillae. What would be the most likely associated HLA marker with this condition?
- a. HLA-DQW2
- b. HLA-DRB1
- c. HLA-DQB1
- d. HLA-DR2

9. Fordyce spots are ectopic:
- a. Salivary glands
- b. Meibomian glands
- c. Sebaceous glands
- d. Gland of moll

10. Mycosis fungoides is also known as:
- a. Cutaneous B cell lymphoma
- b. Extra-mammary Paget's disease
- c. Cutaneous T cell lymphoma
- d. Senile angiomas

11. A 10-year-old child presented with recurrent painful mouth ulcers. On examination, they were found as yellowish elevated spot surrounded by a red halo. They tend to heal within 7-10 days. History and findings is consistent with the diagnosis of:
- a. Measles
- b. Aphthous ulcers
- c. Malignancy
- d. Lichen planus

12. Berloque dermatitis is because of:
- a. Animals
- b. Plants
- c. Cosmetics
- d. Household stuff

13. A 6-month-old baby presented with skin rashes with scaling on face and ante-cubital and popliteal fossa. Most likely diagnosis:
- a. Allergic dermatitis
- b. Contact dermatitis
- c. Atopic dermatitis
- d. Eczema

14. Subepidermal blistering is noticed in:
- a. Pemphigus
- b. Pemphigoid
- c. Both
- d. None

15. Familial benign chronic pemphigus is also known as:
- a. Pemphigus vulgaris
- b. Pemphigus foliaceus
- c. Hailey-Hailey disease
- d. Pemphigus herpetiformis

Ans. 1. a. Gonorrhoea 2. a. Chlamydia trachomatis 3. b. Trichophyton... 4. c. Acanthosis... 5. b. Sarcoptes scabiei 6. c. Psoriasis 7. b. Drugs intake 8. a. HLA-DQW2 9. c. Sebaceous glands 10. c. Cutaneous... 11. b. Aphthous ulcers 12. b. Plants 13. c. Atopic dermatitis 14. b. Pemphigoid 15. c. Hailey-Hailey disease

IMAGE-BASED QUESTIONS

1. Such presentation is seen in:

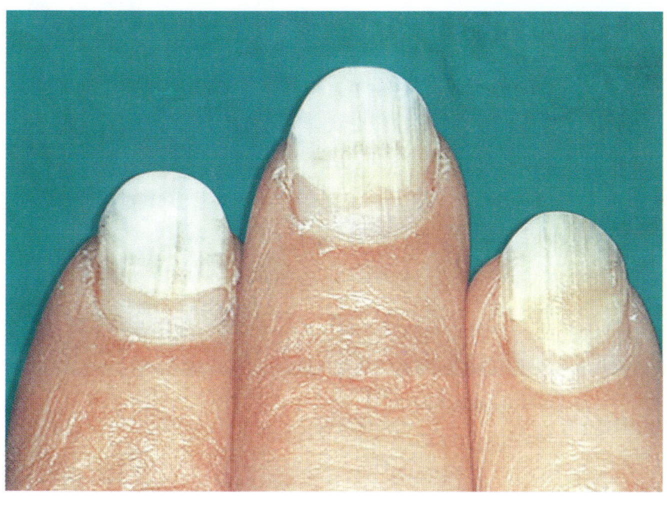

a. Lichen planus
b. Psoriasis
c. Pemphigus vulgaris
d. Arsenic poisoning

Onycholysis refers to the painless separation of distal part of nail plate from nail bed. Separated part of nail plate appears white due to the presence of air. Like pits, onycholysis is most common manifestation of psoriasis.

2. Such a presentation is seen in:

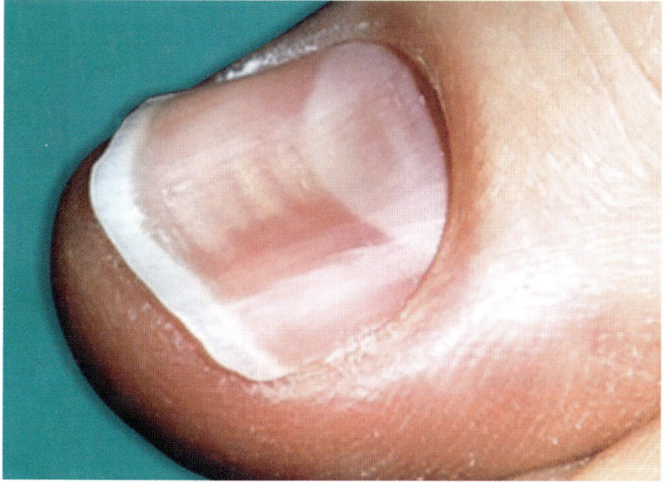

a. Arsenic poisoning
b. Lichen planus
c. Iron deficiency anemia
d. Vitamin B12 deficiency anemia

Koilonychia refers to the concave shape of the nail plate both in transverse and longitudinal axes. Most commonly it is associated with iron deficiency anemia.

3. Drug of choice for this condition:

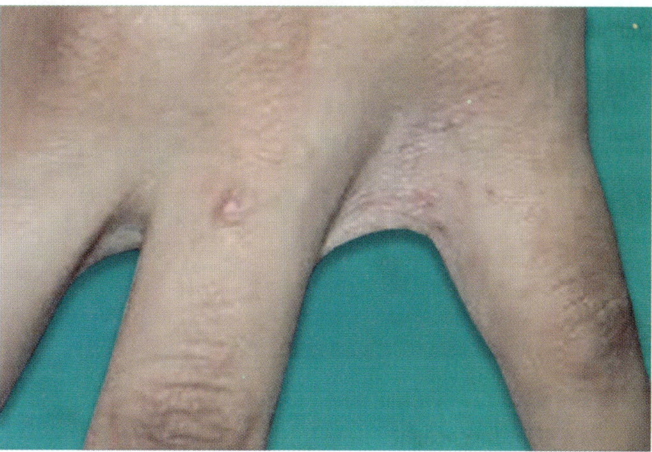

a. Ivermectin
b. Crotamiton
c. 0.5% Malathion
d. 5% Permethrin

Five percent permethrin cream or lotion is ovicidal and is an excellent scabicide. Single application for 8–12 hours, second application a week later. It acts by blocking sodium channel repolarization. Got residual activity for 10 days after application.

4. Management of such a condition:

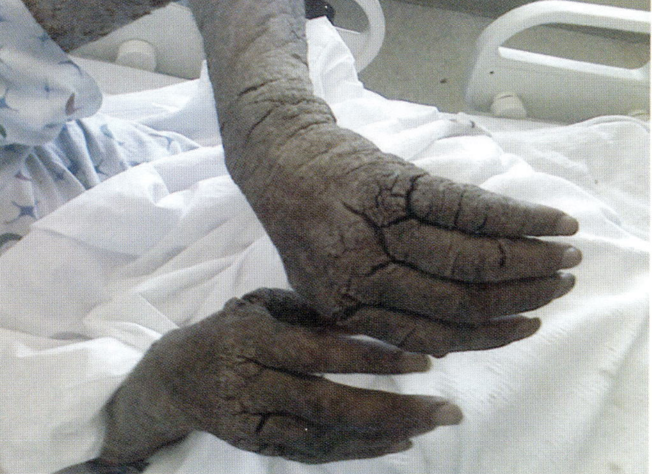

a. Ivermectin
b. Ketoconazole
c. Griseofulvin
d. Penicillin

Ivermectin alone or in combination with topical scabicide is the treatment of choice for crusted/ Norwegian scabies.

5. Spot diagnosis:

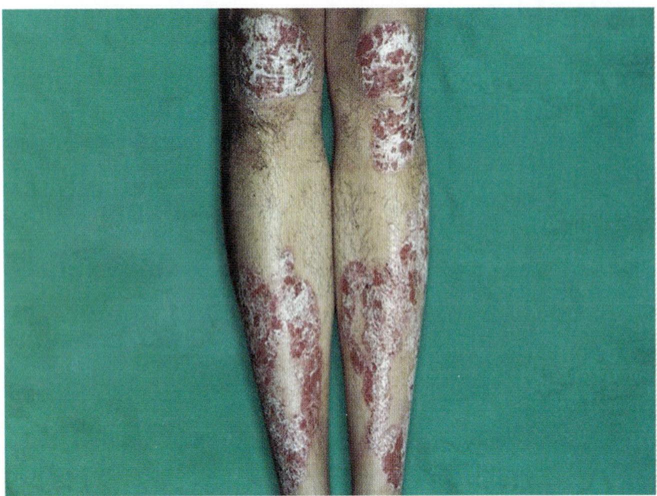

a. Pemphigus
b. Pemphigoid
c. Psoriasis
d. Lichen planus

Well-defined, erythematous raised plaques with silvery white scaling is suggestive of psoriasis.

6. Site of injury develops psoriatic lesions. This is:

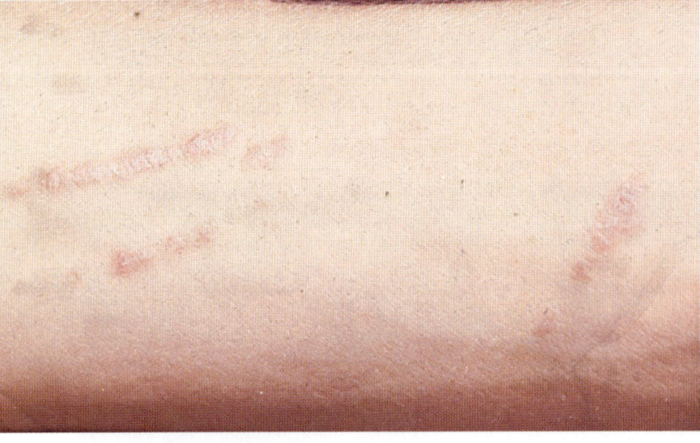

a. Auspitz's sign
b. Grattage test
c. Koebner's phenomenon
d. Nikolsky's sign

Psoriasis exhibit Koebner phenomenon, which refers to the appearance of psoriatic lesions in response to various types of trauma in previously uninvolved skin.

7. Removal of scales leads to bleeding. This is:

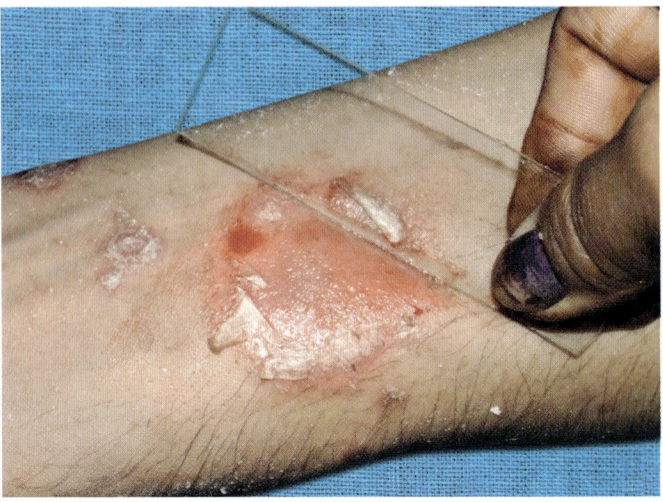

a. Auspitz's sign
b. Grattage test
c. Koebner's phenomenon
d. Nikolsky's sign

Scrapping of scales in psoriasis leads to pinpoint bleeding spots, which has diagnostic value.

8. Management of such a condition:

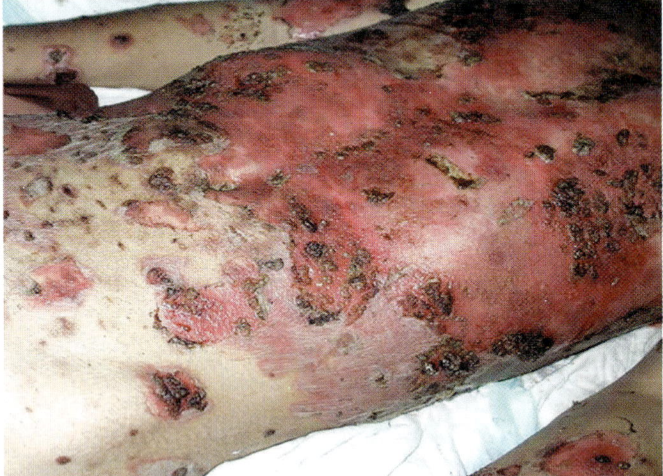

a. Antifungal
b. PUVA
c. Steroids
d. Antibiotics

For mild to moderate cases of pemphigus, 1–1.5 mg/kg/day prednisolone (60-100 mg) is used and 120–240 mg of prednisolone/day is used for severe pemphigus.

MCQ POINTS

S. No.	Question statements	Answers
1.	Acrodermatitis enteropathica is seen with deficiency of:	***Zinc***
2.	Infection of apocrine glands is known as	***Fox Fordyce's spots***
3.	Rhinophyma is	***Hypertrophy of sebaceous glands of nose***
4.	Appearance of hair in alopecia areata	***Exclamation mark hair***
5.	Nail changes in arsenic poisoning	***Mee's line***
6.	Chlamydia trachomatis causes which STD	***Lymphogranuloma venereum***
7.	Burrows is pathognomonic lesion of	***Scabies***
8.	Ivermectin is used in management of	***Scabies***
9.	Removal of scales in psoriasis causes pin point bleeding. This is known as …... sign	***Auspitzs sign***
10.	Clinical sign positive in pemphigus	***Nikolsky sign***
11.	Patch seen in Pityriasis rosea	***Herald patch***
12.	M. furfur causes	***Pityriasis versicolor***
13.	Skin condition associated with gluten sensitive enteropathy	***Dermatitis herpetiformis***
14.	MC cause of acanthosis nigricans	***Type II diabetes mellitus***
15.	2nd MC nerve involved in leprosy	***Median > Posterior auricular***
16.	TB of skin without involvement of underlying structure is known as	***Lupus vulgaris***
17.	HLA associated with Reiter syndrome	***HLA B27***
18.	Dennie Morgan fold is associated with	***Atopic dermatitis***
19.	Important histological feature of tuberculoid leprosy	***Noncaseating granuloma***
20.	Casal's necklace is associated with …. deficiency	***Niacin***
21.	Nail changes in lichen planus	***Pterygium***
22.	Shagreen patches are associated with	***Tuberous sclerosis***
23.	Pautriers micro-abscess is associated with	***Mycosis fungoides***
24.	Civatte bodies are seen in	***Lichen planus***
25.	Koebner's phenomenon is defined as	***Site of injury may develop psoriatic lesion***
26.	Koilonychia is seen in	***Iron deficiency anemia***
27.	Café au lait patches are seen in	***Neurofibromatosis-I***
28.	Lepromin test in lepromatous leprosy	***Negative***
29.	Organism responsible for Chancre	***Treponema pallidum***
30.	Hutchinson teeth is seen in which stage of syphilis	***Late congenital syphilis***
31.	Otomycosis is caused by	***Aspergillus fumigats and candida***
32.	MC cause of chloasma	***Pregnancy***
33.	Honey coloured crust are a feature of	***Impetigo***

S. No.	Question statements	Answers
34.	4 P's suggest the diagnosis of	***Lichen planus (Infact 5 P's: purple, plain topped/ flat, pruritic, polygonal, papule)***
35.	DOC for non-gonococcal urethritis	***Azithromycin/ Doxycycline***
36.	Target lesions are seen in	***Erythema multiforme***
37.	Leonine facies is seen in	***Lepromatous leprosy***
38.	Infectious form of lerosy	***Lepromatous leprosy***
39.	Period of surveillance for lepromatous leprosy	***Paucibacillary: 2 years; Multibacillary: 5 years***
40.	Mycosis fungoides is also known as	***Cutaneous T cell lymphoma***
41.	Chronic ulceration of old burn scars predisposing to squamous cell carcinoma is called .... ulcers	***Marjolins***
42.	Skin sutures on face are usually removed after ..... days	***5th***
43.	Leprosy does not affect which organ of females	***Uterus***
44.	Metal, most likely to cause allergic dermatitis	***Nickel***
45.	DOC for erythema nodosum leprosum	***Steroids (thalidomide can be used)***
46.	Chronic familial benign pemphigus is also known as	***Hailey Hailey disease***
47.	Example of endogenous eczema	***Atopic dermatitis***
48.	.... naevus may lead to melanoma	***Junctional***
49.	MC type of basal cell carcinoma	***Nodulo-ulcerative***
50.	Tinea versicolor is caused by	***Malassezia furfur***
51.	DOC for dermatitis herpetiformis	***Dapsone***
52.	Oral treatment of acne	***Doxycycline***
53.	Dermatophyte which can infect nail is tinea	***Unguum***
54.	Kerion in a .... infection	***Fungal***
55.	MC site of angioedema of skin is of	***Lips***
56.	DOC for severe cystic acne	***Isotretinoin***
57.	Annular herald patch is seen in	***Pityriasis rosea***
58.	Nikolsky sign is seen in	***Pemphigus, toxic shock syndrome etc.***
59.	Verruca vulgaris is caused by .... virus	***Human papilloma virus***
60.	Etiology of pemphigus vulgaris	***Autoimmune***
61.	Partial thickness graft includes which portion of skin	***Epidermis plus some part of dermis***
62.	Layer of skin involved in acantholysis is stratum	***Suprabasal/ intraepidermal***
63.	Hidradenitis suppurativa is a disease of .... glands	***Apocrine***
64.	In sebaceous glands, accumulation of sebum leads to	***Acne***
65.	Pterygium of nail is characteristically seen in	***Lichen planus***
66.	A flat discoloration on skin of 1 cm is known as	***Macule***
67.	A 3 year old child has eczematous dermatitis on extensor surface. His mother has a history of bronchial asthma. Diagnosis	***Atopic dermatitis***
68.	Auspitz sign is related to	***Psoriasis***

S. No.	Question statements	Answers
69.	Itchy, polygonal, violaceous papules are seen in	***Lichen planus***
70.	Itchy, purple papule followed by hyper-pigmentation on resolution is a feature of	***Lichen planus***
71.	Lucio phenomenon is seen in	***Leprosy***
72.	Best diagnostic test for fungal skin infection	***KOH mount***
73.	Soft sore is caused by	***Hemophilus ducreyi***
74.	Condyloma acuminata is caused by	***Human papilloma virus***

CHAPTER

10

ANESTHESIA

KEY POINTS

Order of Sensation Loss in Spinal Anesthesia

- Preganglionic beta fibers
- Cold
- Warm
- Pin prick
- Pain
- Touch
- Pressure
- Motor
- Vibration/proprioception

Contraindications to Spinal Anesthesia

- Vertebral abnormalities
- Local sepsis
- Hypotension and hypovolemia
- Uncooperative and mentally ill person
- Infants

Shortest Acting Muscle Relaxant

- Succinylcholine < Mivacurium

Longest Acting Muscle Relaxant

- Doxacurium > Pipecuronium > Pancuronium > d- Tubocurare

Conditions and Muscle Relaxants

- Carcinoid tumor: Vecuronium
- In renal failure: Vecuronium/Atracurium
- In hepatic failure: Atracurium
- Myasthenia gravis: 1/10th atracurium
- Short cases: Atracurium/ Ropacurium/ Mivacurium
- Obstetrics: All except Gallamine
- Asthmatics: Pancuronium (avoid Metacurine and Succinylcholine)
- Arterial surgery: Pancuronium
- To reduce blood pressure: Tubocurare

Order of Sensation Loss in Local Anesthesia

- Temperature
- Pain
- Touch
- Deep pressure

Shortest Acting Anesthetist

- Chloroprocaine

Longest Acting Local Anesthetist

- Dibucaine > Tetracaine > Bupivacaine

Lignocaine Maximum Dose Without Adrenaline

- 3 mg/kg = 200 mg (average adult)

Lignocaine Maximum Dose with Adrenaline

- 7 mg/ kg = 500 mg (average adult)

Color Coding of Gas Cylinders

- Oxygen: Black body with white shoulders
- Carbon dioxide: Grey
- Cyclopropane: Orange
- Air: Grey body, black and white quartered shoulders

Enflurane

- Contraindicated in epilepsy

Propofol

- Day care surgery

Fentanyl/Droperidol

- Neurolept analgesia
- Used in endoscopy

Trilene

- Not to be used with soda-lime

Etomidate

- Causes adrenal cortex suppression and pain on injection
- Preferred in porphyria
- No analgesic effect

Atracurium

- Undergoes Hoffman elimination
- Used in hepatic and renal failure

Sevoflurane

- Fastest induction
- Used in pediatric surgery
- Not used in closed circuit with soda-lime.

Nitrous oxide

- It inactivates cobalt in vitamin B_{12}
- Irreversibly inactivates enzyme methionine synthetase
- Megaloblastic anemia occurs after exposure for periods of more than 3-12 hours.
- It can be prevented by pretreatment with Folinic acid
- Second gas effect
- Diffusion hypoxia
- Only analgesic effect

Halothane

- Useful in Asthmatics, version, uterine relaxation (hence not used in post-partum hemorrhage as relaxant effect increases bleeding)
- Increases ICT (intracranial tension)
- Sensitizes heart to Catecholamines
- Adverse effects:
  - Hepatitis
  - Malignancy
  - Hyperthermia
  - Shivering
- Should not be used again in next three months

Thiopentone sodium

- Highly lipid soluble
- Contraindicated in acute porphyria

Ether

- Inflammable
- Causes increased blood glucose levels in diabetics

Ketamine

- Dissociative anesthesia
- Used in head, and neck surgery, angiography, cardiac catheterization, burn dressing
- Preferred in asthmatics, porphyria
- Avoided in – MI, hypertension

Cocaine

- Naturally occurring
- Produces vasoconstriction
- Peripheral sympathomimetic action

Prilocaine

- Safest local anesthetic agent
- Produces methemoglobinemia

Succinylcholine

- Used during intubation
- Non- competitive muscle relaxant
- Produces fasciculations and biphasic block
- Significant hyperkalemia with Succinylcholine is seen in burns, paraplegia, tetanus

Isoflurane

- Decreases intracranial tension
- Used in myocardial infarction, neurosurgery, alcoholic cirrhosis.

MCQs WITH SHORT EXPLANATIONS

REGIONAL ANESTHESIA

1. **High spinal anesthesia characterized by:**
   a. Hypertension and tachycardia
   b. Hypertension and bradycardia
   c. Hypotension and bradycardia
   d. Hypotension and tachycardia

   High spinal anesthesia means spinal above the desired level causing problems to the patient. Too high spinal (above cervical) is called very high or total spinal. Management will depend on the level of block.
   i. If it is involving only lower intercostals, the patient will complain of dyspnea. Oxygenation and reassurance is enough.
   ii. If high to block cardioaccelerator fibers the severe bradycardia and hypotension should be treated.
   iii. If too high to involve cervical fibers (diaphragm) then IPPV may be required.

2. **NOT an absolute CONTRAINDICATION for neuraxial blockade:**
   a. Patient refusal
   b. Coagulopathy
   c. Severe hypovolemia
   d. Pre-existing neurological deficits

   Neuropathies are relative contraindication to spinal anesthesia. It is important from medicolegal point. If spinal is to be given in patient already having neuropathies it is mandatory to mention all the deficits in preanesthetic sheet to avoid any litigation.

Local anaesthetics for spinal anaesthesia

Drug	Concentration	Specific gravity
Lignocaine	5% in 7.5% dextrose	1.0333
Bupivacaine	0.5% in 8% dextrose	1.0278
Tetracaine	1% in 5% dextrose	1.0203
Procaine	10% in 5% dextrose	1.0203

3. **Structures pierced in lumbar spinal puncture are all of the following EXCEPT:**
   a. Ligamentum flavum
   b. Duramater
   c. Supraspinous ligament
   d. Posterior Longitudinal ligament

   Vertebral canal is bounded anteriorly by vertebral bodies and intervertebral disc, laterally by pedicles, posteriorly by lamina, ligamentum flavum and roots of vertebral spines. In vertebral canal lies the spinal cord and meninges.

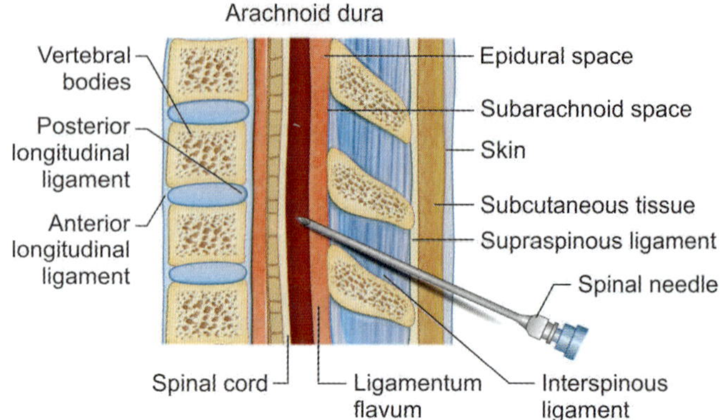

Structures encountered during spinal anaesthesia.

4. **FALSE statement about post-dural puncture headache (PDPH):**
   a. Breech of dura
   b. Onset of headache is usually 12-72 hours following procedure
   c. Commonly occipito-frontal in location
   d. Headache is relieved in sitting/ standing position

   Postspinal headache usually presents after 12-24 hours (corresponds to time when patient starts sitting after operation) and the typical presentation is that pain increases on sitting and relieved on lying down.

5. **Post spinal headache can be prevented by:**
   a. Thinner needle
   b. Early ambulation
   c. Induced hypotension
   d. Decreasing dose of anesthetics

   Single most important factor for PDPH is needle size. Incidence with 16G needle may be 75% while with 25G needle it is 1 to 3%. Use of small bore needle is preventive step.

6. **In spinal anesthesia, first nerve fiber to get blocked is:**
   a. Autonomic preganglionic B fibers
   b. Temperature fibers
   c. Somatic motor fibers
   d. Vibratory and proprioceptive fibers

   Local anesthetic in SA mainly acts on spinal nerves and dorsal ganglia but a small concentration can be detected in substance of spinal cord. Autonomic fibers (mediated by C fibers) are most sensitive and are blocked earliest followed by sensory and then motor fibers. So sequence of block is autonomic → sensory → Motor.

Ans. 1. **c.** Hypotension... 2. **d.** Pre-existing... 3. **d.** Posterior... 4. **d.** Headache... 5. **a.** Thinner needle 6. **a.** Autonomic...

Comparison between spinal and epidural anaesthesia

	Spinal	*Epidural*
1. Cost	Cheaper (Quincke-Babcock type needle cost around ₹ 50 to 60)	Expensive (Epidural set cost around ₹ 600 to 700).
2. Onset of effect	Early (within 2 to 3 minutes with xylocaine and 5 to 6 minutes with bupivacaine).	Delayed (effect take place in 1.5 to 20 minutes).
3. Technically	Easier.	Difficult.
4. Duration of effect	Less (with xylocaine effect last for 45 min to 1 hour and with bupivacaine 2 to 3 hours).	Prolonged and with epidural catheter longer duration surgery can be performed by giving top up doses.
5. Quality of block	Excellent.	Patchy block is very common (due to inconsistent epidural space).
6. Change of level of block	Not possible once the drug is fixed.	Level can be changed by increasing the: dose through ' epidural catheter.
7. Complications		
❑ Post spinal headache	Seen	No post spinal headache (but can occur if dura is punctured accidentally).
❑ Epidural haematoma	Less incidence	More incidence
❑ Total spinal	Rare	High chances if drug is injected in subarachnoid space by accidental dural puncture
❑ Intravascular-injection	Chances are rare	High chances (epidural space have venous plexus of Batson).
❑ Drug toxicity	Less chances	High (because large volume is given).
❑ Catheter complications	Not seen	Present.
8. Block failure rate	Less.	High.
9. Uses	Used for performing surgeries	Used mainly for providing postoperative analgesia.
10.	Performed only at lumbar level (otherwise there are chances of cord injury).	Can be performed at any level (cervical, thoracic).

7. FALSE about lidocaine:

a. Local anesthetic effect
b. Cardiac arrhythmias
c. Ester linked
d. Acts on mucous membranes

Lidocaine (xylocaine, lignocaine) is an aminoamide group of local anesthetic agent and is the MC used LA.

Aminoesters	Aminoamides
❑ Procaine ❑ Chloroprocaine ❑ Tetracaine (Amethocaine) ❑ Benzocaine ❑ Cocaine – Esters are metabolised by pseudocholinesterase (**EXCEPT** cocaine which is metabolised by liver). – High incidence of allergic reactions which are because of para aminobenzoic acid.	❑ Lignocaine ❑ Mepivacaine ❑ Prilocaine ❑ Bupivacaine ❑ Etidocaine ❑ Ropivacaine ❑ Amides are metabolised primarily in liver. ❑ Low incidence of allergic reactions.
– Solutions are not	❑ Solutions are stable (not destroyed even by auto claving).

Contd...

8. Which of the following is NOT used, while giving local anesthesia in the fingers:

a. 2% xylocaine
b. Rubber tourniquet
c. Ring block
d. Adrenaline

Xylocaine should not be used for

i. Ring block of fingers, toes, penis, pinna (absolute contraindication)
ii. When an inhalational agent especially halothane which sensitizes myocardium to adrenaline is used
iii. Myocardial ischemia patients
iv. Hyperthyroid patients
v. Severe hypertensives
vi. Intravenous regional anesthesia (Beir's block)

Drug	*Potency*	*t½*	*Duration of action*		*pKa*	*Maximum safe dose (mg/kg)*	*Comments*
			Without adrenaline	*With adrenaline*			
Esters							
Procaine	+		15-30 minute	30-90 minutes	8.9	12 mg/kg	
Chloroprocaine	+		15-25 minute	30-90 minutes	9.0	12 mg/Kg	Shortest acting
Cocaine	++		—	—	8.7	3 mg/kg	Used for topical anaesthesia ***Potent vaso- constrictor***

Contd...

Ans. **7. c.** Ester linked **8. d.** Adrenaline

Contd...

Tetracanie	++++		2-3 hours	3-5 hours	8.2	3 mg/kg	
Amides ***Lignocaine*** (Xylocaine)	++	1.6 hrs	***45-60 minutes***	2-3 hours	7.8	3 mg/kg (without ailrenaline) 7 mg/kg (with adrenaline)	Most commonly used local anaesthetic
Prilocaine	++		45-60 minutes	2-3 hours	7.8	8 mg/kg	Can cause metha-emoglobinemia
Mepivacaine Etidocaine	++ ++++		45-60 minutes 2-3 hours	2-3 hours 3-5 hours	7.6 7.7	4.5 mg/kg 4 mg/kg	—
Bupivacaine (Sensoricaine,	++++	3.5 hrs	***2-3 hours***	***3-5 hours***	8.1	***2 mg/kg***	Very commonly used local anaesthetic
Marcaine) Ropivacaine	++++		2-3 hours	3-5 hours	8.1	3 mg/kg	Less cardiotoxic than bupivacaine
Dibucaine	++++	4 hrs	2.5-3.5 hours	3.5-5.5 hours	8.8	1 mg/kg	*Longest acting, most potent, most toxic*

SYSTEMIC ANESTHESIA

9. Which nerve is commonly utilized to check for neuromuscular monitoring?

a. Mandibular nerve
b. Ulnar nerve
c. Axillary nerve
d. Median nerve

Most commonly used muscle for neuromuscular monitoring is adductor pollicis supplied by ulnar nerve. Neuromuscular monitoring is required for patients suffering from neuromuscular diseases like myasthenia gravis, Duchenne's muscular dystrophy etc.

10. Purpose of doing Mallampati grading:

a. Assessment of depth of intubation
b. Assessment of airway obstruction
c. Assessment of death due to aspiration
d. Assessment of difficult intubation

Airway assessment is done to rule out difficult intubation. It includes assessment of mouth opening (assessed by Mallampati's grading), denture status and neck movements.

11. Mechanism of degradation of trilene:

a. Chemical degradation
b. Non-enzymatic degradation
c. Enzymatic degradation
d. Hoffman's elimination

Trichlorethylene is metabolized slowly to chloralhydrate (via an epoxide) and then rapidly to 2,3,3-trichloroacetic acid and 2,2,2-trichloroethanol, these latter two metabolites are excreted as urinary glucouronides.

12. General anesthetic agent causing sympathetic stimulation:

a. Thiopental
b. Ketamine
c. Midazolam
d. Etomidate

Ketamine stimulates sympathetic system causing tachycardia and hypertension so it is intravenous anesthetic of choice for shock (but in debilitated patients in which catecholamines have depleted ketamine can cause myocardial depression).

Summary of systemic effects of intravenous anaesthetics

	Cardiovascular system		*Central nervous system*				*Respiratory system*	
Agent	*Heart rate*	*Mean arterial pressure*	*CMO_2*	*CBF*	*ICT*	*IOP*	*Ventilation*	*Bronchial muscles*
Barbiturates Thiopentone	↑ (reflex tachycardia) ↑	↓↓	↓↓↓	↓↓↓	↓↓↓	↓	↓↓	Constriction (++)
Methohexital		↓↓	↓↓	↓↓	↓↓	↓	↓↓	Constriction (+)
Non Barbiturates Ketamine	↑↑	↑↑	↑↑	↑↑	↑↑↑	↑↑	↑/↓	
Propofol	0/↑	↓↓↓	↓↓↓	↓↓↓	↓↓↓	↓	↓↓	Dilatation (+++)
Etomidate	0	↓	↓↓	↓↓	↓↓	↓	↓	O/Dilatation (+)
Opioids Morphine	↓↓	↓↓	↓↓	↓↓	Variable (↓)	↓	↓↓↓	Constriction (because of histamine release)
Fentanyl, Alfentanil and Sufentanil	↓↓	↓↓	↓↓	↓	Variable (↓)	↓	↓↓	Constriction
Pethidine Pentazocine	↑↑ ↑↑	↓ ↑↑	↑	↑	Variable ↑	↓	↓↓ ↓	Constriction/0 0

Contd...

Ans. 9. **b.** Ulnar nerve 10. **d.** Assessment... 11. **c.** Enzymatic degrad... 12. **b.** Ketamine

Contd...

Summary of systemic effects of intravenous anaesthetics

Agent	*Cardiovascular system*		*Central nervous system*				*Respiratory system*	
	Heart rate	*Mean arterial pressure*	*CMO_2*	*CBF*	*ICT*	*IOP*	*Ventilation*	*Bronchial muscles*
Benzodisgepines								
Diazepam	0/ ↑(reflex tachycardia)	↓	↓↓	↓↓	↓	↓	↓↓	0
Midazolam	↑(reflex tachycardia)	↓↓	↓↓	↓↓	↓	↓	↓↓	0
Lorazepam	0/↓	↓	↓↓	↓↓	↓	↓	↓↓	0

0 = no effect, ↓ = decrease ↑ = increase CMO_2 = Cerebral oxygen consumption
CBF = Cerebral blood flow ICT = Intracranial tension IOP = Intraocular pressure

13. Which can increase intraocular pressure:
a. Thiopentone b. Althesin
c. Ketamine d. Barbiturate

Ketamine increases intraocular tension and dilate pupils moderately.

Summary of anaesthetic properties

Agent	*Analgesia*	*Induction*	*Muscle Relaxation*
Thiopentone	Antanal-gesic	Smooth	0
Methohexital	0	Smooth	0
Propofol	0	Smooth	0
Etomidate	0	Smooth	0
Neuroleptanal-gesia (Droperidol + Fentanyl)	++	Only somno-lence	0 (hyperrigidity may be because of fentanyl)
Opioids	++	Slow (usually not used for induction)	0 (hyperrigidity)
Benzodiaz-epines	0	Slow (usually not used for induction)	+ (centrally acting muscle relaxant)
Ketamine	+++	Not smooth	0 (hyperrigidity)

14. In status asthmaticus, anesthetic agent used as bronchodilator:
a. Morphine b. Thiopentone sodium
c. Ketamine d. Halothane

Ketamine is a potent bronchodilator. So it is intravenous anesthetic of choice for asthmatics. Its bronchodilatation properties are excellent so it can be used in the treatment of status asthmaticus which is unresponsive to conventional therapy.

15. Which of the following is drug of choice in shocked individual:
a. Thiopentone sodium b. Propanidid
c. Ketamine d. Althesin

Although ketamine is induction agent of choice for shock (but in chronic/severe shock in which sympathetic depletion has taken place it may produce cardiodepressant effect because ketamine act by sympathetic stimulation).

16. Measure of index of anesthetic potency is:
a. Molecular weight b. Boiling point
c. Minimum alveolar concentration
d. None of the above

Best estimate for determining the potency of inhalational anesthetic is Minimum Alveolar Concentration (MAC) which is defined as minimum concentration of agent required to produce immobility in 50% of the subjects given noxious stimuli which is surgical (skin) incision in human beings and tail clamping in rats.

Agent	*MAC*
Methoxyflurane	0.16%
Trielene	0.2%
Halothane	0.74%
Chloroform	0.8%
Isoflurane	1.15%
Enflurane	1.68%
Ether	1.92%
Sevoflurane	2.05%
Desflurane	6.0%
Cyclopropane	9.2%
Nitrous oxide	104%

17. All are true for ketamine EXCEPT:
a. Hypertension b. Hallucinations
c. Bronchospasm d. Analgesia

Ketamine is a potent bronchodilator.

18. Pin index system is a safety feature adopted in Anesthesia machines is to prevent:
a. Incorrect attachment of anesthesia machines
b. Incorrect attachment of anesthesia face masks
c. Incorrect inhalational agent delivery
d. Incorrect gas cylinder attachment

Pin Index system is the safety mechanism so that one cylinder can not be fitted at the other's position. It consists of 2 pins, 4 mm and 6 mm long on yoke of the anesthesia machine. The pins are so positioned that the cylinder with corresponding hole can only be fitted.

Ans. 13. c. Ketamine 14. c. Ketamine 15. c. Ketamine 16. c. Minimum...
17. c. Bronchospasm 18. d. Incorrect...

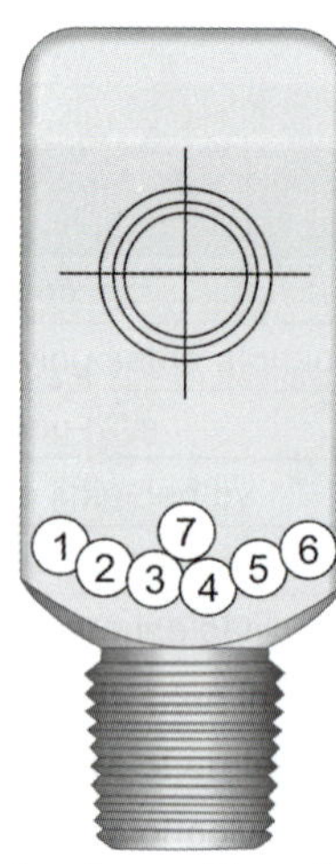

Cylinder valves showing position of holes, these holes correspond to same pins at yoke of machine).

19. Which of the following inhalational anaesthetic agents has rapid onset of action and rapid recovery actions and is most desirous for day care (OPD/outpatient) surgical procedures:

a. Ether
b. Halothane
c. Trichloroethylene
d. Desflurane

Desflurane is the fastest acting induction agent (B/G coefficient 0.42) and its potency is medium (MAC is 6%). It undergoes minimal metabolism (<1%) and does not produce any fluoride. Therefore desflurane is the agent of choice for:

i. Prolonged duration surgeries
ii. Old age patients
iii. Hepatic and renal disease patients

Agent	*Blood gas partition coefficient*
Desflurane	0.42
Cyclopropane	0.44
Nitrous oxide	0.47
Sevoflurane	0.69
Isoflurane	1.38
Enflurane	1.8
Halothane	2.4
Chloroform	8
Trielene	9
Ether	12
Methoxyflurane	15

20. Following statements are true for propofol EXCEPT:

a. Painful intravenous administration
b. Induction agent
c. Contraindicated in porphyria
d. Antiemetic effect

Thiopentone induces enzyme aminolevulenic acid synthetase which stimulates the formation of porphyrin in susceptible individuals. So it is contraindicated in acute intermittent and variegate porphyria (can be used safely in porphyria cutanea tarda).

21. Ketamine should be AVOIDED in:

a. Presence of increased arterial pressure
b. Pregnancy
c. Hypovolemic shock
d. Asthmatic

Ketamine is contraindicated in head injury (as it increases intracranial tension).

22. FALSE for ketamine:

a. Direct myocardial depressant
b. Emergence phenomenon are more likely if anticholinergic premedication is used
c. It may induce cardiac dysarhythmias in patients receiving tricyclic antidepressants
d. Has no effect on intracranial pressure

Ketamine increases brain oxygen consumption and metabolic rate and intracranial tension is highly raised.

23. Pin index for N_2O:

a. 1, 5
b. 1, 6
c. 2, 5
d. 3, 5

Pin index of Nitrous oxide is 3, 5

Oxygen	2, 5
Nitrous oxide	3, 5
Cyclopropane	3, 6
Air	1, 5
Nitrogen	1, 4
Entonox (50% oxygen + 50% nitrous oxide)	7
Carbon dioxide (< 7:6%)	2, 6
Carbon dioxide (> 7.5%)	1, 6

24. Drug which is NOT suitable for patients with acute porphyria for intravenous induction is:

a. Thiopentone sodium
b. Propofol
c. Midazolam
d. Etomidate

Thiopentone is contraindicated in acute intermittent and variegate porphyria (can be used safely in porphyria cutanea tarda).

25. Which of the following inhalational agent is the induction agent of choice in children:

a. Methoxyflurane
b. Sevoflurane
c. Desflurane
d. Isoflurane

Sevoflurane has a faster (Blood/Gas coefficient 0.69), pleasant and smooth induction with no significant systemic toxicity makes the sevoflurane as agent of choice for induction, especially in children.

Ans. **19. d.** Desflurane **20. c.** Contraindicated... **21. a.** Presence... **22. d.** Has no... **23. d.** 3, 5 **24. a.** Thiopentone sodium **25. b.** Sevoflurane

Agent	Induction		Analgesia	Muscle relaxation	Amnesia
	Onset	Smoothness			
Halothane	Intermediate	Very smooth	+.1 0	++	++
Isoflurane	Intermediate	Slightly irritable	++	++	++
Enflurane	Intermediate	Slightly irritable	++	++	++
Nitrous oxide	Fast	Not used for induction	+++	–	++
Sevoflurane	Fast	Very Smooth	++	++	++
Desflurane	Fastest	Slightly irritable	++	++	++
Ether	Slow	Highly irritable	+++	+++	++
Trielene	Slow	Smooth	++++	+	+
Methoxyflurane	Slowest	Smooth	+++	++	++
Cyclopropane	Fast	Smooth	++	++	++
Chloroform	Slow	Smooth	+	++	++

26. A 20-year-old patient presented with early pregnancy for medical termination of pregnancy (MTP) in day care facility. What will be the induction agent of choice:

a. Thiopentone b. Ketamine
c. Propofol d. Diazepam

Because of propofol's (i) early induction (ii) early and smooth recovery (iii) inactive metabolites and (iv) antiemetic effects it is, the IV agent of choice for day care surgery.

MISCELLANEOUS

27. Which of the following is the most effective circuit in spontaneous ventilation?

a. Mapleson D
b. Mapleson C
c. Mapleson B
d. Mapleson A

If type A Mapleson circuit (also called as Magill circuit) is used for controlled ventilation, very high flows (3 times of minute ventilation or 20 L) is required and in spite of such high flows prevention of rebreathing is still unpredictable. So Magill circuit should not be used for controlled ventilation. Therefore type A is circuit of choice for spontaneous ventilation.

28. Murphy's eye is seen in which of the following instrument?

a. Laryngeal mask airway
b. Flexible laryngoscope
c. Endotracheal tube
d. Oxygen cylinder

ETT have two ends, proximal end (machine end) and distal end (patient end). Patient end is bevelled with angle of 45 degree in oral tubes and 30 degrees in nasal tubes.

29. Other than epinephrine, which drug can also be given for ventricular fibrillation postcardiac arrest:

a. Amiodarone b. Amrinone
c. Adenosine d. Atropine

Amiodarone is nowadays considered as drug of choice for ventricular tachycardia (monomorphic). It is preferred over lignocaine.

30. As a muscle relaxant, curonium drugs act by:

a. Inhibition of calcium channels on presynaptic end
b. Repeated stimulation of acetylcholine receptors on muscle end-plate
c. Blocking post-synaptic acetylcholine receptors competitively
d. Neuromuscular junction is persistently depolarized

Non-Depolarizing Muscle Relaxants/ NDMR are the competitive antagonists with acetycholine/ ACh at the Ach receptors and NDMR binds at the same site (alpha subunit) at which Ach binds.

31. FALSE about succinylcholine:

a. Muscle pain
b. Malignant hyperthermia
c. Hyperkalemia
d. Hypokalemia

Suxamethonium causes hyperkalemia due to excessive muscle fasciculations. Ventricular arrhythmias can occur due to hyperkalemia. In a normal subject serum potassium increases by 0.5 mEq/L.

Difference between depolarizing and non-depolarizing block	
Depolarizing	*Nondepolarizing*
1. Also called as phase I block	1. –
2. Block preceded by muscle fasciculations	2. No fasciculations
3. Depolarizing blocking drugs are called as leptocurare	3. Called as pachycurare

Contd...

Ans. 26. c. Propofol 27. d. Mapleson A 28. c. Endotracheal tube 29. a. Amiodarone
30. c. Blocking post... 31. d. Hypokalemia

Contd...

Depolarizing	*Nondepolarizing*
4. No fading is seen (fading can be seen at higher doses, i.e., phase II block)	4. Train of four shows fading
5. Does not require reversal rather cholinesterase inhibitors (neostigmine) can prolong the depolarizing block (because these agents also inhibit the pseudocholinesterase)	5. Reversed by cholinesterase inhibitors like neostigmine

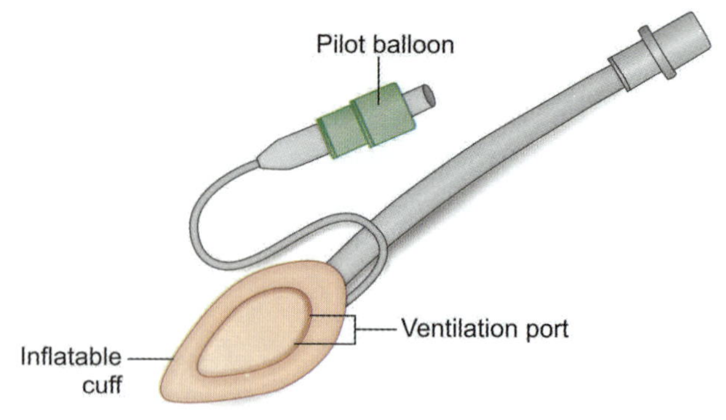

Laryngeal mask airway

32. Laryngeal mask airway is indicated in:

a. Difficult airway
b. To prevent aspiration of stomach contents
c. Short surgical procedure
d. Where endotracheal intubation is contraindicated

Indications of laryngeal mask airway

- As an alternative to intubation where difficult intubation is anticipated.
- Securing airway in emergency where intubation and mask ventilation is not possible
- As an elective method for minor surgeries where anesthetist wants to avoid intubation
- As a conduit for bronchoscopes, small size tubes, gum elastic bougies.

33. Administration of succinylcholine to a paraplegic patient led to the development of dysrhythmia, conduction abnormalities and finally cardiac arrest. The most likely cause is:

a. Hypercalcemia
b. Hyperkalemia
c. Anaphlaxia
d. Hypermagnesemia

Succinylcholine is contraindicated for up to 2-3 months after trauma, up to 6 months after hemiplegia/paraplegia and up to 1 year after burns (the greatest risk is between 1 week to 2 months). In these conditions denervated/regenerating nerve develops extrajunctional receptors which can produce hyperkalemia.

Altered muscle relaxant responses in diseases

Disease	*Response to depolarizers*	*Response to non-depolarizers*	*Comments*
❑ Burns ❑ Hemiplegia ❑ Paraplegia ❑ Denervation muscle injuries	Increased sensitivity and hyperkalemia	Resistance	Extrajunctional receptors in these conditions are sensitive to depolarizing agents and resistant to non-depolarizers
Myasthenia gravis	Resistance	Increased sensitivity	An autoimmune disease destroying acetylcholine receptors, so less competition for nondepolarizers, increasing their sensitivity and less receptors for succinyl- choline to act increasing its resistance.
Myasthenic syndrome	Increased sensitivity	Increased sensitivity	Auto-antibodies against prejunctional calcium channels
Muscle dystrophies like Duchenne	Increased sensitivity and hyperkalemia	Increased sensitivity	Auto-antibodies against prejunctional calcium channels.
Myotonias like dsytrophia, congenita	Hypersensitivity and tonic contractures can develop	Normal or increased sensitivity	
Tetanus	Increased sensitivity and hyperkalemia	Resistance	
Cerebral palsy	Increased sensitivity	Resistance	
Autoimmune diseases like SLE	Increased sensitivity	Increased sensitivity	

34. Transfusion related acute lung injury occurs due to:

a. Citrate toxicity
b. Hypokalemia
c. Mismatch transfusion
d. Hyperkalemia

Causes of ARDS after transfusion

i. Mismatched transfusion reaction.
ii. Anaphylactic reaction.
iii. Pulmonary vasculature obstruction by microaggregates (very rare).

Ans. **32. a.** Difficult airway **33. b.** Hyperkalemia **34. c.** Mismatch...

Blood group	Red cells	Plasma	Can donate blood to	Can receive blood from
A	Antigen A	Anti B anti-bodies	Group A, AB	Group A, O
B	Antigen B	Anti A. anti-bodies	Group B, AB	Group B, O
AB (Universal recipient)	Antigen A and B	Nil	AB	A, B, O, AB
O (Universal donor)	Nil	Anti A & anti B	A, B, O, AB	O

35. Current guidelines for chest compression rate during CPR in adults:

a. 10/min
b. 40/min
c. 80/min
d. 100/min

After advanced airway (i.e. endotracheal tube, laryngeal mask airway or combitube): Compression will be continued at a rate of 100 compressions/minute and breathing rate at a rate of 8-10 breaths/minute with no synchronization i.e. no pause for ventilation.

Cardiopulmonary and Cerebral Resuscitation (CPR)					
	Newborn	*Infant*	*Child*	*Adult*	*Comments*
Age criteria		0-1 year	1-14 years (medical personal) 1-8 yrs (lay rescuers)	> 14 yrs for (medical personal) 1-8 yrs (lay rescuers)	Previously child was 1-8 years for all.
Pulse check	Heart (Auscultation)	Brabcial/ femoral	Carotid	Carotid/femoral	
Compression area	Lower 1/3 of sternum	Midsternum (line below intersection of intermammary line)	Midsternum (line below intersection of intermammary line)	Lower 1/3 sterum (2 finger above xiphisternum)	
Compression method	2 thumb with encircled chest	2-3 fingers	Heel of one hand	Heel of two hand one locked over other	Compression for new born should be started if HR < 60/ min
Sternal depth	½-1 inch	½-1 inch	1-1½ inch	1½-2 inch	
Compression rate	90/min	100/min.	100/min	100/min	
Ventilation rate					
❑ If compression is also provided simultaneously	30/min	8-10/min	8-10/min	8-10/min	
❑ If only veniilation is to be provided i.e. pulses are present	40-60/min	12-20/min	12-20/min	10-12/min	
Compression ventilation ratio					
❑ without advanced airway in place (i.e. vent. by mouth to mouth or nose, bag & mask vent.)	3:1 with pause for ventilation (synchronized) [90 compression with 30 breaths]	30:2-for single resuscitator 15:2-for two resuscitators	30:2-for single resuscitator 6 45:2-for two resuscitators	30:2 irrespective of no. of resuscitators	Previously it 'was 15:2 before intubation
❑ with advanced airway in place (i.e. Encdotracheal tube, LMA, combitube, tracheostomy tube)	—same—	100 compression/ min and 8-10 breath/ min. without any synchronization (i.e. no pause for ventilation)	100 compression and 8-10 breath/ per/min without synchronization	100 Gompression 8-10 breath/ min without any synchrbniltion	Previously it was 5:1 after intubation

36. Ratio of chest compression to breathing while CPR in adults, without advanced airway in place:

a. 15:2
b. 30:2
c. 45:2
d. 60:2

Before advanced airway (i.e. by mouth to mouth, bag and mask ventilation), the ratio should be 30:2 (30 compressions followed by 2 breaths) irrespective of duration of resuscitation (previously this ratio was 15:2). The reason for change in ratio is to minimize interruption in chest compression (this is the most important goal of latest recommendation).

Ans. **35. d.** 100/min **36. b.** 30:2

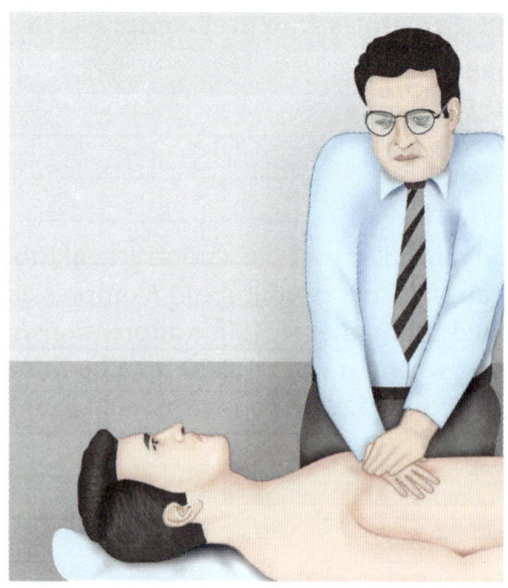

Cardiac massage (note the extension at elbow, pressure exerted from shoulder joint). Patient should lie flat on hard surface

37. Compression ventilation ratio in case of neonatal cardiopulmonary resuscitation:

a. 3:1 b. 15:2
c. 30:2 d. 100:8

Compression ventilation ratio in newborn is 3:1 with pause for ventilation (synchronized) [90 compression with 30 breaths] without advanced or with advanced airway in place.

38. Sternal depth while chest compression in CPR in adults is:

a. 0.5 inch b. 1 inch
c. 1.5 inch d. 2 inch

The force generated during massage should be able to depress sternum by 1.5-2 inches (approx one-third of chest wall diameter). During massage compression relaxation (chest recoil) should be equal.

39. Ratio of chest compression to breathing during cardiopulmonary resuscitation in newborn patient admitted in ICU is:

a. 3:1 b. 5:1
c. 15:2 d. 30:2

C:V ratio in newborn is 3:1 with pause for ventilation (synchronized).

40. Proper technique of endotracheal intubation involves:

a. Flexion of neck
b. Flexion of the neck and extension of the atlanto-occipital joint
c. Extension of the neck
d. Extension of the neck and flexion of the atlanto-occipital joint

Technique of intubation

- The patient should lie supine
- There should be extension at atlanto-occipital joint and flexion at cervical spine
- This position is achieved by putting a 6 to 8 cm thick pillow under the occiput.

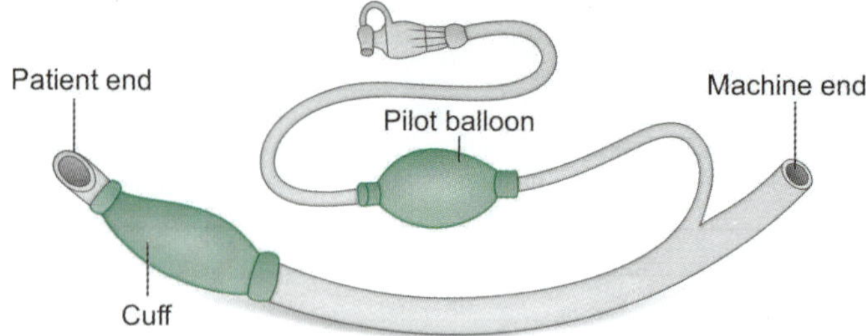

Cuffed endotracheal tube (red rubber)

41. In a severely injured patient, first thing to do is to:

a. Start an intravenous line
b. Give oxygen
c. Maintain airway
d. Vasopressor drug

Basic life support

1. Airway management (manual)
2. Breathing by mouth to mouth, mouth to nose or bag and mask ventilation
3. Circulation by cardiac massage
4. Defibrillation by automatic external defibrillator (AED)

Parameter	*Basic life support (Primary A,B,C,D)*	*Advanced life support (Secondary A,B,C,D)*
Airway management	Manual	With equipments like Guedel's airway, endotracheal tube, laryngeal mask airway (LMA) or tracheostomy tube
Breathing	Mouth to mouth, mouth to nose or bag & mask	Advanced methods like endotracheal tube, LMA, combitube or tracheostomy tube
Circulation	Cardiac massage	Cardiac massage
Defibrillation	Automatic external defibrillator	Manual defibrillator
Drugs	–	+

42. Which drug is used in anaphylactic shock caused by penicillin:

a. Adrenaline b. Noradrenaline
c. Steroids d. Chlorpheniramine

For anaphylaxis, adrenaline is given as 0.5-1 mg subcutaneously to be repeated every 3-5 minutes.

Dose	*Concentration*
1. CPR: 1 mg to be repeated every 3-5 min. Other regimens used in CPR are – High dose (0.1 mg/kg) – Escalating (1 mg, 3 mg and 5 mg) In children: 0.01 mg/kg. Endotracheal dose is 2.5 times of IV dose.	1:10,000 (Available ampoule (1:1,000) is diluted in 10 ml saline.

Contd...

Ans. **37. a.** 3:1 **38. d.** 2 inch **39. a.** 3:1 **40. b.** Flexion...
41. c. Maintain airway **42. a.** Adrenaline

Contd...

Dose	*Concentration*
2. Anaphylaxis: 0.5-1 mg. subcutaneously to be repeated every 3-5 minutes.	1:1,000
3. For producing. vasoconstriction with local anaesthetics	1:10,000
4. For producing local ischemia/to decrease blood loss	
	1:2,00,000
	1:1,00,000

43. Anticoagulant commonly used for blood storage is:
a. Acid citrate dextrose b. CDPA
c. EDTA d. Heparin

CDPA is most commonly used anticoagulant in India. Blood can be stored for 35 days if the preservative anticoagulant solution used is CDPA.

C for citrate as anticoagulant

D for Dextrose as energy source for red cells

P for Phosphate as buffer

A for Adenine to increase the red cell survival

44. Massive transfusion of stored blood results in:
a. Citric acid toxicity b. Hypokalemia
c. Metabolic acidosis d. Hypercalcemia

In massive blood transfusion, alkalosis is more common due to citrate intoxication (one molecule of citrate generates 3 molecules of bicarbonate). Acidic pH of stored blood can cause acidosis as well.

45. Mismatched blood transfusion intra-operatively manifests as:
a. Rise in blood pressure b. Excessive bleeding
c. Dyspnea d. Hematuria

In anesthetized individual, transfusion reaction manifest as tachycardia, hypotension (so minute to minute blood pressure monitoring during early transfusion is necessary) and oozing from surgical site (more specific). The awake patient presents with pain and burning in vein (earliest), fever with chills and rigors, nausea and vomiting, flushing, chest and flank pain, dyspnea.

46. Concentration of adrenaline in CPR is:
a. 1: 10 lakhs b. 1: 1 lakh
c. 1: 10,000 d. 1: 1,000

Concentration of adrenaline for CPR is 1:10,000 (available ampoule of 1:1000 is diluted in 10 mL saline). 1 mg to be repeated every 3-5 min.

47. During abdominal surgery under local anesthetic, patient suddenly felt sharp pain. Injury to which structure is likely:
a. Liver parenchyma
b. Large gut
c. Small gut
d. Parietal peritoneum

The **parietal peritoneum** is supplied by nerves (e.g., phrenic and thoraco-abdominal) to the adjacent body wall, and most of it is very sensitive to **pain**. **Painful** stimuli to the central part of the diaphragmatic **peritoneum** are referred to the shoulder. The visceral **peritoneum** is insensitive.

48. First sign of complication of anesthesia is:
a. Tachycardia b. Bradycardia
c. Hypertension d. Convulsion

Examples of sinus **tachycardia** as a physiologic response include to pain, anxiety, or may indicate inadequate depth of **anesthesia**. It may be a response in order to increase cardiac output to compensate for hypovolemia, anemia, hypoxemia, hypoglycemia, fever, or sepsis.

49. Maximum and minimum score of Glasgow Coma Scale is respectively:
a. 15, 3
b. 15, 0
c. 20, 5
d. 3, 15

Glasgow Coma Scale (**GCS**) is a neurological scale which aims to give a reliable and objective way of recording the conscious state of a person for initial as well as subsequent assessment. A patient is assessed against the criteria of the scale, and the resulting points give a patient score between 3 (indicating deep unconsciousness) and either 14 (original scale) or 15 (the more widely used modified or revised scale).

50. In mouth to mouth respiration during CPR, the oxygen delivered is:
a. 20% b. 10%
c. 25% d. 16%

The efficiency of artificial respiration can be greatly increased by the simultaneous use of oxygen therapy. The amount of oxygen available to the patient in mouth-to-mouth is around 16%. If this is done through a pocket mask with an oxygen flow, this increases to 40% oxygen. If either a bag valve mask or a mechanical ventilator is used with an oxygen supply, this rises to 99% oxygen.

Ans. **43. b.** CDPA **44. a.** Citric... **45. b.** Excessive... **46. c.** 1: 10,000
47. d. Parietal... **48. a.** Tachycardia **49. a.** 15, 3 **50. d.** 16%

ANSWERS WITH REFERENCES

REGIONAL ANESTHESIA

1. **Ans. (c)** Hypotension and bradycardia
Ref: Yadav's Anesthesia 4/e p136

2. **Ans. (d)** Pre-existing neurological deficits
Ref: Yadav's Anesthesia 4/e p138

3. **Ans. (d)** Posterior Longitudinal ligament
Ref: Yadav's Anesthesia 4/e p130

4. **Ans. (d)** Headache is relieved in sitting/standing position
Ref: Yadav's Anesthesia 4/e p136

5. **Ans. (a)** Thinner needle
Ref: Yadav's Anesthesia 4/e p136

6. **Ans. (a)** Autonomic preganglionic B fibers
Ref: Yadav's Anesthesia 4/e p133

7. **Ans. (c)** Ester linked
Ref: Yadav's Anesthesia 4/e p118

8. **Ans. (d)** Adrenaline
Ref: Yadav's Anesthesia 4/e p120

SYSTEMIC ANESTHESIA

9. **Ans. (b)** Ulnar nerve
Ref: Yadav's Anesthesia, 4/e p54

10. **Ans. (d)** Assessment of difficult intubation
Ref: Yadav's Anesthesia, 4/e p45

11. **Ans. (c)** Enzymatic degradation
Ref: Yadav's Anesthesia, 4/e p73

12. **Ans. (b)** Ketamine
Ref: Yadav's Anesthesia 4/e p86

13. **Ans. (c)** Ketamine
Ref: Yadav's Anesthesia 4/e p86

14. **Ans. (c)** Ketamine
Ref: Yadav's Anesthesia 4/e p86

15. **Ans. (c)** Ketamine
Ref: Yadav's Anesthesia 4/e p149

16. **Ans. (c)** Minimum alveolar concentration
Ref: Yadav's Anesthesia 4/e p58

17. **Ans. (c)** Bronchospasm
Ref: Yadav's Anesthesia 4/e p86

18. **Ans. (d)** Incorrect gas cylinder attachment
Ref: Yadav's Anesthesia 4/e p25

19. **Ans. (d)** Desflurane
Ref: Yadav's Anesthesia 4/e p70

20. **Ans. (c)** Contraindicated in porphyria
Ref: Yadav's Anesthesia 4/e p80

21. **Ans. (a)** Presence of increased arterial pressure
Ref: Yadav's Anesthesia 4/e p86

22. **Ans. (d)** Has no effect on intracranial pressure
Ref: Yadav's Anesthesia 4/e p86

23. **Ans. (d)** 3, 5
Ref: Yadav's Anesthesia 4/e p25

24. **Ans. (a)** Thiopentone sodium
Ref: Yadav's Anesthesia 4/e p80

25. **Ans. (b)** Sevoflurane
Ref: Yadav's Anesthesia 4/e p70

26. **Ans. (c)** Propofol
Ref: Yadav's Anesthesia 4/e p82

MISCELLANEOUS

27. **Ans. (d)** Mapleson A
Ref: Yadav's Anesthesia, 4/e p31

28. **Ans. (c)** Endotracheal tube
Ref: Yadav's Anesthesia, 4/e p36

29. **Ans. (a)** Amiodarone
Ref: Yadav's Anesthesia, 4/e p225

30. **Ans. (c)** Blocking post-synaptic acetylcholine receptors competitively
Ref: Yadav's Anesthesia, 4/e p103

31. **Ans. (d)** Hypokalemia
Ref: Yadav's Anesthesia 4/e p97

32. **Ans. (a)** Difficult airway
Ref: Yadav's Anesthesia 4/e p40

33. **Ans. (b)** Hyperkalemia
Ref: Yadav's Anesthesia 4/e p98

34. **Ans. (c)** Mismatch transfusion
Ref: Yadav's Anesthesia 4/e p17

35. **Ans. (d)** 100/min
Ref: Yadav's Anesthesia 4/e p223

36. **Ans. (b)** **30:2**
Ref: Yadav's Anesthesia 4/e p222

37. **Ans. (a)** **3:1**
Ref: Yadav's Anesthesia 4/e p229

38. **Ans. (d)** **2 inch**
Ref: Yadav's Anesthesia 4/e p222

39. **Ans. (a)** **3:1**
Ref: Yadav's Anesthesia 4/e p229

40. **Ans. (b)** **Flexion of the neck and extension of the atlanto-occipital joint**
Ref: Yadav's Anesthesia 4/e p35

41. **Ans. (c)** **Maintain airway**
Ref: Yadav's Anesthesia 4/e p220

42. **Ans. (a)** **Adrenaline**
Ref: Yadav's Anesthesia 4/e p232

43. **Ans. (b)** **CDPA**
Ref: Yadav's Anesthesia 4/e p15

44. **Ans. (a)** **Citric acid toxicity**
Ref: Yadav's Anesthesia 4/e p17

45. **Ans. (b)** **Excessive bleeding**
Ref: Yadav's Anesthesia 4/e p15

46. **Ans. (c)** **1: 10,000**
Ref: Yadav's Anesthesia 4/e p232

47. **Ans. (d)** **Parietal peritoneum**
Ref: Internet resources

48. **Ans. (a)** **Tachycardia**
Ref: Internet resources

49. **Ans. (a)** **15, 3**
Ref: Internet resources

50. **Ans. (d)** **16%**
Ref: Internet resources

PRACTICE QUESTIONS

REGIONAL ANESTHESIA

1. In which of the following blocks, one should NOT use a local anesthetic agent with a vasoconstrictor agent:
- a. Spinal block
- b. Regional block
- c. Epidural block
- d. Ring block

2. BP in hypotensive Anesthesia should be:
- a. Half of the pre-operative value
- b. One-third of the pre-operative value
- c. One-fourth of the pre-operative value
- d. One-fifth of the pre-operative value

3. Which of the following is NOT classified as ester linked local anaesthetic agent:
- a. Prilocaine
- b. Cocaine
- c. Tetracaine
- d. Chlorprocaine

SYSTEMIC ANESTHESIA

4. Induction agent of choice in children:
- a. Desflurane
- b. Isoflurane
- c. Sevoflurane
- d. Ether

5. SCh causes:
- a. Hypokalemia
- b. Hyperkalemia
- c. Hypocalcemia
- d. Hypercalcemia

6. Ketamine is indicated in all of the following conditions EXCEPT:
- a. Full stomach
- b. Increased intracranial pressure
- c. Pediatric patient
- d. Patient with asthma

7. Which of the following is the best agent to control secretions in general anesthetia:
- a. Hyoscine
- b. Glycopyyrolate
- c. Pethidine
- d. Lorazepam

8. A chronic smoker was taken for surgery under general anesthesia. Which of the following will NOT be observed:
- a. Diminished mucosal clearance
- b. Exaggerated mucosal clearance
- c. Atelectasis of lung
- d. Hyporeactive airway

MISCELLANEOUS

9. Calcium is used in CPR in all of the following conditions EXCEPT:
- a. Hypocalcemia
- b. Hyperkalemia
- c. Hypermagnesemia
- d. Overdosage of calcium channel blcokers

10. Tracheostomy tube toilet will help LEAST in:
- a. Pneumothorax
- b. Pulmonary cleaning
- c. Obstruction
- d. Impaired consciousness

11. Capnography detects:
- a. Inspired oxygen
- b. Inspired carbon-di-oxide
- c. Expired carbon-di-oxide
- d. Expired oxygen

Ans. 1. d. Ring block 2. b. One-third... 3. a. Prilocaine 4. c. Sevoflurane 5. b. Hyperkalemia 6. b. Increased... 7. b. Glycopyyrolate 8. b. Exaggerated... 9. c. Hyper... 10. a. Pneumothorax 11. c. Expired...

IMAGE-BASED QUESTIONS

1. Site of this procedure in adults:

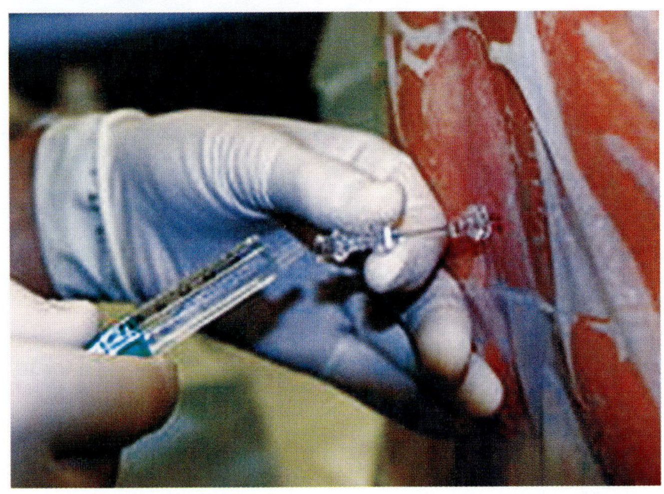

a. L1-L2
b. L2-L3
c. L3-L4
d. D12-L1

Technique of spinal anesthesia

- After cleaning and draping lumbar puncture is done in desired space (usually L3-L4 or L4-L5) and the local anaesthetic drug is injected after confirming the free flow of CSF.

2. The following image shows features of which class of neuromuscular blocking agents:

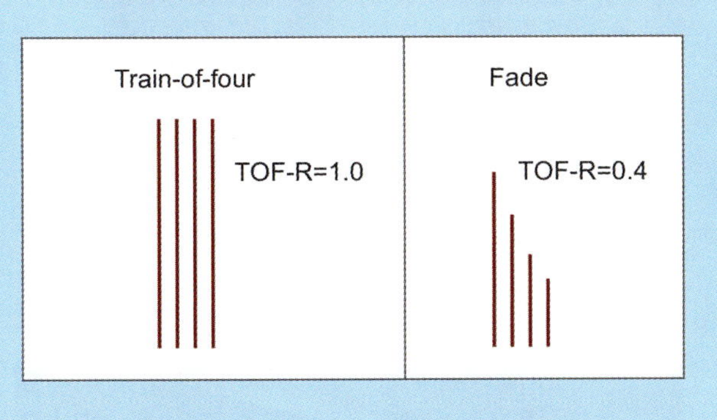

a. Depolarizing
b. Nondepolarizing
c. Centrally acting
d. Variable

TO_4 is best utilized for neuromuscular monitoring during maintenance of Anesthesia. It is best to differentiate between depolarizing and non-depolarizing blocks. Non-depolarizing block shows fading which means T_4 will go first then T_3 and so on but in depolarizing block all four responses decrease simultaneously in amplitude (i.e., T_4/T_1 always remain 1).

3. Which procedure:

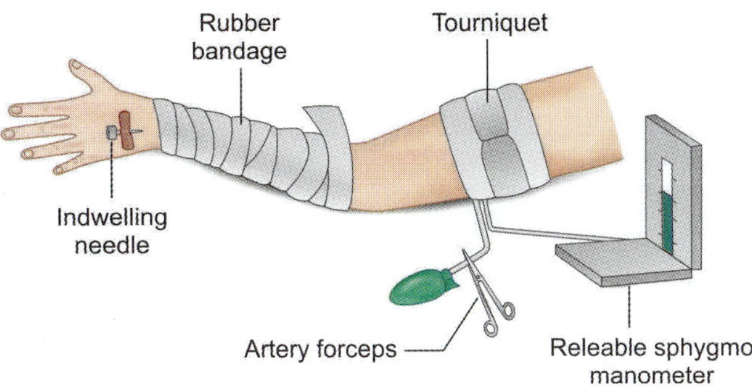

a. Axillary block
b. Brachial block
c. Beir's block
d. Ulnar block

Intravenous regional block (Beir's block) technique

- After applying tourniquet 30 to 40 mL 0.5% xylocaine or prilocaine is injected into a vein
- Adequate tourniquet functioning is most vital in Beir's block.

4. Use of the needles shown below:

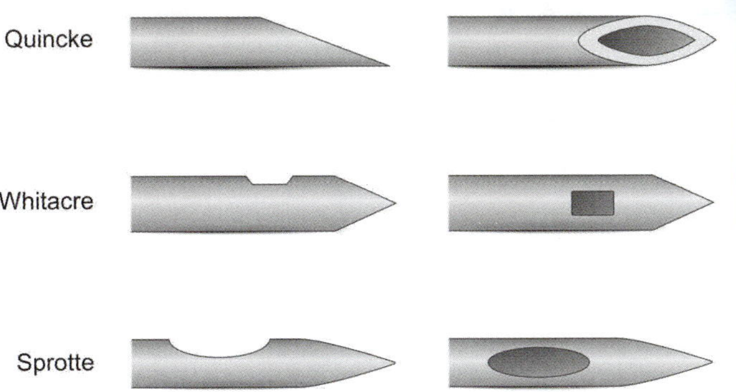

a. Epidural anesthesia
b. Caudal block
c. Spinal anesthesia
d. Beir's block

Spinal needles

- Dura cutting: Standard Quincke-Babcock and Greene needle (incidence of post-spinal headache is high but these needles are cheaper)
- Dura separating: Whitcre, Sporte and Pitkin (incidence of post-spinal headache is less but these needles are expensive)

5. Use of the instrument shown below:

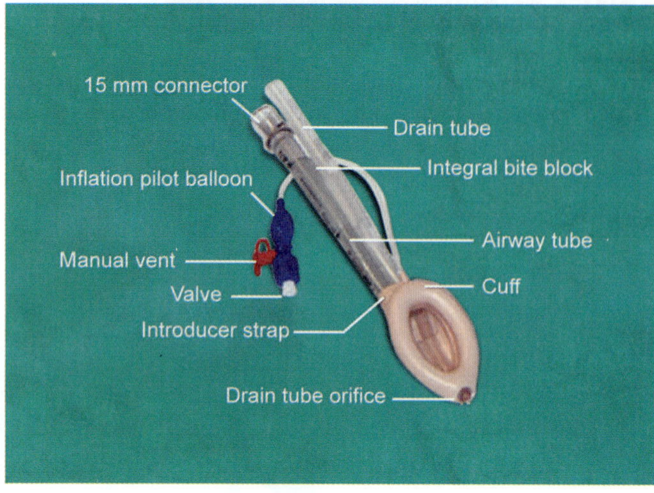

a. Difficult airway
b. To prevent aspiration of stomach contents
c. Short surgical procedure
d. Where endotracheal intubation is contraindicated

Laryngeal mask airways (LMA) was discovered by Archies Brain so also called as Brain Mask. These are special type of airways which are useful in difficult intubation.

6. Percent of oxygen delivered by the instrument shown below:

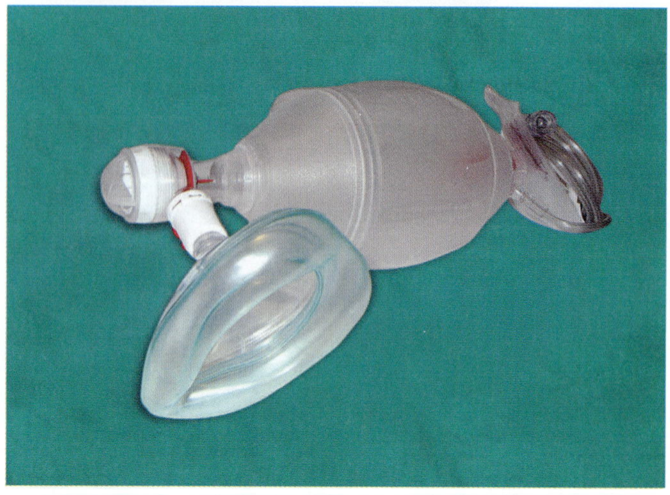

a. 0%
b. 33%
c. 66%
d. 100%

100% oxygen can be delivered by Ambu bag (Artificial Manual Breathing Unit) by attaching oxygen source and oxygen reservoir.

7. Use of the scoring system shown below:

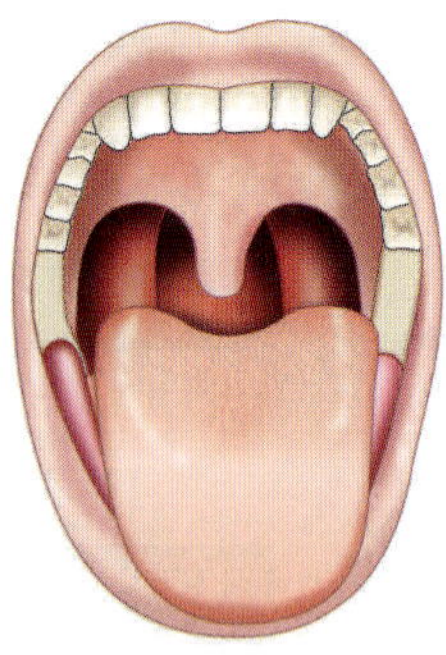

Class 1
Complete visualization of the soft palate

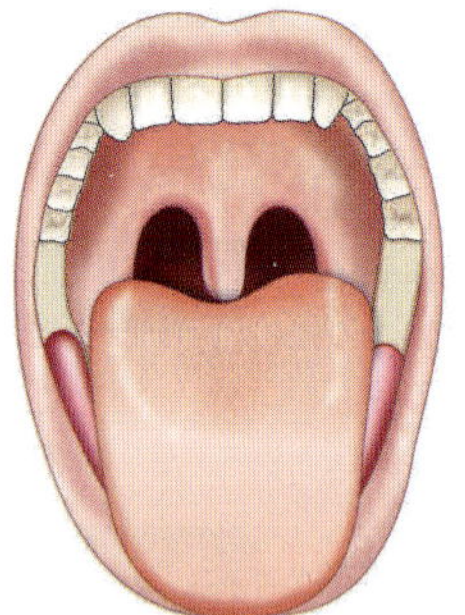

Class 2
Complete visualization of the uvula

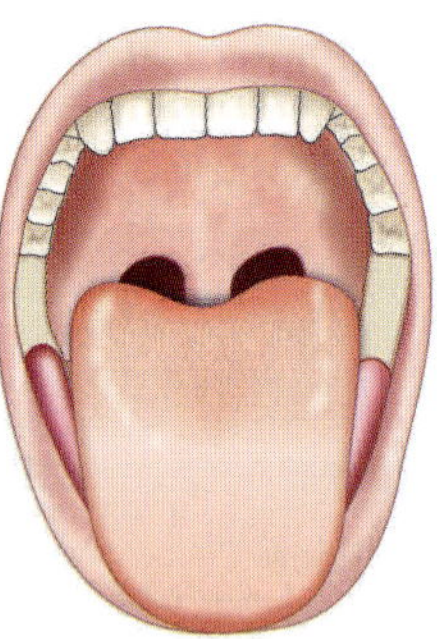

Class 3
Visualization of only the base of the uvula

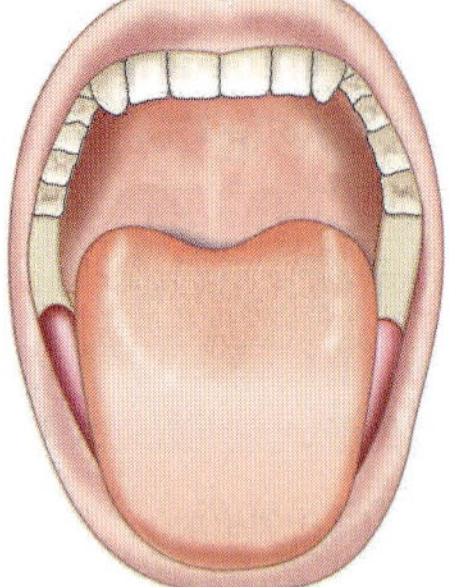

Class 4
Soft palate is not visible at all

a. Disorders of tongue
b. Expecting difficulty in intubation
c. Assessing general condition of the patient
d. Degree of submucosal fibrosis

Airway assessment is done to rule out difficult intubation. It includes assessment of mouth opening, denture status and neck movements. Adequate mouth opening is assessed with Mallampati's grading which is done by asking the patient to open his/her mouth as wide as possible and to protrude the tongue.

8. Use of the instrument shown below:

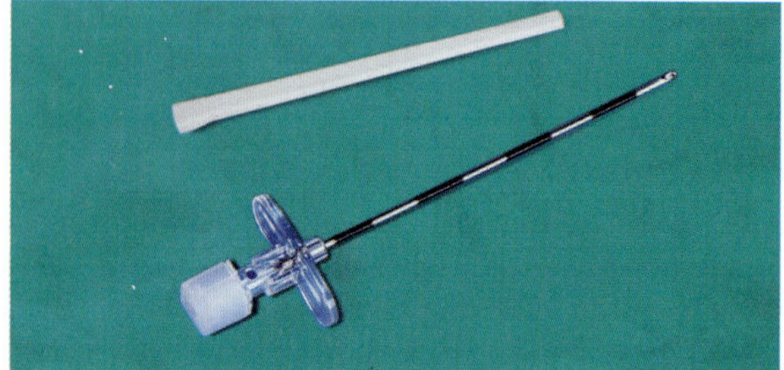

a. Epidural anesthesia
b. Caudal block
c. Spinal anesthesia
d. Beir's block

The most commonly used needle for epidural is Tuohy's needle. It has blunt bevel with curve of 15 to 30 degree at tip. This curved tip is called Huber tip.

9. Length of the instrument needed for use in a 5 year old child:

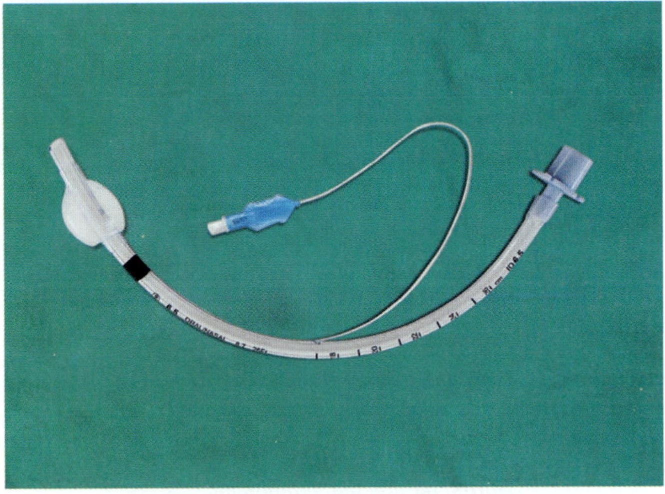

a. 12.5 cm
b. 13.5 cm
c. 14.5 cm
d. 15.5 cm

In children, the length of oral/endotracheal tube is calculated by the formulae:

Age (in years)/ 2 + 12 cm

10. Person shown below is associated with:

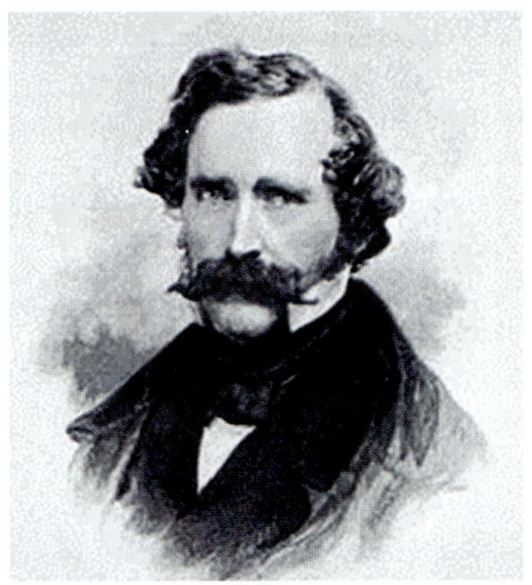

a. Discovery of Nitrous oxide
b. First public demonstration of ether
c. Development of pin index
d. Mallampati's grading

First public demonstration of ether was given by WTG Morton on 16th October 1846, that is why 16th October is celebrated as World anesthesia Day.

MCQ POINTS

S. No.	Question statements	Answers
1.	IVA which precipitates porphyria	*Methohexitone, phenobarbitone*
2.	Site of spinal anesthesia in adults	*L2, 3/ L3, 4*
3.	Shortest acting muscle relaxant	*Succinylcholine*
4.	Hoffman's elimination is related with	*Atracurium*
5.	Local anesthetics block .... channels	*Sodium*
6.	Dissociative anesthesia is related with	*Ketamine*
7.	Agent of choice for day care surgery	*Propofol*
8.	Anesthetic agent causing adrenocortical suppression	*Etomidate*
9.	Surgical anesthesia is stage...	*III*
10.	Anesthetic agent causing post partum hemorrhage	*Halothane*
11.	PIN index of nitrous oxide	*3, 5*
12.	Second gas effect/diffusion hypoxia is seen with	*Nitrous oxide*
13.	Nitric oxide is produced from which amino acid	*Arginine*
14.	Cause of postdural puncture headache	*CSF leak from puncture site*
15.	Color of oxygen cylinder	*Black body, white shoulder*
16.	Mallampatti grading is done for	*Assessment of oral cavity before intubation*
17.	Significant hyperkalemia with succinylcholine is seen with	*Burns, paraplegia, tetanus etc.*
18.	Halothane is useful in	*Asthma*
19.	Site of SA administration in infants	*L4, 5*
20.	Agent of choice for induction in pediatric age group	*Sevoflurane*
21.	Anesthetic agent having low blood and tissue gas partition coefficient	*Desflurane*
22.	Anesthetic agent which sensitizes heart to adrenaline	*Halothane*
23.	Etomidate is contraindicated in	*Adrenal insufficiency*
24.	Anesthetic agent which is cerebroprotective	*Propofol*
25.	Anesthetic agent causing profound analgesia	*Ketamine*
26.	Pin index of nitrous oxide	*3, 5*
27.	Use of laryngeal mask airway	*Maintainance of airway/alternative to intubation*
28.	Position of head and neck during intubation	*Neck flexed, head extended*
29.	MC complication of intubation	*Sore throat*
30.	Indications of hyperbaric oxygen therapy (HBOT)	*CO poisoning, gas gangrene*
31.	ASA classification is used for	*Fitness of patient*
32.	If only hard palate is visible, this is Mallampatti class	*IV*
33.	Aspirin should be stopped .... days before the surgery	*7 days*
34.	A patient is to be taken for surgery. What would you advise him to decrease the chances of aspiration	*Nil orally by mouth for at least 6 hours*
35.	Most potent antiemetic used in premedication	*Hyoscine*
36.	Normal SPO_2 value is ..... %	*80-95*
37.	Best method to detect myocardial ischemia and air embolism in perioperative period	*Transesophageal echocardiography*
38.	CVP is measured most commonly in which vein	*Right Internal Jugular vein*
39.	Swan Ganz catheter is used for	*Arterial catheterization*

S. No.	Question statements	Answers
40.	MC site for intra-arterial cannulation	***Radial***
41.	Larynx extends from Cervical .... to Cervical .... vertebrae	***C3-C6***
42.	Narrowest part of larynx in adults	***Glottis***
43.	Carina is at the level of ..... thoracic vertebrae	***T4***
44.	During endotracheal intubation, endotracheal tube commonly positioned to which sided bronchus:	***Right side***
45.	Location of pneumotaxic center	***Upper pons***
46.	Xylocaine should not be used with adrenaline for blocks in which region	***Ring block, penile block***
47.	Normal V/Q ratio is ..... L/ min	***0.8-0.9***
48.	Normal breath holding time should be more than	***25 seconds***
49.	Directly acting muscle relaxant drug	***Dantrolene***
50.	Succinylcholine is ultra-short acting because	***Destroyed by pseudocholinesterase***
51.	All LA are vasodilators *except*	***Cocaine***
52.	Which muscle relaxant is safer in renal/ hepatic failure patients	***Atracurium***
53.	Best GA in status asthmaticus	***Ketamine***
54.	DOC for Bier's block	***Lidocaine***
55.	Amongst fluranes, fastestacting induction agent is	***Desfluranes***
56.	N_2O is contraindicated in	***Pneumothorax***
57.	Halothane should not be used again in the same patient within a period of ...... months	***3 months***
58.	CVP reflects pressure of which chamber of heart	***Right atrium***
59.	Difference between axillary temperature and core temperature	***0.5***
60.	Safety system developed to discourage incorrect cylinder attachment	***Pin index***
61.	Blue color of cylinder indicates which gas	***Nitrous oxide***
62.	Block used for labor analgesia/ painless labor	***Epidural***
63.	Touhy's needle is employed for administering ...... block	***Epidural***
64.	MC factor related to post dural puncture headache	***Size of needle***
65.	Location of postdural puncture headache	***Occipital or bifrontal***
66.	MC complication of subarachnoid block	***CSF leakage resulting in headache***
67.	Effect of Sch toxicity on heart	***Bradycardia***
68.	Shortest acting non-depolarizing muscle relaxant	***Mivacurium***
69.	Tourniquet time for upper limb	***45 minutes to 1 hour***
70.	Supraclavicular block is employed for surgeries on which part of body	***Upper limb***

CHAPTER

11

PSYCHIATRY

KEY POINTS

Id, Superego and Ego

- Id: Selfish, primitive, childish and pleasure oriented part of the personality with no ability to delay gratification.
- Superego: Internalised societal and parental standards of good, bad, right and wrong behavior.
- Ego: Moderator between the Id and Superego which compromises to pacify both.

Causes of Reversible Dementia

- Hypothyroidism,
- Hypoparathyroidism,
- Hyperparathyroidism, etc.

Causes of Irreversible Dementia

- Alzheimer's dementia (MC cause),
- Multi-infarct dementia, etc.

Asperger's Syndrome

- It is a variant, but without any delay in language or cognitive development;
- Better prognosis

Delusion

- Disorder of thought;
- FALSE unshaken belief NOT amenable to reasoning

Hallucination

- Disorder of perception;
- Perception in the absence of external stimuli;
- Not dependent of will of observer

Illusion

- Misinterpretation of external stimuli

Delusions

- De Clerambault: Delusion that someone from higher socioeconomic is in love with him or her
- Othello syndrome: Delusion of infidelity
- Capgras syndrome: Delusion of doubles
- Cotard's syndrome/Nihilism: Delusion that one has lost everything, including possessions, status, strength and body organs.

Catatonic Schizophrenia

- Defect of conation,
- Negativism,
- Echolalia (repetition of words/phrases),
- Echopraxia,
- Mannerism and grimacing,
- Automatic obedience,
- Cataplexy etc.

Eugen Bleuler's Cardinal Symptoms of Schizophrenia (Four As)

- Blunted Affect
- Loosening of Association
- Ambivalence
- Autism

Kurt Schneider's First Rank Symptoms of Schizophrenia

- Hearing one's thoughts aloud.
- Auditory hallucinations commenting on one's behaviour.
- Thought withdrawal, insertion and broadcasting.
- Somatic hallucinations or the experience of one's thoughts as being controlled or influenced from outside.

Types of Schizophrenia

- Paranoid schizophrenia: Delusions of persecution, Late onset and progressive course.
- Hebephrenic: Marked thought disorder, severe loosening of association, Emotional disturbances. Progressively worse course.
- Catatonic: Acute onset in 2nd to 3rd decade Episodic and complete recovery; Clinical features include - Mutism,

rigidity, negativism, posturing, stupor, echolalia, Echopraxia, waxy flexibility, ambitendency, automatic obedience, verbigeration

- Pseudo neurotic: Initially there are predominant neurotic symptoms. Three classical features are pan anxiety, pan neurosis, and pan sexuality
- Oneiroid: Subtype of schizophrenia with acute onset, clouding of consciousness, disorientation, dream like state and perceptual disturbances with rapid shifting
- Van Gogh syndrome: Schizophrenia with self mutilation
- Propf syndrome: Schizophrenia with mental retardation.

Types of Phobias

- Acrophobia: Fear of high places
- Zoophobia: Fear of animals
- Xenophobia: Fear of strangers
- Claustrophobia: Fear of closed spaces
- Thanatophobia: Fear of death

Delirium Tremens

- MC severe symptom of alcohol withdrawal;
- Disorientation,
- Anxiety,
- Perceptual defect;
- Chlordiazepoxide is used for management

EEG Waves and Sleep Cycles

- Awake and alert: Beta waves
- Awake, result, eyes closed: Alpha
- NREM-1: Theta
- NREM-2: Theta
- NREM-3: Delta
- NREM-4: Delta
- REM: Beta

Lithium

- Side effects: >2 mEq/L
- Life threatening toxicity: >3.5 mEq /L

Drugs of Choice for Psychiatric Disorders

- Generalized anxiety: Benzodiazepines
- Panic attack: Fluoxetine
- Nocturnal enuresis: Imipramine
- Opioid withdrawal: Methadone → 2nd DOC → Clonidine
- Opioid intoxication: Naloxone/Naltrexone
- Alcohol withdrawal: Chlordiazepoxide → 2nd DOC → Diazepam
- Alcohol abstinence; Disulifram
- Benzodiazepines intoxication: Flumazenil
- Obsessive compulsive disorder: Fluoxetine
- Attention deficit hyperactivity disorder: Amphetamine → 2nd DOC → Methylphenidate
- Tic disorder: Haloperidol
- Bulimia nervosa: Fluoxetine
- Alcoholic hallucinations: Diazepam
- Neuroleptic induced urinary retention: Bethanechol
- Neuroleptic induced hyperprolactinemia: Amantadine
- Akathisia: Propranolol

Personality Types

- Schizoid personality type: introverted, withdrawn, solitary and distant.
- Paranoid personality: Interprets the action of others as deliberately threatening. Untrusting, unforgiving, guarded, and prone to aggression. Perceive others as jealous, deceitful and condescending.
- Schizotypal personality: Odd and eccentric manners of dressing and speaking. Strange, paranoid beliefs. Have difficulties forming relations and extreme anxiety in social situations. Display sign of magical thinking.
- Antisocial personality: Impulsive, irresponsible, callous and aggressive. No respect for others and no remorse. High risk for alcohol and substance abuse.
- Borderline personality: Abrupt and extreme mood changes. Unstable Disorder and fluctuating self image. Unpredictable and self Destructive. Fears of abandonment. Excessive Dependency, self mutilation or recurrent suicidal gestures. Impulsive, chronic feeling of boredom, bouts of intense Anger.
- Avoidant personality: Hypersensitive to rejection, excessive social Disorder discomfort, timidity fear of criticism, avoidance of social work.
- Dependant personality: Dependant and submissive behavior, feel fear. No respect, lack self confidence
- Compulsive personality: Compulsive personalities, high levels of aspirations, strive for perfection never satisfied with achievements. Reliable, dependable, orderly, methodical and highly cautious.
- Histrionic personality: Self dramatization, exaggerated expressions suggestibility. Attention seeking attitude, Seductiveness, concerned with Physical appearance.

Neuroleptic Malignant Syndrome

- Muscle rigidity autonomic dysregulation and hyperthermia.
- Idiosyncratic reaction to inhibition of central dopamine receptors that results in increased heat production and failure of heat dissipation.
- Management:
  - Rapid physical cooling.
  - Administration of an antipyretic or acetaminophen bromocriptine and
  - Dantrolene.

MCQs WITH SHORT EXPLANATIONS

PSYCHOACTIVE SUBSTANCE USE DISORDER

1. A heavy alcoholic drinker presents to the psychiatry OPD with irrelevant taking, sweating and tremors. He had not taken alcohol since last three days. Condition is consistent with the diagnosis of:

a. Korsakoff psychosis b. Schizophrenia
c. Delirium tremens d. Dementia

DT is the most severe alcohol withdrawl syndrome. It occurs usually within 2-4 days of complete or significant abstinence from heavy alcohol drinking in about 5% of patients, as compared to acute tremulousness which occurs in about 34% of patients. The course is short, with recovery occurring within 3-7 days. This is an acute organic brain syndrome (delirium).

2. Confabulation is seen in:

a. Mania b. Depression
c. Alcoholism d. Delirium

Clinically, Korsakoff's psychosis presents as an organic amnestic syndrome, characterized by gross memory disturbances, with confabulation.

Some Complications of Alcohol Dependence	
I. Medical Complications	
A. Gastrointestinal System	
i.	Fatty liver, cirrhosis of liver, hepatitis, liver cell carcinoma, liver failure
ii.	Gastritis, reflux oesophagitis, oesophageal varices, Mallory-Weiss syndrome, achlorhydria, peptic ulcer, carcinoma stomach and oesophagus
iii.	Malabsorption syndrome, protein-losing enteropathy
iv.	Pancreatitis: acute, chronic, and relapsing
B. Central Nervous System	
i.	Peripheral neuropathy
ii.	Delirium tremens
iii.	Rum fits (Alcohol withdrawal seizures)
iv.	Alcoholic hallucinosis
v.	Alcoholic jealousy
vi.	Wernicke-Korsakoff psychosis
vii.	Marchiafava-Bignami disease
viii.	Alcoholic dementia
ix.	Suicide
x.	Cerebellar degeneration
xi.	Central pontine myelinosis
xii.	Head injury and fractures.
C. Miscellaneous	
i.	Acne rosacea, palmar erythema, rhinophyma, spider naevi, ascitis, parotid enlargement
ii.	Foetal alcohol syndrome (craniofacial anomalies, growth retardation, major organ system malformations)
iii.	Alcoholic hypoglycaemia and ketoacidosis
iv.	Cardiomyopathy, cardiac beri-beri
v.	Alcoholic myopathy
vi.	Anaemia, thrombocytopenia, Vitamin K factor deficiency, haemolytic anaemia
vii.	Accidental hypothermia
viii.	Pseudo-Cushing's syndrome, hypogonadism, gynaecomastia (in men), amenorrhoea, infertility, decreased testosterone and increased LH levels
ix.	Risk for coronary artery disease
x.	Malnutrition, pellagra
xi.	Decreased immune function and proneness to infections such as tuberculosis
xii.	Sexual dysfunction
II. Social Complications	
i.	Accidents
ii.	Marital disharmony
iii.	Divorce
iv.	Occupational problems, with loss of productive man-hours
v.	Increased incidence of drug dependence
vi.	Criminality
vii.	Financial difficulties.

3. Physical withdrawal symptoms are ABSENT in patients abusing:

a. Pethidine
b. Cannabis
c. Opium
d. Haloperidol

Cannabis produces a very mild physical dependence, with a relatively mild withdrawal syndrome, which is characterized by fine tremors, irritability, restlessness, nervousness, insomnia, decreased appetite and craving. However, some health professionals feel that there is no true physical dependence with cannabis.

Ans. 1. c. Delirium tremens 2. c. Alcoholism 3. b. Cannabis

Psychoactive Substance Use Disorders

Drug	Usual Route of Administration	Physical Dependence	Psychic Dependence	Tolerance
1. Alcohol	Oral	++	++	+
2. Amphetamines	Oral, Parenteral	++	++	+++
3. Barbiturates	Oral, Parenteral	++	++	+++
4. Benzodiazepines	Oral, Parenteral	+	+	+
5. Caffeine	Oral	+	++	+
6. Cannabis (Marihuana)	Smoking, Oral	±	++	+
7. Cocaine	Inhalation, Oral, Smoking, Parenteral	±	++	–
8. Lysergic acid diethylamide (LSD)	Oral	–	+	+
9. Nicotine	Oral, Smoking	+	++	+
10. Opioids	Oral, Parenteral, Smoking	+++	+++	+++
11. Phencyclidine (PCP)	Smoking, Inhalation, Parenteral, Oral	±	+	+
12. Volatile solvents	Inhalation	±	++	+

– = None; ± = Probable/Little; + = Some/Mild; ++ = Moderate; +++ = Severe.
The dependence can be either *psychic*, or *physical*, or both.

4. The characteristic feature of alcohol withdrawal syndrome is:

a. Hallucination b. Delusion
c. Confusion d. Convulsion

Alcoholic hallucinosis is characterized by the presence of hallucinations (usually auditory) during partial or complete abstinence, following regular alcohol intake. It occurs in about 2% of patients.

Classification of Alcoholism

Factors	Type I	Type II
Synonym	Milieu-limited	Male-limited
Gender	Both sexes	Mostly in males
Age of onset	> 25 years	< 25 years
Aetiological factors	Genetic factors important strong *environmental influences* are contributory	*Heritable*; environmental influences are limited
Family history	May be positive	Parental alcoholism and antisocial behaviour usually present
Loss of control	Present	No loss of control
Other features	Psychological dependence; and guilt present	Drinking followed by aggressive behaviour; spontaneous alcohol seeking
Pre-morbid personality traits	Harm avoidance; high reward dependence	Novelty-seeking

5. Jet black tongue with tactile and visual hallucination is a feature of:

a. Heroin b. Opium
c. Alcohol d. Cocaine

The complications of chronic cocaine use include acute anxiety reaction, uncontrolled compulsive behavior, psychotic episodes (with persecutory delusions, and tactile and other hallucinations), delirium and delusional disorder.

6. DOC for delirium tremens:

a. Diazepam b. Chlorpromazine
c. Haloperidol d. Reserpine

The drugs of choice for detoxification are usually benzodiazepines. Chlordiazepoxide (80-200 mg/day in divided doses) and diazepam (40-80 mg/day in divided doses) are the most frequently used benzodiazepines. The higher limit of the normal dose range is used in delirium tremens.

CAGE Questionnaire

The CAGE questionnaire basically consists of four questions:

i.	Have you ever had to **C**ut down on alcohol (amount)?
ii.	Have you ever been **A**nnoyed by people's criticism of alcoholism?
iii.	Have you ever felt **G**uilty about drinking?
iv.	Have you ever needed an **E**ye opener drink (early morning drink)?

A score of 2 or more identifies problem drinkers.

7. NOT a feature of nicotine withdrawal:

a. Anxiety b. Tachycardia
c. Insomnia d. Depression

Ans. 4. **a.** Hallucination 5. **d.** Cocaine 6. **a.** Diazepam 7. **b.** Tachycardia

Nicotine withdrawal can occur 12-14 hours after last smoke and can present with anxiety, restlessness, poor concentration, decreased sleep, increased appetite and exacerbation of psychiatric symptoms in those with pre-existing psychiatric disorder (s).

8. In a patient with history of prolonged alcohol intake, seizures will occur after... of alcohol withdrawal:

a. 4-6 hours
b. 24-48 hours
c. 2-4 days
d. 4-7 days

Generalized tonic-clonic seizures occur in about 10% of alcohol dependence patients, usually 12-48 hours after a heavy bout of drinking. Often these patients have been drinking alcohol in large amounts on a regular basis for many years.

Body Fluid Alcohol Levels		
BAC (mg%)*	*Behavioural Correlates*	
25–100	Excitement	
80	Legal limit for driving (in UK)**	
100–200	Serious intoxication, slurred speech, incoordination, nystagmus	
200–300	Dangerous	
300–350	Hypothermia, dysarthria, cold sweats	
350–400	Coma, respiratory depression	
>400	Death may occur	
Urinary Alcohol (mg%)	*Diagnostic Use*	*Equivalent BAC (mg%)*
>120	Suggestive	80
>200	Diagnostic	150

*BAC - Blood Alcohol Concentration
**30 mg/100 ml in India (Section 185 of the Motor Vehicle Act, 1988)

SCHIZOPHRENIA

9. Kallu, an occasional alcoholic has got a change in his behavior. He has become suspicious that people are trying to conspire against him though his father says that there is no reason for his fears. He is having hallucinations of voices commenting on his actions. Most likely diagnosis is:

a. Delirium tremens
b. Alcohol induced psychosis
c. Schizophrenia
d. Delusional disorder

Schizophrenia is characterized by disturbances in thought and verbal behavior, perception, affect, motor behavior and relationship to the external world. The diagnosis is entirely clinical.

First Rank Symptoms (SFRS) of Schizophrenia	
1.	*Audible thoughts:* Voices speaking out thoughts aloud or 'thought echo'.
2.	*Voices heard arguing:* Two or more hallucinatory voices discussing the subject in third person.
3.	Voices commenting on one's action.
4.	*Thought withdrawal:* Thoughts cease and subject experiences them as removed by an external force.
5.	*Thought insertion:* Experience of thoughts imposed by some external force on person's passive mind.
6.	*Thought diffusion or broadcasting:* Experience of thoughts escaping the confines of self and as being experienced by others around.
7.	*'Made' feelings or affect.*
8.	*'Made' impulses.*
9.	*'Made' volition or acts:* In 'made' affect, impulses and volitions, the person experiences feelings, impulses or acts which are imposed by some external force. In 'made' volition, for example, one's own acts are experienced as being under the control of some external force.
10.	*Somatic passivity:* Bodily sensations, especially sensory symptoms, are experienced as imposed on body by some external force.
11.	*Delusional perception:* Normal perception has a private and illogical meaning.

10. Neurotransmitter in increased quantities in schizophrenia:

a. Noradrenaline
b. Serotonin
c. Dopamine
d. GABA

Schizophrenia is presently thought to be probably due to a functional increase of dopamine at the post-synaptic receptor, though other neurotransmitters such as serotonin (especially 5-HT2 receptors), GABA and acetylcholine are also presumably involved.

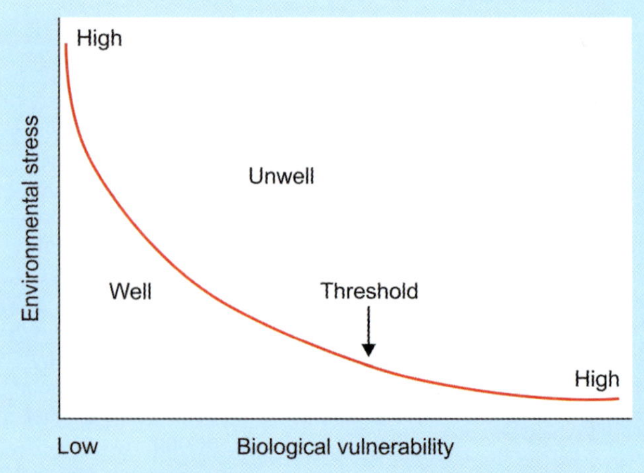

Stress Vulnerability Hypothesis in Schizophrenia.
Ref: Zubin and Spring (1977).

Ans. 8. **b.** 24-48 hours 9. **c.** Schizophrenia 10. **c.** Dopamine

11. Characteristic clinical manifestation of schizophrenia:

a. Confusion b. Anxiety
c. Auditory hallucination d. Visual hallucination

Hallucinations (perceptions without stimuli) are common in schizophrenia. Auditory hallucinations are by far the most frequent. Only the 'third person hallucinations (voices heard arguing, discussing the patient in third person)' are believed to be characteristic of schizophrenia.

Clinical Types of Schizophrenia
1. Paranoid schizophrenia
2. Hebephrenic schizophrenia
3. Catatonic schizophrenia
4. Residual schizophrenia
5. Undifferentiated schizophrenia
6. Simple schizophrenia
7. Post-schizophrenic depression
8. Others

12. NOT a classical symptom of schizophrenia:

a. Autism b. Automatism
c. Association defect d. Ambivalence

4A's of Bleuler include ambivalence, autism, affect disturbance and association disturbance.

Eugen Bleuler's Fundamental Symptoms of Schizophrenia (Also called as 4 A's of Bleuler)	
1.	*Ambivalence*: Marked inability to decide for or against
2.	*Autism*: Withdrawal into self
3.	*Affect disturbances*: Disturbances of affect such as inappropriate affect
4.	*Association disturbances*: Loosening of associations; thought disorder

13. Schizophrenia like picture is a side effect of:

a. Fortwin b. Amphetamine
c. Phenobarbitone d. Morphine

Drugs such as amphetamines and mescaline can cause schizophrenia-like symptoms in normal subjects.

Symptom Clusters in Schizophrenia		
Positive Symptoms	*Negative Symptoms*	*Disorganised Symptoms*
Delusions	Affective flattening	Inappropriate affect
Hallucinations	Alogia (poverty of speech)	Disorganised behaviour
	Anhedonia—asociality	Thought disorder
	Avolition—apathy	Loosening of associations
	Attentional impairment	

14. Tardive dyskinesia is produced by following EXCEPT:

a. Fluphenazine b. Haloperidol
c. Chlorpromazine d. Clozapine

Many patients of schizophrenia require adjuvant antiparkinsonian medication to prevent extrapyramidal side-effects; for example, trihexyphenidyl 6 mg/day, orphenadrine 150 mg/day, procyclidine 7.5-15 mg/day. This is particularly true if the patient is receiving an older, typical antipsychotic (such as haloperidol). However, at times atypical antipsychotics such as risperidone can also cause extrapyramidal symptoms, particularly in higher doses.

Antipsychotic Dose in Schizophrenia

Drug	*Oral Dose Range (mg/day)*	*Parenteral Dose (mg/day)*	*Equivalent Oral Dose* (Equal to 100 mg CPZ)*
A. Typical/Traditional/First Generation Antipsychotics			
1. Chlorpromazine (CPZ)	300-1000	50-100 IM	100
2. Flupentixol	3-18	—	2
3. Haloperidol	5-30	5-10 IM	2-3
4. Loxapine	25-250	—	10
5. Pimozide	4-12	—	2
6. Prochlorperazine	45-150	40-80 IM	15
7. Sulpiride	400-2400	—	200
8. Thioridazine	300-600	—	100
9. Trifluoperazine	15-50	1-5 IM	5
10. Triflupromazine	100-400	30-60 IM	25
11. Zuclopenthixol	25-150	50-100 IM	25
B. Atypical/Second Generation Antipsychotics			
12. Amisulpride	400-1200	—	—

Contd...

Ans. **11. c.** Auditory hall... **12. b.** Automatism **13. b.** Amphetamine **14. d.** Clozapine

Contd...

Drug	Oral Dose Range (mg/day)	Parenteral Dose (mg/day)	Equivalent Oral Dose* (Equal to 100 mg CPZ)
13. Aripiprazole	5-30	5.25-15 IM	—
14. Clozapine	50-900	—	50
15. Olanzapine	5-20	2.5-10 IM	2-3
16. Paliperidone	3-12	—	—
17. Quetiapine	150-800	—	50-100
18. Risperidone	2-16	—	0.5-1.0
19. Ziprasidone	40-160	—	20
20. Zotepine	75-300	—	—

*Equivalent doses are at best approximations only. The dose in a particular patient should be chosen on an individualised basis by the treating professional.

15. NOT a Schneider's first rank symptom of schizophrenia:
a. Passivity phenomenon b. Auditory hallucination
c. Delusion of self reference
d. Delusional perception

Delusion of reference (being referred to by others; e.g. 'people are talking about me') is one of the commonly seen delusions in schizophrenia (but not included in SFRS).

Some Important Clinical Features of Retarded Catatonia	
1.	*Mutism*: Complete absence of speech
2.	*Rigidity*: Maintenance of a rigid posture against efforts to be moved
3.	*Negativism*: An apparently motiveless resistance to all commands and attempts to be moved, or doing just the opposite
4.	*Posturing*: Voluntary assumption of an inappropriate and often bizarre posture for long periods of time
5.	*Stupor*: Akinesis (no movement) with mutism but with evidence of relative preservation of conscious awareness
6.	*Echolalia*: Repetition, echo or mimicking of phrases or words heard
7.	*Echopraxia*: Repetition, echo or mimicking of actions observed
8.	*Waxy flexibility*: Parts of body can be placed in positions that will be maintained for long periods of time, even if very uncomfortable; flexible like wax
9.	*Ambitendency*: Due to ambivalence, conflicting impulses and tentative actions are made, but no goal directed action occurs, e.g. on asking to take out tongue, tongue is slightly protruded but taken back again
10.	Other signs such as *mannerisms*, *stereotypies* (verbal and behavioural), *automatic obedience* (commands are followed automatically, irrespective of their nature) and *verbigeration* (incomprehensible speech).

16. In schizophrenia, FALSE is:
a. 3rd person auditory hallucination
b. Formal thought disorder
c. Inappropriate emotions
d. Sustained mood changes

There is no prominent mood disorder of depressive or maniac type in schizophrenia.

Prognostic Factors in Schizophrenia		
	Good Prognostic Factors	*Poor Prognostic Factors*
1.	Acute or abrupt onset	Insidious onset
2.	Onset >35 years of age (late onset)	Onset <20 years of age (early onset)
3.	Presence of precipitating stressor	Absence of stressor
4.	Good premorbid adjustment	Poor premorbid adjustment
5.	Catatonic subtype (paranoid subtype has an intermediate prognosis)	Disorganised, simple, undifferentiated, or chronic catatonic subtypes
6.	Short duration (< 6 months)	Chronic course (> 2 years)
7.	Presence of depression	Absence of depression
8.	Predominance of positive symptoms	Predominance of negative symptoms
9.	Family history of mood disorder	Family history of schizophrenia
10.	First episode	Past history of schizophrenia
11.	Pyknic (fat) physique	Asthenic (thin) physique
12.	Female sex	Male sex
13.	Good social support	Poor social support or unmarried
14.	Presence of confusion, perplexity, or disorientation in the acute phase	Flat or blunted affect
15.	Proper treatment, good treatment concordance, and good response to treatment	Absence of proper treatment or poor response to treatment
16.	Outpatient treatment	Institutionalisation (long-term hospitalisation)
17.	Normal cranial CT scan	Evidence of ventricular enlargement on cranial CT scan

Ans. **15. c.** Delusion of self reference **16. d.** Sustained mood changes

17. Clozapine is commonly associated with:
a. Hemolytic anemia b. Depression
c. Agranulocytosis d. Tardive dyskinesia

Clozapine is an effective drug; however, as it can cause agranulocytosis and seizures as side-effects, it should be used with caution, with regular WBC and neutrophil counts as advised by the Summary of Product Characteristics (SPC).

18. Clozapine is given in:
a. Mania
b. Depression
c. Obsessive Compulsive disorder
d. Schizophrenia

Clozapine is an atypical (second generation) antipsychotic used in the management of schizophrenia.

19. A young patient of schizophrenia is intolerant to antipsychotic medications. Which drug is most preferred for such a patient:
a. Clozapine b. Olanzapine
c. Risperidone d. Haloperidol

Clozapine, an atypical antipsychotic, is available in the Indian market. The clinical trials have shown that clozapine is effective in about 30% of patients who had no beneficial response to traditional (typical and atypical) antipsychotics.

MOOD DISORDERS

20. Neurotransmitter involved in depression:
a. GABA and dopamine
b. Serotonin and norepinephrine
c. Dopamine and serotonin
d. GABA and norepinephrine

The earlier models of a functional increase (in mania) or decrease (in depression) of amines at the synaptic cleft now appears simplistic; though urinary and CSF levels of amine metabolites indicate decreased norepinephrine and/or 5-HT function in depression, and increased norepinephrine in mania.

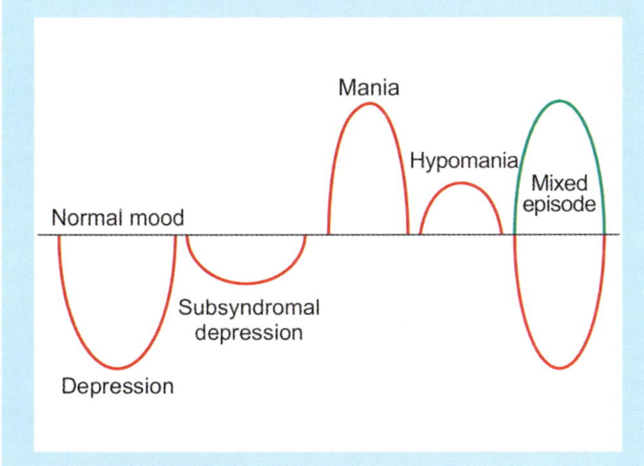

Bipolar disorder: clinical picture.

21. Treatment of choice for endogenous depression with suicidal tendency:
a. Lithium
b. Chlorpromazine
c. Carbamazepine
d. Electroconvulsive therapy

ECT is indicated in major severe depression with suicidal risk. This is the first and most important indication for ECT.

A Brief Early History of Biological Treatments in Psychiatry.

Year	*Treatment*	*Started by*
1785	Camphor-induced seizures	W Oliver
1917	Malarial treatment of GPI	Julius Wagner von Jauregg
1922	Barbiturate coma therapy	Jacob Klaesi
1931	Reserpine (1st drug treatment in psychosis)	Ganesh Sen, Kartik Bose
1933	Insulin coma therapy	Manfred Sakel
1934	Cardiazol (metrazol) induced seizures	LLJ von Meduna
1936	Psychosurgery (prefrontal leucotomy)	Egas Moniz, Almenda Lima
1938	Electroshock (electroconvulsive therapy)	Ugo Cerletti, Lucio Bini
1949	Lithium (for mania)	John F Cade
1952	Chlorpromazine (1st antipsychotic)	Jean PL Delay, Pierre Deniker
1954	Meprobamate	FM Berger
1958	Iproniazid (1st MAO inhibitor)	Nathan Kline
1958	Imipramine (1st tricyclic antidepressant)	Thomas Kuhn
1958	Haloperidol (1st non-phenothiazine antipsychotic)	Janssen
1960	Chlordiazepoxide (1st benzodiazepine)	Hugo Sternbach

22. Mode of action of fluoxetine is:
a. Inhibition of serotonin uptake
b. Inhibition of dopamine uptake
c. Facilitation of adrenergic impulse
d. Facilitation of cholinergic response

Fluoxetine comes under SSRIs (selective serotonin reuptake inhibitors).

Ans. 17. **c.** Agranulocytosis 18. **d.** Schizophrenia 19. **a.** Clozapine 20. **b.** Serotonin and norepine...
21. **d.** Electrocon... 22. **a.** Inhibition of serotonin uptake

Classification and Properties of Antidepressants

Drugs	Oral Dose (mg/d)	Some Common Adverse Effects[#]		
		*Sedation**	*Orthostatic Hypotension**	*Anticholinergic**
I. Cyclic Antidepressants				
A. Tricyclic Tertiary Amines				
1. Amitriptyline	75-300	+++	+++	+++
2. Clomipramine	75-250	++	++	++
3. Dosulepin (Dotheipin)	75-300	+++	+++	++
4. Doxepine	75-300	+++	+++	+
5. Imipramine	75-300	++	++	++
6. Lofepramine	70-210	+	+	+
7. Tri-imipramine	75-300	+++	++	++
B. Tricyclic Secondary Amines				
1. Desipramine	75-300	±	+	++
2. Nortriptyline	75-200	+	++	+
3. Protriptyline	15-60	0	++	++
C. Tetracyclic Antidepressants				
1. Amoxapine	150-400	+	+	++
2. Maprotiline	75-225	++	++	++
3. Mianserin	30-120	+++	±	±
D. Bicyclic Antidepressants				
1. Viloxazine	100-300	±	±	±
II. Selective Serotonin Reuptake Inhibitors (SSRIs)				
1. Citalopram	20-40	±	±	0
2. Escitalopram	10-20	±	±	0
3. Fluoxetine	20-60	±	0	0
4. Fluvoxamine	50-300	±	±	±
5. Paroxetine	20-40	+	0	±
6. Sertraline	50-200	±	±	0
III. Serotonin Norepinephrine Reuptake Inhibitors (SNRIs)				
1. Duloxetine	60	±	±	±
2. Venlafaxine	75-375	+	±	±
IV. Norepinephrine Serotonin Reuptake Enhancers (NSREs)				
1. Tianeptin	37.5	+	0	±
V. Noradrenergic and Specific Serotonergic Antagonists (NaSSAs)				
1. Mirtazapine	15-45	+++	+	±
VI. Norepinephrine Dopamine Reuptake Inhibitors (NDRIs)				
1. Bupropion	150-450	Activating	0	0
VII. Serotonin Antagonists and Reuptake Inhibitors (SARIs)				
1. Nefazodone (withdrawn from market)	200-600	++	+	±

Contd...

Contd...

Drugs	*Oral Dose (mg/d)*	*Some Common Adverse Effects#*		
		*Sedation**	*Orthostatic Hypotension**	*Anticholinergic**
2. Trazodone	150-400	+++	±	±
VIII. Noradrenergic Reuptake Inhibitors (NARIs)				
1. Reboxetine	8-10	±	±	±
IX. Mono-amine Oxidase Inhibitors (MAOIs)				
A. Irreversible Non-selective and Selective MAOIs				
Not available in India				
B. Reversible Selective MAO-B Inhibitors				
1. Selegiline	5-10	Useful in Parkinsonism		
C. Reversible Selective MAO-A Inhibitors (RIMAs)				
1. Moclobemide	300-600	Activating	0	0
X. Melatonin receptor agonist and 5-HT$_{2C}$ antagonist				
1. Agomelatin	25-50	+	0	0

The estimate of common adverse effects in this table is a very rough and empirical guideline to the clinical use of antidepressants. The drug dosage in each patient needs to be individualised based on the clinical symptoms, their severity, response to treatment and several other clinical factors.

* 0 = Absent; ± = Probable/Very little; + = Mild; ++ = Moderate; +++ = Severe.

23. MC symptom of lithium toxicity:

a. Nephrotic syndrome
b. Polyuria
c. ARF
d. Renal calculi

The renal side effects occur in about 10-50% of all patients on maintenance lithium therapy. Some of the features include polyuria, polydypsia, tubular changes, nephrogenic diabetes insipidus and nephrotic syndrome.

Blood Lithium Levels (in treatment of bipolar disorder)
❑ Therapeutic levels = 0.6-1.2 mEq/L (For the treatment of acute mania)
❑ Prophylactic levels = 0.6-1.0 mEq/L (For relapse prevention in bipolar disorder)
❑ Toxic lithium levels > 2.0 mEq/L

24. Commonest complication of modified ECT is:

a. Fracture spine
b. Intracerebral bleeding
c. Amnesia
d. Generalized bodyaches and myopathy

With ECT, memory disturbances (both antegrade and retrograde) are very common. These are usually mild and recovery occurs within 1-6 months after treatment. Unilateral ECTs cause much less memory disturbance than bilateral ECTs.

25. Best indication for ECT is:

a. Depression with suicidal tendencies
b. Mania
c. Hysteria
d. Schizophrenia

Major severe depression with suicidal risk is the first and most important indication for ECT.

Suicidal Risk: Some Important Factors
Suicidal risk is much more in the presence of following factors:
a. Presence of marked hopelessness
b. Males; age>40; unmarried, divorced/widowed
c. Written/verbal communication of suicidal intent and/or plan
d. Early stages of depression
e. Recovering from depression (At the peak of depression, the patient is usually either too depressed or too retarded to commit suicide)
f. Period of 3 months from recovery.

26. True for lithium:

a. Delayed absorption
b. Narrow therapeutic index
c. Protein bound
d. Can be given safely in renal dysfunction

Adverse effects are comsmon with lithium therapy and toxicity can occur easily, if blood levels reach about 2.0 mEq/L; life-threatening intoxication occurs, if levels reach about 3.5 mEq/L. In acute administration, toxicity is primarily neurological whilst during maintenance therapy renal side effects are commonest.

Ans. 23. **b.** Polyuria 24. **c.** Amnesia 25. **a.** Depression with suicidal tendencies
26. **b.** Narrow therapeutic index

27. A patient of maniac depressive psychosis is on lithium, clozapine and fluphenazine. During the course of treatment, he developed seizures and tremors. He is drinking water heavily and had recurrent episodes of urination. Which drug is responsible for these complications:

a. Lithium b. Clozapine
c. Fluphenazine d. None of the above

Polyuria and polydypsia are common renal side-effects of lithium therapy, whereas neurological side effects of lithium therapy include seizures (decreased threshold) and tremors (commonest side effect).

28. DOC for panic disorder:

a. Nitrazepam b. Fluoxetine
c. Diazepam d. Clonidine

Panic disorder is characterized by discrete episodes acute anxiety. The drugs of choice for generalized anxiety disorder have traditionally been benzodiazepines, and for panic disorder, antidepressants. It is useful to begin the treatment of panic disorders with small doses of antidepressants, usually SSRIs (e.g. fluoxetine).

Side Effects of Antidepressants

Category and Side Effect	*Probable Cause*	*Maximum with (For example)*	*Minimum with (For example)*	*Management*
A. Autonomic Side Effects				
1. Dry mouth	Muscarinic Cholinergic blockade	Amitriptyline	Fluoxetine	
2. Constipation	–do–	Amitriptyline	Fluoxetine	
3. Cycloplegia	–do–	Amitriptyline	Fluoxetine	
4. Mydriasis	–do–	Amitriptyline	Fluoxetine	
5. Urinary retention	–do–	Amitriptyline	Fluoxetine	
6. Delirium	–do–	Amitriptyline	Fluoxetine	
7. Aggravation of narrow angle glaucoma	–do–	Amitriptyline	Fluoxetine	Do not use in elderly and in patients with past history. Change or stop drug.
8. Orthostatic hypotension	α_1 Adrenergic blockade	Amitriptyline	Fluoxetine	
B. Sexual Side Effects				
1. Impotence	α_1 Adrenergic blockade	Amitriptyline	Mirtazapine Bupropion	
2. Impaired/retarded ejaculation	α_1 Adrenergic blockade	Amitriptyline Paroxetine	Mirtazapine Bupropion	Cyproheptadine given 1 hour before, can reverse anorgasmia and retarded ejaculation caused by SSRIs.
3. Anorgasmia	5-HT blockade	SSRIs TCAs	Mirtazapine Bupropion	
4. Priapism	Not known	Trazodone	Not known	Stop drug; muscular relaxation; sometimes surgical procedure needed
C. CNS Effects				
1. Sedation	α Adrenergic blockade	Amitriptyline	Protriptyline Fluoxetine	This side effect may be beneficial; Otherwise decrease dose. Change drug. Give single dose only at night.
2. Tremor and Other EPSE	Serotonergic	Amoxapine	Not known	Decrease dose. Change drug.
3. Jitteriness syndrome	Adrenergic; Serotonergic	Imipramine Fluoxetine	MAOI	This is very common in first week of therapy. Add diazepam for first 1-2 weeks. Tolerance occurs.
4. Withdrawal syndrome (mild)	Dependence	Imipramine Paroxetine	Protriptyline Fluoxetine	Slow withdrawal of drug.
5. Seizures	Decreased threshold	Bupropion Amitriptyline	Nomifensine Fluoxetine	Decrease dose. Change drug.

Contd...

Ans. 27. **a.** Lithium 28. **b.** Fluoxetine

Contd...

Category and Side Effect	*Probable Cause*	*Maximum with (For example)*	*Minimum with (For example)*	*Management*
6. Aggravation of psychosis	Sympathomimetic	Not known	Amoxapine	Stop drug. Re-evaluate.
7. Precipitation of mania	Sympathomimetic	Tricyclics	Not known	Stop drug. Use mood stabilisers.
D. Cardiac Side Effects				
1. Tachycardia	Anticholinergic	Amitriptyline	Trazodone	Decrease dosage. Use safer drugs in elderly and those with past history or co-existing heart disease
2. Quinidine-like action (decreased conduction time)	Cardiotoxic	Amitriptyline	Fluoxetine	
3. ECG changes	Cardiotoxic	Amitriptyline	Fluoxetine	
4. Arrhythmias (in overdoses)	Cardiotoxic	Dosulepin Amitriptyline	Fluoxetine	
5. Direct myocardial depression (in overdoses)	Cardiotoxic	Amitriptyline	Fluoxetine	
6. Hypertension	Noradrenegic	Venlafaxine Duloxetine	SSRIs	Close monitoring; ECG and BP check before start (especially on higher doses); treat hypertension
E. Allergic Side Effects				
1. Agranulocytosis (very rare)	Hypersensitivity	Mianserin Mirtazapine	Not known	
2. Cholestatic jaundice (very rare)	Hypersensitivity	Not known	Not known	
3. Skin rashes	Hypersensitivity	Not known	Not known	
4. Systemic vasculitis	Not known	Not known	Not known	
F. Metabolic and Endocrine Side Effects				
1. Weight gain	Not known	Mirtazapine Amitriptyline	Bupropion Fluoxetine can cause weight loss	Change drug. Exercise. Diet control.
G. Miscellaneous Side Effects				
1. Hypertensive crises	Interaction with tyramine in foods (cheese, red wine, chicken liver) and /or sympathomimetic drugs (e.g. amphetamine)	Tranylcypromine	Non-MAOIs	Prevent use of such agents with MAOI. Carry 'warning cards'. When crisis occurs, use alpha (α) blockers like phentolamine.
2. Severe hepatic necrosis (rare)	Toxic or Hypersensitive	Iproniazid	Tranylcypromine	Stop/change drug. Supportive care; Death rate high.
3. Hyperpyrexia	Interaction with tricyclics or meperidine	Not known	Not known	Stop drug. Keep a gap of 1 week between imipramine and MAOI. Supportive care.
4. Bleeding	Decreased platelet serotonin	SSRIs	Not known	Change drug. Do not co-prescribe other drugs that increase risk of bleeding; Gastro-protective drugs such as PPIs can decrease risk to some extent in high-risk patients

Contd...

Contd...

Category and Side Effect	*Probable Cause*	*Maximum with (For example)*	*Minimum with (For example)*	*Management*
5. Hyponatraemia	Probably SIADH	SSRIs SNRIs	Not known; Probably MAOIs	Risk higher in elderly; Avoid co-prescribing other drugs that cause hyponatraemia (such as diuretics); monitor closely

29. Talkativeness and flight of ideas are suggestive of:

a. Schizophrenia b. Hysteria
c. Mania d. Depression

A maniac episode is typically characterized by the following features (which should last for at least one week and cause disruption in occupational and social activities): elevated, expansive or irritable mood (euphoria), psychomotor activity, speech and thought (talkativeness, flight of ideas) and goal directed activity (tries to do many things at one time).

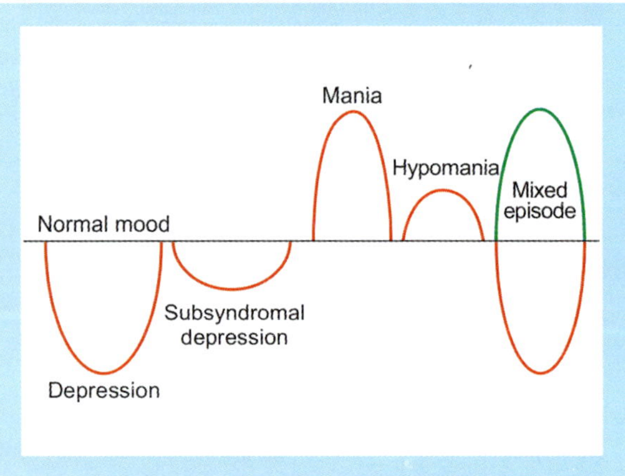

Bipolar disorder: clinical picture.

30. NOT a feature of mania:

a. Insomnia b. Pressure of speech
c. Disorientation d. Delusion of grandeur

Maniac patients are well oriented.

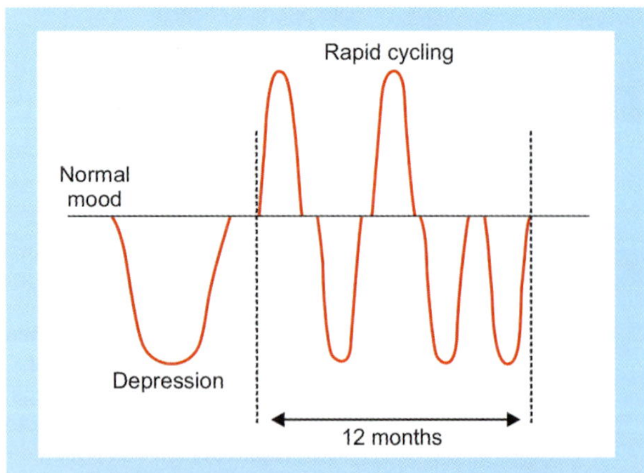

Bipolar Disorder: Rapid Cycling Clinical Picture.

31. Acute mania is managed by:

a. Electroconvulsive therapy
b. Lithium
c. Amitriptyline
d. Diazepam

Lithium has traditionally been the drug of choice for the treatment of manic episodes (acute phase) as well as for prevention of further episodes in bipolar mood disorder.

Some Prognostic Factors in Mood Disorders
Good Prognostic Factors
1. Acute or abrupt onset
2. Typical clinical features
3. Severe depression
4. Well-adjusted premorbid personality
5. Good response to treatment.
Poor Prognostic Factors
1. Co-morbid medical disorder, personality disorder or alcohol dependence
2. Double depression (acute depressive episode superimposed on chronic depression or dysthymia)
3. Catastrophic stress or chronic ongoing stress
4. Unfavourable early environment
5. Marked hypochondriacal features, or mood-incongruent psychotic features
6. Poor drug compliance.

CHILD PSYCHIATRY

32. Down syndrome presents as:

a. Mental instability b. Madness
c. Intellectual disability d. Oligophrenia

DS, also referred to as trisomy 21, is a genetic disorder caused by the presence of all or part of a third copy of chromosome 21. It is typically associated with physical growth delays, characteristic facial features and mild to moderate intellectual disability.

33. As per American Association of Mental Retardation, new term in use for mental retardation:

a. Mental instability
b. Learning disability
c. Feeble mindedness
d. Hyperlexia

Ans. **29. c.** Mania **30. c.** Disorientation **31. b.** Lithium **32. c.** Intellectual disability **33. b.** Learning disability

One to three percent of the general population has mental retardation. In some countries (such as UK), the word learning disability is used instead to avoid the pejorative connotations associated with the word mental retardation.

34. A 10-year-old child is very restless and hyperactive. His activities and running in school are very disturbing to his friends. Likely diagnosis is:

a. Schizophrenia
b. Attention deficit hyperactivity disorder
c. Autistic disorder
d. Conduct disorder

ADHD is commonest type of attention deficit disorder/ADD which is characterized by poor attention span with distractibility (doesn't seem to listen), hyperactivity (moving about here and there and difficulty in sitting still at one place for long) and impulsivity (acts before thinking, on the spur of the moment).

35. Autism is:

a. Neurodevelopmental disorder
b. Social and language communication problem
c. Metabolic disease
d. Mainly due to hypothalamic damage

Autism is one of the PDD (pervasive developmental disorder) characterized by marked impairment in reciprocal social and interpersonal interaction, marked impairment in language and non-verbal communication, abnormal behavioural characteristics (stereotyped behaviours such as head banging) and mental retardation.

36. DOC for attention deficit hyperactivity disorder is:

a. Haloperidol b. Imipramine
c. Methylphenidate d. Lecithin

Stimulant medication like Dextroamphetamine or dexamphetamine (2.5–20 mg/day) and methylphenidate (5–60 mg/day) have been traditionally used for managing ADD. Currently, Methylphenidate is the drug of choice in the treatment of ADD, with a high response rate.

37. A girl with normal milestones spends her time seeing her own hand and do NOT interact with others. Likely diagnosis is:

a. ADHD b. Autism
c. Asperger's syndrome d. Rett's syndrome

Autism is characterized by stereotyped behaviours such as head banging, body-spinning, hand-flicking, lining-up objects, rocking, clapping, twirling etc. and marked impairment in making friends.

38. A child fights with other children frequently. He has disciplinary problem in school and steals things. Most likely diagnosis is:

a. Autism
b. Attention deficit hyperkinetic disorder
c. Conduct disorder
d. Obsessive compulsive disorder

Conduct disorder is characterized by a persistent and significant pattern of conduct, in which the basic rights of others are violated or rules of society are not followed. The diagnosis is only made when the conduct is far in excess of the routine mischief of children and adolescents. The onset occurs much before 18 years of age, usually even before puberty.

NEUROSIS

39. Drug most useful in treatment of obsessive compulsive disorder:

a. Amoxapine b. Fluoxetine
c. Doxepin d. Dothiepin

Some patients of OCD may improve dramatically with specific serotonin reuptake inhibitors (SSRIs). Fluoxetine (20–80 mg/day) is a good alternative to clomipramine and often preferred these days for its better side-effect profile.

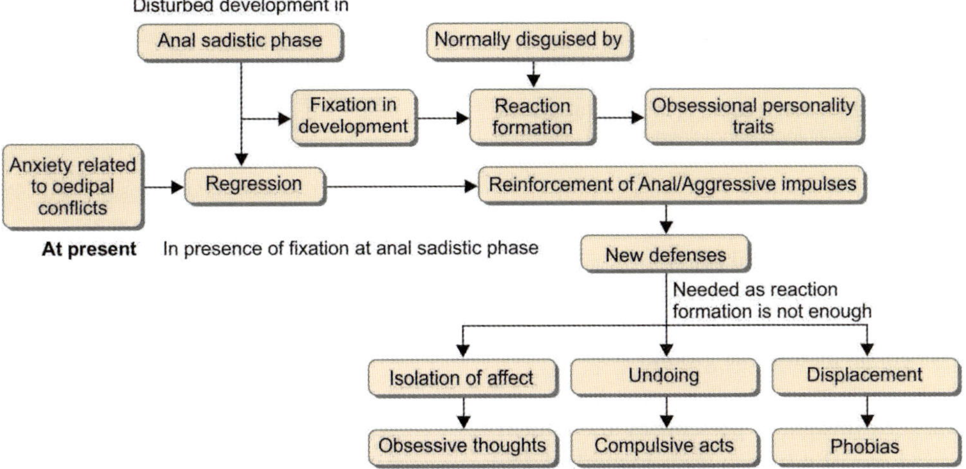

Psychodynamic Theory of Obsessive Compulsive Disorder: A Brief Summary.

Ans. 34. b. Attention deficit... 35. b. Social and language... 36. c. Methylphenidate 37. b. Autism 38. c. Conduct disorder 39. b. Fluoxetine

40. A 40-year-old female had headache for last 6 months. She had several consultations. All her investigations were normal. She still insists that there is something wrong and seeks another consultant. Most likely diagnosis is:

a. Phobia
b. Psychogenic headache
c. Hypochondriasis
d. Depression

Hypochondriasis is defined as a persistent preoccupation with a fear (or belief) of having one (or more) serious disease (s), based on person's own interpretation of normal body function or a minor physical abnormality.

41. A 30-year-old male presented with symptoms of palpitations and sweating on meeting seniors and on making public presentations. This makes him avoid such situations. The diagnosis is:

a. Panic reaction
b. Social phobia
c. Avoidance personality
d. Adjustment disorder

Social phobia is an example of irrational fear of activities of social interaction, characterized by an irrational fear of performing activities in the presence of other people or interacting with others. The patient is afraid of his own actions being viewed by others critically, resulting in embarrassment or humiliation.

Phobia: Some Characteristic Features
1. Presence of the fear of an object, situation or activity.
2. The fear is out of proportion to the dangerousness perceived.
3. Patient recognises the fear as irrational and unjustified (Insight is present).
4. Patient is unable to control the fear and is very distressed by it.
5. This leads to persistent avoidance of the particular object, situation or activity.
6. Gradually, the phobia and the phobic object become a preoccupation with the patient, resulting in marked distress and restriction of the freedom of mobility (afraid to encounter the phobic object; *phobic avoidance*).

42. Which statement differentiates the obsessional idea from delusion:

a. The idea is not a conventional belief
b. The idea is held in spite of contrary evidence
c. The idea is regarded as senseless by patient
d. The idea is held on inadequate ground

An obsession is perceived as ego-alien, recognized as irrational and absurd (insight is present) by the patient and patient tries to resist it (which leads to marked distress), whereas delusion is recognized as one's own idea but is not recognized as ego-alien. In fact, it is strongly believed; hence it is not thought to be irrational and is never resisted.

43. NOT a feature of post traumatic stress disorder:

a. Flashbacks
b. Hyperarousal
c. Hallucination
d. Emotional numbing

According to ICD-10, PTSD arises as a delayed and/or protracted response to an exceptionally stressful or catastrophic life event or situation, which is likely to cause pervasive distress in 'almost any person' (e.g. disasters, war, rape or torture, serious accident). The symptoms of PTSD may develop, after a period of latency, within six months after the stress or may be delayed beyond this period.

44. Female patient presented with acute restlessness and fear of impending doom. Most probable diagnosis is:

a. Schizophrenia
b. Delirium
c. Anxiety neurosis
d. MDP

Anxiety is a 'normal' phenomenon, which is characterized by a state of apprehension or unease arising out of anticipation of danger.

Symptoms of Anxiety
1. Physical Symptoms
A. *Motoric Symptoms:* Tremors; Restlessness; Muscle twitches; Fearful facial expression
B. *Autonomic and Visceral Symptoms:* Palpitations; Tachycardia; Sweating; Flushes; Dyspnoea; Hyperventilation; Constriction in the chest; Dry mouth; Frequency and hesitancy of micturition; Dizziness; Diarrhoea; Mydriasis
2. Psychological Symptoms
A. *Cognitive Symptoms:* Poor concentration; Distractibility; Hyperarousal; Vigilance or scanning; Negative automatic thoughts
B. *Perceptual Symptoms:* Derealisation; Depersonalisation
C. *Affective Symptoms:* Diffuse, unpleasant, and vague sense of apprehension; Fearfulness; Inability to relax; Irritability; Feeling of impending doom (when severe)
D. *Other Symptoms:* Insomnia (initial); Increased sensitivity to noise; Exaggerated startle response.

45. Difference between neurosis and psychosis is in:

a. Severity
b. Insight
c. Clinical features
d. Duration of onset

Symptoms of neurosis are recognized as undesirable (i.e. insight is present).

Ans. **40. c.** Hypochondriasis **41. b.** Social phobia **42. c.** The idea is regarded... **43. c.** Hallucination
44. c. Anxiety neurosis **45. b.** Insight

Definition of Psychosis
The term *psychosis* is defined as:
1. Gross impairment in reality-testing ('not in contact' with reality).
2. Marked disturbance in personality, with impairment in social, interpersonal and occupational functioning.
3. Marked impairment in judgement and absent understanding of the current symptoms and behaviour (loss of insight).
4. Presence of the characteristic symptoms, like delusions and hallucinations.

46. A 20-year-old female presented with complaints of nausea, vomiting and pain in the legs. Her physical examination and lab investigations are normal. What would be the most probable diagnosis:

a. Generalized anxiety disorder
b. Conversion disorder
c. Somatoform pain disorder
d. Somatization disorder

Persistent somatoform pain disorder was previously called as psychogenic pain disorder. In this disorder, persistent, severe, and distressing pain is the main feature, which is, either grossly in excess of what is expected from the physical findings, or inconsistent with the anatomical distribution of nervous system. Preoccupation with pain is common.

47. A 30-year-old lady complained of sudden onset of breathlessness, anxiety, palpitation and feeling of impending doom. Physical examination is normal. What is the diagnosis:

a. Panic attack b. Schizophrenia
c. Conversion disorder d. Acute psychosis

Panic disorder is characterized by discrete episodes of acute anxiety. The onset is usually in early third decade with often a chronic course. The episode is usually sudden, lasts for a few minutes and is characterized by very severe anxiety.

48. Obsessive compulsive disorder with Gilles de la Tourette's syndrome is managed by:

a. Fluoxetine b. Clonidine
c. Haloperidol d. Quetiapine

A special type of chronic tic disorder (abnormal involuntary movements) is Gilles de la Tourette's syndrome or Tourette's disorder. SSRIs (such as fluoxetine) have been used for the treatment of co-morbid obsessive compulsive symptoms.

MISCELLANEOUS

49. All of the following are true statement regarding Alzheimer's disease EXCEPT:

a. Example of dementia causing illnesses
b. Fully curable
c. More common in elderly
d. Memory loss may be seen

At present, Alzheimer's dementia is not considered a treatable disorder. However, Cholinesterase inhibitors such as Rivastigmine, Donepezil, and Galantamine have been used in the recent past for treatment of moderate dementia with Alzheimer's disease.

Dementia vs Pseudodementia

	Dementia	*Pseudodementia (Depressive)*
1.	Patient rarely complains of cognitive impairment	Patient usually always complains about memory impairment
2.	Patient often emphasises achievements	Patient often emphasises disability
3.	Patient often appears unconcerned	Patient very often communicates distress
4.	Usually labile affect	Severe depression on examination
5.	Patient makes errors on cognitive examination	'Do not know' answers are more frequent
6.	Recent memory impairment found on examination	Recent memory impairment rarely found on examination
7.	Confabulation may be present	Confabulation very rare
8.	Consistently poor performance on similar tests	Marked variability in performance on similar tests
9.	History of depression less common	Past history of manic and/or depressive episodes may be present

50. Which of the following is NOT a habit disorder:

a. Teeth grinding b. Temper tantrum
c. Thumb sucking d. Nail biting

A tantrum, temper tantrum, meltdown or hissy fit is an emotional outburst, usually associated with children or those in emotional distress, that is typically characterised by stubbornness, crying, screaming, defiance, anger rating, a resistance to attempts at pacification, and, in some cases, hitting, and other physically violent behaviour. Physical control may be lost.

51. Which of the following is NOT a component of Sigmond Freud's theory of dream:

a. Correlation b. Symbolization
c. Condensation d. Displacement

Ans.
46. **c.** Somatoform pain disorder
47. **a.** Panic attack
48. **a.** Fluoxetine
49. **b.** Fully curable
50. **b.** Temper tantrum
51. **a.** Correlation

According to the theory of dreams, the dream work consists of the following mechanisms: 1. Symbolism, 2. Displacement, 3. Condensation, 4. Projection and 5. Secondary elaboration.

52. A patient complains of accidents in his dreams. There is a past history of road traffic accident 2 months back. Whenever he visited the accident site, he remembers all the episode related to his accident and therefore he is very apprehensive of visiting that place. He is most likely suffering from:

a. Obsessive compulsive disorder
b. Borderline personality disorder
c. Post-traumatic stress disorder
d. Acute delirium

According to ICD-10, PTSD arises as a delayed and/protracted response to an exceptionally stressful or catastrophic life event or situation, which is likely to cause pervasive distress in 'almost any person' (e.g. disasters, was, rape or torture, serious accident). The symptoms of PTSD may develop, after a period of latency, within six months after the stress or may be delayed beyond this period.

53. Squeeze technique is employed in the management of:

a. Antegrade ejaculation
b. Retrograde ejaculation
c. Erectile dysfunction
d. Premature ejaculation

Squeeze technique (Seman's technique) has been used in treatment of PME. The female partner is asked to manually stimulate the penis causing erection. When the male partner experiences 'ejaculatory inevitability', the female partner 'squeezes' the penis on the coronal ridge thus delaying ejaculation.

54. Which of the following differentiates delirium from dementia:

a. Abrupt sudden change
b. Confusion
c. Hallucination
d. Difficulty in communicating

Delirium is characterised by a relatively acute onset.

A Comparison of Delirium and Dementia

	Features	Delirium	Dementia
1.	Onset	Usually acute	Usually insidious
2.	Course	Usually recover in 1 week; may take up to 1 month	Usually protracted, although may be reversible in some cases
3.	Clinical features		
	a. Consciousness	Clouded	Usually normal
	b. Orientation	Grossly disturbed	Usually normal; disturbed only in late stages
	c. Memory	Immediate retention and recall disturbed Recent memory disturbed	Immediate retention and recall normal Recent memory disturbed Remote memory disturbed only in late stages
	d. Comprehension	Impaired	Impaired only in late stages
	e. Sleep-wake cycle	Grossly disturbed	Usually normal
	f. Attention and concentration	Grossly disturbed	Usually normal
	g. Diurnal variation	Marked; sundowning may be present	Usually absent
	h. Perception	Visual illusions and hallucinations very common	Hallucinations may occur
	i. Other features	Asterixis; multifocal myoclonus	Catastrophic reaction; perseveration

55. Which of the following correlates with expression and consequent release of previously repressed emotion:

a. Dissociation
b. Regression
c. Association
d. Abreaction

Abreaction is an important procedure which belongs to conscious awareness, for the first time, unconsciousness conflicts and associated emotions.

56. Subcortical dementia is seen in all EXCEPT:

a. Parkinsonism
b. Alzheimer's disease
c. Wilson's disease
d. Huntington's chorea

Autopsy of Alzheimer's disease shows macroscopic changes such as enlarged cerebral ventricles, widened cerebral sulci and shrinkage of cerebral cortex, as well as microscopic changes such as senile plaques, neurofibrillary tangles, cortical nerve cell loss, and granulovacuolar degeneration.

Ans. **52. c.** Post-traumatic... **53. d.** Premature ejaculation **54. a.** Abrupt sudden... **55. d.** Abreaction **56. b.** Alzheimer's disease

Cortical and Subcortical Dementia		
Features	*Cortical Dementia*	*Subcortical Dementia*
1. Site of lesion	Cortex (frontal and temporoparieto-occipital association areas, and hippocampus)	Subcortical grey matter (thalamus, basal ganglia, and rostral brain stem)
2. Examples	Alzheimer's disease, Pick's disease	Huntingtons' chorea, Parkinson's disease, Progressive supranuclear palsy, Wilson's disease
3. Severity	Severe	Mild to moderate
4. Motor system	Usually normal	Dysarthria, flexed/extended posture, tremors, dystonia, chorea, ataxia, rigidity
5. Other features	Simple delusions; depression uncommon; severe aphasia, amnesia, agnosia, apraxia, acalculia, slowed cognitive speed (bradyphrenia)	Complex delusions; depression common; rarely mania
6. Memory deficit (Short-term)	Recall helped very little by cues	Recall partially helped by cues and recognition tasks

57. Delusion is a disorder of:

a. Thought b. Perception
c. Insight d. Cognition

Delusion is a false unshaken belief which is not amenable to reasoning, and is not in keeping with the patient's socio-cultural and educational background.

58. Circadian rhythm is controlled by:

a. Raphe nuclei b. Suprachiasmatic nuclei
c. Thalamus d. Red nucleus

Suprachiasmatic nuclei of hypothalamus controls circadian rhythm.

59. NOT a feature of paradoxical sleep:

a. Decreased muscle tone
b. Rapid eye movement
c. Brain shows increased metabolism
d. EEG shows decreased activity

One of the most characteristic features of REM-sleep is the presence of REM or rapid (conjugate) eye movements. The other features include generalised muscular atony, penile erection, autonomic hyperactivity (increase in pulse rate, respiratory rate and blood pressure), and movements of small muscle groups, occurring intermittently.

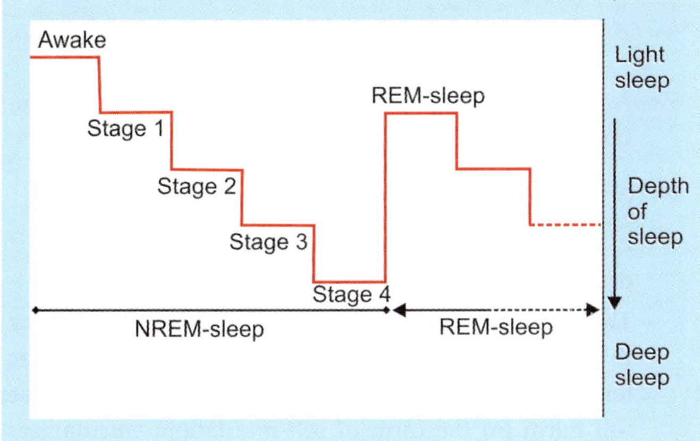

Stages of Sleep.

60. A male of 15 years with a mental age of 9 years has an IQ of:

a. 50 b. 60
c. 70 d. 80

IQ (Intelligence Quotient) which is equal to the mental age, i.e. MA, divided by chronological age, i.e. CA, multiplied by 100, i.e. IQ = MA/CA × 100

Classification of Mental Retardation by IQ	
Mental Retardation Level	*IQ Range*
1. Mild	50-70*
2. Moderate	35-50*
3. Severe	20-35*
4. Profound	<20*

(*As intelligence tests employed to measure IQ generally have an error of measurement of about 5 points, each figure means ± 5 points, e.g. IQ of 50 means an IQ of 50 ± 5, depending on the adaptive behaviour).

61. A 16-year-old male is found to have a mental age of 9 years on IQ testing. He has:

a. Mild mental retardation
b. Moderate mental retardation
c. Severe mental retardation
d. Profound mental retardation

IQ of 50-70 is categorized as mild MR.

Some Causes of Mental Retardation
1. Genetic (probably in 5% of cases)
i. Chromosomal abnormalities (such as Down's syndrome, Fragile-X syndrome, Turner's syndrome, Klinefelter's syndrome)
ii. Inborn errors of metabolism, involving amino-acids (phenylketonuria, homo-cystinuria, Hartnup's disease), lipids (Tay-Sachs disease, Gaucher's disease, Niemann-Pick disease), carbohydrates (galactosaemia, glycogen storage diseases), purines (Lesch-Nyhan syndrome), and mucopolysaccharides (Hurler's disease, Hunter's disease, Sanfilippo's disease).
iii. Single-gene disorders (such as tuberous sclerosis, neurofibromatosis, dystrophia myotonica)
iv. Cranial anomalies (such as microcephaly)

Contd...

Ans. 57. a. Thought 58. b. Suprachiasmatic nuclei 59. d. EEG shows decrea... 60. b. 60
61. a. Mild mental retardation

Contd...

Some Causes of Mental Retardation
2. **Perinatal causes (probably in 10% of cases)** i. Infections (such as rubella, syphilis, toxoplasmosis, cytomegalo-inclusion body disease) ii. Prematurity iii. Birth trauma iv. Hypoxia v. Intrauterine growth retardation (IUGR) vi. Kernicterus vii. Placental abnormalities viii. Drugs during first trimester.
3. **Acquired physical disorders in childhood** (probably in 2-5% of cases) i. Infections, especially encephalopathies ii. Cretinism iii. Trauma iv. Lead poisoning v. Cerebral palsy.
4. **Sociocultural causes** (probably in 15% of cases) i. Deprivation of sociocultural stimulation.

Contd...

Contd...

Some Causes of Mental Retardation
5. **Psychiatric disorders** (probably in 1–2% of cases) i. Pervasive developmental disorders (such as Infantile autism) ii. Childhood onset schizophrenia.

62. FALSE perception without any external stimulus is:

a. Hallucination b. Delusion
c. Illusion d. Mania

A hallucination is a perception experienced in the absence of an external stimulus. The hallucinations can be in the auditory, visual, olfactory, gustatory or tactile domains.

63. Othello syndrome is delusion of:

a. Doubles b. Infidelity
c. Grandeur d. Persecution

When the content of delusions is predominantly jealousy (infidelity) involving the spouse, it is called as Othello syndrome or conjugal paranoia.

Differential Diagnosis of Delusional Disorders

Features	*Paranoid Schizophrenia*	*Delusional Disorder (Paranoid disorder)*	*Paranoid Personality Disorder*
1. General behaviour	Eccentricities, mannerisms, stereotypies, decreased self-care, social withdrawal, guarded and evasive	Eccentricities, decreased social interaction	Restrained social interaction
2. Personality	Disorganised (although deterioration is much less than in other types of schizophrenia)	Disturbed in delusional area, near normal in other areas	No deterioration
3. Thought disorder	Delusions, Schneiderian FRS, loosening of associations, formal thought disorder; delusions may be bizarre	Nonbizarre delusions which are well-systematised, no other thought disorder	No thought disorder
4. Hallucinations	Auditory hallucinations common	Uncommon. If present, are not persistent	Absent
5. Contact with reality	Markedly disturbed	Disturbed in area of delusional belief	Intact
6. Insight	Absent	Absent	Present
7. Affect/mood in relation to thought	Often inappropriate	Usually appropriate	Usually appropriate

64. A patient is depressed for last 3 years, do NOT go out of his house much and is isolated from the society. He is having normal weight and normal sleep. Most probably he is having:

a. No psychiatric illness
b. Chronic fatigue syndrome
c. Dysthymia d. Major depression

If the symptoms consist of persistent mild depression, the disorder is called as dysthymia; and if symptoms consist of persistent instability of mood between mild depression and mild elation, the disorder is called as cyclothymia.

65. A young patient with self mutilating behaviour and impulsivity is having:

a. Paranoid personality disorder
b. Adjustment disorder
c. Borderline personality disorder
d. Dependent personality disorder

The borderline type of personality is also known as borderline personality disorder (DSM-IV-TR), the characteristic features of which include impulsivity, deliberate self harm (in the form of self-mutilation, suicidal gestures, or accident proneness) etc.

Ans. 62. **a.** Hallucination 63. **b.** Infidelity 64. **c.** Dysthymia 65. **c.** Borderline personality...

66. A person confuses rope for snake:

a. Hallucination b. Illusion
c. Delusion d. Depersonalization

An illusion is a misinterpretation of stimuli arising from external object(s).

67. Psychoanalysis was introduced by:

a. Schielder b. Sigmund Freud
c. Dale and De Nicker d. Eugen Beuler

Freudian psychoanalysis typically needs 2-5 visits/week by the patient for a period of 3-5 years (even longer). No detailed history taking, mental status examination, or formalized psychiatric diagnosis is attempted. The patient is allowed to communicate unguided, by using 'free association'.

Psychosocial Therapies

	Therapy/School	*Proponent(s)*
1.	Psychoanalysis	Sigmund Freud
2.	Analytical psychology	Carl Gustav Jung
3.	Behaviourism	John Broadus Watson
4.	Character analysis	Wilhelm Reich
5.	Classical conditioning	Ivan Petrovich Pavlov
6.	Client-centred psycho-therapy	Carl R Rogers
7.	Cognitive behaviour therapy	Donald Meichenbaum
8.	Cognitive therapy	Aaron T Beck
9.	Dual sex therapy	William Masters and Virginia Johnson
10.	Existential logotherapy	Victor E Frankl
11.	Gestalt therapy	Frederich Perls
12.	Group therapy	Joseph Pratt
13.	Hypnosis	James Braid
14.	Operant conditioning	Burrhus Frederic Skinner
15.	Primal therapy	Arthur Janov
16.	Progressive muscular relaxation	E. Jacobson
17.	Psychodrama	Jacob L Moreno
18.	Rational emotive therapy	Albert Ellis
19.	Reciprocal inhibition	Joseph Wolpe
20.	Therapeutic community	Maxwell Jones
21.	Token economy	Ayllon and Azrin
22.	Transactional analysis	Eric Berne
23.	Will therapy	Otto Rank

68. Freud's theory of unconscious, preconscious and the conscious is:

a. Organic theory of mind
b. Structural theory of mind
c. Functional theory of mind
d. Topographic theory of mind

Topographical theory of mind was advanced by Freud in the year 1990, in the book called 'The interpretation of Dreams'. Although it was later on replaced by structural theory, it is still useful in understanding the mental mechanisms. The tripartite division of mind included the unconscious, the preconscious and the conscious.

69. Concept of Id, Ego and Super-ego was given by:

a. Pavlov b. Sigmund Freud
c. Karl Kahlbaum d. Eugen Bleuler

In 1923, in 'The Ego and the Id', Freud divided the mental apparatus into three dynamic structures: the id, the ego and the super-ego.

Commonly used Ego Defense Mechanisms

Defense Mechanism	*Definition*	*Example(s) in Normal life*	*Illustration(s) from Clinical Situations*
A. Primary			
1. Repression	Unconsciously excluding from conscious awareness of anxiety provoking ideas and/or feelings	1. 'Forgetting' 2. Slips of the tongue	Psychogenic amnesia
B. Psychotic/Narcissistic			
1. Regression	Reversion to modes of psychological functioning that are characteristic of earlier life stages, especially childhood years	1. Dreams 2. *Regression in the service of ego* (ability of a mature adult to appropriately indulge periodically in playful childlike activities)	1. Neuroses (mild regression) 2. Psychoses (more pervasive regression) 3. Severe, prolonged physical illness
2. Denial	Involuntary exclusion of unpleasant or painful reality from conscious awareness	1. Grief 2. Children (3-6 year olds)	1. Psychoses 2. Alcohol dependence

Contd...

Ans. 66. **b.** Illusion 67. **b.** Sigmund Freud 68. **d.** Topographic theory of mind 69. **b.** Sigmund Freud

Contd...

Defense Mechanism	*Definition*	*Example(s) in Normal life*	*Illustration(s) from Clinical Situations*
3. Projection	Unconscious attribution of one's own attitudes and urges to other person(s), because of intolerance or painful affect aroused by those attitudes and urges	A universal phenomenon though occurs more commonly in children	Persecutory delusions and hallucinations
4. Distortion	Unconscious gross 'reshaping' of external reality to satisfy inner needs	—	1. Hallucinations 2. Delusions, especially of grandiosity
C. Neurotic/Immature			
1. Conversion	A repressed, forbidden urge is simultaneously kept out of awareness and also expressed in symbolic/ disguised form of some somatic conversion 'reaction' (usually either motor or sensory)	Sometimes seen in normal individuals when exposed to catastrophic stress; otherwise presence always implies psychopathology	Conversion disorder (Hysteria)
2. Dissociation	Involuntary splitting or suppression of a mental function or a group of mental functions from rest of the personality in a manner that allows expression of forbidden unconscious impulses without having any sense of responsibility for actions	Near death experience	Dissociative disorders, e.g. psychogenic amnesia, psychogenic fugue, multiple personality, somnambulism, possession syndrome
3. Displacement	Unconscious shifting of emotions, usually aroused by perceived threat, from an unconscious impulse to a less threatening external object which is then felt to be the source of threat	Normal, day-to-day deflection of 'anger' on a substitute target	1. Phobia (especially in children) 2. OCD
4. Isolation (Isolation of affect)	Separation of the idea of an unconscious impulse from its appropriate affect, thus allowing only the idea and not the associated affect to enter awareness	1. Grief 2. Ability to discuss traumatic events without the associated disturbing emotions, with passage of time	Obsessional thoughts
5. Reaction formation	Unconscious transformation of unacceptable impulses into exactly opposite attitudes, impulses, feelings or behaviours	Normal character formation in childhood (from 3 years onwards)	Obsessive compulsive personality traits and disorder
6. Undoing	Unconsciously motivated acts which magically/symbolically counteract unacceptable thoughts, impulses or acts	1. Checking of gas knobs or locks to ensure safety 2. Automatically saying 'I am sorry' on bumping into somebody	1. Compulsive acts in OCD 2. Compulsive rituals
7. Rationalisation	Providing 'logical' explanations for irrational behaviour motivated by unacceptable unconscious wishes	A universal phenomenon	Usually used to explain behaviours resulting from other defense mechanisms
8. Intellectualisation	Excessive use of intellectual processes (logic) to avoid affective expression (emotion)	When faced with stressful situation, use of logic to focus closely on external reality and avoiding expression of inner feelings (e.g. fear)	—
9. Acting out	Expression of an unconscious impulse, through action, thereby gratifying the impulse	Destruction of any object in a 'fit of rage'	Impulse control disorders
10. Schizoid fantasy	Withdrawal into self to gratify frustrated wishes by fantasy	Seen in adolescence (wish fulfilling daydreams)	Schizoid and schizotypal personality disorder
11. Turning against the self (Retroflexion)	Unconscious deflection of hostility towards another person onto oneself resulting in lowered self-esteem, self-criticism and at times injury to self	1. Head banging in children 2. Destruction of property or self in a fit of rage	1. Suicide 2. Severe depression 3. Any form of deliberate self harm (DSH)

Contd...

Contd...

Defense Mechanism	*Definition*	*Example(s) in Normal life*	*Illustration(s) from Clinical Situations*
12. Introjection	Unconscious internalisation of the qualities of an object or person	1. Identification with the aggressor (e.g. sometimes seen in victims kidnapped by terrorists; also known as *Stockholm syndrome*) 2. Grief reaction	Depression
13. Hypochondriasis	Unconscious transformation of unacceptable impulses into inappropriate somatic concern	Abnormal illness behaviour in physically disordered or normal individuals	Hypochondriasis
14. Inhibition	Involuntary decrease or loss of motivation to engage in some goal-directed activity to prevent anxiety arising out of conflicts with unacceptable impulses	1. Writing 'blocks' or work 'blocks' 2. Social shyness	1. OCD 2. Phobias
15. Compensation (Counter-phobic defense)	Unconscious tendency to deal with a fear or conflict by unusual degree of effort in the opposite direction	1. Involvement in dare-devil activities (e.g. sky diving to counter fear of heights) 2. Excessive pre-occupation with body building to counter feelings of inferiority	1. Nymphomania (to counter a sense of sexual inadequacy) 2. Keeping excessive details in a diary in patients suffering from dementia
16. Splitting	Unconscious viewing of self or others as either good or bad without considering the whole range of qualities	Believing personalities to be either 'black' or 'white' without the shades of 'grey' (e.g. in a 'typical' Bollywood movie, the Hero often is all good and the Villain all bad)	Borderline personality disorder
D. Mature			
1. Sublimation	Unconscious gradual channelisation of unacceptable infantile impulses into personally satisfying and socially valuable behaviour patterns	Channelisation of sexual or aggressive impulses into creative activities (e.g. diverting forbidden sexual impulses into artistic paintings)	—
2. Suppression (Voluntary)	Voluntary postponement of focusing of attention on an impulse which has reached conscious awareness	Voluntary decision not to think about an argument with a close friend while going for an interview	—
3. Anticipation	Realistic thinking and planning about future unpleasurable events	Anticipation is a universal phenomenon occurring in all intelligent individuals	—
4. Humour	Overt expression of unacceptable impulses using humour in a manner which does not produce unpleasantness in self or others	A universal phenomenon	—

No ego defense mechanism is psychotic, neurotic, immature, mature or normal per se. Almost all mechanisms of defense are sometimes used in normal individuals. It is an exclusive or abnormally excessive use that makes a defense mechanism neurotic or psychotic.

70. Mental status examination is:

a. Method to investigate common psychiatric problem
b. 30 point programme to evaluate cognitive function
c. To evaluate schizophrenia
d. Instrument to measure delirium

MSE is a standardized format in which the clinician records the psychiatric signs and symptoms present at the time of the interview.

Mental Status Examination
1. General Appearance and Behaviour
i. General Appearance
ii. Attitude towards Examiner
iii. Comprehension
iv. Gait and Posture
v. Motor Activity
vi. Social Manner
vii. Rapport

Contd...

Ans. 70. b. 30 point programme to evaluate cognitive function

Contd...

Mental Status Examination
2. **Speech** i. Rate and Quantity ii. Volume and Tone iii. Flow and Rhythm
3. **Mood and Affect**
4. **Thought** i. Stream and Form ii. Content
5. **Perception**
6. **Cognition (Higher Mental Functions)** i. Consciousness ii. Orientation
iii. Attention iv. Concentration v. Memory vi. Intelligence vii. Abstract thinking
7. **Insight**
8. **Judgement**

71. Mental status examination does NOT include:

a. Insight b. Cognition
c. Age of the patient d. Motor activity

MSE should describe all areas of mental functioning. Some areas, however, may deserve more emphasis according to the clinical impressions that may arise from the history; for example, mood and affect in depression, and cognitive functions in delirium and depression.

72. Profound mental retardation is defined as:

a. 0-20 b. 21-40
c. 41-60 d. 61-80

IQ less than 20 is considered as profound MR.

73. IQ of 60 falls under which classification of mental retardation:

a. Mild
b. Moderate
c. Severe
d. Profound

IQ range of 50-70 is considered as mild MR.

Normal Developmental Milestones	
Age	*Developmental Milestones*
1. Motor Behaviour	
< 4 weeks	Moves head laterally in prone position
4 weeks	Momentarily lifts head when prone
3 months	Head-holding; Lifts head to 90° when prone
5 months	Sits with support; Rolls over
6 months	Lifts head and upper chest with support of extended arms
8 months	Sits steadily with straight back; Crawls; Early stepping movements when feet are placed on ground, with support
10 months	Pulls from supine to sitting and sitting to standing; Stands holding furniture; Cruises around; Stands without support momentarily; Creeps on ground without support of abdomen
14-15 months	Walks well without support; Walks backwards and sideways
2 years	Runs well; Climbs stairs alone; Kicks a large ball; Throws a ball overhead
2½ years	Walks on tip-toes
3 years	Climbs stairs in a coordinated manner, with alternate feet going up the staircase; Rides a tricycle; Makes a broad jump; Jumps in place
4 years	Stands on one foot for 5 seconds
5 years	Heel-to-toe walk; Jumps on one foot
2. Adaptive Behaviour (includes fine motor movements)	
4 weeks	Momentarily regards close moving objects, close to mid-line
3 months	Follows the moving objects, even away from mid-line; converges and focuses
4-5 months	Grasps objects crudely; Reaches to grasp
6 months	Transfer objects from one hand to other
9-10 months	Claps hands and matches two hand-held objects in mid line; Thumb-finger grasp
1 year	Gives hand-held objects to mother, when asked; Turns 2-3 pages of a book at one time
1½ years	Makes a tower of 3-4 cubes; Scribbles spontaneously, imitating writing; Sometimes may draw a vertical line
2 years	Turns one page of a book at one time; Makes a tower of 6-7 cubes; Draws (copies) a horizontal line
3 years	Makes a tower of 9-10 cubes; Makes a 3-cube bridge; Draws (copies) a circle.

Contd...

Ans. **71. c.** Age of the patient **72. a.** 0-20 **73. a.** Mild

Contd...

Age	*Developmental Milestones*
4 years	Draws (copies) a cross.
5 years	Draws (copies) a square; Draws (copies) a recognisable man
6 years	Draws (copies) a triangle
7 years	Draws (copies) a diamond 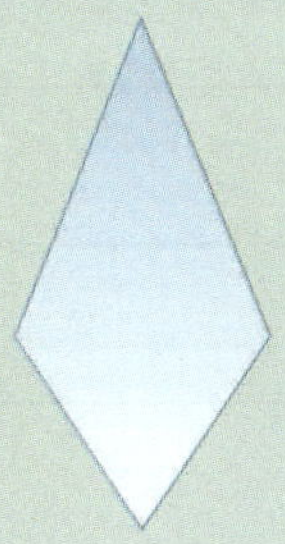
8 years	Draws (copies) the following figures 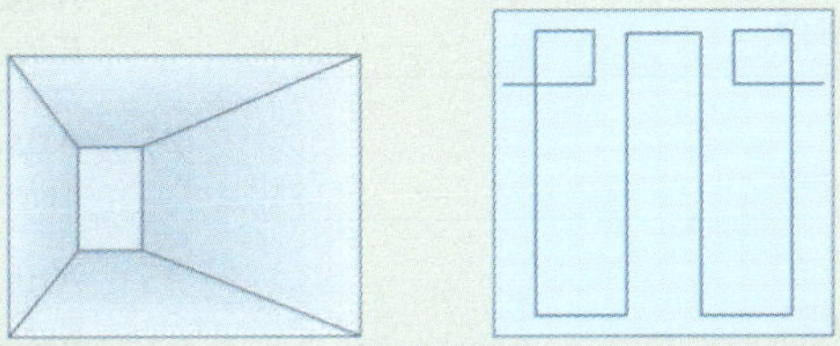
9 years	Draws (copies) the following figure 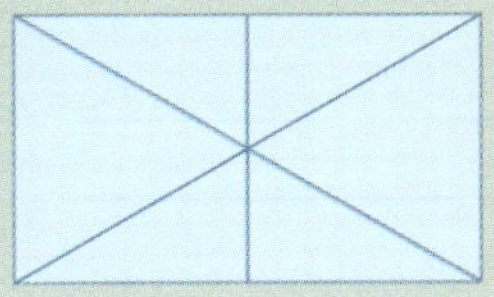
3. Language	
4 weeks	Turns head and responds to sound of a bell; Vocalises (apart from crying)
3 months	Laughs aloud
9 months	Speaks mama, dada, m-m-m, ah (and other vowel sounds); Responds to name
10 months	Understands spoken speech to some extent, e.g. where is 'mama'?
1-1¼ years	Uses 3-5 words meaningfully
18 months	About 10 words spoken including name
2 years	Combines 2 different words; Names at least one object in picture; Points to at least one named body part; Simple sentences made
3 years	Uses plurals; Has a fairly good vocabulary
5 years	Colour naming accurately (primary colours); Defines words
4. Personal and Social Behaviour	
4 weeks	Regards face intently
2-3 months	Social smile
3 months	Recognises mother
6 months	Takes foot to mouth; Smiles back at mirror-image of self
9 months	Responds to social play; Resists pulling away of toy and tries to reach for it; Holds milk-bottle and eats a biscuit all by oneself
1½ years	Feeds oneself with a spoon, with little spilling; Mimics actions of others; Pulls a toy with a string; Toilet training started
2 years	Wears simple garments, socks and shoes
3 years	Unbuttons buttons; Buckles shoes; Can dress and undress, with help
4 years	Buttons the dress well; Washes own face; Plays with other children easily; Separates from mother with little difficulty.
5 years	Dresses without supervision.

ANSWERS WITH REFERENCES

PSYCHOACTIVE SUBSTANCE USE DISORDER

1. **Ans. (c)** Delirium tremens
   Ref: Ahuja's Psychiatry, 7/e p38
2. **Ans. (c)** Alcoholism
   Ref: Ahuja's Psychiatry 7/e p39
3. **Ans. (b)** Cannabis
   Ref: Ahuja's Psychiatry 7/e p35
4. **Ans. (a)** Hallucination
   Ref: Ahuja's Psychiatry 7/e p37
5. **Ans. (d)** Cocaine
   Ref: Ahuja's Psychiatry 7/e p47
6. **Ans. (a)** Diazepam
   Ref: Ahuja's Psychiatry 7/e p39
7. **Ans. (b)** Tachycardia
   Ref: Ahuja's Psychiatry 7/e p52
8. **Ans. (b)** 24-48 hours
   Ref: Ahuja's Psychiatry 7/e p39

SCHIZOPHRENIA

9. **Ans. (c)** Schizophrenia
   Ref: Ahuja's Psychiatry 7/e p55
10. **Ans. (c)** Dopamine
    Ref: Ahuja's Psychiatry 7/e p64
11. **Ans. (c)** Auditory hallucination
    Ref: Ahuja's Psychiatry 7/e p58
12. **Ans. (b)** Automatism
    Ref: Ahuja's Psychiatry 7/e p55
13. **Ans. (b)** Amphetamine
    Ref: Ahuja's Psychiatry 7/e p62
14. **Ans. (d)** Clozapine
    Ref: Ahuja's Psychiatry 7/e p66
15. **Ans. (c)** Delusion of self reference
    Ref: Ahuja's Psychiatry 7/e p59
16. **Ans. (d)** Sustained mood changes
    Ref: Ahuja's Psychiatry 7/e p62
17. **Ans. (c)** Agranulocytosis
    Ref: Ahuja's Psychiatry 7/e p66
18. **Ans. (d)** Schizophrenia
    Ref: Ahuja's Psychiatry 7/e p66
19. **Ans. (a)** Clozapine
    Ref: Ahuja's Psychiatry 7/e p66

MOOD DISORDERS

20. **Ans. (b)** Serotonin and norepinephrine
    Ref: Ahuja's Psychiatry 7/e p73
21. **Ans. (d)** Electroconvulsive therapy
    Ref: Ahuja's Psychiatry 7/e p200
22. **Ans. (a)** Inhibition of serotonin uptake
    Ref: Ahuja's Psychiatry 7/e p183
23. **Ans. (b)** Polyuria
    Ref: Ahuja's Psychiatry 7/e p190
24. **Ans. (c)** Amnesia
    Ref: Ahuja's Psychiatry 7/e p203
25. **Ans. (a)** Depression with suicidal tendencies
    Ref: Ahuja's Psychiatry 7/e p72
26. **Ans. (b)** Narrow therapeutic index
    Ref: Ahuja's Psychiatry 7/e p190
27. **Ans. (a)** Lithium
    Ref: Ahuja's Psychiatry 7/e p190
28. **Ans. (b)** Fluoxetine
    Ref: Ahuja's Psychiatry 7/e p186
29. **Ans. (c)** Mania
    Ref: Ahuja's Psychiatry 7/e p73
30. **Ans. (c)** Disorientation
    Ref: Ahuja's Psychiatry 7/e p74
31. **Ans. (b)** Lithium
    Ref: Ahuja's Psychiatry 7/e p74

CHILD PSYCHIATRY

32. **Ans. (c)** Intellectual disability
    Ref: Internet resources
33. **Ans. (b)** Learning disability
    Ref: Ahuja's Psychiatry, 7/e p155
34. **Ans. (b)** Attention deficit hyperactivity disorder
    Ref: Ahuja's Psychiatry 7/e p166
35. **Ans. (b)** Social and language communication problem
    Ref: Ahuja's Psychiatry 7/e p164
36. **Ans. (c)** Methylphenidate
    Ref: Ahuja's Psychiatry 7/e p167

37. **Ans. (b) Autism**
Ref: Ahuja's Psychiatry 7/e p164

38. **Ans. (c) Conduct disorder**
Ref: Ahuja's Psychiatry 7/e p167

NEUROSIS

39. **Ans. (b) Fluoxetine**
Ref: Ahuja's Psychiatry 7/e p97

40. **Ans. (c) Hypochondriasis**
Ref: Ahuja's Psychiatry 7/e p105

41. **Ans. (b) Social phobia**
Ref: Ahuja's Psychiatry 7/e p92

42. **Ans. (c) The idea is regarded as senseless by patient**
Ref: Ahuja's Psychiatry 7/e p95

43. **Ans. (c) Hallucination**
Ref: Ahuja's Psychiatry 7/e p112

44. **Ans. (c) Anxiety neurosis**
Ref: Ahuja's Psychiatry 7/e p90

45. **Ans. (b) Insight**
Ref: Ahuja's Psychiatry 7/e p83

46. **Ans. (c) Somatoform pain disorder**
Ref: Ahuja's Psychiatry 7/e p109

47. **Ans. (a) Panic attack**
Ref: Ahuja's Psychiatry 7/e p90

48. **Ans. (a) Fluoxetine**
Ref: Ahuja's Psychiatry 7/e p168

MISCELLANEOUS

49. **Ans. (b) Fully curable**
Ref: Ahuja's Psychiatry, 7/e p23

50. **Ans. (b) Temper tantrum**
Ref: Ahuja's Psychiatry, 7/e p170

51. **Ans. (a) Correlation**
Ref: Ahuja's Psychiatry, 7/e p212

52. **Ans. (c) Post-traumatic stress disorder**
Ref: Ahuja's Psychiatry, 7/e p112

53. **Ans. (d) Premature ejaculation**
Ref: Ahuja's Psychiatry, 7/e p131

54. **Ans. (a) Abrupt sudden change**
Ref: Ahuja's Psychiatry, 7/e p22

55. **Ans. (d) Abreaction**
Ref: Ahuja's Psychiatry, 7/e p218

56. **Ans. (b) Alzheimer's disease**
Ref: Ahuja's Psychiatry 7/e p24

57. **Ans. (a) Thought**
Ref: Ahuja's Psychiatry 7/e p246

58. **Ans. (b) Suprachiasmatic nuclei**
Ref: Internet resources

59. **Ans. (d) EEG shows decreased activity**
Ref: Ahuja's Psychiatry 7/e p134

60. **Ans. (b) 60**
Ref: Ahuja's Psychiatry 7/e p156

61. **Ans. (a) Mild mental retardation**
Ref: Ahuja's Psychiatry 7/e p157

62. **Ans. (a) Hallucination**
Ref: Ahuja's Psychiatry 7/e p13

63. **Ans. (b) Infidelity**
Ref: Ahuja's Psychiatry 7/e p84

64. **Ans. (c) Dysthymia**
Ref: Ahuja's Psychiatry 7/e p73

65. **Ans. (c) Borderline personality disorder**
Ref: Ahuja's Psychiatry 7/e p117

66. **Ans. (b) Illusion**
Ref: Ahuja's Psychiatry 7/e p247

67. **Ans. (b) Sigmund Freud**
Ref: Ahuja's Psychiatry 7/e p213

68. **Ans. (d) Topographic theory of mind**
Ref: Ahuja's Psychiatry 7/e p205

69. **Ans. (b) Sigmund Freud**
Ref: Ahuja's Psychiatry 7/e p206

70. **Ans. (b) 30 point programme to evaluate cognitive function**
Ref: Ahuja's Psychiatry 7/e p11

71. **Ans. (c) Age of the patient**
Ref: Ahuja's Psychiatry 7/e p 11

72. **Ans. (a) 0-20**
Ref: Ahuja's Psychiatry 7/e p156

73. **Ans. (a) Mild**
Ref: Ahuja's Psychiatry 7/e p154

PRACTICE QUESTIONS

PSYCHOACTIVE SUBSTANCE USE DISORDERS

1. Most severe manifestation of alcohol withdrawal:
a. Rum fits
b. Alcoholic hallucinosis
c. Delirium tremens
d. Hangover next morning

SCHIZOPHRENIA

2. First episode of schizophrenia should be treated upto:
a. 1 year b. 2-3 years
c. 5 years d. Lifelong

3. Anti-psychotic drug with LEAST extra-pyramidal side effects/EPSE:
a. Fluphenazine b. Haloperidol
c. Flupentixol d. Clozapine

4. Paranoid schizophrenia is a side effect of:
a. Chloroquine
b. Amiodarone
c. Metoclopramide
d. Amphetamine

MOOD DISORDERS

5. Neurotransmitter decreased in depression are all of the following EXCEPT:
a. Norepinephrine b. Dopamine
c. Serotonin d. Dobutamine

6. Nihilistic delusion, delusion of guilt and poverty are suggestive of:
a. Mania b. Phobia
c. Depression d. Neurosis

CHILD PSYCHIATRY

7. Severe mental retardation is an IQ of:
a. 10-20 b. 20-35
c. 35-50 d. 50-70

NEUROTIC DISORDERS

8. All of the following define neurosis EXCEPT:
a. Preserved contact with reality
b. Symptom causing distress to the patient
c. Lack of insight
d. Absence of organic causative factors

MISCELLANEOUS

9. A very sensitive person gets affected quiet easily. He has difficulty in controlling his anger & does NOT like to meet people. Such a personality is defined as:
a. Maniac b. Depressive
c. Borderline d. Paranoid

10. Which of the following is NOT an example of reversible dementia:
a. Parkinson disease b. Alzheimer's disease
c. Low thyroid status d. Multi-infarct dementia

11. Anorexia nervosa may be associated with:
a. Phobia b. Mania
c. OCD d. Schizophrenia

12. Failure to recognize or identify objects despite intact sensory function:
a. Alexithymia b. Anhedonia
c. Agnosia d. Anergia

13. Loss of interest in things which were previously interesting:
a. Anergia b. Anxiety
c. Anhedonia d. Alexithymia

14. Squeeze technique is employed for:
a. Impotence
b. Infertility
c. Loss of erection
d. Premature ejaculation/PME

15. Pseudologia fantastica is a feature of:
a. Delirium tremens
b. Dementia
c. Factitious disorder
d. Schizophrenia

Ans. **1. c.** Delirium tremens **2. a.** 1 year **3. d.** Clozapine **4. d.** Amphetamine
5. d. Dobutamine **6. c.** Depression **7. b.** 20-35 **8. c.** Lack of insight
9. c. Borderline **10. b.** Alzheimer's disease **11. c.** OCD **12. c.** Agnosia
13. c. Anhedonia **14. d.** Premature ejaculation/PME **15. c.** Factitious disorder

IMAGE-BASED QUESTIONS

1. Which of the following term is associated with the person shown below:

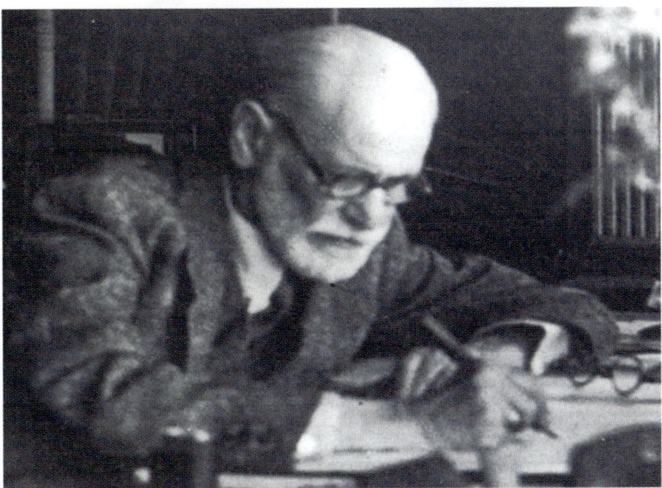

a. Neurosis
b. Schizophrenia
c. Psychoanalysis
d. Psychology

Sigmund Freud coined the term psychoanalysis.

2. Which of the following term is associated with the person shown below:

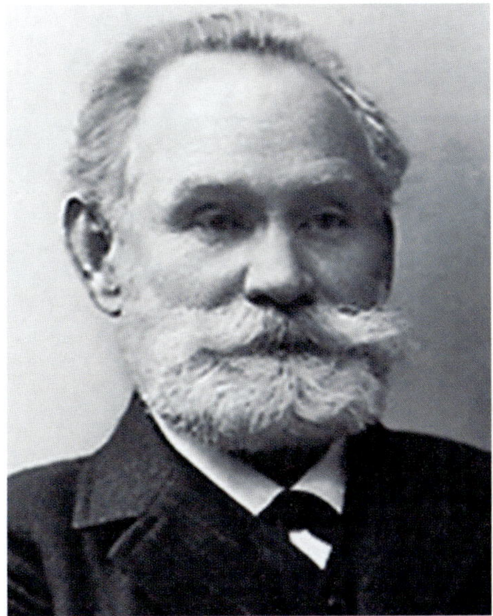

a. Catatonia
b. Sadism
c. Classical conditioning
d. Psychiatry

Ivan Petrovich Pavlov coined the term 'Classical conditioning' which was based on animal studies on conditioned reflexes.

3. Which of the following term is associated with the person shown below:

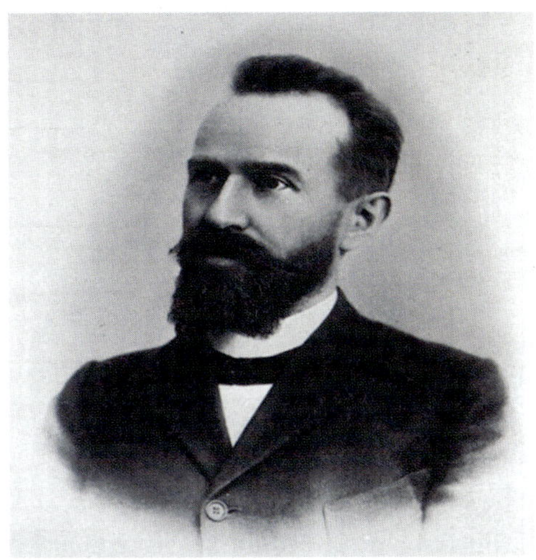

a. Masochism
b. Dementia praecox
c. Hypnosis
d. Schizophrenia

Eugen Bleuler coined the term schizophrenia and described 'cardinal' symptoms of schizophrenia.

4. Which of the following term is associated with the person shown below:

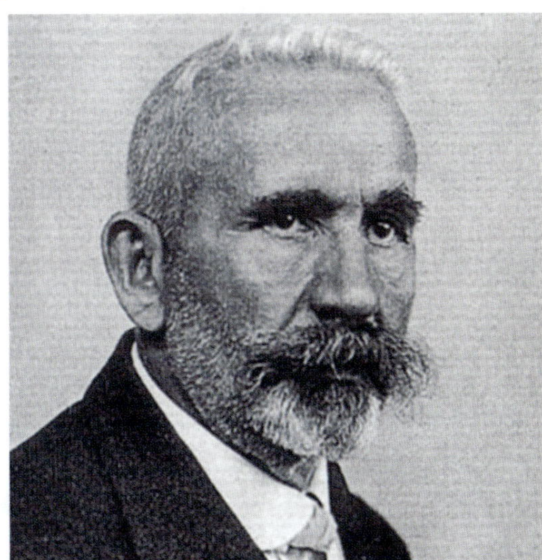

a. Cyclothymia
b. Dementia praecox
c. Moral insanity
d. Onanism

Emil Kraepelin coined the term dementia praecox.

5. Which of the following term is associated with the person shown below:

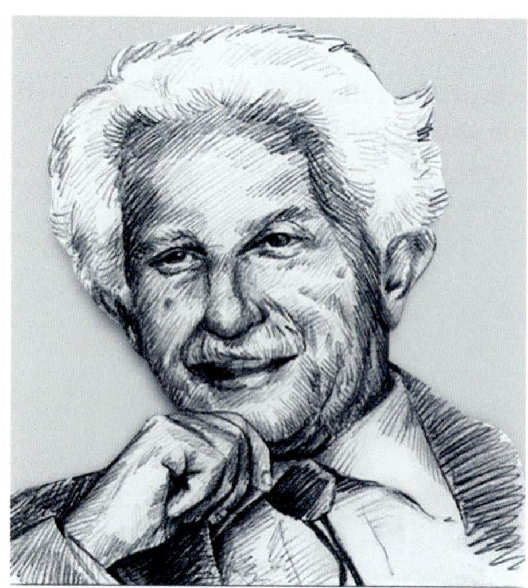

a. Inferiority complex
b. Libido
c. Stages of life
d. Psychosis

Erik H Erikson described the stages of life.

6. Histology of which psychiatric condition:

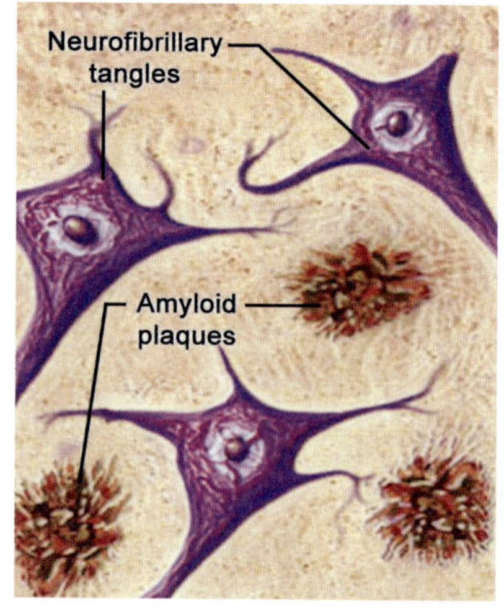

a. Mania
b. Depression
c. Delirium
d. Alzheimer's disease

Microscopy of Alzheimer's disease shows changes such as senile plaques, neurofibrillary tangles, cortical nerve cell loss, and granulovacuolar degeneration.

7. Following picture suggest the diagnosis of:

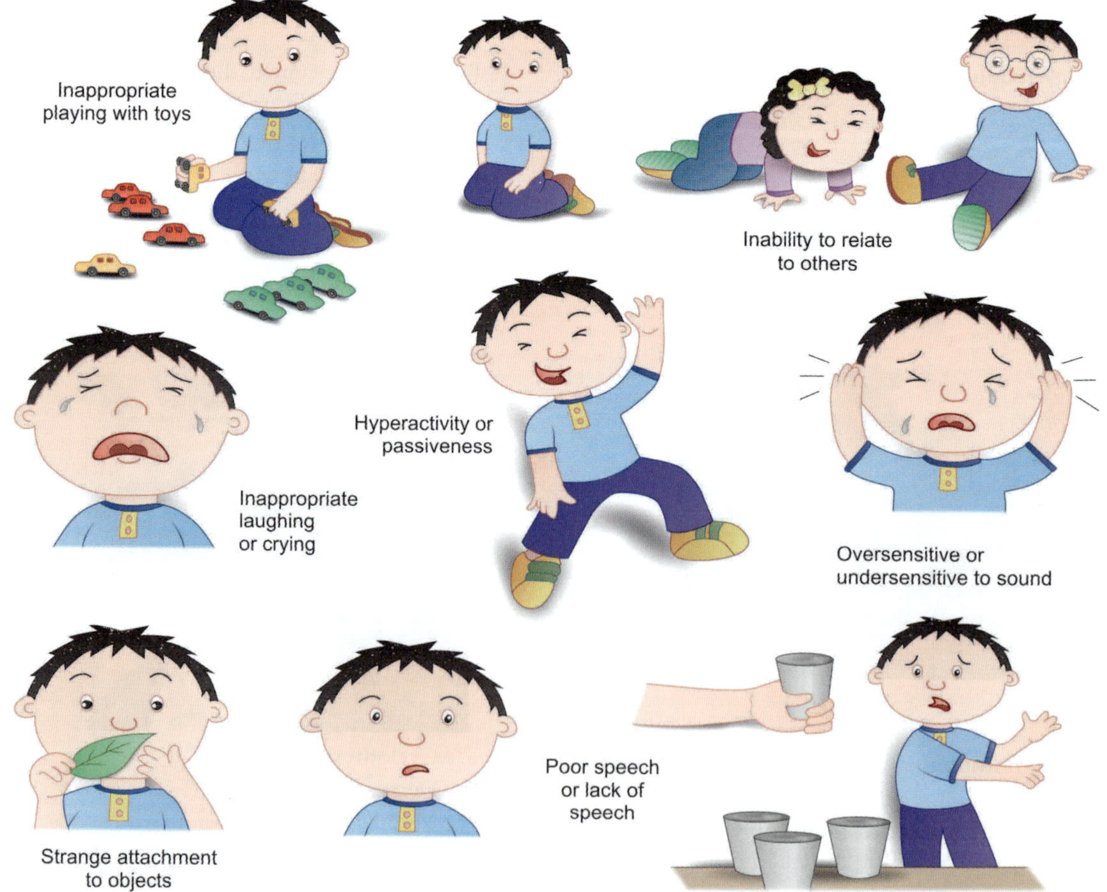

a. Conduct disorder
b. ADHD
c. Autism
d. Childhood schizophrenia

The characteristic features of autism are: (1) autism, (2) marked impairment in language and non-verbal communication, (3) abnormal behavioural characteristics, (4) mental retardation etc.

8. Following image suggest the diagnosis of:

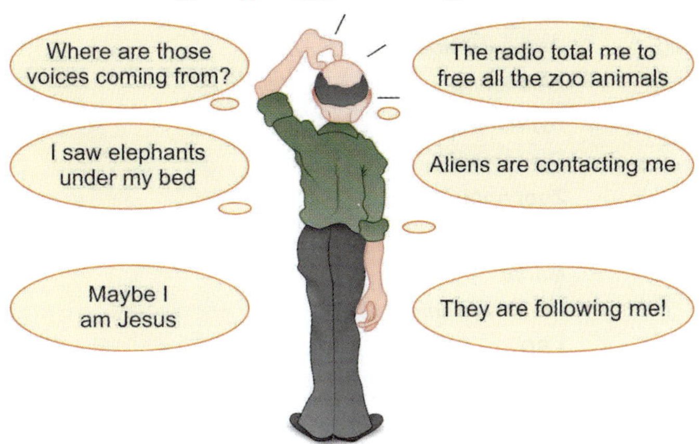

a. Delirium tremens
b. Mania
c. Depression
d. Schizophrenia

First Rank Symptoms (SFRS) of schizophrenia include audible thoughts, voice heard arguing, voice commenting on one's action, thought withdrawl, thought insertion, thought diffusion/broadcasting, 'made' feelings or affect, 'made' impulses, 'made' volition or acts, somatic passivity and delusion perception.

9. Following image suggest the diagnosis of:

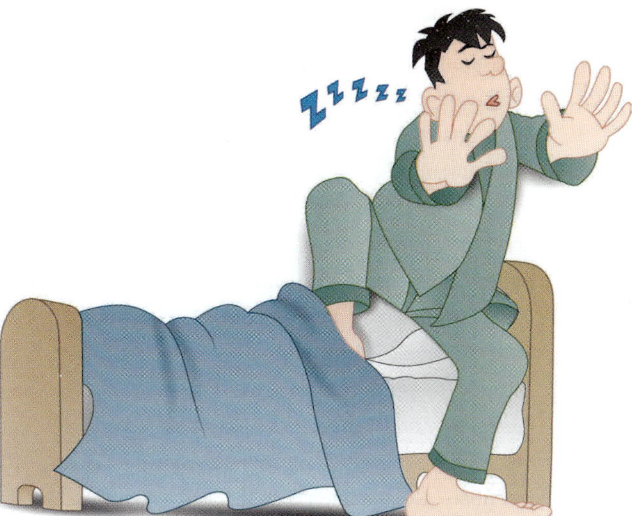

a. Somniloquy
b. Somnambulism
c. Dissociative amnesia
d. Dissociative fugue

In sleep walking/somnambulism, patient carries out automatic motor activities that range from simple to complex. He may leave the bed, walk about or leave the house. Arousal is difficult and accidents may occur during sleep walking. It is a common stage 4 parasomnia.

10. These types of waves are seen in which phase of sleep:

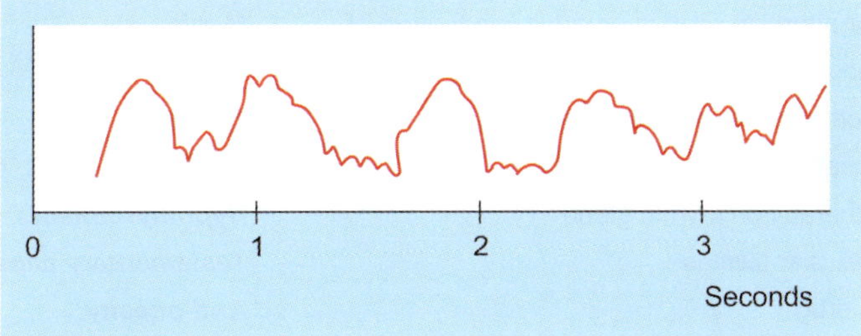

a. REM
b. NREM stage 2
c. NREM stage 3
d. NREM stage 4

Stage 4, NREM-sleep shows predominant delta activity in EEG.

MCQ POINTS

S. No.	Question statements	Answers
1.	Neurotransmitter involved in dementia	***Acetylcholine***
2.	Drug used in ADHD in children	***Methylphenidate***
3.	False unshaken belief not amenable to reasoning is known as	***Delusion***
4.	1st symptom of schizophrenia to go with treatment is	***Auditory hallucination***
5.	Paranoid schizophrenia may be associated with the use of ….drug	***Amphetamine***
6.	Longest acting SSRI	***Fluoxetine***
7.	Abnormal pre-occupation and normal body function is known as	***Hypochondriasis***
8.	Irresistible desire to drink alcohol is known as	***Dipsomania***
9.	Fear of animals is known as	***Zoophobia***
10.	Nihilistic ideas are seen in	***Depression***
11.	Grandiosity and flight of ideas may be a feature of	***Mania***
12.	MC severe symptom of alcohol withdrawal	***Delirium tremens***
13.	Flashback phenomenon is associated with abuse of	***LSD***
14.	Nightmares is seen in which phase of sleep	***REM phase***
15.	Agent of choice for prophylaxis in mania	***Lithium***
16.	Fluoxetine belongs to which group of drug	***SSRI***
17.	DOC for phobia	***Paroxetine***
18.	DOC for OCD	***Fluoxetine***
19.	Value of severe mental retardation	***20-34***
20.	Tactile hallucinations and jet black tongue are associated with abuse of	***Cocaine***
21.	Disorder of content of thought	***Delusion***
22.	Early morning insomnia may be a feature of	***Depression***
23.	Easy distractibility and poor attention span in an adult is a feature of	***Mania***
24.	Child with difficulty in forming social relationships	***Autism***
25.	To diagnose mania, symptoms should be present for at least	***7 days***
26.	Drug used for smoking cessation	***Bupropion***
27.	Effect of long-term lithium therapy on thyroid gland	***Hypothyroidism***
28.	Capacity to make a valid will is known as	***Testamentary capacity***
29.	Sibutramine is which class drug	***Anti-obesity***
30.	Formal thought disorder is considered diagnostic of which disorder	***Schizophrenia***
31.	Drug useful in acute attack of migraine	***Sumatriptan***
32.	Main feature of Korsakoff's psychosis:	***Confabulation***
33.	Sertraline is used in	***Obsessive compulsive disorder***
34.	Neurotransmitter involved in depression	***Serotonin***
35.	Disulfiram-alcohol reaction occurs due to the inhibition of which enzyme	***Aldehyde dehydrogenase***
36.	Characteristic clinical manifestation of Schizophrenia	***Auditory hallucination***
37.	Maximum loss of DALY occurs in which psychiatric disorder	***Depression***
38.	Dementia pugilistica occurs due to	***Trauma***
39.	Bad trip weed is	***LSD***
40.	Nihilistic delusion are seen in	***Depression***
41.	An alteration in perception to self is known as	***Depersonalization***

S. No.	Question statements	Answers
42.	Autism is characterized by onset of symptoms before … years of age	***3 years***
43.	Example of cortical dementia	***Alzheimer's disease***
44.	Amyloid plaques are seen in	***Alzheimer's dementia***
45.	Asperger's syndrome differs from autism in having No delay in development of	***Language***
46.	Othello syndrome is	***Morbid jealousy***
47.	Worst prognosis in which type of schizophrenia	***Hebephrenic***
48.	MC hallucination in schizophrenia	***Auditory***
49.	Irresistible desire to set things on fire	***Pyromania***
50.	Nocturnal enuresis is considered normal upto the age of	***5 years***
51.	DOC for phobia	***SSRI***
52.	Cornerstone of drug therapy for panic disorder	***Antidepressants***
53.	Major depression is defined as depressed mood on daily basis for a minimum duration of	***14 days***
54.	Alcoholic seizures occurs after .... hours of heavy bout of drinking	***24-48 hours***
55.	Delirium tremens occurs within .... days of abstinence from alcohol	***4 days***
56.	Magnan symptoms are seen with abuse of	***Cocaine***
57.	Muscle tone in REM sleep	***Decreased***
58.	Patchy impairment of personal memory is known as	***Dissociative amnesia***
59.	MOA of ondansetron	***5-HT$_3$ antagonist***
60.	Value of profound MR	***Less than 20***
61.	A mentally ill person smells odour when none is present. This is an example of	***Olfactory hallucination***
62.	Undue familiarity to unknown objects is	***Déjà vu***
63.	MC type of hallucination	***Auditory***
64.	Absolute C/I to ECT is	***Raised intracranial tension***
65.	Depressive delusion that the world and everything related cease to exist is delusion of	***Nihilism***
66.	Drug used in opioid dependence to prevent relapse is	***Naloxone***
67.	MC symptom of alcohol withdrawal is	***Tremors***
68.	Delusion is a disorder of	***Content of thought***
69.	A 30-year-old man was started on haloperidol and developed hyperpyrexia, muscle rigidity, akinesia and increased BP. Likely diagnosis	***Neuroleptic malignant syndrome***
70.	A patient often avoids public transport to go to his place of work as he is having fear of being in a crowd. This is	***Claustrophobia***
71.	A person missing from home is found wandering purposefully. Likely diagnosis	***Dissociative fugue***
72.	A 22-year-old lady seeks plastic surgery for her nose which is normal. She rarely meets her friends. Likely diagnosis	***Body dysmorphic disorder***
73.	A 36-year-old woman with a 16-year-old history of vague and chronic physical complaints. She says that she is always been in pain in abdomen, chest, legs etc. Diagnosis	***Somatization disorder***
74.	A 22-year-old lady experiences a sudden loss of vision, after a fight with husband but appears unconcerned (la belle indifference). Diagnosis is	***Conversion disorder***
75.	Waxy flexibility, negativism, echolalia, echopraxia are a feature of .... schizophrenia	***Catatonic***

CHAPTER

12

RADIODIAGNOSIS

KEY POINTS

Expatory Chest Films are Preferred in

- Small pneumothorax
- Early interstitial lung disease
- Along with an inspiratory film in obstructive emphysema

Conditions and Minimum Collection for X-ray Detection

- Pleural effusion: 250 ml
- Pericardial effusion: 200 ml
- Pneumoperitoneum: 1 ml

Remember

- USG is non-ionizing
- Radiation hazard is not a feature of MRI/ Doppler USG

USG

- Activity of transducer of USG are based on the principle of piezoelectric effect
- Absolute barrier to USG is air
- Ultrasound in obstetrics can induce changes in cell migration a an early stage of development

Various Modes of USG

- A mode (Amplitude): Measures axial length of eyeball
- B mode (Brightness): Main mode used for ultrasound imagine
- M mode (Movement): Echocardiography

Remember

- MRI is non-ionizing
- No radiation exposure

Contraindications to MRI

- Pacemakers
- Intracranial clips
- Size and weight above machine limits
- First trimester of pregnancy
- Claustrophobia

Contrasts Used in Various Studies

- Oral cholecystography: Iopanoic acid
- Intravenous cholecystography: Biligraffin (Meglumine)
- Esophageal atresia: Dianosil
- Intravenous pyelogram: Conray 420
- Myelography: Myodil (Iodophendylate), Iohexol (Omnipaque)
- Vertebral angiography: Conray 280

Radiological Signs in Cardiovascular System

- Coeur en sabot/Dutch shoe/Boot- shaped heart: Fallot's tetralogy
- Egg on end appearance: TGA
- Cottage loaf heart: Supracardiac total anomalous pulmonary, venous return, wide mediastinum
- Box-shaped cardiomegaly: Ebstein's anomaly
- Snowman or figure of 8: Supracardiac TAPPVC
- '3' sign: Aortic coarctation, due to stenosis of aorta
- Leather bottle or flask shaped heart: Pericardial effusion
- Double atrial shadow: Left atrial enlargement

Radiological Signs in Respiratory System

- Butterfly/batwing pattern: Pulmonary edema
- Moustache/Antler sign: Prominence or upper lobe veins due to increased left atrial pressure in case of mitral stenosis
- Dirty chest: Chronic bronchitis
- Pneumatoceles: Infection due Staphylococcus and Klebsiella
- Egg shell calcification: Silicosis, Sarcoidosis, Histoplasmosis, Blastomycosis, Scleroderma, Amyloidosis
- Bulging fissure: Klebsiella pneumonia
- Crescent sign: Fungal ball within a cavity

Kerley's Lines

- Kerley's A linen: Seen near the apex
- Kerley's B lines: Seen near the base perpendicular to the pleural surface
- Kerley's C lines: Near the center, interlacing, leading to spider web appearance

Kerley's Lines are Seen in

- Pulmonary edema
- Mitral valve prolapse
- Pneumoconiosis
- Lymphatic metastatic disease

Radiological Signs of Pulmonary Embolism

- Westermark: Pulmonary oligemia
- Hampton's hump: Peripheral wedge-shaped density
- Palla's sign: Enlarged right descending pulmonary artery

Radiological Signs of Hypertrophic Pyloric Stenosis

- String sign: Due to narrowed pyloric canal
- Beak sign: Due to an abrupt cut off of barium point in the pyloric canal
- Tram track sign: Double track of barium

Radiological Signs in Hepatobiliary System

- Floating membrane/Water lily of Camalote sign: Ruptured hydatid cyst
- Rising sun/ Serpent sign: Dry hydatid cyst with crumpled membrane
- Bull's eye lesion in USG of liver: Metastases
- Mercedes Benz sign/sea gull sign: Radiolucent gas in triradiate/ biradiate fissure in a gallbladder
- Pad sign in barium meal: Carcinoma pancreas
- Scrambled egg appearance in ERCP: Carcinoma pancreas
- Reversed 3 sign of Frostburg: Carcinoma head of pancreas
- Beading of bile duct seen in ERCP: Sclerosing cholangitis
- Chain of lakes appearance seen In ERCP: Chronic pancreatitis
- Double duct sign seen in ERCP: Pancreatic carcinoma in conjunction with bile duct obstruction or stricture

Radiological Signs in Gastrointestinal System

- Concertina or stack of coins appearance: Dilated jejunum
- Coffee bean sign: Intestinal obstruction with strangulation
- Cobblestone appearance: Crohn's disease
- Raspberry thorning/Rose thorn ulcers of intestine: Crohn's disease
- Inverted umbrella sign(broad base triangular appearance of ileocecal valve with base towards cecum): Ileocecal junction tuberculosis]
- Sterling's sign (lack of retention of barium in inflamed segment of ileum, caecum and ascending colon): Ileocecal junction tuberculosis, Crohn's disease
- String sign of Kantor (Persistent narrow steam of barium indicating stenosis and strictures): Ileocecal junction tuberculosis, Crohn's disease
- Thumb printing appearance (Due to ulcers and edema): Ulcerative colitis
- Lead pipe appearance (Blunting of haustral folds): Ulcerative colitis
- Omega sign on plain X-ray abdomen: Sigmoid volvulus
- Inverted U appearance of sigmoid colon: Volvulus
- Twisted bird's beak/Ace of spade deformity in barium enema: Sigmoid volvulus
- Bent inner tube or Omega loop sign on straight X-ray of abdomen: Volvulus
- Inverted 3 sign in barium swallow: The impression of aorta on esophagus
- Bird's beak appearance: Achalasia cardia
- Rat tail appearance: Carcinoma esophagus
- Apple core deformity: Carcinoma esophagus
- Cup and spill stomach: Volvulus stomach
- Leather bottle appearance/Linitis plastica:
- Carcinoma, Corrosive gastritis, Cohn's disease, Tuberculosis, Syphilis, Eosinophilic gastritis, Lymphoma
- Double bubble sign: Duodena atresia
- Triple bubble sign: Jejunal atresia
- Barber pole sign/Corkscrew sign/spiral sign in barium studies: Midgut volvulus due to spiraling of superior mesenteric artery
- Whirl sign or peacock tail sign in CT/MRI:
  Midgut volvulus due to spiraling of superior mesenteric artery
- String of beads sign: Small bowel obstruction
- Moulage sign/ Molten wax appearance of intestine in barium studies: Malabsorption

Radiological Signs of Intussusception

- Coiled spring appearance
- Empty Quarter sign (due to empty right iliac fossa)
- Pseudo-kidney sign (Seen on USG)
- Claw sign (in barium meal X-ray)

Radiological Signs of Urinary System

- Crescent sign/ Rim sign in nephrogram: Acquired hydronephrosis
- Mathe's sign (absence of downward displacement of kidney that normally occurs in erect position): Perinephric abscess
- Beak sign in renal arteriogram: Renal cyst

- Flower vase ureters: Horse-shoe kidney
- Spider leg calyces: Polycystic kidney
- Pencil line/Tram line appearance: Acute cortical necrosis
- Egg in cup appearance: Renal papillary necrosis
- Air pyelogram: Emphysematous diabetic pyelonephritis
- Pancake kidney: Failure of both kidney to ascend from the pelvis
- Spoke wheel appearance on angiography: Oncocytoma
- Onion layer appearance on USG: Angiomyolipoma
- Saw toothed, beaded or pipe stem: Ureteric tuberculosis
- Cobra head deformity/Adder head sign: Ureterocele

Radiological Signs in Osteoarthritis

- Osteophytes
- Decreased joint space
- Sclerosis of bone ends forming joints

Commonly Involved Joints in Osteoarthritis

- Major joints of lower limb
- Distal interphalangeal joint
- Proximal interphalangeal joint
- 1st metacarpal joint

Vertebral Signs and Conditions

- Scotty dog appearance: Normal vertebra
- Scotty dog wearing collar: Spondylosis
- Beheaded Scottish terrier: Spondylolisthesis

Radiological Sings in Rheumatoid Arthritis

- Increased joint space
- Periarticular erosion and osteoporosis
- Syndesmophytes
- Bamboo spine
- Tram track sign

Radiological Signs in Musculoskeletal System

- Looser's zone (an area of stress fracture repaired by osteroid in the absence of normal mineralization): Osteomalacia
- Cord fish vertebrae (biconcave): Osteomalacia
- Triradiate pelvis: Osteomalacia
- Pepper pot skull appearance: Hyperparathyroidism
- Aneurysmal sign: Erosion of the anterior surface of vertebral body by tuberculous abscesses, resembling erosions due to aortic aneurysm
- Hot cross bun skull: Congenital syphilis
- Sutural diastases (In children it is the first and the most prominent sign): Raised ICT
- Silver beaten appearance: Raised ICT
- Champagne glass pelvis: Achondroplasia
- Tombstone iliac blades: Achondroplasia
- Saw tooth metaphysis: Congenital syphilis
- Lace work periostitis: Congenital syphilis
- Wimberger's sign (bilateral symmetrical): Perichondritis and osteitis of tibial upper growth plate medially): Congenital syphilis
- Dots and commas/rings and broken rings calcification: Enchondroma or chondrosarcoma
- Tufting of terminal phalanges of fingers and toes: Acromegaly
- Doughnut appearance on radionuclide scan: Avascular necrosis
- Picture frame vertebra: Paget's disease.
- Dural tail sign: Meningiomas
- Licked candy stick appearance (neuropathic resorption of bone): Leprosy

Structures which Calcify Physiologically are

- Pineal gland
- Habenular commissure
- Falx cerebri
- Choroidal plexus
- Dura
- Petroclinoid ligament
- Interclinoid ligament

Intracranial Pathologies which Calcify are

- Gliomas
- Hematomas
- A-V malformations/Aneurysms
- Tuberculomas
- Cysticercosis
- Hydatid disease
- Sturge-Weber syndrome
- Tuberous sclerosis

MCQs WITH SHORT EXPLANATIONS

GENERAL PRINCIPLES

1. **Which of the following structure does NOT form right side of mediastinal shadow?**
   a. Superior vena cava
   b. Right innominate
   c. Right atrium
   d. Right ventricle

   Radiology of heart
   - Right border of heart is formed by:
     – SVC/ Right brachiocephalic vessels,
     – IVC
     – Right atrium
   - Left border of heart is formed by:
     – Left atrial appendage,
     – Left ventricle,
     – Aortic arch
     – Pulmonary artery

2. **Contrast used in MRI:**
   a. Iodine b. Gadolinium
   c. Metrizamide d. Omnipaque

   Contrast agents used in MRI are Gadolinium, Gadodiamide, Gd-BOPTA, Gd-EOB, DTPA, MIONS, SPIO and USPIO.

Radiological procedure	Contrast (Dye) used
Intravenous urography/ pyelography (IVU/ IVP)	Outdated contrast media like Conray 420, i.e. sodium iothalamate and metrizoate (outdated).* Currently used ionic (Sodium or Meglumine salts of Diatrizoate) or nonionic contrast media (Iohexol, iopamidol, iomeprol, ioversol, iodixanol) Nonionic are best preferred
Esophagography (Ba Swallow)	Barium, Gastrografin (outda-ted), water-soluble iodinated contrast agent in suspected case of TO fistula.
Hysterosalpingography	Conray 280, i.e. Meglumine iothalamate (outdated), currently used is Meglumine salt of Diatrizoate (Angiografin 65%)
For intestinal obstruction or perforation Sialography	Gastrografin, water-soluble iodinated contrast agent (preferred) Lipiodol (Neohydiol) is outdated. Use water-soluble ionic/ nonionic contrast agent used
Urethrography	Conray 280, i.e. Meglumine iothalamate (outdated), currently used is water soluble contrast agent like Meglumine salt of Diatrizoate (Angiografin 65%)
Cisternography	Iohexol (Omnipaque)
Myelography	Myodil (outdated), currently used is iohexol (Omnipaque) – outdated study
Lymphangiography	Methylene blue, Lipiodol
Splenoportography	75 percent sodium metrizoate–outdated study
Bronchography	Dianosil (Propylidone)–outdated studies
Intravenous cholangiography	Biligrafin (Meglumine ioglycamate)–outdated studies
DSA/CECT	Water soluble nonionic low osmolar contrast media (LOCM), e.g. iohexol
MRI	Gadolinium, Gadodamide, Gd-BOPTA, Gd-EOB DTPA, MIONS, SPIO, USPIO
Ultrasound	Microbubbles (Echovist, Levovist, Albunex, perfluoropropane microbubbles)

*Currently Conray is completely obsolete from use, and now either ionic or nonionic iodine contrast media are used (nonionic preferred over ionic).

3. **Absolute contraindication of MRI is:**
   a. Pacemaker b. Prosthetic cardiac valves
   c. Insulin pump d. Cochlear implant

   Contraindications to MRI
   - Cochlear implants
   - Intraocular metallic foreign body
   - Aneurysmal clips
   - Cardiac pacemakers (absolute C/I)
   - Prosthetic heart valves
   - Bone implants
   - Claustrophobia (phobia of closed spaces)

Substance	T1 weighted	T2 weighted
Water/Vitreous/CSF	Black	Light gray or white
Fat	White	Light gray
Muscle	Gray	Gray
Air	Black	Black
Fatty bone marrow	White light	Gray
Brain: White matter	Light gray	Gray
Brain: Gray matter	Gray	Very light gray

Ans. 1. **d.** Right ventricle 2. **b.** Gadolinium 3. **a.** Pacemaker

4. Most preferred route to perform cerebral angiography:

a. Transfemoral route b. Transaxillary route
c. Direct carotid puncture d. Transbrachial route

For arteriography, femoral artery is catheterized (large size access to aorta of all its branches).

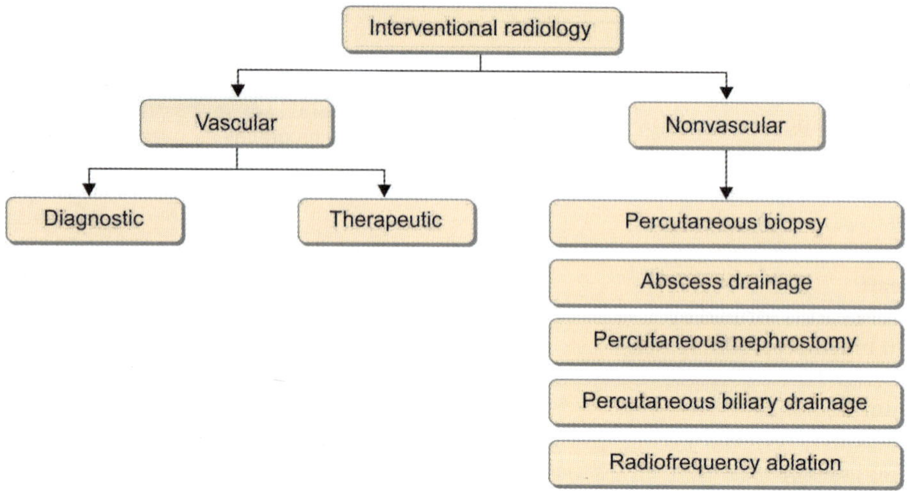

5. False for MRI:

a. Imaging perfusion of brain
b. Presence of hydrogen ions
c. Blood vessels visualized without contrast
d. Superior to CT for bone scanning

CT scan is best to detect cortical bony lesions and fine osseous details.

Generation of CT	CT machine
First generation CT (Outdated)	EMI scanner
Second generation CT (Going out of use)	Conventional CT
Third generation CT (Most common type in India at present, but rapidly being superceded by MDCT)	Spiral helical CT (It can be single or multislice CT)
Fourth generation CT (No beam-hardening artefacts)	MDCT (Multidetector CT)
Electron beam CT/Ultrafast CT/Real-time CT/mSec CT	EBCT

Points of difference	X-rays	*γ-rays*
Origin	Extranuclear ❑ X-ray tube ❑ Linear accelerator	Intranuclear Radioactive isotopes like Co-60, 99mTc
Penetrating power	Intermediate	Highest
Ionization potential	Intermediate	Least
Diagnostic use	❑ Radiography ❑ Mammography ❑ Contrast radiography (IVU, Ba studies, etc.) ❑ Xeroradiography (Outdated) ❑ Fluoroscopy ❑ CT scan ❑ DEXA	Nuclear scan/ Scintigraphy/ Gamma-imaging
Therapeutic use	Teletherapy (Ortho < Super < Megavoltage X-ray therapy)	Tele- as well as brachytherapy

6. "Target material" which produces X-rays in a diagnostic X-rays tube is made of:

a. Lead b. Tungsten
c. Cobalt d. Copper

X-rays are produced whenever stream of fast-moving electrons undergo rapid deceleration and these conditions prevail during operation of special thermionic vacuum tube called hot filament or Coolidge X-ray tube. A typical X-ray tube is a thermionic diode consisting of a tungsten filament cathode, a tungsten target anode, an evacuated glass tube enclosure (Pyrex glass) and 2 circuits to heat the filament and to drive the space charge electrons to anode.

7. Photosensitive material used in X-rays films consists of:

a. Cellulose b. Silver bromide
c. Zinc sulphide d. Cadmium tungstate

Layers of X-ray film

- Supportive base made up of polyester plastic
- Adhesive or scrubbing layer for proper binding of the emulsion to the base
- Emulsion containing silver halide (most commonly used is silver bromide). Crystals are suspended in gelatin (photosensitive layer) – the key component of a X-ray film.
- Protective anti-abrasive supercoat of pure gelatin

Ans. 4. **a.** Transfemoral route 5. **d.** Superior to CT for... 6. **b.** Tungsten 7. **b.** Silver bromide

- Non-curl backing (only in single coated film) to prevent curling of the film
- Antihalation layer of dye added to non-curl backing or to the base to prevent reflection and unsharpness.

Diagnostic imaging modality and resolution

Modality	*Resolution*	*Typical imaging time*	*Radiation dose*
Plane X-ray	<mm	<1 sec	Low
Mammography	<mm	<1 sec	High
Compound tomography (CT)	mm	Few seconds	High
SPECT and PET	0.5–1 cm	10–30 minutes	High
Digital radiography	mm	<1 sec	Low
MRI and MRS	mm	10–40 minutes	Nil

8. In USG machines, the principle is:

a. Piezoelectric crystal excitation
b. Very low frequency radio waves
c. Microwaves
d. None of the above

The piezoelectric crystals in the ultrasound probe are nothing but innumerable dipoles arranged in geometric pattern and electric field causes sudden change in their physical dimensions (shape) by realigning them, thereby starting a series of vibrations that produce sound waves. Thus by virtue of piezoelectric effect in the ultrasound probe one form of energy (electric energy) is converted in to another form (sound energy) the body/organs parts are imaged.

Key indications for various radiological investigations

Radiological tool	*Prime indications*
IVP/IVU	Renal tuberculosis
	Renal anomalies
Esophagography	TO fistula (Water-soluble contrast study)
	Motility disorders (initial evaluation)
	Dysphagia
HSG	Infertility[Q]
(Postmenstrual-	Congenital uterine anomalies
preovulatory period)	Tubal block
Urethrography	PU valves (RGU)
	VUR (RGU)
	Trauma
	Stricture
Ultrasound	Hydrocephalus in infants[Q]
	Thyroid nodule
	Initial evaluation of rotator cuff injury/ subacromial bursitis/bicipital tendinitis[Q]
	Synovial cysts
	Pleural/Pericardial effusion[Q]
	First investigation done for acute abdomen and obstructive jaundice[Q]
	Congenital hypertrophic pyloric stenosis and intussusception
	Gallstones[Q]
	Adenomyomatosis of Gallbladder ("Comet tail" sign)
	Initial evaluation of focal liver lesions
	Initial evaluation of blunt trauma abdomen (FAST protocol)[Q]
	Minimal ascites[Q]
	Cystic hygroma
	Prostatic pathologies (TRUS)
	Seminal vesicle pathologies (TRUS)
	Staging of early rectal/pancreatic head malignancies (EUS)
	Neuroectodermal pancreatic tumors—insulinoma and gastrinoma (EUS)
	Scrotal pathologies
	Developmental dysplasia of Hip[Q]
CT Scan	***HRCT (Bone algorithm)***
	Lungs: ❑ ILD ❑ Bronchiectasis ❑ Emphysema
	Temporal bone: ❑ Petrositis ❑ Mastoiditis ❑ Ossicular chain disruption ❑ Cogenital anomalies [e.g. Mondani's malformation] ❑ EAC osteoma ❑ Cholesteatoma ❑ Fracture facial canal
	Noncontrast CT (NCCT) ❑ *Initial test of choice for acute stroke* ❑ *Fractures:* – Skull (Head injury) – Facial bones – Vertebral – Pelvis – Talus – Scaphoid

Contd...

Ans. 8. **a.** Piezoelectric crystal excitation

Contd...

Radiological tool	*Prime indications*
	❑ *Acute hemorrhage:* – Intratumoral – Intracerebral – Intraventricular – EDH/SDH – Acute SAH ❑ *Minimum air:* – Pneumoperitoneum – Pneumocephalus – Pneumomediastinum ❑ Calcification anywhere in body ❑ Ureteric calculi
	CTA (CT angiography) ❑ Screening of intracranial internal carotid (ICA) lesions ❑ Screening of circle of Willi's lesions ❑ Chronic abdominal angina ❑ Pulmonary embolism ❑ Noninvasive coronary angiography ❑ Coronary anomalies ❑ Pulmonary sequestration ❑ Rapid screening tool for aortic lesions ❑ Sensitive and specific screening tool for renal artery stenosis
	CT brain ❑ Oligodendroglioma ❑ Screening for cortical venous thrombosis (Empty delta sign in lateral sinus thrombosis) ❑ Evaluation of an acute change in mental status ❑ Evaluation of an focal neurologic findings ❑ Conductive hearing loss ❑ Craniopharyngioma ❑ Craniosynostosis ❑ Krabbe's disease (Globoid cell dystrophy)
	CECT neck ❑ Staging of ca larynx ❑ Staging of ca thyroid ❑ Cold abscess ❑ Nodal characterization
	CT PNS ❑ Chronic recurrent sinusitis (NCCT) ❑ Noninvasive fungal sinusitis (NCCT) ❑ Sinonasal polyps (NCCT) ❑ Pre-FESS CT (NCCT) ❑ Neoplasms of maxilla (CECT) ❑ Juvenile angiofibroma (CECT) ❑ Screening for Glomus jugulare (Phlep sign) ❑ CSF rhinorrhea (CT cisternography)
	CT orbit ❑ Metallic foreign body (NCCT) ❑ Optic drusen ❑ Retinoblastoma (CECT)

Contd...

Contd...

Radiological tool	*Prime indications*
	CECT chest ❑ Screening detection and staging of lung cancer ❑ Lung hamartoma ❑ Pleural lesions ❑ Diaphragmatic hernia ❑ Anterior and middle mediastinal lesions ❑ Congenital labor emphysema ❑ Congenital adenomatoid lung malformation ❑ Morgagni's hernia ❑ Mediastinal lymph node characterization ❑ Tubercular pericarditis ❑ Calcified cardiac tumors
	CECT abdomen ❑ Blunt trauma abdomen (FAST USG for screening only) ❑ Abdominal lump ❑ Abdominal wall hematoma ❑ Advanced rectal/esophagus/stomach/bladder cancer ❑ Detection and staging of ca gallbladder and small bowel tumors ❑ Focal hepatic lesions ❑ Adrenal imaging (Nonfunctional lesions) ❑ Renal carcinoma detection and staging ❑ Oncocytoma (Central stellate scar) ❑ Renal and perirenal infections ❑ Complicated ADPKD ❑ Mesenteric cyst ❑ Enteric duplication cyst ❑ Abdominal lymph node and peritoneal TB ❑ Diverticulitis and diverticular abcess ❑ Subdiaphragmatic abscess ❑ Bowel obstruction evaluation ❑ Complicated appendicitis ❑ Appendicitis epiploicae
	CECT pelvis ❑ Adnexal mass ❑ Ovarian dermoid ❑ Ca urinary bladder ❑ Advanced prostatic cancer staging ❑ Sacrococcygeal teratoma
MRI	***MRI advantages*** ❑ Superior soft tissue contrast resolution—excellent pathological discrimination ❑ No ionizing radiation ❑ Direct multiplanar imaging (transverse, coronal, sagittal, any oblique) ❑ Noninvasive—vascular studies can be performed without contrast

Contd...

Contd...

Radiological tool	*Prime indications*
	MRI disadvantages ❑ Expensive ❑ Long scan times ❑ Audible noise (65–115 dB) ❑ Isolation of patient (cloustrophobia monitoring of ill patients) ❑ Exclusion of patients with pacemakers and certain implants
	Cranial MRI ❑ Chronic hemorrhage (GRE < FLAIR) ❑ Sensitive most for acute and hyperacute ischemic stroke (DWMRI) ❑ Demyelinating disorders (e.g. MS, ALS, SSPE, SACD, SMON, CPM, ADEM, PML, PVL, PRES, etc.) ❑ Infectious processes (encephalitis, meningitis) ❑ Abscesses ❑ Brain neoplasms (supra as well as infratentorial) ❑ Neurofibromatosis ❑ DAI ❑ Vascular disorders (AVM's, aneurysms, vasculitis, Moya-moya disease) ❑ Metastasis ❑ Internal auditory canal pathology ❑ Pituitary pathology ❑ Hydrocephalus especially in adults ❑ Cranial nerve pathology (e.g. vestibular Schwannoma) ❑ Congenital anomalies (for anatomical review) ❑ Epilepsy (seizures in general) ❑ Parameningeal tumors ❑ Low CSF volume headache
	Spine MRI ❑ Cauda equina syndrome ❑ Tethered cord ❑ Arachnoiditis ❑ Marrow-replacing processes ❑ Degeneration disk disease ❑ Discitis ❑ Congenital anomalies ❑ Radiculopathy ❑ Spinal cord tumors ❑ Trauma/contusion ❑ Syringomyelia ❑ Metastasis ❑ Vascular disorders ❑ Cord edema ❑ MS plaques ❑ Traumatic paraplegia ❑ Retroperitoneal tumor with spine extension ❑ Pott's spine ❑ Myelomalacia

Contd...

Contd...

Radiological tool	*Prime indications*
	Musculoskeletal MRI ❑ Meniscal pathology ❑ Ligament/tendon injury ❑ PVNS ❑ Muscle/nerve impingement ❑ Rotator cuff tear ❑ Avascular necrosis ❑ Labral tears (shoulder, hip) ❑ Chondromalacia ❑ Inflammation (acute osteomyelitis) ❑ Primary bone tumors ❑ Spinal metastases ❑ Soft tissue tumors ❑ Perthe's disease ❑ Cartilage injury
	Breast MRI ❑ Screening in young females (as glandular tissue is more than fat in young breasts)[Q] ❑ Breast with silicone implants (Augmented breast) ❑ Sensitive most investigation to detect DCIS
	Chest MRI ❑ Imaging of Pancoast's tumor (superior sulcus tumor)[Q] ❑ Imaging of posterior mediastinal masses ❑ Demonstration of vascular sling[Q] ❑ Investigation of choice in aortic dissection[Q] ❑ Best diagnosis for dissecting aorta (aortic dissection)[Q]
	Cardiac MRI ❑ Vascular rings (e.g. Double aortic arch; Aberrant right subclavian; Pulmonary sling) ❑ Post-up complex cyanotic congenital heart diseases[Q] ❑ ARVD ❑ Coarctation of aorta ❑ Cardiomyopathies (*in general*) ❑ Malignant cardiac tumors ❑ Pericardial malignancies
	Abdominal MRI ❑ Investigation of choice for a pregnant lady with upper abdominal mass[Q] ❑ The most sensitive and specific investigation for renal artery stenosis ❑ Preoperative staging of endometrial and cervical cancer[Q] ❑ Anorectal sepsis, anorectal malformation and anorectal tumors ❑ RCC with suspected RV or IVC invasion ❑ Fetal cranial abnormalities ❑ Liver pathologies
MRA (Gd-enhanced MRA > PC or ToF MRA)	
❑ Best for circle of Willis	❑ Renal artery stenosis lesions

Contd...

Contd...

Radiological tool	*Prime indications*
❑ AVMS	❑ Acute mesenteric ischemia (Laparotomy test)
❑ Aneurysms	❑ Cortical venous thrombosis (MR venography)
❑ Aortic lesions	❑ Vertebral artery dissection/thrombosis
– Aneurysms	
– Dissection	
– Takayasu's	
❑ Vascular rings	❑ Corticocavernous fistula (Pulsatile exophthalmos)
❑ Carotid lesions	❑ Coronary artery aneurysms
❑ Carotid body tumors	
❑ Paragangliomas (South Peeper appearance)	

Note: 'Q' as a superscript indicates 'vital indications'

THORAX

9. Egg on side appearance is seen in:

a. TOF
b. TAPVC
c. Uncorrected TGA
d. Truncus arteriosus

"Egg on Side" heart ("Egg in cup" heart) is seen in TGA

Increased pulmonary perfusion (Plethora)	Decreased pulmonary perfusion (Oligemia)
ASD (Primum and secundum defect)	Tricuspid atresia/stenosis
Anomalous pulmonary venous connection	Ebstein's anomaly
Membranous/bulbar VSD	Pulmonary infundibular/valvular stenosis
PDA	Tetralogy of Fallot (TOF)
Sinus venous defect	Pulmonary artery atresia
Gerbode defect	Peripheral pulmonary artery stenosis
DORV	Persistent truncus (type IV)
Single ventricle	Uncorrected transposition with PVS
Aortopulmonary window	Eisenmenger reaction (lung periphery only)
Persistent truncus arteriosus	
Coronary artery to right heart fistula	
TGA with ASD or VSD	
Endocardial cushion defect	

10. IOC to differentiate pericardial effusion and dilation of heart is:

a. Echocardiography b. Angiocardiography
c. MRI d. CT

Echocardiography is a safe, painless, portable and relatively inexpensive method of acquiring high quality tomographic images of the heart in a variety of patients. It is "first-test" of choice in the noninvasive examination of cardiac anatomy and function. Echocardiography is most commonly used method for diagnosing pericardial effusions.

Cardiovascular imaging protocols

	Echocardiography	*Nuclear scan*	*CT*	*MRI*
IV Size/ function	Initial modality of choice Provides ancillary structural and hemodynamic information)	Available from gated SPECT stress imaging	Best resolution Highest cost	Best resolution Highest cost
Valve disease	Initial modality of choice Valve motion and morphology studied. Doppler hemodynamics assessed	—	—	Visualize valve motion Delineate abnormal flow
Pericardial disease	Pericardial effusion	—	Pericardial thickening and calcification	Pericardial thickening and malignancies
Aortic disease	TEE rapid diagnosis Acute dissection of thoracic aorta can be diagnosed rapidly	—	Image entire aorta rapidly Acute dissection of any part of aorta can be diagnosed rapidly	Image entire aorta in 15-30 minutes Dissection of any part of aorta can be diagnosed with maximum accuracy
			Acute aneurysm screening Best for acute aortic dissection, especially when time is a concern as in hemodynamically unstable patient	Aortic aneurysm confirmation and evaluation Best for chronic dissection

Contd...

Ans. 9. c. Uncorrected TGA 10. a. Echocardiography

Contd...

	Echocardiography	*Nuclear scan*	*CT*	*MRI*
Cardiac masses	First/initial investigation to detect: ❑ TTE—large intracardiacmasses ❑ TEE—smaller intracardiac masses	—	Extracardiac masses Myocardial masses	Extracardiac masses Myocardiac masses
Vascular rings	May sometimes be useful	—	Excellent for screening	Best for diagnosing Best for diagnosing compression of adjacent airways esophagus

11. High resolution CT is the imaging modality for:

a. Pleural effusion
b. Interstitial lung disease
c. Lung mass
d. Mediastinal adenopathy

Clinical applications of HRCT

- Lung diseases
  - Bronchiectasis
  - Interstitial and diffuse lung diseases
  - Emphysema
- Temporal bone imaging
  - Ossicular chain disruption
  - Cholesteatoma
  - Mastoiditis and petrositis
  - Fracture of facial canal

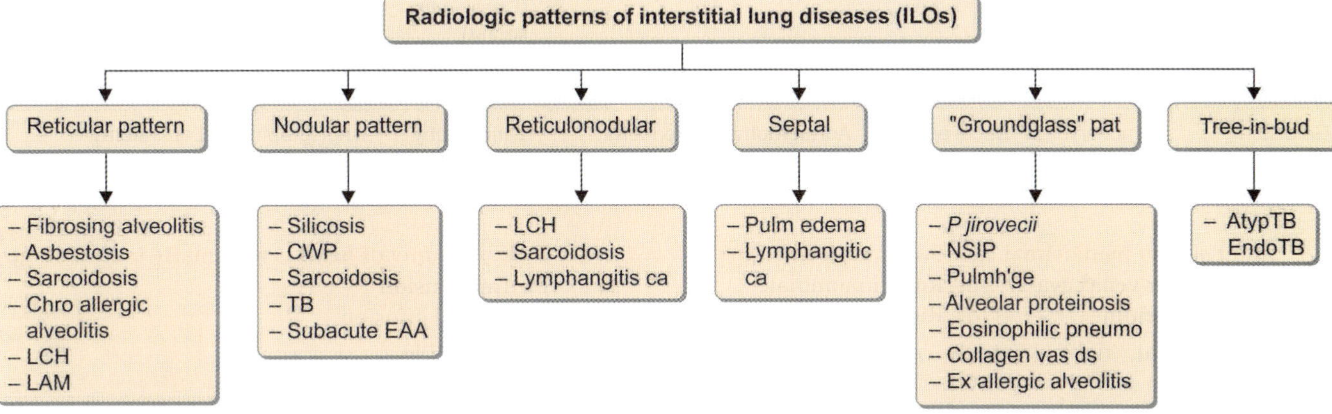

12. Floating water lily sign is seen in:

a. Lung hydatid
b. Bronchial adenoma
c. Lung abscess
d. Aspergilloma

Completely collapsed crumpled cyst membrane (of Hydatid Disease of Lung) floating on the cyst fluid produce Water Lily sign of Camelot.

Note
Bull's eye calcification (Dense central nidus or laminated calcification) → granuloma (Granulomatous lesion).
Popcorn calcification → hamartoma.
Eggshell nodal calcification → Silicosis, sarcoidosis, histoplasmosis, blastomycosis, scleroderma and amyloidosis.
Bronchogenic carcinoma (6–7%) → Granular calcification in larger tumors and amorphous or cloud like calcification especially in small peripheral tumors.
Pulmonary metastasis calcification is very unusual except in metastasis from osteosarcoma, chondrosarcoma.

13. Which shows rib notching on chest radiography:

a. PDA
b. ASD
c. Ebstein's anomaly
d. Coarctation of aorta

Rib notching, a feature of COA (bilateral but asymmetric, and best seen on inferior aspects of posterior thirds of the upper ribs, sparing 1st two) usually takes several years to develop, and is caused by pressure erosion of adjacent ribs by enlarged tortuous intercostals arteries. So rib notching is rare in young children, even in severe coarctation.

Investigations preference for chest diseases	
Diseases	*Investigations of choice*
Congenital heart disease	Transesophageal echocardiography
Portal hypertension	Color Doppler
Mitral value disease	Echocardiography with Doppler

Contd...

Ans. 11. **b.** Interstitial lung... 12. **a.** Lung hydatid 13. **d.** Coarctation of aorta

Contd...

Diseases	*Investigations of choice*
Mediastinal fibrosis	CECT, magnetic resonance imaging
COPD	Pulmonary function tests
Obstructive sleep apnea	Sleep apnea study
Pulmonary fibrosis	HRCT
Interstitial pneumonitis	Transbronchial or open-lung biopsy >HRCT
Pulmonary thromboembolic disease	Contrast-enhanced spiral CT (CTA)

14. HRCT is the investigation of choice for all except:

a. Pulmonary artery aneurysm
b. Interstitial fibrosis
c. Miliary TB
d. Sarcoidosis

Investigations for Aneurysm in General

- Angiography/ DSA: First choice for final confirmation and evaluation of the aneurysm
- MRI: Most sensitive and specific investigation. It is best/ preferred/ diagnostic/ investigation of choice.

Imaging preferences for vascular pathologies

Disease	*Pulmonary embolism*	*Renal artery stenosis*	*Aortic dissection*	*Vertebral artery dissection*	*DVT*	*Chronic abdominal angina (Venous occlusion)*	*Acute mesenteric ischemia (Arterial)*
Screening tool of choice	D-dimer	Doppler/CTA	CTA>TEE	CTA	Doppler (Duplex ultrasound)	Doppler	Doppler
Investigation of choice	CTA	3D-dynamic CEMRA	MRI	MRA	Doppler> MRI	CTA	Angiography (MRA >CTA)
Gold standard investigation	Pulmonary arteriography	Renal arteriography	Aortography	Vertebral angiography	Venography	Angiography	Laparotomy

15. Right side of mediastinal shadow is not formed by:

a. Superior vena cava b. Right innominate
c. Right atrium d. Right ventricle

The normal right ventricle makes virtually no contribution to the cardiac silhouette in frontal view, although infundibulum lies close to left upper heart border.

Structure of silhouetted	Pathology
Right heart border	Right middle lobe pathology
Left heart border	Lingular lobe pathology
Aortic knuckle	Apicoposterior segment of LU
Right aortic border	Right middle lobe
Hemidiaphragm	Basal segments of lower lobe

16. Snowman sign is seen in:

a. TGA
b. TAPVC
c. ASD
d. VSD

Mixed radiographic features of TAPVC (esp. the supradiaphragmatic variety) include: Overall heart size notably normal. Dilated SVC and left vertical vein giving "Figure of-8 or Snowman" or "Cottage-loaf" heart configuration of cardiac silhouette and pretracheal density on lateral film.

17. On X-ray, shadow of heart is maximally increased in:

a. Pleural effusion
b. Pericardial effusion
c. Hiatus hernia
d. Thymoma

Radiographic features of pericardial effusion includes cardiomegaly (with narrow pedicle), producing a classical 'flask shaped' heart ("Water-bottle" or "Money-bag" heart).

18. Radiographic finding of Ebstein's anomaly:

a. Shrunken heart
b. Atrialization of right ventricle
c. Pulmonary plethora
d. All of the above

Ebstein's anomaly is a congenital heart defect in which the septal and posterior leaflets of the tricuspid valve are displaced towards the apex of the right ventricle of the heart. The annulus of the valve is still in the normal position. The valve leaflets, however, are to a varying degree, attached to the walls and septum of the right ventricle. A subsequent 'atrialization' of a portion of the morphologic right ventricle (which is then contiguous with the right atrium) is seen. This causes the right atrium to be large and the anatomic right ventricle to be small in size.

Ans. **14. a.** Pulmonary arte... **15. d.** Right ventricle **16. b.** TAPVC **17. b.** Pericardial effusion
18. b. Atrialization of right ventricle

19. Floating lily sign on X-ray is seen in:
a. Aspergilloma
b. Hydatid lung
c. Primary tuberculosis
d. Secondary tuberculosis

Radiological features of Hydatid disease of lung
- Meniscus/ double arch/ moon/ crescent sign
- Combo sign
- Serpent sign
- Water lily sign
- Cyst-in-cyst sign

Key signs in chest film pathologies	
Sign	*Disease*
Thumb sign	Epiglottitis
Steeple sign	Croup
Air crescent sign	Aspergilloma
Bulging fissure sign	Klebsiella pneumonia
Golden 'S' sign	Right upper lobe collapse
Stag antlers sign/Hands-up signs/Inverted	Earliest radiological sign of pulmonary venous
Mustache sign	hypertension

20. Investigation of choice for detection and characterization of interstitial lung disease is:
a. MRI
b. Chest X-ray
c. High resolution CT scan
d. Ventilation perfusion scan

HRCT is of proven value in the diagnosis of diffuse lung disease (like interstitial lung diseases), particularly in the early stages when the chest radiograph is normal and for follow-up.

Important facts	
HRCT	*Disease*
Reticular pattern	Many ILDs
Multiple cysts	Lymphangioleiomyomatosis (LAM) Pulmonary histiocytosis
Lepidote growth	Bronchoalveolar cancer
Crazy paving	Alveolar proteinosis > silicosis
"Tree-in-bud" appearance	Endobronchial TB and
	Atypical mycobacterial TB

ABDOMINAL

21. Adder head appearance on intravenous pyelography is seen in:
a. Hydronephrosis
b. Horse shoe kidney
c. Ureterocele
d. Tubercular cystitis

Intravenous urography (IVU) shows early filling of bulbous terminal ureter ("cobra head" appearance) and a radiolucent halo (ureteral wall + adjacent bladder urothelium) giving "spring onion" appearance.

Various radiological studies in GUT		
Radiological study	*Clinical utility*	*Key comments*
KUB X-ray	❑ Commonly done study for calculus diseases, but is of no vital use compared to CT and IVU ❑ The topography of staghorn calculi is well-assessed with X-ray KUB.	❑ Noncontrast helical/spiral CT is today the most sensitive and practical technique for a case of ureteric colic ❑ X-ray KUB is of no use for renal infections and tumors
IVU	❑ Pelvicalyceal anatomy is most reliably assessed by IVU ❑ Best for diagnosing renal TB ❑ Best for diagnosing renal papillary necrosis ❑ Urorenal anomalies ❑ Second line investigation for assessing renal function ❑ Second line investigation for renal and ureteric calculi ❑ Part of FIGO staging for cervical cancer	❑ IVU is a better term than IVP ❑ DTPA/MAG_3 scan is best for assessing renal function ❑ Iohexol (Low osmolar non-ionic iodinated contrast media) is the ideal contrast agent for IVU (Conray is outdated)
USG	❑ Screening tool for focal renal lesions ❑ Best for diagnosing vesical calculus ❑ Highly sensitive for diagnosing hydronephrosis ❑ Excellent for diagnosing urinoma ❑ USG with renal Doppler is one of the best studies for follow-up of transplanted kidney ❑ USG is tool of choice for follow-up of patients with ADPKD	❑ Air in bowel interferes with imaging of ureters ❑ It cannot assess renal function ❑ Color Doppler is initial screening tool of choice for renal artery stenosis. But in obese individuals, in patients who do not cooperate with respect to breath-holding its not of much use

Contd...

Ans. **19. b.** Hydatid lung **20. c.** High resolution CT scan **21. c.** Ureterocele

Contd...

Radiological study	*Clinical utility*	*Key comments*
CT scan (Multislice helical or spiral CT)	❑ Ureteric calculi (Noncontrast CT) ❑ Renal and perirenal infections ❑ Renal trauma ❑ Renal tumors: including RCC and oncocytoma (central satellite scar)	❑ Multislice CT with contrast is the best protocol ❑ Phasic CECT is required for detecting small RCCs ❑ CTA scores over color Doppler as most sensitive and specific test for screening of renal artery stenosis ❑ CT urography is not very popular
MRI	❑ RCC with renal vein and IVC invasion ❑ To differentiate bland from tumor thrombus ❑ 3D dynamic CE MRA is the most sensitive and specific investigation to detect renal artery stenosis	❑ MRU (MR urography is possible today but yet not very popular except for ureteric strictures and congenital anomalies, even for which it is not very cost-effective ❑ MRU is possible by two techniques: – By using heavily T2 weighted turbo spin echo MR sequences – Gadolinium-enhanced excretory MR urography ❑ The main advantage of MRU is no use of ionizing radiation
Nuclear scan	❑ Assessing renal function (GFR) by MAG_3 or DTPA scan ❑ Renal morphology assessment and detecting renal cortical scars ❑ Iodohippurate is outdated	❑ DTPA scan is also useful the VUR, PUJO, RAS ❑ The disadvantage of nulcear scans is anatomical delineations is not possible ❑ Captopril enhanced DTPA/MAG_3 renogram is secondline study for renovascular hypertension (RAS)

22. Functional analysis of kidney is best done by:

a. Radionuclide scanning b. IVP
c. USG d. MRI

The most accurate method of measuring GFR is by 99mTc DTPA/ MAG3 scan.

Definitive diagnosis of patency of renal arteries: Chronical renal disease associated with normal or increased kidney size are:	Contrast angiography ❑ Polycystic kidney disease ❑ Amyloidosis ❑ Diabetes ❑ HIV ars. renal disease
Investigation of bladder – neck obstruction in male is done by:	Cystourethrography (MCU)
Investigation of choice after acute renal trauma is:	CECT
Vesicoureteric reflux is best demonstrated:	Micturating Cystogram
The dye used for IVP:	Iohexol (300 mg/kg)
Isotopes used for scanning kidney:	^{99m}Tc DMSA/DTPA/MAG_3 (DTPA – for GFR, DMSA – for cortex)
Rapid sequence IVP is done in:	Renovascular hypertension
Whitaker's test is done to know:	Ureteropelvic junction obstruction
Maximum dose of contrast medium administered is:	600 mg of Iodine/kg body weight in a well hydrated patient
Choke urethrogram is done for:	Demonstration of anatomy of urethral stricture
Internal spermatic venography is an extremely accurate method of demonstrating the location of:	Undescended testis
The most accurate method of measuring GFR is by:	^{99m}Tc DTPA/MAG3 scan
Renal scarring is best shown by:	DMSA scan
Static renal scans are performed using DMSA, dynamic using DTPA DTPA is excreted by glomerular filtration, while Mag_3 is handled by filtration and tubular secretion. ^{99m}Tc DTPA captopril stress test is used for diagnosis of renovascular hypertension as second line study (MRA is first line).	

Contd...

Ans. 22. **a.** Radionuclide scanning

Contd...

Bead cystography which measures the posterior urethro vesical angle, is used to evaluate:	Stress incontinence
In pregnancy the ureter above the pelvic brim gets dilated, right more than left, this dilation persists for a month after delivery and predisposes to infection.	
Combined synchronous video cystometrography (VCMG):	Indications Symptoms of outflow obstruction in men below 35 years Urinary incontinence <35 years age Possible outflow obstruction in females Problems following pelvic or plastic surgery Some neuropathic bladder problems
Initial screening test for Renal artery stenosis/ischemic renal: disease	Doppler ultrasonography
Most sensitive and specific test for diagnosis of RAS:	MRA
Most definitive diagnostic procedure for RAS:	Contrast enhanced arteriography

23. String sign is seen in:

a. Crohn's disease
b. TB of ileocaecal region
c. Idiopathic hypertrophic pyloric stenosis
d. All of the above

Crohn's disease (Regional ileitis) shows "String sign" of Kantor on barium enema.

X-ray appearance	Diagnosis
❑ 'String of beads' sign	❑ Small bowel obstruction
❑ Cupola sign	❑ Pneumoperitoneum
❑ Rigler's (double-wall) sign	❑ Pneumoperitoneum
❑ Foot-ball sign	❑ Pneumoperitoneum
❑ Coffee bean sign	❑ Sigmoid volvulus (Strangulated bowel obstruction)
❑ 'Bird of prey' sign	❑ Sigmoid volvulus
❑ 'Coiled-spring' appearance	❑ Intussusception
❑ 'Claw' sign	❑ Intussusception
❑ 'Saw-toothed' appearance	❑ Diverticulosis
❑ Hat sign	❑ Colonic polyp
❑ 'Apple core' appearance	❑ Carcinoma colon
❑ 'Thumb-print' sign	❑ Ischemic colitis
❑ Reverse '3' sign of Frostburg	❑ Carcinoma head of pancreas

Contd...

Contd...

X-ray appearance	Diagnosis
❑ Moulage sign	❑ Malabsorption (Celiac disease)
❑ String sign of Kantor	❑ Crohn's disease
❑ String sign	❑ CHPS
❑ 'Pseudobiloth' appearance and	❑ Crohn's disease
❑ 'Ram's horn' stomach	
– String sign	❑ Ileocecal TB
– Fleishner's sign	
– Inverted umbrella sign	
– Widened ileocecal angle	
– "Contracted-pulled" cecum	
– Amputed cecum	
❑ Bull's eye lesion	❑ Leiomyoma (GIST) on Ba
	❑ Liver metastases and hepatic candidiasis on USG
❑ Mucosal granularity	❑ Earliest sign of ulcerative colitis on Ba enema

24. Pipe stem appearance in barium enema is seen in:

a. Crohn's disease
b. Ulcerative colitis
c. Schistosomiasis
d. Ca colon

'Lead pipe' colon is a chronic change of ulcerative colitis.

Type of abnormality	Radiological feature	Ulcerative colitis	Crohn's disease
Mucosal	Granularity	++	±
	Cobble-stoning	–	+
	Aphthoid ulcers	–	++
Configuration of	Fissuring ulcers	–	++
bowel wall	Haustra blunted	++	+
	Gen. narrowing and shortening	++	–

Contd...

Ans. 23. **a.** Crohn's disease 24. **b.** Ulcerative colitis

Contd...

	(hose-pipe)		
	String sign of Kantor	–	+
	Widened postrectal space	++	±
Distribution of lesions	Transmural	+	–
	Pseudodiverticuli	–	++
	Rectum involved	++	+
	Continuity	++	±
	Skip areas	–	+
	Backwash ileitis	+	–
	Multiple anal fistulas	–	+
Complications	Enteroenteric fistula	–	+
	Perforation	+	–
	Toxic megacolon	+	±
	Carcinoma	+	±

25. IOC to demonstrate vesico-ureteric reflex:

a. IVP b. USG

c. Contrast MCU d. Cystoscopy

Voiding cystourethrogram/Micturating cystoure-throgram (VCUG/ MCU) is the investigation of choice for evaluation of VUR. Renal nuclear scan preferred for follow up.

26. Rim sign is seen in:

a. Massive hydronephrosis

b. Polycystic kidney

c. Chronic pyelonephritis

d. Hypernephroma

Features of Hydronephrosis on IVU

- Large kidney with wasted parenchyma
  - Diminished nephrographic density
  - Moderate to marked widening or dilatation of PC system
- Rim sign – 'thin band of radiodensity surrounding calyces' in advanced cases
  - Delayed opacification of collection system
  - Faint nephrogram around the ballooned calyces, may produce 'soap-bubble' appearance.

27. Spider leg appearance is seen in:

a. Polycystic kidney b. Pyelonephritis

c. Hydronephrosis d. Renal artery stenosis

Intravenous urography (IVU) in ADPKD (autosomal dominant polycystic kidney disease) typically shows classical stretched appearance of calyces with sometimes spider leg appearance.

Inherited cystic kidney diseases

Disease	*Renal abnormalities*	*Extra-renal abnormalities*
Autosomal dominant polycystic kidney disease	Cortical and medullary cysts	Cerebral aneurysms, liver cysts (MC) Pancreatic cysts, colonic diverticuli, and mitral valve prolapse.
Autosomal recessive polycystic kidney disease	Distal tubule and collecting duct cysts (Bilateral large kidneys with multiple radially arranged microcysts)	Hepatic fibrosis: Caroli syndrome
Nephronophthisis I (Juvenile/Adolescent)	Small fibrotic kidneys; medullary cysts	Retinitis pigmentosa
Nephronophthisis II (Infantile)	Large kidneys; widespread cysts	Situs inversus
Nephronophthisis III (Juvenile/Adolescent)	Small fibrotic kidneys; medullary cysts	Retinitis pigmentosa, hepatic fibrosis
Nephronophthisis IV (Juvenile/Adolescent)	Small fibrotic kidneys; medullary cysts	Retinitis pigmentosa
Medullary cystic kidney disease	Small fibrotic kidneys; medullary cysts	Hyperuricemia and gout
Tuberous sclerosis	Renal cystis; angiomyolipomas; renal cell carcinoma	Adenoma sebaceum; CNS hamartomas. Kaenan's tumor, subependymal giant cell astrocytoma
Von Hippel-Lindau disease	Renal cysts; renal cell carcinoma	Retinal angiomas; CNS hemangioblastomas; Pheochromocytomas

Ans. **25. c.** Contrast MCU **26. a.** Massive hydroneph... **27. a.** Polycystic kidney

28 Earliest finding of renal tuberculosis on IVP:
a. Golf holes ureter b. Hydronephrosis
c. Feathery appearances of calyces
d. Cortical scar

Distinctive features of renal TB on IVU
- Putty kidney
- Autonephrectomy
- Nonfunctioning kidney
- Dystrophic calcification
- "Moth-eaten" calyx smudged papillae (earliest sign)
- Cavities communicating with collecting system
- Hydrocalycosis with infundibular strictures (most common sign).

MUSCULOSKELETAL

29. "Champagne glass pelvis" is seen in:
a. Achondroplasia
b. Cretinism
c. Down's syndrome
d. Congenital dislocation of hip

Radiological features of achondroplasia (pelvis)
- Small square shaped iliac bone with 'tombstone' appearance
- Small pelvis with narrow pelvic inlet resembling a 'champagne glass'.

Diagnostic imaging techniques for musculoskeletal disorders

Method	*Current indications*
Ultrasound	Synovial cysts Rotator cuff tears Tendon injury
^{99m}Tc scintigraphy	Metastatic bone survey Evaluation of Paget's disease Acute and chronic osteomyelitis
^{111}In-WBc scintigraphy	Acute infection Prosthetic infection Acute osteomyelitis
^{67}Ga scintigraphy	Acute and chronic infection Acute osteomyelitis
Computed tomography	Herniated intervertebral disk Sacroiliitis Spinal stenosis Spinal trauma Osteoid osteoma Stress fracture
Magnetic resonance imaging	Avascular necrosis Osteomyelitis Intra-articular derangement and soft tissue injury Derangements of axial skeleton and spinal cord Herniated intervertebral disk Pigmented villonodular synovitis Inflammatory and metabolic muscle pathology

30. Acro-osteolysis is seen in:
a. Frostbite b. Leprosy
c. Scleroderma d. Hypoparathyroidism

Vascular causes of acro-osteolysis are scleroderma with Raynaud's phenomenon and occlusive vascular disease.

Rheumatoid arthritis	Marginal bony erosions (bare area affected)
Scleroderma	Most common site of bone erosion is distal phalanx and erosion + subluxation of thumb carpo-metacarpal joint is characteristic
Dermatomyositis/polymyositis	Bone erosions very rare
SLE	Nonerosive arthritis
Jaccoud's arthritis (classically develops following rheumatic fever)	Late in the disease, "hook-erosions" may be seen
Multicentric reticulohistiocytosis	Large "punched-out" erosions
Psoriatic	Erosions similar as in RA and seen at DIP, "mouse-ears" marginal erosion and cup-like erosions
Gout	Punched out erosions with sclerotic margins and overhanging bony edge
Reiter's disease	Calcaneal erosions (Lover's heel)

31. IOC for traumatic paraplegia:
a. MRI b. CT scan
c. Myelography d. Spine X-ray

MRI is the investigation of choice for all spinal cord pathologies (e.g. Prolpased intervertebral disc, metastases, spinal cord tumours, traumatic paraplegia, transverse myelitis).

Modalities	Comment	Use (Prototype)
Plain X-ray (Radiograph)	Digital > Conventional	Routine fractures
Ultrasound (not for bone per se)	High frequency probe 7–15 mHz	Screening of rotator cuff tear, popliteal cysts
CT scan (for fine osseous details)	Multislice $\bar{c}$3D Recon	Complex fractures cortical lesions
MRI	STIR, T1, T2, Fatsat sequences	The best tool for many lesions

Contd...

Ans. 28. c. Feathery appear... 29. a. Achondroplasia 30. c. Scleroderma 31. a. MRI

Contd...

Modalities	Comment	Use (Prototype)
Bone scan (Triple phase)	^{99m}Tc-MDP is ideal agent	Highly sensitive for infection and metastases
Ga-67 ro Indium–111 WBC scan	Indium^{111} > Ga^{67}	Osteomyelitis
PET scan (18 FDG agent of choice)	Better than SPECT	Oncoimaging – FTU and recurrence

32. Beheaded scottish terrier sign is seen in:

a. Spondylosis
b. Spondylolisthesis
c. Fracture transverse process of lumbar vertebra
d. Fracture rib

Must know

- Scotty dog with Collar or broken neck = spondylolysis
- Beheaded scotty dog = spondylolisthesis

33. Dead bone on an X-ray looks:

a. More radio-opaque b. Radiolucent
c. Less radio-opaque d. Not seen at all

Sequestra is detached necrotic cortical bone fragments if surrounded by pus, are not absorbed and remain as sequestra, seen as more radiopaque densities than the surrounding bone (develops after 30 days).

Type of study	Comments
Plain radiographs	Insensitive, especially in early osteomyelitis May show perfosteal elevation after 10 days, lytic changes after 2–6 weeks.[Q]
Three-phase bone scan (^{99m}Tc-MDP)	Characteristic finding in osteomyelitis increased uptake in all three phases of scan Highly sensitive (~95%) in acute infection[Q]
^{67}Ga-citrate, ^{111}In-labeled	^{111}In-WBCs more specific than gallium but not always available[Q]
WBCs scans	Lack of consensus over role; often supplanted by MRI when the latter is available
MRI	As sensitive as ^{99m}Tc-MDP bone scan for acute osteomyelitis (~95%)[Q] High specificity (~87%), with better anatomic detail than nuclear studies

Note: 'Q' as a superscript indicates 'vital indications'

34. Not a feature of scurvy:

a. Epiphyseal widening b. Metaphyseal porosis
c. Metaphyseal infarction d. Pelkan spur

Widening and irregularity of epiphyseal plates is a radiographical feature of rickets.

35. Splaying and cupping of metaphysis is seen in:

a. Rickets b. Scurvy
c. Paget's disease d. Lead poisoning

Radiological features of rickets

- Poorly mineralized epiphyseal centers with delayed appearance
- Widening and lengthening of growth plate (zone of provisional calcification affected) is earliest radiographic features of rickets
- Increased distance between end of shaft and epiphyseal center
- Epiphyseal plates widening and irregularity
- Fraying, splaying and cupping of metaphyses.

36. Gold standard for diagnosing osteoporosis is:

a. Dual energy X-ray absorptiometry
b. Single energy X-ray absorptiometry
c. USG
d. Quantitative CT

Bone densitometry is currently the most accurate bone density measurement technique or a method for predicting patients at risk of osteoporotic fracture (Gold standard). DXA has superseded DPA (dual photon absorptiometry) and is now the most commonly used technique for measuring BMD throughout the world.

37. A 40-year-old female patient on long term steroid therapy presents with recent onset of severe pain in the right hip. IOC of choice:

a. CT b. Bone scan
c. MRI d. Plain X-ray

MRI is IOC for

- Empty sella syndrome
- Hyperacute and acute infarct
- Chronic SAH
- To detect cerebral metastases
- Demyelinating and dysmyelinating diseases of brain (e.g. Multiple sclerosis, SSPE, motor neuron disease, central pontine myelinolysis, etc.)
- Congenital brain anomalies (e.g. Arnold Chiari malformation, etc.)
- To differentiate between arachnoid cyst and epidermoid cyst
- All brain tumours, especially the posterior fossa tumours
- All spinal cord pathologies
- Imaging of breast with silicon implants
- Juvenile angiofibroma
- Ca nasopharynx (CT better for delineating skull base/bony erosion)
- All bone tumours (except osteoid osteoma, for which CT is better)
- Avascular necrosis (may occur on long term steroid use).

Ans. 32. **b.** Spondylolisthesis 33. **a.** More radio-opaque 34. **a.** Epiphyseal widening 35. **a.** Rickets 36. **a.** Dual energy X-ray absorptiometry 37. **c.** MRI

Best investigation for imaging of a bone tumor	MRI
Most sensitive investigation for bone metastases	Bone scan
Best investigation for bone metastases	MRI
Ideal agent for bone scan (scintigraphy)	^{99m}Tc MDP
Double density sign on bone scintigraphy	Osteoid osteoma
"Doughnut sign" on bone scan	Osteosarcoma

SKULL

38. Best investigation to study presence of calcification on an intracranial lesion:

a. MRI
b. USG
c. CT scan
d. Contrast study

CNS: Radiological signs & conditions

- IOC for subarachnoid hemorrhage (SAH): Non-contrast CT
- Intracranial calcification is seen in:
  - Cystecercosis,
  - Pineal & dural calcification
- Basal ganglia calcification is seen in: Hypoparathyroidism
- Suprasellar calcification is seen in:
  - Craniopharyngioma,
  - Meningioma
- Rail road/Tram track calcification: Sturge Weber syndrome
- Periventricular calcification is seen in: CMV infection
- Bracket calcification in skull is seen in: Corpus callosum lipoma
- Separation of sutures in a child is radiological sign of: Raised intra-cranial tension

39. CT scan findings of extradural hematoma:

a. Hypodense biconves lesion
b. Hyperdense biconvex lesion
c. Concavo-convex hyperdense lesion
d. Low attenuated biconvex lesion

CT scan findings in EDH

- Biconvex, displaced gray white interface
- 2/3 hyperdense, 1/3 mixed.

	EDH	SDH
Incidence	1–4 percent overall	10–20 percent overall
Etiology	Associated # in 85-95 percent cases. Stretching, tearing of bridging cortical veins in 70–85 percent cases and venous "OOZE" or MMA tear without # in 15 percent cases only	Stretching, tearing of bridging cortical veins
Location	Between skull and dura. Cross dural attachments but not sutures. 95 percent supratentorial, 5 percent bilateral	Between dura and arachnoid. Cross sutures but not dural attachment. 95 percent supratentorial, 15 percent bilateral
Imaging	CT: Biconvex displaced gray white interface. 2/3 hyperdense, 1/3 mixed	CT: a. Acute SDH: Crescentic. 60 percent hyperdense, 40 percent mixed b. Subacute SDH: May be nearly isodense with cortex neomembrane, underlying vessels may enhance. c. Chronic SDH: Hypodense with enhancing membrane. May be loculated. Rehemorrhage can cause mixed density. 1–2 percent of very old SDH calcify.

40. IOC in case of subarachnoid hemorrhage:

a. CT
b. MRI
c. MRI angiography
d. Carotid angiogram

NCCT is 60 to 90 percent accurate for diagnosing SAH, even higher within first 4-5 days of the onset (pseudodelta sign and cortical vein sign). MRI is relatively insensitive in acute SAH (first 48 hours of onset).

Guidelines for CT, ultrasound and MRI in neuroimaging	
Condition	*Recommended technique*
Hemorrhage	
❑ Acute parenchymal	CT > MR
❑ Subacute/chronic	MRI
❑ Subarachnoid hemorrhage	CT, CTA, lumbar puncture → angiography
Aneurysm	Angiography > CTA, MRA

Contd...

Ans. **38. c.** CT scan **39. b.** Hyperdense biconvex... **40. a.** CT

Contd...

Condition	*Recommended technique*
Ischemic infarction	
❑ Hemorrhagic infarction	CT
❑ Bland infarction	MRI > CT
❑ Carotid or vertebral dissection	MRI/MRA
❑ Vertebral basilar insufficiency	CTA, MRI/MRA
❑ Carotid stenosis	CTA > Doppler ultrasound, MRA
Suspected mass lesion	
❑ Neoplasm, primary or metastatic	MRI + contrast
❑ Infection/abscess	MRI + contrast
❑ Immunosuppressed with focal findings	MRI + contrast
Vascular malformation	MRI ± contrast
White matter disorders	MRI
Demyelinating disease	MRI ± contrast
Dementia	MRI
Trauma	
❑ Acute trauma	CT (noncontrast)
❑ Shear injury/chronic hemorrhage	MRI
Headache/migraine	CT (noncontrast)/MRI
Seizure	
❑ First time, no focal neurologic deficits	CT as screen
❑ Partial complex/refractory	MRI with coronal T2W imaging
Cranial neuropathy	MRI with contrast
Meningeal disease	MRI with contrast
Spine	
Low back pain	
❑ No neurologic deficits	MRI or CT after 4 weeks
❑ With focal deficits	MRI > CT
Spinal stenosis	MRI or CT
Cervical spondylosis	MRI or CT myelography
Infection	MRI + contrast, CT
Myelopathy	MRI + contrast > myelography
Arteriovenous malformation	MRI, myelography/angiography

Note: CT: Computed tomography; MRI: Magnetic resonance imaging; MRA: MR angiography; CTA: CT angiography; T2W: T2-weighted.

41. Multiple punched out lesions in skull is seen in:
a. Acute leukemia
b. Thalassemia
c. Multiple myeloma
d. Ca prostate

Radiographic features of multiple myeloma include multiple punched out widespread osteolytic lesions in skull, however, classic 2-3 mm 'rain drop' circular lytic defects are not always evident.

42. Earliest sign of raised intracranial tension in adults:
a. Copper beaten appearance
b. Widening of sella
c. Pineal displacement
d. Erosion of dorsum sella

Radiographic signs of increased intracranial tension in adults
- Erosion of posterior clinoid process (earliest sign)
- Interruption of the lamina dura at the base of the dorsum sellae (earliest sign)
- Slight porosis of anterior cortex followed by loss of lamina dura/cortex/compact bone

Ans. 41. c. Multiple myeloma **42. d.** Erosion of dorsum sella

- Frank erosion of dorsum sellae (other causes may be hyperparathyroidism, nutritional, and local causes)
- Pineal displacement.

43. Hyperostosis and prominent vascular markings is a radiographic feature of:

a. Corpus callosum lipoma
b. Meningioma
c. Craniopharyngioma
d. Raised intracranial tension

X-ray skull in meningioma

- Hyperostosis at site close to or within bone
- Calcification (psammomatous)
- Enlarged meningeal grooves and marked vascular markings
- Enlarged foramen spinosum
- Blistering of paranasal sinuses with or without sclerosis (pneumosinus dilatans).

MISCELLANEOUS

44. Most serious complication of myelogram is:

a. Allergy
b. Transient neurological deficit
c. Headache
d. Thinned out vault

Because a contrast dye is used during the procedure, there is risk of allergic reaction to the substance.

45. In stricture esophagus due to corrosive poisoning, investigation of choice is:

a. X-rays
b. Pharyngoscopy
c. Barium meal
d. Endoscopy

Esophageal stricture can be diagnosed with an X-ray while the patient swallows barium (called a barium study of the esophagus), by a computerized tomography scan, a biopsy, or by an endoscopy (best).

Ans. **43. b.** Meningioma **44. a.** Allergy **45. d.** Endoscopy

ANSWERS WITH REFERENCES

GENERAL PRINCIPLES

1. **Ans. (d)** Right ventricle
Ref: Chest X-ray Made Easy by J. Corne, p-20

2. **Ans. (b)** Gadolinium
Ref: Daga's Radiodiagnosis 1/e p62

3. **Ans. (a)** Pacemaker
Ref: Daga's Radiodiagnosis 1/e p45

4. **Ans. (a)** Transfemoral route
Ref: Daga's Radiodiagnosis 1/e p530

5. **Ans. (d)** Superior to CT for bone scanning
Ref: Daga's Radiodiagnosis 1/e p38

6. **Ans. (b)** Tungsten
Ref: Daga's Radiodiagnosis 1/e p5

7. **Ans. (b)** Silver bromide
Ref: Daga's Radiodiagnosis 1/e p6

8. **Ans. (a)** Piezoelectric crystal excitation
Ref: Daga's Radiodiagnosis 1/e p53

THORAX

9. **Ans. (c)** Uncorrected TGA
Ref: Daga's Radiodiagnosis 1/e p137

10. **Ans. (a)** Echocardiography
Ref: Daga's Radiodiagnosis 1/e p132

11. **Ans. (b)** Interstitial lung disease
Ref: Daga's Radiodiagnosis 1/e p116

12. **Ans. (a)** Lung hydatid
Ref: Daga's Radiodiagnosis 1/e p94

13. **Ans. (d)** Coarctation of aorta
Ref: Daga's Radiodiagnosis 1/e p130

14. **Ans. (a)** Pulmonary artery aneurysm
Ref: Daga's Radiodiagnosis 1/e p149

15. **Ans. (d)** Right ventricle
Ref: Daga's Radiodiagnosis 1/e p98

16. **Ans. (b)** TAPVC
Ref: Daga's Radiodiagnosis 1/e p137

17. **Ans. (b)** Pericardial effusion
Ref: Daga's Radiodiagnosis 1/e p147

18. **Ans. (b)** Atrialization of right ventricle
Ref: Internet resources

19. **Ans. (b)** Hydatid lung
Ref: Daga's Radiodiagnosis 1/e p129

20. **Ans. (c)** High resolution CT scan
Ref: Daga's Radiodiagnosis 1/e p121

21. **Ans. (c)** Ureterocele
Ref: Daga's Radiodiagnosis 1/e p228

22. **Ans. (a)** Radionuclide scanning
Ref: Daga's Radiodiagnosis 1/e p226

23. **Ans. (a)** Crohn's disease
Ref: Daga's Radiodiagnosis 1/e p167

24. **Ans. (b)** Ulcerative colitis
Ref: Daga's Radiodiagnosis 1/e p198

25. **Ans. (c)** Contrast MCU
Ref: Daga's Radiodiagnosis 1/e p223

26. **Ans. (a)** Massive hydronephrosis
Ref: Daga's Radiodiagnosis 1/e p235

27. **Ans. (a)** Polycystic kidney
Ref: Daga's Radiodiagnosis 1/e p230

28. **Ans. (c)** Feathery appearances of calyces
Ref: Daga's Radiodiagnosis 1/e p237

MUSCULOSKELETAL

29. **Ans. (a)** Achondroplasia
Ref: Daga's Radiodiagnosis 1/e p249

30. **Ans. (c)** Scleroderma
Ref: Daga's Radiodiagnosis 1/e p303

31. **Ans. (a)** MRI
Ref: Daga's Radiodiagnosis 1/e p249

32. **Ans. (b)** Spondylolisthesis
Ref: Daga's Radiodiagnosis 1/e p278

33. **Ans. (a)** More radio-opaque
Ref: Daga's Radiodiagnosis 1/e p272

34. **Ans. (a)** Epiphyseal widening
Ref: Daga's Radiodiagnosis 1/e p265

35. **Ans. (a)** Rickets
Ref: Daga's Radiodiagnosis 1/e p265

36. **Ans. (a) Dual energy X-ray absorptiometry**
Ref: Daga's Radiodiagnosis 1/e p50

37. **Ans. (c) MRI**
Ref: Daga's Radiodiagnosis 1/e p302

SKULL

38. **Ans. (c) CT scan**
Ref: Grainger's Radiology, 4th/ed, p-2327

39. **Ans. (b) Hypodense biconves lesion**
Ref: Daga's Radiodiagnosis 1/e p365

40. **Ans. (a) CT**
Ref: Daga's Radiodiagnosis 1/e p322

41. **Ans. (c) Multiple myeloma**
Ref: Daga's Radiodiagnosis 1/e p283

42. **Ans. (d) Erosion of dorsum sella**
Ref: Daga's Radiodiagnosis 1/e p318

43. **Ans. (b) Meningioma**
Ref: Daga's Radiodiagnosis 1/e p360

MISCELLANEOUS

44. **Ans. (a) Allergy**
Ref: Internet resources

45. **Ans. (d) Endoscopy**
Ref: Internet resources

PRACTICE QUESTIONS

GENERAL PRINCIPLES

1. Which of the following carries MINIMUM radiation exposure:

a. Plane X-ray
b. CT scan
c. PET scan
d. MRI

THORAX

2. Reverse 3 sign is seen in:

a. Transposition of great arteries
b. Infracardiac TAPVC
c. Supracardiac TAPVC
d. Coarctation of aorta

3. McConnell's sign is seen in:

a. Pulmonary artery stenosis
b. Acute pulmonary embolism
c. Miliary TB
d. Pneumothorax

ABDOMINAL

4. A 30 years old female presented with slight fever and pain in right hypochondrium. Which of the following investigation is best to investigate the case?

a. CT scan
b. Abdominal plain film
c. Ultrasound
d. Oral cholecystography

MUSCULOSKELETAL

5. In acute osteomyelitis, early visible X-ray changes is noticed on what day:

a. 5th day
b. 10th day
c. 15th day
d. 20th day

SKULL

6. Which of the following is the investigation of choice for acute parenchymal haemorrhage in brain:

a. MRI
b. USG
c. X-ray
d. CT scan

MISCELLANEOUS

7. Which of the following condition commonly predisposes to contrast induced nephropathy?

a. Diabetes mellitus
b. Malignant hypertension
c. Benign hypertension
d. Sarcoidosis

Ans. 1. **d.** MRI 2. **d.** Coarctation of aorta 3. **b.** Acute pulmonary embolism
4. **c.** Ultrasound 5. **b.** 10th day 6. **d.** CT scan
7. **a.** Diabetes mellitus

IMAGE-BASED QUESTIONS

1. Following X-ray is suggestive of:

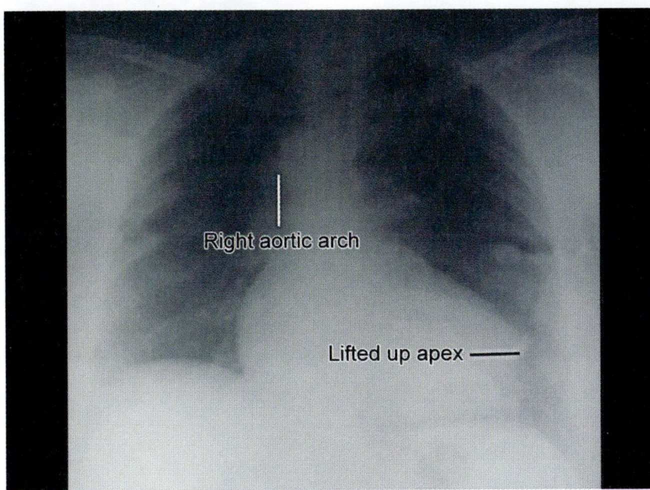

a. ASD
b. TOF
c. TGA
d. TAPVC

The characteristic elevation of the apex of heart or 'Cœur en sabot' or 'boot shaped' heart, the appearance of right ventricular enlargement, is seen in untreated tetralogy of Fallot and in pulmonary atresia with ASD. The large right ventricle probably causes it.

2. Following X-ray is suggestive of:

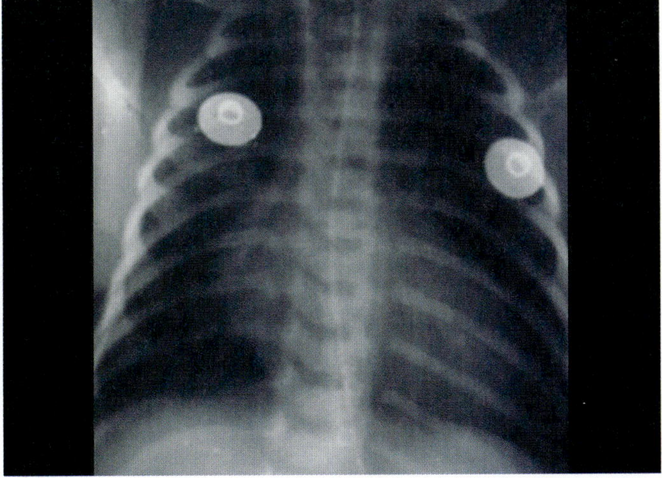

a. TAPVC
b. TOF
c. TGA
d. VSD

"Egg on Side" heart ("Egg in Cup" heart) is seen in TGA.

3. Following X-ray is suggestive of:

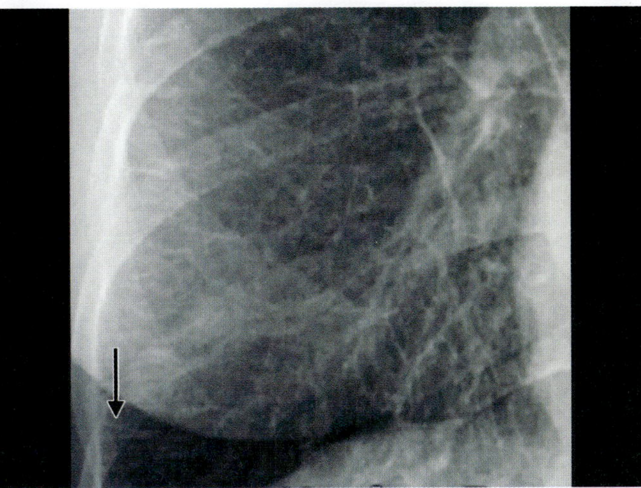

a. Pulmonary embolism
b. Pulmonary edema
c. Pulmonary TB
d. Asbestosis

Interstitial pulmonary edema (in congestive cardiac failure) is characterized by loss of sharp definition of vascular marking; thickening of interlobular septa, i.e. Kerley B-lines (shown in figure); pulmonary venous pressure 17-20 mm Hg; interlobar fissural thickening poorly defined increased bronchial wall thickness.

4. Following X-ray is suggestive of:

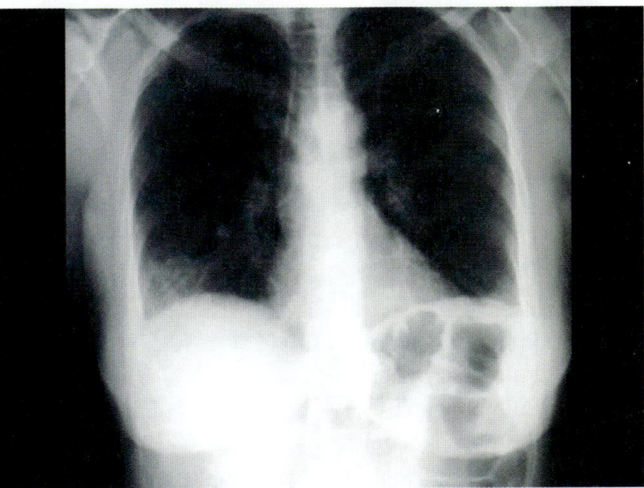

a. Pulmonary embolism
b. Pulmonary edema
c. Pulmonary TB
d. Asbestosis

A peripheral wedge-shaped density above the diaphragm (Hampton's hump) is a radiological feature of pulmonary embolism.

5. Following CT scan is suggestive of:

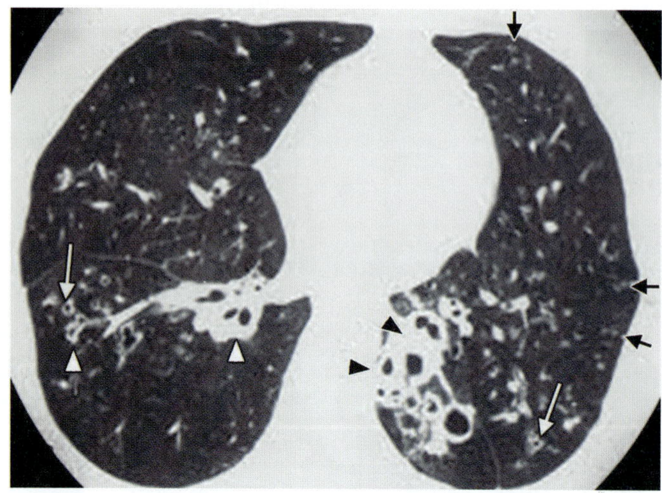

a. Pulmonary embolism
b. Pulmonary edema
c. Pulmonary TB
d. Bronchiectasis

Signet ring sign on HRCT is suggestive of bronchiectasis.

6. Following CT scan is suggestive of:

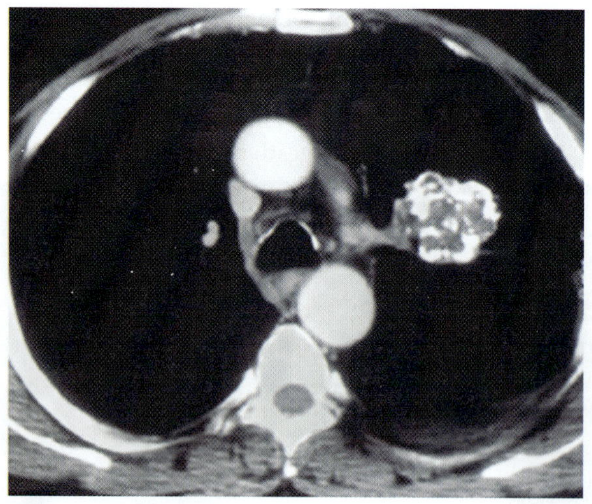

a. Pulmonary embolism
b. Pulmonary edema
c. Pulmonary TB
d. Pulmonary hamartoma

Popcorn calcification on CT scan is virtually diagnostic (only DD is a chondrosarcoma) and central fat density, if present also establishes the diagnosis.

7. Following X-ray is suggestive of:

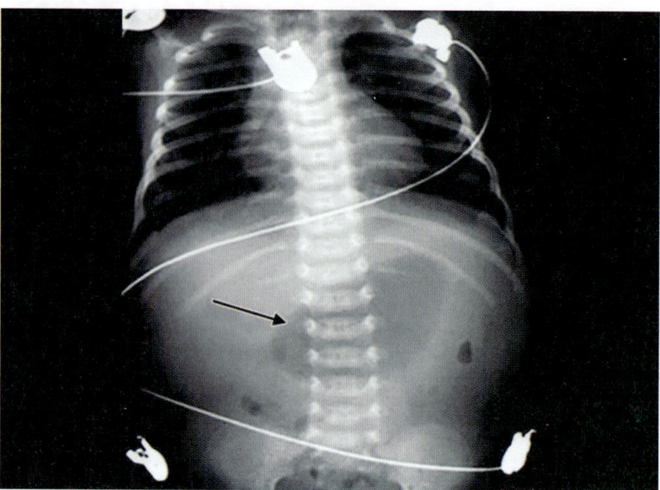

a. Esophageal atresia
b. Pyloric stenosis
c. Duodenal atresia
d. Jejunal atresia

An abdominal radiography in neonate with hypertrophic pyloric stenosis shows a distended air-filled stomach with a relative paucity of bowel gas distally.

8. Following X-ray is suggestive of:

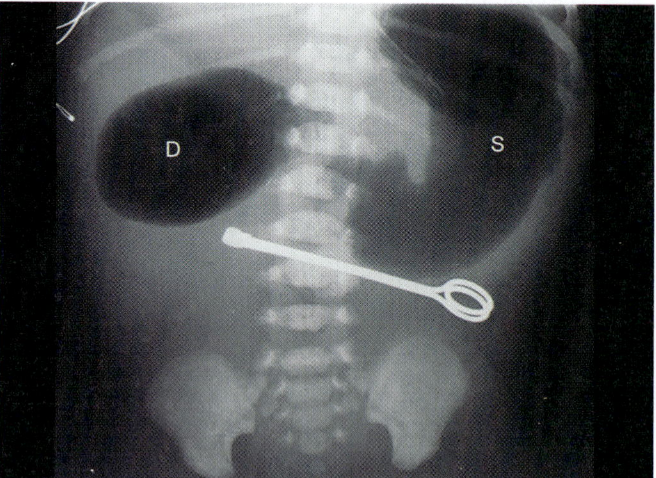

a. Esophageal atresia
b. Pyloric stenosis
c. Duodenal atresia
d. Jejunal atresia

Abdominal radiography in duodenal atresia demonstrates the classic 'double-bubble' sign with the absence of distal air.

9. Following X-ray is suggestive of:

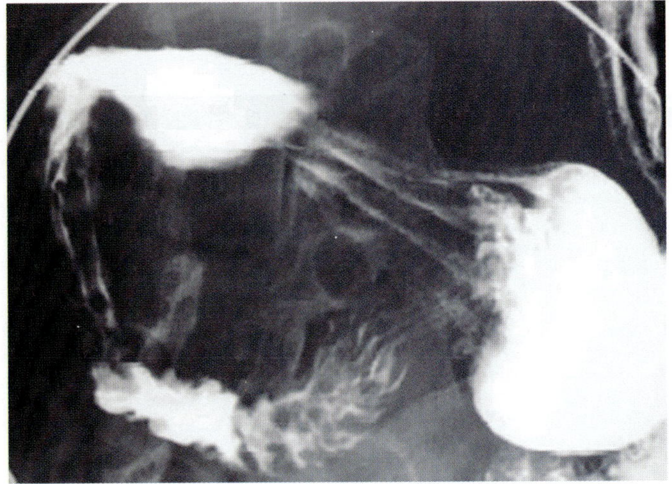

a. Duodenal atresia
b. Duodenal blowout
c. Ca head of pancreas
d. Ca duodenum

Carcinoma head of the pancreas frequently causes changes in the duodenal loop. There may be widening of duodenal loop double contour, irregularity of the inner border, and structuring or distortion of the valvulae conniventes.

10. Following X-ray is suggestive of:

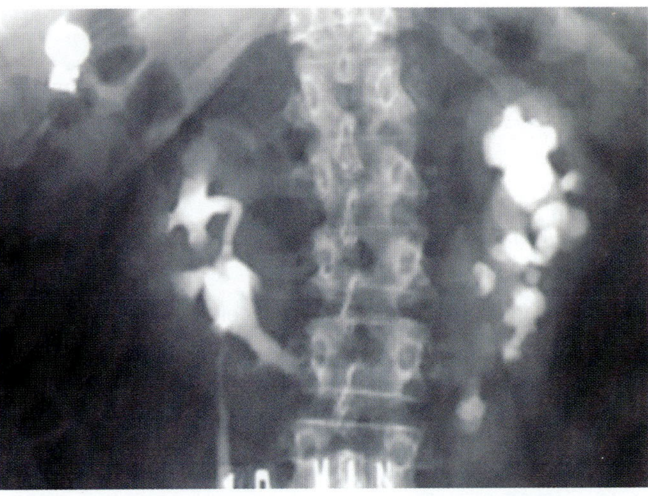

a. Ureteric calculi
b. Renal calculi
c. Polycystic kidney
d. Horseshoe kidney

Ureters in horseshoe kidneys had characteristically vase-like curves ('flower vase' ureters).

MCQ POINTS

S. No.	Question statements	Answers
1.	Substance having same atomic mass and different atomic number is	***Isobars***
2.	Most penetrating rays	***Neutron followed by gamma rays***
3.	MRI rooms are shielded by	***Copper/Aluminium***
4.	Sugar used in PET scan	***Glucose***
5.	Tram track appearance of skull on CT scan is seen in	***Sturge-Weber syndrome***
6.	Triple bubble sign is seen in	***Jejunal atresia***
7.	Radiological feature of ureterocele	***Adder head appearance***
8.	Radiological feature of polycystic kidney disease	***Spider leg appearance***
9.	Investigation of choice for chronic subarachnoid hemorrhage	***MRI***
10.	Investigation of choice for Perthe's disease	***MRI***
11.	Best method to detect minimal pleural effusion on right side	***USG***
12.	Radiological feature of ankylosing spondylitis	***Bamboo spine***
13.	Claw sign is seen in	***Intussusception***
14.	Measure of activity of radiation	***Becquerel (SI unit)/ Curie (non-SI unit)***
15.	Half life of Radium	***1600 years***
16.	Most radiosensitive phase of cycle	***G2M***
17.	Radioactive Iodine Uptake/ RAIU test is done by using	***Iodine-123***
18.	Use of gamma knife	***Stereo-tactic radiosurgery***
19.	Radiological feature of pulmonary hamartoma	***Popcorn calcification***
20.	Radiological feature of osteoclastoma	***Soap bubble appearance***
21.	Frostburg's reverse 3 sign is seen in	***Ca head of pancreas***
22.	Investigation of choice for interstitial lung disease	***High resolution CT scan***
23.	'Coeur en sabot' heart is seen in	***Tetralogy of Fallot***
24.	Rays having maximum ionizing power	***Alpha rays***
25.	Robert's sign is suggestive of	***Intrauterine fetal death***
26.	Earliest radiological change of mitral stenosis on radiography	***Straightening of left border of heart***
27.	Double atrial shadow is suggestive of	***Mitral stenosis***
28.	Snowman heart/figure of 8 is radiological feature of	***TAPVC***
29.	Investigation, which itself can lead to acute pancreatitis	***ERCP***
30.	Radiological finding in a case of duodenal stenosis	***Double bubble sign***
31.	Air crescent sign is seen in which lung pathology	***Aspergilloma***
32.	Signet ring sign is associated with which lung pathology	***Bronchiectasis***
33.	Hampton hump is a radiological feature of	***Pulmonary embolism***
34.	IOC for osteoporosis	***DEXA scan***
35.	Shepherd crook deformity of femur is a radiological feature of	***Fibrous dysplasia***
36.	'Figure of 3' on chest X-ray is suggestive of	***Coarctation of aorta***
37.	'Dropping flower' sign is suggestive of	***Ectopic/duplication of ureter***
38.	'Water lily' sign is suggestive of	***Hydatid cyst of lung***
39.	Straightening of left border of heart is seen in	***Mitral stenosis***

S. No.	Question statements	Answers
40.	Right border of heart (on X-ray) is formed by	***Superior vena cava, right atrium and inferior vena cava***
41.	Frog eye appearance in USG is suggestive of	***Anencephaly***
42.	IOC for renal vein thrombosis and IVC thrombosis	***Doppler USG***
43.	Linear accelerator produces which rays	***X-rays***
44.	X-ray for closed pneumothorax is done in which stage of respiration	***Expiration***
45.	Double bubble appearance is seen in	***Duodenal atresia and annular pancreas***
46.	Figure of 8 appearance is seen in	***TAPVC***
47.	DTPA and DMSA scans are used for which organ	***Kidney***
48.	IOC for kidney morphology is	***DMSA***
49.	Half life of radioiodine is	***8 days***
50.	IOC for remnant spleen is	***Tc99 labelled RBC***
51.	Si unit of radiation absorbed dose is	***Gray***
50.	Cystic lesion with suprasellar calcification is a feature of	***Craniopharyngioma***
53.	Corkscrew esophagus is seen in	***Diffuse esophageal spasm***
54.	Egg shell calcification in hilar node suggests	***Silicosis, sarcoidosis***
55.	Subperiosteal resorption and thickness of skull is increased in	***Hyperparathyroidism***
56.	Renal calculi associated with proteus infection	***Struvite/staghorn/triple phosphate***
57.	String of beads/sausage appearance of the renal artery is seen in	***Fibromuscular dysplasia***
58.	Meckel's diverticulum is best diagnosed by	***Tc99***
59.	Dye used for myelography	***Metrizamide***
60.	Epiphyseal dysgenesis is a pathognomic feature of	***Hypothyroidism***
61.	Gold standard investigation in a case of acute cholecystitis	***HIDA scan***
62.	IOC for vestibular schwannoma	***Gadolinium enhanced MRI***
63.	On radiography, widened duodenal C loop with irregular mucosal pattern on upper gastrointestinal barium series is a feature of	***Ca head of pancreas***
64.	Osteoclastic bone metastasis is found most commonly in which carcinoma	***Renal cell ca***
65.	Shield used in radiology are made up of which metal	***Lead***
66.	Appearance of dead bone on X-ray	***Radio-opaque (more white)***
67.	Fetus is most radiosensitive at what gestational age	***3 weeks***
68.	Angiographic findings in Buerger's disease	***Corkscrew vessels***
69.	IOC for minimal ascites is	***USG***
70.	Solitary hypoechoic lesion of liver with septa and debris is seen in	***Hydatid cyst***
71.	Snowman sign is seen in	***TAPVC***
72.	Gamma knife is used in	***Stereotactic radiosurgery***
73.	Apple core sign n barium enema is seen in carcinoma	***Ca colon***
74.	PET scan uses which trace material	***FDG***
75.	Chain of lake appearance is seen in	***Chronic pancreatitis***

CHAPTER

13

RADIOTHERAPY

KEY POINTS

Radionuclides in Nuclear Medicine

- Tc-99m medronate (MDP): Bone scanning
- Tc-99m Pentetate (DTPA): Renal imaging and function studies; radioaerosol ventilation imaging
- Tc-99m RBCs: Imaging of GI bleeds, cardiac chambers
- Tc-99m Succimer (DMSA): Renal imaging
- Tc-99m Lidofenin (HIDA): Hepatobiliary imaging

Ionizing Radiation

- Order of ionizing and damaging power: Gamma rays < X-rays < beta particles < Alpha particles
- Order of penetrating power: Alpha particles < Beta particles < X-rays < Gamma rays

Radiotherapy

- Systemic radiotherapy
  - Iodine-131 in papillary Ca of thyroid
- Teletherapy (external beam radiotherapy)
  - Source of radiation is distant from the patient
  - Gamma rays: Cobalt-60 or Cesium-137
- Brachytherapy (internal radiotherapy)
  - Radiation source is in close contact with tumour
  - Interstitial: Iridium-192
  - Intracavitary: Cesium-137
  - Mould: Iridium-192

Radiation Units

Quantity measured	SI unit	Old unit
Dose equivalent	Sievert	Rem
Absorbed dose	Gray	Rad
Radiation exposure	Columb/cm	Roentgen
Radioactivity	Becquerel	Curie

Most Radiosensitive Tumors of

- Kidney: Wilms tumor
- Brain: Lymphoma > medulloblastoma
- Lung: Small cell Ca
- Ovary: Dysgerminoma
- Testes: Seminoma
- Bone: Ewing's sarcoma

Most Radiosensitive

- Mucosa: Intestinal mucosa
- Abdominal organ: Kidney
- Body tissue: Bone marrow
- Blood cell: Lymphocyte
- Phase of cell cycle: G2M

MCQs WITH SHORT EXPLANATIONS

RADIOSENSITIVITY OF TISSUES

1. **Most radiosensitive tumour in the body:**
   a. Seminoma
   b. Squamous cell carcinoma of lung
   c. Rectal carcinoma
   d. Soft-tissue sarcoma

   Highly radiosensitive tumor include seminoma, lymphoma, etc.

Radiosensitivity of different tumors

Highly radiosensitive	*Moderately radiosensitive*	*Relatively resistant*	*Highly resistant*
Lymphoma	Small cell lung cancer	Squamous cell carcinoma of lung	Melanoma
Seminoma	Breast cancer	RCC	Osteosarcoma
Myeloma	Basal cell carcinoma	Rectal carcinoma	Pancreatic carcinoma
Ewing's sarcoma	Medulloblastoma	Bladder carcinoma	HCC
Wilms' tumors	Teratoma	Soft tissue sarcoma	Malignant fibrous
	Ovarian cancer	Cervical cancer	Histiocytoma

2. **Most radiosensitive female tumour:**
   a. Teratoma
   b. Dysgerminoma
   c. Ovarian carcinoma
   d. Breast cancer

   Dysgerminoma is one of the highly radiosensitive malignancies in females.

Type of RT	Indications
Whole body RT	❑ Mycosis fungoides ❑ Before bone marrow transplant
Mantle RT	❑ Hodgkin's lymphoma
Prophylactic craniospinal RT	❑ ALL
	❑ Small cell lung cancer
	❑ NHL
CHART	❑ Nonsmall cell lung cancer
Accelerated RT	❑ Head and neck cancer
Hyperfractionated RT	❑ Lung cancer
	❑ Head and neck cancer
Emergency RT	❑ SVC obstruction due to lung cancer
	❑ Cardiac tamponade due to pericardial invasion by malignancy
	❑ Spinal cord compression by metastases
Intraoperative RT (electrons > X-rays)	❑ Breast cancer
	❑ Pancreatic cancer
	❑ Lung carcinoma
	❑ Skull base
	❑ Melanoma
Postoperative RT	❑ Tumor margins positive
	❑ Tumor margins within 5 mm
	❑ LN metastases
	❑ Peritumoral invasion
	❑ Deep lobe involvement of parotid

Contd...

Ans. 1. **a.** Seminoma 2. **b.** Dysgerminoma

Contd...

Type of RT	Indications
	❑ Endocervical involvement
	❑ More than 50% of uterine wall involved
	❑ Recurrent tumor
	❑ High grade malignancies
IMRT	❑ Ca prostate
	❑ Head and neck cancer
	❑ Oral cancers
3D CRT	❑ Head and neck cancer
	❑ Lung cancer
	❑ Thyroid cancer
	❑ Breast cancer
Stereotactic radiosurgery	❑ Brain metastases (<4 in number)
– Co-60 (Gamma-knife)	❑ AVMs
– Linear accelerator (X-ray knife)	❑ Small meningioma
– Cyclotron (Proton beam)	❑ Small acoustic neuroma
	❑ Pituitary adenoma
Neutron therapy	❑ Salivary gland tumor
	❑ Cystic gliomas of brain
Proton therapy	❑ Stereotactic RT
	❑ Skin cancer
Concurrent chemotherapy	❑ Head and neck cancer
	❑ Ca cervix stage IIb/IIIA onwards
	❑ Ca anal canal
	❑ Ca nasopharynx
Intracavitary brachytherapy	❑ Treatment of gynecological malignancies, particularly those of the cervix, vagina, and uterus
Interstitial brachytherapy	❑ Oral cavity
	❑ Oropharynx
	❑ Nasopharynx
	❑ Neck nodes
	❑ Skin cancer
	❑ Carcinoma of the prostate
	❑ Anal canal
	❑ Penis
	❑ Carcinoma of the breast as salvage for local recurrence
	Please note contraindications to interstitial brachytherapy:
	– Tumor infiltrating or attached to bone.
	– Presence of active infection within the potential implant volume.
	– Target volume not definable
	– Tumor not properly accessible
Brachytherapy for benign disease	❑ Keloid scars are not only unsightly but often itchy and painful
	❑ Pterygium is a condition where a pad of connective tissue with blood vessels grows over the cornea
	❑ Peripheral vascular disease
	❑ Following balloon angioplasty of stenosed peripheral arteries

Contd...

Contd...

Type of RT	Indications
	❑ Coronary artery disease
Systemic RT	❑ I-131-Ca thyroid
	❑ Strontium-89 and Samarium-132 = painful bone metastases **(8 Gy in single fraction)**
	❑ Yttrium
	❑ Phosphorus-32 = Polycythemia rubra vera

DIAGNOSTIC

3. For diagnosing ectopic gastric mucosa in Meckel's diverticulum, which of the following is used?

a. Gallium citrate
b. Thallium
c. Selenium
d. Technetium-99 pertechnate

Uses of radioisotopes

- Gallium citrate is useful for tumours/ abscess
- Thallium scan is used to study myocardial perfusion
- Selenium is useful in thyroid malignancy
- For detection of ectopic gastric mucosa in Meckel's diverticulum, Tc-99 pertechnate is used

Uses of radiotherapy

- Hot spot in MI is detected by: Technetium scan
- Pancreatic scanning is done by: Selenium 75
- Scan used for parathyroid gland: Sestamibi scan
- Scan for measurement of renal GFR: Tc99-DTPA scan
- Vesicourethral reflex (VUR) is seen by: MAG3-tc99 scan
- Isotope used in thyroid scan: I-131
- 99Tc scan shows hot spot in: Adenolymphoma (Salivary gland tumour)
- PACS/ picture archiving & communication system: New system (completely computerized network) to replace conventional analogue film & paper clinical request forms & reports
- Brachytherapy: Radiation therapy in which sources are placed within or near tumour for therapy
- Gamma knife (using gamma rays) is used in: Stereotactic surgery (cuts tumour in different location/ 3D)
- Mantle irradiation is done in: Hodgkin's disease
- Hyper-fractionation radiotherapy is used to treat: Lung cancer
- Intra-operative radiotherapy is used to treat: Pancreatic Ca
- Emergency radiotherapy is given in:
  - SVC syndrome,
  - Pericardial tamponade
- RAIU/ (RadioActive Iodine Uptake test) is done mostly using: I-123
- Photodynamic therapy with hemato-porphyrins & light is used in the treatment of:
  - Colon Ca,
  - Skin Ca

4. MIBG scan is done for:

a. Gastrointestinal stromal tumours
b. Acute pancreatitis
c. Pheochromocytoma
d. Meckel's diverticulum

MIBG is accumulated by pheochromocytoma and neuroblastoma.

Radiopharmaceutical	Critical organ/Disease (imaged)
Salivary gland	^{99m}Tc pertechnetate
PET-sestamibi fusion scan	Parathyroid
^{99m}Tc-sestamibi	
^{99m}Tc-thalium^{201} subtraction scan	
^{131}I, ^{125}I, ^{123}I	Thyroid
^{99m}Tc-MDP	Bone
^{99m}Tc pertechnetate	Meckel's diverticulum, gastric mucosa, Intestine, thyroid, choroid plexus
^{99m}Tc DTPA	Renal GFR
^{99m}Tc DMSA	Renal cortical function
Xe-127, Xe-133, Kr-81m	Lung (VP scan), trachea
Tc-tagged RBCs	Spleen, GI bleeding
^{99m}Tc HMPAO	Brain scan
Stress induced thalium-201	Reversible myocardial ischemia
^{99m}Tc Stannous pyrophosphate > Tetrofosmin	Acute myocardial infarction (Heart)
HIDA/DISIDA	Biliary scintigraphy
^{99m}Tc sulfur colloid	Liver pathologies
Ga^{67}/Indium^{111} labeled WBC	Intra-abdominal abscess and inflammatory bowel disease
DOPA-PET > MIBG/MRI	Extra-adrenal pheochromocytoma
Selenium methionine	Pancreas
SRS (Octreoscan)	Pancreatic neuroendocrine tumors

5. Isotope used in bone scans:

a. Technetium
b. Gallium
c. Selenium
d. Chromium

Ans. 3. **d.** Technetium-99... 4. **c.** Pheochromocytoma 5. **a.** Technetium

Radionuclides considered for bone scanning

- 45Ca Calcium
- 85Sr Strontium
- 131Ba Barium
- 157Dy Dysprosium
- 67Ga Gallium
- 32P Phosphate
- 18F Fluorine
- Technetium ^{99m}Tc

Tumors on Bone Scans
Intense
Fibrous dysplasia
Giant cell tumor
Aneurysmal bone cyst
Osteoblastoma
Osteoid osteoma
Moderate
Adamantinoma
Chondroblastoma
Enchondroma

Contd...

Contd...

Tumors on Bone Scans
Mild or Isointense
Fibrous cortical defect
Bone island
Cortical desmoid
Nonossifying fibroma
Osteoma
Cold
Bone cyst without fracture
Multiple myeloma
Variable
Hemangioma
Multiple hereditary exostosis

THERAPEUTIC

6. **Which of the following is used in both teletherapy as well as brachytherapy:**
   a. Radium-226 b. Iodine-125
   c. Gold-198 d. Caesium-137

   Cesium emits gamma rays.

Some useful radionuclides used in clinical radiotherapy

Sr No	Radionuclide	Energy	Half-life	Medical uses
1.	Radium-226	0.83 MV	1625 years	For brachytherapy but not used nowadays
2.	Cobalt-60	1.25 MV	5.4 years	Teletherapy and brachytherapy (T > B)
3.	Caesium-137	0.666 MV	30 years	Teletherapy and brachytherapy
4.	Iridium-192	0.380 MV	72 days	Brachytherapy only
5.	Iodine-125	0.030 MV	60 days	Brachytherapy
6.	Iodine-131	0.61 MV	8 days	Unsealed radioiodine for thyroid cancer Rx
7.	Gold-198	0.412 MV	2.7 days	Brachytherapy
8.	Strontium-90	2.24 MV	30 years	For shield (mold) in eye tumors
9.	Phosphorous-32	1.71 MV	14 days	Intraperitoneal

MISCELLANEOUS

7. **Which of the following is the SI unit of radioactivity?**
   a. Rem
   b. Rad
   c. Becquerel
   d. Curie

   Remember RBC:

   *Radioactivity; SI unit - **Becquerel**; Non-SI unit - **Curie***

Measure of radiation

- Measure of activity of radiation: Becquerel
- Measure of absorbed dose: Gray, (1 gray = 100 rads)
- Measure of radioactivity: Curie;
- Radioactivity was discovered by Curie (1896)

8. **What dose of radiation would affect hematological system:**
   a. 0-250 cGY
   b. 250-500 cGY
   c. 500-750 cGY
   d. 750-1000 cGY

   250-500 cGY of radiation affects hemopoietic system and death can occur in weeks post-exposure. Hemopoietic and gastrointestinal syndromes are reversible with good symptomatic and supportive care.

Ans. 6. **d.** Caesium-137 7. **c.** Becquerel 8. **b.** 250-500 cGY

Sr No	*Dose (cgy)*	*Time of post-exposure to death*	*System affected*	*Presentation*
1.	250–500	Weeks	*Hemopoietic syndrome*	Mitotically active precursor cells are sterilized by radiation. This prevents replenishment of these cells. Time of crisis is seen after all the circulating cells in the body reach the minimum value.
				Prodromal symptoms: Nausea and vomiting.
				Infection and chills, fatigue, petechial hemorrhages and ulceration of mouth
				These symptoms are the manifestation of depression of blood elements
2.	500–1200	Days	*Gastrointestinal syndrome*	*Nausea, vomiting and prolonged diarrhea. Loss of appetite, sluggishness and lethargy*
				Symptoms and death are due to depopulation of the epithelial lining of the GIT
3.	>10,000	24–48 hrs	*Cerebrovascular*	*No prodromal symptoms*
			syndrome	❑ Severe nausea and vomiting within minutes
				❑ Disorientation
				❑ Loss of coordination of muscular movement
				❑ Respiratory distress
				❑ Diarrhea
				❑ Convulsions
				❑ Coma and finally *death*.
				At this dose all other systems are also seriously damaged. But cerebrovascular damage brings death so fast, that the failure of the other systems does not become obvious.

Hemopoietic and *gastrointestinal syndromes* are reversible with good symptomatic and supportive care.

ANSWERS WITH REFERENCES

RADIOSENSITIVITY OF TISSUES

1. **Ans. (a) Seminoma**
   Ref: Daga's Radiodiagnosis 1/e p509

2. **Ans. (b) Dysgerminoma**
   Ref: Daga's Radiodiagnosis 1/e p509

DIAGNOSTIC

3. **Ans. (d) Tecnetium-99 pertechnate**
   Ref: Internet resources

4. **Ans. (c) Pheochromocytoma**
   Ref: Daga's Radiodiagnosis 1/e p437

5. **Ans. (a) Technetium**
   Ref: Daga's Radiodiagnosis 1/e p451

THERAPEUTIC

6. **Ans. (d) Caesium-137**
   Ref: Daga's Radiodiagnosis 1/e p454

MISCELLANEOUS

7. **Ans. (c) Becquerel**
   Ref: Grainger & Allison's Diagnostic Radiology, 3/e p101

8. **Ans. (b) 250-500 cGY**
   Ref: Daga's Radiodiagnosis 1/e p506

PRACTICE QUESTIONS

RADIOSENSITIVITY OF TISSUES

1. DNA can be damaged by:
a. USG
b. Ionizing radiation
c. MRI
d. All of the above

DIAGNOSTIC

2. Strontium is used for:
a. Teletherapy
b. Brachytherapy
c. Diagnosing thyroid carcinoma
d. Bone scan

THERAPEUTIC

3. Concurrent chemoradiotherapy is commonly given for carcinoma of:
a. Liver b. Lung
c. Head and neck region d. Ovary

MISCELLANEOUS

4. A patient was posted for radiotherapy. Which of the following drug will reduce the toxicity of radiation:
a. Cisplatin b. Gemcitabine
c. Amifostine d. Actinomycin D

5. Which of the following is used as a source in permanent brachytherapy:
a. Cesium-137 b. Iridium-198
c. Iodine-131 d. Gold

Ans. 1. **b.** Ionizing radiation 2. **d.** Bone scan 3. **c.** Head and neck region
4. **c.** Amifostine 5. **d.** Gold

IMAGE-BASED QUESTIONS

1. Identify the following scientist:

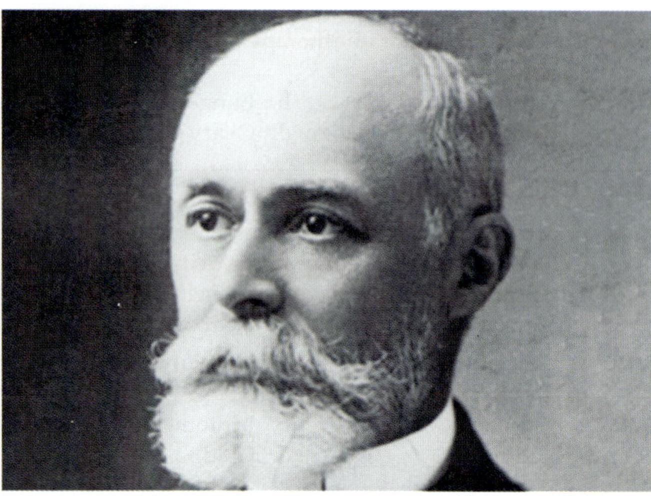

a. Gray b. Roentgen
c. Henri Becquerel d. Hounsefield

Antoine Henri Becquerel (15 December 1852 – 25 August 1908) was a French Physicist, Nobel laureate, and the first person to discover evidence of radioactivity. For work in this field, he, along with Marie Skłodowska-Curie and Pierre Curie, received the 1903 Nobel Prize in Physics. The SI unit, for radioactivity, the becquerel (Bq), is named after him.

2. Madam Curie is associated with:

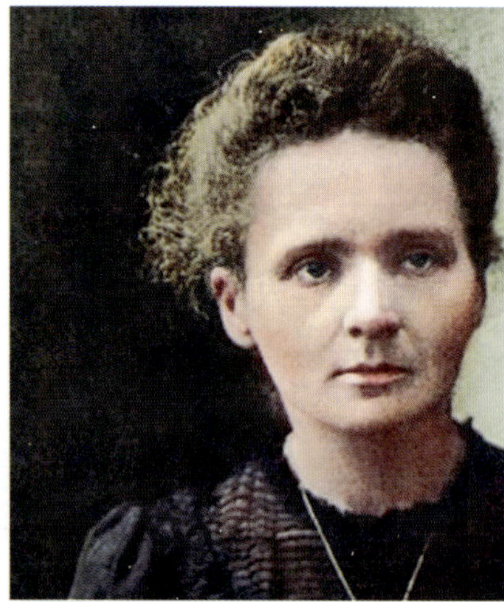

a. Discovery of radium b. Radiation exposure
c. Radiation absorbed dose d. Discovery of cesium

Her achievements included the development of the theory of *radioactivity* (a term that she coined), techniques for isolating radioactive isotopes, and the discovery of two elements, polonium and radium.

3. The following image is an example of:

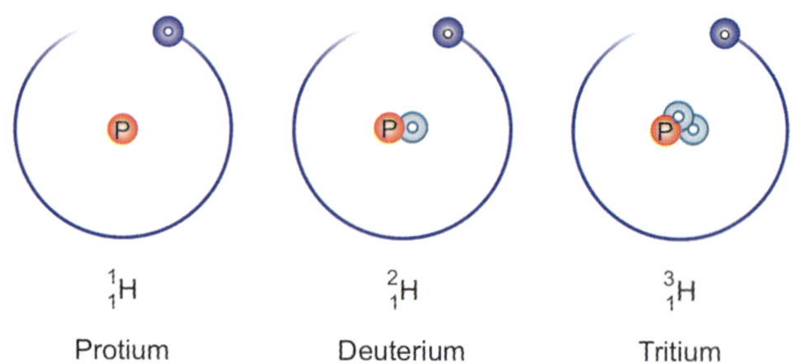

a. Isobars
b. Isotopes
c. Isomers
d. Isozymes

Isotopes are variants of a particular chemical element which differ in neutron number. All isotopes of a given element have the same number of protons in each atom.

4. Which procedure:

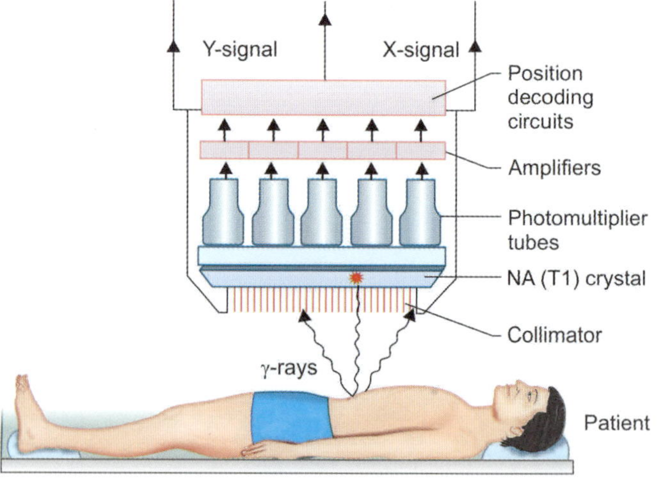

a. X-ray
b. Gamma scintillator camera
c. CT scan
d. MRI scan

A gamma camera converts photons emitted by the radionuclide in the patient into a light pulse and subsequently into a voltage signal. This signal is used to form an image of the distribution of the radionuclide (organ imaging).

5. **Identify the sign:**

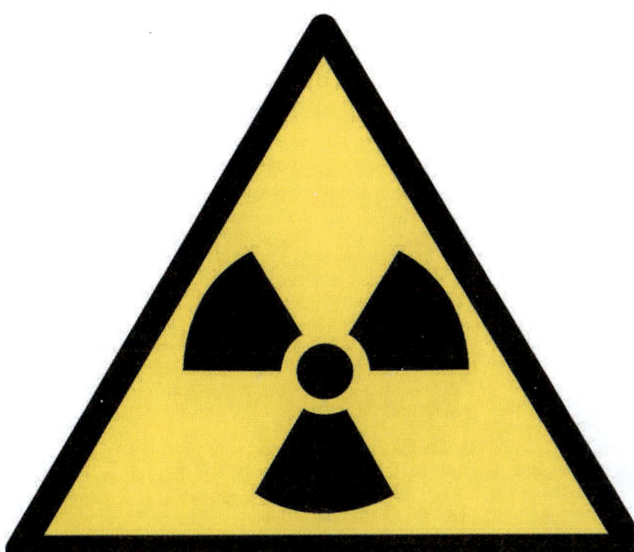

a. Hospital waste management
b. Radioactive warning sign
c. Recyclable matter
d. Non-ionizing radiation

The trefoil symbol used to indicate ionising radiation.

6. **Which study:**

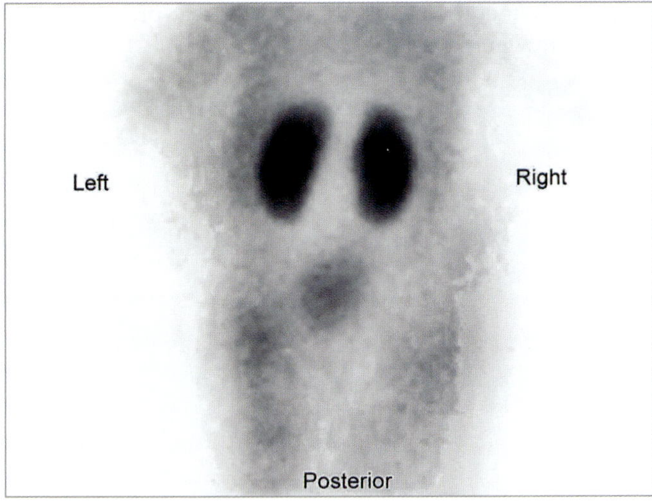

a. DTPA
b. DMSA
c. Thallium scan
d. Sestamibi scan

A **DMSA scan** is a radionuclide scan that uses dimercaptosuccinic acid (as a radioactive tracer) in assessing renal morphology, structure (static scan), and function.

7. **Substance used in such scan:**

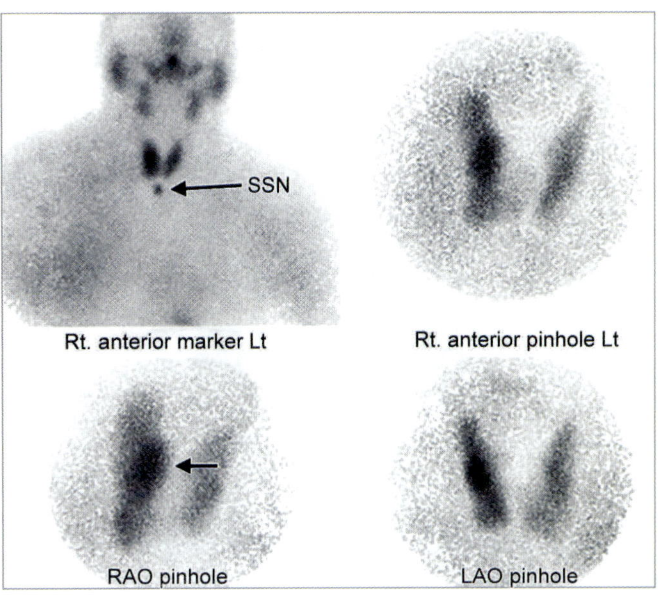

a. I-115 b. I-123
c. I-125 d. I-131

^{123}I has a shorter half-life than ^{131}I (a half day vs 8.1 days), so use of ^{123}I exposes the body to less radiation, at the expense of less time to evaluate delayed scan images. Furthermore, ^{123}I emits gamma radiation, while ^{131}I emits gamma and beta radiation.

8. **Spot diagnosis:**

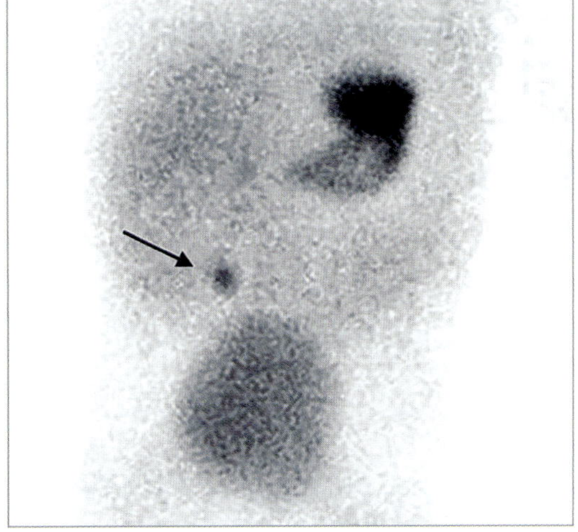

a. Ureteric calculi b. Urinary bladder calculi
c. Meckel's diverticulum d. Gall stones

A technetium-99m (99mTc) pertechnetate scan, also called Meckel scan, is the investigation of choice to diagnose Meckel's diverticula in children. This scan detects gastric mucosa; since approximately 50% of symptomatic Meckel's diverticula have ectopic gastric or pancreatic cells contained within them, this is displayed as a spot on the scan distant from the stomach itself.

9. Substance common used in such scan:

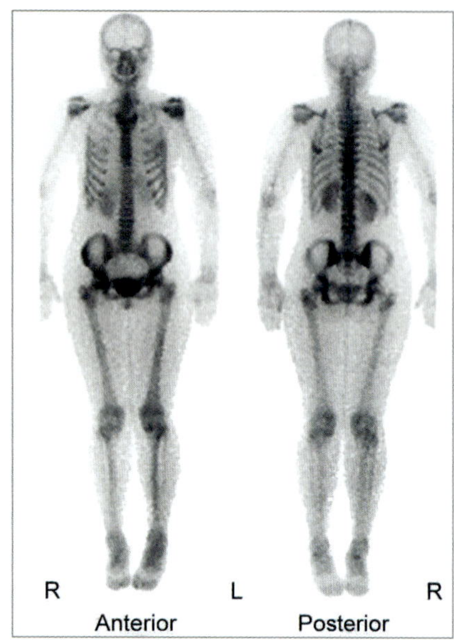

a. Thallium
b. Gallium
c. Technetium
d. Strontium

In the nuclear medicine technique (bone scan), the patient is injected (usually into a vein in the arm or hand, occasionally the foot) with a small amount of radioactive material such as 740 MBq of technetium-99m-MDP and then scanned with a gamma camera, a device sensitive to the radiation emitted by the injected material.

10. Spot diagnosis:

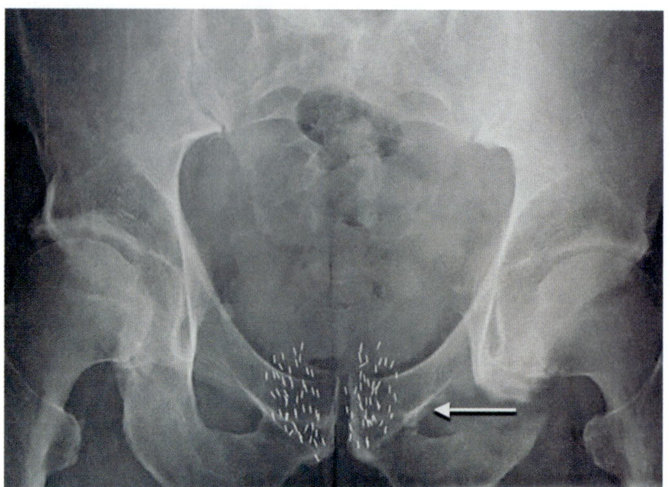

a. Pellet injury
b. Artefacts
c. Interstitial brachytherapy
d. Maggots

Brachytherapy beads are used to treat prostate cancer (Arrow marks beads).

MCQ POINTS

S. No.	Question statements	Answers
1.	MC used radionuclide for skeletal imaging	***Tc-99-MDP***
2.	Radionuclide studies for GFR estimation	***Tc-99-DTPA***
3.	Radionuclide used for static renal scintigraphy	***Tc-99-DMSA***
4.	Isotope used for spleen diseases	***Tc-99 RBC***
5.	Same atomic number but different atomic mass of same element	***Isotopes***
6.	SI unit of absorbed dose	***Gray***
7.	MC radioisotope used for HDR (high dose rate) brachytherapy	***Iridium-192***
8.	Linear accelerator produces	***Electrons and X-rays***
9.	Craniospinal irradiation is used for	***Medulloblastoma***
10.	Earliest effect of radiation on skin	***Erythema***